NURSING DIAGNOSIS MANUAL:
Planning, Individualizing, and Documenting Client Care

MARILYNN E. DOENGES, RN, BSN, MA, CS

Clinical Specialist, Adult Psychiatric/Mental Health Nursing, Retired

Adjunct Faculty, Beth-El College of Nursing and Health Sciences, CU-Springs
Colorado Springs, Colorado

MARY FRANCES MOORHOUSE, RN, BSN, CRRN, LNC

Nurse Consultant
TNT-RN Enterprises, Adjunct Nursing Faculty, Pikes Peak Community College
Colorado Springs, Colorado

ALICE C. MURR, RN, BSN, LNC

Legal Nurse Consultant
Telephone Triage Nurse
Colorado Springs, Colorado

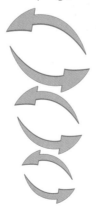

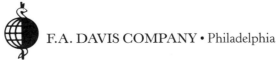
F.A. DAVIS COMPANY • Philadelphia

F. A. Davis Company
1915 Arch Street
Philadelphia, PA 19103
www.fadavis.com

Printed in the United States of America

Last digit indicates print number: 10 9 8 7 6 5 4 3 2 1

Publisher, Nursing: Robert G. Martone
Design Manager: Joan Wendt
Developmental Editor: Alan Sorkowitz
Project Editor: Danielle J. Barsky

As new scientific information becomes available through basic and clinical research, recommended treatments and drug therapies undergo changes. The author(s) and publisher have done everything possible to make this book accurate, up to date, and in accord with accepted standards at the time of publication. The author(s), editors, and publisher are not responsible for errors or omissions or for consequences from application of the book, and make no warranty, expressed or implied, in regard to the contents of the book. Any practice described in this book should be applied by the reader in accordance with professional standards of care used in regard to the unique circumstances that may apply in each situation. The reader is advised always to check product information (package inserts) for changes and new information regarding dose and contraindications before administering any drug. Caution is especially urged when using new or infrequently ordered drugs.

Library of Congress Cataloging-in-Publication Data

Doenges, Marilynn E., 1922-
 Nursing diagnosis manual : planning, individualizing, and documenting client care / Marilynn E. Doenges, Mary Frances Moorhouse, Alice C. Geissler-Murr.
  p. ; cm.
  Includes bibliographical references and index.
  ISBN 0-8036-1156-0 (softcover : alk. paper)
  1. Nursing diagnosis—Handbooks, manuals, etc. 2. Nursing assessment—Handbooks, manuals, etc. 3. Nursing—Planning—Handbooks, manuals, etc.
  [DNLM: 1. Nursing Diagnosis. 2. Nursing Records. 3. Patient Care Planning. WY 100.4 D649n 2005] I. Moorhouse, Mary Frances, 1947- II. Geissler-Murr, Alice, 1946- III. Title.
RT48.6.D643 2005
610.73—dc22
2004014155

To our spouses, children, parents, and friends, who much of the time have had to manage without us while we work and dream as well as cope with our struggles and frustrations.

The Doenges families: the late Dean, Jim; Barbara and Bob Lanza; David, Monita, Matthew and Tish, Tyler; John, Holly, Nicole, and Kelsey; and the Daigle family, Nancy, Jim, Jennifer, Brandon and Annabelle Smith-Daigle, and Jonathan and Kim.

The Moorhouse family: Jan; Paul; Jason, Alexa, and Mary Isabella.

To my large, extended family: Thank you all for having patience and giving me help and time. I love each one of you. *Alice*

To our FAD family, especially Bob Martone; and to Alan Sorkowitz, whose support, "acupressure," and encouragement were so vital to the completion of a project of this magnitude.

To the nurses we are writing for, who daily face the challenge of caring for the acutely ill patient and are looking for a practical way to organize and document this care. We believe that nursing diagnosis and these guides will help.

And to NANDA and the International nurses who are developing and using nursing diagnoses—we continue to champion your efforts and the work of promoting standardized languages.

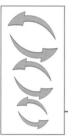

Preface

The American Nurses Association (ANA) Social Policy Statement of 1980 was the first to define nursing as the diagnosis and treatment of human responses to actual and potential health problems. This definition, when combined with the ANA Standards of Practice, has provided impetus and support for the use of nursing diagnosis. Defining nursing and its effect on client care supports the growing awareness that nursing care is a key factor in client survival and in the maintenance, rehabilitative, and preventive aspects of healthcare. Changes and new developments in healthcare delivery in the last decade have given rise to the need for a common framework of communication to ensure continuity of care for the client moving between multiple healthcare settings and providers.

This book is designed to aid the student nurse and the practitioner in identifying interventions commonly associated with specific nursing diagnoses as proposed by NANDA International (formerly the North American Nursing Diagnosis Association). These interventions are the activities needed to implement and document care provided to the individual client and can be used in varied settings from acute to community/home care.

Chapter 1 presents a brief discussion of the nursing process and introduces the concept of evidence-based practice. Standardized nursing languages (SNLs) are discussed in Chapter 2, with a focus on NANDA (nursing diagnoses), NIC (interventions), and NOC (outcomes). NANDA has 167 diagnosis labels with definitions, defining characteristics, and related or risk factors used to define a client need or problem. NIC is a comprehensive standardized language providing 514 direct and indirect intervention labels with definitions and a list of activities a nurse might choose to carry out each intervention. NOC language provides 330 outcome labels with definitions, a set of indicators describing a specific client, caregiver, family, or community states related to the outcome, and a 5-point Likert-type measurement scale that can demonstrate client progress even when outcomes are not fully met. Chapter 3 addresses the assessment process using a nursing framework for data collection such as the Diagnostic Divisions Assessment Tool.

A creative approach for developing and documenting the planning of care is demonstrated in Chapter 4. Mind Mapping is a new technique or learning tool provided to assist you in achieving a holistic view of your client, enhancing your critical thinking skills, and facilitating the creative process of planning client care. For more in-depth information and inclusive plans of care related to specific medical/psychiatric conditions (with rationales and the application of the diagnoses), the nurse is referred to the larger works, all published by the F. A. Davis Company: *Nursing Care Plans: Guidelines for Individualizing Patient Care*, ed 6 (Doenges, Moorhouse, & Geissler-Murr, 2002); *Psychiatric Care Plans: Guidelines for Individualizing Care*, ed 3 (Doenges, Townsend, & Moorhouse, 1998); and *Maternal/Newborn Plans of Care: Guidelines for Individualizing Care*, ed 3 (Doenges & Moorhouse, 1999).

Chapter 6 contains over 800 disorders/health conditions reflecting all specialty areas, with associated nursing diagnoses written as client problem/need statements to aid you in validating the assessment and diagnosis steps of the nursing process.

In Chapter 5, the heart of the book, all the nursing diagnoses are listed alphabetically for ease of reference and include the diagnoses accepted for use by NANDA through 2004. The alphabetization of diagnoses follows NANDA's own sequencing, whereby diagnoses are alphabetized first by their key term, which is capitalized. Subordinate terminology or descriptors of the diagnosis are presented in lowercase words and are alphabetized secondarily to the key term (for example, chronic Pain is alphabetized under P). Each approved diagnosis includes its definition and information divided into the NANDA categories of Related or Risk Factors and Defining Characteristics. Related/Risk Factors information reflects causative or contributing factors that can be useful for determining whether the diagnosis is applicable to a particular client. Defining Characteristics (signs and symptoms or cues) are listed as subjective and/or objective and are used to confirm actual diagnoses, aid in formulating outcomes, and provide additional data for choosing appropriate interventions. We have not deleted or altered NANDA's listings; however, on occasion, we have added to their definitions and suggested additional criteria to provide clarification and direction. These additions are denoted with brackets [].

NANDA nursing diagnosis labels are designed to be multiaxial with 7 axes or descriptors. An axis is defined as a dimension of the human response that is considered in the diagnostic process (see the Appendix). Sometimes, an axis may be included in the diagnostic concept, such as ineffective community coping, in which the unit of care (i.e., community) is named. Some are implicit, such as activity intolerance, in which the individual is the unit of care. At times, an axis may not be pertinent to a particular diagnosis and will not be a part of the nursing diagnosis label. For example, the time frame (e.g., acute, intermittent) or body part (e.g., cerebral, oral, skin) may not be relevant to each diagnostic situation.

Desired Outcomes/Evaluation Criteria are identified to assist you in formulating individual client outcomes and to support the evaluation process. Suggested NOC linkages to the nursing diagnosis are provided.

Nursing priorities are used to group the suggested interventions, which are directed primarily to adult care, although interventions designated as across the life span do include pediatric and geriatric considerations and are designated by an icon. In general, the interventions can be used in multiple settings—acute care, rehabilitation, community clinics, or home care. Most interventions are independent or nursing-originated; however, some interventions are collaborative orders (e.g., medical, psychiatric), and you will need to determine when this is necessary and take the appropriate action. Icons are also used to differentiate collaborative interventions, diagnostic studies, and medications as well as transcultural considerations. All of these "specialized" interventions are presented with icons, rather than being broken out under separate headings, to maintain their sequence within the prioritization of all nursing interventions for the diagnosis. Although all defining characteristics are listed, interventions that address specialty areas outside the scope of this book are not routinely presented (e.g., obstetrics/gynecology/pediatrics), except for diagnoses that are infancy-oriented, such as ineffective Breastfeeding, disorganized Infant Behavior, and risk for impaired parent/infant/child Attachment. For example, when addressing deficient Fluid Volume, isotonic (hemorrhage), the nurse is directed to stop blood loss; however, specific direction to perform fundal massage is not listed. Additionally, in support of evidenced-based practice, rationales are provided for the interventions, and references for these rationales are cited.

The inclusion of Documentation Focus suggestions is to remind you of the importance and necessity of recording the steps of the nursing process.

As noted, with few exceptions, we have presented NANDA's recommendations as formulated. We support the belief that practicing nurses and researchers need to study, use, and evaluate the diagnoses as presented. Nurses can be creative as they use the standardized language, redefining and sharing information as the diagnoses are used with individual clients. As new nursing diagnoses are developed, it is important that the data they encompass are added to the current data base. As part of the process by clinicians, educators, and researchers across practice specialties and academic settings to define, test, and refine nursing diagnosis, nurses are encouraged to share insights and ideas with NANDA at the following address: North American Nursing Diagnosis Association, 1211 Locust Street, Philadelphia, PA 19107; e-mail: info@nanda.org

Marilynn E. Doenges
Mary Frances Moorhouse
Alice C. Murr

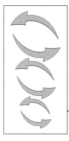

Contributors

Diane Bligh, RN, MS, CNS
Associate Professor, Nursing
Front Range Community College
Westminster, Colorado
Co-author of Chapter 4: *Results of the Nursing Process: Documenting the Plan of Care*

Mary F. Johnston, RN, MSN
Program Director, Nursing
Front Range Community College
Westminster, Colorado
Co-author of Chapter 4: *Results of the Nursing Process: Documenting the Plan of Care*

Sheila Marquez, RN, BSN, PNP
Executive Director
Vice President/Chief Operating Officer
The Colorado SIDS Program, Inc.
Denver, Colorado
Contributor of Chapter 5 monograph on *Risk for Sudden Infant Death Syndrome*

Susan Moberly, RNC, BSN, ICCE
Childbirth Educator
Obstetric Nursing and Lactation Consultant
Colorado Springs, Colorado
Contributor of Chapter 5 monographs related to *Breastfeeding*

Alma Mueller, RN, MEd
Retired Chair and Professor of Nursing
Front Range Community College
Westminster, Colorado
Co-author of Chapter 4: *Results of the Nursing Process: Documenting the Plan of Care*

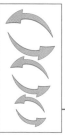

Contents

Chapter 1

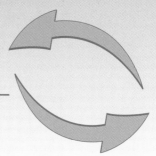

The Nursing Process: The Foundation of Quality Client Care

↳ Defining the Profession

In the world of healthcare, nursing has long struggled to establish itself as a profession. Dictionary terms describe nursing as "a calling requiring specialized knowledge and often long and intensive academic preparation; a principal calling, vocation, or employment; the whole body of persons engaged in a calling."[1] Throughout the history of nursing, unfavorable stereotypes (based on the view of nursing as subservient and dependent on the medical profession) have negatively affected the view of nursing as an independent entity. In its early developmental years, nursing did not seek or have the means to control its own practice. Florence Nightingale, in discussing the nature of nursing in 1859, observed that "nursing has been limited to signify little more than the administration of medicines and the application of poultices."[2] Although this attitude may still persist to some degree, the nursing profession has defined what makes nursing unique and identified a body of professional knowledge. As early as 1896, nurses in America banded together to seek standardization of educational programs and laws governing their practice. The task of nursing since that time has been to create descriptive terminology reflecting not only specific nursing functions but also levels of competency.[3] Erickson, Tomlin, and Swain believe "Nursing will thrive as a unique and valued profession when nurses present a theory and rationalistic model for their practice, correct misleading stereotypes, locate control with clients, and actively participate in processes for change."[4]

In the past several decades, more than a dozen prominent nursing scholars (e.g., Rogers, Parse, Henderson) have developed conceptualizations to define the nature of nursing. Because much of nursing is nonphenomenalogical or nonobservable, the nature of nursing cannot be explained using the usual parameters of scientific investigation. In her article, Kikuchi proposes that conceptualizations about nursing are philosophic in nature and as such are still testable.[5] As nursing research continues the work of establishing the profession as independent in its own right, the value of nursing goals is understood and the difference between nursing and other professions is being delineated. Nursing is now recognized as both a science and an art concerned with the physical, psychological, sociological, cultural, and spiritual concerns of the individual. The science of nursing is based on a broad theoretical framework; its art depends on the caring skills and abilities of the individual nurse. The importance of the nurse within the healthcare system is noted in many positive ways, and the profession of nursing is itself acknowledging the need for its practitioners to act professionally and be accountable for the care they provide.

Barely a century after Miss Nightingale noted that "the very elements of nursing are all but unknown," the American Nurses Association (ANA) developed their first Social Policy Statement in 1980, defining nursing as "the diagnosis and treatment of *human responses* to actual or potential health problems."[6] Human responses (defined as people's experiences with and responses to health, illness, and life events) are nursing's phenomena of concern. In 1995, this statement was revisited, updated, and titled *Nursing's Social Policy Statement*. The new policy statement acknowledged that since the release of the original statement, "nursing has been influenced by many social and professional changes, as well as by the science of caring."[7]

The new statement delineates four essential features of today's contemporary nursing practice:

1. Attention to the full range of human experiences and responses to health and illness without restriction to a problem-focused orientation
2. Integration of objective data with knowledge gained from an understanding of the client's or group's subjective experience
3. Application of scientific knowledge to the processes of diagnosis and treatment
4. Provision of a caring relationship that facilitates health and healing[7]

Thus, nursing's role includes promotion of health as well as performance of activities that contribute to recovery from, or adjustment to illness. Also, nurses support the right of clients to define their own health-related goals and to engage in care that reflects their personal values. Emphasis is placed on the mind-body-spirit connection with a holistic view of the individual as nurses facilitate the client's efforts in striving for growth and development.

In your readings you will likely encounter other definitions of nursing. As your knowledge and experience develops, your definition of nursing may change to reflect your personal nursing philosophy, focus on a particular care setting or population, or your specific role. For example, although the definition of nursing developed by Erickson, Tomlin, and Swain is 20 years old, it remains viable and timely because it incorporates the concepts noted previously with today's holistic approach to care. Their definition includes what nursing is, how it is accomplished, and the goals of nursing—"Nursing is the holistic helping of persons with their self-care activities in relation to their health. This is an interactive, interpersonal process that nurtures strengths to enable development, release, and channeling of resources for coping with one's circumstances and environment. The goal is to achieve a state of perceived optimum health and contentment."[4]

An understanding of human nature is certainly important in the development of a philosophy of nursing. Understanding that "needs motivate behavior" helps the nurse to determine the client's needs at a particular moment in time. Maslow's hierarchy of needs[20] provides a basis for understanding that unmet needs can interfere with an individual's holistic growth and may even result in physical/mental distress or illness. Other theorists have also studied how people are similar, providing the nurse with more information to help understand the client. For example, Erikson's observations on the stages of psychological development suggest that the individual is a "work in progress" accomplishing age-specific maturational tasks throughout the life span. Piaget's cognitive stages address how thinking develops and the individual adapts to and organizes his/her environment intellectually.[4] However, in the end the individual is the primary source of information about himself/herself. The nurse needs to listen to what the client is relating with an open mind and empathic unconditional acceptance. Knowing how people are alike provides a basis to understand human nature. However, each person is unique, and the nurse needs to look for the client's model of the world and how this relates to the client's own situation.

The nursing profession is further defined by fundamental philosophical beliefs that have been identified over time as essential to the practice of nursing and recently expanded by the update of the ANA's Nursing's Social Policy Statement. These values and assumptions offer guidance to the nurse and need to be kept in mind to enhance the quality of nursing care provided:

- The client is a human being who has worth and dignity.
- Humans manifest an essential unity of mind/body/spirit.[7]
- There are basic human needs that must be met (Maslow's hierarchy).
- When these needs are not met, problems arise that may require intervention by another person until the individuals can resume responsibility for themselves.
- Human experience is contextually and culturally defined.[7]
- Health and illness are human experiences.[7]
- Clients have a right to quality health and nursing care delivered with interest, compassion, and competence with a focus on wellness and prevention.
- The presence of illness does not preclude health nor does optimal health preclude illness.[7]
- The therapeutic nurse-client relationship is important in the nursing process.

Finally, the Code of Ethics for Nurses[8] addresses the need for nurses to respect human dignity, acknowledge the uniqueness of each client, and honor the client's right to privacy. The Code also calls on nurses to assume responsibility for individual nursing judgments and actions and for the delegation of nursing activities to others. Nurses are encouraged to maintain competence in nursing, contribute to the ongoing development of the profession, and participate in implementation and improvement of standards. This last goal can be accomplished by using the results of nursing research to engage in evidence-based nursing practice.

The roots of evidence-based practice lie in the efforts of many in the past. Hippocrates described the symptoms and course of illnesses and related them to the seasons, geographical area, and types of people associated with each. These hypotheses founded the rational approach to the understanding of disease. As knowledge grew and the germ theory of disease was accepted, epidemiology began to count disease events, leading to the establishment of a central government agency to collect and record data. This led to the posing of questions in the form of testable hypotheses, the collection of data to support or refute hypotheses, and the development of statistical tools to summarize numerical data.[9] The work of Pasteur and Koch expanded the understanding of causal relationships between bacterial causes of many diseases, leading to reducing illness and mortality.

Florence Nightingale used statistics to measure health, identify causes of mortality, evaluate health services, and reform institutions. After the Crimean War, she began organizing committees, assembling data, and preparing reports and hearings on how administrative inadequacies affected patients' health. Her work resulted in British Army Hospital and government reform in the interest of preventing death and disease. She became an honorary member of the American Statistical Association in 1874, and her papers were read at a National Social Science Congress in 1863 and at the nurses' congress of the Chicago World's Fair in 1893. The efforts of these pioneers laid the groundwork for the development of evidence-based practice.

Barnsteiner and Provost note "the current definition [of evidence-based practice] is the integration of best research evidence with clinical expertise and patient values."[10] That is, both research and nonresearch components are combined to create evidence-based practice. Quantitative research is invaluable in measuring the effectiveness of nursing interventions while qualitative studies capture the preferences, attitudes, and values of healthcare consumers. But the nurses' clinical judgment and individual client needs and perspective must also be included. "The most important requirement for practicing nurses in the 21st century will be to utilize appropriate evidence available to improve practice."[11]

ᕼ Administering Nursing Care

Nursing leaders have identified a process that "combines the most desirable elements of the art of nursing with the most relevant elements of systems theory, using the scientific method."[12] This *nursing process* incorporates an interactive/interpersonal approach with a problem-solving and decision-making process which serves as a framework for the delivery of nursing care.[13–15]

The concept of nursing process was first introduced in the 1950s as a three-step process of assessment, planning, and evaluation based on the scientific method of observing, measuring, gathering data, and analyzing the findings. Years of study, use, and refinement have led nurses to expand the nursing process to five distinct steps that provide an efficient method of organizing thought processes for clinical decision making, problem solving, and delivery of higher quality, individualized client care. The nursing process now consists of:

- *assessment* or the systematic collection of data relating to clients;
- *diagnosis/need identification* involving the analysis of collected data to identify the client's needs or problems;
- *planning,* which is a two-part process of identifying goals and the client's desired outcomes to address the assessed health and wellness needs along with the selection of appropriate nursing interventions to assist the client in attaining the outcomes;
- *implementation* or putting the plan of care into action; and
- *evaluation* by determining the client's progress toward attaining the identified outcomes, and the client's response to and effectiveness of the selected nursing interventions for the purpose of altering the plan as indicated.

Because these five steps are central to nursing actions in any setting, the nursing process is now included in the conceptual framework of nursing curricula and is accepted as part of the legal definition of nursing in the Nurse Practice Acts of most states.

When a client enters the healthcare system, whether as an inpatient, clinic outpatient, or a home care client, the steps of the nursing process are set into motion. The nurse collects data, identifies client needs (nursing diagnoses), establishes goals, creates measurable outcomes, and selects nursing interventions to assist the client in achieving these outcomes and goals. Finally, after the interventions have been implemented, the nurse evaluates the client's responses and the effectiveness of the plan of care in reaching the desired outcomes and goals to determine whether or not the needs or problems have been resolved and the client is ready to be discharged from the care setting. If the identified needs or problems remain unresolved, further assessment, additional nursing diagnoses, alteration of outcomes and goals, and/or changes of interventions are required.

Although we use the terms assessment, diagnosis/need identification, planning, implementation, and evaluation as separate, progressive steps, in reality they are interrelated. Together these steps form a continuous circle of thought and action, which recycles throughout the client's contact with the healthcare system. Figure 1–1 depicts a model for visualizing this process. You can see that the nursing process uses the nursing diagnosis (the clinical judgment product of critical thinking). Based on this judgment, nursing interventions are selected and implemented. Figure 1–1 also shows how the progressive steps of the nursing process create an

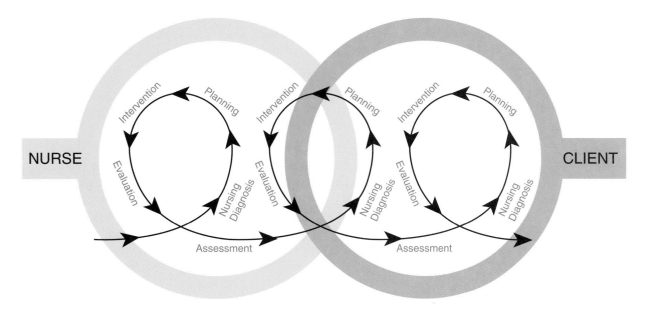

FIGURE 1–1 • Diagram of the nursing process. The steps of the nursing process are interrelated, forming a continuous circle of thought and action that is both dynamic and cyclic.

understandable model of both the products and processes of critical thinking contained within the nursing process. The model graphically emphasizes both the dynamic and cyclic characteristics of the nursing process.

↳ Application of the Nursing Process

The scientific method of problem solving introduced in the previous section is used almost instinctively by most people, without conscious awareness.

> **FOR EXAMPLE:** While studying for your semester finals you snack on pepperoni pizza. After going to bed you are awakened by a burning sensation in the center of your chest. You are young and in good health and note no other symptoms (Assessment). You decide that your pain is the result of the spicy food you have eaten (Diagnosis). You then determine that before you will be able to achieve your goal of returning to sleep, you first need to relieve the discomfort with an over-the-counter preparation (Planning). You take a liquid antacid for your discomfort (Implementation). Within a few minutes, you note the burning sensation is relieved, and you return to bed without further concern (Evaluation).

As you see, this is a process you routinely use to solve problems in your life that can be readily applied to client-care situations. You only need to learn the new terms describing the nursing process, rather than having to think about each step (assessment, diagnosis/need identification, planning, implementation, and evaluation) in an entirely new way.

To effectively use the nursing process, there are some basic abilities that the nurse must possess and apply. Particularly important is a thorough knowledge of science and theory, not only as applied in nursing but also in other related disciplines such as medicine and psychology. Creativity is needed in the application of nursing knowledge as well as adaptability in handling change and the many unexpected happenings that occur. As a nurse, you must make a commitment to practice your profession in the best possible way, trusting in yourself and your ability to do your job well and displaying the necessary leadership to organize and supervise as your position requires. In addition, intelligence, well-developed interpersonal skills, and competent technical skills are essential.

FOR EXAMPLE: A diabetic client's irritable behavior could be the result of low serum glucose or the effects of excessive caffeine intake. However, it could also arise from a sense of helplessness regarding life events. A single behavior may have varied causes. It is important that your nursing assessment skills identify the underlying etiology to provide appropriate care.

The practice responsibilities presented in the definitions of nursing and the nursing process are explained in detail in the publication *Standards of Clinical Nursing Practice*.[16] The standards provide workable guidelines to ensure that the practice of nursing can be carried out by each individual nurse. Table 1–1 presents an abbreviated description of the standards of clinical practice. With the ultimate goal of quality healthcare, the effective use of the nursing process will result in a viable nursing-care system that is recognized and accepted as nursing's body of knowledge and that can be shared with other healthcare professionals.

 TABLE 1–1

ANA STANDARDS OF CLINICAL NURSING PRACTICE

Standards of Care

Describes a competent level of nursing care as demonstrated by the nursing process that encompasses all significant actions taken by the nurse in providing care, and forms the foundation of clinical decision making.

1. Assessment: the nurse collects client health data.
2. Diagnosis: the nurse analyzes the assessment data in determining diagnoses.
3. Outcome Identification: the nurse identifies expected outcomes individualized to the client.
4. Planning: the nurse develops a plan of care that prescribes interventions to attain expected outcomes.
5. Implementation: the nurse implements the interventions identified in the plan of care.
6. Evaluation: the nurse evaluates the client's progress toward attainment of outcomes.

Standards of Professional Performance

Describes roles expected of all professional nurses appropriate to their education, position, and practice setting.

1. Quality of Care: the nurse systematically evaluates the quality and effectiveness of nursing practice.
2. Performance Appraisal: the nurse evaluates his/her own nursing practice in relation to professional practice standards and relevant statutes and regulations.
3. Education: the nurse acquires and maintains current knowledge in nursing practice.
4. Collegiality: the nurse contributes to the professional development of peers, colleagues, and others.
5. Ethics: the nurse's decisions and actions on behalf of clients are determined in an ethical manner.
6. Collaboration: the nurse collaborates with the client, significant others, and healthcare providers in providing client care.
7. Research: the nurse uses research findings in practice.
8. Resource Utilization: the nurse considers factors related to safety, effectiveness, and cost in planning and delivering client care.

Source: American Nurses' Association (1991). Standards of Clinical Nursing Practice. Kansas City, MO: Author.

↳ Advantages of Using the Nursing Process

There are many advantages to the use of the nursing process:

- The nursing process provides an organizing framework for meeting the individual needs of the client, the client's family/significant other(s), and the community.
- The steps of the nursing process focus the nurse's attention on the "individual" human responses of a client/group to a given health situation, resulting in a holistic plan of care addressing the specific needs of the client/group.
- The nursing process provides an organized, systematic method of problem solving (while still allowing for creative solutions) that may minimize dangerous errors or omissions in caregiving and avoid time-consuming repetition in care and documentation.
- The use of the nursing process promotes the active involvement of the client in his or her healthcare, enhancing consumer satisfaction. Such participation increases the client's sense of control over what is happening to him or her, stimulates problem solving, and promotes personal responsibility, all of which strengthen the client's commitment to achieving the identified goals.
- The use of the nursing process enables you as a nurse to have more control over your practice. This enhances the opportunity for you to use your knowledge, expertise, and intuition constructively and dynamically to increase the likelihood of a successful client outcome. This, in turn, promotes greater job satisfaction and your professional growth.
- The use of the nursing process provides a common language (nursing diagnosis) for practice, unifying the nursing profession. Using a system that clearly communicates the plan of care to coworkers and clients enhances continuity of care, promotes achievement of client goals, provides a vehicle for evaluation, and aids in the developing of nursing standards. In addition, the structure of the process provides a format for documenting the client's response to all aspects of the planned care.
- The use of the nursing process provides a means of assessing nursing's economic contribution to client care. The nursing process supplies a vehicle for the quantitative and qualitative measurement of nursing care that meets the goal of cost-effectiveness and still promotes holistic care.

↳ Summary

Nursing is continuing to evolve into a well-defined profession with a more clearly delineated definition and phenomena of concern. Fundamental philosophical beliefs and qualities have been identified that are important for the nurse to possess to provide quality care.

The nursing profession has developed a body of knowledge that contributes to the growth and well-being of the individual and the community, the prevention of illness, and the maintenance and/or restoration of health (or relief of pain/discomfort and provision of support when a return to health is not possible). The nursing process is the basis of all nursing actions and is the essence of nursing providing a flexible, orderly, logical problem-solving approach for administering nursing care so that client (whether individual, community, or population) needs for such care are met comprehensively and effectively. It can be applied in any healthcare or educational setting, in any theoretical or conceptual framework, and within the context of any nursing philosophy.

Each step of the nursing process builds on and interacts with the other steps, ensuring an effective practice model. Inclusion of the standards of clinical nursing practice provides additional information to reinforce understanding and opportunities to apply knowledge.

Please note, the term *client* is used in this book rather than *patient* to reflect the philosophy that the individuals or groups you work with are legitimat members of the decision-making process with some degree of control over the planned regimen and as able, active participants in the planning and implementation of their care.[4]

Next, we will introduce the language described in the nursing process. This includes NANDA International Inc.'s (formerly the North American Nursing Diagnosis Association) classification of nursing diagnoses[17] and the Iowa Intervention and Outcome Projects: Nursing Intervention Classification (NIC)[18] and the Nursing Outcomes Classification (NOC).[19] NANDA, NIC, and NOC have combined their classification systems (NNN Alliance) to provide a comprehensive nursing language.

References

1. Merriam-Webster Online Dictionary. Available at: http://www.m-w.com/dictionary.htm. Accessed on May 7, 2003.
2. Nightingale, F. (1859). Notes on Nursing: What It Is and What It Is Not (Facsimile edition). Philadelphia: J.B. Lippincott, 1946.
3. Jacobi, E. M. (1976). Foreword. In Flanigan, L. (ed.): One Strong Voice: The Story of the American Nurses' Association. Kansas City, Missouri: American Nurses' Association.
4. Erickson, H. C., Tomlin, E. M., Swain, M. A. P. (1983). Modeling and Role-Modeling. Englewood Cliffs, NJ: Prentice-Hall.
5. Kikuchi, J. F. (1999). Clarifying the nature of conceptualizations about nursing. Canadian J Nurs Research, 30(4), 115–128.
6. American Nurses Association. (1980). Nursing: A Social Policy Statement. Kansas City, MO: Author.
7. American Nurses Association. (1995). Nursing's Social Policy Statement. Washington, DC: Author.
8. American Nurses Association. (2001). Code of Ethics for Nurses. Washington, DC: Author.
9. Stolley, P. D., Lasky, T. (1995). Investigating Disease Patterns: The Science of Epidemiology (Scientific American Library, no. 57). New York: WH Freeman.
10. Barnsteiner, J., Provost, S. (2002). How to implement evidence-based practice: Some tried and true pointers. Reflections on Nursing Leadership, 28(2), 18.
11. Amarsi, Y. (2002). Evidence-based nursing: Perspective from Pakistan. Reflections on Nursing Leasership, 28(2), 28.
12. Shore, L. S. (1988). Nursing Diagnosis: What It Is and How to Do It, a Programmed Text. Richmond, VA: Medical College of Virginia Hospitals.
13. Peplau, H. E. (1952). Interpersonal Relations in Nursing: A Conceptual Frame of Reference for Psychodynamic Nursing. New York: Putnam.
14. King, L. (1971). Toward a Theory for Nursing: General Concepts of Human Behavior. New York: Wiley.
15. Yura, H., Walsh, M. B. (1988). The Nursing Process: Assessing, Planning, Implementing, Evaluating, ed 5. Norwalk, CT: Appleton & Lange.
16. American Nurses Association. (1991). Standards of Clinical Nursing Practice. Kansas City, MO: Author.
17. Johnson, M., Maas, M., Moorhead, S. (2000). Nursing Outcomes Classification (NOC), 2nd ed,.St. Louis: Mosby.
18. North American Nursing Diagnosis Association (2001). Nursing Diagnoses: Definitions & Classification. Philadelphia: Author.
19. McCloskey, J. C., Bulecheck, G. M. (2000). Nursing Intervention Classification (NIC), 3rd ed. St. Louis: Mosby.
20. Maslow, A.H. (1970). Motivation and Personality, ed 2. New York: Harper & Row.

Chapter 2

The Language of Nursing: NANDA, NIC, NOC, and other Standardized Nursing Languages

In this chapter, we will look at the process and progress of describing the work of nursing. At first glance, it would seem to be a simple task. However, over many years the profession has struggled with it. The struggle, in part, is a result of changes in healthcare delivery and financing, the expansion of nursing's role, and the dawning of the computer age. Gordon reminds us that classification system development parallels knowledge development in a discipline.[1] As theory development and research have begun to define nursing, it has become a necessity for nursing to find a common language to describe what nursing is, what nursing does, and how to codify it. Thus, the terms "classification systems" and "standardized language" were born, and the work continues.

Changes in the healthcare system occur at an ever-increasing rate. One of these changes is the movement toward a paperless (computerized or electronic) client record. The use of electronic healthcare information systems is rapidly expanding, and the focus has shifted from its original uses—financial and personnel management functions—to the efficient documentation of the client encounter, whether that is a single office visit or a lengthy hospitalization. The move to electronic documentation is being fueled by changes in healthcare delivery and reimbursement as well as the advent of alternative healthcare settings (outpatient surgeries, home health, rehabilitation or subacute units, extended or long-term care facilities, etc.), all of which increase the need for a commonality of communication to ensure continuity of care for the client, who moves from one setting or level of care to another.

These changes in the business and documentation of healthcare require the industry to generate data about its operations and outcomes. Evaluation and improvement of provided services are important to the delivery of cost-effective client care. Therefore, providers and consumers interested in outcomes of care benefit from accurate documentation of the care provided and the client's response. With the use of language or terminology that can be coded, healthcare information can be recorded in terms that are universal and easily entered into an electronic database and that can generate meaningful reporting data about its operation and outcomes. In short, standardized language is required.

A standardized language contains formalized terms with definitions and guidelines for use. For example, if the impact of nursing care on financial and clinical outcomes is to be analyzed, coding of this information is essential. While it has been relatively easy to code medical procedures, nursing is more of an enigma, because its work has not been so clearly defined.

Since the 1970s, nursing leaders have been working to define the profession of nursing, to develop a commonality of words describing practice (a framework of communication and documentation), so that nursing's contribution to healthcare is captured, is visible in healthcare databases, and is thereby recognized as essential. Therefore, the focus of the profession has been on the effort to classify tasks and to develop standardized nursing languages (SNLs) to better demonstrate what nursing is and what nursing does.

Around the world, nursing researchers continue their efforts to identify and label people's experiences with (and responses to) health and illness as they relate to the scope of nursing practice. The use of universal nursing terminology directs our focus to the central content and process of nursing care by identifying, naming, and standardizing the "what" and "how" of the work of nursing—including both direct and indirect activities. This wider application for a standardized language has spurred its development.

A recognized pioneer in SNL is NANDA International's (formerly North American Nursing Diagnosis Association) "Nursing Diagnosis."[2] Simply stated, a nursing diagnosis is defined as a clinical judgment about individual, family, or community responses to actual or potential health problems/life processes. Nursing diagnoses provide the basis for selection of nursing interventions to achieve outcomes for which the nurse is accountable.[3] NANDA nursing diagnoses currently include 167 labels with definitions, defining characteristics, and related or risk factors used to define a client need or problem. Once the client's need is defined, outcomes can be developed and nursing interventions chosen to achieve the desired outcomes.

The linkage of client problems or nursing diagnoses to specific nursing interventions and client outcomes has led to the development of a number of other SNLs, including Home Health Care Classification (HHCC),[4] Nursing Interventions Classifications (NIC),[5] Nursing Outcome Classifications (NOC),[6] Omaha System (OS),[7] Patient Care Data Set,[8] and Perioperative Nursing Data Set.[9]

Whereas some of these languages are designed for a specific client population (e.g., OS, HHCC, Patient Care Data Set, and PNDS), the NANDA, NIC, and NOC languages are comprehensively designed for use across systems and settings and at individual, family, and community or population levels.[10]

NIC is a comprehensive standardized language providing 514 direct and indirect intervention labels with definitions (Table 2–1). A list of activities a nurse might choose to carry out each intervention is also provided and can be modified as necessary to meet the specific needs of the client. These research-based interventions address general practice and specialty areas.

⤺ TABLE 2–1

NURSING INTERVENTIONS CLASSIFICATION LABELS

Abuse Protection Support	Abuse Protection Support: Religious	Acid-Base Management: Respiratory Acidosis	Acupressure
Abuse Protection Support: Child	Acid-Base Management	Acid-Base Management: Respiratory Alkalosis	Admission Care
Abuse Protection Support: Domestic Partner	Acid-Base Management: Metabolic Acidosis	Acid-Base Monitoring	Airway Insertion and Stabilization
Abuse Protection Support: Elder	Acid-Base Management: Metabolic Alkalosis	Active Listening	Airway Management
		Activity Therapy	Airway Suctioning
			Allergy Management

Amnioinfusion
Amputation Care
Analgesic Administration
Analgesic Administration:
   Intraspinal
Anaphylaxis Management
Anesthesia Administration
Anger Control Assistance
Animal-Assisted Therapy
Anticipatory Guidance
Anxiety Reduction
Area Restriction
Aromatherapy
Art Therapy
Artificial Airway
   Management
Aspiration Precautions
Assertiveness Training
Asthma Management
Attachment Promotion
Autogenic Training
Autotransfusion

Bathing
Bed Rest Care
Bedside Laboratory
   Testing
Behavior Management
Behavior Management:
   Overactivity/Inattention
Behavior Management:
   Self-Harm
Behavior Management:
   Sexual
Behavior Modification
Behavior Modification: Social
   Skills
Bibliotherapy
Biofeedback
Bioterrorism Preparedness
Birthing
Bladder Irrigation
Bleeding Precautions
Bleeding Reduction
Bleeding Reduction:
   Antepartum Uterus
Bleeding Reduction:
   Gastrointestinal
Bleeding Reduction: Nasal
Bleeding Reduction:
   Postpartum Uterus
Bleeding Reduction: Wound

Blood Products
   Administration
Body Image Enhancement
Body Mechanics
   Promotion
Bottle Feeding
Bowel Incontinence Care
Bowel Incontinence Care:
   Encopresis
Bowel Irrigation
Bowel Management
Bowel Training
Breast Examination
Breastfeeding Assistance

Calming Technique
Capillary Blood Sample
Cardiac Care
Cardiac Care: Acute
Cardiac Care:
   Rehabilitation
Cardiac Precautions
Caregiver Support
Care Management
Cast Care: Maintenance
Cast Care: Wet
Cerebral Edema
   Management
Cerebral Perfusion
   Promotion
Cesarean Section Care
Chemical Restraint
Chemotherapy
   Management
Chest Physiotherapy
Childbirth Preparation
Circulatory Care: Arterial
   Insufficiency
Circulatory Care:
   Mechanical Assist Device
Circulatory Care: Venous
   Insufficiency
Circulatory Precautions
Circumcision Care
Code Management
Cognitive Restructuring
Cognitive Stimulation
Communicable Disease
   Management
Communication
   Enhancement: Hearing
   Deficit

Communication
   Enhancement: Speech
   Deficit
Communication
   Enhancement: Vision
   Deficit
Community Disaster
   Preparedness
Community Health
   Development
Complex Relationship
   Building
Conflict Mediation
Constipation/Impaction
   Management
Consultation
Contact Lens Care
Controlled Substance
   Checking
Coping Enhancement
Cost Containment
Cough Enhancement
Counseling
Crisis Intervention
Critical Path Development
Culture Brokerage
Cutaneous Stimulation

Decision-Making Support
Delegation
Delirium Management
Delusion Management
Dementia Management
Dementia Management:
   Bathing
Deposition/Testimony
Developmental Care
Developmental
   Enhancement: Adolescent
Developmental
   Enhancement: Child
Dialysis Access
   Maintenance
Diarrhea Management
Diet Staging
Discharge Planning
Distraction
Documentation
Dressing
Dying Care
Dysreflexia Management
Dysrhythmia Management

Ear Care
Eating Disorders
   Management
Electroconvulsive Therapy
   Management
Electrolyte Management
Electrolyte Management:
   Hypercalcemia
Electrolyte Management:
   Hyperkalemia
Electrolyte Management:
   Hypermagnesemia
Electrolyte Management:
   Hypernatremia
Electrolyte Management:
   Hyperphosphatemia
Electrolyte Management:
   Hypocalcemia
Electrolyte Management:
   Hypokalemia
Electrolyte Management:
   Hypomagnesemia
Electrolyte Management:
   Hyponatremia
Electrolyte Management:
   Hypophosphatemia
Electrolyte Monitoring
Electronic Fetal Monitoring:
   Antepartum
Electronic Fetal Monitoring:
   Intrapartum
Elopement Precautions
Embolus Care: Peripheral
Embolus Care: Pulmonary
Embolus Precautions
Emergency Care
Emergency Cart Checking
Emotional Support
Endotracheal Extubation
Energy Management
External Tube Feeding
Environmental Management
Environmental Management:
   Attachment Process
Environmental Management:
   Comfort
Environmental Management:
   Community
Environmental Management:
   Home Preparation
Environmental Management:
   Safety

(Continued)

NURSING INTERVENTIONS CLASSIFICATION LABELS *(Continued)*

Environmental Management: Violence Prevention
Environmental Management: Worker Safety
Environmental Risk Protection
Examination Assistance
Exercise Promotion
Exercise Promotion: Strength Training
Exercise Promotion: Stretching
Exercise Therapy: Ambulation
Exercise Therapy: Balance
Exercise Therapy: Joint Mobility
Exercise Therapy: Muscle Control
Eye Care

Fall Prevention
Family Integrity Promotion
Family Integrity Promotion: Childbearing Family
Family Involvement Promotion
Family Mobilization
Family Planning: Contraception
Family Planning: Infertility
Family Planning: Unplanned Pregnancy
Family Presence Facilitation
Family Process Maintenance
Family Support
Family Therapy
Feeding
Fertility Preservation
Fever Treatment
Financial Resource Assistance
Fire-Setting Precautions
First Aid
Fiscal Resource Management

Flatulence Reduction
Fluid/Electrolyte Management
Fluid Management
Fluid Monitoring
Fluid Resuscitation
Foot Care
Forgiveness Facilitation

Gastrointestinal Intubation
Genetic Counseling
Grief Work Facilitation
Grief Work Facilitation: Perinatal Death
Guilt Work Facilitation

Hair Care
Hallucination Management
Healthcare Information Exchange
Health Education
Health Policy Monitoring
Health Screening
Health System Guidance
Heat/Cold Application
Heat Exposure Treatment
Hemodialysis Therapy
Hemodynamic Regulation
Hemofiltration Therapy
Hemorrhage Control
High-Risk Pregnancy Care
Home Maintenance Assistance
Hope Instillation
Hormone Replacement Therapy
Humor
Hyperglycemia Management
Hypervolemia Management
Hypnosis
Hypoglycemia Management
Hypothermia Treatment
Hypovolemia Management

Immunization/Vaccination Management

Impulse Control Training
Incident Reporting
Incision Site Care
Infant Care
Infection Control
Infection Control: Intraoperative
Infection Protection
Insurance Authorization
Intracranial Pressure (ICP) Monitoring
Intrapartal Care
Intrapartal Care: High-Risk Delivery
Intravenous (IV) Insertion
Intravenous (IV) Therapy
Invasive Hemodynamic Monitoring

Kangaroo Care

Labor Induction
Labor Suppression
Labor Data Interpretation
Lactation Counseling
Lactation Suppression
Laser Precautions
Latex Precautions
Learning Facilitation
Learning Readiness Enhancement
Leech Therapy
Limit Setting
Lower Extremity Monitoring

Malignant Hyperthermia Precautions
Mechanical Ventilation
Mechanical Ventilatory Weaning
Medication Administration
Medication Administration: Ear
Medication Administration: Enteral
Medication Administration: Eye

Medication Administration: Inhalation
Medication Administration: Interpleural
Medication Administration: Intramuscular (IM)
Medication Administration: Intraosseous
Medication Administration: Intraspinal
Medication Administration: Intravenous (IV)
Medication Administration: Nasal
Medication Administration: Oral
Medication Administration: Rectal
Medication Administration: Skin
Medication Administration: Subcutaneous
Medication Administration: Vaginal
Medication Administration: Ventricular Reservoir
Medication Management
Medication Prescribing
Meditation Facilitation
Memory Training
Milieu Therapy
Mood Management
Multidisciplinary Care Conference
Music Therapy
Mutual Goal Setting

Nail Care
Nausea Management
Neurologic Monitoring
Newborn Care
Newborn Monitoring
Nonnutritive Sucking
Normalization Promotion
Nutrition Management
Nutrition Therapy
Nutritional Counseling
Nutritional Monitoring

Oral Health Maintenance
Oral Health Promotion
Oral Health Restoration
Order Transcription
Organ Procurement
Ostomy Care
Oxygen Therapy

Pain Management
Parent Education:
    Adolescent
Parent Education:
    Childbearing Family
Parent Education: Infant
Parenting Promotion
Patient Contracting
Patient-Controlled Analgesia
    Assistance
Patient Rights Protection
Peer Review
Pelvic Muscle Exercise
Perineal Care
Peripheral Sensation
    Management
Peripherally Inserted
    Central Catheter Care
Peritoneal Dialysis Therapy
Pessary Management
Phlebotomy: Arterial Blood
    Sample
Phlebotomy: Blood Unit
    Acquisition
Phlebotomy: Cannulated
    Vessel
Phlebotomy: Venous Blood
    Sample
Phototherapy: Mood/Sleep
    Regulation
Phototherapy: Neonate
Physical Restraint
Physician Support
Pneumatic Tourniquet
    Precautions
Positioning
Positioning: Intraoperative
Positioning: Neurologic
Positioning: Wheelchair
Postanesthesia Care
Postmortem Care
Postpartal Care
Preceptor: Employee

Preceptor: Student
Preconception Counseling
Pregnancy Termination Care
Premenstrual Syndrome
    Management
Prenatal Care
Preoperative
    Coordination
Preparatory Sensory
    Information
Presence
Pressure Management
Pressure Ulcer Care
Pressure Ulcer Prevention
Product Evaluation
Program Development
Progressive Muscle
    Relaxation
Prompted Voiding
Prosthesis Care
Pruritus Management

Quality Monitoring

Radiation Therapy
    Management
Rape-Trauma Treatment
Reality Orientation
Recreation Therapy
Rectal Prolapse
    Management
Referral
Religious Addiction
    Prevention
Religious Ritual
    Enhancement
Relocation Stress
    Reduction
Reminiscence Therapy
Reproductive Technology
    Management
Research Data Collection
Resiliency Promotion
Respiratory Monitoring
Respite Care
Resuscitation
Resuscitation: Fetus
Resuscitation: Neonate
Risk Identification
Risk Identification:
    Childbearing Family

Risk Identification: Genetic
Role Enhancement

Seclusion
Security Enhancement
Seduction Management
Seizure Management
Seizure Precautions
Self-Awareness
    Enhancement
Self-Care Assistance:
Self-Care Assistance:
    Bathing/Hygiene
Self-Care Assistance:
    Dressing/Grooming
Self-Care Assistance:
    Feeding
Self-Care Assistance: IADL
Self-Care Assistance:
    Toileting
Self-Care Assistance:
    Transfer
Self-Esteem Enhancement
Self-Hypnosis Facilitation
Self-Modification Assistance
Self-Responsibility
    Facilitation
Sexual Counseling
Shift Report
Shock Management
Shock Management: Cardiac
Shock Management:
    Vasogenic
Shock Management: Volume
Shock Prevention
Sibling Support
Simple Guided Imagery
Simple Massage
Simple Relaxation Therapy
Skin Care: Donor Site
Skin Care: Graft Site
Skin Care: Topical
    Treatments
Skin Surveillance
Sleep Enhancement
Smoking Cessation
    Assistance
Socialization Enhancement
Specimen Management
Spiritual Growth Facilitation
Spiritual Support

Splinting
Sports-Injury Prevention
Staff Development
Staff Supervision
Subarachnoid Hemorrhage
    Precautions
Substance Use Prevention
Substance Use Treatment
Substance Use Treatment:
    Alcohol Withdrawal
Substance Use Treatment:
    Drug Withdrawal
Substance Use Treatment:
    Overdose
Suicide Prevention
Supply Management
Support Group
Support System
    Enhancement
Surgical Assistance
Surgical Precautions
Surgical Preparation
Surveillance
Surveillance: Community
Surveillance: Late Pregnancy
Surveillance: Remote
    Electronic
Surveillance: Safety
Sustenance Support
Suturing
Swallowing Therapy

Teaching: Disease Process
Teaching: Foot Care
Teaching: Group
Teaching: Individual
Teaching: Infant Nutrition
Teaching: Infant Safety
Teaching: Infant Stimulation
Teaching: Preoperative
Teaching: Prescribed
    Activity/Exercise
Teaching: Prescribed Diet
Teaching: Prescribed
    Medication
Teaching:
    Procedure/Treatment
Teaching: Psychomotor Skill
Teaching: Safe Sex
Teaching: Sexuality
Teaching: Toddler Nutrition

(Continued)

NURSING INTERVENTIONS CLASSIFICATION LABELS *(Continued)*

Teaching: Toddler Safety	Traction/Immobilization	Ventriculostomy/Lumbar	Values Clarification
Teaching: Toilet Training	Care	Drain	Vehicle Safety Promotion
Technology	Transcutaneous Electrical	Ultrasonography: Limited	Venous Access Device
Management	Nerve Stimulation	Obstetric	(VAD) Maintenance
Telephone Consultation	Transport	Unilateral Neglect	Ventilation Assistance
Telephone Follow-Up	Trauma Therapy: Child	Management	Visitation Facilitation
Temperature Regulation	Triage: Disaster	Urinary Bladder Training	Vital Signs Monitoring
Temperature Regulation:	Triage: Emergency Center	Urinary Catheterization	Vomiting Management
Intraoperative	Triage: Telephone	Urinary Catheterization:	
Temporary Pacemaker	Truth Telling	Intermittent	Weight Gain Assistance
Management	Tube Care	Urinary Elimination	Weight Management
Therapeutic Play	Tube Care: Chest	Management	Weight Reduction
Therapeutic Touch	Tube Care:	Urinary Habit Training	Assistance
Therapy Group	Gastrointestinal	Urinary Incontinence Care	Wound Care
Total Parenteral	Tube Care: Umbilical Line	Urinary Incontinence Care:	Wound Care: Closed
Nutrition Administration	Tube Care: Urinary	Enuresis	Drainage
Touch	Tube Care:	Urinary Retention Care	Wound Irrigation

From Dochterman, J., Bulecheck, G. (2004). Nursing Interventions Classifications (NIC), 4th ed. St. Louis: Mosby.

NOC is also a comprehensive standardized language providing 330 outcome labels (Table 2–2) with definitions; a set of indicators describing specific client, caregiver, family, or community states related to the outcome; and a 5-point Likert-type measurement scale that facilitates tracking clients across care settings and that can demonstrate client progress even when outcomes are not fully met. The outcomes are research-based and are applicable in all care settings and clinical specialties.

In addition, NIC and NOC have been linked to the Omaha System problems, to resident assessment protocols (RAPs) used in extended/long-term care settings, and to NANDA. This last linkage created the NANDA, NIC, NOC (NNN) Taxonomy of Nursing Practice. The combination of NANDA nursing diagnoses, NOC outcomes, and NIC interventions in a common unifying structure provides a comprehensive nursing language recognized by the American Nurses Association (ANA) and is coded in the Systematized Nomenclature of Medicine (SNOMED) in support of the electronic client record.

The use of a SNL entered into international coded terminology not only allows nursing to describe the care received by the client and to document the effects of that care on client outcomes but also facilitates the comparison of nursing care across worldwide settings and diverse databases. In addition, it supports research by comparing client care delivered by nurses with that delivered by other providers, which is essential if nursing's contribution is to be recognized and nurses are to be reimbursed for the care they provide.

Today, more than nine versions of SNLs are recognized by the ANA and have been submitted to the National Library of Medicine for inclusion in the Unified Medical Language System Metathesaurus. The Metathesaurus provides a uniform, integrated distribution format from over 100 biomedical vocabularies and classifications (the majority in English and some in multiple languages) and links many different names for the same concepts, establishing new relationships between terms from different source vocabularies.

NURSING OUTCOMES CLASSIFICATION LABELS

Abuse Cessation
Abuse Protection
Abuse Recovery Status
Abuse Recovery: Emotional
Abuse Recovery: Financial
Abuse Recovery: Physical
Abuse Recovery: Sexual
Abusive Behavior Self-
Restraint
Acceptance: Health Status
Activity Tolerance
Adaptation to Physical
Disability
Adherence Behavior
Agression Self-Control
Allergic Response: Localized
Allergic Response: Systemic
Ambulation
Ambulation: Wheelchair
Anxiety Level
Anxiety Self-Control
Appetite
Aspiration Prevention
Asthma Self-Management

Balance
Blood Coagulation
Blood Glucose Level
Blood Loss Severity
Blood Transfusion Reaction
Body Image
Body Mechanics
Performance
Body Positioning: Self-
Initiated
Bone Healing
Bowel Continence
Bowel Elimination
Breastfeeding Establishment:
Infant
Breastfeeding Establishment:
Maternal
Breastfeeding
Maintenance
Breastfeeding Weaning

Cardiac Disease Self-
Management

Cardiac Pump Effectiveness
Caregiver Adaptation to
Patient Institutionalization
Caregiver Emotional Health
Caregiver Home Care
Readiness
Caregiver Lifestyle
Disruption
Caregiver-Patient
Relationship
Caregiver Performance:
Direct Care
Caregiver Performance:
Indirect Care
Caregiver Physical Health
Caregiver Stressors
Caregiver Well-Being
Caregiving Endurance
Potential
Child Adaptation to
Hospitalization
Child Development: 1
Month
Child Development: 2
Months
Child Development: 4
Months
Child Development: 6
Months
Child Development: 12
Months
Child Development: 2 Years
Child Development: 3 Years
Child Development: 4 Years
Child Development:
Preschool
Child Development: Middle
Childhood
Child Development:
Adolescence
Circulation Status
Client Satisfaction: Access to
Care Resources
Client Satisfaction: Caring
Client Satisfaction:
Communication
Client Satisfaction:
Continuity of Care

Client Satisfaction: Cultural
Needs Fulfillment
Client Satisfaction:
Functional Assistance
Client Satisfaction:
Physical Care
Client Satisfaction:
Physical Environment
Client Satisfaction:
Protection
of Rights
Client Satisfaction:
Psychological Care
Client Satisfaction: Safety
Client Satisfaction: Symptom
Control
Client Satisfaction:
Teaching
Client Satisfaction: Technical
Aspects of Care
Cognition
Cognitive Orientation:
Ability to identify person,
place, and time
Comfort Level
Comfortable Death
Communication
Communication: Expressive
Community Competence
Community Disaster
Readiness
Community Health Status
Community Health Status:
Immunity
Community Risk Control:
Chronic Disease
Community Risk Control:
Communicable Disease
Community Risk Control:
Lead Exposure
Community Risk Control:
Violence
Community Violence
Level
Compliance Behavior
Concentration
Coordinated Movement
Coping

Decision Making
Depression Level
Depression Self-Control
Diabetes Self-Management
Dignified Life Closure
Discharge Readiness:
Independent Living
Discharge Readiness:
Supported Living
Distorted Thought Self-
Control

Electrolyte and Acid/Base
Balance
Endurance
Energy Conservation

Fall Prevention Behavior
Falls Occurrence
Family Coping
Family Functioning
Family Health Status
Family Integrity
Family Normalization
Family Participation in
Professional Care
Family Physical
Environment
Family Resiliency
Family Social Climate
Family Support During
Treatment
Fear Level
Fear Level: Child
Fear Self-Control
Fetal Status: Antepartum
Fetal Status: Intrapartum
Fluid Balance
Fluid Overload Severity

Grief Resolution
Growth

Health Beliefs
Health Beliefs: Perceived
Ability to Perform
Health Beliefs: Perceived
Control

(Continued)

NURSING OUTCOMES CLASSIFICATION LABELS *(Continued)*

Health Beliefs: Perceived
   Resources
Health Beliefs: Perceived
   Threat
Health Orientation
Health-Promoting Behavior
Health-Seeking Behavior
Hearing Compensation
   Behavior
Hemodialysis Access
Hope
Hydration
Hyperactivity Level

Identity
Immobility Consequences:
   Physiological
Immobility Consequences:
   Psycho-Cognitive
Immune Hypersensitivity
   Response
Immune Status
Immunization Behavior
Impulse Self-Control
Infection Severity
Infection Severity: Newborn
Information Processing

Joint Movement: Ankle
Joint Movement: Elbow
Joint Movement: Fingers
Joint Movement: Hip
Joint Movement: Knee
Joint Movement: Neck
Joint Movement: Passive
Joint Movement: Shoulder
Joint Movement: Spine
Joint Movement: Wrist

Kidney Function
Knowledge: Body Mechanics
Knowledge: Breastfeeding
Knowledge: Cardiac Disease
   Management
Knowledge: Child Physical
   Safety
Knowledge: Conception
   Prevention

Knowledge: Diabetes
   Management
Knowledge: Diet
Knowledge: Disease Process
Knowledge: Energy
   Conservation
Knowledge: Fall Prevention
Knowledge: Fertility
   Promotion
Knowledge: Health Behavior
Knowledge: Health
   Promotion
Knowledge: Health
   Resources
Knowledge: Illness Care
Knowledge: Infant Care
Knowledge: Infection
   Control
Knowledge: Labor and
   Delivery
Knowledge: Medication
Knowledge: Ostomy Care
Knowledge: Parenting
Knowledge: Personal
   Safety
Knowledge: Postpartum
   Maternal Health
Knowledge: Preconception
   Maternal Health
Knowledge: Pregnancy
Knowledge: Prescribed
   Activity
Knowledge: Sexual
   Functioning
Knowledge: Substance
   Abuse Control
Knowledge: Treatment
   Procedure(s)
Knowledge: Treatment
   Regimen

Leisure Participation
Loneliness Severity

Maternal Status:
   Antepartum
Maternal Status:
   Intrapartum

Maternal Status: Postpartum
Mechanical Ventilation
   Response: Adult
Mechanical Ventilation
   Weaning Response: Adult
Medication Response
Memory
Mobility
Mood Equilibrium
Motivation

Nausea and Vomiting
   Control
Nausea and Vomiting:
   Disruptive Effects
Nausea and Vomiting
   Severity
Neglect Cessation
Neglect Recovery
Neurological Status
Neurological Status:
   Autonomic
Neurological Status:
   Central Motor Control
Neurological Status:
   Consciousness
Neurological Status:
   Cranial Sensory/Motor
   Function
Neurological Status: Spinal
   Sensory/Motor Function
Newborn Adaptation
Nutritional Status
Nutritional Status:
   Biochemical Measures
Nutritional Status: Energy
Nutritional Status: Food &
   Fluid Intake
Nutritional Status: Nutrient
   Intake

Oral Hygiene
Ostomy Self-Care

Pain: Adverse Psychological
   Response
Pain Control
Pain: Disruptive Effects

Pain Level
Parent-Infant Attachment
Parenting: Adolescent
   Physical Safety
Parenting: Early/Middle
   Childhood Physical Safety
Parenting: Infant/Toddler
   Physical Safety
Parenting Performance
Parenting: Psychological
   Safety
Participation in Health Care
   Decisions
Personal Autonomy
Personal Health Status
Personal Safety Behaviors
Personal Well-Being
Physical Aging
Physical Fitness
Physical Injury Severity
Physical Maturation: Female
Physical Maturation: Male
Play Participation
Post-Procedure Recovery
   Status
Parental Health Behavior
Preterm Infant Organization
Psychomotor Energy
Psychosocial Adjustment:
   Life Change

Quality of Life

Respiratory Status: Airway
   Patency
Respiratory Status: Gas
   Exchange
Respiratory Status:
   Ventilation
Rest
Risk Control
Risk Control: Alcohol Use
Risk Control: Cancer
Risk Control: Cardiovascular
   Health
Risk Control: Drug Use
Risk Control: Hearing
   Impairment

Risk Control: Sexual Transmitted Diseases (STD)
Risk Control: Tobacco Use
Risk Control: Unintended Pregnancy
Risk Control: Visual Impairment
Risk Detection
Role Performance

Safe Home Environment
Self-Care Status
Self-Care: Activities of Daily Living (ADL)
Self-Care: Bathing
Self-Care: Dressing
Self-Care: Eating
Self-Care: Hygiene
Self-Care: Instrumental Activities of Daily Living (IADL)
Self-Care: Non-Parenteral Medications
Self-Care: Oral Hygiene

Self-Care: Parenteral Medication
Self-Care: Toileting
Self-Direction of Care
Self-Esteem
Self-Mutilation Restraint
Sensory Function Status
Sensory Function: Cutaneous
Sensory Function: Hearing
Sensory Function: Proprioception
Sensory Function: Taste and Smell
Sensory Function: Vision
Sexual Functioning
Sexual Identity
Skeletal Function
Sleep
Social Interaction Skills
Social Involvement
Social Support
Spiritual Health
Stress Level
Student Health Status

Substance Addiction: Consequences
Suffering Severity
Suicide Self-Restraint
Swallowing Status
Swallowing Status: Esophageal Phase
Swallowing Status: Oral Phase
Swallowing Status: Pharyngeal Phase
Symptom Control
Symptom Severity
Symptom Severity: Perimenopause
Symptom Severity: Premenstrual Syndrome
Systemic Toxic Clearance: Dialysis

Thermoregulation
Thermoregulation: Newborn
Tissue Integrity: Skin and Mucous Membrane

Tissue Perfusion: Abdominal Organs
Tissue Perfusion: Cardiac
Tissue Perfusion: Cerebral
Tissue Perfusion: Peripheral
Tissue Perfusion: Pulmonary
Transfer Performance
Treatment Behavior: Illness or Injury

Urinary Continence
Urinary Elimination
Vision Compensation Behavior

Vital Signs

Weight: Body Mass
Weight Control
Will to Live
Wound Healing: Primary Intention
Wound Healing: Secondary Intention

Moorhead, S., Johnson, M., Maas, M. (Eds). (2004). Nursing Outcomes Classifications (NOC), 3rd ed., St. Louis: Mosby.

Indexing of the entire medical record supports disease management activities (including decision support systems), research, and analysis of outcomes for quality improvement for all healthcare disciplines. Coding also supports telehealth (the use of telecommunications technology to provide medical information and healthcare services over distance) and facilitates access to healthcare data across care settings and different computer systems.

So to those who stated "Nursing will thrive as a unique and valued profession when nurses present a theory and rationalistic model for their practice…and actively participate in processes for change,"[11] we answer, "We are actively participating in processes for change, and as a profession, we will continue."

References

1. Gordon, M. (1998). Nursing nomenclature and classification system development. Online Journal of Issues in Nursing. Available at: http://nursingworld.org/ojin/tpc7/tpc7_1.htm. Accessed 2004.
2. NANDA International (2003). Nursing Diagnoses: Definitions & Classifications 2003–2004. Philadelphia: Author.
3. Carroll-Johnson, R. M. (Ed). (1991). Classification of Nursing Diagnoses: Proceedings of the Ninth Conference. Philadelphia: J. B. Lippincott.
4. Saba, V. K. (1994). Home Health Care Classification (HHCC) of Nursing Diagnoses and Interventions. (Revised). Washington, DC: Author.
5. McCloskey, J. C., Bulechek, G. M. (Eds). (2004). Nursing Interventions Classification (NIC), 4th ed., St. Louis: Mosby.

6. Moorhead, S., Johnson, M., Maas, M. (Eds). (2004). Nursing Outcomes Classification (NOC), 3rd ed., St. Louis: Mosby.

7. Martin, K. S., Scheet, N. J. (Eds). (1992). The Omaha System: Applications for Community Health Nursing. Philadelphia: W. B. Saunders.

8. Ozboldt, J. G. (1996). From minimum data to maximum impact: Using clinical data to strengthen patient care. Advanced. Practice Nursing Quarterly, 1, 62–69.

9. Beyea, S. (2002). Preioperative Nursing Data Set (PNDS), 2nd ed. Denver: AORN.

10. Johnson, M., Bulechek, G., Dochterman, J. M., Maas, M., Moorhead, S. (Eds). (2001). Nursing Diagnoses, Outcomes, and Interventions: NANDA, NOC, and NIC Linkages. St. Louis: Mosby.

11. Erickson, H. C., Tomlin, E. M., Swain, M. A. P. (1983). Modeling and Role-Modeling. Englewood Cliffs, NJ: Prentice-Hall.

Chapter 3

The Assessment Process: Developing the Client Database

The Standard of Clinical Nursing Practice[1] addresses the assessment process. The standard stipulates the data collection process is systematic and ongoing. The nurse collects client health data from the client, significant others, and healthcare providers when appropriate. The priority of the data collection activities is determined by the client's immediate condition or needs. Pertinent data are collected using appropriate assessment techniques and instruments. Relevant data are documented in a retrievable form.

↳ The Client Database

The assessment step of the nursing process is focused on eliciting a profile of the client that allows the nurse to identify client problems or needs and corresponding nursing diagnoses, plan care, implement interventions, and evaluate outcomes. This profile, or *client database,* supplies a sense of the client's overall health status, providing a picture of the client's physical, psychological, sociocultural, spiritual, cognitive, and developmental levels; economic status, functional abilities, and lifestyle. It is a combination of data gathered from the history-taking interview (a method of obtaining SUBJECTIVE information by talking with the client and/or significant other(s) and listening to their responses), the physical examination (a "hands-on" means of obtaining OBJECTIVE information), and data gathered from the results of laboratory/diagnostic studies. To be more specific, subjective data are what the client/significant others perceive and report, and objective data are what the nurse observes and gathers from other sources.

Assessment involves three basic activities:

* Systematically gathering data
* Organizing or clustering the data collected
* Documenting the data in a retrievable format

↳ Gathering Data—The Interview

Information in the client database is obtained primarily from the client (who is the most important source) and then from family members/significant others (secondary sources), as appropriate, through conversation and by observation during a structured interview. Clearly, the interview involves more than simply exchanging and processing data. Nonverbal communication is as important as the client's choice of words in providing the data. The ability to collect data that are meaningful to the client's health concerns depends heavily on the nurse's knowledge base; the choice and sequence of questions; and the ability to give meaning to the client's responses, integrate the data gathered, and prioritize the resulting information. Insight into the nature and behavior of the client is essential as well.

The nurse's initial responsibility is to observe, collect, and record data without drawing conclusions or making judgments/assumptions. Personal self-awareness is a crucial factor in the interaction, because perceptions, judgments, and assumptions can easily color the assessment findings unless they are recognized.

The quality of a history improves with experience with the interviewing process. Tips for obtaining a meaningful history include:

- Be a good listener.
- Listen carefully and attentively for whole thoughts and ideas, not merely isolated facts.
- Use skills of active listening, silence, and acceptance to provide ample time for the person to respond. Be as objective as possible.
- Identify only the client's and/or significant others' contributions to the history.

The interview question is the major tool used to obtain information. How the question is phrased is a skill that is important in obtaining the desired results and getting the information necessary to make accurate nursing diagnoses. Note: Some questioning strategies to be avoided include closed-ended and leading questions, probing, and agreeing or disagreeing that implies the client is "right" or "wrong." It is important to remember, too, that the client has the right to refuse to answer any question at all, no matter how reasonably phrased.

Nine effective data collection questioning techniques include:

1. Open-ended questions allow the client maximum freedom to respond in his or her own way, impose no limitations on how the question may be answered, and can produce considerable information.
2. Hypothetical questions pose a situation and ask the client how it might be handled.
3. Reflecting or "mirroring responses" are useful techniques in getting at underlying meanings that might not be verbalized clearly.
4. Focusing consists of eye contact (within cultural limits), body posture, and verbal responses.
5. Giving broad openings encourages the client to take the initiative in what is to be discussed.
6. Offering general leads encourages the client to continue.
7. Exploring pursues a topic in more depth.
8. Verbalizing the implied gives voice to what has been suggested.
9. Encouraging evaluation helps the client to consider the quality of his or her own experiences.

The client's medical diagnosis can provide a starting point for gathering data. Knowledge of the anatomy and physiology of the specific disease process/severity of condition also helps in choosing and prioritizing specific portions of the assessment. For example, when examining a client with severe chest pain, it may be wise to evaluate the pain and the cardiovascular system in a focused assessment before addressing other areas, possibly at a later time. Likewise, the duration and length of any assessment depend on circumstances such as the condition of the client and the urgency of the situation.

The data collected about the client and/or significant others contain a vast amount of information, some of which may be repetitious. However, some of it will be valuable for eliciting information that was not recalled or volunteered previously. Enough material needs to be noted in the history so that a complete picture is presented, and yet not so much that the information will not be read or used.

↳ Gathering Data—The Physical Examination

The physical examination is performed to gather objective information and also as a screening device. Four common methods used during the physical examination are inspection, palpation, percussion, and auscultation. These techniques incorporate the senses of sight, hearing, touch, and smell. For the data collected during the physical examination to be meaningful, it is vital to know the normal physical and emotional characteristics of human beings sufficiently well enough to be able to recognize deviations. To gain as much information as possible from the assessment procedure, the same format should be used each time a physical examination is performed to lessen the possibility of omissions.

↳ Gathering Data—Laboratory Tests/Diagnostic Procedures

Laboratory and other diagnostic studies are a part of the information-gathering stage providing supportive evidence. These studies aid in the management, maintenance, and restoration of health. In reviewing and interpreting laboratory tests, it is important to remember that the origin of the test material does not always correlate to an organ or body system (e.g., a urine test to detect the presence of bilirubin and urobilinogen could indicate liver disease, biliary obstruction, or hemolytic disease). In some cases the results of a test are *nonspecific* because they only indicate a disorder or abnormality and do not indicate the location of the cause of the problem (e.g., an elevated erythrocyte sedimentation rate suggests the presence but not the location of an inflammatory process).

In evaluating laboratory tests, it is advisable to consider which medications (e.g., heparin, promethazine) are being administered to the client, including over-the-counter and herbal supplements (e.g., vitamin E), because these have the potential to alter, blur, or falsify results, creating a misleading diagnostic picture.

↳ Documenting and Clustering the Data

Data gathered during the interview, the physical examination, and from other records/sources are organized and recorded in a concise systematic way and clustered into similar categories. Various formats have been used to accomplish this, including a review of body systems. This approach has been used by both medicine and nursing for many years, but was initially developed to aid the physician in making medical diagnoses. Currently nursing is developing and fine-tuning its own tools for recording and clustering data. Several nursing models available to guide data collection include Doenges and Moorhouse Diagnostic Divisions (Table 3–1),[2,3] Gordon's Functional Health Patterns,[4] and Guzzetta's Clinical Assessment Tool.[5]

The use of a nursing model as a framework for data collection (rather than a body-systems approach [assessing the heart, moving on to the lungs] or the commonly known head-to-toe approach) has the advantage of focusing data collection on the nurse's phenomena of concern—the human responses to health and illness.[6] This facilitates the identification and validation of *nursing* diagnosis labels to describe the data accurately.

GENERAL ASSESSMENT TOOL

This is a suggested guideline/tool applicable in most care settings for creating a client database. It provides a nursing focus (Doenges & Moorhouse' Diagnostic Divisions of Nursing Diagnoses) that will facilitate planning client care. Although the sections are alphabetized here for ease of presentation, they can be prioritized or rearranged to meet individual needs.

Adult Medical/Surgical Assessment Tool

General Information

Name: _____ Age: _____ DOB: _____ Gender: _____ Race: _____

Admission Date: _____ Time: _____ From: _____

Source of Information: _____ Reliability (1–4 with 4 = very reliable): _____

Activity/Rest

Subjective (Reports)

Occupation: _____ Able to participate in usual activities/hobbies: _____ Leisure time/diversional activities: _____

Ambulatory status: _____ Gait (describe): _____ Activity level (sedentary to very active): _____ Daily exercise (type): _____

History of problems/limitations imposed by condition (e.g. immobility, weakness, breathlessness, fatigue): _____

_____

Feelings of boredom, dissatisfaction: _____

Developmental factors (describe): _____

Sleep: Hours: _____ Naps: _____ Aids: _____ Insomnia: _____ Related to: _____

    Difficulty falling asleep: _____ Difficulty staying asleep: _____

    Rested on awakening: _____ Excessive grogginess: _____

Bedtime rituals: _____ Relaxation techniques: _____

Sleeps on more than one pillow: _____ Use of oxygen (type): _____ When used: _____

Medications: _____ Herbals: _____

Objective (Exhibits)

Observed response to activity: Heart rate: _____ Rhythm (reg/irreg): _____

    Blood pressure: _____ Respiratory rate: _____ Pulse oximetry: _____

Mental status (i.e., withdrawn/lethargic): _____

Neuromuscular assessment:

    Muscle mass/tone: _____ Posture (e.g., normal, stooped): _____ Tremors: _____

    ROM: _____ Strength: _____ Deformity: _____

    Mobility aids (list): _____

Circulation

Subjective (Reports)

History of/treatment for: High blood pressure: _____ Brain injury/stroke: _____

    Heart condition/surgery: _____ Rheumatic fever: _____ Palpitations: _____ Syncope: _____

    Claudication: _____ Ankle/leg edema: _____ Blood clots/bleeding tendencies/episodes: _____

    Dysreflexia episodes: _____ Slow healing: _____

Extremities: Numbness: _____ Tingling: _____

Cough (describe)/hemoptysis: _____

Change in frequency/amount of urine: _____

Other: _____

Medications: _____ Herbals: _____

Objective (Exhibits)

Skin color (e.g., pale, cyanotic, jaundiced, mottled, ruddy): _____ Mucous membranes: _____

Lips: _____ Nailbeds: _____ Conjunctiva: _____ Sclera: _____

Skin moisture: (e.g., dry, diaphoretic): _____

BP: (R and L): Lying: _____ Sitting: _____ Standing: _____

Pulse pressure: _____ Auscultatory gap: _____

Pulses (Palpated 1–4 strength): Carotid: _____ Temporal: _____ Jugular: _____ Radial: _____

Femoral: _____ Popliteal: _____ Post-tibial: _____ Dorsalis pedis: _____

Cardiac (palpation): Thrill: _____ Heaves: _____

Heart sounds (auscultation): Rate: _____ Rhythm: _____ Quality: _____ Friction rub: _____

Murmur (describe location & sounds): _____

Vascular bruit: _____ Jugular vein distention: _____

Breath sounds (describe location & sounds): _____

Extremities: Temperature: _____ Color: _____ Capillary refill (1–3 sec): _____ Homan's sign (+

or –): _____ Varicosities: _____ Nail abnormalities: _____ Edema: _____ Distribution/quality

of hair: _____ Trophic skin changes: _____

Ego Integrity

Subjective (Reports)

Expression of concerns (e.g., financial, relationships; recent or anticipated lifestyle or role changes (specify): _____

_____

Expression of feelings of: Anger: _____ Anxiety: _____ Fear: _____ Grief: _____

Helplessness: _____ Hopelessness: _____ Powerlessness: _____

Stress factors: _____ Usual ways of handling stress: _____

Cultural factors/ethnic ties: _____

Religious affiliation: _____ Active/practicing: _____ Practices prayer/mediation: _____

Religious/Spiritual concerns: _____ Desires clergy visit: _____

Expression of sense of connectedness/harmony with self and others: _____

Medications/herbals: _____

Objective (Exhibits)

Emotional status (check those that apply):

Calm: _____ Anxious: _____ Angry: _____ Withdrawn: _____ Fearful: _____ Irritable: _____

Restive: _____ Euphoric: _____

Observed body language: _____ Observed physiological responses

(e.g., crying, change in voice quality/volume): _____

Changes in energy field:

Temperature: _____ Color: _____ Distribution: _____ Movement: _____ Sounds: _____

(Continued)

GENERAL ASSESSMENT TOOL (Continued)

Elimination

Subjective (Reports)

Usual bowel elimination pattern and character of stool (e.g., hard, soft, liquid): _____

Stool color (e.g., brown, black, yellow, clay colored, tarry): _____ Last BM and

character of stool: _____ History of bleeding: _____ Hemorrhoids/fistula: _____

Constipation (acute/chronic): _____ Diarrhea (acute/chronic): _____ Incontinence: _____

Laxative use: _____ How often: _____ Enema/suppository: _____ How often: _____

Usual voiding pattern and character of urine: _____

Incontinence (type & time of day): _____ Urgency: _____ Overflow: _____ Frequency: _____

Retention: _____ Bladder spasms: _____ Pain/burning: _____ Difficulty voiding: _____

History of kidney/bladder disease: _____

Diuretic use: _____ Other medications/herbals: _____

Objective (Exhibits)

Abdomen (palpation): Soft/firm: _____ Tenderness/pain (quadrant location): _____

Distention: _____ Palpable mass: _____ Size/girth: _____

Abdomen (auscultation): Bowel sounds (Location/type): _____

Bladder palpable: _____ Overflow voiding: _____

Rectal sphincter tone: (describe): _____ Hemorrhoids/fistulas: _____ Stool

in rectum: _____ Impaction: _____

Occult blood: (+ or –): _____

Presence/use of catheter, continence devices, ostomy appliances (describe appliance and location): _____

_____

Food/Fluid

Subjective (Reports)

Usual diet (type): _____ # of meals daily: _____ Snacks (#. daily, time consumed

& type): _____

Usual appetite: _____ Change in appetite: _____

Usual weight: _____ Unexpected or undesired weight loss or gain: _____

Nausea/vomiting: _____ related to? _____ Heartburn/indigestion: _____ related to? _____

relieved by? _____

Food preferences: _____ Food allergies/intolerances: _____

Cultural or religious food preparations/prohibitions: _____

Dietary pattern/content: (usual calorie, carbohydrate, protein, fat intake): B: _____ L: _____

D: _____ Last meal/intake: _____

Chewing/swallowing problems: _____ Gag/swallow reflex (present/absent): _____ Facial

injury/surgery: _____ Stroke/other neurologic deficit: _____

Teeth: Normal: _____ Dentures (full, partial): _____ Sore mouth, gums: _____

Dental hygiene: _____ Professional dental care: _____

Vitamin/food supplement use: _____ Other medications/herbals: _____

Objective (Exhibits)

Current weight: _____ Height: _____ Body build: _____ Body fat %: _____

Skin turgor (e.g. firm, supple, dehydrated): _____ Mucous membranes (moist/dry): _____

Edema (describe): Generalized: _____ Dependent: _____ Feet/ankles: _____ Periorbital: _____

   Abdominal/ascites: _____

Jugular vein distention: _____

Breath sounds (auscultation): Faint/distant: _____ Crackles: _____ Wheezes: _____

Condition of teeth/gums: _____ Appearance of tongue: _____ Mucous membranes: _____

Abdomen: Bowel sounds (quadrant location and type): _____

   Hernia/masses: _____

Urine S/A or Chemstix: _____ Serum glucose (Glucometer): _____

Hygiene

Subjective (Reports)

Ability to carry out activities of daily living: Independent/dependent (level 1, no assistance needed; to level 4, completely dependent):

   Mobility: _____ Needs assistance (describe): _____ Assistance provided by: _____

   Equipment/prosthetic devices required: _____

   Feeding: _____ Needs assistance (describe): _____ Assist devices: _____

   Hygiene: _____ Needs assistance (describe): _____ Preferred time of

   personal care/bath: _____

   Dressing/grooming: _____ Needs assistance (describe): _____

   Toileting: _____ Needs assistance with (describe): _____

Objective (Exhibits)

General appearance (e.g., cognition, alertness, orientation, strength, grooming, manner of dress): _____

_____

Personal habits: _____ Body odor: _____ Condition of hair/scalp: _____

   Presence of vermin: _____

Neurosensory

Subjective (Reports)

History of brain injury, trauma, stroke (residual effects): _____

Fainting spells/dizziness: _____ Headaches: _____ Location: _____ Frequency: _____

Tingling/numbness/weakness (location): _____

Seizures: _____ Type: _____ History/onset: _____ Frequency: _____ Aura

   (describe): _____ Postictal state: _____ How controlled: _____

Eyes: Vision loss/changes: _____ Glasses/contacts: _____ Last exam: _____

   Glaucoma: _____ Cataract: _____ Eye surgery: _____

Ears: Hearing loss/changes in hearing: _____ Hearing aids: _____ Last exam: _____

Epistaxis: _____ Sense of smell (changes): _____ Sense of taste (changes): _____

Other: _____

(Continued)

GENERAL ASSESSMENT TOOL *(Continued)*

Objective (Exhibits)

Mental status (note duration of change):

    Oriented/disoriented: Time: _____ Place: _____ Person: _____ Situation: _____

    Check all that apply: Alert: _____ Drowsy: _____ Lethargic: _____ Stuporous: _____ Comatose: _____

    Cooperative: _____ Follows commands: _____ Agitated/Restless: _____ Combative: _____

    Delusions (describe): _____ Hallucinations (describe): _____

    Affect (describe): _____

    Memory: Recent: _____ Remote: _____

Pupil shape: _____ Size/reaction: R/L: _____

Facial droop: _____ Swallowing: _____

Handgrasp/release, R/L: _____ Deep tendon reflexes: _____

Coordination: _____ Balance: _____ Walking: _____

Tremors: _____ Posturing: _____ Paralysis (L/R): _____

Pain/Discomfort

Subjective (Reports)

Primary focus: _____ Location: _____

    Intensity (use pain scale or pictures): _____ Frequency: _____ Duration: _____

    Quality (e.g., stabbing, aching, burning,) _____ Radiation: _____

How relieved (including nonpharmaceuticals/therapies): _____

Precipitating/aggravating factors: _____

Associated symptoms (e.g., nausea, sleep problems, crying): _____

Effect on activities of daily living: _____ Relationships: _____ Job: _____

    Enjoyment of life: _____

Cultural expectations regarding pain perception and expression: _____

Objective (Exhibits)

Facial grimacing: _____ Guarding affected area: _____ Posturing: _____

    Behaviors: _____ Narrowed focus: _____

Emotional response (e.g., crying, withdrawal, anger): _____

Vitals sign changes (acute pain): BP: _____ Pulse: _____ Respirations: _____

Respiration

Subjective (Reports)

Dyspnea/related to: _____ Worse with: _____ Better with: _____

Cough/type (e.g., hard, persistent, croupy): _____ Produces sputum (describe

    color/character): _____ Requires suctioning: _____

History of Bronchitis: _____ Asthma: _____ Emphysema: _____ Tuberculosis: _____

    Recurrent pneumonia: _____

Exposure to noxious fumes/allergens, infectious agents/diseases, poisons: _____

Smoker, packs/day: _____ no. of pack years: _____

Use of respiratory aids: _____ Oxygen (type & frequency): _____

Medications/herbals: _____

Objective (Exhibits)

Respirations (spontaneous/assisted): _____ Rate: _____ Chest excursion: Depth: _____
   equal/symmetrical: _____

   Use of accessory muscles: _____ Nasal flaring: _____ Fremitus: _____

   Breath sounds (describe): _____ Egophony: _____

Skin/mucous membrane color (e.g., pale, cyanotic): _____ Clubbing of fingers: _____

Sputum characteristics: _____

Mentation: (anxiety, restlessness): _____

Safety

 Subjective (Reports)

Allergies/sensitivity (medications, foods, environment, latex, etc.): _____

  Type of reaction: _____

Exposure to infectious diseases (e.g. measles, influenza, pink eye): _____

Exposure to toxins, poisons, biologic agents (list and describe reactions): _____

Geographic areas lived in/recent travel: _____

Immunization History: Tetanus: _____ MMR: _____ Polio: _____ Hepatitis: _____ Pneumonia: _____
  Influenza: _____ Other: _____

   Altered/suppressed immune system (list cause): _____

   History of sexually transmitted disease (date/type): _____ Testing: _____

Blood transfusion/number: _____ When: _____ Reaction (describe): _____

Work place safety: Occupation: _____ Rate working conditions (e.g., safety, noise, heating,
  water, ventilation, etc.): _____

Uses seat belt regularly: _____ Uses helmets/other safety devices: _____

High-risk behaviors (specify): _____

History of accidental injuries: _____ Fractures/dislocations: _____

Arthritis/unstable joints: _____ Back problems: _____

Skin problems (e.g., rashes, lesions, moles, breast lumps, enlarged nodes, delayed healing)/describe: _____
_____

Cognitive limitations (e.g., disorientation, confusion, etc. describe): _____

Sensory limitations (e.g., impaired vision, detecting heat/cold, taste, smell, hearing, touch, etc.): _____
_____

Prosthesis: _____ Ambulatory/mobility devices: _____

Violence (episodes or tendencies): _____

 Objective (Exhibits)

Body temperature: (where measured/method): _____

Skin integrity (mark location on diagram): _____ Scars: _____ Rashes: _____ Lacerations: _____
  Ulcerations: _____ Bruises: _____ Blisters: _____ Drainage: _____ Other: _____

  Burns: (describe area/degree/percent of body surface, using diagram): _____

Musculoskeletal: General strength: _____ Muscle tone: _____ Gait: _____ ROM: _____
  Paresthesia/paralysis: _____

Results of cultures: _____ Immune system testing: _____ Tuberculosis: _____ Hepatitis: _____

(Continued)

GENERAL ASSESSMENT TOOL *(Continued)*

Sexuality [Component of Social Interaction]
Subjective (Reports)

Sexually active: _____ Monogamous/Committed relationship: _____

Birth control method: _____ Use of condoms: _____

Sexual concerns/difficulties: _____

Recent change in frequency/interest: _____

Pain/discomfort: _____

Medications/herbals: _____

Objective: (exhibits)

Comfort level with subject matter: _____

Female: Subjective (Reports)

Age at menarche: _____ Length of cycle: _____ Duration: _____ Number of pads used/day: _____

Last menstrual period: _____ Bleeding between periods: _____

Infertility concerns: _____ Type of therapy: _____

Pregnant now: _____ Para: _____ Gravida: _____ Due date: _____

Menopausal: _____ Last period: _____ Hot flashes: _____ Vaginal lubrication: _____

Vaginal discharge: _____ Hormonal therapy: _____ Supplemental calcium: _____

Surgeries (type and date): _____

Practices breast self-examination: _____ Last mammogram: _____ Last Pap smear: _____

Objective: (exhibits)

Breast examination: _____

Genital warts/lesions: _____ Vaginal bleeding: _____ Discharge: _____

STD results: _____

Male: Subjective (Reports)

Penis: Circumcised: _____ Lesions/discharge: _____ Vasectomy: _____

Prostate disorder: _____

Practice self-exam: Breast: _____ Testicles: _____

Last proctoscopic/prostate examination: _____ Last PSA: _____

Objective (Exhibits)

Penis (lesions/discharge): _____ Testicles (descended, lumps, etc.): _____ Genital

warts/lesions: _____ Prostate: _____

Breast examination: _____

Social Interactions
Subjective (Reports)

Relationship status: Single: _____ Married: _____ Living with partner: _____

Divorced: _____ Widowed: _____

Years in relationship: _____ Perception of relationship: _____

Concerns/stresses: _____

Role within family structure: _____ Caregiver (to whom & how long): _____

Number & age of children: _____ Individuals living in home: _____

Extended family/availability: _____ Other support

person(s): _____

Perception of relationship with family members: _____

Ethnic affiliation: _____ Strength of ethnic identity: _____ Lives in ethnic community: _____

Feelings of: Mistrust: _____ Rejection: _____ Unhappiness: _____ Loneliness/isolation: _____

Describe: _____

Problems related to illness/condition: _____

Problems with communication (e.g., speech, another language, brain injury): _____

Use of communication aids (list): _____ Requires interpreter: _____

Genogram: (complete on separate form)

Objective (Exhibits)

Speech: Clear: _____ Slurred: _____ Unintelligible: _____ Aphasic: _____

Unusual speech pattern/impairment: _____

Use of speech/communication aids: _____ Laryngectomy present: _____

Verbal/nonverbal communication with family/SO(s): _____

Family interaction (behavioral) pattern: _____

Teaching/Learning
Subjective (Reports)

Dominant language (specify): _____ Second language: _____ Literate: _____

Education level: _____ Learning disabilities (specify): _____

Cognitive limitations: _____

Where born: _____ If immigrant, how long in this country: _____

Health and illness beliefs/practices/customs: _____

What family member makes healthcare decisions/is spokesperson for client: _____

Special healthcare concerns (e.g., impact of religious/cultural practices): _____

Health goals: _____

Presence of Advance Directives/Durable Medical Power of Attorney: _____

Client understanding of current problem: _____

Familial risk factors (indicate relationship): Diabetes: _____ Thyroid (specify): _____

Tuberculosis: _____ Heart disease: _____ Strokes: _____ High BP: _____ Epilepsy: _____

Kidney disease: _____ Cancer: _____ Mental illness: _____ Other: _____

Prescribed medications (list each separately):

Drug: _____ Dose: _____ Times (circle last dose): _____

Take regularly: _____ Purpose: _____ Side effects/problems: _____

Nonprescription drugs:

OTC drugs: _____ Vitamins: _____ Herbals: _____ Street

drugs: _____

Tobacco: _____ Smokeless tobacco: _____ Alcohol (amount/frequency): _____

Admitting diagnosis per provider: _____

Reason for hospitalization per client: _____

Client expectations of this hospitalization: _____

Will this admission cause any lifestyle changes (describe): _____

(Continued)

GENERAL ASSESSMENT TOOL *(Continued)*

History of current complaint: _____

Previous illnesses and/or hospitalizations/surgeries: _____

Evidence of failure to improve: _____

Last complete physical examination: _____

Discharge Plan Considerations

DRG projected mean length of stay: _____ Anticipated date of discharge: _____

  Date information obtained: _____

Resources available: Persons: _____ Financial: _____ Community

  supports: _____ Groups: _____

Areas that may require alteration/assistance: Food preparation: _____ Shopping: _____

  Transportation: _____ Ambulation: _____ Medication/IV therapy: _____ Treatments: _____

  Wound care: _____ Supplies: _____ Self-care (specify): _____ Homemaker/maintenance

  (specify): _____ Socialization: _____

  Physical layout of home (specify): _____

Anticipated changes in living situation after discharge: _____ Living facility

  other than home (specify): _____

Referrals (date, source, services): Social services: _____ Rehab services: _____

  Dietary: _____ Home care: _____ Resp/O$_2$: _____ Equipment: _____

  Supplies: _____ Other: _____

↳ Reviewing and Validating Findings

The nurse's initial responsibility is to observe, collect, and record data without drawing conclusions or making judgments/assumptions. Personal self-awareness is a crucial factor in this interaction, because perceptions, judgments, and assumptions can easily color the assessment findings.

Validation is an ongoing process that occurs during the data collection phase and upon its completion, when the data are reviewed and compared. The nurse should review the data to be sure that what is recorded is factual, to identify errors of omission, and to compare the objective and subjective data for congruencies and/or inconsistencies that require additional investigation, or a more focused assessment. Data that are grossly abnormal are rechecked, and any temporary factors that may affect the data are identified/noted. Validation is particularly important when the data are conflicting, when the source of the data may not be reliable, or when serious harm to the client could result from any inaccuracies. Validating the information can avoid the possibility of making wrong inferences or conclusions that could result in inaccurate nursing diagnoses, incorrect outcomes, and/or inappropriate nursing actions. This can be done by sharing the assumptions with the individuals involved and having them verify the accuracy of those conclusions. Sharing pertinent data with other healthcare professionals, such as the physician, dietician, or physical therapist can aid in collaborative planning of care. Data given in confidence should not be shared with other individuals (unless withholding that information would hinder appropriate evaluation or care of the client).

↳ Summary

The assessment step of the nursing process emphasizes and should provide a holistic view of the client. The generalized assessment done during the overall gathering of data creates a profile of the client. A focused, or more detailed, assessment may be warranted given the client's condition or emergent time constraints, or may be done to obtain more information about a specific issue that needs expansion or clarification. Both types of assessments provide important data that complement each other. A successfully completed assessment creates a picture of the client's state of wellness, response to health concerns or problems, and individual risk factors that is the foundation for identifying appropriate nursing diagnoses, developing client outcomes, and choosing relevant interventions necessary for providing individualized care.

References

1. American Nurses Association. (1991). Standards of Clinical Nursing Practice. St. Louis, MO: Author.
2. Doenges, M. E., Moorhouse, M. F., & Geissler-Murr, A. C. (2004). Nurse's Pocket Guide: Diagnoses, Interventions, and Rationales, ed 9. Philadelphia: F.A. Davis.
3. Doenges, M. E., Moorhouse, M. F., & Geissler-Murr, A. C. (2002). Nursing Care Plans: Guidelines for Individualizing Patient Care, ed 6. Philadelphia: F.A. Davis.
4. Gordon, M. (1994). Nursing Diagnosis: Process and Application, ed 3. St. Louis, MO: Mosby.
5. Guzzetta, C. E. et al. (1989). Clinical Assessment Tools for Use with Nursing Diagnoses. St. Louis, MO: Mosby.
6. American Nurses Association. (1995). Nursing's Social Policy Statement. Washington, DC: Author.

Chapter 4

Mind Mapping to Create
and Document the Plan of Care

The plan of care may be recorded on a single page or in a multiple-page format, with one page for each nursing diagnosis or client diagnostic statement. The format for documenting the plan of care is determined by agency policy. As a practicing professional, you might use a computer with a plan-of-care database, preprinted standardized care plan forms, or clinical pathways. Whichever form you use, the plan of care enables visualization of the nursing process and must reflect the basic nursing standards of care; personal client data; nonroutine care; and qualifiers for interventions and outcomes, such as time, frequency, or amount.

As students, you are asked to develop plans of care that often contain more detail than what you see in the hospital plans of care. This is to help you learn how to apply the nursing process and create individualized client care plans. However, even though much time and energy may be spent focusing on filling the columns of traditional clinical care plan forms, some students never develop a holistic view of their clients and fail to visualize how each client need interacts with other identified needs. A new technique or learning tool has been developed to assist you in visualizing the linkages, enhance your critical thinking skills, and facilitate the creative process of planning client care.

↰ Mind Mapping Client Care

Have you ever asked yourself whether you are more right-brained or left-brained? Those of us who think more naturally with our left brains are more linear in our thinking. Right-brain thinkers see more in pictures and illustrations. It is best for nurses to use the whole brain (right and left) when thinking about providing the broad scope of nursing care to clients.

No More Columns!

Traditional nursing care plans are linear—that is, they are designed in columns. They speak almost exclusively to the left brain. The traditional nursing care plan is organized according to the nursing process, which guides us in problem-solving the nursing care we give. However, the linear nature of the traditional plan does not facilitate interconnecting data from one "row" to another or between parts in a column. Mind mapping allows us to show the interconnections between various client symptoms, interventions or problems as they impact each other.

You can keep the parts that are great about traditional care plans (problem solving and categorizing) but change the linear/columnar nature of the plan to a design that uses the whole brain—a design that brings left-brained, linear problem-solving thinking together with the free-wheeling, interconnected, creative right brain. Joining mind mapping and care planning enables you to create a whole picture of a client with all the interconnections identified.

There are several diverse and innovative ways to mind map or to concept map nursing care plans.[1] The examples in this chapter use mind mapping and require placement of the client at the center, all ideas on one page (for a whole picture), color coding, and creative energy.[2,3] When doing a large mapped plan of care, a light posterboard is often used so that all ideas fit on one page.

Components of a Mind Map

Tony Buzan developed the idea of mind mapping, a way to depict how ideas about a main subject are related. Mapping represents, in a graphic manner, the relationships and interrelationships of ideas and concepts.[4] It fosters and encourages critical thinking through brainstorming about a particular subject.

Instead of starting at the top of the page, mind mapping starts in the center of the page. The main concept of our thinking goes in this center stage place.

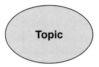

From that central thought, you simply begin thinking of other main ideas that relate to the central topic. These ideas radiate out from the central idea likes spokes of a wheel (see subsequent discussion); however, they do not have to be added in a balanced manner; it does not have to be a round "wheel".

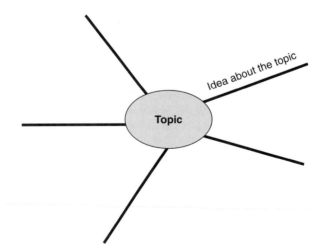

You will generate further ideas related to each spoke (see subsequent discussion); and your mind will race with even more ideas from those thoughts, which can be represented through pictures or words.

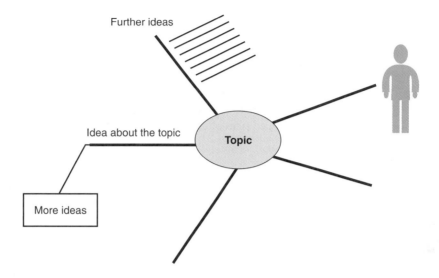

As you think of new ideas, write them down immediately. This may require going back and forth from one area of the page to another. Writing your mind map by hand allows you to move faster. Avoid using a computer to generate a map because this hinders the fast-paced process. You can group different concepts together by color-coding or by placement on the page (see subsequent discussion).

As you see connections and interconnections between groups of ideas, use arrows or lines to connect those concepts (refer to the dotted lines).

You can also add defining phrases that explain how the interconnected thoughts relate to one another as in the following figure.

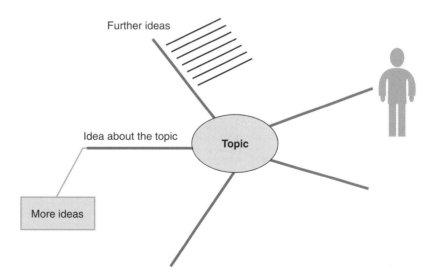

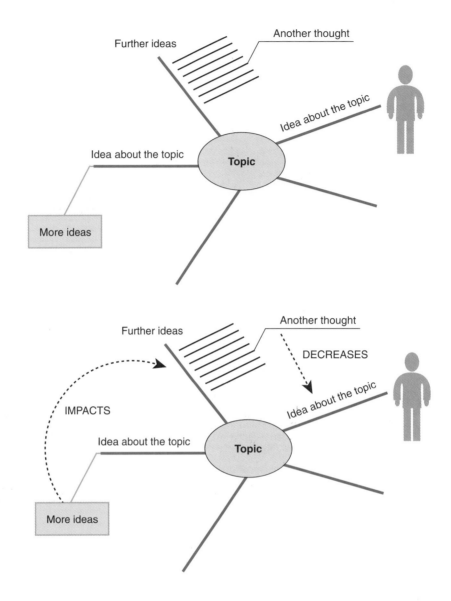

Some people are strongly linear, left-brain thinkers. They find it very difficult to start their ideas in the middle of a page. If you are this type of thinker, try starting at the top of the page (see subsequent discussion), but you must still represent your ideas in illustration form, not in paragraphs.

Mind maps created by different people look different. They are unique to the mind's eye picture. So don't expect your map to be the same as someone else's.

ᕇ Mind Mapping a Plan of Care

Mind mapping is an exciting alternative format for illustrating a written plan of care. A mapped care plan will look very different from traditional plans of care, which are usually completed on linear forms.

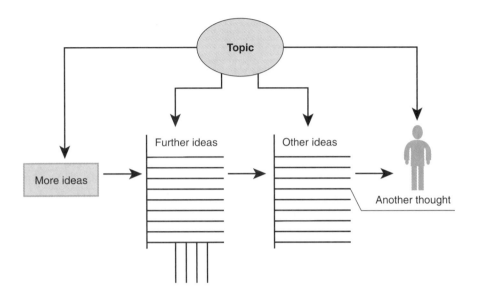

To begin mapping a client plan of care, you must begin with the central topic—the client. Now, you are thinking like a nurse. Create a shape that signifies "client" to you and place that at the center of your map. If your hand just can't start at the center, then put the shape at the top. This will help you keep in mind that the client is the focus of your plan, not the medical diagnosis or condition. All other pieces of the map will be connected in some manner to the client. Many different pieces of information *about* the client can be connected directly *to* the client. For example, each of the following pieces of critical client data could stem from the center (Fig. 4–1):

- 78-year-old widower
- no family in the state
- obese
- medical diagnosis of recurrent community-acquired pneumonia

Now, you must do a bit of thinking about how you think. To create the rest of your map, you must ask yourself how *you* plan client care. For example, which of these items do you see first or think of first in your mind's eye as the basis for your plan: the clustered assessment data, nursing diagnoses, or outcomes? Whichever piece you choose becomes your first layer of connections. Suppose when thinking about a plan of care for a female client with heart failure, you think first in terms of all the nursing diagnoses about that woman and her condition. Then your map would start with the diagnoses featured as the first "branches," each one being listed separately in some way on the map (Fig. 4–2).

Completing the map then becomes a matter of adding the rest of the pieces of the plan using the nursing process and your own way of thinking/planning as your guide. If your map was begun using nursing diagnoses, you might think to yourself, "What signs and symptoms or data support these diagnoses?" Then, you would connect clusters of supporting data to the related nursing diagnosis. Or your thought might be, "What client outcomes am I trying to achieve when I address this nursing diagnosis?" In that case, you would next connect client outcomes (or NOC labels) to the nursing diagnoses.

To keep your map clear, as suggested previously, use different colors and maybe a different shape/spoke/line for each piece of the care plan that you are adding. For example:

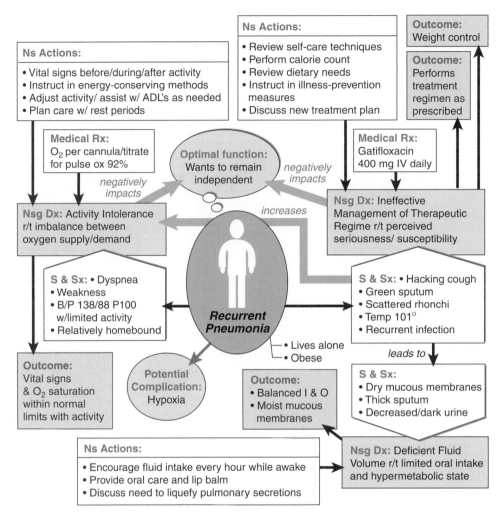

FIGURE 4–1 • Mind map of a plan of care for a client with pneumonia.

- Red—for signs and symptoms (to signify danger)
- Yellow—for nursing diagnoses (for "stop and think what this is")
- Green—for nursing interventions/NIC labels (for "go")
- Black (or some other color)—for outcomes/NOC labels

When all the pieces of the nursing process are represented, each "branch" of the map is complete. There should be a nursing diagnosis (supported by subjective and objective assessment data), nursing interventions, desired client outcome/s and any evaluation data, all connected in a manner that shows there is a relationship between them.

It is critical to understand that there is no pre-set order for the pieces, because one cluster is not more or less important than another (or one is not "subsumed" under another). It is important, however, that those pieces within a branch be in the same order in each branch.

So, you might ask, how is this different than writing out information in a linear manner? What makes mapping so special? One of the things you may have discovered about caring for clients is that the care you deliver is very interconnected. Taking care of one problem often

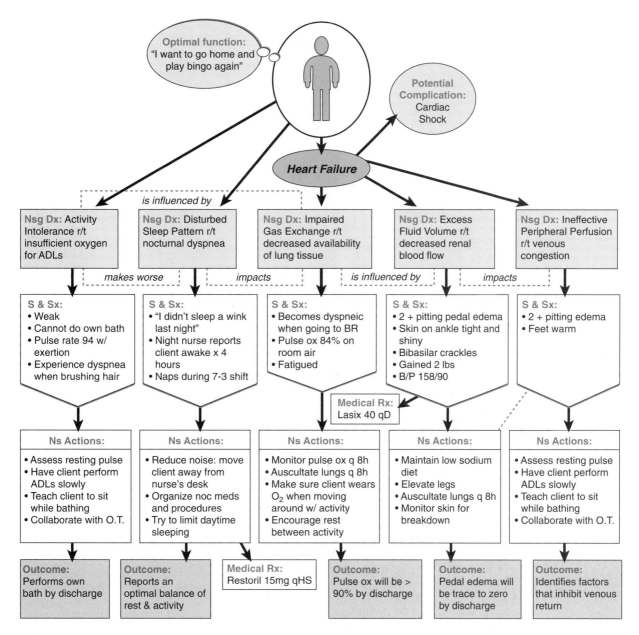

FIGURE 4–2 • Mind map of a plan of care for a client with heart failure.

results in the correction of another at the same time. For example, if you resolve a fluid volume problem in a client with heart failure, you will also positively impact the client's gas exchange and decrease their anxiety. These kinds of interconnections cannot be shown on linear care plans, yet they are what practicing nurses see in their mind's eye picture all the time. These interconnections can be represented on a map with arrows or dotted or dashed lines that tie related ideas together.

Defining phrases that explain the nature of the interconnection can be added to further clarify the relationship, as shown subsequently (as follows).

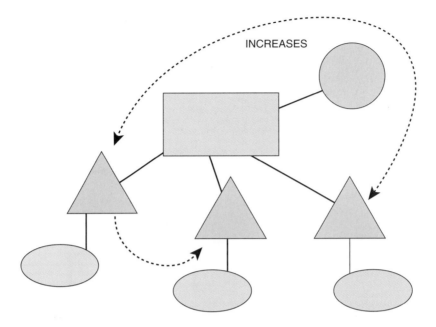

INCREASES

In addition to the pieces of the nursing process, there are other components of care that can be illustrated on a map. Nurses have certain responsibilities when clients have diagnostic tests (such as an angiography or a bronchoscopy). These tests can be connected to the appropriate piece of your map, along with the correct nursing interventions related to those tests. Another item to be added would be potential complications (collaborative problems).

Taking your client's needs one step further, try asking every client you have medical/surgical or otherwise, "What is the most important thing to you now in relation to why you are here?" Obtaining this information builds an alliance between you and your client, and together you can work toward that desired outcome. Add it to your map and see how your care plan becomes more client-centered (refer to Fig. 4–1).

↻ Summary

Mind maps allow you to do something that is different and creative. Mind maps require you to think (and learn), make connections, and use colors and shapes. They help you to focus on the client; and having the map on one page helps you to understand the "whole picture" better. They also help you to become better organized and to develop your own unique approach to "thinking like a nurse" much sooner.

A student who had written many traditional care plans in her previous nursing program wrote the following about mind-mapped care plans: "Mind mapping is painting a picture using colors of the rainbow on blank paper to tell the story of your client using 'NANDA' nursing diagnoses and the nursing process. Previously, I was a student in prison (my mind) who hated the words 'CARE PLAN,' writing page after page in narrative form. It was laborious to do and boring to read. There was no life or heartbeat.

Mind mapping opened the prison doors, and my care plan took on human from with a VOICE, a beating HEART, and COLOR while still incorporating the nursing process and standardized nursing language. My mind now took on the professional thought process that NANDA, NIC, and NOC were created to facilitate nursing; however, the magic was in mind mapping, which removed all my fears, and the client became a beautiful painting with a heart beat."

References

1. Schuster, P. (2002). Concept Mapping: A Critical-Thinking Approach to Care Planning. Philadelphia: F. A. Davis.
2. Mueller, A., Johnston, M., Bligh, D. (2001). Mind-mapped care plans, a remarkable alternative to traditional nursing care plans. Nurse Educator 26(2), 75–80.
3. Mueller, A., Johnston, M., Bligh, D. (2002). Viewpoint: joining mind mapping and care planning to enhance student critical thinking and achieve holistic nursing care. Nursing Diagnosis: The International Journal of Nursing Language and Classification 13(1).
4. Buzan T. (1995). The MindMap Book, 2nd ed. London: BBC Books.

Chapter 5

Nursing Diagnoses in Alphabetical Order

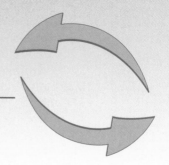

Activity Intolerance [specify level]

Definition: Insufficient physiologic or psychological energy to endure or complete required or desired daily activities

RELATED FACTORS
Generalized weakness
Sedentary lifestyle
Bed rest or immobility
Imbalance between oxygen supply and demand
[Cognitive deficits/emotional status; secondary to underlying disease process/depression]
[Pain, vertigo, extreme stress]

DEFINING CHARACTERISTICS

Subjective
Report of fatigue or weakness
Exertional discomfort or dyspnea
[Verbalizes no desire and/or lack of interest in activity]

Objective
Abnormal heart rate or blood pressure response to activity
Electrocardiographic changes reflecting dysrhythmias or ischemia [Pallor, cyanosis]

FUNCTIONAL LEVEL CLASSIFICATION (GORDON, 1987):
Level I: Walk, regular pace, on level indefinitely; one flight or more but more short of breath than normally
Level II: Walk one city block [or] 500 ft on level; climb one flight slowly without stopping

Information that appears in brackets has been added by the authors to clarify and enhance the use of nursing diagnoses.

Level III: Walk no more than 50 ft on level without stopping; unable to climb one flight of stairs without stopping

Level IV: Dyspnea and fatigue at rest

SAMPLE CLINICAL APPLICATIONS: Anemias, angina, aortic stenosis, bronchitis, emphysema, diabetes mellitus, dysmenorrhea, heart failure, human immunodeficiency virus/acquired immunodeficiency disease (HIV/AIDS), labor/preterm labor, leukemias, mitral stenosis obesity, pain, pericarditis, peripheral vascular disease, preterm labor, rheumatic fever, thrombocytopenia, tuberculosis, uterine bleeding

DESIRED OUTCOMES/EVALUATION CRITERIA

Sample **NOC** linkages:

Activity Tolerance: Responses to energy-conserving body movements involved in required or desired daily activities

Energy Conservation: Extent of active management of energy to initate and sustain activity

Endurance: Extent that energy enables a person to sustain activity

Client Will (Include Specific Time Frame)

- Identify negative factors affecting activity tolerance and eliminate or reduce their effects when possible.
- Use identified techniques to enhance activity tolerance.
- Participate willingly in necessary/desired activities.
- Report measurable increase in activity tolerance.
- Demonstrate a decrease in physiological signs of intolerance (e.g., pulse, respirations, and blood pressure remain within client's normal range).

ACTIONS/INTERVENTIONS

Sample **NIC** linkages:

Activity Therapy: Prescription of and assistance with specific physical, cognitive, social, and spiritual activities to increase the range, frequency, or duration of an individual's (or group's) activity

Energy Management: Regulating energy use to treat or prevent fatigue and optimize function

Exercise Promotion: Facilitation of regular physical exercise to maintain or advance to a higher level of fitness and health

NURSING PRIORITY NO. **1.** To identify causative/precipitating factors:

- Note presence of acute or chronic illness, such as heart failure, hypothyroidism, diabetes mellitus, AIDS, cancers, acute and chronic pain, etc. *Many factors cause or contribute to fatigue, but acitivity intolerance implies that the client cannot endure or adapt to increased energy or oxygen demands caused by an actvity.*[1]
- Assess cardiopulmonary response to physical activity by measuring vital signs, noting heart rate/regularity and blood pressure before, during, and after activity. Note progression/accelerating degree of fatigue. *Dramatic changes in heart rate and rhythm, changes in usual blood pressure and progressively worsening fatigue result from imbalance of oxygen supply and demand. These changes are potentially greater in the elderly population.*[1-3]
- Note treatment-related factors such as side effects/interactions of medications. *Can influence presence and degree of fatigue.*
- Determine if patient is receiving medications such as vasodilators, diuretics, or beta-block-

 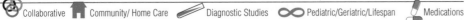

ers. *Orthostatic hypotension can occur with activity because of medication effects (vasodilation), fluid shifts (diuresis), or compromised cardiac pumping function.*[4]

- Note client reports of difficulty accomplishing tasks or desired activities. Evaluate current limitations/degree of deficit in light of usual status and what the client percieves causes, exacerbates, and helps the problem. *Provides comparative baseline and influences choice of interventions and may reveal causes that the client is unaware of affecting energy, such as sleep deprivation, smoking, poor diet, or lack of support.*[2]
- Ascertain ability to sit, stand, and move about as desired. Note degree of assistance necessary, and/or use of assistive equipment. *Helps to differentiate between problems relating to movement, and problems with oxyygen supply and demand characterized by fatigue and weakness.*[2]
- Identify activity needs versus desires (e.g., client barely able to walk upstairs but states would like to play racquetball). *Assists caregiver in dealing with reality of situation, as well as the feasibility of goals client wants to achieve,to find a place to start in developing a realistic activity goal.*[4]
- Assess emotional/psychological factors affecting the current situation. *Stress and/or depression may be exacerbating the effects of an illness, or depression may be the result of therapy/limitations.*

NURSING PRIORITY NO. 2. To assist client to deal with contributing factors and manage activities within individual limits:

- Monitor vital signs, before and during activity, watching for changes in blood pressure, heart and respiratory rate, as well as post-activity vital sign response. *Vital signs increase during activity and should return to baseline within 5 to 7 minutes after activity if response to activity is normal.*[1]
- Observe respiratory rate, noting breathing pattern, breath sounds, skin color, and mental status. *Pallor and/or cyanosis, presence of respiratory distresss, or confusion may be indicative of need for oxygen during activities, especially if respiratory infection or compromise is present.*[4]
- Plan care with rest periods between activities *to reduce fatigue.*
- Assist with self-care activities. Adjust activities/reduce intensity level, or discontinue activities that cause undesired physiologic changes. *Prevents overexertion.*
- Increase exercise/activity levels gradually; encourage stopping to rest for 3 minutes during a 10-minute walk, sitting down instead of standing to brush hair, etc. *Methods of conserving energy.*
- Encourage expression of feelings contributing to/resulting from condition. Provide positive atmosphere, while acknowledging difficulty of the situation for the client. *Helps to minimize frustration, rechannel energy.*
- Involve client/significant others (SOs) in planning of activities as much as possible. *May give client opportunity to perform desired/essential activities during periods of peak energy.*
- Assist with activities and provide/monitor client's use of assistive devices. Enables client to maintain mobility while *protecting from injury.*
- Promote comfort measures and provide for relief of pain. *Feeling comfortable can enhance client's ability and desire to participate in activities.* (Refer to NDs acute Pain, chronic Pain.)
- Provide referral to collaborative disciplines such as exercise physiologist, psychological counseling/therapy, occupational/physical therapy, and recreation/leisure specialists. *May be needed to develop individually appropriate therapeutic regimens.*
- Prepare for/assist with and monitor effects of exercise testing. *May be performed to determine degree of oxygen desaturation and/or hypoxemia that occurs with exertion; or to optimize titration of supplemental oxygen when used.*[5]

- Implement graded exercise/rehabilitation program under direct medical supervision. *Gradual increase in activity avoids excessive myocardial workload/excessive oxygen demand.*[4]
- Administer supplemental oxygen, medications, prepare for surgery, as indicated. *Type of therapy or medication is dependent on the underlying condition, and might include medications (such as antiarrythmics) or surgery (e.g.,stents or CABG) to improve myocardial perfusion and systemic circulation. Other treatments might include iron preparations or blood transfusion to treat severe anemia, or use of oxygen and bronchodialators to improve respiratory function.*[6,7]

NURSING PRIORITY NO. 3. To promote wellness (Teaching/Discharge Considerations):

- Review expectations of client/SO(s)/providers and explore conflicts/differences. *Helps to establish goals and to reach agreement for the most effective plan.*
- Assist/direct client/SO to plan for progressive increase of activity level aiming for maximal activity within the client's ability. *Promotes improved or more normal activity level, stamina, and conditioning.*
- Instruct client/SOs in monitoring response to activity and in recognizing signs/symptoms that indicate need to alter activity level. *Increases likelihood that client will stick with plan when doing well within guidelines and understanding of reportable problems.*
- Give client information that provides evidence of daily/weekly progress *to sustain motivation.*
- Assist client to learn and demonstrate appropriate safety measures *to prevent injuries.*
- Provide information about proper nutrition to meet metabolic and energy needs, obtaining or mantaining normal body weight. *Energy is improved when nutrients are maximal to meet metabolic demands.*[1]
- Encourage client to use relaxation techniques such as visualization/guided imagery as appropriate. *Useful in maintaining positive attitude and enhancing sense of well-being.*
- Encourage participation in recreation/social activities and hobbies appropriate for situation. (Refer to ND deficient Diversional Activity.)
- Monitor laboratory values (such as for anemia) and pulse oximetry.

DOCUMENTATION FOCUS

Assessment/Reassessment
- Level of activity as noted in Functional Level Classification.
- Causative/precipitating factors.
- Client reports of difficulty/change.

Planning
- Plan of care and who is involved in planning.

Implementation/Evaluation
- Response to interventions/teaching and actions performed.
- Implemented changes to plan of care based on assessment/reassessment findings.
- Teaching plan and response/understanding of teaching plan.
- Attainment/progress toward desired outcome(s).

Discharge Planning
- Referrals to other resources.
- Long-term needs and who is responsible for actions.

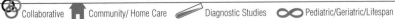

References

1. Cox, H. C., et al. (2002). Clinical Applications of Nursing Diagnosis: Adult, Child, Womens's, Psychiatric, Gerontic, and Home Health Considerations, ed 4. Philadelphia: F. A. Davis, pp 231–237.
2. Blair, K. A. (1999). Immobility and activity intolerance in older adults. In Stanley, M. & Beare, P. G., (eds): Gerontological Nursing: A Health Promotion/Protection Approach, ed 2. Philadelphia: F.A. Davis, pp 193–202.
3. Gordon, M. (2002). Manual of Nursing Diagnosis, ed 10. St. Louis: Mosby, p 223.
4. Hypertension: severe; Heart failure: chronic; Myocardial infarction; and Pneumonia: microbial. In Doenges, M. E., Moorhouse, M. F., & Geissler-Murr, A. C. (2002). Nursing Care Plans: Guidelines for Individualizing Patient Care, ed 6. Philadelphia: F. A. Davis, pp 37, 51, 75, 133.
5. Exercise testing for evaluation of hypoxemia and /or desaturation. (2001). Revision & Update. Resp Care, 46 (5), 514–522.
6. Gibbons, R. J., et al. (1999). ACC/AHA/ACP-ASIM: Guidelines for the management of patients with chronic stable angina: A report of the American College of Cardiology/American Heart Association Task Force on Practice Guidelines. J Am Coll Cardiol 33(7), 2092.
7. Congestive heart failure in adults. (2002). Bloomington, MN: Institute for Clinical Systems Improvement (ICSI).

risk for Activity Intolerance

Definition: At risk of experiencing insufficient physiological or psychological energy to endure or complete required or desired daily activities

RISK FACTORS

History of intolerance

Presence of circulatory/respiratory problems

Deconditioned status

Inexperience with the activity

[Diagnosis of progressive disease state/debilitating condition, such as cancer, multiple sclerosis (MS); extensive surgical procedures]

[Verbalized reluctance/inability to perform expected activity]

NOTE: A risk diagnosis is not evidenced by signs and symptoms as the problem has not occurred and nursing interventions are directed at prevention.

SAMPLE CLINICAL APPLICATIONS: Anemias, angina aortic stenosis, bronchitis, emphysema, dysmenorrhea, heart failure, HIV/AIDS, labor/preterm labor, leukemias, mitral stenosis, obesity, pain, pericarditis, peripheral vascular disease, preterm labor, rheumatic fever, thrombocytopenia, tuberculosis, uterine bleeding

DESIRED OUTCOMES/EVALUATION CRITERIA

Sample NOC linkages:

Endurance: Extent that energy enables a person to sustain activity

Energy Conservation: Extent of activity management of energy to initiate and sustain activity

Circulation Status: Extent to which blood flows unobstructed, unidirectionally, and at an appropriate pressure through large vessels of the systemic and pulmonary circuits.

Client Will (Include Specific Time Frame)
- Verbalize understanding of potential loss of ability in relation to existing condition.
- Participate in conditioning/rehabilitation program to enhance ability to perform.
- Identify alternative ways to maintain desired activity level (e.g., if weather is bad, walking in a shopping mall could be an option).
- Identify conditions/symptoms that require medical reevaluation.

ACTIONS/INTERVENTIONS

Sample NIC linkages:

Energy Management: Regulating energy use to treat or prevent fatigue and optimize function

Exercise Promotion: Facilitation of regular physical exercise to maintain or advance to a higher level of fitness and health

Pain Management: Alleviation of pain or a reduction in pain to a level of comfort that is acceptable to the patient

NURSING PRIORITY NO. 1. To assess factors affecting current situation:

- Note age, medical diagnosis, and/or therapeutic regimen for conditions such as heart failure, lung diseases, arthritis, and climate or weather changes. *Factors that can affect desired level of activity. Many factors cause or contribute to fatigue, but acitivity intolerance implies that individual cannot endure or adapt to increased energy or oxygen demands caused by an actvity.*[1]
- Determine baseline activity level and physical condition. *Influences choice of interventions and provides opportunity to track changes.*

NURSING PRIORITY NO. 2. To develop/investigate alternative ways to remain active within the limits of the disabling condition/situation:

- Implement physical therapy/exercise program in conjunction with the client and other team members such as physical and/or occupational therapist, exercise/rehabilitation physiologist. *Collaborative program with short-term achievable goals enhances likelihood of success and may motivate client to adopt a lifestyle of physical exercise for enhancement of health.*[2]
- Promote/implement conditioning program and support inclusion in exercise/activity groups *to prevent/limit deterioration.*
- Instruct client in proper performance of unfamiliar activities and/or alternate ways of doing familiar activities. *To learn methods of conserving energy and promote safety in performing activities.*

NURSING PRIORITY NO. 3. To promote wellness (Teaching/ Discharge Considerations):

- Discuss relationship of illness/debilitating condition to inability to perform desired activity(ies). *Clients may not know that certain conditions are associated with fatigue and imbalance between their oxygen demand and supply.*[1–5]
- Provide information regarding potential interferences to activity.
- Assist client/SO with planning for changes that may become necessary. *Education and anticipatory guidance is essential to preventing problems associated with oxygen and energy need imbalance and may include counseling for smoking cessation, weight management, compliance with treatment regimens, shiftng of family responsibilities, changes in dietary patterns, early intervention if symptoms occur.*[3,4]
- Identify and discuss symptoms for which client needs to seek medical assistance/ evaluation, *providing for timely intervention.*
- Refer to appropriate sources for assistance and/or equipment as needed *to sustain or improve activity level and to promote client safety.*

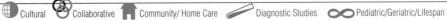 Cultural   Collaborative   Community/ Home Care   Diagnostic Studies   ∞ Pediatric/Geriatric/Lifespan   Medications

Assessment/Reassessment
- Identified/potential risk factors for individual.
- Current level of activity tolerance and blocks to activity.

Planning
- Treatment options, including physical therapy/exercise program, other assistive therapies and devices.
- Lifestyle changes that are planned, who is to be responsible for each action, and monitoring methods.

Implementation/Evaluation
- Responses to interventions/teaching and actions performed.
- Attainment/progress toward desired outcome(s).
- Modification of plan of care.

Discharge Planning
- Referrals for medical assistance/evaluation.

References

1. Cox, H. C., et al. (2002). Clinical Applications of Nursing Diagnosis: Adult, Child, Womens's, Psychiatric, Gerontic, and Home Health Considerations, ed 4. Philadelphia: F. A. Davis, pp 231–237.
2. Blair, K. A. (1999). Immobility and activity intolerance in older adults. In Stanley, M. & Beare, P. G. (eds): Gerontological Nursing: a Health Promotion/Protection Approach, ed 2. Philadelphia: F. A. Davis, pp 193–202.
3. Congestive heart failure in adults. (2002). Bloomington, MN: Institute for Clinical Systems Improvement (ICSI).
4. Meleski, D. D. (2002). Families with chronically ill children. AJN 102(5), 47.
5. Borroso, J. (2002). HIV-related fatigue. AJN, 102(5), 83.

impaired Adjustment

Definition: Inability to modify lifestyle/behavior in a manner consistent with a change in health status

RELATED FACTORS
Disability or health status requiring change in lifestyle
Multiple stressors; intense emotional state
Low state of optimism; negative attitudes toward health behavior; lack of motivation to change behaviors
Failure to intend to change behavior
Absence of social support for changed beliefs and practices
[Physical and/or learning disability]

DEFINING CHARACTERISTICS

Subjective
Denial of health status change
Failure to achieve optimal sense of control

Objective
Failure to take actions that would prevent further health problems
Demonstration of nonacceptance of health status change

SAMPLE CLINICAL APPLICATIONS: New diagnosis/life changes for client, Alzheimer's disease, brain injury, personality or psychotic disorders, postpartum depression/psychosis, substance use/abuse

DESIRED OUTCOMES/EVALUATION CRITERIA

Sample **NOC** linkages:

Acceptance: Health Status: Reconciliation to health circumstances

Psychosocial Adjustment: Life Change: Psychosocial adaptation of an individual to a life change

Treatment Behavior: Illness or Injury: Personal actions to palliate or eliminate pathology

Client Will (Include Specific Time Frame)
- Demonstrate increasing interest/participation in self-care.
- Develop ability to assume responsibility for personal needs when possible.
- Identify stress situations leading to impaired adjustment and specific actions for dealing with them.
- Initiate lifestyle changes that will permit adaptation to present life situations.
- Identify and use appropriate support systems.

ACTIONS/INTERVENTIONS

Sample **NIC** linkages:

Coping Enhancement: Assisting a patient to adapt to perceived stressors, changes, or threats that interfere with meeting life demands and roles

Counseling: Use of an interactive helping process focusing on the needs, problems, or feelings of the patient and significant others to enhance or support coping, problem-solving, and interpersonal relationships

Teaching: Disease Process: Assisting the patient to understand information related to a specific disease process

NURSING PRIORITY NO. 1. To assess degree of impaired function:

- Perform a physical and/or psychosocial assessment. *Determines the extent of the limitation(s) of the present condition.*[1]
- Listen to the client's perception of inability/reluctance to adapt to situations that are occurring at present. *Perceptions are reality to the client and need to be identified so they may be addressed and dealt with.*[3]
- 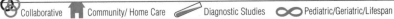 Survey (with the client) past and present significant support systems (family, church, groups, and organizations). *Identifies helpful resources that may be needed in current situation/change in health status.*[2]
- Explore the expressions of emotions signifying impaired adjustment by client/SO(s). *Overwhelming anxiety, fear, anger, worry, passive and/or active denial can be experienced by the client who is having difficulty adjusting to change in health, feared diagnosis.*[4]
- Note child's interaction with parent/care provider. *Interactions can be indicative of problems when family is dealing with major health problems and change in family functioning. Development of coping behaviors is limited at this age, and primary care providers provide support for the child and serve as role-models.*[5]

- Determine whether child displays problems with school performance, withdraws from family/peers, or demonstrates aggressive behavior toward others/self. *Indicators of poor coping and need for specific interventions to help child deal with own health issues and/or what is happening in the family.*[6]

NURSING PRIORITY NO. 2. To identify the causative/contributing factors relating to the impaired adjustment:

- Listen to client's perception of the factors leading to the present impairment, noting onset, duration, presence/absence of physical complaints, social withdrawal. *Change often creates a feeling of disequilibrium, and the individual may respond with fears that are irrational or unfounded. Client may benefit from feedback that corrects misperceptions about how life will be with the change in health status.*[7]
- Review with client previous life situations and role changes to determine coping skills used. *Identifies the strengths that may be used to facilitate adaptation to change or loss that has occurred.*[8]
- Identify possible cultural beliefs/values influencing client's response to change. *Different cultures deal with change of health issues, such as cancer, chronic obstructive pulmonary disease, diabetes mellitus in different ways, (i.e., American Indians believe they should be sick, quiet, and stoic; Chinese are passive and expect the family to care for the client; Americans may be assertive and direct their care more frequently).*[14]
- Assess affective climate within family system and how it determines family members response to adjustment to major health challenge. *Families who are high strung and nervous may interfere with client's dealing with illness in a rational manner while those who are more sedate and phlegmatic may be more helpful to the client in accepting the current circumstances.*[2]
- Determine lack of/inability to use available resources. *The high degree of anxiety that usually accompanies a major lifestyle change often interferes with ability to deal with problems created by the change or loss. Helping client learn to use these resources enables her or him to take control of own illness.*[8]
- Discuss normalcy of anger as life is being changed and encourage channeling anger to healthy activities. *The increased energy of anger can be used to accomplish other tasks and enhance feelings of self-esteem.*[2]
- Reinforce structure in daily life. Include exercise as part of routine. *Routines help the client focus. Exercise improves sense of wellness and enhances immune response.*[10]
- Review available documentation and resources to determine actual life experiences (e.g., medical records, statements of SOs, consultants' notes). *In situations of great stress, physical and/or emotional, the client may not accurately assess occurrences leading to the present situation.*[9]

NURSING PRIORITY NO. 3. To assist client in coping/dealing with impairment:

- Organize a team conference (including client and ancillary services). *Individuals who are involved and knowledgeable can focus on the contributing factors that are affecting client's adjustment to the current situation and plan for management as indicated.*[11]
- Acknowledge client's efforts to adjust: "Have done your best." *Avoids feelings of blame/guilt and defensive response.*[12]
- Share information with adolescent's peers with client's permission and involvement when illness/injury affects body image. *Peers are primary support for this age group and sharing information promotes understanding and compassion.*[5]

- Explain disease process/causative factors and prognosis as appropriate, promote questioning, and provide written/other materials. *Enhances understanding, clarifies information, and provides opportunity to review information at individual's leisure.*[10]
- Provide an open environment encouraging communication. *Supports expression of feelings concerning impaired function so they can be dealt with realistically.*[2]
- Use therapeutic communication skills (Active-listening, acknowledgment, silence, I-statements). *Promotes open relationship in which client can explore possibilities and solutions for changing lifestyle situation.*[15]
- Discuss/evaluate resources that have been useful to the client in adapting to changes in other life situations. *Vocational rehabilitation, employment experiences, psychosocial support services may be useful in current situation.*[12]
- Develop a plan of action with client to meet immediate needs (e.g., physical safety and hygiene, emotional support of professionals and SOs) and assist in implementation of the plan. *Provides a starting point to deal with current situation for moving ahead with plan for adjusting to change in life circumstances and for evaluation of progress toward goals.*[13]
- Explore previously used coping skills and application to current situation. Refine/develop new strategies as appropriate. *Identifying skills that the client already has provides a starting point for dealing with change in health/lifestyle.*[10]
- Identify and problem-solve with the client frustrations in daily care. *Focusing on the smaller factors of concern gives the individual the ability to perceive the impaired function from a less threatening perspective, one-step-at-a-time concept. Also promotes sense of control over situation.*[10]
- Involve SO(s) in long-range planning for emotional, psychological, physical, and social needs. *Change that is occuring when illness is long-term/permanent indicates that lifestyle changes will need to be made and dealt with on an ongoing basis which may be difficult for client and family to adjust to.*[14]
- Refer for individual/family counseling as indicated. *May need additional assistance to cope with current situation.*[13]

NURSING PRIORITY NO. 4. To promote wellness (Teaching/Discharge Considerations):

- Identify strengths the client perceives in present life situation. Keep focus on the present. *Unknowns of the future may be too overwhelming when diagnosis/injury means permanent changes in lifestyle/management.*[13]
- Refer to other resources in the long-range plan of care. *Occupational therapy, vocational rehabilitation may be useful for making indicated changes in life, assisting with adjustment to new situation as needed.*[2]
- Assist client/SO(s) to see appropriate alternatives and potential changes in locus of control. *Often major change in health status results in loss of sense of control and client needs to begin to look at possibilities for managing illness and what abilities can make life go on in a positive manner.*[10]
- Assist SOs to learn methods of managing present needs. (Refer to NDs specific to client's deficits.) *Promotes internal locus of control and helps develop plan for long-term needs with changes required by illness/changes in health status.*[2]
- Pace and time learning sessions to meet client's needs, providing for feedback during and after learning experiences (e.g., self-catheterization, range of motion exercises, wound care, therapeutic communication). *Promotes skill and enhances retention, improving confidence.*[1]

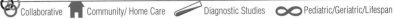 Cultural   Collaborative   Community/ Home Care   Diagnostic Studies   Pediatric/Geriatric/Lifespan   Medications

Assessment/Reassessment
- Reasons for/degree of impairment.
- Client's/SO(s) perception of the situation.
- Effect of behavior on health status/condition.

Planning
- Plan for adjustments and interventions for achieving the plan and who is involved.
- Teaching plan.

Implementation/Evaluation
- Client responses to the interventions/teaching and actions performed.
- Attainment/progress toward desired outcome(s).
- Modifications to plan of care.

Discharge Planning
- Resources that are available for the client and SO(s) and referrals that are made.

References

1. Doenges, M. E., Moorhouse, M. F., & Geissler-Murr, A. C. (2002). Nursing Care Plans: Guidelines for Individualizing Patient Care, ed 6. Philadelphia: F. A. Davis.
2. Doenges, M. E., & Townsend, M. C., & Moorhouse, M. F., (1998). Psychiatric Care Plans: Guidelines for Individualizing Care, 3rd ed. Philadelphia: F. A. Davis.
3. Locher, J, et al. (2002). Effects of age and casual attribution to aging on health-related behaviors associated with urinary incontinence in older women. Gerontologist, 42(4), 525–521.
4. Cox, H, et al. (2002). Clinical Applications of Nursing Diagnoses, 4th ed. Philadelphia: F. A. Davis.
5. Pinhas-Hamiel, O., Dolan, L. M., et al. (1996). Increased incidence of non-insulin-dependent diabetes mellitus among adolescents. J Pediatr, 128(8), 608.
6. Deckelbaum, R. J., & Williams, C. L. (2001). Childhood obesity: The health issue. Obesity Res, 9(5) 239s.
7. Badger, J. M. (2001). Burns: The psychological aspect. AJN, 101(11) 38–41.
8. Bartol, T. (2002). Putting a patient with diabetes in the driver's seat. Nursing2002, 32(2), 53–55.
9. Konigova, R. (1992). The psychological problems of burned patients. The Rudy Hermans Lecture 1991. Burns, 18(3), 189–199.
10. Townsend, M. C. (2000). Psychiatric Mental Health Nursing: Concepts of Care, 3rd ed. Philadelphia: F. A. Davis.
11. Konstam, M., et al. (1994). Heart failure: Evaluation and care of patients with left-ventricular systolic dysfunction. Rockville (MD): Agency for Health Care Policy and Research; Clinical Practice Guideline No. 11. AHCPR Pub. No 94–0612. Available at http://www.gerweb.com/HeartDSS/hpract.htm.
12. Rolland, J.S. (1994a). Families, Illness, and Disability. New York: Harper Collins.
13. Wright, L.M., & Leahey, M. (1987). Families and Chronic Illness. Springhouse, PA: Springhouse.
14. Lipson, J., Dibble, S., & Minarik, P. (1996). Culture & Nursing Care: A Pocket Guide. San Francisco: UCSF Nursing Press, School of Nursing, University of California.
15. Gordon, T. (2000). Parent Effectiveness Training, updated edition. New York: Three Rivers Press.

ineffective Airway Clearance

Definition: Inability to clear secretions or obstructions from the respiratory tract to maintain a clear airway

Environmental
Smoking; second-hand smoke; smoke inhalation

Obstructed airway
Retained secretions; secretions in the bronchi; exudate in the alveoli; excessive mucus; airway spasm
Foreign body in airway; presence of artificial airway

Physiologic
Chronic obstructive pulmonary disease (COPD); asthma
Allergic [Reactive] airways; hyperplasia of the bronchial walls
Neuromuscular dysfunction [Neurological disorders]
[Immobility]
Infection

DEFINING CHARACTERISTICS

Subjective
Dyspnea

Objective
Diminished or adventitious breath sounds (rales, crackles, rhonchi, wheezes)
Cough, ineffective or absent; sputum
Changes in respiratory rate and rhythm
Difficulty vocalizing
Wide-eyed; restlessness
Orthopnea
Cyanosis

SAMPLE CLINICAL APPLICATIONS: Chronic obstructive pulmonary disease (COPD), pneumonia, influenza, acute respiratory distress syndrome (ARDS), cancer of lung/head and neck, congestive heart failure (CHF), cystic fibrosis, neuromuscular diseases, inhalation injuries

DESIRED OUTCOMES/EVALUATION CRITERIA
Sample **NOC** linkages:
Respiratory Status: Airway Patency: Extent to which the tracheobronchial passages remain open
Aspiration Control: Personal actions to prevent the passage of fluid and solid particles into the lung
Cognitive Ability: Ability to execute complex mental processes

Client Will (Include Specific Time Frame)
- Maintain airway patency.
- Expectorate/clear secretions readily.
- Demonstrate absence/reduction of congestion with breath sounds clear, respirations noiseless, improved oxygen exchange (e.g., absence of cyanosis, ABG results within client norms).
- Verbalize understanding of cause(s) and therapeutic management regimen.

 Cultural Collaborative Community/ Home Care 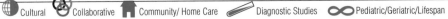 Diagnostic Studies Pediatric/Geriatric/Lifespan Medications

- Demonstrate behaviors to improve or maintain clear airway.
- Identify potential complications and how to initiate appropriate preventive or corrective actions.

ACTIONS/INTERVENTIONS

Sample NIC linkages:

Airway Management: Facilitation of patency of air passages

Respiratory Monitoring: Collection and analysis of patient data to ensure airway patency and adequate gas exchange

Cough Enhancement: Promotion of deep inhalation by the patient with subsequent generation of high intrathoracic pressures and compression of underlying lung parenchyma for the forceful expulsion of air

NURSING PRIORITY NO. 1. To maintain adequate, patent airway:

- Identify client populations at risk. *Persons with impaired ciliary function (e.g., cystic fibrosis, status post heart-lung transplantation); those with excessive or abnormal mucus production (e.g., asthma, emphysema, bronchiectasis, mechanical ventilation); those with impaired cough function (e.g., neuromuscular diseases such as muscular dystrophy; neuromotor conditions such as cerebral palsy, spinal cord injury); those with swallowing abnormalities (e.g., post stroke, disorders of esophagus, seizures, coma, tracheostomy) and immobility (e.g., spinal cord injury, severe cerebral palsy and developmental delay); infant/child (e.g., feeding intolerance, abdominal distention, and emotional stressors that may compromise airway) are all at risk for problems with maintenance of open airways.[1,2]*
- Assess level of consciousness/cognition and ability to protect own airway. *Information essential for identifying potential for airway problems, providing baseline level of care needed and influencing choice of interventions.*
- Evaluate respiratory rate/depth and breath sounds. *Tachypnea is usually present to some degree and may be pronounced during respiratory stress. Respirations may be shallow. Some degree of bronchospasm is present with obstruction in airways and may/may not be manifested in adventitious breath sounds, such as scattered moist crackles (bronchitis), faint sounds with expiratory wheezes (emphysema) or absent breath sounds (severe asthma).[2]*
- Position head appropriate for age and condition/disorder. *Repositioning head may at times be all that is needed to open or maintain open airway in at-rest or compromised individual, such as one with sleep apnea.*
- ∞ Insert oral airway, using correct size for adult or child, when indicated. Have appropriate emergency equipment at bedside (such as tracheostomy equipment, ambu bag, suction apparatus) to *restore or maintain an effective airway.[3,4]*
- Evaluate amount and type of secretions being produced. *Excessive and/or sticky mucus can make it difficult maintain effective airways, especially if client has impaired cough function, is very young or old, developmentally delayed, has restrictive or obstructive lung disease, or is mechanically ventilated.[5]*
- Note ability/effectiveness of cough. *Cough function may be weak or ineffective in diseases and conditions such as extremes in age (e.g., premature infant or elderly) cerebral palsy, muscular dystrophy, spinal cord injury, brain injury, post-surgery, and/or mechanical ventilation due to mechanisms affecting muscles of throat, chest, and lungs.[5,6]*
- ∞ Suction (nasal/tracheal/oral) when indicated, using correct size catheter and suction timing for child or adult *to clear airway when secretions are blocking airways, client is unable to clear airway by coughing, cough is ineffective, infant is unable to take oral feedings because of secretions, or ventilated patient is showing desaturation of oxygen by oximetry or ABGs.[2,5,7]*

- Assist with/prepare for appropriate testing (e.g., pulmonary function/sleep studies) *to identify causative/precipitating factors.*

- Assist with procedures (e.g., bronchoscopy, tracheostomy) *to clear/maintain open airway.*
- Keep environment free of smoke, dust, and feather pillows according to individual situation. *Precipitators of allergic type of respiratory reactions that can trigger/exacerbate acute episode.*[3]

NURSING PRIORITY NO. 2. To mobilize secretions:

- Elevate head of the bed/change position as needed. *Elevation/upright position facilitates respiratory function by use of gravity; however, the client in severe distress will seek position of comfort.*[3]
- Encourage/instruct in deep-breathing and directed coughing exercises; teach (presurgically) and reinforce (postsurgically) breathing and coughing while splinting incision *to maximize cough effort, lung expansion and drainage, and reduce pain impairment.*
- Mobilize client as soon as possible. *Reduces risk or effects of atelectasis, enhancing lung expansion and drainage of different lung segments.*[5]

- Administer analgesics, as indicated. *Analgesics may be needed to improve cough effort when pain is inhibiting (Caution—overmedication, especially with opioids, can depress respirations and cough effort).*

- Give expectorants, anti-inflammatory agents, bronchodilators and mucolytic agents as ordered *to relax smooth respiratory musculature, reduce airway edema and mobilize secretions.*[8]
- Encourage/provide warm versus cold liquids, as appropriate. Increase fluid intake to at least 2000 to 3000 mL/day within level of cardiac tolerance (may require intravenous line). *Improvement of hydration status can help liquefy secretions.*[4,5]
- Provide ultrasonic nebulizer, room humidifier as needed *to deliver supplemental humidification, helping to reduce viscosity of secretions.*

- Assist with respiratory treatments (intermittent positive-pressure breathing [IPPB], incentive spirometry) *to enhance oxygen diffusion and to deliver aerosolized/nebulized medications.*[3]

- Perform/assist client in learning airway clearance techniques, particularly when airway clearance is a chronic/long term condition. *Numerous techniques may be used including (and not limited to) postural drainage and percussion (CPT), positive expiratory pressure (PEP), high-pressure PEP, flutter devices; high-frequency chest compression with an inflatable vest, intrapulmonary percussive ventilation administered by a percussinator, and active cycle breathing (ACB), as indicated. Many of these techniques are the result of research in treatments of cystic fibrosis and muscular dystrophy as well as other chronic lung diseases.*[9]

NURSING PRIORITY NO. 3. To assess changes, note complications:

- Auscultate breath sounds, noting changes in air movement *to ascertain current status/effects of treatments to clear airways.*
- Monitor vital signs, noting blood pressure/pulse changes. Observe for increased rate, restlessness/anxiety, and use of accessory muscles for breathing *suggesting advancing respiratory distress.*

- Monitor/document serial chest radiographs, ABGs, pulse oximetry readings. *Identifies baseline status, influences interventions and monitors progress of condition and/or treatment response.*
- Evaluate changes in sleep pattern, noting insomnia or daytime somnolence. *May be evidence of nighttime airway incompetence or sleep apnea.* (Refer to ND disturbed Sleep Pattern.)

 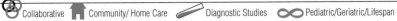

- Document response to drug therapy and/or development of adverse reactions or side effects with antimicrobial agents, steroids, expectorants, bronchodilators. *Pharmacologic therapy is used to prevent and control symptoms, reduce severity of exacerbations, and improve health status. The choice of medications depends on availability of the medication and the client's decision-making about medication regimen and response to any given medication.*[10]
- Observe for signs/symptoms of infection (e.g., increased dyspnea, onset of fever, increase in sputum volume, change in color or character) *to identify infectious process/promote timely intervention.*[10]
- Obtain sputum specimen, preferably before antimicrobial therapy is initiated, *to verify appropriateness of therapy. Note: the presence of purulent sputum during an exacerbation of symptoms is sufficient indication for starting antibiotic, but a sputum culture and antibiogram (antibiotic sensitivity) may be done if the illness is not responding to the initial antibiotic.*[10]

NURSING PRIORITY NO. 4. To promote wellness (Teaching/Discharge Considerations):

- Assess client's/caregiver's knowledge of contributing causes, treatment plan, specific medications, and therapeutic procedures *to determine educational needs.*
- Provide information about the necessity of raising and expectorating secretions versus swallowing them *to examine and report changes in color and amount.*
- Demonstrate/reinforce pursed-lip or diaphragmatic breathing (huffing) techniques if indicated *to maintain airway pressure and enhance expiration.*
- Review breathing exercises, effective cough, use of adjunct devices (e.g., IPPB or incentive spirometry) in preoperative teaching *to facilitate postoperative recovery, reduce risk of pneumonia.*
- Instruct client's caregiver in use of inhalers and other respiratory drugs. Include expected effects and information regarding possible side effects and interactions with other medications/OTC/ herbals. Discuss symptoms requiring medical followup. *Clients are often taking multiple medications that have similar side effects and potential for interactions. It is important to understand the difference between nuisance side effects (such as fast heart beat after albuterol inhaler) and adverse effect (such as chest pain, hallucinations, or uncontrolled cardiac arrhythmia).*[9]
- Encourage/provide opportunities for rest; limit activities to level of respiratory tolerance. *Prevents/lessens fatigue associated with underlying condition or efforts to clear airways.*
- Urge reduction/cessation of smoking. *Smoking is known to increase production of mucus and paralyzes (or causes loss of) cilia needed to move secretions to clear airway and improve lung function.*[10]
- Refer to appropriate support groups (e.g., stop-smoking clinic, COPD exercise group, weight reduction, American Lung Association, Cystic Fibrosis Foundation, Muscular Dystrophy Association).
- Instruct in use of nocturnal positive pressure airflow for treatment of sleep apnea. (Refer to NDs disturbed Sleep Pattern, Sleep Deprivation.)

DOCUMENTATION FOCUS

Assessment/Reassessment
- Related Factors for individual client.
- Breath sounds, presence/character of secretions, use of accessory muscles for breathing.
- Character of cough/sputum.

Planning
- Plan of care and who is involved in planning.
- Teaching plan.

Implementation/Evaluation
- Client's response to interventions/teaching and actions performed.
- Attainment/progress toward desired outcome(s).
- Modifications to plan of care.

Discharge Planning
- Long-term needs and who is responsible for actions to be taken.
- Specific referrals made.

References

1. Impaired Airway Clearance: Information for Patients and Information for Health Plans: The Vest Airway Clearance System. Advanced Respiratory, Inc., 2002. Available at www.abivest.com.
2. Seay, S. J., Gay, S. L. & Strauss, M. (2002). Tracheostomy emergencies. AJN 102(3): 59.
3. Doenges, M. E., Moorhouse, M. F. & Geissler-Murr, A. C. (2002). Nursing Care Plans: Guidelines for Individualizing Patient Care, ed 6. Philadelphia: F. A. Davis, pp 118–120.
4. Cox, H. C., et al. (2002). Clinical Applications of Nursing Diagnosis: Adult, Child, Psychiatric, Gerontic, and Home Health Considerations, ed 4. Philadelphia: F. A. Davis, pp 244–249.
5. Fink, J. B., & Hess D. R. (2002). Secretion clearance techniques. In Hess, D. R. et al., (eds): Respiratory Care: Principles and Practices. Philadelphia: W. B. Saunders.
6. Blair, K. A. (1999). The aging pulmonary system. In Stanley, M. & Beare, P. G. (eds): Gerontological Nursing, ed 2. Philadelphia: F. A. Davis.
7. Suctioning of the patient in the home. American Association for Respiratory Care (AARC) Clinical Practice Guidelines. Respir Care 41(7): 647–653, 1996.
8. Deglin, J. H., & Vallerand, A. H. (2003). Davis's Drug Guide for Nurses, ed 8. Bronchodilators: Pharmacolgic Profile G56. Philadelphia: F. A. Davis.
9. Yngsdal-Krenz, R. (1999, Spring). Airway Clearance Techniques. Center Focus, newsletter of the University of Wisconsin, Madison.
10. Global strategy for the diagnosis, management, and prevention of chronic obstructive pulmonary disease. Developers: World Health Organization (WHO); National Heart, Lung and Blood Institute (NHLBI); Global Imitative for Chronic Obstructive Lung Disease (GOLD). National Guideline Clearinghouse, May 2001. Available at www.ngc.com.

latex Allergy Response

Definition: An allergic response to natural latex rubber products

RELATED FACTORS

No immune mechanism response [although this is true of irritant and allergic contact dermatitis, type I/immediate reaction is a true allergic response]

DEFINING CHARACTERISTICS

Type I reactions [hypersensitivity; IgE-mediated reaction]: immediate reaction (<1 hour) to latex proteins (can be life-threatening); contact urticaria progressing to generalized symptoms; edema of the lips, tongue, uvula, and/or throat; shortness of breath, tightness in chest, wheezing, bronchospasm leading to respiratory arrest; hypotension, syncope, cardiac arrest. May also include: Orofacial characteristics—edema of sclera or eyelids; erythema and/or itching of the eyes; tearing of the eyes; nasal congestion, itching, and/or erythema; rhinorrhea; facial erythema; facial itching; oral itching.

 Cultural Collaborative Community/ Home Care Diagnostic Studies 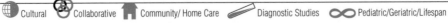 Pediatric/Geriatric/Lifespan Medications

Gastrointestinal characteristics—abdominal pain; nausea. Generalized characteristics—flushing; general discomfort; generalized edema; increasing complaint of total body warmth; restlessness

Type IV reactions [irritant and delayed-type hypersensitivity]: irritant [contact dermatitis] reactions: erythema [dry, crusty, hard bumps], chapped or cracked skin. Delayed onset (hours): eczema, irritation, blisters, reaction to additives (e.g., thiurams, carbamates); causes discomfort, redness

SAMPLE CLINICAL APPLICATIONS: multiple allergies, neural tube defects (e.g., spina bifida, myelomeningoceles), multiple surgeries at early age, chronic urologic conditions (e.g., neurogenic bladder, exstrophy of bladder), spinal cord trauma

DESIRED OUTCOMES/EVALUATION CRITERIA

Sample NOC linkages:

Immune Hypersensitivity Control: Extent to which inappropriate immune responses are suppressed

Symptom Severity: Extent of perceived adverse changes in physical, emotional, and social functioning

Knowledge: Treatment Regimen: Extent of understanding conveyed about a specific treatment regimen

Client Will (Include Specific Time Frame)
- Be free of signs of hypersensitive response.
- Verbalize understanding of individual risks/responsibilities in avoiding exposure.
- Identify signs/symptoms requiring prompt intervention.

ACTIONS/INTERVENTIONS

Sample NIC linkages:

Latex Precautions: Reducing the risk of a systemic reaction to latex

Allergy Management: Identification, treatment, and prevention of allergic responses to food, medications, insect bites, contrast material, blood, or other substances

Environmental Risk Protection: Preventing and detecting disease and injury in populations at risk from environmental hazards

NURSING PRIORITY NO. 1. To assess contributing factors:

- Identify persons in high-risk categories: 1) history of allergies, and food allergies (particularly bananas); 2) skin rashes including eczema/other dermatitis; 3) routinely exposed to natural rubber latex products (e.g. healthcare workers, police/firefighters, emergency medical technicians [EMTs], food handlers, hairdressers, cleaning staff, factory workers in plants that manufacture latex-containing products); 4) individuals with neural tube defects (e.g., spina bifida, myelomeningoceles); 5) children having multiple surgeries at early age (e.g., repeated placement of ventriculo-peritoneal shunts); 6) urologic conditions requiring frequent surgeries and/or catheterizations (e.g., exstrophy of the bladder, spinal cord trauma, neurogenic bladder).
- Question new client regarding latex allergy upon admission to healthcare facility, especially when procedures are anticipated, e.g., laboratory, emergency department, operating room, wound care management, one-day surgery, dentist. *Basic safety information to help healthcare providers prevent/prepare for safe environment for client and themselves while providing care.*[2,4,7]

- Discuss history of exposure, e.g., client works in environment where latex is manufactured or latex gloves used frequently; child was blowing up balloons (this might be an acute reaction to the powder); use of condoms (may affect either partner), individual requires frequent catheterizations. *Finding cause of reaction may be simple or complex, but often requires diligent investigation and history taking from multiple people and places.*

- Administer or note presence of positive skin-prick test (SPT), when performed. *Sensitive indicator of IgE sensitivity reflecting immune system activation.*
- Note response to radioallergosorbent test (RAST). *Performed to measure the quantity of IgE antibodies in serum after exposure to specific antigens, and has generally replaced skin tests and provocation tests, which are inconvenient, often painful, and/or hazardous to the client.*[1]

NURSING PRIORITY NO. 2. To take measures to reduce/limit allergic response/ avoid exposure to allergens:

- Ascertain client's current symptoms, noting rash, hives, itching, eye symptoms, edema, diarrhea, nausea, and feeling of faintness. *Baseline for determining where the client is along a continuum of symptoms, so that appropriate treatments can be initiated.*
- Assess skin (usually hands, but may be anywhere) for dry, crusty, hard bumps, horizontal cracks *caused by irritation from chemicals used in/on the latex item (e.g., latex or powder used in latex gloves, condoms, etc). Dry itchy rash (contact irritation) is the most common response, and is not a true allergic reaction, but can progress to a delayed type of allergic contact dermatitis with oozing blisters and spread in a way similar to poison ivy.*[2–5]
- Assist with treatment of contact dermatitis/type IV reaction:
  Wash affected skin with mild soap and water
  Wash hands between glove changes and after each glove removal
  Avoid oil-based salves or lotions when using latex gloves
  Consider application of topical steroid ointment
  Inform client that the most common cause is latex gloves, but that many other products contain latex, and could aggravate condition
- Monitor closely for signs of systemic reactions *because type IV response can lead to/progress to type I anaphylaxis.* Be watchful for onset of difficulty breathing or swallowing, hoarseness, wheezing, stridor, hypotension, tachycardia, dysrhythmias, edema of face, eyelids, lips, tongue and mucous membranes. Note behavior such as agitation, restlessness, and expressions of fearfulness. *Indicative of severe allergic response that can result in anaphylactic reaction and lead to respiratory/cardiac arrest.*[6]
- Administer treatment as appropriate if type I reaction occurs:
  Stop treatment or procedure if needed
  Support airway, administer 100% oxygen, mechanical ventilation if needed
  Administer emergency medications and treatments per protocol: e.g., antihistamines, epinephrine, corticosteroids and IV fluids
  Document allergy to latex in client's file
- Post latex-sensitive precaution signs in client's environment. Survey and routinely monitor client's environment for latex-containing products and remove them promptly.
- Notify physicians, colleagues, and employers of diagnosis and need for latex avoidance.
- Inform medical products providers of condition (e.g., pharmacy *so that medications can be prepared in latex-free environment*, homecare oxygen company *to provide latex-free cannulas*).
- Encourage client to wear medical ID bracelet *to alert providers to condition if client unresponsive.*[3,4,7]

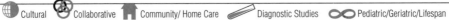

NURSING PRIORITY NO. 3. To promote wellness (Teaching/Learning):

- Emphasize the critical importance of taking immediate action for type I reaction *to limit life-threatening symptoms.*
- Demonstrate procedure and recommend client carry auto-injectable epinephrine *to provide timely emergency treatment as needed.*
- Instruct client/family/SO about latex exposure. *Occurs through contact with skin or mucous membrane, by inhalation, parenteral injection, or wound inoculation.*
- Provide client/SO with printed lists or Web sites *for identifying common household products that contain latex (e.g, carpet backing, diapers, shoes, rubber toys, pacifiers, and much more) and where to obtain latex-free products and supplies.*[4,7]
- Provide resource and assistance numbers for emergencies. *When allergy is suspected or the potential for allergy exists, protection must begin with identification and removal of possible sources of latex.*
- Instruct in signs of reaction and emergency treatment needs. *Reactions range from skin irritation to anaphylaxis. Reaction may be gradual but progressive, affecting multiple body systems, or may be sudden, requiring lifesaving treatment. Allergy can result in chronic illness, disability, career loss, hardship and death. There is no cure except complete avoidance of latex.*
- Provide worksite review/recommendations to prevent exposure. *Latex allergy can be a disabling occupational disease.*[4] *Education about the problem promotes prevention of allergic reaction, facilitates timely intervention and helps nurse to protect patients, latex-sensitive colleagues and themselves.*[3,4]
- Recommend full medical workup for client presenting with hand dermatitis, especially if job tasks include use of latex.[8]
- Contact suppliers *to verify that latex-free, equipment, products and supplies are available, including (and not limited to) low-allergen/powder-free synthetic gloves, airways, masks, stethoscope tubings, IV tubing, tape, thermometers, urinary catheters, stomach and intestinal tubes, electrodes, oxygen cannulas, pencil erasers, wrist name bands, and rubber bands.*[7]
- Ascertain that procedures are in place to identify and resolve problems with medical devices relevant to allergic reactions or glove performance.[4]
- Refer to resources, including and not limited to, ALERT (Allergy to Latex Education & Resource Team, Inc), Latex Allergy News, Spina Bifida Assoc., National Institute for Occupational Safety and Health (NIOSH), Kendall's Healthcare Products [Web site], Hudson RCI [Web site]) *for further information about common latex products in the home, latex-free products and assistance.*

DOCUMENTATION FOCUS

Assessment/Reassessment
- Assessment findings/pertinent history of contact with latex products/frequency of exposure.
- Type/extent of symptoms.

Planning
- Plan of care and interventions and who is involved in planning.
- Teaching plan.

Implementation/Evaluation
- Response to interventions/teaching and actions performed.

- Attainment/progress toward desired outcome(s).
- Modifications to plan of care.

Discharge Planning
- Discharge needs/referrals made, additional resources available.

References

1. Cavanaugh, B. M. (1999). Nurse's Manual of Diagnostic Tests, ed 3. Philadelphia: F. A. Davis.
2. Latex Allergy: Protect yourself, protect your patients. Nursing World: Workplace Issues: Occupational Safety and Health. ANA pub No.WP-7, 1996.
3. Preventing Allergic Reactions to Natural Rubber Latex in the Workplace, National Institutes for Occupational Safety and Health (NIOSH) Alert. June 1997. DHHS (NIOSH) Pub No. 97–135.
4. ANA Position Statement: Latex Allergy [online]. Effective September 1997. Available at www.nursingworld.org.
5. Truscott, W., & Roley, L. (1995). Glove-associated reactions: Addressing an increasing concern. Dermatol Nurs 7(5): 283.
6. Urticaria and angioedema. In Sommers, M. S. & Johnson, S. A. (eds): (1997). Davis's Manual of Nursing Therapeutics for Diseases and Disorders. Philadelphia: F. A. Davis.
7. AANA Latex Protocol. Certified Registered Nurse Anesthetists (CRNA), American Association of Nurse Anesthetists. Developed 1993, Revised and Approved July 1998. Available at www.aana.com.
8. Worthington, K., & Wilburn, S. (2001). Latex allergy: What's the facility's responsibility and what's yours? AJN 101(7):88.

risk for latex Allergy Response

Definition: At risk for allergic response to natural latex rubber products

RISK FACTORS

History of reactions to latex (e.g., balloons, condoms, gloves); allergies to bananas, avocados, tropical fruits, kiwi, chestnuts, poinsettia plants

History of allergies and asthma

Professions with daily exposure to latex (e.g., medicine, nursing, dentistry)

Conditions associated with continuous or intermittent catheterization

Multiple surgical procedures, especially from infancy (e.g., spina bifida)

NOTE: A risk diagnosis is not evidenced by signs and symptoms, as the problem has not occurred and nursing interventions are directed at prevention.

SAMPLE CLINICAL APPLICATIONS: multiple allergies, neural tube defects (e.g., spina bifida, myelomeningoceles), multiple surgeries at early age, chronic urologic conditions (e.g., neurogenic bladder, exstrophy of bladder), spinal cord trauma

DESIRED OUTCOMES/EVALUATION CRITERIA

Sample NOC linkages:

Immune Hypersensitivity Control: Extent to which inappropriate immune responses are suppressed

Risk Control: Actions to eliminate or reduce actual, personal, and modifiable health threats

Knowledge: Health Behaviors: Extent of understanding conveyed about the promotion and protection of health

Client Will (Include Specific Time Frame)
- Identify and correct potential risk factors in the environment.
- Demonstrate appropriate lifestyle changes to reduce risk of exposure.

 Cultural Collaborative Community/ Home Care  Diagnostic Studies Pediatric/Geriatric/Lifespan Medications
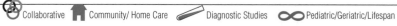

- Identify resources to assist in promoting a safe environment.
- Recognize need for/seek assistance to limit response/complications.

ACTIONS/INTERVENTIONS

Sample NIC linkages:

Latex Precautions: Reducing the risk of a systemic reaction to latex

Allergy Management: Identification, treatment, and prevention of allergic responses to food, medications, insect bites, contrast material, blood, or other substances

Risk Identification: Analysis of potential risk factors, determination of health risks, and prioritization of risk reduction strategies for an individual or group

NURSING PRIORITY NO. **1.** To assess causative/contributing factors:

- Identify persons in high-risk categories (e.g., those with history of allergies, eczema and other dermatitis); those routinely exposed to [natural rubber] latex products: healthcare workers, police/firefighters, emergency medical technicians (EMTs), food handlers (restaurants, grocery stores, cafeterias), hairdressers, cleaning staff, factory workers in plants that manufacture latex-containing products; those with neural tube defects (e.g., spina bifida, myelomeningoceles), multiple surgeries at early age, such as repeated placement of ventriculo-peritoneal shunts, persons with multiple food allergies, particularly to bananas, or urologic conditions requiring frequent surgeries and/or catheterizations (e.g., exstrophy of the bladder, spinal cord trauma, neurogenic bladder).
- Question client regarding latex allergy upon admission to healthcare facility, especially when procedures are anticipated, (e.g., laboratory, emergency department, operating room, wound care management, one-day surgery, dentist). *Current information indicates that natural latex is found in thousands of medical supplies; however, many manufacturers are now using synthetic SB latex. These products have never been associated with allergic reactions, even among individuals that are sensitive to natural latex.*[1]

NURSING PRIORITY NO. **2.** To assist in correcting factors that could lead to latex allergy:

- Discuss necessity of avoiding latex exposure. Recommend/assist client/family to survey environment and remove any medical or household products containing latex. *Avoidance of latex is the only way to prevent the allergy.*[2]
- Substitute nonlatex products, such as natural rubber gloves, PCV IV tubing, latex-free tape, thermometers, electrodes, oxygen cannulas, etc. *Reduces risk of exposure.*
- Provide client/SO with printed lists or Web sites *for obtaining latex-free products and supplies.*
- Ascertain that facilities have established policies and procedures. Promote awareness in the workplace *to address safety and reduce risk to workers and client.*[3]

NURSING PRIORITY NO. **3.** To promote wellness (Teaching/Discharge Considerations):

- Instruct client/care providers about types of potential reactions. *Reaction may be gradual and progressive (e.g., irritant contact rash with gloves); can be progressive, affecting multiple body systems; or may be sudden and anaphylactic and require life-saving treatment.*[1,3]

• Identify measures to take if reactions occur and ways to avoid exposure to latex products *to reduce risk of injury.* (Refer to ND latex Allergy Response.)

 • Refer to allergist for testing as appropriate. *Testing may include challenge test with latex gloves, skin patch test, or blood test for IgE.*

 • Refer to resources (e.g., Latex Allergy News, National Institute for Occupational Safety and Health (NIOSH), Kendall's Healthcare Products [Web site], Hudson RCI [Web site]) *for further information about common latex products in the home, latex-free products and assistance.*

DOCUMENTATION FOCUS

Assessment/Reassessment
• Assessment findings, pertinent history of contact with latex products and frequency of exposure.

Planning
• Plan of care and who is involved in planning.
• Teaching plan.

Implementation/Evaluation
• Response to interventions/teaching and actions performed.
• Attainment/progress toward desired outcome(s).
• Modifications to plan of care.

Discharge Planning
• Long-term needs and who is responsible for actions to be taken.
• Specific referrals made.

References

1. American Nurses Association (ANA) Position Statement: Latex Allergy [online]. Effective September 1997. Available at www.nursingworld.org.
2. Statement on natural latex allergies and SB latex. Occupational Hazards, retrieved 02/11/03. Available at www.occupationalhazards.com.
3. Latex Allergy: Protect yourself, protect your patients. Nursing World: Workplace Issues: Occupational Safety and Health. ANA Pub No. WP-7, 1996.
4. Preventing allergic reactions to natural rubber in the workplace. National Institutes for Occupational Safety and Health (NIOSH) Alert. DHHS Pub No. 97–135, June, 1997.

Anxiety [mild, moderate, severe, panic]

Definition: Vague uneasy feeling of discomfort or dread accompanied by an autonomic response (the source often nonspecific or unknown to the individual); a feeling of apprehension caused by anticipation of danger. It is an altering signal that warns of impending danger and enables the individual to take measures to deal with threat.

RELATED FACTORS
Unconscious conflict about essential [beliefs]/goals and values of life

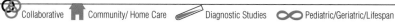 Cultural   Collaborative   Community/ Home Care   Diagnostic Studies   Pediatric/Geriatric/Lifespan   Medications

Situational/maturational crises

Stress

Familial association/heredity

Interpersonal transmission/contagion

Threat to self-concept [perceived or actual]; [unconscious conflict]

Threat of death [perceived or actual]

Threat to or change in health status [progressive/debilitating disease, terminal illness], interaction patterns, role function/status, environment [safety], economic status

Unmet needs

Exposure to toxins

Substance abuse

[Positive or negative self-talk]

[Physiologic factors, such as hyperthyroidism, pheochromocytoma, drug therapy including steroids, etc.]

DEFINING CHARACTERISTICS

Subjective

Behavioral

Expressed concerns due to change in life events

Affective

Regretful; scared; rattled; distressed; apprehension; uncertainty; fearful; feelings of inadequacy; anxious; jittery; [sense of impending doom]; [hopelessness]

Cognitive

Fear of unspecific consequences; awareness of physiologic symptoms

Physiologic

Shakiness, worried, regretful, dry mouth (s), tingling in extremities (p), heart pounding (s), nausea (p), abdominal pain (p), diarrhea (p), urinary hesitancy (p), urinary frequency (p), faintness (p), weakness (s), decreased pulse (p), respiratory difficulties (s), fatigue (p), sleep disturbance (p), [chest, back, neck pain]

Objective

Behavioral

Poor eye contact, glancing about, scanning and vigilance, extraneous movement (e.g., foot shuffling, hand/arm movements), fidgeting, restlessness, diminished productivity, [crying/tearfulness], [pacing/purposeless activity], [immobility]

Affective

Increased wariness, focus on self, irritability, overexcited, anguish, painful and persistent increased helplessness

Physiologic

Voice quivering, trembling/hand tremors, increased tension, facial tension, increased pulse, increased perspiration, cardiovascular excitation (s), facial flushing (s), superficial vasoconstriction (s), increased blood pressure (s), twitching (s), increased reflexes (s), urinary urgency (p), decreased blood pressure (p), insomnia, anorexia (s), increased respiration (s)

Cognitive

Preoccupation, impaired attention, difficulty concentrating, forgetfulness, diminished ability to problem-solve, diminished learning ability, rumination, tendency to blame others, blocking of thought, confusion, decreased perceptual field

DESIRED OUTCOMES/EVALUATION CRITERIA

Sample NOC linkages:

Anxiety Control: Personal actions to eliminate or reduce feelings of apprehension and tension from an unidentifiable source

Coping: Actions to manage stressors that tax an individual's resources

Impulse Control: Self-restraint of compulsive or impulsive behaviors

---

Client Will (Include Specific Time Frame)

- Appear relaxed and report anxiety is reduced to a manageable level.
- Verbalize awareness of feelings of anxiety.
- Identify healthy ways to deal with and express anxiety.
- Demonstrate problem-solving skills.
- Use resources/support systems effectively.

ACTIONS/INTERVENTIONS

Sample NIC linkages:

Anxiety Reduction: Minimizing apprehension, dread, foreboding, or uneasiness related to an unidentified source or anticipated danger

Dementia Management: Provision of a modified environment for the patient who is experiencing a chronic confusional state

Calming Technique: Reducing anxiety in patient experiencing acute distress

NURSING PRIORITY NO. 1. To assess level of anxiety:

- Review familial/physiologic factors, current prescribed medications and recent drug history (e.g., genetic depressive factors, history of thyroid problems; metabolic imbalances, pulmonary disease, anemia, dysrhythmias; use of steroids, thyroid, appetite control medications, substance abuse). *May be related to/or cause of anxious feelings.*[1]
- Identify client's perception of the threat represented by the situation. *Distorted perceptions of the situation may magnify feelings. Understanding client's point of view promotes a more accurate plan of care.*[2]
- Note cultural factors that may influence anxiety. *Individual responses are influenced by the cultural values/beliefs and culturally learned patterns of family of origin. (For instance, Arab-Americans are very expressive about feelings, while Chinese are more reticent).*[4] *Biologic factors may also be involved.*[3]
- Monitor physical responses; for example, palpitations/rapid pulse, repetitive movements, pacing. *Changes in vital signs may suggest degree of anxiety client is experiencing or reflect the impact of physiologic factors, (e.g., endocrine imbalances, medications).*[1]
- Observe behavior indicative of anxiety *which can be a clue to the client's level of anxiety:*
  Mild:
  Alert, more aware of environment, attention focused on environment and immediate events.
  Restless, irritable, wakeful, reports of insomnia.
  Motivated to deal with existing problems in this state.
  Moderate:
  Perception narrower, concentration increased and able to ignore distractions in dealing with problem(s).

 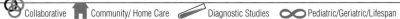

Voice quivers or changes pitch.

Trembling, increased pulse/respirations.

Severe:

Range of perception is reduced; anxiety interferes with effective functioning.

Preoccupied with feelings of discomfort/sense of impending doom.

Increased pulse/respirations with reports of dizziness, tingling sensations, headache, and so on.

Panic:

Ability to concentrate is disrupted; behavior is disintegrated; the client distorts the situation and does not have realistic perceptions of what is happening. The individual may be experiencing terror or confusion or be unable to speak or move (paralyzed with fear).

- Note own feelings of anxiety or uneasiness. *Feelings of anxiety are circular and those in contact with the client may find themselves feeling more anxious.*[3]
- Note use of drugs (alcohol), insomnia or excessive sleeping, limited/avoidance of interactions with others, *which may be behavioral indicators of use of drugs/withdrawal to deal with problems.*[5]
- Be aware of defense mechanisms being used (client may be in denial, regression, and so forth) *May be dealing well with the situation at the moment; (e.g., denial and regression may be helpful coping mechanisms for a time). However, continued use of such mechanisms diverts energy client needs for healing, and problems need to be dealt with at some point.*[6]
- Identify coping skills the individual is using currently, such as anger, daydreaming, forgetfulness, eating, smoking, lack of problem-solving. *These may be useful for the moment, but may eventually interfere with resolution of current situation.*[6]
- Review coping skills used in past. *Can determine those that might be helpful in current circumstances.*[6]

NURSING PRIORITY NO. 2. To assist client to identify feelings and begin to deal with problems:

- Establish a therapeutic relationship, conveying empathy and unconditional positive regard. *Enables client to become comfortable, begin to look at feelings and deal with situation.*[3]
- Be available to client for listening and talking. *Establishes rapport, promotes expression of feelings, and helps client/SO look at realities of the illness/treatment without confronting issues they are not ready to deal with.*[3]
- Encourage client to acknowledge and to express feelings, for example, crying (sadness), laughing (fear, denial), swearing (fear, anger), using Active-listening, reflection. *Often acknowledging feelings enables client to accept and deal more appropriately with situation, relieving anxiety.*[8]
- Assist client to develop self-awareness of verbal and nonverbal behaviors. *Becoming aware helps client to control these behaviors and begin to deal with issues that are causing anxiety.*[9]
- Clarify meaning of feelings/actions by providing feedback and checking meaning with the client. *Validates meaning and ensures accuracy of communication.*[10]
- Acknowledge anxiety/fear. Do not deny or reassure client that everything will be all right. *Validates reality of feelings. False reassurances may be interpreted as lack of understanding or honesty, further isolating client.*[3]
- Provide accurate information about the situation. *Helps client to identify what is reality based and provides opportunity for client to feel reassured.*[11]
- Be truthful with child, avoid bribing, and provide physical contact (e.g., hugging, rocking). *Soothes fears and provides assurance. Children need to recognize that their feelings are not different from others.*[5]

- Provide comfort measures (e.g., calm/quiet environment, soft music, warm bath, back rub: Therapeutic Touch). *Aids in meeting basic human need, decreasing sense of isolation, and assisting client to feel less anxious. Therapeutic Touch requires the nurse to have specific knowledge and experience to use the hands to correct energy field disturbances by redirecting human energies to help or heal.*[3,11]

 - Modify procedures as possible (e.g., substitute oral for intramuscular medications, combine blood draws/use fingerstick method). *Limits degree of stress, avoids overwhelming child or anxious adult.*[2]

- Manage environmental factors such as harsh lighting and high traffic flow, excessive noise. *May be confusing/stressful to older individuals. Managing these factors can lessen anxiety, especially when client is in strange and unusual circumstances.*[2]

- Accept client as is. *The client may need to be where he or she is at this point in time, such as in denial after receiving the diagnosis of a terminal illness.*[3]

- Allow the behavior to belong to the client; do not respond personally. *Reacting personally can escalate the situation promoting a non-therapeutic situation and increasing anxiety.*[1]

- Assist client to use anxiety for coping with the situation if helpful. *Moderate anxiety heightens awareness and can help client to focus on dealing with problems.*[9]

- Encourage awareness of negative self-talk and discuss replacing with positive statements, using can instead of can't, etc. *Negative self-talk promotes feelings of anxiety and self-doubt. Becoming aware and replacing these thoughts can enhance sense of self-worth and reduce anxiety.*[9]

- Discuss the use of music, accommodating client's preferences. *Promotes calming atmosphere alleviating anxiety.*[3]

PANIC STATE

- Stay with client, maintaining a calm, confident manner. *Presence communicates caring and helps client to calm down.*[1]

- Speak in brief statements using simple words. *Client is not able to comprehend complex information at this time.*[1]

- Provide for nonthreatening, consistent environment/atmosphere. Minimize stimuli and monitor visitors and interactions with others. *Lessens effect of transmission of anxious feelings.*[1]

- Set limits on inappropriate behavior and help client to develop acceptable ways of dealing with anxiety. Note: Staff may need to provide safe controls/environment until client regains control. *Behavior may result in damage or injury that client will regret when control is regained diminishing sense of self-worth.*[1]

- Gradually increase activities/involvement with others as anxiety is decreased. *Regaining normal activities will help control feelings of anxiety.*[1]

- Use cognitive therapy to focus on/correct faulty catastrophic interpretations of physical symptoms. *Thoughts of dying, etc. increase anxiety and feelings of panic. Controlling these thoughts allows client to look at situation more realistically and begin to deal appropriately with what is happening.*[1]

- Give antianxiety medications (antianxiety agents/sedatives) as ordered. *Appropriate medication can be helpful in enabling the client to regain control.*[1]

NURSING PRIORITY NO. 3. To promote wellness (Teaching/Discharge Considerations):

- Assist client to identify/deal with precipitating factors and learn new methods of coping with disabling anxiety. *Avoids possibility of repeat episodes.*[9]

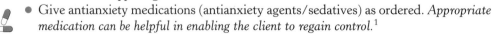

- Review happenings, thoughts, and feelings preceding the anxiety attack. *Identifies factors that led to onset of attack, promoting opportunity to prevent reoccurrences.*[2]
- Identify things the client has done previously to cope successfully when feeling nervous/anxious. *Realizing that they already have coping skills that can be applied in current and future situations can relieve anxiety.*[2]
- List helpful resources/people, including available "hotline" or crisis managers. *Provides ongoing/timely support.*[2]
- Encourage client to develop an exercise/activity program; *may be helpful in reducing level of anxiety by relieving tension. Has been shown to raise endorphin levels to enhance sense of well-being.*[2]
- Assist in developing skills (e.g., awareness of negative thoughts, saying "Stop" and substituting a positive thought*). Eliminating negative self-talk can lead to feelings of positive self-esteem. (Note: Mild phobias seem to respond better to behavioral therapy.)*[10]
- Review strategies such as role playing, use of visualizations to practice anticipated events, prayer/meditation. *These activities can help the client practice behaviors to enable him or her to manage anxiety-provoking situations.*[10]
- 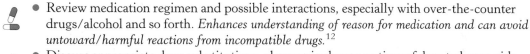 Review medication regimen and possible interactions, especially with over-the-counter drugs/alcohol and so forth. *Enhances understanding of reason for medication and can avoid untoward/harmful reactions from incompatible drugs.*[12]
- Discuss appropriate drug substitutions, changes in dosage or time of dose to lessen side effects. *Ensures proper dosage and avoids untoward side effects. This is especially important in the elderly who are particularly susceptible to multi-drug complications.*[12]
- Refer to physician for drug management program/alteration of prescription regimen. (Drugs that often cause symptoms of anxiety include aminophylline/theophylline, anticholinergics, dopamine, levodopa, salicylates, steroids.) *Reviews and corrects possible undesirable effects of these drugs.*[12]
- Refer to individual and/or group therapy as appropriate. *May be useful to help client deal with chronic anxiety states.*[2]

DOCUMENTATION FOCUS

Assessment/Reassessment
- Level of anxiety and precipitating/aggravating factors.
- Description of feelings (expressed and displayed).
- Awareness/ability to recognize and express feelings.
- Related substance use, if present.

Planning
- Treatment plan and individual responsibility for specific activities.
- Teaching plan.

Implementation/Evaluation
- Client involvement and response to interventions/teaching and actions performed.
- Attainment/progress toward desired outcome(s).
- Modifications to plan of care.

Discharge Planning
- Referrals and follow-up plan.
- Specific referrals made.

References

1. Doenges, M., Moorhouse, M., & Murr, A. (2002). Nursing Care Plans, Guidelines for Individualizing Patient Care, ed 6. Philadelphia: F. A. Davis.
2. Doenges, M., Townsend, M., & Moorhouse, M. (1998). Psychiatric Care Plans: Guidelines for Individualizing Care, ed 3. Philadelphia: F. A. Davis.
3. Townsend, M. (2003). Psychiatric Mental Health Nursing: Concepts of Care, ed 4. Philadelphia: F. A. Davis.
4. Lipson, J. G., Dibble, S. L., & Minarik, P. A. (1996). Culture & Nursing Care: A Pocket Guide. School of Nursing. San Francisco: UCSF Nursing Press.
5. National Institute of Mental Health (2000). Anxiety Disorders, NIH Publication No. 00–3879. Rockville, Md: author. Available at www.nimh.nih.gov.anxiety/anxiety.cfm.
6. Stuart, G. W. (2001). Anxiety responses and anxiety disorders. In Stuart, G. W. & Laraia, M. T. (eds): Principles and Practice of Psychiatric Nursing, ed 7. St. Louis: Mosby.
7. Kunert, P. K. (2002). Stress and adaptation. In Porth, C. M. (ed): Pathophysiology: Concepts of Altered Health States. Philadelphia: Lippincott.
8. Moller, M. D., & Murphy, M. F. (1998). Recovering from Psychosis: A Wellness Approach. Nine Mile Falls, WA: Psychiatric Rehabilitation Nurses Inc.
9. Bohrer, G. J. (March 18, 2002). Anxiety, emotional and physical discomfort. NurseWeek (Mountain West edition), 3(1):21–22.
10. Burns, D. D. (1999). Feeling Good: The New Mood Therapy. New York: Avon.
11. Krieger, D. O. (1979). The Therapeutic Touch: How to Use Your Hands to Heal. Englewood Cliffs, NJ: Prentice Hall.
12. Townsend, M. (2001). Nursing Diagnoses in Psychiatric Nursing: Care Plans and Psychotropic Medications, ed 5. Philadelphia: F. A. Davis.

death Anxiety

Definition: Apprehension, worry, or fear related to death or dying

RELATED FACTORS

To be developed by nurse researchers and submitted to NANDA

DEFINING CHARACTERISTICS

Subjective

Fear of developing a terminal illness, the process of dying, loss of physical and/or mental abilities when dying, premature death because it prevents the accomplishment of important life goals, leaving family alone after death, delayed demise

Negative death images or unpleasant thought about any event related to death or dying, anticipated pain related to dying

Powerlessness over issues related to dying, total loss of control over any aspect of one's own death

Worrying about: the impact of one's death on SOs, being the cause of other's grief and suffering

Concerns of overworking the caregiver as terminal illness incapacitates self

Concern about meeting one's creator or feeling doubtful about the existence of God or higher being

Denial of one's mortality or impending death

Objective

Deep sadness

(Refer to ND anticipatory Grieving.)

SAMPLE CLINICAL APPLICATIONS: chronic debilitating health conditions, cancer, hospital admission, impending major surgery

 Cultural Collaborative Community/ Home Care Diagnostic Studies Pediatric/Geriatric/Lifespan Medications

DESIRED OUTCOMES/EVALUATION CRITERIA

Sample NOC linkages:

Dignified Dying: Maintaining personal control and comfort with the approaching end of life

Fear Control: Personal actions to eliminate or reduce disabling feelings of alarm aroused by an identifiable source

Acceptance: Health Status: Reconciliation to health circumstances

---

Client Will (Include Specific Time Frame)

- Identify and express feelings (e.g., sadness, guilt, fear) freely/effectively.
- Look toward/plan for the future 1 day at a time.
- Formulate a plan dealing with individual concerns and eventualities of dying.

ACTIONS/INTERVENTIONS

Sample NIC linkages:

Dying Care: Promotion of physical comfort and psychological peace in the final phase of life

Spiritual Support: Assisting the patient to feel balance and connection with a greater power

Grief Work Facilitation: Assistance with the resolution of a significant loss

NURSING PRIORITY NO. 1. To assess causative/contributing factors:

- Determine how client sees self in usual lifestyle role functioning and perception and meaning of anticipated loss to him or her and SO(s). *Provides information that can be compared to changes that are occurring. Understanding of these factors is helpful for planning.*[1]
- Ascertain current knowledge of situation. *Identifies misconceptions, lack of information, other pertinent issues and determines accuracy of knowledge. Death may not be anticipated by healthcare providers in current situation.*[1]
- Determine client's role in family constellation. Observe patterns of communication in family and response of family/SO to client's situation and concerns. *In addition to identifying areas of need/concern, also reveals strengths useful in addressing the current concerns.*[3]
- Assess impact of client reports of subjective experiences and experience with death (or exposure to death), for example, witnessed violent death or as a child viewed body in casket, and so on. *Identifies possible feelings that may be affecting current situation and promote accurate planning.*[2]
- Identify cultural factors/expectations and impact on current situation/feelings. *These factors affect client attitude toward events and impending loss. For instance, in Russia, the head of the family is informed first of the impending death, who may not want the client to know so they will have a peaceful death. Many cultures prefer to keep the client at home instead of in a nursing home or hospital, and growth of the hospice movement in the United States provides palliative care and comfort during the client's final days.*[4]
- Note age, physical/mental condition, complexity of therapeutic regimen. *May affect ability to handle current situation. Younger people may handle stress of illness in more positive ways. Older people may be more accepting of possibility of death. Individual/s of any age will deal with situation in own way, depending on diagnosis and condition.*[1]
- Determine ability to manage own self-care, end-of-life and other affairs, awareness/use of available resources. *Information will be necessary for planning care.*[1]
- Observe behavior indicative of the level of anxiety present (mild to panic). *The level of anxiety affects client's/SO's ability to process information/participate in activities.*[5]

 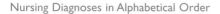

- Identify coping skills currently used, and how effective they are. Be aware of defense mechanisms being used by the client. *Provides a starting point to plan care and assist client to acknowledge reality and deal more effectively with what is happening.*[3]

- Note use of drugs (including alcohol), presence of insomnia, excessive sleeping, avoidance of interactions with others. *Indicators of withdrawal and need for intervention to deal with symptoms and help client deal realistically with diagnosis/illness.*[6]
- Note client's religious/spiritual orientation, involvement in religious/church activities, presence of conflicts regarding spiritual beliefs. *May benefit by referral to appropriate resource to help client resolve these issues if desired.*[7]
- Listen to client/SO reports/expressions of anger/concern, alienation from God, belief that impending death is a punishment for wrongdoing, and so on. *Allows client to freely express feelings and concerns without judgment and opportunity to work toward individual solution.*[7]
- Determine sense of futility, feelings of hopelessness, helplessness, lack of motivation to help self. *Indicators of depression and need for early intervention to help client acknowledge and deal with impending death.*[7]
- Active-listen comments regarding sense of isolation. *Active-listening acknowledges reality of feelings and encourages client to find own solutions.*[2]
- Listen for expressions of inability to find meaning in life or suicidal ideation. *Signs of depression indicating need for referral to therapist/psychiatrist and possible pharmacologic treatment to help client deal with terminal illness/situation.*[7]

NURSING PRIORITY NO. 2. To assist client to deal with situation:

- Provide open and trusting relationship. *Promotes opportunity to explore feelings about impending death.*[2]
- Include family in discussions and decision-making as appropriate. *Involved family members can provide support and ideas for problem-solving.*[7]
- Use therapeutic communication skills of Active-listening, silence, acknowledgment. Respect client desire/request not to talk. Provide hope within parameters of the individual situation. *Promotes open environment that encourages client to talk freely about thoughts and feelings. Client may not be ready to talk about situation/concerns about death or may be denying reality of what is happening.*[1]
- Encourage expressions of feelings (anger, fear, sadness, etc.). Acknowledge anxiety/fear. Do not deny or reassure client that everything will be all right. Be honest when answering questions/providing information. *Enhances trust and therapeutic relationship.*[2]
- Provide information about normalcy of feelings and individual grief reaction. *Most individuals question their reactions and whether they are normal or not and information can provide reassurance for them.*[3]
- Make time for nonjudgmental discussion of philosophical issues/questions about spiritual impact of illness/situation. *Can help client clarify own position on these issues.*[3]
- Review life experiences of loss and use of coping skills, noting client strengths and successes. *Provides opportunity to identify and use previously successful skills.*[2]
- Provide calm, peaceful setting and privacy as appropriate. *Promotes relaxation and enhances ability to deal with situation.*[1]
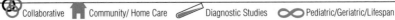
- Assist client to engage in spiritual growth activities, experience prayer/meditation and forgiveness to heal past hurts. Provide information that anger with God is a normal part of the grieving process. *Reduces feelings of guilt/conflict, allowing client to move forward toward resolution.*[1]

 Cultural   Collaborative Community/ Home Care   Diagnostic Studies Pediatric/Geriatric/Lifespan Medications

- Refer to therapists, spiritual advisors, counselors. *Promotes facilitation of grief work.*[1]
- Refer to community agencies/resources. *Assists client/SO in planning for eventualities (legal issues, funeral plans, etc.)*[1]

NURSING PRIORITY NO. 3. To promote independence:

- Support client's efforts to develop realistic steps to put plans into action. *Provides sense of control over situation in which client does not have much control.*[1]
- Direct client's thoughts beyond present state to enjoyment of each day and the future when appropriate. *Being in the moment can help client enjoy this time rather than dwelling on what is ahead.*[1]
- Provide opportunities for client to make simple decisions. *Enhances sense of control.*[1]
- Develop individual plan using client's locus of control. *Identifying locus of control (internal or external) and using that information to assist client/family through the process will promote effective management of the situation.*[2]
- Treat expressed decisions and desires with respect and convey to others as appropriate. *Expresses regard for the individual and enhances sense of control in situation that is not controllable.*[1]
- Assist with completion of Advance Directives and cardiopulmonary resuscitation (CPR) instructions. *Provides opportunity for client to understand options and express desires.*[1]
- Refer to palliative, hospice, or end-of-life care resources as appropriate. *Provides support and assistance to client and SO/family through potentially complex and difficult process. Choice of type of care is dependent on timing of care (e.g., palliative care interfaces with curative treatment which hospice does not allow).*[1]

DOCUMENTATION FOCUS

Assessment/Reassessment
- Assessment findings, including client's fears and signs/symptoms being exhibited.
- Responses/actions of family/SOs.
- Availability/use of resources.

Planning
- Plan of care and who is involved in planning.

Implementation/Evaluation
- Client's response to interventions/teaching and actions performed.
- Attainment/progress toward desired outcome(s).
- Modifications to plan of care.

Discharge Planning
- Identified needs and who is responsible for actions to be taken.
- Specific referrals made.

References

1. Doenges, M., Moorhouse, M., & Murr, A. C. (2002). Nursing Care Plans, Guidelines for Individualizing Patient Care, ed 6. Philadelphia: F. A. Davis.
2. Doenges, M., Townsend, M., & Moorhouse, M. (1998). Psychiatric Care Plans: Guidelines for Individualizing Care, ed 3. Philadelphia: F. A. Davis.

3. Townsend, M. (2003). Psychiatric Mental Health Nursing: Concepts of Care, ed 4. Philadelphia: F. A. Davis.
4. Lipson, J. G., Dibble. S. L., & Minarik, P. A. (1996). Culture & Nursing Care: A Pocket Guide. San Francisco: School of Nursing, UCSF Nursing Press.
5. Doenges, M., Moorhouse, M., Murr, A. C. (2004). Nurse's Pocket Guide Diagnoses, Interventions, and Rationales, ed 9. Philadelphia: F. A. Davis.
6. Bruera, E., et al. (1995). The frequency of alcoholism among patients with pain due to terminal cancer. J Pain Symptom Manage, 10(8):599–603.
7. Paice, J. (2002). Managing psychological conditions in palliative care. AJN, 102(11):36–43.

risk for Aspiration

Definition: At risk for entry of gastrointestinal secretions, oropharyngeal secretions, or [exogenous food] solids or fluids into tracheobronchial passages [due to dysfunction or absence of normal protective mechanisms]

RISK FACTORS

Reduced level of consciousness

Depressed cough and gag reflexes

Impaired swallowing

Facial/oral/neck surgery or trauma, wired jaws

Situation hindering elevation of upper body [weakness, paralysis]

Incompetent lower esophageal sphincter [hiatal hernia or other esophageal disease affecting stomach valve function], delayed gastric emptying, decreased gastrointestinal motility, increased intragastric pressure, increased gastric residual

Presence of tracheostomy or endotracheal (ET) tube [inadequate or overinflation of tracheostomy/ET tube cuff]

[Presence of] gastrointestinal tubes, tube feedings/medication administration

NOTE: A risk diagnosis is not evidenced by signs and symptoms, as the problem has not occurred and nursing interventions are directed at prevention.

SAMPLE CLINICAL APPLICATIONS: surgery, vomiting/bulimia nervosa, presence of nasogastric tube, brain injury, spinal cord injury, enteral feedings.

DESIRED OUTCOMES/EVALUATION CRITERIA

Sample NOC linkages:

Risk Control: Actions to eliminate or reduce actual, personal, and modifiable health threats

Neurologic Status: Extent to which the peripheral and central nervous system receive, process, and respond to internal and external stimuli

Respiratory Status: Airway Patency: Extent to which the tracheobronchial passages remain open

Client Will (Include Specific Time Frame)

- Experience no aspiration as evidenced by noiseless respirations, clear breath sounds; clear, odorless secretions.
- Identify causative/risk factors.
- Demonstrate techniques to prevent and/or correct aspiration.

ACTIONS/INTERVENTIONS

Sample NIC linkages:

Aspiration Precautions: Prevention or minimization of risk factors in the patient at risk for aspiration

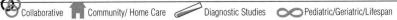 Cultural Collaborative Community/ Home Care Diagnostic Studies Pediatric/Geriatric/Lifespan Medications

Artificial Airway Management: Facilitation of patency of air passages

Postanesthesia Care: Monitoring and management of the patient who has recently undergone general or regional anesthesia

NURSING PRIORITY NO. **1.** To assess causative/contributing factors:

- Assess for age-related risk factors potentiating risk of aspiration (e.g., prematurity and elderly infirm).
- Note level of consciousness/awareness of surroundings, cognitive impairment. *Aspiration is common in coma patients, owing to inability to cough, to swallow well and/or presence of mechanical ventilation and tube feedings.*[1]
- Evaluate presence of conditions/diseases causing neuromuscular weakness, noting muscle groups involved, degree of impairment, and whether acute or of a progressive nature (e.g., stroke, cerebral palsy, Parkinson's disease, Guillain-Barré syndrome, amyotrophic lateral sclerosis [ALS], psychiatric client following electric shock therapy).
- Observe for neck and facial edema, for example, client with head/neck surgery, tracheal/bronchial injury (upper torso burns, inhalation/chemical injury). *Problems with swallowing and maintenance of airways can be expected in these clients and the potential is high for aspiration and aspiration pneumonia.*
- Assess amount and consistency of respiratory secretions, breath sounds, and rate/depth of respirations, as well as client's coughing and swallowing abilities. *Helps differentiate the potential cause for risk of aspiration. The major pathophysiological dysfunction is the inability of the epiglottis and true vocal cords to move to close the trachea (e.g. changes in the structures themselves, or because messages to the brain are absent, decreased or impaired). Problems with coughing (clearing airways) and swallowing (pooling of saliva, liquids) increase risk of aspiration and respiratory complications.*[2–4]
- Auscultate lung sounds periodically (especially in client who is coughing frequently or not coughing at all; ventilator client being tube-fed, immediately following extubation) and observe chest radiographs *to determine presence of aspirated food or secretions, and "silent aspiration."*[5]
- Evaluate for/note presence of gastrointestinal pathology and motility disorders. *Nausea with vomiting (associated with metabolic disorders, or following surgery, certain medications) and gastroesophageal reflux disease (GERD) can be a cause for aspiration.*[3,6]
- Note administration of enteral feedings, which may be initiated when oral nutrition is not possible, such as in head injury, stroke/other neurologic disorders, head and neck surgery, esophageal obstruction, and discontinuous gastrointestinal tract. *Potential exists for regurgitation and aspiration, even with proper tube placement, and/or misplacement of tube. The client at high risk for aspiration associated with nasogastroenteral feedings should be evaluated for enteral feedings into the jejunum.*[7]
- Ascertain lifestyle habits (chronic use of alcohol and drugs, alcohol intoxication, tobacco, and other CNS suppressant drugs). *Can affect awareness, as well as impair gag and swallow mechanisms.*[5]

NURSING PRIORITY NO. **2.** To assist in correcting factors that can lead to aspiration:

- Place client in proper position for age and condition/disease affecting airways. *Adult and child should be upright for meals, or placed on right side to decrease likelihood of drainage into trachea rather than esophagus, to reduce reflux, and to improve gastric emptying.*[2] *Prone*

position may provide shorter gastric emptying time and decreased incidence of regurgitation and subsequent aspiration in premature infants.[8]

- Encourage client to cough as able *to clear secretions. May simply need to be reminded or encouraged to cough, such as might occur in elderly person with delayed gag reflex or in postoperative, sedated client.*[2]
- Provide close monitoring for use of oxygen masks in clients at risk for vomiting. Refrain from using oxygen mask for comatose individuals.

- Keep wire cutters/scissors with client at all times when jaws are wired/banded *to facilitate clearing airway in emergencies.*
- In client requiring suctioning *to manage secretions:*
  Maintain operational suction equipment at bedside/chairside
  Suction (oral cavity, nose, and ET/tracheostomy tube) as needed, using correct size of catheter and timing for adult or child *to clear secretions in client with more frequent or congested sounding cough; presence of coarse rhonchi and expiratory wheezing (audible with or without auscultation); visible secretions, increased peak pressures during volume-cycled ventilation; indication from client that suctioning is necessary; suspected aspiration of gastric or upper airway secretions; or otherwise unexplained increases in shortness of breath, respiratory rate or heart rate.* [2,9,10]
  Avoid triggering gag mechanism when performing suction or mouth care.
- Assist with postural drainage and other respiratory therapies *to mobilize thickened secretions that may interfere with swallowing.*

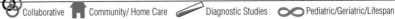
- Refer to speech therapist for specific exercises *to strengthen muscles and techniques to enhance swallowing.*

- For a verified swallowing problem[3,5]:
  Elevate client to highest or best possible position for eating and drinking
  Feed slowly, instruct client to take small bites, to chew thoroughly
  Give semisolid foods; avoid pureed foods and mucus-producing foods (milk). Use soft foods that stick together/form a bolus (e.g., casseroles, puddings, stews) *to aid swallowing effort.*
  Provide very warm or very cold liquids *(activates temperature receptors in the mouth that help to stimulate swallowing).* Add thickening agent to liquids as appropriate.
  Avoid washing solids down with liquids *to prevent bolus of food pushing down too rapidly, increasing risk of aspiration.*

  Provide oral medications in elixir form or crush, if appropriate. Have client self-medicate when possible. Time medications to coincide with meals when possible.
- When feeding tube is in place[3,11]:
  Note radiograph and/or measurement of aspirate pH following placement of feeding tube *to verify correct position.*
  Measure residuals during intermittent feeding, when appropriate *to prevent overfeeding.*

  Elevate head of bed 30 degrees during and for at least 30 minutes after bolus feeding.
  Add food coloring (per protocol) to feeding *to identify regurgitation.*

- Determine best position for infant/child (e.g., with the head of bed elevated 30 degrees and infant propped on right side after feeding. *Upper airway patency is facilitated by upright position and turning to right side decreases likelihood of drainage into trachea.*

NURSING PRIORITY NO. 3. To promote wellness (Teaching/Discharge Considerations):

- Review individual risk or potentiating factors with client/care provider. Provide informa-

 Cultural   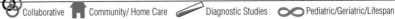 Collaborative   Community/ Home Care   Diagnostic Studies   Pediatric/Geriatric/Lifespan   Medications tion about the effects of aspiration on the lungs. *Increases awareness of potential severity of problem.*

- Instruct in safety concerns when feeding oral or tube feeding. Refer to ND impaired Swallowing.
- Train client to suction self or train family members in suction techniques (especially if client has constant or copious oral secretions) *to enhance safety/self-sufficiency.*
- Instruct individual/family member to avoid/limit activities that increase intra-abdominal pressure (straining, strenuous exercise, tight/constrictive clothing). *May slow digestion/increase risk of regurgitation.*

DOCUMENTATION FOCUS

Assessment/Reassessment
- Assessment findings/conditions that could lead to problems of aspiration.
- Verification of tube placement, observations of physical findings.

Planning
Interventions to prevent aspiration or reduce risk factors and who is involved in the planning.
Teaching plan.

Implementation/Evaluation
- Client's responses to interventions/teaching and actions performed.
- Foods/fluids client handles with ease/difficulty.
- Amount/frequency of intake.
- Attainment/progress toward desired outcome(s).
- Modifications to plan of care.

Discharge Planning
- Long-term needs and who is responsible for actions to be taken.

References

1. Dimancescu, M. D. (Fall, 1989). Aspiration pneumonia. Coma Recovery Institute, Newsletter.
2. Cox, H. C., et al. (2002). Clinical Applications of Nursing Diagnosis: Adult, Child, Women's Psychiatric, Gerontic, and Home Health Considerations, ed 4. Philadelphia: F.A. Davis.
3. Altered nutritional status. Clinical Practice Guidelines. American Medical Directors Association (AMDA). December, 2002. Available at www.amda.com.
4. American Gastroenterological Association. (1999). Medical position statement: Management of oropharyngeal dysphagia. 116(2):452.
5. Galvan, T. J. (2001). Dysphagia: Going down and staying down. AJN, 101(1): 37.
6. Clinical consensus statement: Managing cough as a defense mechanism and as a symptom. (Quick Reference Guide for Clinicians) Northbrook, IL: American College of Chest Physicians, 1998.
7. Practice management guidelines for nutritional support of the trauma patient. Eastern Association for the Surgery of Trauma (EAST). March 1998. EAST Web site.
8. Apnea of prematurity. Clinical Practice Guideline, National Association of Neonatal Nurses (NANN), February 1999.
9. Removal of the endotracheal tube. The ARC Clinical Practice Guidelines. American Association for Respiratory Care (ARC), April 1999. Available at www.aarc.org.
10. Suctioning of the patient in the home. The ARC Clinical Practice Guidelines. American Association for Respiratory Care (ARC), April 1999. Available at www.aarc.org.
11. Metheny, N. A. & Titler, M. G. (2001). Assessing placement of feeding tubes. AJN 101(5): 36.

Definition: Disruption of the interactive process between parent/SO and infant that fosters the development of a protective and nurturing reciprocal relationship

RISK FACTORS

Inability of parents to meet the personal needs

Anxiety associated with the parent role

Substance abuse

Premature infant; ill infant/child who is unable to effectively initiate parental contact due to altered behavioral organization

Separation; physical barriers

Lack of privacy

[Parents who themselves experienced altered attachment]

[Uncertainty of paternity; conception as a result of rape/sexual abuse]

[Difficult pregnancy and/or birth (actual or perceived)]

NOTE: A risk diagnosis is not evidenced by signs and symptoms, as the problem has not occurred and nursing interventions are directed at prevention.

SAMPLE CLINICAL APPLICATIONS: prematurity, genetic/congenital conditions, autism, attention deficit disorder, developmental delay (parent or child), substance abuse (parent), bipolar disorder (parent)

DESIRED OUTCOMES/EVALUATION CRITERIA

Sample NOC linkages:

Parent-Infant Attachment: Behaviors that demonstrate an enduring affectionate bond between parent and infant

Parenting: Provision of an environment that promotes optimum growth and development of dependent children

Child Development: [specify age group]: Milestones of physical, cognitive, and psychosocial progression by [specify] months/years of age

---

Parent Will (Include Specific Time Frame)
- Identify and prioritize family strengths and needs.
- Exhibit nurturant and protective behaviors toward child.
- Identify and use resources to meet needs of family members.
- Demonstrate techniques to enhance behavioral organization of the infant/child.
- Engage in mutually satisfying interactions with child.

ACTIONS/INTERVENTIONS

Sample NIC linkages:

Attachment Promotion: Facilitation of the development of the parent-infant relationship

Parenting Promotion: Providing parenting information, support, and coordination of comprehensive services to high-risk families

Environmental Management: Attachment Process: Manipulation of the patient's surroundings to facilitate the development of the parent-infant relationship

NURSING PRIORITY NO. 1. To identify causative/contributing factors:

- Interview parents, noting their perception of situation, individual concerns. *Identifies problem areas/strengths to formulate appropriate plans to change situation that is currently creating problems for the parents.*[8]

 Cultural Collaborative Community/ Home Care Diagnostic Studies 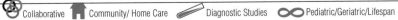 Pediatric/Geriatric/Lifespan Medications

- Assess parent/child interactions. *Identifies relationships, communication skills and feelings about one another. The way in which a parent responds to a child and how the child responds to the parent largely determines how the child develops. Identifying the way in which this family responds to one another is crucial to determining the need for and type of interventions required.*[8]
- Ascertain availability/use of resources to include extended family, support groups, and financial. *Lack of support from or presence of extended family, lack of involvement in groups such as church or specific resources, such as La Leche League and financial stresses can affect family negatively, interfering with ability to deal effectively with parenting responsibilities. Parents need support from both inside and outside of the family.*[9,12]
- Determine emotional and behavioral problems of the child. *Attachment-disordered children are unable to give and receive love and affection, defy parental rules and authority, and are physically and emotionally abusive, creating ongoing stress and turmoil in the family.*[12]
- Evaluate parent's ability to provide protective environment, participate in reciprocal relationship. *Parents may be immature, may be substance abusers, or may be mentally ill and unable or unwilling to assume the task of parenting. The way in which the parent responds to the child is critical to the child's development, and intervention needs to be directed at helping the parents to deal with own issues and learn positive parenting skills.*[1,7]
- Note attachment behaviors between parent and child(ren), recognizing cultural background. *For example, lack of eye contact and touching may indicate bonding problems. Behaviors such as eye-to-eye contact, use of en face positon, talking to the infant in a high-pitched voice are indicative of attachment behaviors in American culture but may not be appropriate in another culture. Failure to bond effectively is thought to affect subsequent parent-child interaction.*[4,5]
- Assess parenting skill level, considering intellectual, emotional, and physical strengths and limitations. *Identifies areas of need for further education, skill training, and factors that might interfere with ability to assimilate new information.*[1,2]

NURSING PRIORITY NO. 2. To enhance behavioral organization of infant/child:

- Identify infant's strengths and vulnerabilities. *Each child is born with his or her temperament that affects interactions with caregivers and when these are known, actions can be taken to assist parents/caregivers to parent appropriately.*[3,7,11]
- Educate parent regarding child growth and development, addressing parental perceptions. *Parents often have misconceptions about the abilities of their children, and providing correct information clarifies expectations and is more realistic.*[6]
- Assist parents in modifying the environment. *The environment can be changed to provide appropriate stimulation; to diminish stimulation, for example, before bedtime; to simplify when the environment is too complex to handle; and to provide life space where the child can play unrestricted, resulting in freedom for the child to meet his or her needs. (Refer to ND: readiness for enhanced organized Infant Behavior.)*[2,7]
- Model caregiving techniques that best support behavioral organization, such as attachment parenting. *Recognizing that the child deserves to have his or her needs taken seriously and responding to those needs in a loving fashion promotes trust, and children learn to model their behavior after what they have seen the parents do.*[9,11]
- Respond consistently with nurturance to infant/child. *Babies come wired with an ability to signal their needs by crying, and when parents respond to these signals they develop a sensitivity that in turn develops parental intuition providing the infant with gratification of their needs and trust in their environment.*[10]

NURSING PRIORITY NO. 3. To enhance best functioning of parents:

• Develop therapeutic nurse-client relationship. Provide a consistently warm, nurturant, and nonjudgmental environment. *Parents are often surprised to find that this tiny infant can cause so many changes in their lives and need help to adjust to this new experience. The warm, caring relationship of the nurse can help with this adjustment and provide the information and empathy they need at this time.*[1]

• Assist parents in identifying and prioritizing family strengths and needs. *Promotes positive attitude by looking at what they already do well and using those skills to address needs.*[2]

• Support and guide parents in process of assessing resources. *Outside support is important at this time and making sure that parents receive the help they need will help them in this adjustment period.*[12]

• Involve parents in activities with the infant/child that they can accomplish successfully. *Activities, such as Baby Gymboree and baby yoga, enable the parents to get to know their infant/child and themselves, which enhances their confidence and self-concept.*[12]

• Recognize and provide positive feedback for nurturant and protective parenting behaviors. *Using I-messages to let parents know their behaviors are effective reinforces continuation of desired behaviors and promotes feelings of confidence in their abilities.*[2,12]

• Minimize number of professionals on team with whom parents must have contact. *Parents begin to know the individuals they are dealing with on a regular basis, which fosters trust in these relationships and provides opportunities for modeling and learning.*[3]

NURSING PRIORITY NO. 4. To support parent/child attachment during separation:

• Provide parents with telephone contact as appropriate. *Knowing there is someone they can call if they have a problem provides a sense of security.*[3]

• Establish a routine time for daily phone calls/initiate calls as indicated when child is hospitalized. *Provides sense of consistency and control; allows for planning of other activities so parents can maintain contact and get information on a regular basis.*[1]

• Invite parents to use Ronald McDonald House or provide them with a listing of a variety of local accommodations, restaurants. *When child is hospitalized out of town, parents need to have a place to stay so they can have ready access to the hospital and be able to rest and refresh from time to time.*[3]

• Arrange for parents to receive photos, progress reports from the child. *Provides information and comfort as the infant/child progresses, allowing the parents to continue to have hope for a positive resolution.*[3]

• Suggest parents provide a photo and/or audiotape of themselves for the child. *Provides a connection during the separation sustaining attachment between parent and child.*[1]

• Consider use of contract with parents. *Clearly communicating expectations of both family and staff serves as a reminder of what each person has committed to and as tool to evaluate whether expectations are being maintained.*[3]

• Suggest parents keep a journal of infant/child progress. *Serves as a reminder of the progress that is being made, especially when they become discouraged and believe infant/child is "never" going to be better.*[3]

• Provide "homelike" environment for situations requiring supervision of visits. *An environment that is comfortable supports the family as they work toward resolving conflicts and promotes a sense of hopefulness enabling them to experience success when family is involved with a legal situation.*[12]

 Cultural   Collaborative   Community/ Home Care Diagnostic Studies Pediatric/Geriatric/Lifespan   Medications

NURSING PRIORITY NO. 5. To promote wellness (Teaching/Discharge Considerations):

 • Refer to addiction counseling/treatment, individual counseling, or family therapies as indicated. *May need additional assistance when situation is complicated by drug abuse (including alcohol), mental illness, disruptions in caregiving, parents who are burned out with caring for child with attachment difficulties.*[12]

 • Identify services for transportation, financial resources, housing, and so forth. *Assistance with these needs can help families focus on therapeutic regimen and on issues of parenting to improve family dynamics.*[9]

• Develop support systems appropriate to situation. *Depending on individual situation, support from extended family, friends, social worker, or therapist can assist family to deal with attachment disorders.*[10]

• Explore community resources available to family. *Church affiliations, volunteer groups, day/respite care can help parents who are overwhelmed with care of a child with attachment disorder.*[12]

DOCUMENTATION FOCUS

Assessment/Reassessment
• Identified behaviors of both parents and child.
• Specific risk factors, individual perceptions/concerns.
• Interactions between parent and child.

Planning
• Plan of care and who is involved in planning.
• Teaching plan.

Implementation/Evaluation
• Parents'/child's responses to interventions/teaching and actions performed.
• Attainment/progress toward desired outcomes.
• Modifications to plan of care.

Discharge Planning
• Long-term needs and who is responsible.
• Plan for home visits to support parents and to ensure infant/child safety and well-being.
• Specific referrals made.

References

1. Townsend, M. C. (2003). Psychiatric Mental Health Nursing Concepts of Care, ed 4. Philadelphia: F. A. Davis.
2. Gordon, T. (2000). Parent Effectiveness Training, (updated ed). New York: Three Rivers Press.
3. Cox, H. C., et al. (2002). Clinical Applications of Nursing Diagnosis: Adult, Child, Women's, Psychiatric, Gerontic, and Home Health Considerations, ed 4. Philadelphia: F. A. Davis.
4. Lipson, J. G., Dibble, S. L., & Minarik, P. A. (1996). Culture & Nursing Care: A Pocket Guide. San Francisco: UCSF Nursing Press.
5. Doenges, M. E., Townsend, M. C., & Moorhouse, M. F. (1998). Psychiatric Care Plans Guidelines for Individualizing Care, ed 3. Philadelphia: F. A. Davis.
6. Gordon, T. (1989). Teaching Children Self-discipline: At Home and At School. New York: Random House.
7. Gordon, T. (2000). Family Effectiveness Training Video. Solana Beach, CA: Gordon Training Intnl.
8. Doenges, M. E., Moorhouse, M. F., & Murr, A. C. (2004). Nurse's Pocket Guide Diagnoses, Interventions, and Rationales, ed 9. Philadelphia: F. A. Davis.

9. Henningsen, M. (1996). Attachment Disorder, Theory, Parenting, and Therapy. Evergreen, CO: Evergreen Family Counseling Center.
10. Sears, W. (1999). Attachment Parenting: A Style that Works. Excerpted from Nighttime Parenting – How to Get Your Baby and Child to Sleep (La Leche League International Book), (revised ed). Plume.
11. Hunt, J. What is Attachment Parenting? The Natural Child Project. Available at http://www.naturalchild.com/jan_hunt/attachment_parenting.html. Accessed February 2004.
12. Corrective Attachment Parenting. Evergreen, CO: Evergreen Psychotherapy Center Attachment Treatment and Training Institute.

Autonomic Dysreflexia

Definition: Life-threatening, uninhibited sympathetic response of the nervous system to a noxious stimulus after a spinal cord injury (SCI) at T7 or above [has been demonstrated in clients with injuries at T8 and occasionally lower]

RELATED FACTORS

Bladder or bowel distention; [catheter insertion, obstruction, irrigation]
Skin irritation
Lack of client and caregiver knowledge
[Sexual excitation]
[Environmental temperature extremes]

DEFINING CHARACTERISTICS

Subjective
Headache (a diffuse pain in different portions of the head and not confined to any nerve distribution area)
Paresthesia, chilling, blurred vision, chest pain, metallic taste in mouth, nasal congestion

Objective
Paroxysmal hypertension (sudden periodic elevated blood pressure in which systolic pressure >140 mm Hg and diastolic >90 mm Hg)
Bradycardia or tachycardia (heart rate 60 or 100 beats per minute, respectively)
Diaphoresis (above the injury), red splotches on skin (above the injury), pallor (below the injury)
Horner's syndrome (contraction of the pupil, partial ptosis of the eyelid, enophthalmos and sometimes loss of sweating over the affected side of the face); conjunctival congestion
Pilomotor reflex (gooseflesh formation when skin is cooled)

SAMPLE CLINICAL APPLICATIONS: spinal cord injury

DESIRED OUTCOMES/EVALUATION CRITERIA
Sample NOC linkages:
Neurologic Status: Autonomic: Extent to which the autonomic nervous system coordinates visceral function
Knowledge: Disease Process: Extent of understanding conveyed about a specific disease process
Symptom Severity: Extent of perceived adverse changes in physical, emotional, and social functioning

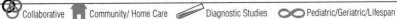 Cultural Collaborative Community/ Home Care Diagnostic Studies Pediatric/Geriatric/Lifespan Medications

Client/Caregiver Will (Include Specific Time Frame)
- Identify risk factors.
- Recognize signs/symptoms of syndrome.
- Demonstrate corrective techniques.
- Experience no episodes of dysreflexia or will seek medical intervention in a timely manner.

ACTIONS/INTERVENTIONS

Sample NIC linkages:

Dysreflexia Management: Prevention and elimination of stimuli that cause hyperactive reflexes and inappropriate autonomic responses in a patient with a cervical or high thoracic cord lesion

Urinary Elimination/Bowel Management: Maintenance of an optimum urinary elimination pattern/establishment and maintenance of a regular pattern of bowel elimination

Anxiety Reduction: Minimizing apprehension, dread, foreboding, or uneasiness related to an unidentified source or anticipated danger

NURSING PRIORITY NO. 1. To assess precipitating risk factors:

- Assess for bladder distention (most common cause), presence of bladder spasms/stones or infection.
- Evaluate for bowel distention, fecal impaction, and problems with bowel management program.
- Assess skin/tissue for pressure areas, especially following prolonged sitting.
- Monitor environmental temperature for extremes/drafts.
- Monitor closely during procedures/diagnostics that manipulate bladder or bowel.

NURSING PRIORITY NO. 2. To provide for early detection and immediate intervention:

- Investigate associated complaints/syndrome of symptoms (e.g., severe pounding headache, [blood pressure may be > 200/100 mm Hg], chest pain, irregular heart rate/dysrhythmias, blurred vision, nausea, facial flushing, metallic taste, severe anxiety; or minimal symptoms or expressed complaints in presence of significantly elevated blood pressure—silent autonomic dysreflexia [AD]). *Body's reaction to misinterpreted sensations from below the injury site, resulting in an autonomic reflex, which can cause blood vessels to constrict and increase blood pressure. This is a potentially life-threatening condition, requiring immediate and correct action.*[1-3]
- Note onset of crying, irritability, or somnolence in infant or child *(may present with nonspecific symptoms, not be able to verbalize discomforts).*[1]
- Locate/eliminate causative stimulus, moving in step-wise fashion (Note: cause can be anything that would normally cause pain or discomfort below level of injury)[1-6]

  Assess for bladder distention *(most common cause of AD):*

  Empty bladder by voiding or catheterization—applying local anesthetic ointment *to prevent exacerbation of AD by procedure.*

  Ascertain that urine is free flowing if Foley or suprapubic catheter in place, empty drainage bag, straighten tubing if kinked, lower drainage bag if it is higher than bladder.

  Irrigate gently or change catheter, if not draining freely. Note color, character and odor of urine *(infection can cause AD).*

Check for distended bowel *(if urinary problem is not causing AD):*

Perform digital stimulation, checking for constipation/impacted stool. (If symptoms first appear while performing digital stimulation, stop procedure.)

Apply local anesthetic ointment to rectum; remove impaction after symptoms subside *to remove causative problem without causing additional symptoms.*

Check for skin pressure/irritation *(if bowel problem is not causing AD):*

Do a pressure release if sitting.

Check for tight clothing, straps, belts.

Note whether pressure sore has developed or changed.

Observe for bruising, signs of infection.

Check for ingrown toenail or other injury to skin, tissue (e.g. burns, sunburn) or fractured bones.

Check for other possible causes *(if skin pressure is not causing AD):*

Menstrual cramps, sexual activity, labor and delivery

Abdominal conditions (e.g. colitis, ulcer)

Environmental temperature extremes

- Take steps to reduce blood pressure *and reduce potential for stroke (primary concern)*[1-6]:

Elevate head of bed immediately, or place in sitting position with legs hanging down. *Lowers blood pressure by pooling of blood in legs.*

Loosen any clothing or restrictive devices. *May allow pooling of blood in abdomen and lower extremities.*

Monitor vital signs frequently during acute episode. *(Blood pressures may fluctuate quickly due to impaired autonomic regulation.)* Continue to monitor blood pressure at intervals during procedures to remove cause of AD and after acute episode symptoms subside *to evaluate effectiveness of interventions and antihypertensives.*

 Administer medications as indicated. *If an episode is particularly severe, and/or persists after removal of suspected cause, antihypertensive medications with rapid onset and short duration (such as nifedipine, hydralazine, clonidine) may be used to block excessive autonomic nerve transmission, normalize heart rate, and reduce hypertension.*[1,4]

Carefully adjust dosage of antihypertensive medications for child, elderly, and pregnant woman. *(To prevent complications, such as systemic hypotension or seizure activity, and to maintain blood pressure within optimal range.)*[1]

NURSING PRIORITY NO. 3. To promote wellness (Teaching/Discharge Considerations):

- Discuss with client/caregivers warning signs of AD, as listed previously. Be aware of client's communication abilities. *AD can occur at any age from infant to very old, and the individual may not be able to verbalize a pounding headache, which is often the first symptom during onset of AD.*[1]

- Ascertain that client/caregivers understand ways to avoid onset or treat syndrome as noted previously. Provide with information card and instruct/reinforce teaching as needed regarding[1,2,5,6]:

Indwelling catheter care—keep tubing free of kinks, keep bag empty and situated below bladder level; check daily for deposits (bladder grit) inside catheter.

Intermittent catheterization program—catheterize as often as necessary to prevent overfilling/distension.

Spontaneous voiding—monitor for adequate voiding frequency and amount.

Maintain a regular and effective bowel evacuation program.

Perform routine skin assessments.

 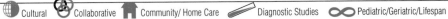

Monitor all systems for signs of infection and report promptly *for timely medical treatment.* Scheduling routine medical evaluations.

  • Instruct family member/caregiver in proper blood pressure monitoring. Note: A spinal cord–injured client's (both adult and child) baseline blood pressure is lower than non-injured person so advise frequent measurements during acute episodes.

• Review proper use/administration of medications, when used. *Some clients are on medications routinely, and if so, should receive instructions for routine administration, as well as symptoms to report for immediate or emergent care, when blood pressure is not responsive.*[1]

• Recommend wearing Medic Alert bracelet/necklace and carrying information card about signs/symptoms of AD, and usual methods of treatment. *Provides vital information in emergency.*

 • Assist client/family in identifying emergency referrals (e.g., physician, rehabilitation nurse/home care supervisor). Place telephone number(s) in prominent place.

DOCUMENTATION FOCUS

Assessment/Reassessment
• Individual findings, noting previous episodes, precipitating factors, and individual signs/symptoms.

Planning
• Plan of care and who is involved in planning.
• Teaching plan.

Implementation/Evaluation
• Client's responses to interventions and actions performed, understanding of teaching.
• Attainment/progress toward desired outcome(s).
• Modifications to plan of care.

Discharge Planning
• Long-term needs and who is responsible for actions to be taken.

References

1. Acute management of autonomic dysreflexia: Individuals with spinal cord injury presenting to health-care facilities. Paralyzed Veterans of America/Consortium for Spinal Cord Medicine. Washington DC, Paralyzed Veterans of America (PVA) July 2001. Available at www.pva.org. Accessed September 2003.
2. Acuff, M. Autonomic dysreflexia: What it is, what it does, and what to do if you experience it. The Missouri Model Spinal Cord Injury System. Columbia, MO: University of Missouri-Columbia, School of Health Professions.
3. Christopher & Dana Reeve Paralysis Resource Center: Health: Autonomic Dysreflexia. Available at www.paralysis.org. Accessed 2002.
4. Deglan, J. H. & Vallerand, A. H. (2003). Davis's Drug Guide for Nurses, ed 8. Philadelphia: F. A. Davis.
5. Other complications of spinal cord injury: Autonomic dysreflexia (hyperreflexia) treatment. RehabTeamSite. Available at http://www.calder.med.miami.edu.
6. SCI Complications Resource: National Spinal Cord Injury Association (NSCIA). Update January 2003. Available at www.spinalcord.org.

risk for Autonomic Dysreflexia

Definition: At risk for life-threatening, uninhibited response of the sympathetic nervous system post spinal shock, in an individual with a SCI or lesion at T6 or above (has been demonstrated in clients with injuries at T7 and T8)

Musculoskeletal—integumentary stimuli

Cutaneous stimulations (e.g., pressure ulcer, ingrown toenail, dressing, burns, rash); sunburns; wounds

Pressure over bony prominences or genitalia; range of motion exercises; spasms

Fractures; heterotrophic bone

Gastrointestinal stimuli

Constipation; difficult passage of feces; fecal impaction; bowel distention; hemorrhoids

Digital stimulation; suppositories; enemas

Gastrointestinal system pathology; esophageal reflux; gastric ulcers; gallstones

Urologic stimuli

Bladder distention/spasm

Detrusor sphincter dyssynergia

Instrumentation or surgery; calculi

Urinary tract infection; cystitis; urethritis; epididymitis

Regulatory stimuli

Temperature fluctuations; extreme environmental temperatures

Situational stimuli

Positioning; surgical procedure

Constrictive clothing (e.g., straps, stockings, shoes)

Drug reactions (e.g., decongestants, sympathomimetics, vasoconstrictors, narcotic withdrawal)

Neurologic stimuli

Painful or irritating stimuli below the level of injury

Cardiac/pulmonary stimuli

Pulmonary emboli; deep vein thrombosis

Reproductive [and sexual] stimuli

Sexual intercourse; ejaculation

Menstruation; pregnancy; labor and delivery; ovarian cyst

NOTE: A risk diagnosis is not evidenced by signs and symptoms, as the problem has not occurred and nursing interventions are directed at prevention.

SAMPLE CLINICAL APPLICATIONS: spinal cord injury

Desired Outcomes/Evaluation Criteria

Sample NOC linkages:

Risk Control: Actions to eliminate or reduce actual, personal, and modifiable health threats

Knowledge: Disease Process: Extent of understanding conveyed about a specific disease process

Caregiver Home Care Readiness: Preparedness to assume responsibility for the health care of a family member or significant other in the home

Client Will (Include Specific Time Frame)

- Identify risk factors present.
- Demonstrate preventive/corrective techniques.
- Be free of episodes of dysreflexia.

ACTIONS/INTERVENTIONS

Sample NIC linkages:

Dysreflexia Management: Prevention and elimination of stimuli that cause hyperactive reflexes and inappropriate autonomic responses in a patient with a cervical or high thoracic cord lesion

 Cultural   Collaborative Community/ Home Care Diagnostic Studies 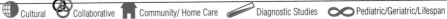 Pediatric/Geriatric/Lifespan Medications

Surveillance: Purposeful and ongoing acquisition, interpretation, and synthesis of patient data for clinical decision making

Medication Management: Facilitation of safe and effective use of prescription and over-the-counter drugs

NURSING PRIORITY NO. 1. To assess risk factors present:

- Monitor all clients with SCI at T8 and above for potential risk factors listed previously.

NURSING PRIORITY NO. 2. To prevent occurrence:

- Monitor vital signs routinely, noting changes in blood pressure, heart rate, and temperature, especially during times of physical stress *to identify trends and intervene in a timely manner.* Recognize that baseline blood pressure in spinal cord-injured client (adult and child) is lower than general population; *therefore an elevation of > 15 mm Hg above baseline may be indicative of AD.*[1]
- Instruct all caregivers in safe bowel and bladder care, and in interventions for long-term prevention of skin stress/breakdown *to reduce risk of AD episode.*[1-5]
- Instruct client/caregivers in additional preventive interventions (e.g., appropriate padding for skin and tissue, proper positioning, temperature control) *to reduce risk of AD episode.*[1-5]

- Administer antihypertensive medications as indicated. *At-risk client may be placed on routine "maintenance dose," such as when noxious stimuli cannot be removed (e.g., presence of chronic sacral pressure ulcer, fracture, or acute postoperative pain).*[1]
- Refer to ND Autonomic Dysreflexia.

NURSING PRIORITY NO. 3. To promote wellness (Teaching/Discharge Considerations):

- Review warning signs of AD as listed previously with client/caregivers. *Early signs can develop rapidly (in minutes), requiring quick intervention.*

- Be aware of client's communication abilities. *AD can occur at any age from infant to very old, and the individual may not be able to verbalize a pounding headache, which is often the first symptom during onset of AD.*[1]

- Ascertain that client/caregivers understand ways to avoid onset of syndrome. Provide with information card and instruct/reinforce teaching as needed[1-5].
- Indwelling catheter: keep tubing free of kinks, keep bag empty and situated below bladder level; check daily for deposits (bladder grit) inside catheter:

  Intermittent catheterization program: catheterize as often as necessary to prevent overfilling.

  Spontaneous voiding, monitor for adequate voiding frequency and amount.

  Maintain a regular and effective bowel evacuation program.

  Perform routine skin assessments.

  Monitor all systems for signs of infection and report early *for timely medical treatment*

  Schedule routine medical evaluations.

- Instruct family member/caregivers in blood pressure monitoring.
- Review proper use/administration of medications, when used. *Some clients are on medications routinely, and if so, should receive instructions for routine administration, as well as symptoms to report for immediate or emergent care, when blood pressure is not responsive.*[1]

• Recommend wearing Medic Alert bracelet/necklace with information card about signs/symptoms of AD, and usual methods of treatment. *Provides vital information in emergencies.*

 • Assist client/family in identifying emergency referrals (e.g., physician, rehabilitation nurse/home care supervisor). Place telephone number(s) in prominent place.

DOCUMENTATION FOCUS

Assessment/Reassessment
• Individual findings, noting previous episodes, precipitating factors, and individual signs/symptoms.

Planning
• Plan of care and who is involved in planning.
• Teaching plan.

Implementation/Evaluation
• Client's responses to interventions and actions performed, understanding of teaching.
• Attainment/progress toward desired outcome(s).
• Modifications to plan of care.

Discharge Planning
• Long-term needs and who is responsible for actions to be taken.

References

1. Acute management of autonomic dysreflexia: Individuals with spinal cord injury presenting to health-care facilities. (2001). Retrieved: September, 2003, Paralyzed Veterans of America/Consortium for Spinal Cord Medicine. Washington DC: Paralyzed Veterans of America (PVA). Available at www.pva.org.
2. Acuff, M: Autonomic dysreflexia: What it is, what it does, and what to do if you experience it. The Missouri Model Spinal Cord Injury System. Columbia, MO: University of Missouri-Columbia, School of Health Professions.
3. Christopher and Dana Reeve Paralysis Resource Center: Health: Autonomic Dysreflexia. Available at www.paralysis.org. Accessed 2002.
4. Other complications of spinal cord injury: Autonomic dysreflexia (hyperreflexia) treatment. RehabTeamSite. Available at http://www.calder.med.miami.edu.
5. SCI Complications Resource: National Spinal Cord Injury Association (NSCIA). Update January 2003. Available at www.spinalcord.org.

disturbed Body Image

Definition: Confusion in mental picture of one's physical self

RELATED FACTORS

Biophysical illness; trauma or injury; surgery; [mutilation, pregnancy]; illness treatment [change caused by biochemical agents (drugs), dependence on machine]

Psychosocial

Cultural or spiritual

Cognitive/perceptual; developmental changes

[Significance of body part or functioning with regard to age, sex, developmental level, or basic human needs]

[Maturational changes]

Cultural Collaborative Community/ Home Care Diagnostic Studies 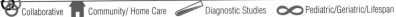Pediatric/Geriatric/Lifespan Medications

Subjective

Verbalization of feelings/perceptions that reflect an altered view of one's body in appearance, structure, or function; change in lifestyle

Fear of rejection or of reaction by others

Focus on past strength, function, or appearance

Negative feelings about body (e.g., feelings of helplessness, hopelessness, or powerlessness); [depersonalization/ grandiosity]

Preoccupation with change or loss

Refusal to verify actual change

Emphasis on remaining strengths, heightened achievement

Personalization of part or loss by name

Depersonalization of part or loss by impersonal pronouns

Objective

Missing body part

Actual change in structure and/or function

Nonverbal response to actual or perceived change in structure and/or function; behaviors of avoidance, monitoring, or acknowledgment of one's body

Not looking at/not touching body part

Trauma to nonfunctioning part

Change in ability to estimate spatial relationship of body to environment

Extension of body boundary to incorporate environmental objects

Hiding or overexposing body part (intentional or unintentional)

Change in social involvement

[Aggression; low frustration tolerance level]

SAMPLE CLINICAL APPLICATIONS: eating disorders (anorexia/bulimia nervosa), traumatic injuries, amputation, ostomies, aging process, arthritis, pregnancy, chronic renal failure/ dialysis, burns

DESIRED OUTCOMES/EVALUATION CRITERIA

Sample NOC linkages:

Body Image: Positive perception of own appearance and body functions

Self-Esteem: Personal judgment of self-worth

Distorted Thought Control: Self-restraint of disruption in perception, thought processes, and thought content

Client Will (Include Specific Time Frames)

- Verbalize acceptance of self in situation (e.g., chronic progressive disease, amputee, decreased independence, weight as is, effects of therapeutic regimen).
- Verbalize relief of anxiety and adaptation to actual/altered body image.
- Verbalize understanding of body changes.
- Recognize and incorporate body image change into self-concept in accurate manner without negating self-esteem.
- Seek information and actively pursue growth.
- Acknowledge self as an individual who has responsibility for self.
- Use adaptive devices/prosthesis appropriately.

ACTIONS/INTERVENTIONS

Sample NIC linkages:

Body Image Enhancement: Improving a patient's conscious and unconscious perceptions and attitudes toward his/her body

Developmental Enhancement: Adolescent: Facilitating optimal physical, cognitive, social, and emotional growth of individuals during the transition from childhood to adulthood

Self-Esteem Enhancement: Assisting a patient to increase his/her personal judgment of self-worth

NURSING PRIORITY NO. 1. To assess causative/contributing factors:

- Discuss pathophysiology present and/or situation affecting the individual and refer to additional NDs as appropriate. *For example, when alteration in body image is related to neurologic deficit (e.g., cerebrovascular accident [CVA]), refer to ND unilateral Neglect; in the presence of severe, ongoing pain, refer to chronic Pain; or in loss of sexual desire/ability, refer to Sexual Dysfunction.*

- Determine whether condition is permanent/no hope for resolution. (May be associated with other NDs such as Self-Esteem [specify], or risk for impaired parent/infant/child Attachment when child is affected.) *Identifies appropriate interventions based on reality of situation and need to plan for long or short-term prognosis.*[1]

- Assess mental/physical influence of illness/condition on the client's emotional state (e.g., diseases of the endocrine system, use of steroid therapy, and so on). *Some diseases can have a profound effect on one's emotions and need to be considered in the evaluation and treatment of the individual's behavior and reaction to the current situation.*[1]

- Evaluate level of client's knowledge of and anxiety related to situation. Observe emotional changes. *Provides information about starting point for providing information about illness. Emotional changes may indicate level of anxiety and need for intervention to lower anxiety before learning can take place.*[1]

- Recognize behavior indicative of overconcern with body and its processes. *May interfere with ability to engage in therapy and indicate need to provide interventions to deal with concern before beginning therapy.*[3]

- Assume all individuals are sensitive to changes in appearance but avoid stereotyping. *Not all individuals react to body changes in the same way and it is important to determine how this person is reacting to changes.*[2]

- Have client describe self, noting what is positive and what is negative. Be aware of how client believes others see self. *Identifies self-image and whether there is a discrepancy between own view and how clients believe others see them, which may have an effect on how client perceives changes that have occurred.*[3]

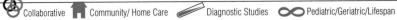 - Discuss meaning of loss/change to client. *A small (seemingly trivial) loss may have a big impact (such as the use of a urinary catheter or enema for bowel continence). A change in function (such as immobility) may be more difficult for some to deal with than a change in appearance. Permanent facial scarring of child may be difficult for parents to accept.*[1]

- Use developmentally appropriate communication techniques for determining exact expression of body image in child (e.g., puppet play or constructive dialogue for toddler). *Developmental capacity must guide interaction to gain accurate information.*[4]

- Note signs of grieving/indicators of severe or prolonged depression. *May require evaluation of need for counseling and/or medications.*[3]

- Determine ethnic background and cultural/religious perceptions and considerations. *Understanding how these factors affect the individual in this situation is necessary to develop appropriate interventions.*[5]

 Cultural   Collaborative   Community/ Home Care   Diagnostic Studies   Pediatric/Geriatric/Lifespan   Medications

- Identify social aspects of illness/disease. *Sexually transmitted diseases, sterility, chronic conditions may affect how client views self and functions in social settings and how others view them.*[2]
- Observe interaction of client with SO(s). *Distortions in body image may be unconsciously reinforced by family members, and/or secondary gain issues may interfere with progress.*[2]

NURSING PRIORITY NO. 2. To determine coping abilities and skills:

- Assess client's current level of adaptation and progress. *Client may have already adapted somewhat and information provides starting point for developing plan of care.*[2]
- Listen to client's comments and note responses to the situation. *Different situations are upsetting to different people, depending on individual coping skills, severity of the perceived changes in body image and past experiences with similar illnesses/conditions.*[4]
- Note withdrawn behavior and the use of denial. *May be normal response to situation or may be indicative of mental illness (e.g., depression, schizophrenia). (Refer to ND ineffective Denial.)*[6]
- Note use of addictive substances/alcohol. *May reflect dysfunctional coping as client turns to use of these substances to deal with changes that are occurring to body or ability to function in their accustomed manner.*[4]
- Identify previously used coping strategies and effectiveness. *Familiar coping strategies can be used to begin adaptation to current situation.*[2]
- Determine individual/family/community resources. *Can provide efficient assistance and support to enable the client to adapt to changing circumstances.*[4]

NURSING PRIORITY NO. 3. To assist client and SO(s) to deal with/accept issues of self-concept related to body image:

- Establish therapeutic nurse-client relationship. *Conveys an attitude of caring and develops a sense of trust in which client can discuss concerns and find answers to issues confronting him or her in new situation.*[2]
- Visit client frequently and acknowledge the individual as someone who is worthwhile. *Provides opportunities for listening to concerns and questions to promote dealing positively with individual situation and change in body image.*[1]
- Assist in correcting underlying problems when possible. *Promotes optimal healing/ adaptation to individual situation, (i.e., amputation, presence of colostomy, mastectomy, and impotence).*[1]
- Provide assistance with self-care needs/measures as necessary while promoting individual abilities/independence. *Client needs support to achieve the goal of independence and positive return to managing own life.*[4]
- Work with client's self-concept without moral judgments regarding client's efforts or progress (e.g., "You should be progressing faster; you're weak/lazy/not trying hard enough"). *Such statements diminish self-esteem and are counterproductive to progress.*[2]
- Discuss concerns about fear of mutilation, prognosis, and rejection when client is facing surgery or potentially poor outcome of procedure/illness. *Addresses realities and provides emotional support to enable client to be ready to deal with whatever the outcome may be.*[1]
- Acknowledge and accept feelings of dependency, grief, and hostility. *Conveys a message of understanding.*[1]
- Encourage verbalization of and role-play anticipated conflicts *to enhance handling of potential situations. Provides an opportunity to imagine and practice how different situations can be dealt with, promoting confidence.*[4]

- Encourage client and SO(s) to communicate feelings to each other and discuss situation openly. *Enhances relationship improving sense of self-worth and sense of support.*[2]
- Alert staff to monitor own facial expressions and other nonverbal behaviors. *Important to convey acceptance and not revulsion especially when the client's appearance is affected. Clients are very sensitive to reactions of those around them, and negative reactions will affect self-esteem and may retard adaptation to situation.*[1]
- Encourage family members to treat client normally and not as an invalid. *Helps client return to own routine and begin to gain confidence in ability to manage own life.*[1]
- Encourage client to look at/touch affected body part *to begin to incorporate changes into body image. Acceptance will enhance self-esteem and enable client to move forward in a positive manner.*[1,4]
- Allow client to use denial without participating (e.g., client may at first refuse to look at a colostomy; the nurse says "I am going to change your colostomy now" and proceeds with the task). *Provides individual time to adapt to situation.*[2]
- Set limits on maladaptive behavior. *Self-esteem will be damaged if client is allowed to continue behaviors that are destructive or not helpful and adaptation to new image will be delayed.* Assist client to identify positive behaviors. *Aids in recovery and acceptance of new body image.*[2]
- Provide accurate information as desired/requested. Reinforce previously given information. *Accurate knowledge helps client make better decisions for the future.*[4]
- Discuss the availability of prosthetics, reconstructive surgery, and physical/occupational therapy or other referrals as dictated by individual situation. *Provides hope that situation is not impossible and the future does not look so bleak.*[1]
- Help client to select and use clothing/makeup *to minimize body changes and enhance appearance.*[1]
- Discuss reasons for infectious isolation and procedures when used, and make time to sit down and talk/listen to client while in the room. *Promotes understanding and decreases sense of isolation/loneliness.*[1]

NURSING PRIORITY NO. 4. To promote wellness (Teaching/Discharge Considerations):

- Begin counseling/other therapies (e.g., biofeedback/relaxation) as soon as possible. *Provides early/ongoing sources of support to promote rehabilitation in a timely manner.*[1]
- Provide information at client's level of acceptance and in small segments. *Allows for easier assimilation.* Clarify misconceptions and reinforce explanations given by other health team members. *Ensures client is hearing factual information to make the best decisions for own situation.*[1]
- Include client in decision-making process and problem-solving activities. *Promotes adherence to decisions and plans that are made.*[1]
- Assist client to incorporate therapeutic regimen into activities of daily living (ADLs) (e.g., including specific exercises, housework activities). *Promotes continuation of program by helping client see that progress can be made within own daily activities.*[1]
- Identify/plan for alterations to home and work environment/activities when necessary. *Accommodates individual needs and supports independence.*[1]
- Assist client in learning strategies for dealing with feelings/venting emotions. *Helps individual move toward healing and optimal recuperation.*[1]
- Offer positive reinforcement for efforts made (e.g., wearing makeup, using prosthetic device). *Client needs to hear that what he or she is doing is helping.*[1]
- Refer to appropriate support groups. *May need additional help to adjust to new situation and life changes.*[1]

 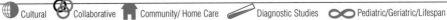

Assessment/Reassessment

- Observations, presence of maladaptive behaviors, emotional changes, stage of grieving, level of independence.
- Physical wounds, dressings; use of life-support–type machine (e.g., ventilator, dialysis machine).
- Meaning of loss/change to client.
- Support systems available (e.g., SOs, friends, groups).

Planning

- Plan of care and who is involved in planning.
- Teaching plan.

Implementation/Evaluation

- Client's response to interventions/teaching and actions performed.
- Attainment/progress toward desired outcome(s).
- Modifications of plan of care.

Discharge Planning

- Long-term needs and who is responsible for actions.
- Specific referrals made (e.g., rehabilitation center, community resources).

References

1. Doenges, M., Moorhouse, M., & Murr, A. (2002). Nursing Care Plans, Guidelines for Individualizing Patient Care, ed 6. Philadelphia: F. A. Davis.
2. Doenges, M., Townsend, M., & Moorhouse, M. (1998). Psychiatric Care Plans: Guidelines for Individualizing Care, ed 3. Philadelphia: F. A. Davis.
3. Townsend, M. (2003). Psychiatric Mental Health Nursing: Concepts of Care, ed 4. Philadelphia: F. A. Davis.
4. Cox, H.; Hinz, M., Lubno, M. A., Newfield, S., Scott-Tilley, D., Slater, M., & Sridaromont, K. (2002). Clinical Applications of Nursing Diagnosis Adult, Child, Women's Psychiatric, Gerontic and Home Health Considerations, ed 4. Philadelphia: F. A. Davis.
5. Lipson, J. G., Dibble, S. L., & Minarik, P. A. (1996). Culture & Nursing Care: A Pocket Guide. School of Nursing. San Francisco: UCSF Nursing Press.
6. Townsend, M. (2001). Nursing Diagnoses in Psychiatric Nursing: Care Plans and Psychotropic Medications, ed 5. Philadelphia: F. A. Davis.

risk for imbalanced Body Temperature

Definition: At risk for failure to maintain body temperature within normal range

RISK FACTORS

Extremes of age, weight

Exposure to cold/cool or warm/hot environments

Dehydration

Inactivity or vigorous activity

Medications causing vasoconstriction/vasodilation, altered metabolic rate, sedation, [use or overdose of certain drugs or exposure to anesthesia]

Inappropriate clothing for environmental temperature

Illness or trauma affecting temperature regulation [e.g., infections, systemic or localized; neoplasms, tumors; collagen/vascular disease]

NOTE: A risk diagnosis is not evidenced by signs and symptoms, as the problem has not occurred and nursing interventions are directed at prevention.

SAMPLE CLINICAL APPLICATIONS: any infectious process, surgical procedures, brain injuries, hypo/hyperthyroidism, prematurity

DESIRED OUTCOMES/EVALUATION CRITERIA

Sample NOC linkages:

Risk Control: Actions to eliminate or reduce actual, personal, and modifiable health threats

Infection Status: Presence and extent of infection

Hydration: Amount of water in the intracellular and extracellular compartments of the body

---

Client Will (Include Specific Time Frame)

- Maintain body temperature within normal range.
- Verbalize understanding of individual risk factors and appropriate interventions.
- Demonstrate behaviors for monitoring and maintaining appropriate body temperature.

ACTIONS/INTERVENTIONS

Sample NIC linkages:

Fever Treatment: Management of a patient with hyperpyrexia caused by nonenvironmental factors

Temperature Regulation: Attaining and/or maintaining body temperature within a normal range

Temperature Regulation: Intraoperative: Attaining and/or maintaining desired intraoperative body temperature

NURSING PRIORITY NO. 1. To identify causative/risk factors present:

- Monitor for factors noted previously that can impair body's heat production and heat dissipation
- Determine if present illness/condition results from exposure to environmental factors, surgery, infection, or trauma. *Helps to determine the scope of interventions that may be needed, (e.g., simple addition of warm blankets after surgery, or hypothermia therapy following brain trauma).*[1]
- Monitor laboratory values (e.g., tests indicative of infection, thyroid/other endocrine tests, drug screens) *to identify potential internal causes of temperature imbalances.*
- Note client's age (e.g., premature neonate, young child, or aging individual), *as it can directly impact ability to maintain/regulate body temperature and respond to changes in environment.*[2]
- Assess nutritional status *to determine metabolism effect on body temperature and to identify foods or nutrient deficits that affect metabolism.*[1,2]

NURSING PRIORITY NO. 2. To prevent occurrence of temperature alteration:

- Monitor temperature regularly (e.g., q 1–4 h) measuring core body temperature, whenever needed to observe this vital sign. *Traditionally, temperature measurements have been taken orally (good in alert, oriented adult), rectally (accurate, but not always easy to obtain), or axillary (readings may be lower than core temperature), with each site offering advantages and disadvantages in terms of accuracy and safety. Newer technologies allow temperatures to be instantly and accurately measured. Tympanic temperature measurement is a noninvasive way to measure core temperature as blood is supplied to the tympanic membrane by the carotid artery. This method is preferred by healthcare providers and parents, as it is the most noninvasive method, although some pediatricians may still prefer rectal temperature measurements in sick newborns or infants.*[3]

 Cultural   Collaborative   Community/ Home Care   Diagnostic Studies   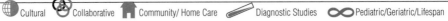 Pediatric/Geriatric/Lifespan   Medications

- Maintain comfortable ambient environment to reduce risk of body temperature alterations[1,2,4]:
  Provide heating/cooling measures as needed such as space heater or air conditioner/fans. Ascertain that cooling and warming equipment and supplies are available during/following procedures and surgery.
- Supervise use of heating pads, electric blankets, ice bags, and hypothermia blankets, especially in those clients who cannot protect their own temperature regulation.
- Dress or discuss with client/caregivers dressing appropriately:
  Wear layers of clothing that can be removed or added. Wear hat and gloves in cold weather, wear light loose protective clothing in hot weather, and wear water-resistant outer gear to protect from wet weather chill.
- Cover infant's head with knit cap, use layers of lightweight blankets. Place newborn infant under radiant warmer. Teach parents to dress infant appropriately for weather and home environment. *Newborns/infants can have temperature instability. Heat loss is greatest through head and by evaporation and convection.*[5]
- Maintain adequate fluid intake. Offer cool or warm liquids as appropriate. *Hydration assists in maintaining normal body temperature.*[1,2,4]
- Restore/maintain core temperature within client's normal range. (If temperature is below or above normal range, or parameters defined by physician, refer to NDs Hypothermia or Hyperthermia for additional interventions.)
- Recommend lifestyle changes, such as cessation of substance use, normalization of body weight, nutritious meals, regular exercise *to maximize metabolism and health.*[1,2]
- Refer at-risk persons to appropriate community resources (e.g., home care, social services, Foster Adult Care, housing agencies) *to provide assistance to meet individual needs.*[1]

NURSING PRIORITY NO. 3. To promote wellness (Teaching/Discharge Considerations):

- Review potential problem/individual risk factors with client/SO(s).
- Instruct in measures to protect from identified risk factors. *Understanding ways to manage lifestyle and environment (e.g., clothing, shelter, nutritional status), possible effects of medication regimen/drug use such as depression of cerebral function, alteration of the body's ability to regulate temperature, changes in circulation, or possibility of hyperthermic or hypothermic effects (e.g., certain antipsychotic agents or anesthesia) enhances self-care abilities.*[1,2]
- Review with client/caregivers ways to prevent accidental thermoregulation problems *(e.g., hypothermia can result from overzealous cooling to reduce fever; or maintaining too warm an environment when client has lost the ability to perspire).*

DOCUMENTATION FOCUS

Assessment/Reassessment
- Identified individual causative/risk factors.
- Record of core temperature, initially and PRN.
- Results of diagnostic studies/laboratory tests.

Planning
- Plan of care and who is involved in planning.
- Teaching plan, including best ambient temperature, and ways to prevent hypothermia or hyperthermia.

Implementation/Evaluation
- Response to interventions/teaching and actions performed.
- Attainment/progress toward desired outcome(s).
- Modifications to plan of care.

Discharge Planning
- Long-term need and who is responsible for actions.
- Specific referrals made.

References

1. Surgical Intervention. In Doenges, M. E., Moorhouse, M. F., & Geissler-Murr, A. C. (2002). Nursing Care Plans: Guidelines for Individualizing Patient Care, ed 6. Philadelphia: F. A. Davis.
2. Cox, H. C., et al. (2002). Clinical Applications of Nursing Diagnosis: Adult, Child, Women's, Psychiatric, Gerontic, and Home Health Considerations, ed 4. Philadelphia: F. A. Davis.
3. Nicoll, L. H. (2002). Heat in motion: Evaluating and managing temperature. Nursing2002, 32(5):s1–s12.
4. Guidelines for the pediatric perioperative anesthesia environment. (1999). American Academy of Pediatrics (AAP) Section on Anesthesiology Pediatrics. 103(2): 515.
5. Early discharge of the term newborn. (1999). Guideline from National Association of Neonatal Nurses. Glenview, IL. Retrieved from National Guideline Clearinghouse Web site. Available at www.guideline.gov.

Bowel Incontinence

Definition: Change in normal bowel habits characterized by involuntary passage of stool

RELATED FACTORS

Self-care deficit—toileting; impaired cognition; immobility; environmental factors (e.g., inaccessible bathroom)

Dietary habits; medications; laxative abuse

Stress

Colorectal lesions

Incomplete emptying of bowel; impaction; chronic diarrhea

General decline in muscle tone; abnormally high abdominal or intestinal pressure

Impaired reservoir capacity

Rectal sphincter abnormality; loss of rectal sphincter control; lower/upper motor nerve damage

DEFINING CHARACTERISTICS

Subjective
Recognizes rectal fullness but reports inability to expel formed stool

Urgency

Inability to delay defecation

Self-report of inability to feel rectal fullness

Objective
Constant dribbling of soft stool

Fecal staining of clothing and/or bedding

Fecal odor

Red perianal skin

Inability to recognize/inattention to urge to defecate

 Cultural Collaborative Community/ Home Care Diagnostic Studies Pediatric/Geriatric/Lifespan Medications

SAMPLE CLINICAL APPLICATIONS: hemorrhoids, rectal prolapse, anal/gynecological surgery, childbirth injuries/uterine prolapse, spinal cord injury, stroke, multiple sclerosis, ulcerative colitis, dementia

DESIRED OUTCOMES/EVALUATION CRITERIA

Sample NOC linkages:

Bowel Continence: Control of passage of stool from the bowel

Bowel Elimination: Ability of the gastrointestinal tract to form and evacuate stool effectively

Neurologic Status: Extent to which the peripheral and central nervous system receive, process, and respond to internal and external stimuli

Client Will (Include Specific Time Frame)

- Verbalize understanding of causative/controlling factors.
- Identify individually appropriate interventions.
- Participate in therapeutic regimen to control incontinence.
- Establish/maintain as regular a pattern of bowel functioning as possible.

ACTIONS/INTERVENTIONS

Sample NIC linkages:

Bowel Incontinence Care: Promotion of bowel continence and maintenance of perineal skin integrity

Bowel Incontinence Care: Encopresis: Promotion of bowel continence in children

Bowel Training: Assisting the patient to train the bowel to evacuate at specific intervals

NURSING PRIORITY NO. 1. To assess causative/contributing factors:

- Identify pathophysiologic factors present. *The client's age and gender is a factor; e.g., more common in children and elderly adults (difficulty responding to urge in a timely manner, problems walking or undoing zippers); more common in boys than girls, but women more than men in elderly. Common causes include 1) structural changes in the sphincter muscle (e.g., hemorrhoids, rectal prolapse, anal or gynecological surgery, childbirth injuries); 2) injuries to sensory nerves (e.g., spinal cord injury, trauma, stroke, tumor, radiation treatments, multiple sclerosis); 3) strong urge diarrhea (e.g., ulcerative colitis, Crohn's disease, infectious diarrhea); 4) constipation from holding stool (especially in children); 5) dementia (e.g., acute or chronic cognitive impairment, not necessarily related to sphincter control); 6) certain medications; e.g., laxative abuse, drugs with side effects of diarrhea (e.g., antibiotics) or constipation (e.g., sedatives, hypnotics, narcotics, muscle relaxants); 7) result of toxins (e.g., salmonella); and 7) effects of improper diet or enteral feedings.*[1–6]

- Assist with physical evaluation and diagnostic studies. *Pelvic and/or anal ultrasound (may be used to identify structural abnormalities), endoscopy (to visualize lower gastrointestinal tract), manometry (measures pressure and strength of anal muscles), nerve studies (checks for nerve damage). Blood tests and stool cultures may be done to identify bacteria and toxins.*[1,2,3,5]
- Refer to NDs Diarrhea, when incontinence is due to uncontrolled diarrhea; Constipation if diarrhea is due to impaction.

NURSING PRIORITY NO. 2. To determine current pattern of elimination:

- Ascertain timing and characteristic aspects of incontinent occurrence, noting preceding/precipitating events. *Helps to identify patterns and/or worsening trends.*

Interventions are different for sudden acute accident than for chronic long-term incontinence problems. Person may have passive incontinence being unaware that stool is being passed (related to poorly functioning sphincter muscle) or urge incontinence in which person is aware but unable to prevent passage of stool (sphincter muscle normal). Problem may have been present for a long time, either because of client/caregiver sense of embarrassment, or failure to realize that effective treatment may be available.[2,5]

 ● Determine stool characteristics including consistency (may be liquid, hard formed, or hard at first and then soft), amount (may be a small amount of liquid or entire solid bowel movement), and frequency. *Provides information that can help differentiate type of incontinence present and provides comparative baseline for response to interventions.[4,6]*

 ● Note where bowel accidents occur and what client is experiencing at the time. *Changes in usual routines or surrounding environment, general health condition, and addition of emotional stressors such as new baby in the home, increased confusion in dementia client can cause or exacerbate incontinence behaviors.[5]*

● Palpate abdomen for masses and auscultate for presence/location and characteristics of bowel sounds.

NURSING PRIORITY NO. 3. To promote control/management of incontinence:

● Assist in treatment of underlying causative/contributing factors (e.g., as listed in the Related Factors and Defining Characteristics). *While incontinence is a symptom and not a disease, appropriate treatment can often correct the problem or at least improve the client's quality of life.[2]*

● Administer medications as indicated: stool softeners/bulk formers and laxatives *when cause is constipation,* antidiarrheal drugs, including cholinergic medications *may be used to decrease intestinal secretions and bowel motility if diarrhea is cause for incontinence.[1,2,4]*

 ● Establish toileting program as early as possible *to maximize success of program and preserve comfort and self-esteem*[1–6]:
Take client to the bathroom/place on commode or bedpan at specified intervals, taking into consideration individual needs and incontinence patterns
Use the same type of facility for toileting as much as possible
Make sure bathroom is safe for impaired person (good lighting, support rails, good height for getting on to and up from stool)
Provide time and privacy for elimination
Demonstrate techniques/assist client/caregiver to practice contracting abdominal muscles, leaning forward on commode *to increase intra-abdominal pressure during defecation,* and left to right abdominal massage *to stimulate peristalsis.*
Provide meticulous skin care and incontinence aids/pads until control is obtained *to reduce deleterious effects to skin and perineal tissue*

● Encourage and instruct client/caregiver in providing diet high in natural bulk/fiber, with fruits, vegetables and grains and reduced fatty foods. *Identify/eliminate problem foods to avoid diarrhea, constipation or gas formation.[2,4,6]*

● Adjust enteral feedings and/or change formula as indicated *to reduce diarrhea effect.[4]*

● Encourage adequate fluid intake (at least 2000 mL/d) within client's need and tolerance, including fruit juices *to help manage constipation.* Encourage warm fluids after meals *to promote intestinal motility.* Avoid caffeine and alcohol *to reduce diarrhea.[4,6]*

 ● Recommend walking and regular exercise program, pelvic floor exercises and biofeedback as individually indicated, *to improve abdominal and pelvic muscles, and strengthen rectal sphincter tone.[2,4,6]*

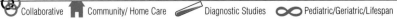

NURSING PRIORITY NO. 4. To promote wellness (Teaching/Discharge Considerations):

- Review and encourage continuation of successful interventions as individually identified.
- Instruct in use of laxatives or stool softeners if indicated, *to stimulate timed defecation.*
- Identify foods that promote bowel regularity and avoidance of problem foods.
- Refer client/caregivers to outside resources when condition is long-term or chronic *to obtain care assistance, emotional support and respite.*
- Encourage scheduling of social activities within time frame of bowel program as indicated (e.g., avoid a 4-hour excursion with no access to appropriate facilities if bowel program requires toileting every 3 hours) *to maximize social functioning and success of bowel program.*

DOCUMENTATION FOCUS

Assessment/Reassessment
- Current and previous pattern of elimination/physical findings, character of stool, actions tried.

Planning
- Plan of care and who is involved in planning.
- Teaching plan.

Implementation/Evaluation
- Client's/caregiver's responses to interventions/teaching and actions performed.
- Changes in pattern of elimination, characteristics of stool.
- Attainment/progress toward desired outcome(s).
- Modifications to plan of care.

Discharge Planning
- Identified long-term needs, noting who is responsible for each action.
- Specific bowel program at time of discharge.

References

1. Whitehead, W. E. (2002). Understanding fecal incontinence. Patient Information Page. Chapel Hill, NC: The UNC School of Medicine Center for functional GI and Motility Disorders Website. Available at http://www.med.unc.edu/medicine/fgidc.
2. What is bowel incontinence? Cleveland Clinic Health System, May 2001. Available at www.cchs.net.
3. Bowel Incontinence. Patient Brochure. (1996). Arlington Heights, IL: American Society of Colon and Rectal Surgeons.
4. Doenges, M. E., Moorhouse, M. F., & Geissler-Murr, A. C. (2002). Spinal cord injury (acute rehabilitative phase). In: Nursing Care Plans: Guidelines for Individualizing Patient Care, ed 6. Philadelphia: F. A. Davis, p 276.
5. Monicken, D. Special care problems, part 5: Bowel incontinence. In: What to do? A Guide for Families Caring for Persons with Dementia-Related Diseases. Geriatric Research. Minneapolis: Education and Clinical Center (GRECC) of the Dept of Veterans Affairs Medical Center.
6. Cox, H. C., et al. (2002). Clinical Applications of Nursing Diagnosis: Adult. Child, Women's, Psychiatric, Gerontic, and Home Health Considerations, ed 4. Philadelphia: F. A. Davis.

effective Breastfeeding [Learning Need]*

Definition: Mother-infant dyad/family exhibits adequate proficiency and satisfaction with breastfeeding process

RELATED FACTORS

Basic breastfeeding knowledge
Normal [maternal] breast structure
Normal infant oral structure
Infant gestational age greater than 34 weeks
Support sources [available]
Maternal confidence

DEFINING CHARACTERISTICS

Subjective
Maternal verbalization of satisfaction with the breastfeeding process

Objective
Mother able to position infant at breast to promote a successful latch-on response
Infant is content after feedings
Regular and sustained suckling/swallowing at the breast [e.g., 8 to 10 times/24 h]
Appropriate infant weight patterns for age
Effective mother/infant communication pattern (infant cues, maternal interpretation and response)
Signs and/or symptoms of oxytocin release (letdown or milk ejection reflex)
Adequate infant elimination patterns for age; [stools soft; more than 6 wet diapers/day of unconcentrated urine]
Eagerness of infant to nurse [breastfeed]

SAMPLE CLINICAL APPLICATIONS: wellness diagnosis associated with pre/postnatal client

DESIRED OUTCOMES/EVALUATION CRITERIA

Sample NOC linkages:

Breastfeeding Establishment: Infant: Proper attachment of an infant to and sucking from the mother's breast for nourishment during the first 2 to 3 weeks

Breastfeeding Establishment: Maternal: Maternal establishment of proper attachment of an infant to and sucking from the breast for nourishment during the first 2 to 3 weeks

Breastfeeding Maintenance: Continued nourishment of an infant through breastfeeding

Client Will (Include Specific Time Frame)
- Verbalize understanding of breastfeeding techniques.
- Demonstrate effective techniques for breastfeeding.
- Demonstrate family involvement and support.
- Attend classes/read appropriate materials as necessary.

---

*This is difficult to address, because the Related Factors and Defining Characteristics are in fact the outcome/evaluation criteria that would be desired. We believe that normal breastfeeding behaviors need to be learned and supported, with interventions directed at learning activities.

 Cultural Collaborative Community/ Home Care  Diagnostic Studies Pediatric/Geriatric/Lifespan Medications

ACTIONS/INTERVENTIONS

Sample NIC linkages:

Lactation Counseling: Use of an interactive helping process to assist in maintenance of successful breastfeeding

Anticipatory Guidance: Preparation of patient for an anticipated developmental and/or situational crisis

Teaching: Infant Nutrition: Instruction on nutrition and feeding practices during the first year of life

NURSING PRIORITY NO. 1. To assess individual learning needs:

- Assess mother's knowledge and previous experience with breastfeeding. *Provides information for developing plan of care. Accurate knowledge and previous experience can lead to a positive breastfeeding experience.*[1]
- Monitor effectiveness of current breastfeeding efforts. *Determining the actions client is taking provides information about measures that may enhance efforts to be successful in endeavor.*[1]
- Determine support systems available to mother/family. *Presence of adequate support can provide encouragement to mother who may be feeling nervous and unsure about new role.*[1]

NURSING PRIORITY NO. 2. To promote effective breastfeeding behaviors:

- Initiate breastfeeding within first hours after birth. *The time of the first feeding is determined by the physiological and behavioral cues. Throughout the first 2 hours after birth, the infant is usually alert and ready to nurse. Early feedings are of great benefit to mother and infant because oxytocin release is stimulated helping to expel the placenta and prevent excessive maternal blood loss; the infant receives the immunological protection of colostrum, peristalsis is stimulated; lactation is accelerated; and maternal-infant bonding is enhanced.*[2]
- Demonstrate how to support and position infant. *The mother should be made as comfortable as possible and specific instructions given for positioning self and baby depending on the type of birth; (e.g., cesarean section or vaginal).*[1]
- Observe mother's return demonstration. *Provides practice and the opportunity to correct misunderstandings and add additional information to promote optimal experience for breastfeeding.*[1]
- Keep infant with mother for unrestricted breastfeeding duration and frequency. *Rooming-in offers opportunity for spontaneous encounters for the family to practice handling skills and increase confidence in own ability. It also encourages feeding in response to cues from the baby.*[1]
- Note how culture and society influences infant feeding and choice of breast or bottle-feeding. *In Western cultures, the breast has taken on a sexual connotation and some mothers may be embarrassed to breastfeed. While breastfeeding may be accepted, in some cultures certain beliefs may affect specific feeding practices; (e.g., in Mexican American, Navajo, Filipino, and Vietnamese colostrum is not offered to the newborn, breastfeeding begins only after the milk flow is established).*[3]
- Encourage mother to follow a well-balanced diet containing an extra 500 calories a day. The breastfeeding mother requires extra fluids and should be encouraged to drink at least 2000 to 3000 mL of fluid per day. *There is an increased need for maternal energy, protein, minerals and vitamins during lactation to restore what the mother loses in secreting milk to provide adequate nutrients for the nourishment of the infant and protect the mother's own stores.*[4]

Nursing Diagnoses in Alphabetical Order

- Provide information as needed. *Having adequate information about the nutritional, psychological, immunologic advantages, contraindications and disadvantages of breastfeeding helps the parents to make a decision that is best for the family. Many mothers indicate that if they had had adequate information they would have chosen breastfeeding.*[1]

NURSING PRIORITY NO. 3. To promote wellness (Teaching/Discharge Considerations):

 - Provide for follow-up contact/home visit 48 hours after discharge; repeat visit as necessary. *Provides opportunity to assess adequacy of home situation and breastfeeding efforts as well as support and assistance with problem solving if needed.*[1]

 - Recommend monitoring number of infant's wet diapers (at least six wet diapers suggests adequate hydration). *Often mothers who are breastfeeding worry about whether infant is getting adequate nutrition because they cannot measure the amount of milk being received and having this information can allay these fears.*[1]

- Encourage mother/other family members to express feelings/concerns, and Active-listen to determine nature of concerns. *Identifying the concerns of the parents promotes problem solving and alleviation of worries and fears. When individuals do not express these concerns, they can create frustration and interfere with successful breastfeeding.*[1]

- Review techniques for expression and storage of breast milk to help sustain breastfeeding activity. *Having this information enables the mother to successfully manage continuation of breastfeeding while engaging in activities outside the home for specified periods of time.*[1]

- Problem-solve return-to-work issues or periodic infant care requiring bottle-feeding. *Enables mothers who need or desire to return to work for economic or personal reasons, or simply want to attend activities without the infant to deal with these issues allowing more freedom while maintaining adequate breastfeeding.*[1]

- Refer to support groups, such as La Leche League, as indicated. *While the father or SO is the most important support person, in Western society family support systems may be lacking other support systems, such as nurses, mother to mother support groups, are needed.*[1]

- Refer to ND ineffective Breastfeeding for more specific information as appropriate.

DOCUMENTATION FOCUS

Assessment/Reassessment
- Identified assessment factors (maternal and infant).
- Number of daily wet diapers and periodic weight.

Planning
- Plan of care/interventions and who is involved in the planning.
- Teaching plan.

Implementation/Evaluation
- Mother's response to interventions/teaching plan and actions performed.
- Effectiveness of infant's efforts to feed.
- Attainment/progress toward desired outcome(s).
- Modifications to plan of care.

Discharge Planning
- Long-term needs/referrals and who is responsible for follow-up actions.

 Cultural   Collaborative   Community/ Home Care 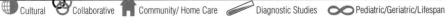 Diagnostic Studies  Pediatric/Geriatric/Lifespan   Medications

References

1. Ladewig, P., London, M., Moberly, S., & Olds, S. (2002). Contemporary Maternal-Newborn Care, ed 5. Upper Saddle River, NJ: Prentice Hall.
2. Riodan, J., & Auerbach, K. (1993). Breastfeeding and Human Lactation. Boston: Jones & Bartlett.
3. Lipson, J., Dibble, S., & Minarik, P. (1996). Culture & Nursing Care: A Pocket Guide. UCSF Nursing Press.
4. Lowdermilk, D., Perry, S., & Bobak, I. (2001). Maternity & Women's Health Care, ed 6. St. Louis: Mosby.

ineffective Breastfeeding

Definition: Dissatisfaction or difficulty a mother, infant, or child experiences with the breastfeeding process

RELATED FACTORS

Prematurity; infant anomaly; poor infant sucking reflex

Infant receiving [numerous or repeated] supplemental feedings with artificial nipple

Maternal anxiety or ambivalence

Knowledge deficit

Previous history of breastfeeding failure

Interruption in breastfeeding

Nonsupportive partner/family

Maternal breast anomaly; previous breast surgery; [painful nipples/breast engorgement]

DEFINING CHARACTERISTICS

Subjective

Unsatisfactory breastfeeding process

Persistence of sore nipples beyond the first week of breastfeeding

Insufficient emptying of each breast per feeding

Actual or perceived inadequate milk supply

Objective

Observable signs of inadequate infant intake [decrease in number of wet diapers, inappropriate weight loss/or inadequate gain]

Nonsustained or insufficient opportunity for suckling at the breast; infant inability [failure] to attach onto maternal breast correctly

Infant arching and crying at the breast; resistant latching on

Infant exhibiting fussiness and crying within the first hour after breastfeeding; unresponsive to other comfort measures

No observable signs of oxytocin release

SAMPLE CLINICAL APPLICATIONS: prematurity, cleft lip/palate, child abuse/neglect, failure to thrive, diseases of the breast

DESIRED OUTCOMES/EVALUATION CRITERIA

Sample NOC linkages: Knowledge:

Knowledge: Breastfeeding: Extent of understanding conveyed about lactation and nourishment of infant through breastfeeding

Breastfeeding Establishment: Maternal or Infant: Maternal establishment of/proper attachment of an infant to and sucking from the breast for nourishment during the first 2 to 3 weeks

Breastfeeding Maintenance: Continued nourishment of an infant through breastfeeding

Client Will (Include Specific Time Frame)
- Verbalize understanding of causative/contributing factors.
- Demonstrate techniques to improve/enhance breastfeeding.
- Assume responsibility for effective breastfeeding.
- Achieve mutually satisfactory breastfeeding regimen with infant content after feedings and gaining weight appropriately.

ACTIONS/INTERVENTIONS
Sample NIC linkages:

Lactation Counseling: Use of an interactive helping process to assist in maintenance of successful breastfeeding

Breastfeeding Assistance: Preparing a new mother to breastfeed her infant

Support Group: Use of a group environment to provide emotional support and health-related information for members

NURSING PRIORITY NO. 1. To identify maternal causative/contributing factors:

- Assess client knowledge about breastfeeding and extent of instruction that has been given. *Provides baseline information for identifying needs and developing plan of care.*[1,7]
- Encourage discussion of current/previous breastfeeding experience(s). *Identifies current needs and problems encountered to develop a plan of care.*[5]
- Note previous unsatisfactory experience (including self or others). *Often unsolved problems and stories told by others may cause doubt about chance for success.*[1]
- Perform physical assessment, noting appearance of breasts/nipples, marked asymmetry of breasts, obvious inverted or flat nipples, minimal or no breast enlargement during pregnancy. *Identifies existing problems that may interfere with successful breastfeeding experience and provides opportunity to correct them when possible.*[1,7]
- Determine whether lactation failure is primary (i.e., maternal prolactin deficiency/serum prolactin levels, inadequate mammary gland tissue, breast surgery that has damaged the nipple, areola enervation) or secondary (i.e., sore nipples, severe engorgement, plugged milk ducts, mastitis, inhibition of letdown reflex, maternal/infant separation with disruption of feedings). *Primary failure may be irremedial and alternate plans need to be made. Secondary failure can be remedied so breastfeeding efforts can be successful.*[5]
- Note history of pregnancy, labor and delivery (vaginal or cesarean section), other recent or current surgery; preexisting medical problems (e.g., diabetes mellitus, epilepsy, cardiac diseases, or presence of disabilities). *While some conditions may preclude breastfeeding and alternate plans need to be made, others will need specific plans for monitoring and treatment to ensure successful breastfeeding.*[5]
- Identify maternal support systems; presence and response of SO(s), extended family, friends. *Having sufficient support enhances opportunity for a successful breastfeeding experience. Negative attitudes and comments interfere with efforts and may cause client to abandon attempt to breastfeed.*[5]
- Ascertain mother's age, number of children at home, and need to return to work. *These factors may have a detrimental effect of desire to breastfeed. Immaturity may influence mother to avoid breastfeeding, believing that it will be inconvenient, or being insensitive to the infant's needs. The stress of the responsibility of other children or the need to return to work can affect the ability to manage effective breastfeeding; mother will need support and information to be successful.*[6]
- Determine maternal feelings (e.g., fear/anxiety, ambivalence, depression). *Indicators of underlying emotional state that may suggest need for intervention and referral.*[1]

- Ascertain cultural expectations/conflicts. *Understanding impact of culture and idiosyncrasies of specific feeding practices is important to determine the effect on infant feeding. The practice may be different but not inferior. For example, in many cultures, such as Mexican American, Navajo, and Vietnamese, colostrum is not offered to the newborn. Intervention is only necessary if the practice/belief is harmful to the infant.*[1,3]

NURSING PRIORITY NO. 2. To assess infant causative/contributing factors:

- Determine suckling problems, as noted in Related Factors/Defining Characteristics. *These factors, prematurity, infant anomaly, poor sucking reflex, indicate need for interventions directed at correcting individual situation.*[1]
- Note prematurity and/or infant anomaly (e.g., cleft palate). *Degree of prematurity will dictate type of interventions needed to deal with situation. Infant may be put to breast if sufficiently developed, or mother may pump breast and the breast milk given via gavage. Conditions such as cleft palate need evaluation for correction and individualized instruction in holding infant upright and using special nipple or feeding device.*[2]
- Review feeding schedule, to note increased demand for feeding (at least eight times/day, taking both breasts at each feeding for more than 15 minutes on each side) or use of supplements with artificial nipple. *Provides opportunity to evaluate infant's growth, determine whether sufficient nourishment is provided, and make adjustments as needed.*[2]
- Evaluate observable signs of inadequate infant intake. *Baby latches onto mother's nipples with sustained suckling but minimal audible swallowing/gulping noted, infant arching and crying at the breasts with resistance to latching on, decreased urinary output/frequency of stools, inadequate weight gain indicate need for evaluation and intervention.*[1,7]
- Determine whether baby is content after feeding, or exhibits fussiness and crying within the first hour after breastfeeding. *Suggests unsatisfactory breastfeeding process.*[1]
- Note any correlation between maternal ingestion of certain foods and "colicky" response of infant. *Certain foods may seem to result in reaction by the infant and identification and elimination may correct the problem.*[2]

NURSING PRIORITY NO. 3. To assist mother to develop skills of adequate breastfeeding:

- Provide emotional support to mother. Use 1:1 instruction with each feeding during hospital stay/clinic visit. *New mothers say they would like more support, encouragement, and practical information, especially when they are discharged early. Contact during each feeding provides the opportunity to develop nurse-client relationship in which these goals can be attained.*[1]
- Inform mother that some babies do not cry when they are hungry; instead some make "rooting" motions and suck their fingers. *New mothers may not be aware that these behaviors indicate hunger and may not respond appropriately.*[1]
- Recommend avoidance or overuse of supplemental feedings and pacifiers (unless specifically indicated). *These can lessen infant's desire to breastfeed. The shape of the mouth and lips and the sucking mechanism is different for breast and bottle and the infant may be confused by the difference, causing interference in the breastfeeding process.*[1]
- Restrict use of breast shields (i.e., only temporarily to help draw the nipple out), then place baby directly on nipple. *These have been found to contribute to lactation failures. Shields prevent the infant's mouth from coming into contact with the mother's nipple, which is necessary for continued release of prolactin (promoting milk production), and can interfere with or prevent establishment of adequate milk supply. Temporary use of shield may be beneficial in the presence of severe nipple cracking.*[6]

- Demonstrate use of electric piston-type breast pump with bilateral collection chamber when necessary to maintain or increase milk supply. *The need to use a pump to store milk for feedings while the mother is away (i.e., going back to work, or simply to allow time away from the infant), demands some degree of proficiency in the use of the pump.*[1]
- Encourage frequent rest periods, sharing household/child-care duties. *The new mother may feel overwhelmed with taking care of infant and other household duties and having assistance can limit fatigue and facilitate relaxation at feeding times.*[6]
- Suggest abstinence/restriction of tobacco, caffeine, alcohol, drugs, excess sugar. *May affect milk production/letdown reflex or be passed on to the infant.*[1]
- Promote early management of breastfeeding problems. *Dealing with problems in a timely manner will promote successful breastfeeding.*[1,7]

For example:

Engorgement: Heat and/or cool applications to the breasts, massage from chest wall down to nipple; use synthetic oxytocin nasal spray to enhance letdown reflex; soothe "fussy baby" before latching on the breast, properly position baby on breast/nipple, alternate the side baby starts nursing on, nurse round-the-clock and/or pump with piston-type electric breast pump with bilateral collection chambers at least eight to 12 times/day.

Sore nipples: Wear 100% cotton fabrics, do not use soap/alcohol/drying agents on nipples, avoid use of nipple shields or nursing pads that contain plastic; cleanse and then air dry, use thin layers of lanolin (if mother/baby not sensitive to wool); provide exposure to sunlight/sunlamps with extreme caution; administer mild pain reliever as appropriate, apply ice before nursing; soak with warm water before attaching infant to soften nipple and remove dried milk, begin with least sore side or begin with hand expression to establish letdown reflex, properly position infant on breast/nipple, and use a variety of nursing positions.

Clogged ducts: Use larger bra or extender to avoid pressure on site; use moist or dry heat, gently massage from above plug down to nipple; nurse infant, hand express, or pump after massage; nurse more often on affected side.

Inhibited letdown: Use relaxation techniques before nursing (e.g., maintain quiet atmosphere, assume position of comfort, massage, apply heat to breasts, have beverage available); develop a routine for nursing, concentrate on infant; administer synthetic oxytocin nasal spray as appropriate.

Mastitis: Promote bedrest (with infant) for several days; administer antibiotics; provide warm, moist heat before and during nursing; empty breasts completely, continuing to nurse baby at least eight to 12 times/day, or pumping breasts for 24 hours; then resuming breastfeeding as appropriate.

NURSING PRIORITY NO. 4. To condition infant to breastfeed:

- Scent breast pad with breast milk and leave in bed with infant along with mother's photograph when separated from mother for medical purposes (e.g., prematurity).
- Increase skin-to-skin contact.
- Provide practice times at breast.
- Express small amounts of milk into baby's mouth.
- Have mother pump breast after feeding to enhance milk production.
- Use supplemental nutrition system cautiously when necessary.
- Identify special interventions for feeding in presence of cleft lip/palate. *These measures promote optimal interaction between mother and infant and provide adequate nourishment for the infant, enhancing successful breastfeeding.*[1]

 Cultural Collaborative  Community/ Home Care 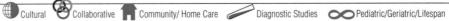 Diagnostic Studies ∞ Pediatric/Geriatric/Lifespan Medications

NURSING PRIORITY NO. 5. To promote wellness (Teaching/Discharge Considerations):

- Schedule follow-up visits with healthcare provider 48 hours after hospital discharge and 2 weeks after birth. *Provides opportunity to evaluate milk intake/breastfeeding process and adequacy of home situation.*[2]
- Recommend monitoring number of infant's wet diapers. *At least six wet diapers a day suggests adequate hydration and provides reassurance that infant is receiving sufficient intake.*[6]
- Weigh infant at least every third day as indicated and record. *Provides record of appropriate weight gain verifying adequacy of nutritional intake or indicates need for evaluation of insufficient weight gain.*[1]
- Encourage spouse education and support when appropriate. Review mother's need for rest, relaxation, and time together with spouse and with other children as appropriate. *Involving spouse and family promotes understanding of mother's needs and cooperation with incorporation of new member into family. Spouse and children feel included when they have time alone with mother and are more willing to allow mother time with infant and for herself.*[4]
- Discuss importance of adequate nutrition/fluid intake, prenatal vitamins, or other vitamin/mineral supplements, such as vitamin C as indicated. *During lactation there is an increased need for energy, and supplementation of protein, minerals, and vitamins is necessary to provide nourishment for the infant and protect mother's stores, along with extra fluid intake. Alternating different types of fluid, water, juices, decaffeinated tea, and milk can help mother promote sufficient intake. Beer or wine are not recommended for increasing lactation.*[4]
- Address specific problems (e.g., suckling problems, prematurity/anomalies). *Individualized planning can enhance mother's understanding and ability to manage situation.*[1,7]
- Inform mother that the return of menses varies in nursing mothers and usually averages 3 to 36 weeks with ovulation returning in 17 to 28 weeks. *Return of menstruation does not affect breastfeeding and is not a reliable method of birth control.*[1]
- Refer to support groups (e.g., La Leche League, parenting support groups, stress reduction, or other community resources as indicated). *Provides information and visible support for ensuring an effective outcome.*[5]
- Provide bibliotherapy for further information. *Additional resources to assist mother and family learn and apply new skills.*[1]

DOCUMENTATION FOCUS

Assessment/Reassessment
- Identified assessment factors, both maternal and infant (e.g., is engorgement present, is infant demonstrating adequate weight gain without supplementation).

Planning
- Plan of care/interventions and who is involved in planning.
- Teaching plan.

Implementation/Evaluation
- Mother's/infant's responses to interventions/teaching and actions performed.
- Attainment/progress toward desired outcome(s).
- Modifications to plan of care.

Discharge Planning
- Referrals that have been made and mother's choice of participation.

References

1. Ladewig, P., London, M., Moberly, S., & Olds, S. (2002). Contemporary Maternal-Newborn Nursing Care, ed 5. Upper Saddle River, NJ: Prentice Hall.
2. Riodan, J., & Auerbach, K. (1993). Breastfeeding and Human Lactation. Boston: Jones & Bartlett.
3. Lipson, J., Dibble, S., & Minarik, P. (1996). Culture & Nursing Care: A Pocket Guide. San Francisco: UCSF Nursing Press.
4. Lowdermilk, D., Perry, S., & Bobak, I. (2001). Maternal & Women's Health Care, ed 6. St. Louis: Mosby.
5. Doenges, M., & Moorhouse, M. (1999). Maternal/Newborn Plans of Care Guidelines for Individualizing Care, ed 3. Philadelphia: F. A. Davis.
6. Phillips, C. (1996). Family-Centered Maternity and Newborn Care, ed 4. St. Louis: Mosby.
7. London, M., Ladewig, P., Ball, J., & Bindler, R. (2003). Maternal-Newborn and Child Nursing: Family Centered Care. Upper Saddle River, NJ: Prentice Hall.

interrupted Breastfeeding

Definition: Break in the continuity of the breastfeeding process as a result of inability or inadvisability to put baby to breast for feeding

RELATED FACTORS

Maternal or infant illness
Prematurity
Maternal employment
Contraindications to breastfeeding (e.g., drugs, true breast milk jaundice)
Need to abruptly wean infant

DEFINING CHARACTERISTICS

Subjective

Maternal desire to maintain lactation and provide (or eventually provide) her breast milk for her infant's nutritional needs
Lack of knowledge regarding expression and storage of breast milk

Objective

Separation of mother and infant
Infant does not receive nourishment at the breast for some or all of feedings

SAMPLE CLINICAL APPLICATIONS: prematurity, postpartum depression, conditions requiring hospitalization of infant or mother, occasionally maternal medication/drug use

DESIRED OUTCOMES/EVALUATION CRITERIA

Sample NOC linkages:

Knowledge: Breastfeeding: Extent of understanding conveyed about lactation and nourishment of infant through breastfeeding

Breastfeeding Maintenance: Continued nourishment of an infant through breastfeeding

Parent-Infant Attachment: Behaviors that demonstrate an enduring affectionate bond between parent and infant

Client Will (Include Specific Time Frame)

- Identify and demonstrate techniques to sustain lactation until breastfeeding is reinitiated.

 Cultural Collaborative  Community/ Home Care Diagnostic Studies 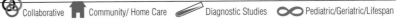 Pediatric/Geriatric/Lifespan Medications

- Achieve mutually satisfactory feeding regimen with infant content after feedings and gaining weight appropriately.
- Achieve weaning and cessation of lactation if desired or necessary.

ACTIONS/INTERVENTIONS

Sample NIC linkages:

Lactation Counseling: Use of an interactive helping process to assist in maintenance of successful breastfeeding

Emotional Support: Provision of reassurance, acceptance, and encouragement during times of stress

Bottle Feeding: Preparation and administration of fluids to an infant via a bottle

NURSING PRIORITY NO. 1. To identify causative/contributing factors:

- Assess client knowledge and perceptions about breastfeeding and extent of instruction that has been given. *Provides baseline information to develop plan of care for individual situation.*[1,8]
- Encourage discussion of current/previous breastfeeding experience(s). *Identifying knowledge and experience is useful for determining efforts needed to continue breastfeeding, if desired, while circumstances interrupting process are resolved if possible.*[2]
- Determine maternal responsibilities, routines, and scheduled activities. *Caretaking of siblings, employment in/out of home, work/school schedules of family members may affect ability to visit hospitalized infant when this is the reason for mother/infant separation.*[7]
- Note contraindications to breastfeeding (e.g., maternal illness, drug use); desire/ need to wean infant. *Interruptions do not necessarily mean that mother will be unable to resume breastfeeding. Capabilities can be maintained by planning for time that mother and infant need to be separated. The use of medications needs to be evaluated on an individual basis as most drugs pass into breast milk, and some are contraindicated for breastfeeding women.*[1,8]
- Ascertain cultural expectations/conflicts. *The dominant culture in America has sexualized women's breasts and mother may be embarrassed by breastfeeding or mate may not want mother to breastfeed. Mother may believe her independence will be curtailed by breastfeeding. Some cultures, such as Arab American, may believe that modernization means giving up breastfeeding.*[1,3]

NURSING PRIORITY NO. 2. To assist mother to maintain or conclude breastfeeding as desired/required:

- Give emotional support to mother and accept decision regarding cessation/continuation of breastfeeding. *Many women are ambivalent about breastfeeding, and providing information about the pros and cons of both breast- and bottle-feeding along with support for the mother's/ couple's decision will promote a positive experience.*[1,8]
- Demonstrate use of manual and/or electric piston-type breast pump. *When circumstances dictate that mother and infant are separated for a time, whether by illness, prematurity, or returning to work, the milk supply can be maintained by use of the pump. Storing the milk for future use enables the infant to continue to receive the value of breast milk. Learning the correct technique is important to successful use of the pump.*[1]
- Suggest abstinence/restriction of tobacco, caffeine, alcohol, drugs, excess sugar as appropriate when breastfeeding is reinitiated. *These substances may affect milk production/ letdown reflex or may be passed on to the infant.*[1]

● Provide information (e.g., wearing a snug, well-fitting brassiere, avoiding stimulation, and using medication for discomfort. *When weaning becomes necessary, these measures can support the process.*[1,8]

NURSING PRIORITY NO. 3. To promote successful infant feeding:

 ● Review techniques for storage/use of expressed breast milk. *Provides safety and optimal nutrition, promoting continuation of the breastfeeding process.*[1]

 ● Discuss proper use and choice of supplemental nutrition and alternate feeding method (e.g., bottle/syringe). *When by choice or necessity, infant is not receiving sufficient nourishment, other means for supplementing intake must be taken and mother needs to be given information regarding method chosen.*[1]

 ● Review safety precautions when bottle-feeding is necessary/chosen. *Identifying importance of proper flow of formula from nipple, frequency of burping, holding bottle instead of propping, techniques of formula preparation, and sterilization techniques are necessary for successful bottle-feeding.*[1]

● Determine if a routine visiting schedule or advance warning can be provided. *When infant remains in the hospital or when working mother continues to nurse, it helps to make preparations so that infant will be hungry/ready to feed when the mother arrives. A sleepy baby can be gently played with to arouse him or her, clothing can be loosened, exposing infant to room air, or if infant is hungry and upset, a calm voice and gentle rocking can calm the infant and prepare him or her to nurse.*[1]

● Provide privacy, calm surroundings when mother breastfeeds in hospital setting.

 ● Recommend/provide for infant sucking on a regular basis, especially if gavage feedings are part of the therapeutic regimen. *Reinforces that feeding time is pleasurable and enhances digestion.*[1]

NURSING PRIORITY NO. 4. To promote wellness (Teaching/Discharge Considerations):

 ● Encourage mother to obtain adequate rest, maintain fluid and nutritional intake, and schedule breast pumping every 3 hours while awake, as indicated. *Sustains adequate milk production and enhances breastfeeding process when mother and infant are separated for any reason.*[1,8]

● Identify other means of nurturing/strengthening infant attachment. *Activities that provide comfort, consolation, and play activities help mother become comfortable with handling infant, enhancing relationship.*[7]

  ● Refer to support groups (e.g., La Leche League, Lact-Aid), community resources (e.g., public health nurse, lactation specialist, WIC program). *Additional support may provide assistance and education to promote a successful outcome. WIC and other federal programs support breastfeeding through education and enhanced nutritional intake.*[5]

 ● Promote use of bibliotherapy. *Provides an additional source of information.*[5]

DOCUMENTATION FOCUS

Assessment/Reassessment
● Baseline findings maternal/infant factors.
● Number of wet diapers daily/periodic weight.

 Cultural Collaborative Community/ Home Care Diagnostic Studies 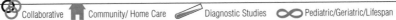 Pediatric/Geriatric/Lifespan Medications

Planning
- Plan of care and who is involved in planning.
- Teaching plan.

Implementation/Evaluation
- Maternal response to interventions/teaching and actions performed.
- Infant's response to feeding and method.
- Whether infant appears satisfied or still seems to be hungry.
- Attainment/progress toward desired outcome(s).
- Modifications to plan of care.

Discharge Planning
- Referrals, plan for follow-up, and who is responsible.
- Specific referrals made.

References

1. Ladewig, P., London, M., Moberly, S., & Olds, S. (2002). Contemporary Maternal-Newborn Nursing Care. Upper Saddle River, NJ: Prentice Hall.
2. Riodan J., & Auerbach K. (1993). Breastfeeding and Human lactation. Boston: Jones & Bartlett.
3. Lipson, J., Dibble, S., & Minarik, P. (1996). Culture & Nursing Care: A Pocket Guide. San Francisco: UCSF Nursing Press.
4. Lowdermilk, D., Perry, S., & Bobak, I. (2001). Maternity and Woman's Health Care, ed 6. St. Louis: Mosby.
5. Doenges, M., & Moorhouse, M. (1999). Maternal/Newborn Plans of Care Guidelines for Individualizing Care, ed 3. Philadelphia: F. A. Davis.
6. Phillips, C. (1996). Family-Centered Maternity and Newborn Care, ed 4. St. Louis: Mosby.
7. Cox, H., Hinz, M., Lubno, M., Newfield, S., Ridenour, N., Slater, M., & Sridaromont, K. (2002). Clinical Applications of Nursing Diagnosis Adult, Child, Women's, Psychiatric, Gerontic and Home Health Considerations, ed 4. Philadelphia: F. A. Davis.
8. London, M., Ladewig, P., Ball, J., & Bindler, R. (2003). Maternal-Newborn and Child Nursing: Family Centered Care. Upper Saddle River, NJ: Prentice Hall.

ineffective Breathing Pattern

Definition: Inspiration and/or expiration that does not provide adequate ventilation

RELATED FACTORS

Neuromuscular dysfunction; SCI; neurologic immaturity

Musculoskeletal impairment; bony/chest wall deformity

Anxiety

Pain

Perception/cognitive impairment

Decreased energy/fatigue; respiratory muscle fatigue

Body position; obesity

Hyperventilation; hypoventilation syndrome; [alteration of client's normal O_2:CO_2 ratio (e.g., O_2 therapy in COPD)]

DEFINING CHARACTERISTICS

Subjective
Shortness of breath

Objective

Dyspnea; orthopnea

Respiratory rate:

Adults (age 14 or greater)	equal to or <11 or >24
Children 1 to 4 yr	<20 or >30
5 to 14 yr	<14 or >25
Infants 0 to 12 mo	<25 or >60

Adult tidal volume (VT) 500 mL at rest

Infants 6 to 8 mL/kg

Timing ratio, prolonged expiration phases, decreased minute ventilation, vital capacity

Decreased inspiratory/expiratory pressure

Use of accessory muscles to breathe, pursed-lip breathing

Assumption of three-point position

Altered chest excursion [paradoxical breathing patterns]

Nasal flaring [grunting]

Increased anterior-posterior diameter

SAMPLE CLINICAL APPLICATIONS: chronic obstructive pulmonary disease (COPD), emphysema, asthma, pneumonia, chest trauma/surgery, SCI, Guillain-Barré syndrome, cystic fibrosis, drug/alcohol toxicity

DESIRED OUTCOMES/EVALUATION CRITERIA

Sample NOC linkages:

Respiratory Status: Ventilation: Movement of air in and out of the lungs

Respiratory Status: Airway Patency: Extent to which the tracheobronchial passages remain open

Asthma Control: Personal actions to reverse inflammatory condition resulting in bronchial constriction of the airways

Client Will (Include Specific Time Frame)

- Establish a normal/effective respiratory pattern.
- Be free of cyanosis and other signs/symptoms of hypoxia with ABGs within client's normal/acceptable range.
- Verbalize awareness of causative factors and initiate needed lifestyle changes.
- Demonstrate appropriate coping behaviors.

ACTIONS/INTERVENTIONS

Sample NIC linkages:

Ventilation Assistance: Promotion of an optimal spontaneous breathing pattern that maximizes oxygen and carbon dioxide exchange in the lungs

Airway Management: Facilitation of patency of air passages

Respiratory Monitoring: Collection and analysis of patient data to ensure airway patency and adequate gas exchange

NURSING PRIORITY NO. 1. To identify etiology/precipitating factors:

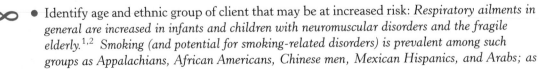 • Identify age and ethnic group of client that may be at increased risk: *Respiratory ailments in general are increased in infants and children with neuromuscular disorders and the fragile elderly.*[1,2] *Smoking (and potential for smoking-related disorders) is prevalent among such groups as Appalachians, African Americans, Chinese men, Mexican Hispanics, and Arabs; as*

 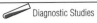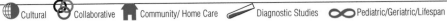

well as persons living in highly polluted environments (both children and adults). [3,4] *People most at risk for infectious pneumonias include the very young and fragile elderly, those suffering from chronic respiratory or circulatory problems, those with compromised immune systems from congenital deficiencies, AIDS, cancers and cancer medications.* [2,5]

- Ascertain if client has history of underlying or new conditions with potential for breathing problems (e.g., asthma, other acute or chronic respiratory diseases, neuromuscular disorders, heart disease, sepsis, burns, acute chest or brain trauma) *important in pointing to cause for current problems.* [6]
- Discuss current symptoms with client/SO and how they relate to past history. *Assessing current illness should include history of 1) onset and duration of symptoms; 2) how they are similar to/different from past symptoms; 3) precipitating, relieving, and exacerbating factors; and 4) exposures (e.g., environmental toxins, alcohol/other drugs, source of infection) may help in selecting the correct diagnosis.*
- Evaluate client's respiratory status:
- ∞ Note rate and depth of respirations, counting for full one minute, if rate is irregular. *Rate may be greater or less than usual. In infants and younger children, rate increases dramatically relative to anxiety, crying, fever, or disease. Depth may be difficult to evaluate, but is usually described as shallow, normal or deep.* [7,8]
- Note client's reports/perceptions of breathing ease: *Client may report a range of symptoms (e.g., air hunger, shortness of breath with speaking, activity, or at rest) and demonstrate wide range of signs (e.g., tachypnea, gasping, wheezing, coughing).*
- ∞ Observe type breathing pattern. *May see use of accessory muscles for breathing, sternal retractions (infants and young children) nasal flaring, pursed-lip breathing. Client may change position in effort to breathe easier. Irregular patterns may be pathologic (e.g., prolonged expiration, periods of apnea, obvious agonal breathing) with pronounced alterations in conditions such as severe asthma attack, brain stem damage, or impending respiratory failure.* [6,7]
- Auscultate and percuss chest, describing presence, absence and character of breath sounds. *Air should be moving freely through air passages (differs from ineffective airway clearance) but ventilatory effort is insufficient to bring in enough oxygen or to exchange sufficient amounts of carbon dioxide. Abnormal breath sounds are indicative of numerous problems (e.g., obstruction by foreign object, hypoventilation such as might occur with chest or spinal cord injury, atelectasis, or presence of secretions, improper endotracheal tube placement, collapsed lung) and must be evaluated and reported for further intervention.* [8,9]
- Observe chest size, shape, and symmetry of movement. *Changes in movement of chest wall (such as might occur with chest trauma, chest wall deformities) can impair breathing patterns.*
- Note color of skin and mucous membranes. *If pallor, duskiness, and/or cyanosis are present, oxygen and/or other interventions may be required.* (Refer to ND impaired Gas Exchange.)
- Assess for pregnancy, other abdominal distention and muscle guarding. *Distended abdomen and muscle tension can impede diaphragmatic excursion and reduce lung expansion.* [8]
- ∞ Note presence and character of cough. *Cough function may be weak or ineffective in diseases and conditions such as extremes in age (e.g., premature infant or elderly), cerebral palsy, muscular dystrophy, SCI, brain injury, after surgery, and/or mechanical ventilation due to mechanisms affecting muscles of throat, chest, and lungs. Cough that is persistent and constant can interfere with breathing (such as can occur with asthma, acute bronchitis, cystic fibrosis, croup, whooping cough).* [1,6–10] Refer to ND ineffective Airway clearance.
- Assess client's awareness and cognition. *Affects ability to manage own airway and cooperate with interventions such as controlling breathing and managing secretions.* [2,8,9]

- Note emotional state. *Gasping, crying, anxiety, irritability, struggling, look of fear, report of tingling lips/fingers, withdrawal, and self-focus are responses often associated with respiratory distress. Emotional changes can accompany a condition, or precipitate or aggravate ineffective breathing patterns.*[6-9]

 - Assist with/monitor results of necessary testing (e.g., pulmonary/cardiac function studies, neuromuscular evaluation, sleep studies) *to diagnose presence/severity of lung diseases and degree of respiratory compromise.*

 - Review chest radiographs and laboratory data (e.g., arterial blood gases [ABGs], pulse oximetry at rest and activity, drug screens, white blood cell count, blood and sputum culture tests for viruses and bacteria).

NURSING PRIORITY NO. 2. To provide for relief of causative factors:

- Assist with measures to promote breathing ease[6-12]:

    Assist in treatment of underlying conditions, administering medications and therapies as ordered.

    Suction airway *to clear secretions* as needed. Refer to ND impaired Airway Clearance for additional interventions.

    Maintain emergency equipment in readily accessible location, and include age/size appropriate airway/ET/trach tubes (e.g., infant, child, adolescent, or adult).

    Administer oxygen (by cannula, mask, mechanical ventilation) at lowest concentration needed (per ABGs, pulse oximetry) for underlying pulmonary condition and current respiratory problem. Refer to ND impaired Gas Exchange for additional interventions.

    Elevate HOB, support with pillows *to prevent slumping and promote rest*; or place in position of comfort. as appropriate *to promote maximal inspiration*. In ventilated client, place in prone position for short periods when indicated *to improve pulmonary perfusion and increase oxygen diffusion*

    Reposition client frequently *to enhance respiratory effort and ventilation of all lung segments especially if immobility is a factor.*

    Encourage early ambulation, using assistive devices, as individually indicated *to prevent onset or reduce severity of respiratory complications.*

    Direct client in breathing efforts as needed. Encourage slower/deeper respirations, use of pursed-lip technique, *to assist client in "taking control" of the situation, especially when condition is associated with anxiety and air hunger.*

    Coach client in effective coughing techniques. Place in appropriate position for clearing airways. Splint rib cage/surgical incisions as appropriate. Medicate for pain, as indicated. *Promotes breathing that is more effective and airway management when client is guarding, as might occur with chest, ribcage or abdominal injuries or surgeries.* Refer to NDs acute Pain; chronic Pain for additional interventions.

    Provide and assist with use of respiratory therapy adjuncts such as spirometry.

    Maintain calm attitude while working with client/SOs. Provide quiet environment, instruct/reinforce client in the use of relaxation techniques, and administer antianxiety medications as indicated *to reduce intensity of anxiety/deal with fear that may be present.* Refer to NDs Fear; Anxiety for additional interventions.

    Avoid overfeeding, such as might occur with young infant, or client on tube feedings. *Abdominal distention can interfere with breathing as well as increase risk of aspiration.*

    Assist with bronchoscopy or chest tube insertion as indicated.

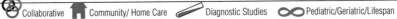

NURSING PRIORITY NO. 3. To promote wellness (Teaching/Discharge Considerations):

- Review with client/SO: client's type of respiratory condition, treatments, rehabilitation measures, and quality of life issues. *Many conditions with impaired breathing are associated with chronic conditions that require lifetime management.*[9]
- Teach/reinforce breathing retraining. *Education may include many measures including conscious control of respiratory rate, effective use of accessory muscles, breathing exercises (diaphragmatic, abdominal breathing, inspiratory resistive, and pursed-lip), assistive devices such as rocking bed.*[6]
- Discuss relationship of smoking to respiratory function. Stress importance of smoking cessation and smoke-free environment.
- Encourage client/SO(s) to develop a plan for smoking cessation. Provide appropriate referrals.
- Encourage self-assessment and symptom management[6–12]:
  Use of equipment to identify respiratory decompensation, such as peak flow meter.
  Appropriate use of oxygen (dosage, route, and safety factors).
  Medication regimen, including actions, side effects, and potential interactions of medications, over-the-counter (OTC) drugs, vitamins, and herbal supplements.
  Adhere to home treatments such as metered-dose inhalers (MDIs), compressor, nebulizer, chest physiotherapies.
  Dietary patterns and needs; access to foods and nutrients supportive of health and breathing.
  Management of personal environment, including stress reduction, rest and sleep, social events, travel, and recreation issues.
  Avoidance of known irritants, allergens, and sick persons.
  Immunizations against influenza and pneumonia.
  Early intervention when respiratory symptoms occur, and what symptoms require reporting to medical providers, seeking emergency care.
- Discuss benefits of exercise for endurance, muscle strengthening, and flexibility training *to improve general health and respiratory muscle function.* Refer to physical therapy and rehabilitation resources as indicated.
- Review energy conservation techniques (e.g., sitting instead of standing to wash dishes, pacing activities, taking short rest periods between activities) *to limit fatigue and improve endurance.*
- Reinforce instruction in proper use and safety concerns for home oxygen therapy, and/or use of respirator/diaphragmatic stimulator, rocking bed, apnea monitor, when used. *Protects client's safety, especially when used in the very young, fragile elderly, or when cognitive or neuromuscular impairment present.*
- Discuss impact of respiratory condition on occupational performance, as well as work environment issues that affect client.
- Provide referrals as indicated by individual situation. *May include a wide variety of services and providers, including support groups, comprehensive rehabilitation program, occupational nurse, oxygen and DME companies for supplies, home health services, occupational and physical therapy, transportation, assisted/alternate living facilities, local and national Lung Association chapters, and Web sites for educational materials.*

DOCUMENTATION FOCUS

Assessment/Reassessment
- Relevant history of problem.

- Respiratory pattern, breath sounds, use of accessory muscles.
- Laboratory values.
- Use of respiratory supports, ventilator settings, and so forth.

Planning
- Plan of care/interventions and who is involved in the planning.
- Teaching plan.

Implementation/Evaluation
- Response to interventions/teaching, actions performed, and treatment regimen.
- Mastery of skills, level of independence.
- Attainment/progress toward desired outcome(s).
- Modifications to plan of care.

Discharge Planning
- Long-term needs, including appropriate referrals and action taken, available resources.
- Specific referrals provided.

References

1. Evidence-based Clinical Practice Guideline of Community-acquired Pneumonia in Children 60 days to 17 years of age. (2000). Cincinnati Children's Hospital Medical Center. HPCE@chmcc.org.
2. Stanley, M., & Beare, P. G. (1999). Gerontological Nursing: A Health Promotion/Protection Approach, ed 2. Philadelphia: F. A. Davis.
3. Lung Disease in Minorities in 1999. Focus Asthma. Available at www.stateoftheair.org.
4. Purnell, L. D., & Paulanka, B. J. (1998). Transcultural Health Care: A Culturally Competent Approach. Philadelphia: F. A. Davis.
5. Minority Lung Disease Data-Major Acute Infections: Influenza and Pneumonia. American Lung Association: State of the Air 2002. Available at www.stateoftheair.org.
6. Global strategy for the diagnosis, management, and prevention of chronic obstructive pulmonary disease. Global Initiative for Chronic Obstructive Lung Disease (GOLD), World Health Organization, National Heart, Lung, and Blood Institute, 2001, National Guideline Clearinghouse [NGC 2205].
7. Engel, J. (2002). Mosby's Pocket Guide to Pediatric Assessment, ed 4. St Louis: Mosby.
8. Cox, H. C., et al. (2002). Clinical Applications of Nursing Diagnosis: Adult, Child, Women's, Gerontic, and Home Health Considerations, ed 4. Philadelphia: F. A. Davis, pp 256–261.
9. Doenges, M. E., Moorhouse, M. F., & Geissler-Murr, A. C. (2002). Nursing Care Plans: Guidelines for Individualizing Patient Care, ed 6. Philadelphia: F. A. Davis, p 167.
10. Irwin, R. S., et al. (1998). Managing cough as a defense mechanism and as a symptom: A Clinical Reference Guide. Northbrook, IL: American College of Chest Physicians (ACCP).
11. Marion, B. S. (2001). A turn for the better: "Prone positioning" of patients with ARDS. AJN 101(5): 26–33.
12. Pulmonary Rehabilitation. America Association for Respiratory Care (AARC): Clinical Practice Guideline. National Guideline Clearinghouse [NGC: 2437] 2002.

decreased Cardiac Output

Definition: Inadequate blood pumped by the heart to meet the metabolic demands of the body. [Note: In a hypermetabolic state, although cardiac output may be within normal range, it may still be inadequate to meet the needs of the body's tissues. Cardiac output and tissue perfusion are interrelated, although there are differences. When cardiac output is decreased, tissue perfusion problems will develop; however, tissue perfusion problems can exist without decreased cardiac output.]

 Cultural Collaborative 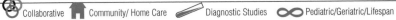 Community/ Home Care Diagnostic Studies ∞ Pediatric/Geriatric/Lifespan Medications

Altered heart rate/rhythm, [conduction]

Altered stroke volume: altered preload [e.g., decreased venous return]; altered afterload [e.g., systemic vascular resistance]; altered contractility [e.g., ventricular-septal rupture, ventricular aneurysm, papillary muscle rupture, valvular disease]

DEFINING CHARACTERISTICS

Subjective
Altered heart rate/rhythm: Palpitations
Altered preload: Fatigue
Altered afterload: Shortness of breath/dyspnea
Altered contractility: Orthopnea/paroxysmal nocturnal dyspnea [PND]
Behavioral/emotional: Anxiety

Objective
Altered heart rate/rhythm: [Dys] arrhythmias (tachycardia, bradycardia); ECG changes
Altered preload: Jugular vein distention (JVD), edema, weight gain, increased/decreased central venous pressure (CVP), increased/decreased pulmonary artery wedge pressure (PAWP), murmurs
Altered afterload: Cold, clammy skin; skin [and mucous membrane] color changes [cyanosis, pallor]; prolonged capillary refill; decreased peripheral pulses; variations in blood pressure readings; increased/decreased systemic vascular resistance (SVR)/pulmonary vascular resistance (PVR); oliguria; [anuria]
Altered contractility: Crackles; cough; cardiac output <4 L/min; cardiac index <2.5 L/min; decreased ejection fraction/stroke volume index (SVI), left ventricular stroke work index (LVSWI); S3 or S4 sounds [gallop rhythm]
Behavioral/emotional: Restlessness

SAMPLE CLINICAL APPLICATIONS: myocardial infarction, CHF, valvular heart disease, dysrhythmias, cardiomyopathy, cardiac contusions/trauma, pericarditis, ventricular aneurysm

DESIRED OUTCOMES/EVALUATION CRITERIA
Sample NOC linkages:
Cardiac Pump Effectiveness: Extent to which blood is ejected from the left ventricle per minute to support systemic perfusion pressure
Circulation Status: Extent to which blood flows unobstructed, unidirectionally, and at an appropriate pressure through large vessels of the systemic and pulmonary circuits
Energy Conservation: Extent of active management of energy to initiate and sustain activity

Client Will (Include Specific Time Frame)
- Display hemodynamic stability (e.g., blood pressure, cardiac output, urinary output, peripheral pulses).
- Report/demonstrate decreased episodes of dyspnea, angina, and dysrhythmias.
- Demonstrate an increase in activity tolerance.
- Verbalize knowledge of the disease process, individual risk factors, and treatment plan.
- Participate in activities that reduce the workload of the heart.
- Identify signs of cardiac decompensation, alter activities, and seek help appropriately.

ACTIONS/INTERVENTIONS

Sample NIC linkages:

Hemodynamic Regulation: Optimization of heart rate, preload, afterload, and contractility

Cardiac Care: Limitation of complications resulting from an imbalance between myocardial oxygen supply and demand for a patient with symptoms of impaired cardiac function

Circulatory Care: Mechanical Assist Devices: Temporary support of the circulation through the use of mechanical devices or pumps

NURSING PRIORITY NO. 1. To identify causative/contributing factors:

- Review clients at risk as noted in *Related Factors and Defining Characteristics. In addition to individuals obviously at risk with known cardiac problems, look for potential cardiac output problems in persons with trauma, hemorrhage, alcohol and other drug intoxication/chronic use/overdose; pregnant women with hypertensive states; individuals with chronic renal failure; with brainstem trauma, or spinal cord injuries at T8 or above.*[1]

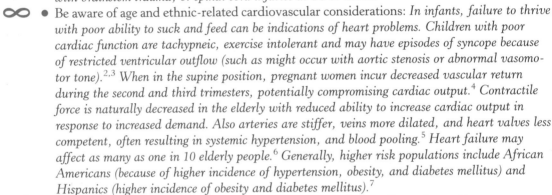

- Be aware of age and ethnic-related cardiovascular considerations: *In infants, failure to thrive with poor ability to suck and feed can be indications of heart problems. Children with poor cardiac function are tachypneic, exercise intolerant and may have episodes of syncope because of restricted ventricular outflow (such as might occur with aortic stenosis or abnormal vasomotor tone).*[2,3] *When in the supine position, pregnant women incur decreased vascular return during the second and third trimesters, potentially compromising cardiac output.*[4] *Contractile force is naturally decreased in the elderly with reduced ability to increase cardiac output in response to increased demand. Also arteries are stiffer, veins more dilated, and heart valves less competent, often resulting in systemic hypertension, and blood pooling.*[5] *Heart failure may affect as many as one in 10 elderly people.*[6] *Generally, higher risk populations include African Americans (because of higher incidence of hypertension, obesity, and diabetes mellitus) and Hispanics (higher incidence of obesity and diabetes mellitus).*[7]
- Review diagnostic studies (including/not limited to: chest radiograph, cardiac stress testing, ECG, echocardiogram, cardiac output/ventricular ejection studies, and heart scan/catheterization). *For example, EGG may show previous or evolving MI, left ventricular hypertrophy, and valvular stenosis. Ventricular function studies with ejection fraction <40% is indicative of systolic dysfunction, and cardiac output <4 L/m is indicative of heart failure. Additional cardiac studies (e.g., radionuclide scans or catheterization) may be indicated to assess left ventricular function, valvular function and coronary circulation. Chest radiography may show enlarged heart, pulmonary infiltrates.*[8–10]
- Review laboratory data, including/not limited to: complete blood cell (CBC) count, electrolytes, blood gases (ABGs), cardiac enzymes, kidney, thyroid and liver function studies, cultures (e.g., blood/wound/secretions), bleeding and coagulation studies to *identify imbalances, disease processes and effects of interventions.*[1,8]

NURSING PRIORITY NO. 2. To assess degree of debilitation:

- Assess for signs of poor ventricular function and or impending cardiac failure/shock[1–5,9]:
  Client reports/evidence of extreme fatigue, intolerance for activity, sudden or progressive weight gain, swelling of extremities, and progressive shortness of breath.
  Reports of chest pain. *May indicate evolving heart attack, can also accompany congestive heart failure. Chest pain may be atypical in women experiencing an MI and is often atypical in the elderly owing to altered pain pathways.*
  Mental status changes. *Confusion, agitation, decreased cognition and coma may occur due to decreased brain perfusion.*

 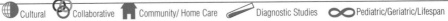

Heart rate/rhythm: Tachycardia at rest, bradycardia, atrial fibrillation, or multiple dysrhythmias may be noted. *Heart irritability is common, reflecting conduction defects and/or ischemia.*

Heart sounds may be distant, with irregular rhythms; murmurs—systolic *(valvular stenosis and shunting)* and diastolic *(aortic or pulmonary insufficiency)* or gallop rhythm (S_3, S_4) noted *when heart failure is present and ventricles are stiff.*

Peripheral pulses may be weak and thready *reflecting hypotension, vasoconstriction, shunting, and venous congestion.*

 Changes in skin color, moisture, temperature, and capillary refill time. *Pallor or cyanosis, cool moist skin, and slow capillary refill time may be present because of peripheral vasoconstriction and decreased oxygen saturation. Note: Children with chronic heart failure and adults with COPD often show clubbing of fingertips.*

Blood pressure: *Hypertension may be chronic, and/or blood pressure elevated initially in client with impending cardiogenic, hypovolemic, or septic shock. Later, as cardiac output decreases, profound hypotension can be present, often with narrowed pulse pressure.*

Breath sounds may reveal bilateral crackles and wheezing *associated with congestion. Respiratory distress/failure often occurs as shock progresses.*

Edema with neck vein distention often present and pitting edema noted in extremities and dependent portions of body *because of impaired venous return.* Other veins in trunk and extremities can be prominent *owing to venous congestion.*

 Urinary output may be decreased or absent reflecting *poor perfusion of kidneys. Note: output < 30 mL/h (adult) or <10 mL/h (child) indicates inadequate renal perfusion.*

NURSING PRIORITY NO. 3. To minimize/correct causative factors, maximize cardiac output:

Acute/severe phase[1–3,9–12]:

- Keep client on bed or chair rest in position of comfort. In congestive state, semi-Fowler's position is preferred. May raise legs 20 to 30 degrees in shock situation. *Decreases oxygen consumption/demand, reducing myocardial workload and risk of decomposition.*
- Administer supplemental oxygen as indicated (by cannula, mask, ET/trach tube with mechanical ventilation) *to improve cardiac function by increasing available oxygen and reducing oxygen consumption. Critically ill client may be on ventilator to support cardiopulmonary function.*
- Monitor vital signs frequently *to evaluate response to treatments and activities.* Perform periodic hemodynamic measurements as indicated (e.g., arterial, central venous pressure (CVP), pulmonary artery wedge pressure (PAWP), and left atrial pressures; cardiac output/cardiac index and oxygen saturation). *These measurements (via central line monitoring) are commonly used in the critically ill to provide continuous, accurate assessment of cardiac function and response to inotropic and vasoactive medications that affect cardiac contractility, and systemic circulation (preload and afterload).*
- Monitor cardiac rhythm continuously *to note changes, and evaluate effectiveness of medications and/or devices (e.g., implanted pacemaker/defibrillator)*
- Administer or restrict fluids as indicated. *Replacement of blood and large amounts of IV fluids may be needed if low output state is due to hypovolemia. If fluid overload is present, monitor IV rates closely, using infusion pumps to prevent bolus and exacerbation of fluid overload.*
- Assess hourly or periodic urinary output and daily weight, noting 24-hr total fluid balance *to evaluate kidney function and effects of interventions, as well as to allow for timely alterations in therapeutic regimen.*
- Administer medications as indicated: (e.g., inotropic drugs *to enhance cardiac contractility*, antiarrhythmics *to improve cardiac output*, diuretics *to reduce congestion by improving*

urinary output, vasopressors, and/or dilators as indicated *to manage systemic effects of vaso-constriction and low cardiac output;* pain medications and antianxiety agents *to reduce oxygen demand and myocardial workload;* anticoagulants *to improve blood flow and prevent thromboemboli.*

- Note reports of anorexia/nausea and limit/withhold oral intake as indicated. *Symptoms may be systemic reaction to low cardiac output, visceral congestion, or reaction to medications or pain.*

- Assist with preparations for/monitor response to support procedures/devices as indicated (e.g. cardioversion, pacemaker, angioplasty, coronary artery bypass-graft (CABG) or valve replacement, intra-aortic balloon pump (IABP), left ventricular assist device (LVAD). *Any number of interventions may be required to correct a condition causing heart failure, or support a failing heart during recovery from myocardial infarction, while awaiting transplantation or for long-term management of chronic heart failure.*

- Promote rest *to reduce catecholamine-induced stress response and cardiac workload*[1,13]:
  Decrease stimuli, providing quiet environment.
  Schedule activities/assessments to maximize sleep periods.
  Assist with or perform self-care activities for client.
  Avoid the use of restraints whenever possible if client is confused.

  Use sedation and analgesics as indicated with caution *to achieve desired rest state (without compromising hemodynamic responses).*

- Postacute/chronic phase[1]:
- Provide for adequate rest, positioning client for maximum comfort.
- Encourage changing positions slowly, dangling legs before standing *to reduce risk of ortho-static hypotension.*
- Increase activity levels gradually as permitted by individual condition noting vital sign response to activity.

- Administer medications as appropriate, and monitor cardiac responses.
- Encourage relaxation techniques *to reduce anxiety.*

- Refer for nutritional needs assessment and management *to provide for supportive nutrition while meeting diet restrictions (e.g., IV nutrition [TPN], sodium-restricted or other type diet with frequent small feedings).*
- Monitor intake/output and calculate 24-hour fluid balance. Provide/restrict fluids as indicated *to maximize cardiac output and improve tissue perfusion.*

NURSING PRIORITY NO. 4. To enhance safety/prevent complications:

- Promote safety[1]:
  Wash hands before and after client contacts, maintain aseptic technique during invasive procedures, and provide site care as indicated *to prevent nosocomial infection.*
  Maintain patency of invasive intravascular monitoring/infusion lines and tape connections *to prevent air embolus and/or exsanguination.*
  Provide antipyretics/fever control actions as indicated.
  Minimize activities that can elicit Valsalva response (e.g., rectal straining, vomiting, spas-modic coughing with suctioning, prolonged breath holding during pushing stage of labor) and encourage client to breathe deeply in/out during activities that increase risk of Valsalva effect. *Valsalva response to breath holding causes increased intrathoracic pressure, reducing cardiac output and blood pressure.*
  Avoid prolonged sitting position for all clients, and supine position for sleep/exercise for gravid clients (second/third trimesters) *to maximize vascular return*[4]
  Provide skin care, special bed or mattress (e.g. air, water, gel, foam) and assist with frequent position changes *to avoid the development of pressure sores.*

 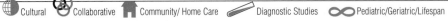

Elevate legs when in sitting position and also edematous extremities when at rest. Apply antiembolic hose or sequential compression stockings when indicated, being sure they are individually fitted and appropriately applied. *Devices limit venous stasis, improve venous return and reduce risk of thrombophlebitis.*

Manage client's temperature and ambient environmental temperature *to maintain body temperature in near-normal range.*

Refer to NDs: risk for Infection; ineffective Tissue Perfusion for additional interventions.

Provide psychological support *to reduce anxiety and its adverse effects on cardiac function:*

Maintain calm attitude and limit stressful stimuli

Provide/encourage use of relaxation techniques: massage therapy, soothing music, quiet activities.

Promote visits from family/SO(s) that provide positive input/encouragement.

Provide information about testing procedures and client participation.

Explain limitations imposed by condition, dietary and fluid restrictions.

Share information about positive signs of improvement.

NURSING PRIORITY NO. 6. To promote wellness (Teaching/Discharge Considerations)[1,13]:

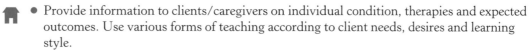

- Provide information to clients/caregivers on individual condition, therapies and expected outcomes. Use various forms of teaching according to client needs, desires and learning style.

- Direct client and/or caregivers to resources for emergency assistance, financial help, durable medical supplies, psychosocial support and respite, especially when client has impaired functional capabilities, or requires supporting equipment, (such as pacemaker, LVAD, or 24-hour oxygen).

- Emphasize importance of regular medical follow up *to monitor client's condition and response to treatment and provide most effective care.*

- Educate client/caregivers about drug regimen, including indications, dose and dosing schedules, potential adverse side effects, or drug/drug interactions. *Client is often on multiple medications, which can be difficult to manage, increasing potential that medications can be dropped or incorrectly used.*

- Emphasize reporting of adverse effects of medications *so that adjustments can be made in dosing or another class of medication considered.*

- Discuss significant signs/symptoms that need to be reported to healthcare provider: Unrelieved or increased chest pain, dyspnea, fever, swelling of ankles, sudden unexplained cough. *"Danger signs" that may require immediate intervention, change of usual therapies.* Muscle cramps, headaches, dizziness, skin rashes or unexplained symptoms that *may be signs of drug toxicity and/or mineral loss, especially potassium.*

- Teach home monitoring of weight, pulse, and/or blood pressure as appropriate *to detect change and allow for timely intervention.*

- Recommend annual influenza vaccination.

- Discuss individual's particular risk factors (e.g., smoking, stress, obesity, recent MI) and specific resources for assistance (e.g., written information sheets, direction to helpful Web sites, formalized rehabilitation programs, and home interventions for management of identified factors for:

Smoking cessation

Stress management techniques

Energy conservation techniques

Nutrition education regarding needs (e.g., to improve general health status, reduce or gain weight, lower blood fat levels, manage sodium, etc.)

Exercise/activity plan *to systematically increase endurance*
- Refer to NDs Activity Intolerance, deficient Diversional Activity, ineffective Coping, compromised family Coping, Sexual Dysfunction, acute/chronic Pain, imbalanced Nutrition, deficient/excess Fluid Volume, as indicated.

DOCUMENTATION FOCUS

Assessment/Reassessment
- Baseline and subsequent findings and individual hemodynamic parameters, heart and breath sounds, ECG pattern, presence/strength of peripheral pulses, skin/tissue status, renal output, and mentation.

Planning
- Plan of care and who is involved in planning.
- Teaching plan.

Implementation/Evaluation
- Client's responses to interventions/teaching and actions performed.
- Status and disposition at discharge.
- Attainment/progress toward desired outcome(s).
- Modifications to plan of care.

Discharge Planning
- Discharge considerations and who will be responsible for carrying out individual actions.
- Long-term needs.
- Specific referrals made.

References

1. Doenges, M. E., Moorhouse, M. F., & Geissler-Murr, A. C. (2002). Nursing Care Plans: Guidelines for Individualizing Patient Care, ed 6. Philadelphia: F. A. Davis.
2. Cox, H. C., et al. (2002). Clinical Applications of Nursing Diagnosis: Adult, Child, Women's Psychiatric, Gerontic, and Home Health Considerations, ed 4. Philadelphia: F. A. Davis, pp 262–269.
3. Pathophysiologic interpretation of cardiac symptoms and signs. Pediatric Cardiology for Parents and Patients, Rush Children's Heart Center, Chicago, IL. Available at: www.rchc.rush.edu/rmawebfiles/HP.htm.
4. Ladewig, P., London, M., Moberly, S., & Olds, S. (2002). Contemporary Maternal-Newborn Nursing Care, ed 5. Upper Saddle River, NJ: Prentice Hall.
5. Stanley, M., & Beare, P. G. (1999). Gerontological Nursing: A Health Promotion/Protection Approach, ed 2. Philadelphia: F. A. Davis.
6. Heidenreich, P. A., Ruggerico, C. M., & Massie, B. M. (2000). Effect of a home-based monitoring system on hospitalization and resource use for patients with heart failure. Pilot study supported by Agency for Healthcare Research and Quality (National Research Service Award Training Grant T32 HS00028). Available at www.ahrq.gov.
7. Purnell, L. D., & Paulanka, B. J. (1998). Transcultural Health Care: A Culturally Competent Approach. Philadelphia: F. A. Davis.
8. Cavanaugh, B. M. (1999). Nurse's Manual of Laboratory and Diagnostic Tests, ed 3. Philadelphia: F. A. Davis, pp. 654–659.
9. Heart failure. Clinical Practice Guideline. (2002). Columbia, MD: American Medical Directors Association (AMDA), NGC: 2529.
10. The pharmacologic management of chronic heart failure. (2001). Washington DC: Department of Veterans Affairs (U.S.), Veterans Health Administration (VHA).
11. Bond, A.E., et al. (2003). The left ventricular assist device, AJN 103(1):33–40.

 Cultural Collaborative Community/ Home Care Diagnostic Studies 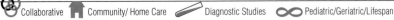 Pediatric/Geriatric/Lifespan Medications

12. Gawlinski, A., & McAtee, M. E. (May, 2002). Biventricular pacing: New treatment for patients with heart failure: Important nursing implications. AJN Suppl. Critical Care Update 102(5): 4–7.
13. Clinical Practice Guidelines: Cardiac Rehabilitation Guidelines. Cosponsored by the National Heart, Lung, and Blood Institute and Agency for Healthcare Policy and Research (AHCPR), Oct, 1995. Available at: www.ahrq.gov.

Caregiver Role Strain

Definition: Difficulty in performing caregiver role

RELATED FACTORS

Care receiver health status

Illness severity/chronicity
Unpredictability of illness course; instability of care receiver's health
Increasing care needs and dependency
Problem behaviors; psychological or cognitive problems
Addiction or codependency of care receiver

Caregiving activities

Discharge of family member to home with significant care needs (e.g., premature birth/congenital defect)
Unpredictability of care situation; 24-hour care responsibility; amount/complexity of activities
Ongoing changes in activities; years of caregiving

Caregiver health status

Physical problems; psychological or cognitive problems
Inability to fulfill one's own or others' expectations; unrealistic expectations of self
Marginal coping patterns
Addiction or codependency

Socioeconomic

Competing role commitments
Alienation from family, friends, and coworkers; isolation from others
Insufficient recreation

Caregiver—care receiver relationship

Unrealistic expectations of caregiver by care receiver
History of poor relationship
Mental status of elder inhibits conversation
Presence of abuse or violence

Family processes

History of marginal family coping/dysfunction

Resources

Inadequate physical environment for providing care (e.g., housing, temperature, safety)
Inadequate equipment for providing care; inadequate transportation
Insufficient finances

Inexperience with caregiving; insufficient time; physical energy; emotional strength; lack of support

Lack of caregiver privacy

Lack of knowledge about or difficulty accessing community resources; inadequate community services (e.g., respite care, recreational resources); assistance and support (formal and informal)

Caregiver is not developmentally ready for caregiver role

[NOTE: The presence of this problem may encompass other numerous problems/high-risk concerns such as deficient Diversional Activity, disturbed Sleep Pattern, Fatigue, Anxiety, ineffective Coping, compromised/disabled family Coping, ineffective Denial, Hopelessness, Powerlessness, ineffective Health Maintenance, ineffective Sexuality Patterns, readiness for enhanced family Coping, interrupted Family Processes, Social Isolation. Careful attention to data gathering will identify and clarify the client's specific needs, which can then be coordinated under this single diagnostic label.]

DEFINING CHARACTERISTICS

Subjective

Caregiving activities

Apprehension about possible institutionalization of care receiver, the future regarding care receiver's health and caregiver's ability to provide care, care receiver's care if caregiver becomes ill or dies

Caregiver health status—physical

Gastrointestinal (GI) upset (e.g., mild stomach cramps, vomiting, diarrhea, recurrent gastric ulcer episodes)

Weight change, rash, headaches, hypertension, cardiovascular disease, diabetes, fatigue

Caregiver health status—emotional

Feeling depressed; anger; stress; frustration; increased nervousness

Disturbed sleep

Lack of time to meet personal needs

Caregiver health status—socioeconomic

Changes in leisure activities; refuses career advancement

Caregiver-care receiver relationship

Difficulty watching care receiver go through the illness

Grief/uncertainty regarding changed relationship with care receiver

Family processes—caregiving activities

Concern about family members

Objective

Caregiving activities

Difficulty performing/completing required tasks

Preoccupation with care routine

Dysfunctional change in caregiving activities

Caregiver health status—emotional

Impatience; increased emotional lability; somatization

Impaired individual coping

Caregiver health status—socioeconomic

Low work productivity; withdraws from social life

Family processes

Family conflict

 Cultural   Collaborative   Community/ Home Care   Diagnostic Studies 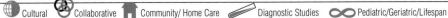 Pediatric/Geriatric/Lifespan   Medications

SAMPLE CLINICAL APPLICATIONS: chronic conditions (e.g., severe brain injury, spinal cord injury, severe developmental delay), progressive debilitating conditions (e.g., muscular dystrophy, multiple sclerosis, dementia/Alzheimer's disease, end-stage COPD, renal failure/dialysis), substance abuse, end-of-life care, psychiatric conditions (e.g., schizophrenia, personality disorders)

DESIRED OUTCOMES/EVALUATION CRITERIA
Sample NOC linkages:
Caregiver Lifestyle Disruption: Disturbances in the lifestyle of a family member due to caregiving
Caregiver Stressors: The extent of biopsychosocial pressure on a family care provider caring for a family member or significant other over an extended period of time
Caregiver Well-Being: Primary care provider's satisfaction with health and life circumstances

Caregiver Will (Include Specific Time Frame)
- Identify resources within self to deal with situation.
- Provide opportunity for care receiver to deal with situation in own way.
- Express more realistic understanding and expectations of the care receiver.
- Demonstrate behavior/lifestyle changes to cope with and/or resolve problematic factors.
- Report improved general well-being, ability to deal with situation.

ACTIONS/INTERVENTIONS
Sample NIC linkages:
Caregiver Support: Provision of the necessary information, advocacy, and support to facilitate primary patient care by someone other than a health care professional
Family Involvement Promotion: Facilitating family participation in the emotional and physical care of the patient
Parenting Promotion: Providing parenting information, support, and coordination of comprehensive services to high-risk families

NURSING PRIORITY NO. 1. To assess degree of impaired function:

- Inquire about/observe physical condition of care receiver and surroundings as appropriate. *Important to determine factors that may indicate problems that can interfere with ability to continue caregiving.*[4]
- Assess caregiver's current state of functioning (e.g., hours of sleep, nutritional intake, personal appearance, demeanor). *Provides basis for determining needs that indicate caregiver is having difficulty dealing with role.*[4]
- Determine use of prescription/OTC drugs, alcohol. *Caregiver may turn to using these substances to deal with situation.*[1]
- Identify safety issues concerning caregiver and receiver. *The stress and anxiety of caregiving situations can lead to inattention and by identifying these issues an opportunity is provided to correct problems before injury can occur.*[1]
- Assess current actions of caregiver and how they are received by care receiver. *Caregiver may be trying to be helpful but is not perceived as helpful; may be too protective or may have unrealistic expectations of care receiver, which can lead to misunderstanding and conflict.*[4]

• Note choice/frequency of social involvement and recreational activities. *Caregiver needs to take time away from situation to maintain own sense of self and ability to continue in role.*[1]

• Determine use/effectiveness of resources and support systems. *May not be aware of what is available or may need help in using them to the best advantage.*[4]

NURSING PRIORITY NO. 2. To identify the causative/contributing factors relating to the impairment:

• Note presence of high risk situations. *Elderly client with total self-care dependence, or caregiver with several small children with one child requiring extensive assistance due to physical condition/developmental delays may necessitate role reversal resulting in added stress or placing excessive demands on parenting skills.*[4]

• Determine current knowledge of the situation, noting misconceptions, lack of information. *May interfere with caregiver/care receiver's response to illness/condition.*[2]

• Identify relationship of caregiver to care receiver (e.g., spouse/lover, parent/child, sibling, friend). *Close relationships may make it more difficult to remain separate when caring for care receiver.*[2]

• Ascertain proximity of caregiver to care receiver. *There is added stress in maintaining own life and responsibilities when caregiver has to travel some distance to provide care.*[4]

• Note physical/mental condition, complexity of therapeutic regimen of care receiver. *Contributes to difficulty of caregiving, leading to possibility of 'burn-out' sooner.*[7]

• Determine caregiver's level of responsibility, involvement in and anticipated length of care. *Information needed to develop plan of care that takes into consideration who will provide care, timing and any other factors to maintain coverage for situation.*[4]

• Ascertain developmental level/abilities and additional responsibilities of caregiver. *Critical information to plan care that takes these factors into consideration in developing plan that meets the needs of all involved.*[1]

• Use assessment tool, such as Burden Interview, when appropriate, to further determine caregiver's abilities. *Provides additional information to aid in planning.*[4]

• Identify individual cultural factors and impact on caregiver. *Helps clarify expectations of caregiver/receiver, family, and community. Many cultures, such as American Indian, Cuban, believe strongly in keeping care receiver in the home and caring for them.*[5]

• Identify presence/degree of conflict between caregiver/care receiver/family. *Stressful situations can exacerbate underlying feelings of anger and resentment, resulting in difficulty managing caregiving needs.*[2]

• Determine preillness/current behaviors that may be interfering with the care/recovery of the care receiver. *Underlying personality of care receiver may create situation in which old conflicts interfere with current treatment regimen.*[2] Note codependency needs/enabling behaviors of caregiver. *These behaviors can interfere with competent caregiving and contribute to caregiver burn-out.*[2]

NURSING PRIORITY NO. 3. To assist caregiver to identify feelings and begin to deal with problems:

• Establish a therapeutic relationship, conveying empathy and unconditional positive regard. *Promotes positive environment in which problems and solutions can be identified.*[2]

• Acknowledge difficulty of the situation for the caregiver/family. *Communicates understanding promoting sense of acceptance.*[2]

• Discuss caregiver's view of and concerns about situation. *Important to identify issues so planning and solutions can be developed.*[7]

 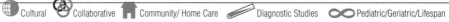

- Encourage caregiver to acknowledge and express negative feelings. Discuss normalcy of the reactions without using false reassurance. *There are no bad feelings and individual needs to understand that all are acceptable to be expressed, dealt with but not acted on in the situation.*[2]
- Discuss caregiver's/family members' life goals, perceptions and expectations of self. *Clarifies unrealistic thinking and identifies potential areas of flexibility or compromise.*[4]
- Discuss impact of and ability to handle role changes necessitated by situation. *May not initially realize the changes that will be encountered as situation develops and it helps to identify and deal with changes as they arise.*[1]

NURSING PRIORITY NO. 4. To enhance caregiver's ability to deal with current situation:

- Identify strengths of caregiver and care receiver. *Bringing these to the individual's awareness promotes positive thinking and helps with problem-solving to deal more effectively with circumstances.*[4]
- Discuss strategies to coordinate caregiving tasks and other responsibilities (e.g., employment, care of children/dependents, housekeeping activities). *Managing these tasks will reduce the stress associated with performing the activities of daily living.*[1]
- Facilitate family conference to share information and develop plan for involvement in care activities as appropriate. *Involving everyone promotes sense of control and willingness to follow-through on responsibilities.*[1]
- Identify classes and/or needed specialists (e.g., first aid/cardiopulmonary resuscitation classes, enterostomal/physical therapist). *Provides information needed to manage tasks of caregiving more effectively, giving individuals more sense of control.*[1]
- Determine need for/sources of additional resources (e.g., financial, legal, respite care). *Can help to resolve problems that arise in the course of caregiving that are out of the knowledge/abilities of the individual. Solving these issues can relieve caregiver of anxiety and concern.*[4]
- Provide information and/or demonstrate techniques for dealing with acting out/violent or disoriented behavior. *Presence of dementia may result in such behaviors requiring learning these techniques/skills to enhance safety of caregiver and receiver.*[2]
- Identify equipment needs/resources, adaptive aids. *Enhances the independence and safety of the care receiver and makes the task of caregiving easier.*[1]
- Provide contact person/case manager to coordinate care, provide support, assist with problem solving. *Promotes more effective caregiving, thereby preventing burn-out.*[2]

NURSING PRIORITY NO. 5. To promote wellness (Teaching/Discharge Considerations):

- Assist caregiver to plan for changes that may be necessary (e.g., home care providers, eventual placement in long-term care facility). *As caregiving tasks become more difficult, other options need to be considered and planning ahead can promote acceptance of necessary changes.*[8]
- Discuss/demonstrate stress management techniques and importance of self-nurturing (e.g., pursuing self-development interests, personal needs, hobbies, and social activities). *Being involved in activities such as these can prevent caregiver burnout.*[4]
- Encourage involvement in support group. *Having others to share concerns and fears is therapeutic, provides ideas of different ways to manage problems, helping caregivers deal more effectively with the situation.*[1]

• Refer to classes/other therapies as indicated. *Provides additional information as needed.*[1]

 • Identify available 12-step program when indicated to provide tools to deal with enabling/codependent behaviors that impair level of function. *Provides a more structured environment to learn how to deal with problems of caregiving situation.*[2]

 • Refer to counseling or psychotherapy as needed. *Intensive treatment may be needed in very stressful situations.*[2]

• Provide bibliotherapy of appropriate references for self-paced learning and encourage discussion of information. *Further information can help individuals understand what is happening and manage more effectively.*[9]

DOCUMENTATION FOCUS

Assessment/Reassessment
• Assessment findings, functional level/degree of impairment, caregiver's understanding/perception of situation.
• Identified risk factors.

Planning
• Plan of care and individual responsibility for specific activities.
• Needed resources, including type and source of assistive devices/durable equipment.
• Teaching plan.

Implementation/Evaluation
• Caregiver's/receiver's response to interventions/teaching and actions performed.
• Identification of inner resources, behavior/lifestyle changes to be made.
• Attainment/progress toward desired outcome(s).
• Modifications to plan of care.

Discharge Planning
• Plan for continuation/follow-through of needed changes.
• Referrals for assistance/evaluation.

References

1. Doenges, M., Moorhouse, M., & Murr, A. (2002). Nursing Care Plans, Guidelines for Individualizing Patient Care, ed 6. Philadelphia: F. A. Davis.
2. Doenges, M., Townsend, M., & Moorhouse, M. (1998). Psychiatric Care Plans: Guidelines for Individualizing Care, ed 3. Philadelphia: F. A. Davis.
3. Townsend, M. (2003). Psychiatric Mental Health Nursing: Concepts of Care, ed 4. Philadelphia: F. A. Davis.
4. Cox, H., Hinz, M., Lubno, M. A., Newfield, S., Scott-Tilley, D., Slater, M., & Sridaromont, K. (2002). Clinical Applications of Nursing Diagnosis Adult, Child, Women's Psychiatric, Gernontic and Home Health Considerations, ed 4. Philadelphia: F. A., Davis.
5. Lipson, J. G., Dibble, S. L., & Minarik, P. A. (1996). Culture & Nursing Care: A Pocket Guide. San Francisco: School of Nursing, UCSF Nursing Press.
6. Townsend, M. (2001). Nursing diagnoses in Psychiatric Nursing: Care Plans and Psychotropic Medications, ed 5. Philadelphia: F. A. Davis.
7. Hareven, T. K., & Adams, K. J. (eds). (1982). Aging and Life Course Transitions: An Interdisciplinary Perspective. New York: Guilford.
8. Liken, M. A. (2001b). Caregivers in crisis: Moving a relative with Alzheimer's to assisted living. Clin Nurs Res, 10(1):53–69.
9. Liken, M. A. Experiences of family caregivers of a relative with Alzheimer's disease. J Psychosoc Nurs, 39(12):33–37.

 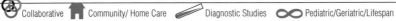

risk for Caregiver Role Strain

Definition: Caregiver is vulnerable for felt difficulty in performing the family caregiver role

RISK FACTORS

Illness severity of the care receiver; psychological or cognitive problems in care receiver; addiction or codependency

Discharge of family member with significant home-care needs; premature birth/congenital defect

Unpredictable illness course or instability in the care receiver's health

Duration of caregiving required; inexperience with caregiving; complexity/amount of caregiving tasks; caregiver's competing role commitments

Caregiver health impairment

Caregiver is female/spouse

Caregiver not developmentally ready for caregiver role (e.g., a young adult needing to provide care for middle-aged parent); developmental delay or retardation of the care receiver or caregiver

Presence of situational stressors that normally affect families (e.g., significant loss, disaster or crisis, economic vulnerability, major life events [such as birth, hospitalization, leaving home, returning home, marriage, divorce, change in employment, retirement, death])

Inadequate physical environment for providing care (e.g., housing, transportation, community services, equipment)

Family/caregiver isolation

Lack of respite and recreation for caregiver

Marginal family adaptation or dysfunction prior to the caregiving situation

Marginal caregiver's coping patterns

History of poor relationship between caregiver and care receiver

Care receiver exhibits deviant, bizarre behavior

Presence of abuse or violence

NOTE: A risk diagnosis is not evidenced by signs and symptoms, as the problem has not occurred and nursing interventions are directed at prevention.

SAMPLE CLINICAL APPLICATIONS: chronic conditions (e.g., severe brain injury, SCI, severe developmental delay), progressive debilitating conditions (e.g., muscular dystrophy, multiple sclerosis, dementia/Alzheimer's disease, end-stage COPD, renal failure/dialysis), substance abuse, end-of-life care, psychiatric conditions (e.g., schizophrenia, personality disorders)

DESIRED OUTCOMES/EVALUATION CRITERIA

Sample NOC linkages:

Caregiver Home Care Readiness: Preparedness to assume responsibility for the health care of a family member or significant other in the home

Caregiving Endurance Potential: Factors that promote family care provider continuance over an extended period of time

Family Functioning: Ability of the family to meet the needs of its members through developmental transitions

Caregiver Will (Include Specific Time Frame)
- Identify individual risk factors and appropriate interventions.
- Demonstrate/initiate behaviors or lifestyle changes to prevent development of impaired function.

- Use available resources appropriately.
- Report satisfaction with current situation.

ACTIONS/INTERVENTIONS

Sample NIC linkages:

Caregiver Support: Provision of the necessary information, advocacy, and support to facilitate primary patient care by someone other than a healthcare professional

Family Support: Promotion of family values, interests, and goals

Parenting Promotion: Providing parenting information, support, and coordination of comprehensive services to high-risk families

NURSING PRIORITY NO. 1. To assess factors affecting current situation:

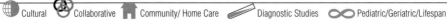

- Note presence of high risk situations (e.g., elderly client with total self-care dependence or several small children with one child requiring extensive assistance due to physical condition/developmental delays). *May necessitate role reversal resulting in added stress or place excessive demands on parenting skills. Identification of high-risk situations can help in planning and resolving problems before they can become unmanageable.*[1]
- Identify relationship and proximity of caregiver to care receiver (e.g., spouse/lover, parent/child, friend). *There is added stress in maintaining own life and responsibilities when caregiver has to travel some distance to provide care.*[4] *Close relationships may create problems of co-dependency and identification that can be counterproductive to caregiving.*[3]
- Determine current knowledge of the situation, noting misconceptions, lack of information. *May interfere with caregiver/care receiver's response to illness/condition.*[2]
- Compare caregiver's and receiver's view of situation. *Different views need to be openly expressed so each person understands how other sees situation.*[1]
- Note therapeutic regimen and physical/mental condition of care receiver. *Complexity of regimen and caregiver who is elderly, or physically or mentally impaired, will have difficulty managing care giving. Knowledge of these factors is necessary for planning adequate care for the individual. Plans for additional help my be necessary to prevent caregiver role strain.*[1]
- Determine caregiver's level of responsibility, involvement in and anticipated length of care. *Information that may indicate level of stress that may be anticipated for the situation. Progressive debilitation taxes caregiver and may alter ability to meet client/own needs.*[1]
- Identify individual cultural factors and impact on caregiver. *Helps clarify expectations of caregiver/receiver, family, and community. Many cultures, such as American Indian, Cuban, believe strongly in keeping care receiver in the home and caring for them.*[5]
- Ascertain developmental level/abilities and additional responsibilities of caregiver. *Factors indicative of ability of the individual to take on the task of caregiver.*[4]
- Use assessment tool, such as Burden Interview, when appropriate. *Provides additional information to further determine caregiver's abilities.*[1]
- Identify strengths/weaknesses of caregiver and care receiver. *Caregiver may not be aware of demands that will be expected. Knowing these factors helps to determine how to use them to advantage in planning and delivering care.*
- Verify safety of caregiver/receiver. *Identifying and correcting unsafe situations is crucial so both individuals can be assured of safety in dealing with difficult situation.*[2]
- Determine available supports and resources currently used. *Helplful to identify if they are being used effectively.*[4]
- Note any codependency needs of caregiver and plan for dealing appropriately with them. *Can contribute to burn-out unless identified and dealt with.*[2]

NURSING PRIORITY NO. 2. To enhance caregiver's ability to deal with current situation:

- Establish a therapeutic relationship, conveying empathy and unconditional positive regard. *Promotes positive environment in which needs and concerns can be discussed and proactive solutions identified.*[2]

- Discuss strategies to coordinate care and other responsibilities (e.g., employment, care of children/dependents, housekeeping activities). *Such planning can prevent chaos and resultant burnout.*[8]

- Facilitate family conference as appropriate. *To share information and develop plan for involvement in care activities. When everyone is involved and listened to, each person is more likely to carry out his or her responsibilities.*[4]

- Refer to classes and/or specialists (e.g., first aid/CPR classes, enterostomal/physical therapist) for special training as indicated. *Additional information that can help individuals involved feel more competent and able to deal with situation more effectively.*[1]

- Identify additional resources to include financial, legal, respite care. *Can help to resolve problems that arise in the course of caregiving that are out of the knowledge/abilities of the individual. Solving these issues can relieve caregiver of associated anxiety and concern.*[4]

- Identify equipment needs/resources, adaptive aids. *Enhances the independence and safety of the care receiver and reduces chances for untoward incidents.*[1]

- Identify contact person/case manager as needed. *Coordinates care, provides support, assists with problem solving. Assistance with planning minimizes problems that could arise.*[10]

- Provide information and/or demonstrate techniques for dealing with acting out/violent or disoriented behavior. *Planning ways to deal with these behaviors before they occur promotes safety and enhances positive outcomes.*[2]

- Assist caregiver to recognize codependent behaviors (i.e., doing things for others that others are able to do for themselves) and how these behaviors affect the situation. *Provides options for changing behaviors in ways that enhance the caregiving situation.*[2]

NURSING PRIORITY NO. 3. To promote wellness (Teaching/Discharge Considerations):

- Stress importance of self-nurturing (e.g., pursuing self-development interests, personal needs, hobbies, and social activities). *Improves/maintains quality of life for caregiver.*

- Discuss/demonstrate stress-management techniques. *As caregiver learns how to take care of self, chances for burnout are lessened.*[4]

- Encourage involvement in specific support group(s). *Opportunity to be with others in similar situations and discuss different ways to handle problems helps caregiver deal with difficult role in positive ways.*[3]

- Provide bibliotherapy of appropriate references and encourage discussion of information. *Promotes retention of new information that can help caregiver manage more effectively.*[3]

- Assist caregiver to plan for changes that may become necessary for the care receiver (e.g., home care providers, eventual placement in long-term care facility, use of palliative/hospice services). *Getting information and thinking about possibilities will help with decisions when they become necessary.*[8]

- Refer to classes/therapists as indicated. *May need additional support and information.*[3]

- Identify available 12-step program when indicated to provide tools to deal with codependent behaviors that impair level of function. *This type of program can help caregiver learn ways to deal with these behaviors in positive ways.*[1]

- Refer to counseling or psychotherapy as needed. *May need additional help to resolve issues that are interfering with caregiving responsibilities.*[4]

Assessment/Reassessment

- Identified risk factors and caregiver perceptions of situation.
- Reactions of care receiver/family.

Planning

- Treatment plan and individual responsibility for specific activities.
- Teaching plan.

Implementation/Evaluation

- Caregiver/receiver response to interventions/teaching and actions performed.
- Attainment/progress toward desired outcome(s).
- Modifications to plan of care.

Discharge Planning

- Long-term needs and who is responsible for actions to be taken.
- Specific referrals provided for assistance/evaluation.

References

1. Doenges, M., Moorhouse, M., Murr, A. (2002). Nursing Care Plans, Guidelines for Individualizing Patient Care, ed 6. Philadelphia: F. A. Davis.
2. Doenges, M., Townsend, M., & Moorhouse, M. (1998). Psychiatric Care Plans: Guidelines for Individualizing Care, ed 3. Philadelphia: F. A. Davis.
3. Townsend, M. (2003). Psychiatric Mental Health Nursing: Concepts of Care, ed 4. Philadelphia: F. A. Davis.
4. Cox, H., Hinz, M., Lubno, M. A., Newfield, S., Scott-Tilley, D., Slater, M., & Sridaromont, K. (2002). Clinical Applications of Nursing Diagnosis Adult, Child, Women's Psychiatric, Gernontic and Home Health Considerations, ed 4. Philadelphia: F. A. Davis.
5. Lipson, J. G., Dibble, S. L., & Minarik, P. A. (1996). Culture & Nursing Care: A Pocket Guide. San Francisco: School of Nursing, UCSF Nursing Press.
6. Townsend, M. (2001). Nursing diagnoses in Psychiatric Nursing: Care Plans and Psychotropic Medications, ed 5. Philadelphia: F. A. Davis.
7. Hareven, T. K., & Adams, K. J. (eds) (1982). Aging and Life Course Transitions: An Interdisciplinary Perspective. New York: Guilford.
8. Liken, M. A. (2001b). Caregivers in crisis: Moving a relative with Alzheimer's to assisted living. Clin Nurs Res, 10(1):53–69.
9. Liken, M. A. Experiences of family caregivers of a relative with Alzheimer's disease. J Psychosoc Nurs, 39(12):33–37.
10. Halper, J., et. al. (2000). Multiple Sclerosis: Best Practices in Nursing Care (mongraph). Columbia, MD: Medicallance.

impaired verbal Communication

Definition: Decreased, delayed, or absent ability to receive, process, transmit, and use a system of symbols

RELATED FACTORS

Decrease in circulation to brain, brain tumor

Anatomic deficit (e.g., cleft palate, alteration of the neurovascular visual system, auditory system, or phonatory apparatus)

Difference related to developmental age

Physical barrier (tracheostomy, intubation)

 Cultural Collaborative  Community/ Home Care Diagnostic Studies Pediatric/Geriatric/Lifespan Medications

Physiologic conditions [e.g., dyspnea]; alteration of CNS; weakening of the musculoskeletal system

Psychological barriers (e.g., psychosis, lack of stimuli); emotional conditions [depression, panic, anger]; stress

Environmental barriers

Cultural differences

Lack of information

Side effects of medication

Alteration of self-esteem or self-concept

Altered perceptions

Absence of SOs

DEFINING CHARACTERISTICS

Subjective
[Reports of difficulty expressing self]

Objective
Unable to speak dominant language

Speaks or verbalizes with difficulty

Does not or cannot speak

Disorientation in the three spheres of time, space, person

Stuttering; slurring

Dyspnea

Difficulty forming words or sentences (e.g., aphonia, dyslalia, dysarthria)

Difficulty expressing thoughts verbally (e.g., aphasia, dysphasia, apraxia, dyslexia)

Inappropriate verbalization, [incessant, loose association of ideas, flight of ideas]

Difficulty in comprehending and maintaining the usual communicating pattern

Absence of eye contact or difficulty in selective attending; partial or total visual deficit

Inability or difficulty in use of facial or body expressions

Willful refusal to speak

[Inability to modulate speech]

[Message inappropriate to content]

[Use of nonverbal cues (e.g., pleading eyes, gestures, turning away)]

[Frustration, anger, hostility]

SAMPLE CLINICAL APPLICATIONS: brain injury/stroke, facial trauma, head/neck cancer, radical neck surgery/laryngectomy, cleft lip/palate, dementia, Tourette's syndrome, autism, schizophrenia

DESIRED OUTCOMES/EVALUATION CRITERIA
Sample NOC linkages:

Communication Ability: Ability to receive, interpret, and express spoken, written, and nonverbal messages

Communication: Expressive Ability: Ability to express and interpret verbal and/or nonverbal messages

Information Processing: Ability to acquire, organize, and use information

Client Will (Include Specific Time Frame)
- Verbalize or indicate an understanding of the communication difficulty and plans for ways of handling.

- Establish method of communication in which needs can be expressed.
- Participate in therapeutic communication (e.g., using silence, acceptance, restating reflecting, Active-listening, and I-messages).
- Demonstrate congruent verbal and nonverbal communication.
- Use resources appropriately.

ACTIONS/INTERVENTIONS

Sample NIC linkages:

Communication Enhancement: Speech Deficit: Assistance in accepting and learning alternative methods for living with impaired speech

Communication Enhancement: Hearing Deficit: Assistance in accepting and learning alternative methods for living with diminished hearing

Active Listening: Attending closely to and attaching significance to a patient's verbal and nonverbal messages

NURSING PRIORITY NO. **1.** To assess causative/contributing factors:

- Review results of diagnostic studies (e.g., speech/language and hearing evaluations, brain function studies, psychological evaluations) as needed *to assess/delineate underlying conditions affecting verbal communication.*
- Note new onset or diagnosis of deficits that will progress/permanently affect speech.
- Determine age/developmental considerations: 1) child too young for language, or has developmental delays affecting speech and language skills/comprehension; 2) autism or other mental impairments; 3) older client doesn't or isn't able to speak, verbalizes with difficulty, has difficulty hearing or comprehending language or concepts.[1–3]
- Note parent/caregiver's speech patterns and interactive manner of communicating, including gestures.
- Obtain history of hearing/speech related pathophysiology or trauma (e.g., cleft lip/palate, traumatic brain injury/shaken baby syndrome, frequent ear infections affecting hearing, or sensorineural changes associated with aging, etc.).
- Identify dominant language spoken. *Knowing the language spoken and fluency in English is important to understanding. While some individuals may be fluent in English, they may still have limited understanding of the language, especially the language of health professionals, and may have difficulty answering questions, describing symptoms, or following directions.*[17]
- Ascertain whether client is recent immigrant/country of origin and what cultural, ethnic group client identifies as own *(e.g., recent immigrant may identify with home country, and its people, beliefs and healthcare practices).*[6]
- Determine cultural factors affecting communication such as beliefs concerning touch and eye contact *(certain cultures may prohibit client from speaking directly to healthcare provider; some Native Americans, Appalachians, or young African Americans may interpret direct eye contact as disrespectful, impolite, an invasion of privacy, or aggressive; Latinos, Arabs, and Asians may shout and gesture when excited, etc.*[4]*; silence and tone of voice has various meanings, and slang words can cause confusion/misunderstandings)*[5]*; and conditions/factors of high prevalence in certain groups/populations (e.g., middle ear infection high among Native Americans with potential for hearing deficits).*
- Note presence of physical barriers including tracheostomy/intubation, wired jaws; or problem resulting in failure of voice production or "problem voice" *(pitch, loudness, or quality calls attention to voice rather than what speaker is saying as might occur with electronic voice box or "talking valves" when tracheostomy in place).*[7,8]
- Note physiologic/neurologic conditions impacting speech such as severe shortness of

 Cultural Collaborative Community/ Home Care 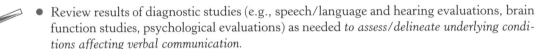 Diagnostic Studies 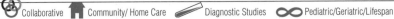 Pediatric/Geriatric/Lifespan Medications

breath, cleft palate, facial trauma, neuromuscular weakness, stroke, brain tumors/infections, dementia, brain trauma, deafness/hard of hearing.

- Review results of neurologic testing such as electroencephalogram (EEG), computed tomography (CT) scan.
- Identify environmental barriers: recent or chronic exposure to hazardous noise in home, job, recreation and healthcare setting (e.g., rock music, jackhammer, snowmobile, lawnmower, truck traffic/busy highway, heavy equipment, medical equipment). *Noise not only affects hearing, it increases blood pressure and breathing rate, can have negative cardiovascular effects, disturbs digestion, increases fatigue, causes irritability, and reduces attention to tasks.*[9]
- Investigate client reports of problems such as constantly raising voice to be heard, can't hear someone 2 feet away, conversation in room sounds muffled/dull, too much energy required to listen, or pain/ringing in ears after exposure to noise.[9]
- Determine if client with communication impairment has a speech or language problem, or both. *Language is code made up of rules (e.g., what words mean, how to make new words, combine words and what combinations work in what situations). When a person cannot understand the language code, there is a receptive problem. When a speech problem is present, the language code can be correct, but words might be garbled, person may stutter, or there may be problems with voice. Language and speech problems can exist together or by themselves.*[10]
- Determine presence of psychological/emotional barriers: history/presence of psychiatric conditions (e.g., manic-depressive illness, schizoid/affective behavior); high level of anxiety, frustration, or fear; presence of angry, hostile behavior. Note effect on speech and communication.[1,4]
- Identify information barriers such as lack of knowledge/need of information or misunderstanding of terms related to client's medical conditions, procedures, treatments and equipment.[4]
- Assess level of understanding in a sensitive manner. *Individual may be reluctant to say they don't understand or be embarrassed to ask for help. Head nodding and smiles do not always mean comprehension.*[17]

NURSING PRIORITY NO. 2. To assist client to establish a means of communication to express needs, wants, ideas, and questions:

- Establish rapport with the client, initiate eye contact, shake hands, address by preferred name, meet family members present; ask simple questions, smile, engage in brief social conversation if appropriate. *Helps establish a trusting relationship with client/family, demonstrating caring about the client as a person.*[2–4]
- Provide glasses, hearing aids, dentures, electronic speech devices as needed *to maximize sensory perception and improve speech patterns.*[2,4]
- Maintain a calm, unhurried manner, sit at client's eye level if possible. Provide sufficient time for client to respond. *Sitting down conveys that nurse has time and interest in communicating.*
- Pay attention to speaker. Be an active listener.
- Begin conversation with elderly individual with casual and familiar topics (e.g., weather, happenings with family members) *to convey interest and stimulate conversation and reminiscence.*[2,15]
- Reduce distractions and background noise (e.g., close the door, turn down the radio/television).[15]
- Refrain from shouting when directing speech to confused, deaf or hearing-impaired client. Speak slowly and clearly, pitching voice low *to increase likelihood of being understood.*[2,16]

 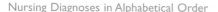

- Be honest and let speaker know when you have difficulty understanding. Repeat part of message that you do understand, *so speaker doesn't have to repeat entire message.*[11]
- Clarify type and special features of aphasia, when present. *Aphasia is a temporary, permanent or progressive impairment of language, affecting production or comprehension of speech and the ability to read or write.*[11] *Some people with aphasia have problems primarily with expressive language (what is said), others with receptive language (what is understood). Aphasia can also be global (person understands almost nothing that is said, and says little or nothing).*[4,11]
- Note diagnosis of apraxia *(impairment in carrying out purposeful movements affecting rhythm and timing of speech),* dysarthria *(language code can be correct but the right body parts do not move at the right time to produce the right message),* or dementia *(defect is in decline in mental functions, including memory, attention, intellect, and personality)* to help clarify individual needs, appropriate interventions.[11,12]
- Determine meaning of words used by the client and congruency of communication and nonverbal messages.
- Evaluate the meaning of words that are used/needed to describe aspects of healthcare (e.g., pain) and ascertain how to communicate important concepts.[5]
- Observe body language, eye movements, and behavioral clues. *For example, when pain is present, client may react with tears, grimacing, stiff posture, turning away, angry outbursts.*[14]
- Use confrontation skills, when appropriate, within an established nurse-client relationship *to clarify discrepancies between verbal and nonverbal cues.*[4,16]
- Point to objects, or demonstrate desired actions, when client has difficulty with language. *Speaker's own body language can be used to assist client's understanding.*
- Work with confused, brain injured, mentally disabled or sensory deprived client *to correctly interpret his/her environment.* Establish understanding/convey to others meaning of symbolic speech *to reduce frustration.* Teach basic signs such as "eat," "toilet," "more," "finished" *to communicate basic needs.*[4,16]
- Provide reality orientation by responding with simple, straightforward, honest statements. Associate words with objects using repetition and redundancy *to improve communication patterns.*[2,4,16]
- Assess psychological response to communication impairment, willingness to find alternate means of communication.
- Identify family member who can speak for client, and who is the family decision-maker regarding healthcare decisions.[5,17]
- Obtain interpreter with language or signing abilities and preferably with medical knowledge when needed. *Federal law mandates that interpretation services be made available. Trained, professional interpreter who translates precisely and possesses a basic understanding of medical terminology and healthcare ethics is preferred (over a family member) to enhance client and provider interactions.*[6,18]
- Evaluate ability to read/write and musculoskeletal status including manual dexterity (e.g., ability to hold a pen and write); and need/desire for pictures or written communications and instructions as part of treatment plan.
  Plan for/provide alternative methods of communication[2–4,18]:
  Provide pad and pencil, slate board *if client able to write but cannot speak.*
  Use letter/picture board *if client can't write and picture concepts are understandable to both parties.*
  Establish hand/eye signals *if client can understand language, but cannot speak or has physical barrier to writing.*

Remove isolation mask *if client is deaf and reads lips.*
Obtain/provide access to typewriter/computer *if communication impairment is long-standing/or client is used to this method.*

- Consider form of communication when placing IV. *IV positioned in hand/wrist may limit ability to write or sign.*
- Answer call bell promptly. Anticipate needs and avoid leaving client alone with no way to summon assistance. *Reduces fear and conveys caring to client and protects nurse from problems associated with failure to provide due care.*[13]
- Refer for appropriate therapies/support services. *Client and family may have multiple needs (e.g., sources for further examinations and rehabilitation services, local community/national support groups and services for disabled, financial assistance with obtaining necessary aids for improving communication).*[4,13]

NURSING PRIORITY NO. 3. To promote wellness (Teaching/Discharge Considerations):

- Encourage family presence and use of touch. Involve them in plan of care as much as possible. *Enhances participation and commitment to plan, assists in normalizing family role patterns, and provides support and encouragement when learning new patterns of communicating.*[4]
- Review information about condition, prognosis, and treatment with client/SO(s).
- Reinforce that loss of speech does not imply loss of intelligence.
- Teach client and family the needed techniques for communication, whether it be speech/language techniques or alternate modes of communicating. Encourage family to involve client in family activities using enhanced communication techniques. *Reduces stress of difficult situation and promotes earlier return to more normal life patterns.*[4]
- Assess family for possible role changes resulting from client's impairment. Discuss methods of dealing with impairment.
- Use and assist client/SOs to learn therapeutic communication skills of acknowledgment, active-listening, and I-messages. *Improves general communication skills, emphasizes acceptance and conveys respect.*
- Discuss ways to provide environmental stimuli as appropriate *to maintain contact with reality;* or reduce environmental stimuli/noise. *Unwanted sound affects physical health, increases fatigue, reduces attention to tasks, and makes speech communication more difficult.*[9,15]
- Refer to appropriate resources (e.g., speech therapist, group therapy, individual/family and/or psychiatric counseling) *to address long-term needs, enhance coping skills.*
- Refer to NDs ineffective Coping, disabled family Coping, Anxiety, Fear for additional interventions.

DOCUMENTATION FOCUS

Assessment/Reassessment
- Assessment findings/pertinent history information (i.e., physical/psychological/cultural concerns).
- Meaning of nonverbal cues, level of anxiety client exhibits.

Planning
- Plan of care and interventions (e.g., type of alternative communication/translator).
- Teaching plan.

Implementation/Evaluation
- Response to interventions/teaching and actions performed.
- Attainment of/progress toward desired outcomes.
- Modifications to plan of care.

Discharge Planning
- Discharge needs/referrals made, additional resources available.

References

1. Szymanski, L., & King, B. (1999). Practice parameters for the assessment and treatment of children, adolescents, and adults with mental retardation and comorbid mental disorders. American Academy of Child and Adolescent Psychiatry (AACAP) Working Group on Quality Issues. J Am Acad Child Adolesc Psychiatry, 38(12 suppl).
2. Stanley, M., & Beare, P. G. (1999). Gerontological Nursing: A Health Promotion Approach, ed 2. Philadelphia: F. A. Davis.
3. Cox, H. C., et al. (2002). Clinical Applications of Nursing Diagnosis: Adult, Child, Women's, Psychiatric, Gerontic, and Home Health Considerations, ed 4. Philadelphia: F. A. Davis.
4. Doenges, M. E., Moorhouse, M. F., & Geissler-Murr, A. C. (2002). Nurse's Pocket Guide: Diagnoses, Interventions, and Rationales, ed 8. Philadelphia: F. A. Davis, pp 134–138.
5. Purnell, L., & Paulanka, B. (1998). Transcultural Health Care: A Culturally Diverse Approach, ed 2. Philadelphia: F. A. Davis.
6. Enslein, J., et al. (2002). Evidence-based protocol. Interpreter facilitation for persons with limited English proficiency. University of Iowa Gerontological Nursing Interventions Research Center. Retrieved September 2003, from National Guidelines Clearinghouse. Available at: www. guideline.gov.
7. Questions/Answers about Voice Problems. (Information sheet). Retrieved September 2003, from American Speech-Language-Hearing Association (ASHA). Available at: www.asha.org.
8. Speech for Patients with Tracheostomies or Ventilators. (Information Sheet). Retrieved September 2003, from American Speech-Language-Hearing Association (ASHA). Available at: www.asha.org.
9. Noise. Retrieved September 2003, from American Speech-Language-Hearing Association (ASHA). Available at: www.asha.org.
10. What is Language? What is Speech? Retrieved September 2003, from American Speech-Language-Hearing Association (ASHA). Available at www.asha.org.
11. Aphasia Fact Sheet. (Revised June 1999). Retrieved September 2003, from National Aphasia Association (NAA). Available at: www.aphasia.org.
12. Understanding Primary Progressive Aphasia. (Revised January 2001). Retrieved September 2003, from National Aphasia Association. Available at: www.aphasia.org.
13. Doenges, M. E., Moorhouse, M. F., & Geissler-Murr, A. C. (2002). Nursing Care Plans: Guidelines for Individualizing Patient Care, ed 6. Philadelphia: F. A. Davis.
14. Hahn, J. (1999). Cueing in to patient language. Reflections, 25(1), 8–11.
15. Tip Sheet: "I can hear, but I can't understand what's being said." (2000). Retrieved September 2003, from American Speech-Language-Hearing Association (ASHA). Available at: www.asha.org.
16. Research Dissemination Core: Acute Confusion/delirium. (1998). Iowa City, IA: University of Iowa Gerontological Nursing Interventions Research Center.
17. Lipson, J. G., Dibble, S. L., & Minarik, P. A. (1996). Culture & Nursing Care: A Pocket Guide. San Francisco: UCSF Nursing Press.
18. Harquez-Rebello, M. C., & Tornel-Costa M. C. (1997). Design of a non-verbal method of communication using cartoons. Rev Neurol, 25(148), 2027–2045.

readiness for enhanced Communication

Definition: A pattern of exchanging information and ideas with others that is sufficient for meeting one's needs and life' goals and can be strengthened.

RELATED FACTORS

To be developed by nurse researchers and submitted to NANDA

 Cultural Collaborative Community/ Home Care Diagnostic Studies 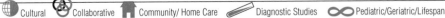 Pediatric/Geriatric/Lifespan Medications

Subjective
Expresses willingness to enhance communication
Expresses thoughts and feelings
Expresses satisfaction with ability to share information and ideas with others

Objective
Able to speak or write a language
Forms words, phrases, and language
Uses and interprets nonverbal cues appropriately

SAMPLE CLINICAL APPLICATIONS: brain injury/stroke, head/neck cancer, facial trauma, cleft lip/palate, Tourette's syndrome, autism

DESIRED OUTCOMES/EVALUATION CRITERIA
Sample NOC Linkages:

Communication Ability: Ability to receive, interpret, and express spoken, written, and non-verbal messages
Information Processing: Ability to acquire, organize, and use information

Client/SO/Caregiver Will (Include Specific Time Frame)
- Verbalize or indicate an understanding of the communication difficulty and ways of handling
- Be able to express information, thoughts and feelings in a satisfactory manner

ACTIONS/INTERVENTIONS
Sample NIC Linkages:

Communication Enhancement: Speech Deficit: Assistance in accepting and learning alternative methods for living with impaired speech
Communication Enhancement: Hearing Deficit: Assistance in accepting and learning alternative methods for living with diminished hearing
Active Listening: Attending closely to and attaching significance to a patient's verbal and nonverbal messages

NURSING PRIORITY NO. 1. Assess how client is managing communication and potential difficulties:

- Ascertain circumstances that result in client's desire to improve communication. *Many factors are involved in communication and identifying specific needs/expectations helps in developing realistic goals and determining likelihood of success.*
- Evaluate mental status. *Disorientation, psychotic conditions may be affecting speech and the communication of thoughts, needs and desires.*
- Determine client's developmental level of speech and language comprehension. *Provides baseline information for developing plan for improvement.*
- Determine ability to read/write. *Evaluating grasp of language as well as musculoskeletal states, including manual dexterity (e.g., ability to hold a pen and write) provides information about nature of client's situation. Educational plan can address language skills. Neuromuscular deficits will require individual physical/occupational therapeutic program to correct.*
- 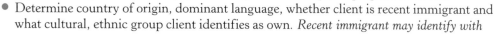 Determine country of origin, dominant language, whether client is recent immigrant and what cultural, ethnic group client identifies as own. *Recent immigrant may identify with*

home country and its people, language, beliefs and healthcare practices affecting desire to learn language and improve ability to interact in new country.[1]

- Ascertain if interpreter is needed/desired. *Law mandates that interpretation services be made available. Trained, professional interpreter who translates precisely and possesses a basic understanding of medical terminology and healthcare ethics is preferred over family member to enhance client and provider interaction and sharing of information.*[1]
- Determine comfort level in expression of feelings and concepts in nonproficient language. *Anxiety about language difficulty can interfere with ability to communicate effectively.*
- Note any physical barriers to effective communication (e.g. hearing impairment, talking tracheostomy apparatus, wired jaws) or physiological/neurological conditions (e.g. severe shortness of breath, neuromuscular weakness, stroke, brain trauma, deafness, cleft palate, facial trauma). *Client may be dealing with speech/language comprehension or have voice production problems (pitch, loudness or quality), which calls attention to voice rather than what speaker is saying. These barriers will need to be addressed to enable client to improve communication skills.*[2,3]
- Clarify meaning of words used by the client to describe important aspects of life and health/well-being (e.g., pain, sorrow, anxiety). *Words can easily be misinterpreted when sender and receiver have different ideas about their meanings. This can affect the way both client and caregivers communicate important concepts. Restating what one has heard can clarify whether an expressed statement has been understood or misinterpreted.*[4]
- Evaluate level of anxiety, frustration, or fear; presence of angry, hostile behavior. *Emotional/psychiatric issues can affect communication and interfere with understanding.*
- Evaluate congruency of verbal and nonverbal messages. *It is estimated that 65% to 95% of communication is nonverbal and communication is enhanced when verbal and nonverbal messages are congruent.*
- Determine lack of knowledge or misunderstanding of terms related to client's specific situation. *Indicators of need for additional information, clarification to help client improve ability to communicate.*
- Evaluate need/desire for pictures or written communications and instructions as part of treatment plan. *Alternative methods of communication can help client feel understood and promote feelings of satisfaction with interaction.*

NURSING PRIORITY NO. 2. To improve client's ability to communicate thoughts, needs and ideas:

- Maintain a calm, unhurried manner. Provide sufficient time for client to respond. *An atmosphere in which client is free to speak without fear of criticism provides the opportunity to explore all the issues involved in making decisions to improve communication skills.*[10]
- Pay attention to speaker. Be an active listener. *The use of active listening communicates acceptance and respect for the client, establishing trust and promoting openness and honest expression. It communicates a belief that the client is a capable and competent person.*
- Sit down, maintain eye contact, preferably at client's level and spend time with the client. *Conveys; message that the nurse has time and interest in communicating.*[10]
- Observe body language, eye movements, and behavioral clues. *May reveal unspoken concerns; for example, when pain is present, client may react with tears, grimacing, stiff posture; turning away, and angry outbursts.*[5]
- Help client identify and learn to avoid use of nontherapeutic communication. *These barriers are recognized as detriments to open communication and learning to avoid them maximizes the effectiveness of communication between client and others.*

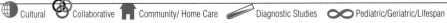 Cultural   Collaborative   Community/ Home Care   Diagnostic Studies   Pediatric/Geriatric/Lifespan   Medications

- Establish hand/eye signals if indicated. *Neurological impairments may allow client to understand language, but not be able to speak and/or has a physical barrier to writing.*[6]
- Obtain interpreter with language or signing abilities as needed. *May be needed to enhance understanding of words, language concepts, or needs, enabling accurate interpretation of communication.*[6,10]
- Encourage use of pad and pencil, slate board, letter/picture board, as indicated. *When client has physical impairments that interfere with spoken communication, alternate means can provide concepts that are understandable to both parties.*[4,10]
- Obtain/provide access to typewriter/"talking" computer. *Use of these devices may be more helpful when impairment is long-standing or when client is used to using them.*[1]
- Respect client's cultural communication needs. *Different cultures can dictate beliefs of what is normal or abnormal, (i.e., in some cultures, eye-to-eye contact is considered disrespectful, impolite, or an invasion of privacy; silence and tone of voice have various meanings, and slang words can cause confusion).*[4]
- Provide glasses, hearing aids, dentures, electronic speech devices, as needed. *These devices maximize sensory perception and can improve understanding and enhance speech patterns.*[7]
- Reduce distractions and background noises (e.g., close the door, turn down the radio/television). *A distracting environment can interfere with communication limiting attention to tasks, and makes speech and communication more difficult. Reducing noise can help both parties hear clearly, improving understanding.*[8]
- Associate words with objects using repetition and redundancy, point to objects, or demonstrate desired actions. *Speaker's own body language can be used to enhance client's understanding when neurological conditions result in difficulty understanding language.*[9]
- Use confrontation skills carefully when appropriate, within an established nurse-client relationship. *Can be used to clarify discrepancies between verbal and nonverbal cues enabling client to look at areas that may require change.*[10]

NURSING PRIORITY NO. 3. To promote optimum communication:

- Discuss with family/SO and other caregivers effective ways in which the client communicates. *Identifying positive aspects of current communication skills enables family members to learn and move forward in desire to enhance ways of interacting.*[10]
- Encourage client and family use of successful techniques for communication, whether it is speech/language techniques or alternate modes of communicating. *Enhances family relationships and promotes self-esteem for all members as they are able to communicate clearly regardless of the problems which have interfered with ability to interact.*[10]
- Reinforce client/SOs learning and use of therapeutic communication skills of acknowledgment, Active-listening, and I-messages. *Improves general communication skills, emphasizes acceptance and conveys respect enabling family relationships to improve.*
- Refer to appropriate resources (e.g., speech therapist, language classes, individual/family and/or psychiatric counseling). *May need further assistance to overcome problems that are preventing family from reaching desired goal of enhanced communication.*

DOCUMENTATION FOCUS

Assessment/Reassessment
- Assessment findings/pertinent history information (i.e., physical/psychological/cultural concerns).
- Meaning of nonverbal cues, level of anxiety client exhibits.

Planning
- Plan of care and interventions (e.g., type of alternative communication/translator).
- Teaching plan.

Implementation/Evaluation
- Progress toward desired outcome(s).
- Modifications to plan of care.

Discharge Planning
- Discharge needs/referrals made, additional resources available.

References

1. Enslein, J., et al: Evidence-based protocol. Interpreter facilitation for persons with limited English proficiency. (2002). University of Iowa Gerontological Nursing Interventions Research center. From National Guidelines Clearinghouse. Available at: http://www.guideline.gov. Accessed June 2003.
2. Questions/Answers about Voice Problems. Information Sheet. American Speech-Language-Hearing Association (ASHA). Available at: http://www.asha.org. Accessed June 2003.
3. Speech for Clients with Tracheostomies or Ventilators. Information Sheet. American Speech-Language-Hearing Association (ASHA). Available at: http://www.asha.org. Accessed June 2003.
4. Purnell, L. & Paulanka, B. (1998). Transcultural Health Care: A Culturally Diverse Approach, ed 2. Philadelphia: F. A. Davis.
5. Hahn, J. (1999). Cueing in to client language. Reflections, 25(1):8–11.
6. What is Language? What is Speech? Information Sheet. American Speech-Language-Hearing Association (ASHA). Available at: http://www.asah.org. Accessed June 2003.
7. Stanley, M., & Beare, P. G. (1999). Gerontological Nursing: A Health Promotion Approach, ed 2. Philadelphia: F. A. Davis.
8. Noise. Information Sheet. American Speech-Language-Hearing Association (ASHA). Available at: http://www.asha.org. Accessed June 2003.
9. Acute Confusion/delirium. (1998). Research Dissemination Core University of Iowa Gerontological Nursing Interventions Research Center. Iowa City, IA.
10. Cox, H. C., et al. (2002). Clinical Applications of Nursing Diagnosis: Adult, Child, Women's, Psychiatric, Gerontic, and Home Health Considerations, ed 4. Philadelphia: F. A. Davis.

Helpful Resources

- Gordon, T. (2000). Parent Effectiveness Training, updated edition. New York: Three Rivers Press.
- Doenges, M. E., Moorhouse, M. F., & Geissler-Murr, A. C. (2004). Nurse's Pocket Guide: Diagnoses, Interventions, and Rationales, ed 9. Philadelphia: F. A. Davis.
- Townsend, M. C. (2003). Psychiatric Mental Health Nursing Concepts of Care, ed 4. Philadelphia: F. A. Davis.
- Szymanski, L., & King, B. (1999). Practice parameters for the assessment and treatment of children, adolescents, and adults with mental retardation and comorbid mental disorders. J Am Acad Child Adolesc Psychiatry, Dec, 38 (12 suppl).

decisional Conflict [specify]

Definition: Uncertainty about course of action to be taken when choice among competing actions involves risk, loss, or challenge to personal life values

 Cultural Collaborative Community/ Home Care  Diagnostic Studies Pediatric/Geriatric/Lifespan Medications

RELATED FACTORS

Unclear personal values/beliefs; perceived threat to value system
Lack of experience or interference with decision making
Lack of relevant information, multiple or divergent sources of information
Support system deficit
[Age, developmental state]
[Family system, sociocultural factors]
[Cognitive, emotional, behavioral level of functioning]

DEFINING CHARACTERISTICS

Subjective

Verbalized uncertainty about choices or of undesired consequences of alternative actions being considered
Verbalized feeling of distress or questioning personal values and beliefs while attempting a decision

Objective

Vacillation between alternative choices; delayed decision making
Self-focusing
Physical signs of distress or tension (increased heart rate; increased muscle tension; restlessness; and so on)

SAMPLE CLINICAL APPLICATIONS: therapeutic options with undesired side effects (e.g., amputation, visible scarring)/conflicting with belief system (e.g., blood transfusion, termination of pregnancy), chronic disease states, dementia/Alzheimer's disease, terminal/end-of-life situations

DESIRED OUTCOMES/EVALUATION CRITERIA

Sample NOC linkages:

Decision Making: Ability to choose between two or more alternatives
Health Beliefs: Personal convictions that influence health behaviors
Psychosocial Adjustment: Life Change: Psychosocial adaptation of an individual to a life change

Client Will (Include Specific Time Frame)

- Verbalize awareness of positive and negative aspect of choices/alternative actions.
- Acknowledge/ventilate feelings of anxiety and distress associated with choice/related to making difficult decision.
- Identify personal values and beliefs concerning issues.
- Make decision(s) and express satisfaction with choices.
- Meet psychological needs as evidenced by appropriate expression of feelings, identification of options, and use of resources.
- Display relaxed manner/calm demeanor, free of physical signs of distress.

ACTIONS/INTERVENTIONS

Sample NIC linkages:

Decision-Making Support: Providing information and support for a person who is making a decision regarding healthcare

Values Clarification: Assisting another to clarify her/his own values in order to facilitate effective decision making

Coping Enhancement: Assisting a patient to adapt to perceived stressors, changes, or threats that interfere with meeting life demands and roles

NURSING PRIORITY NO. 1. To assess causative/contributing factors:

• Determine usual ability to manage own affairs. Clarify who has legal right to intervene on behalf of child (e.g., parent, other relative, or court-appointed guardian/advocate). *Family disruption/conflicts can complicate decision-making process. Unimpaired individuals have the right to make their own decisions.*[4]

• Note expressions of indecision, dependence on others, availability/involvement of support persons (e.g., lack of/conflicting advice). Ascertain dependency of other(s) on client and/or issues of codependency. *Influence of others may lead client to make decision that is not what is really wanted.*[1]

• Actively listen/identify reason for indecisiveness. *Helps client to clarify problem and begin looking for resolution.*[2]

• Determine effectiveness of current problem-solving techniques. *Provides information about client's ability to make decisions that are needed/desired.*[1]

• Note presence/intensity of physical signs of anxiety (e.g., increased heart rate, muscle tension). *Client may be conflicted about the decision that is required and may need help to deal with anxiety to begin to deal with reality of situation.*[2]

• Listen for expressions of inability to find meaning in life/reason for living, feelings of futility, or alienation from God and others around them. (Refer to ND Spiritual Distress, as indicated.) *May need to talk about reasons for feelings of alienation to resolve concerns.*[7]

NURSING PRIORITY NO. 2. To assist client to develop/effectively use problem-solving skills:

• Promote safe and hopeful environment, as needed. *Client needs to be protected while he or she regains inner control.*[8]

• Encourage verbalization of conflicts/concerns. *Helps client to clarify these issues so he or she can come to a resolution of the situation.*[8]

• Accept verbal expressions of anger/guilt, setting limits on maladaptive behavior. *Promotes client safety. Such expressions are to be expected and need to be allowed. If negative behavior were allowed, client would regret actions and self-esteem would suffer.*[2]

• Clarify and prioritize individual goals, noting where the subject of the "conflict" falls on this scale. *Helps to identify importance of problems client is addressing, enabling realistic problem-solving.*[2]

• Identify strengths and presence of positive coping skills (e.g., use of relaxation technique, willingness to express feelings). *Helpful for developing solutions to current situation.*[1]

• Identify positive aspects of this experience and assist client to view it as a learning opportunity. *Enables client to develop new and creative solutions. Reframing the situation can help the client see things in a different light.*[1]

• Correct misperceptions client may have and provide factual information. *Promotes understanding and enables client to make better decisions for own situation.*[1]

• Provide opportunities for client to make simple decisions regarding self-care and other daily activities. Accept choice not to do so. Advance complexity of choices as tolerated.

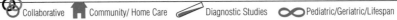 Cultural  Collaborative   Community/ Home Care Diagnostic Studies   Pediatric/Geriatric/Lifespan   Medications

Acceptance of what client wants to do, with gentle encouragement to progress, enhances self-esteem and ability to try more.[1]

- Encourage child to make developmentally appropriate decisions concerning own care. *Fosters child's sense of self-worth, enhances ability to learn/exercise coping skills.*[4]
- Discuss time considerations, setting time line for small steps and considering consequences related to not making/postponing specific decisions to facilitate resolution of conflict. *When time is a factor in making a decision, these strategies can promote movement toward solution.*[4]
- Have client list some alternatives to present situation or decisions, using a brainstorming process. Include family in this activity as indicated (e.g., placement of parent in long-term care facility, use of intervention process with addicted member). Refer to NDs interrupted Family Processes; dysfunctional Family Processes: alcoholism; compromised family Coping. *Involving family and looking at different options can promote successful resolution of decision to be made.*[8]
- Practice use of problem-solving process with current situation/decision. *Promotes identification of different possibilities that may not have been thought of otherwise.*[1]
- Discuss/clarify spiritual concerns, accepting client's values in a nonjudgmental manner. *Client will be willing to consider own situation when accepted as an individual of worth.*[1]

NURSING PRIORITY NO. 3. To promote wellness (Teaching/Discharge Considerations):

- Promote opportunities for using conflict-resolution skills, identifying steps as client does each one. *Learning this process can help to solve current problem and provide the person with skills they can use in the future.*[3]
- Provide positive feedback for efforts and progress noted. *Client needs to hear he or she is doing well and this feedback promotes continuation of efforts.*[2]
- Encourage involvement of family/SO(s) as desired/available. *Provides support for the client and facilitates resolution when client has this support.*[10]
- Support client for decisions made, especially if consequences are unexpected, difficult to cope with. *Positive feedback promotes feelings of success even when difficult situations occur.*[10]
- Encourage attendance at stress reduction, assertiveness classes. *Learning these skills can help client achieve lowered stress level which can promote ability to make decisions.*[4]
- Refer to other resources as necessary (e.g., clergy, psychiatric clinical nurse specialist/psychiatrist, family/marital therapist, addiction support groups). *May need this additional help to deal with current problems and facilitate problem-solving and decision making.*[2]

DOCUMENTATION FOCUS

Assessment/Reassessment
- Assessment findings/behavioral responses, degree of impairment in lifestyle functioning.
- Individuals involved in the conflict.
- Personal values/beliefs.

Planning
- Plan of care/interventions and who is involved in the planning process.
- Teaching plan.

Implementation/Evaluation
- Client's and involved individual's responses to interventions/teaching and actions performed.
- Ability to express feelings, identify options; use of resources.
- Attainment/progress toward desired outcome(s).
- Modifications to plan of care.

Discharge Planning
- Long-term needs/referrals, actions to be taken, and who is responsible for doing.
- Specific referrals made.

References

1. Doenges, M., Moorhouse, M., & Murr, A. (2002). Nursing Care Plans, Guidelines for Individualizing Patient Care, ed 6. Philadelphia: F. A. Davis.
2. Doenges, M., Townsend, M., & Moorhouse, M. (1998). Psychiatric Care Plans: Guidelines for Individualizing Care, ed 3. Philadelphia: F. A. Davis.
3. Townsend, M. (2003). Psychiatric Mental Health Nursing: Concepts of Care, ed 4. Philadelphia: F. A. Davis.
4. Cox, H., Hinz, M., Lubno, M. A., Newfield, S., Scott-Tilley, D., Slater, M., & Sridaromont, K. (2002). Clinical Applications of Nursing Diagnosis Adult, Child, Women's Psychiatric, Gerontic and Home Health Considerations, ed 4. Philadelphia: F. A. Davis.
5. Lipson, J. G., Dibble, S. L., & Minarik, P. A. (1996). Culture & Nursing Care: A Pocket Guide. San Francisco: School of Nursing, UCSF Nursing Press.
6. Townsend, M. (2001). Nursing Diagnoses in Psychiatric Nursing: Care Plans and Psychotropic Medications, ed 5. Philadelphia: F. A. Davis.
7. Hareven, T. K., & Adams, K. J. (eds). (1982). Aging and Life Course Transitions: An Interdisciplinary Perspective. New York: Guilford.
8. Liken, M. A. (2001b). Caregivers in crisis: Moving a relative with Alzheimer's to assisted living. Clin Nurs Res, 10(1), 53–69.
9. Liken, M. A. (2001). Experiences of family caregivers of a relative with Alzheimer's disease. J Psychosoc Nurs, 39(12), 33–37.
10. Halper, J, et. al. Multiple sclerosis: Best practices in nursing care (monograph). Columbia, MD: Medicallance.

parental role Conflict

Definition: Parent experience of role confusion and conflict in response to crisis

RELATED FACTORS
Separation from child because of chronic illness [/disability]

Intimidation with invasive or restrictive modalities (e.g., isolation, intubation); specialized care centers, policies

Home care of a child with special needs (e.g., apnea monitoring, postural drainage, hyperalimentation)

Change in marital status

Interruptions of family life because of home-care regimen (treatments, caregivers, lack of respite)

DEFINING CHARACTERISTICS

Subjective
Parent(s) express(es) concerns/feeling of inadequacy to provide for child's physical and emotional needs during hospitalization or in the home

 Cultural Collaborative Community/ Home Care Diagnostic Studies 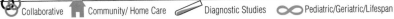 Pediatric/Geriatric/Lifespan Medications

Parent(s) express(es) concerns about changes in parental role, family functioning, family communication, family health

Expresses concern about perceived loss of control over decisions relating to child

Verbalizes feelings of guilt, anger, fear, anxiety and/or frustrations about effect of child's illness on family process

Objective

Demonstrates disruption in caretaking routines

Reluctant to participate in usual caretaking activities even with encouragement and support

Demonstrates feelings of guilt, anger, fear, anxiety, and/or frustrations about the effect of child's illness on family process

SAMPLE CLINICAL APPLICATIONS: prematurity, genetic/congenital conditions, chronic illness (parent/child)

DESIRED OUTCOMES/EVALUATION CRITERIA

Sample NOC linkages:

Parenting: Provision of an environment that promotes optimum growth and development of dependent children

Role Performance: Congruence of an individual's role behavior with role expectations

Caregiver Home Care Readiness: Preparedness to assume responsibility for the health-care of a family member or significant other in the home

Parent(s) Will (Include Specific Time Frame)

- Verbalize understanding of situation and expected parent's/ child's role.
- Express feelings about child's illness/situation and effect on family life.
- Demonstrate appropriate behaviors in regard to parenting role.
- Assume caretaking activities as appropriate.
- Handle family disruptions effectively.

ACTIONS/INTERVENTIONS

Sample NIC linkages:

Parenting Promotion: Providing parenting information, support, and coordination of comprehensive services to high-risk families

Role Enhancement: Assisting a patient, significant other, and/or family to improve relationships by clarifying and supplementing specific role behaviors

Family Process Maintenance: Minimization of family process disruption effects

NURSING PRIORITY NO. 1. To assess causative/contributory factors:

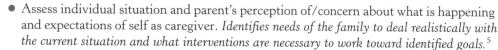

- Assess individual situation and parent's perception of/concern about what is happening and expectations of self as caregiver. *Identifies needs of the family to deal realistically with the current situation and what interventions are necessary to work toward identified goals.*[5]

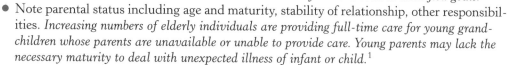

- Note parental status including age and maturity, stability of relationship, other responsibilities. *Increasing numbers of elderly individuals are providing full-time care for young grandchildren whose parents are unavailable or unable to provide care. Young parents may lack the necessary maturity to deal with unexpected illness of infant or child.*[1]

- Ascertain parent's understanding of child's developmental stage and expectations for the future to identify misconceptions/strengths. *Parents often have no information regarding developmental stages and have unrealistic expectation of abilities of the child. Identifying what the parents know and providing information can help them deal more realistically with the situation.*[1]

- Note coping skills currently being used by each individual as well as how problems have been dealt with in the past. *Provides basis for comparison and reference for client's coping abilities in current situation.*[1]
- Determine use of substances (e.g., alcohol, other drugs, including prescription medications). *May interfere with individual's ability to cope/problem-solve and manage current illness/situation and indicate need for additional interventions.*[8]
- Determine availability/use of resources, including extended family, support groups, and financial. *Factors that may affect ability to manage illness, unexpected expenses/caregiving, etc.*[1]
- Perform testing such as Parent-Child Relationship Inventory (PCRI) for further evaluation as indicated. *Provides information on which to develop plan of care and appropriate interventions.*[1]
- Determine cultural/religious influences on parenting expectations of self and child, sense of success/failure. *Parenting is one of the most important jobs an individual will have and one for which they are least prepared. Family of origin practices an beliefs will influence parents in how they parent and this information is crucial to developing a plan of care that meets their needs.*[4]

NURSING PRIORITY NO. 2. To assist parents to deal with current crisis:

- Encourage free verbal expression of feelings (including negative feelings of anger and hostility), setting limits on inappropriate behavior. *Verbalization of feelings enables parent(s) to sift through situation and begin to deal with reality of what is happening. Behavior that is inappropriate is not helpful to dealing with the situation and will lead to feelings of guilt and low self-worth.*[2]
- Acknowledge difficulty of situation and normalcy of feeling overwhelmed and helpless. Encourage contact with parents who experienced similar situation with child and had positive outcome. *Parents feel listened to when feelings are acknowledged and hearing how other parents have dealt with situation can give them hope.*[2]
- Provide information in an honest and forthright manner at level of understanding of the client, including technical information when appropriate. *Helping client understand what is happening corrects misconceptions and helps to make decisions that meet individual needs.*[3]
- Promote parental involvement in decision making and care as much as possible/desired. *When family members are involved in the process it enhances their sense of control and they are more likely to follow through on plans that have been made.*[2]
- Encourage interaction/facilitate communication between parent(s) and children. *Sometimes people who find themselves in difficult/distressful situations tend to withdraw because they don't know what to do. Encouraging these interactions enables them to connect with one another to facilitate dealing with situation.*[2]
- Promote use of assertiveness, relaxation skills. *Providing information and helping individuals learn these skills will help them to deal more effectively with situation/crisis.*[6]
- Assist parent to learn proper administration of medications/treatments as indicated. *May need to be involved in care and knowing how to do these activities enhances their sense of control and comfort in their ability to handle situation.*[5]
- Provide for/encourage use of respite care, parent time off. *Parents may believe they are being "selfish" if they take time out for themselves, that they have to remain with the child. However, parents are important, children are important, and the family is important and when parents take time for themselves it enhances their emotional well-being and promotes ability to deal with ongoing situation.*[7]

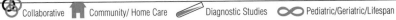

Cultural   Collaborative   Community/ Home Care   Diagnostic Studies   Pediatric/Geriatric/Lifespan   Medications

NURSING PRIORITY NO. 3. To promote wellness (Teaching/Discharge Considerations):

- Provide anticipatory guidance relevant to the situation/long-term expectations of the illness. *Encourages making plans for future needs, provides feelings of hope, and promotes sense of control over difficult situation.*[3]
- Encourage setting realistic and mutually agreed-on goals. *As family members work together they can feel empowered and are more apt to follow through on decisions that they have been involved in making.*[2]
- Provide/identify learning opportunities specific to needs. *Activities such as parenting classes, information about equipment use and methods of troubleshooting can enhance knowledge and ability to deal with situation.*[3]
- Refer to community resources as appropriate (e.g., visiting nurse, respite care, social services, psychiatric care/family therapy, well-baby clinics, special needs support services). *Provides additional assistance as needed to handle individual situation/illness.*[5]
- Refer to ND impaired Parenting for additional interventions.

DOCUMENTATION FOCUS

Assessment/Reassessment
- Findings, including specifics of individual situation/parental concerns, perceptions, expectations.

Planning
- Plan of care and who is involved in the planning.
- Teaching plan.

Implementation/Evaluation
- Parent's responses to interventions/teaching and actions performed.
- Attainment/progress toward desired outcome(s).
- Modifications to plan of care.

Discharge Planning
- Long-term needs and who is responsible for each action to be taken.
- Specific referrals made.

References

1. Townsend, M. C. (2003). Psychiatric Mental Health Nursing Concepts of Care, ed 4. Philadelphia: F. A. Davis.
2. Gordon, T. (2000). Parent Effectiveness Training, (updated ed). New York: Three Rivers Press.
3. Cox, H. C., et al. (2002). Clinical Applications of Nursing Diagnosis: Adult, Child, Women's, Psychiatric, Gerontic, and Home Health Considerations, ed 4. Philadelphia: F. A. Davis.
4. Lipson, J. G., Dibble, S. L., & Minarik, P. A. (1996). Culture & Nursing Care: A Pocket Guide. San Francisco: UCSF Nursing Press.
5. Doenges, M. E., Townsend, M. C., & Moorhouse, M. F. (1998). Psychiatric Care Plans Guidelines for Individualizing Care, ed 3. Philadelphia: F. A. Davis.
6. Gordon, T. (1989). Teaching Children Self-discipline: At Home and At School. New York: Random House.
7. Gordon, T. (2000). Family Effectiveness Training Video. Solana Beach, CA: Gordon Training Intn'l.
8. Townsend, M. (2001). Nursing Diagnoses in Psychiatric Nursing: Care Plans and Psychotropic Medications, ed 5. Philadelphia: F. A. Davis.

acute Confusion

Definition: Abrupt onset of a cluster of global, transient changes and disturbances in attention, cognition, psychomotor activity, level of consciousness, and/or sleep/wake cycle

RELATED FACTORS

Over 60 years of age
Dementia
Alcohol abuse, drug abuse
Delirium [including febrile epilepticus (following or instead of an epileptic attack), toxic and traumatic]
[Medication reaction/interaction; anesthesia/surgery; metabolic imbalances]
[Exacerbation of a chronic illness, hypoxemia]
[Severe pain]
[Sleep deprivation]

DEFINING CHARACTERISTICS

Subjective
Hallucinations [visual/auditory]
[Exaggerated emotional responses]

Objective
Fluctuation in cognition
Fluctuation in sleep/wake cycle
Fluctuation in level of consciousness
Fluctuation in psychomotor activity [tremors, body movement]
Increased agitation or restlessness
Misperceptions [inappropriate responses]
Lack of motivation to initiate and/or follow through with goal-directed or purposeful behavior

SAMPLE CLINICAL APPLICATIONS: brain injury/stroke, respiratory conditions with hypoxia, medication adverse reactions, drug/alcohol intoxication, hyperthermia/infectious processes, malnutrition/eating disorders, fluid and electrolyte imbalances, chemical exposure

DESIRED OUTCOMES/EVALUATION CRITERIA

Sample NOC linkages:
Cognitive Ability: Ability to execute complex mental processes
Information Processing: Ability to acquire, organize, and use information
Distorted Thought Control: Self-restraint of disruption in perception, thought processes, and thought content

Client Will (Include Specific Time Frame)
- Regain/maintain usual reality orientation and level of consciousness.
- Verbalize understanding of causative factors when known as able.
- Initiate lifestyle/behavior changes to prevent or minimize recurrence of problem.

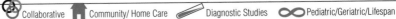 Cultural   Collaborative   Community/ Home Care   Diagnostic Studies   Pediatric/Geriatric/Lifespan   Medications

ACTIONS/INTERVENTIONS

Sample NIC linkages:

Delirium Management: Provision of a safe and therapeutic environment for the patient who is experiencing an acute confusional state

Reality Orientation: Promotions of patient's awareness of personal identity, time, and environment

Surveillance: Safety: Purposeful and ongoing collection and analysis of information about the patient and the environment for use in promoting and maintaining patient safety

NURSING PRIORITY NO. 1. To assess causative/contributing factors:

- Identify potential contributing factors present, such as diabetes mellitus, recent surgery, recent stroke, alcohol or drug intoxication/withdrawal; use of large numbers of medications/polypharmacy (four or more); dehydration/volume depletion (e.g., vomiting/diarrhea, failure to eat); fever/presence of acute infection (especially urinary tract infection or pneumonia in elderly client), exposure to toxic substances, significant pain, recent fall or traumatic event; electroconvulsive therapy (ECT treatments); person with dementia experiencing sudden change in environment, including unfamiliar noises, excessive visitors. *Helps identify causes of acute confusion/delirium that might be easily reversed or treated.*[1]

- Assess mental status. *Typical symptoms of delirium include anxiety, disorientation, tremors, hallucinations, delusions and incoherence. Onset is usually sudden, coming on over a few hours or days.*[2]

- Evaluate vital signs. *Signs of poor tissue perfusion (i.e., hypotension, tachycardia, tachypnea or fever) may identify underlying cardiovascular or infectious cause for mental status changes.*[2]

- Determine current medications/drug use (especially antianxiety agents, barbiturates, lithium, methyldopa, disulfiram, cocaine, alcohol, amphetamines, hallucinogens, opiates) *Use, misuse, overdose and withdrawal of many drugs is associated with high risk of confusion, disorientation, and delirium.*[1]

- Investigate possibility of drug withdrawal or medication interactions. *Noncompliance with regimen, sudden discontinuation or overuse of drug, and certain drug combinations increase risk of toxic reactions and adverse reactions/interactions.*[1,2]

- Evaluate for exacerbation of psychiatric conditions (e.g., mood disorder, dissociative disorders, dementia). *Identification of the presence of mental illness provides opportunity for correct treatment and medication.*[10]

- Assess diet/nutritional status. *Failure to eat (forgetfulness or lack of food) or deficiencies in essential nutrients (e.g., vitamin B-12 foliate, thiamine, iron) can contribute to acute confusion.*[2]

- Evaluate sleep/rest status, noting deprivation/oversleeping. *Discomfort, worry and lack of sleep and rest can cause/exacerbate confusion.* Refer to ND disturbed Sleep Pattern, as appropriate.

- Monitor laboratory values, (e.g. ABGs, oxygen saturation, electrolytes, glucose, thyroid, renalytes, CBC and drug levels [including peak/trough as appropriate]). Review chest radiograph, ECG/rhythm strip. *Can point to underlying causes for confusion and monitor response to therapies.*[1-7]

NURSING PRIORITY NO. 2. To determine degree of impairment:

- Talk with client/SOs to determine client's physical, functional, cognitive and behavioral baseline, observed changes, and onset/precipitator of changes *to understand and clarify the current situation.*[1]

- Collaborate with medical and psychiatric providers *to evaluate extent of impairment in orientation, attention span, ability to follow directions, send/receive communication, appropriateness of response.*[1]
- Note occurrence/timing of agitation, hallucinations, and violent behaviors *(e.g., delirium may occur as early as 1 or 2 days after last drink in an alcoholic; or "Sundown syndrome" may occur in ICU, with client oriented during daylight hours but confused during night).*[1,3]
- Determine threat to safety of client/others. *Delirium can cause client to become verbally and physically aggressive resulting in behavior threatening to safety of self and others.*

NURSING PRIORITY NO. 3. To maximize level of function, prevent further deterioration:

- Assist with treatment of underlying problem *(e.g., establish/maintain normal fluid and electrolyte balance and oxygenation; treat infectious process or pain; detoxify from alcohol and other drugs; withdraw medications causing adverse reaction; provide psychological interventions, etc).*[1–7,9]
- Implement helpful communication measures, e.g.[1–7,9]:
  Use short simple sentences. Speak slowly and clearly.
  Call client by name and identify yourself at each contact.
  Tell client what you want done, not what to do
  Orient to surroundings, staff, and necessary activities as often as needed.
  Acknowledge client's fears and feelings. *Confusion can be very frightening, especially when client knows thinking is not normal.*[4]
  Listen to what client says, try to identify message, emotion or need being communicated.
  Limit choices and decisions until client is able to make them.
  Give simple directions. Allow sufficient time for client to respond, to communicate, and to make decisions.
  Present reality concisely and briefly. Avoid challenging illogical thinking. *Defensive reactions may result.*[1]
  Refer to ND impaired Communication for additional interventions.
- Manage environment, e.g.[1–7,9]:
  Provide undisturbed rest periods. Eliminate extraneous noise/stimuli. *Preventing overstimulation can help client relax and can result in reduced level of confusion.*[10]
  Provide calm and comfortable environment with good lighting. Encourage client to use vision/hearing aids when needed *to reduce disorientation and discomfort* from sensory overload or deprivation.
  Observe client on regular basis, informing client of this schedule.
  Provide adequate supervision (may need one-to-one during severe episode); removing harmful objects from environment; providing siderails, seizure precautions, placing call bell within reach, positioning needed items within reach/clearing traffic paths, ambulating with devices *to meet client's safety needs.*
  Provide clear feedback on appropriate and inappropriate behavior.
  Remove client from situation; provide time out, seclusion as indicated *for protection of client/others.*
  Encourage family/SO(s) to participate in reorientation and provide ongoing normal life input (e.g., current news and family happenings). Provide normal levels of essential sensory/tactile stimulation—include personal items/pictures. *Client may respond positively to well-known person and familiar items.*
- Note behavior that may be indicative of potential for violence and take appropriate actions *to prevent client/caregiver injury.* Refer to NDs risk for self-/other- directed Violence.

 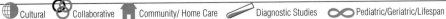

• Administer medication cautiously to control restlessness, agitation, hallucinations. *In acute confusion, the short-term goal is to calm the person down quickly. Sedation with conventional antipsychotic agent (e.g. haloperidol, lorazepam) may be used, although many other medications can be used, depending on the underlying cause of the delirium.*[1,5–7]

• Avoid/limit use of restraints. *May worsen agitation, increase likelihood of untoward complications.*[5]

 • Mobilize elderly client (especially after orthopedic injury) as soon as possible. *Older person with low level of activity prior to crisis is at particular risk for acute confusion and may do better when out of bed.*[4]

• Establish and maintain elimination patterns. *Disruption of elimination may be a cause for confusion or changes in elimination may also be a symptom of acute confusion.*[5]

 • Consult with psychiatric clinical nurse specialist or psychiatrist for additional interventions related to disruptive behaviors, psychosis and unresolved symptoms.

• Refer also to NDs disturbed Thought Processes and disturbed Sensory Perception for additional interventions.

NURSING PRIORITY NO. 4. To promote wellness (Teaching/Discharge Considerations):

 • Explain to client/SO reason for confusion, if known, what interventions are being implemented, and how best to approach client. Discuss situation with family and involve in planning to meet identified needs. *Reduces fear of unknown and provides support system to client/SO/ caregivers.*[1]

• Educate SO/caregivers to monitor client at home for sudden change in cognition and behavior. *An acute change is a classic presentation of delirium and should be considered a medical emergency. Early intervention can often prevent long-term complications.*[8]

 • Encourage periodic review of client's drug regimen. *Medications are frequent precipitant of acute confusion, especially in very young or old.*[8,9]

 • Provide appropriate referrals. *Additional assistance may be required for client with confusion, (e.g., cognitive retraining, substance abuse support groups, medication monitoring program, Meals on Wheels, home health, and adult day care).*[1]

DOCUMENTATION FOCUS

Assessment/Reassessment
• Nature, duration, frequency of problem.
• Current and previous level of function, effect on independence/lifestyle (including safety concerns).

Planning
• Plan of care and who is involved in planning.
• Teaching plan.

Implementation/Evaluation
• Response to interventions and actions performed.
• Attainment/progress toward desired outcomes.
• Modifications to plan of care.

Discharge Planning
• Long-term needs and who is responsible for actions to be taken.
• Available resources and specific referrals.

References

1. Doenges, M. E., Moorhouse, M. F. & Geissler-Murr, A. C. (2002). Nurse's Pocket Guide: Diagnoses, Interventions and Rationales, ed 8. Philadelphia: F. A. Davis, pp. 142–145.
2. Altered mental states. (1998). Columbia, MD: American Medical Directors Association (AMDA). Available at the AMDA Web site, http://www.amda.com. or National Guidelines Clearinghouse Web site, www.guideline.gov.
3. Stanley, M. & Bear, P. G. (1999). Gerontological Nursing: A Health Promotion/Protection Approach, ed 2. Philadelphia: F.A Davis, pp. 342–349.
4. Matthiesen, V., et al. (1994). Acute confusion: Nursing intervention in older patients, Orthop Nurs, 13, 25.
5. Rapp, C. (1997). Acute confusion/delirium, Iowa Veterans Affairs Nursing Research Consortium: Iowa City: University of Iowa.
6. American Psychiatric Association. (1999). Practice guideline for the treatment of patients with delirium. Am J Psychiatry, 156(5 Suppl), 1–20.
7. Expert Consensus Guideline Series: Agitation in older persons with dementia: A guide for families and caregivers. Available at www.psychguides.com/gahe.html.
8. Ackley, B. J. & Ladwig, G.B. (2002). Nursing Diagnosis Handbook: A Guide to Planning Care, ed 5. St Louis: Mosby.
9. Cox, H. C., et al. (2002). Clinical Applications of Nursing Diagnosis: Adult, Child, Women's, Psychiatric, Gerontic and Home Health Considerations, ed 4. Philadelphia: F. A. Davis, pp 391–397.
10. Doenges, M. E., Townsend, M. C., & Moorhouse, M. F. (1999). Psychiatric Care Plans Guidelines for Individualizing Care, ed 3. Philadelphia: F. A. Davis.

chronic Confusion

Definition: Irreversible, long-standing, and/or progressive deterioration of intellect and personality characterized by decreased ability to interpret environmental stimuli; decreased capacity for intellectual thought processes; and manifested by disturbances of memory, orientation, and behavior

RELATED FACTORS

Alzheimer's disease [dementia of the Alzheimer's type]
Korsakoff's psychosis
[AIDS dementia]
[Depression]
Multi-infarct dementia
Cerebral vascular accident; head injury

DEFINING CHARACTERISTICS

Objective
Clinical evidence of organic impairment
Altered interpretation/response to stimuli
Progressive/long-standing cognitive impairment
No change in level of consciousness [disorientation, difficulties with attention, concentration, judgment, behavior]
Impaired socialization [withdrawal from social interaction, inability to maintain employment]
Impaired memory [usually progressive] (short-term, long-term)
[Decreased ability to function independently]
Altered personality

 Cultural Collaborative  Community/ Home Care  Diagnostic Studies Pediatric/Geriatric/Lifespan Medications

SAMPLE CLINICAL APPLICATIONS: brain injury/stroke, dementia/Alzheimer's disease, medication adverse reactions, drug/alcohol abuse, malnutrition/eating disorders, chemical exposure

DESIRED OUTCOME/EVALUATION CRITERIA
Sample NOC linkage:
Safety Status: Physical Injury: Severity of injuries from accidents and trauma

Client Will (Include Specific Time Frame)
- Remain safe and free from harm.

    Sample NOC linkages:
    Cognitive Ability: Ability to execute complex mental processes
    Knowledge: Disease Process: Extent of understanding conveyed about a specific disease process

Family/SO Will (Include Specific Time Frame)
- Verbalize understanding of disease process/prognosis and client's needs.
- Identify/participate in interventions to deal effectively with situation.
- Provide for maximal independence while meeting safety needs of client.

ACTIONS/INTERVENTIONS
Sample NIC linkages:
Dementia Management: Provision of a modified environment for the patient who is experiencing a chronic confusional state
Calming Technique: Reducing anxiety in patient experiencing acute distress
Surveillance: Purposeful and ongoing acquisition, interpretation, and synthesis of patient data for clinical decision making

NURSING PRIORITY NO. 1. To assess degree of impairment:

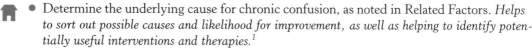
- Determine the underlying cause for chronic confusion, as noted in Related Factors. *Helps to sort out possible causes and likelihood for improvement, as well as helping to identify potentially useful interventions and therapies.[1]*

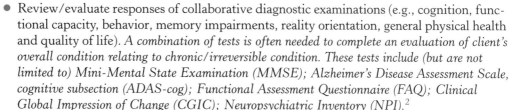
- Review/evaluate responses of collaborative diagnostic examinations (e.g., cognition, functional capacity, behavior, memory impairments, reality orientation, general physical health and quality of life). *A combination of tests is often needed to complete an evaluation of client's overall condition relating to chronic/irreversible condition. These tests include (but are not limited to) Mini-Mental State Examination (MMSE); Alzheimer's Disease Assessment Scale, cognitive subsection (ADAS-cog); Functional Assessment Questionnaire (FAQ); Clinical Global Impression of Change (CGIC); Neuropsychiatric Inventory (NPI).[2]*

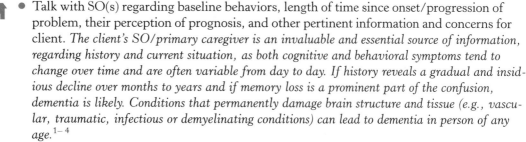
- Talk with SO(s) regarding baseline behaviors, length of time since onset/progression of problem, their perception of prognosis, and other pertinent information and concerns for client. *The client's SO/primary caregiver is an invaluable and essential source of information, regarding history and current situation, as both cognitive and behavioral symptoms tend to change over time and are often variable from day to day. If history reveals a gradual and insidious decline over months to years and if memory loss is a prominent part of the confusion, dementia is likely. Conditions that permanently damage brain structure and tissue (e.g., vascular, traumatic, infectious or demyelinating conditions) can lead to dementia in person of any age.[1–4]*

- Obtain information regarding recent changes or disruptions in client's health or routine. *Decline in physical health or disruption in daily living situation (e.g., hospitalization, change in medications or moving to new home) can exacerbate agitation or bring on acute confusion.* Refer to ND, acute Confusion.

- Evaluate client's response to primary care providers as well as receptiveness to interventions. *Awareness of these dynamics is helpful for evaluation of ongoing needs for both client and caregiver, as client becomes increasingly dependent on caregivers and/or resistant to interventions.*

- Determine client and caregiver anxiety level in relation to situation. Note behavior that may be indicative of potential for violence. *The diagnosis of irreversible condition, the organic brain changes and the day-to-day problems of living with it causes great stress and can potentiate violence.*[3]

NURSING PRIORITY NO. 2. To limit effects of deterioration/maximize level of function:

- Monitor for treatable conditions (e.g. depression, infections, malnutrition, electrolyte imbalances, and adverse medication reactions) *that may contribute to or exacerbate distress, discomfort and agitation.*[1–6]

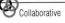 - Implement behavioral and environmental management interventions such as: *Promotes orientation, provides opportunity for client interaction using current cognitive skills, and preserves client's dignity and safety.*[2–6]
  Ascertain interventions previously used/tried and evaluate effectiveness.
  Provide calm environment, eliminate extraneous noise/stimuli *that may increase client's level of agitation/confusion.*
  Introduce yourself at each contact if needed. Call client by preferred name.
  Use touch judiciously. Tell client what is being done before touching *to reduce sense of surprise/negative reaction.*
  Be supportive and sensitive to fears, misperceived threats and frustration with expressing what is wanted.
  Be open and honest when discussing client's disease, abilities and prognosis.
  Maintain continuity of caregivers and care routines as much as possible.
  Use positive statements, offer guided choices between two options.
  Avoid speaking in loud voice, crowding, restraining, shaming, demanding or condescending actions toward client.
  Set limits on acting-out behavior *for safety of client/others.*
  Remove from stressors and agitation triggers or danger; move client to quieter place; offer privacy.
  Simplify client's tasks and routines *to reduce agitation associated with multiple options/demands.*
  Provide for/assist with daily care activities, including bathing, dressing, grooming, toileting, exercise. *Client may "forget" how to perform ADLs.*
  Monitor and assist with meeting nutritional needs, feeding and fluid intake; monitor weight. Provide finger food if client has problems with eating utensils or is unable to sit to eat.
  Assist with toileting and perineal care as needed. Provide incontinence supplies.
  Allow adequate rest between stimulating events.
  Use lighting and visual aids to reduce confusion.
  Encourage family/SO(s) to provide ongoing orientation/input to include current news and family happenings.
  Maintain reality-oriented relationship/environment (clocks, calendars, personal items, seasonal decorations).

 Cultural Collaborative Community/ Home Care 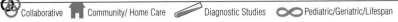 Diagnostic Studies Pediatric/Geriatric/Lifespan Medications

Encourage participation in resocialization groups.

Allow client to reminisce, exist in own reality if not detrimental to well-being.

Avoid challenging illogical thinking *because defensive reactions may result.*

Provide appropriate safety measures. *Client who is confused needs close supervision. Measures such as use of identification bracelet, alarms on unlocked exits; toxic substances and medication lockup, supervision of outdoor activities and wandering, removal of car or car keys, lowered temperature on hot water tank can prevent injuries.*[5]

- Administer medications as ordered (e.g., antidepressants, anxiolytics, antipsychotics) at lowest possible therapeutic dose. Monitor for expected and/or adverse responses, side effects and interactions. *May be used to manage symptoms of psychosis and aggressive behavior but need to be used cautiously.*[5]

- Implement complementary therapies as indicated/desired (e.g. music therapy, hand massage, Therapeutic Touch—if touch is tolerated—aromatherapy, bright-light treatment. *Use of alternative therapies can be calming and provide relaxation enabling care to be provided with less difficulty.*[7]

- Refer to NDs, acute Confusion, impaired Memory, disturbed Thought Processes, impaired verbal Communication for additional interventions

NURSING PRIORITY NO. 3. To assist SO(s) to develop coping strategies[2–6]:

- Determine family dynamics, cultural values, resources, availability and willingness to participate in meeting client's needs. Evaluate SO's attention to own needs including health status, grieving process, and respite. *Primary caregiver and other members of family will suffer from the stress that accompanies caregiving and will require ongoing information and support.* Refer to ND risk for Caregiver Role Strain.[5]

- Involve SO(s) in care and discharge planning. Maintain frequent interactions with SOs *in order to relay information, to change care strategies, try different responses, or implement other problem-solving solutions.*[6]

- Teach the family about caregiver burden (if appropriate). Provide educational materials (responding to their needs and learning styles) and list of available resources, such as newsletters, books, Web sites, telephone help lines, etc.

- Identify appropriate community resources (e.g., Alzheimer's Disease and Related Disorders Association [ADRDA]; stroke or other brain injury support groups; senior support groups, respite care, clergy, social services, therapists, attorney services for advance directives and durable power of attorney) *to provide support for client and SOs, and assist with problem solving.*[5]

NURSING PRIORITY NO. 4. To promote wellness (Teaching/Discharge Considerations)[2–6]:

- Discuss how client's condition may progress, ongoing treatment needs and appropriate follow-up. *Intermittent evaluations are needed to determine client's general health, any deterioration in cognitive function, required adjustment in medication regimen, etc., to maintain the client at the highest possible level of functioning.*[6]

- Ascertain that caregiver(s) understand all medications, including dosage, route, action, expected and reportable side effects and potential drug interactions *to prevent/limit complications associated with multiple psychiatric and CNS medications.*[5]

- Develop plan of care with family to meet client's and SO individual needs. *The individual plan is dependent on cultural and belief patterns, as well as family (personal, emotional, and financial) resources.*[6]

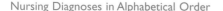

- Instruct SO/caregivers to share information about client's condition, functional status and medications whenever encountering new providers. *Clients often have multiple doctors, each of whom may prescribe medications, with potential for adverse affects and overmedication.*[7]
- Provide appropriate referrals (e.g., Meals on Wheels, adult day care, home care agency, nursing home placement, respite care for family member). *May need additional assistance to maintain the client in the home setting or make arrangements for placement if necessary.*[6]

DOCUMENTATION FOCUS

Assessment/Reassessment
- Individual findings including current level of function and rate of anticipated changes.

Planning
- Plan of care and who is involved in planning.

Implementation/Evaluation
- Response to interventions and actions performed.
- Attainment/progress toward desired outcomes.
- Modifications to plan of care.

Discharge Planning
- Long-term needs/referrals and who is responsible for actions to be taken.
- Available resources, specific referrals made.

References

1. Bostwick, J. M. (2000). The many faces of confusion: Timing and collateral history often holds the key to diagnosis. Postgrad Med, 108 (6), 60–72.
2. About Alzheimer's. Physicians and Care Professionals, Various Educational Materials. Alzheimer's Disease and Related Disorders Association (ADRDA) 2003. Available at: www.alz.org.
3. Doenges, M. E., Moorhouse, M. F., & Geissler-Murr, A. C. (2002). Nurse's Pocket Guide: Diagnoses, Interventions, and Rationales, ed 8. Philadelphia: F. A. Davis, pp 145–147.
4. Expert Consensus Guideline Series: Agitation in older persons with dementia: A guide for families and caregivers. Expert Knowledge Systems, LLC. Ross Editorial Services, April 1998. Available at: www.psychguides.com.
5. Sommers, M.S. & Johnson, S.A. (1997). Alzheimer's disease and delirium/dementia. In Davis's Manual of Nursing Therapeutics for Diseases and Disorders. Philadelphia: F. A. Davis.
6. Kovach, C.R. & Wilson, S.A. (1999). Dementia in older adults. In Stanley, M. & Beare P. G. (eds): Gerontologic Nursing: A Health Promotion/Protection Approach, ed 2. Philadelphia: F. A. Davis.
7. Burns, A., Byrne, J., & Ballard, C. (2002). Sensory stimulation in dementia: An effective option for managing behavioral problems. BMJ, 325, 1312–1313. Summarized on Dementia Center Health and Age Website. www.healthandage.com

Constipation

Definition: Decrease in normal frequency of defecation accompanied by difficult or incomplete passage of stool and/or passage of excessively hard, dry stool

RELATED FACTORS

Functional
Irregular defecation habits; inadequate toileting (e.g., timeliness, positioning for defecation, privacy)

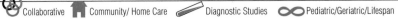 Cultural Collaborative  Community/ Home Care Diagnostic Studies Pediatric/Geriatric/Lifespan Medications

Insufficient physical activity; abdominal muscle weakness
Recent environmental changes
Habitual denial/ignoring of urge to defecate
[Colonic inertia, delayed transit, anorectal dysfunction]

Psychological
Emotional stress; depression; mental confusion

Pharmacologic
Antilipemic agents; laxative overdose; calcium carbonate; aluminum-containing antacids; nonsteroidal anti-inflammatory agents; opiates; anticholinergics; diuretics; iron salts; phenothiazides; sedatives; sympathomimetics; bismuth salts; antidepressants; calcium channel blockers

Mechanical
Hemorrhoids; pregnancy; obesity
Rectal abscess or ulcer, anal fissures, prolapse; anal strictures; rectocele
Prostate enlargement
Postsurgical obstruction
Neurological impairment; megacolon (Hirschsprung's disease); tumors
Electrolyte imbalance

Physiologic
Poor eating habits; change in usual foods and eating patterns; insufficient fiber intake; insufficient fluid intake, dehydration
Inadequate dentition or oral hygiene
Decreased motility of gastrointestinal tract

DEFINING CHARACTERISTICS

Subjective
Change in bowel pattern, unable to pass stool, decreased frequency, decreased volume of stool
Change in usual foods and eating patterns; increased abdominal pressure, feeling of rectal fullness or pressure
Abdominal pain, pain with defecation; nausea and/or vomiting, headache, indigestion, generalized fatigue

Objective
Dry, hard, formed stool
Straining with defecation
Hypoactive or hyperactive bowel sounds; change in abdominal growling (borborygmi)
Distended abdomen; abdominal tenderness with or without palpable muscle resistance
Percussed abdominal dullness
Presence of soft paste like stool in rectum, oozing liquid stool, bright red blood with stool, dark or black or tarry stool
Severe flatus, anorexia
Atypical presentations in older adults (e.g., change in mental status, urinary incontinence, unexplained falls, and elevated body temperature)

SAMPLE CLINICAL APPLICATIONS: abdominal surgeries, hemorrhoids/anal lesions, irritable bowel syndrome, diverticulitis, spinal cord injury, multiple sclerosis, enteral/parenteral feedings, hypothyroidism, iron deficiency anemia, uremia/renal dialysis, Alzheimer's disease/dementia

DESIRED OUTCOMES/EVALUATION CRITERIA

Sample NOC linkages:

Bowel Elimination: Ability of the gastrointestinal tract to form and evacuate stool effectively

Nutritional Status: Food and fluid intake: Amount of food and fluid taken into the body over a 24-hour period

Self-Care: Non-parenteral medications: Ability to administer oral and topical medications to meet therapeutic goals

Client Will (Include Specific Time Frame)
- Establish/regain normal pattern of bowel functioning.
- Verbalize understanding of etiology and appropriate interventions/solutions for individual situation.
- Demonstrate behaviors or lifestyle changes to prevent recurrence of problem.
- Participate in bowel program as indicated.

ACTIONS/INTERVENTIONS

Sample NIC linkages:

Constipation/Impaction Management: Prevention and alleviation of constipation/impaction

Bowel Management: Establishment and maintenance of a regular pattern of bowel elimination

Ostomy Care: Maintenance of elimination through a stoma and care of surrounding tissue

NURSING PRIORITY NO. 1. To identify causative/contributing factors:

- Review medical/surgical history. *Problems with colon or rectum (e.g., obstruction scar tissue, diverticulitis, tumors, irritable bowel syndrome), metabolic or endocrine disorders (e.g., diabetes mellitus, hypothyroidism, uremia), primary diseases of colon (e.g., cancers, stricture, anal fissure), limited physical activity (e.g., bedrest, poor mobility, chronic disability), chronic pain problems (especially when client is on pain medications), pregnancy and childbirth, recent abdominal or perianal surgery, neurologic disorders (e.g., Parkinsonism, multiple sclerosis, spinal cord abnormalities are all conditions commonly associated with constipation.*[1,2,4,5,7–10]
- Note client's age. *Constipation is more likely to occur in individuals older than 55 years of age,*[1] *but can occur in any age from infant to elderly. A bottle-fed infant is more prone to constipation than breastfed infant, especially when formula contains iron.*[2,5] *Toddlers are at risk because developmental factors (e.g., too young, too interested in other things, rigid schedule during potty training), and children and adolescents are at risk because of unwillingness to take break from play, poor eating and fluid intake habits, and withholding because of perceived lack of privacy.*[3] *Many older adults experience constipation as a result of duller nerve sensations, incomplete emptying of the bowel or failing to attend to signals to defecate.*[4]
- Review daily dietary regimen. *Imbalanced nutrition influences the amount and consistency of feces.*[2] *Inadequate dietary fiber (vegetable, fruits, and whole grains); highly processed foods contribute to poor intestinal function. Loss of teeth can force individuals to eat soft foods, mostly lacking in fiber.*[1,4,5,8]

 Cultural   Collaborative   Community/ Home Care   Diagnostic Studies   Pediatric/Geriatric/Lifespan   Medications

- Determine fluid intake *to note deficits. Most individuals do not drink enough fluids, even when healthy, reducing the speed at which stool moves through the colon. Active fluid loss through sweating, vomiting, diarrhea, or bleeding can greatly increase chances for constipation.*[1,2,4,5,7–10]

- Evaluate medication/drug usage and note interactions or side effects (e.g., narcotics, antacids, chemotherapy, iron, contrast media such as barium, steroids*). Many medications can slow passage of bowel movements.*[1,2,4,5,7–10]
- Note energy/activity level and exercise pattern. *Lack of physical activity and/or regular exercise is often a factor in constipation.*[1–4,7,8,10]
- Identify areas of life changes/stressors. *Factors such as pregnancy, travel, traumas, and changes in personal relationships, occupational factors, or financial concerns can cause or exacerbate constipation.*[7,10]
- Determine access to bathroom, privacy, and ability to perform self-care activities.
- Investigate reports of pain with defecation. *Hemorrhoids, fissures, skin breakdown, or other abnormal findings may be hindering passage of stool or causing client to hold stool.*[1,5–8]
- Discuss laxative/enema use. Note signs/reports of laxative abuse. *This is most common among older adults preoccupied with having daily bowel movement.*[5,7]
- Assist with diagnostic evaluation, as indicated (e.g., barium enema, colonoscopy, and anorectal function tests) *for identification of other possible causative factors.*

NURSING PRIORITY NO. 2. To determine usual pattern of elimination:

- Discuss usual elimination pattern and problem. *Helps to identify/clarify client's perception of problem. For example, constipation has been defined as not only infrequent stools (less than three per week), but also straining with bowel movements, hard stools, unproductive urges and feeling of incomplete evacuation.*[8]
- Ascertain presence of associated symptoms. *Bloating, abdominal pain, loss of appetite, and feeling of being unwell often accompany constipation and are present between infrequent stools.*[8]
- Note factors that usually stimulate bowel activity and any interferences present. *Client may describe having to sit in a particular position, or needing to apply perineal pressure or digital stimulation to start stool. Interferences can include not wanting to use a particular facility or not wanting to interrupt play or an activity.*[8]

NURSING PRIORITY NO. 3. To assess current pattern of elimination:

- Note color, odor, consistency, amount, and frequency of stool following each bowel movement during assessment phase. *Provides a baseline for comparison, promoting recognition of changes. If usual number of weekly bowel movements is decreased; stool is hard formed, or client is straining, constipation is likely present.*[2,10]
- Ascertain duration of current problem and degree of concern (e.g., long-standing condition that client has "lived with" or an acute postsurgical event that causes great distress) *as client's response may/may not be congruent with the severity of condition.*[10]
- Auscultate abdomen for presence, location, and characteristics of bowel sounds *reflecting intestinal activity.*
- Palpate abdomen for hardness, distention, and masses *indicating possible obstruction or retention of stool.*
- Perform digital rectal examination as indicated, *to evaluate rectal tone, detect tenderness, blood or fecal impaction.*

NURSING PRIORITY NO. 4. To facilitate return to usual/acceptable pattern of elimination:

- Promote lifestyle changes[1–10]:
  Instruct in/encourage balanced fiber and bulk in diet *to improve consistency of stool and facilitate passage through colon.*
  Limit foods with little or no fiber (e.g., ice cream, cheese, meat, and processed foods)
  Promote adequate fluid intake, including water, high-fiber fruit and vegetable juices. Suggest drinking warm, stimulating fluids (e.g., decaffeinated coffee, hot water, tea) *to promote moist/soft stool, and increase rate of passage.*
  Encourage daily activity/exercise within limits of individual ability *to stimulate contractions of the intestines.*
  Encourage client to not ignore urge. Provide privacy and routinely scheduled time for defecation (bathroom or commode preferable to bedpan) *to promote psychological readiness and comfort.*
- Administer medications as indicated: stool softeners *(to provide moisture to stool)*, mild stimulants *(to cause rhythmic muscle contractions)*, lubricants *(to enable stool to move more easily)*; saline laxatives *(to draw water into colon)* or bulk-forming agents *(to absorb water in intestine)* as ordered, and/or routinely when appropriate (e.g., client receiving opiates, decreased level of activity/immobility).[1–3,7–10]
- Administer enemas/suppositories, digitally remove impacted stool, when indicated. Apply lubricant/anesthetic ointment to anus *to soften impaction and decrease rectal pain if needed, especially when manual removal is required.*[7,8]
- Provide sitz bath before stools *to relax sphincter,* and after stools *for soothing effect to rectal area.*[5,10]
- Establish bowel program to provide predictable and effective elimination and reduce evacuation problems when long-term or permanent bowel dysfunction is present (such as with spinal cord injury). *Program may include dietary and fluid management, abdominal massage, Valsalva maneuver, deep breathing, ingestion of warm fluids, digital stimulation, and medications/enemas, use of particular position for defecation.*[9,10]
- Support/assist with treatment of underlying medical cause where appropriate (e.g., discontinuing certain medications, surgery to repair rectal prolapse, thyroid treatment) *to improve body and bowel function.*[1–10]

NURSING PRIORITY NO. 5. Promote wellness (Teaching/Discharge Considerations)[1,8,10]:

- Discuss anatomy and physiology of bowel, and acceptable variations in elimination.
- Provide information and resources to client/SO about relationship of diet, exercise, fluid, and appropriate use of laxatives as indicated.
- Provide social and emotional support *to help client manage actual or potential disabilities associated with long-term bowel management.* Discuss rationale for and encourage continuation of successful interventions.
- Encourage client to maintain elimination diary if appropriate *to facilitate monitoring of long-term problem.*
- Design bowel management program to be easily replicated in home and community setting.
- Identify specific actions to be taken if problem does not resolve *to promote timely intervention, enhancing client's independence.*

 Cultural Collaborative Community/ Home Care 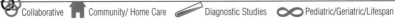 Diagnostic Studies Pediatric/Geriatric/Lifespan Medications

Assessment/Reassessment

- Usual and current bowel pattern, duration of the problem, and individual contributing factors.
- Characteristics of stool.
- Underlying dynamics.

Planning

- Plan of care/interventions and changes in lifestyle that are necessary to correct individual situation, and who is involved in planning.
- Teaching plan.

Implementation/Evaluation

- Responses to interventions/teaching and actions performed.
- Change in bowel pattern, character of stool.
- Attainment/progress toward desired outcomes.
- Modifications to plan of care.

Discharge Planning

- Individual long-term needs, noting who is responsible for actions to be taken.
- Recommendations for follow-up care.
- Specific referrals made.

References

1. Hert, M., Huseboe, J. (1998). Management of constipation. University of Iowa Gerontological Nursing Interventions Research Center, Research Dissemination Core. Iowa City (IA). [NGC: 543]. Retrieved from National Guideline Clearinghouse. Available at: http://www.guideline.gov.
2. Cox, H. C., et al. (2002). Clinical Applications of Nursing Diagnosis: Adult, Child, Women's Psychiatric, Gerontic, and Home Health Considerations, ed 3. Philadelphia: F. A. Davis, pp 192–205.
3. Streeter, B. L. (2002). Teenage constipation: A case study. Gastroenterol Nurs 25(6), 253–256.
4. Stanley, M. (1999). The aging gastrointestinal system, with nutritional considerations. In Stanley, M. & Beare, P. G. (eds): Gerontological Nursing: A Health Promotion/Protection Approach, ed 7. Philadelphia: F. A. Davis, pp 180–181.
5. Constipation in Children. NIH Publication No. 02–4633, October 2001, National Digestive Diseases Information Clearinghouse (NDDIC), Bethesda, MD. Available at: nddic@info.niddk.nih.gov.
6. Idiopathic constipation and soiling in children. University of Michigan Medical Center. Ann Arbor, 1997. [NCG 1011]. Available at: www.guidline.gov.
7. Constipation. NIH Publication No. 95–2754, July, 1995. National Digestive Diseases Information Clearinghouse (NDDIC), Bethesda MD. Available at: nddic@info.niddk.nih.gov.
8. Locke, G. R., Pemberton, J. H., & Phillips, S. F. (2000). American Gastroenterological Association: Medical position statement: Guidelines on constipation. Gastroenterology, 119(6), 1761–1766.
9. Neurogenic bowel management in adults with spinal cord injury. (1998). Paralyzed Veterans of America, Consortium for Spinal Cord Medicine: Clinical Practice Guidelines. Washington DC.
10. Doenges, M. E., Moorhouse, M. F., & Geissler-Murr, A. C. (2002). Nurse's Pocket Guide: Diagnoses, Interventions, and Rationales, ed 8. Philadelphia: F. A. Davis, p. 151.

perceived Constipation

Definition: Self-diagnosis of constipation and abuse of laxatives, enemas, and suppositories to ensure a daily bowel movement

Cultural/family health beliefs
Faulty appraisal [long-term expectations/habits]
Impaired thought processes

DEFINING CHARACTERISTICS

Subjective
Expectation of a daily bowel movement with the resulting overuse of laxatives, enemas, and suppositories
Expected passage of stool at same time every day

SAMPLE CLINICAL APPLICATIONS: irritable bowel, confused states/dementia, hypochondriasis

DESIRED OUTCOMES/EVALUATION CRITERIA
Sample NOC linkages:
Health Beliefs: Personal convictions that influence health behaviors
Bowel Elimination: Ability of the gastrointestinal tract to form and evacuate stool effectively
Knowledge: Health Behaviors: Extent of understanding conveyed about the promotion and protection of health

Client Will (Include Specific Time Frame)
- Verbalize understanding of physiology of bowel function.
- Identify acceptable interventions to promote adequate bowel function.
- Decrease reliance on laxatives/enemas.
- Establish individually appropriate pattern of elimination.

ACTIONS/INTERVENTIONS
Sample NIC linkages:
Bowel Management: Establishment and maintenance of a regular pattern of bowel elimination
Counseling: Use of an interactive helping process focusing on the needs, problems, or feelings of the patient and SOs to enhance or support coping, problem-solving, and interpersonal relationships
Medication Management: Facilitation of safe and effective use of prescription and over-the-counter drugs

NURSING PRIORITY NO. 1. To identify factors affecting individual beliefs:

- Determine client's understanding of a "normal" bowel pattern. Compare with client's current bowel functioning. *Helps to identify areas for discussion and/or intervention. For example, what is considered "normal" varies with the individual and geographic area, with differences in cultural expectations and dietary habits of that area.[1] In addition, individuals can think they are constipated when, in fact, their bowel movments are regular and soft, possibly revealing a problem with thought processes/perception. Some people believe they are constipated, or irregular, if they do not have a bowel movement every day because of ideas instilled from childhood.[2] The elderly client may believe that laxatives or purgatives are necessary for elimination, when in fact the problem may be long-standing habits, e.g., insufficient fluids, lack of exercise and/or fiber in the diet.[3]*

 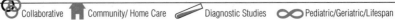

- Identify interventions used by client to correct perceived problem *to establish needed changes/interventions or points for discussion/teaching.*

NURSING PRIORITY NO. 2. To promote wellness (Teaching/Discharge Considerations):

- Discuss the following with client/SO/caregiver: (*to clarify issues regarding actual and perceived bowel functioning, and to provide support during behavior modification/bowel retraining*[3,4])
  Review anatomy and physiology of bowel function, and acceptable variations in elimination.

  Identify detrimental effects of long-term laxitive/enema use.
  Provide information and resources to client/SO about relationship of diet, exercise, fluid, regular time for elimination, and appropriate use of laxatives.
  Encourage client to maintain elimination calendar or diary if appropriate.
  Discuss rationale for and encourage continuation of successful interventions.
  Provide support by actively listening and discussing client's concerns/fears.
  Provide social and emotional support to help client manage actual or potential disabilities associated with long-term bowel management.
  Encourage use of stress reduction activities/refocusing of attention while client works to establish individually appropriate pattern.

DOCUMENTATION FOCUS

Assessment/Reassessment
- Assessment findings/client's perceptions of the problem.
- Current bowel pattern, stool characteristics.

Planning
- Plan of care/interventions and who is involved in the planning.
- Teaching plan.

Implementation/Evaluation
- Client's responses to interventions/teaching and actions performed.
- Changes in bowel pattern, character of stool.
- Attainment/progress toward desired outcome(s).
- Modifications to plan of care.

Discharge Planning
- Referral for follow-up care.

References

1. Pieken, S.R. (1999). Constipation. In Gastrointestinal Health. New York: HarperCollins.
2. Constipation. HIH Publication No. 95–2745, July, 1995. Bethesda, MD: National Digestive Diseases Information Clearinghouse (NDDIC).
3. Stanley, M. (1999). The aging gastrointestinal system with nutritional considerations. In Stanley, M., & Beare, P. G. (eds): Gerontological Nursing: A Health Promotion/Protection Approach, ed 7. Philadelphia: F. A. Davis, pp 180–181.
4. Hert, M., & Hueboe, J. (1998). Management of constipation. Iowa City (IA): University of Iowa Gerontological Nursing Interventions Research Center, Research Dissemination Core:[NGC 543]. Available at: www.guideline.gov. Accessed June 2003.

risk for Constipation

Definition: At risk for a decrease in normal frequency of defecation accompanied by difficult or incomplete passage of stool and/or passage of excessively hard, dry stool

RISK FACTORS

Functional
Irregular defecation habits; inadequate toileting (e.g., timeliness, positioning for defecation, privacy)
Insufficient physical activity, abdominal muscle weakness
Recent environmental changes
Habitual denial/ignoring of urge to defecate

Psychological
Emotional stress, depression, mental confusion

Physiologic
Change in usual foods and eating patterns, insufficient fiber/fluid intake, dehydration, poor eating habits
Inadequate dentition or oral hygiene
Decreased motility of gastrointestinal tract

Pharmacologic
Phenothiazides, nonsteroidal anti-inflammatory agents, sedatives, aluminum-containing antacids, laxative overuse, iron salts, anticholinergics, antidepressants, anticonvulsants, antilipemic agents, calcium channel blockers, calcium carbonate, diuretics, sympathomimetics, opiates, bismuth salts

Mechanical
Hemorrhoids, pregnancy; obesity
Rectal abscess or ulcer, anal stricture, anal fissures, prolapse, rectocele
Prostate enlargement, postsurgical obstruction
Neurologic impairment, megacolon (Hirschsprung's disease), tumors
Electrolyte imbalance
NOTE: A risk diagnosis is not evidenced by signs and symptoms, as the problem has not occurred and nursing interventions are directed at prevention.

SAMPLE CLINICAL APPLICATIONS: abdominal surgeries, hemorrhoids/anal lesions, irritable bowel syndrome, diverticulitis, spinal cord injury, multiple sclerosis, enteral/parenteral feedings, hypothyroidism, iron deficiency anemia, uremia/renal dialysis, Alzheimer's disease/dementia

DESIRED OUTCOMES/EVALUATION CRITERIA
Sample NOC linkages:
Bowel Elimination: Ability of the gastrointestinal tract to form and evacuate stool effectively
Risk Control: Actions to eliminate or reduce actual, personal, and modifiable health threats
Knowledge: Medication: Extent of understanding conveyed about the safe use of medication

 Cultural  Collaborative Community/ Home Care 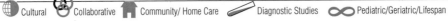 Diagnostic Studies Pediatric/Geriatric/Lifespan Medications

Client/Caregiver Will (Include Specific Time Frame)
- Maintain effective pattern of bowel functioning.
- Verbalize understanding of risk factors and appropriate interventions/solutions related to individual situation.
- Demonstrate behaviors or lifestyle changes to prevent developing problem.

ACTIONS/INTERVENTIONS

Sample NIC linkages:

Constipation/Impaction Management: Prevention and alleviation of constipation/impaction

Bowel Management: Establishment and maintenance of a regular pattern of bowel elimination

Medication Management: Facilitation of safe and effective use of prescription and OTC drugs

NURSING PRIORITY NO. 1. To identify individual risk factors/needs:

- Review medical/surgical history. *Problems with colon or rectum (e.g., obstruction, scar tissue, diverticulitis, tumors, irritable bowel syndrome), metabolic or endocrine disorders (e.g., diabetes mellitus, hypothyroidism, uremia), primary diseases of colon (e.g., cancers, stricture, anal fissure), limited physical activity (e.g., bedrest, poor mobility, chronic disability), chronic pain problems (especially when client is on pain medications), pregnancy and childbirth, recent abdominal or perianal surgery, neurologic disorders (e.g., parkinsonism, multiple sclerosis, spinal cord abnormalities) are all commonly associated with constipation.*[1,2,4,5,7–10]
- Note client's age. *Constipation is more likely to occur in individuals older than 55 years of age,*[1] *but can occur in any age from infant to elderly. A bottle-fed infant is more prone to constipation than breastfed infant, especially when formula contains iron.*[2,5] *Toddlers are at risk because developmental factors (e.g., too young, too interested in other things, rigid schedule during potty training), and children and adolescents are at risk because of unwillingness to take break from play, poor eating and fluid intake habits, and withholding because of perceived lack of privacy.*[3] *Many older adults experience constipation as a result of duller nerve sensations, incomplete emptying of the bowel or failing to attend to signals to defecate.*[4]
- Discuss usual elimination pattern and use of laxatives *to establish baseline and identify possible areas for intervention/instruction.*
- Ascertain client's beliefs and practices about bowel elimination, such as "must have a bowel movement every day or I need an enema." *These factors reflect familial and/or cultural thinking about elimination, which affect client's lifetime patterns.*
- Review daily dietary regimen. *Imbalanced nutrition influences the amount and consistency of feces.*[2] *Inadequate dietary fiber (vegetable, fruits, and whole grains) highly processed foods contribute to poor intestinal function. Loss of teeth can force individuals to eat soft foods, mostly lacking in fiber.*[1,4,5,8]
- Determine fluid intake *to note deficits. Most individuals do not drink enough fluids, even when healthy, reducing the speed at which stool moves through the colon. Active fluid loss through sweating, vomiting, diarrhea, or bleeding can greatly increase chances for constipation.*[1,2,4,5,7–10]
- Evaluate medication/drug usage and note interactions or side effects (e.g., narcotics, antacids, chemotherapy, iron, contrast media such as barium, steroids). *Many medications can slow passage of bowel movements.*[1,2,4,5,7–10]
- Note energy/activity level and exercise pattern. *Lack of physical activity and/or regular exercise is often a factor in constipation.*[1–4,7,8,10]

- Identify areas of life changes/stressors. *Factors such as pregnancy, travel, traumas, and changes in personal relationships, occupational factors, or financial concerns can cause or exacerbate constipation.*[7,10]
- Auscultate abdomen for presence, location, and characteristics of bowel sounds *reflecting bowel activity.*

NURSING PRIORITY NO. 2. To facilitate normal bowel function:

 Promote healthy lifestyle for elimination[1–10]:

Instruct in/encourage balanced fiber and bulk in diet *to improve consistency of stool and facilitate passage through colon.*

Limit foods with little or no fiber (e.g., ice cream, cheese, meat, and processed foods).

Promote adequate fluid intake, including water, high-fiber fruit, and vegetable juices. Suggest drinking warm, stimulating fluids (e.g., decaffeinated coffee, hot water, tea) *to promote moist/soft stool and increase rate of passage.*

Encourage daily activity/exercise within limits of individual ability *to stimulate contractions of the intestines.*

Encourage client to not ignore urge. Provide privacy and routinely scheduled time for defecation (bathroom or commode preferable to bedpan) *to promote psychological readiness and comfort.*

- Administer medications (stool softeners, mild stimulants, or bulk-forming agents) prn and/or routinely when appropriate *to prevent constipation (e.g., client taking pain medications, especially opiates, or who is inactive, immobile, or unconscious).*

NURSING PRIORITY NO. 3. Promote wellness (Teaching/Discharge Considerations)[1,8,10]:

- Discuss physiology and acceptable variations in elimination. *May help reduce concerns/anxiety about situation.*
- Review individual risk factors/potential problems and specific interventions *for prevention of constipation*
- Review appropriate use of medications, including laxatives *to manage elimination and prevent complications*
- Encourage client to maintain elimination diary if appropriate *to help monitor bowel pattern.*
- Refer to NDs Constipation; perceived Constipation.

DOCUMENTATION FOCUS

Assessment/Reassessment
- Current bowel pattern, characteristics of stool, medications.

Planning
- Plan of care and who is involved in planning.
- Teaching plan.

Implementation/Evaluation
- Responses to interventions/teaching and actions performed.
- Attainment/progress toward desired outcomes.
- Modifications to plan of care.

 Cultural   Collaborative 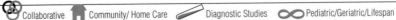 Community/ Home Care Diagnostic Studies Pediatric/Geriatric/Lifespan   Medications

Discharge Planning

- Individual long-term needs, noting who is responsible for actions to be taken.
- Specific referrals made.

References

1. Hert. M., Huseboe, J. (1998). Management of constipation. University of Iowa Gerontological Nursing Interventions Research Center, Research Dissemination Core. Iowa City (IA). [NGC: 543]. Retrieved from National Guideline Clearinghouse. Available at: http://www.guideline.gov.
2. Cox, H. C., et al. (2002). Clinical Applications of Nursing Diagnosis: Adult, Child, Women's Psychiatric, Gerontic, and Home Health Considerations, ed 3. Philadelphia: F. A. Davis, pp 192–205.
3. Streeter, B. L. (2002). Teenage constipation: A case study. Gastroenterol Nurs, 25(6), 253–256.
4. Stanley, M. (1999). The Aging Gastrointestinal System, with Nutritional Considerations. In Stanley, M., & Beare, P. G. Gerontological Nursing: A Health Promotion/Protection Approach, ed 7. Philadelphia: F. A. Davis, pp 180–181.
5. Constipation in Children. NIH Publication No. 02–4633, October 2001, National Digestive Diseases Information Clearinghouse (NDDIC), Bethesda, MD. Contact: nddic@info.niddk.nih.gov.
6. Idiopathic constipation and soiling in children. (1997). Ann Arbor: University of Michigan Medical Center. [NCG 1011]. Available at: www.guidline.gov.
7. Constipation. NIH Publication no. 95–2754, July, 1995. National Digestive Diseases Information Clearinghouse (NDDIC), Bethesda, MD. Contact: nddic@info.niddk.nih.gov.
8. Locke, G. R., Pemberton, J. H., & Phillips, S. F. (2000). American Gastroenterological Association: Medical position statement: Guidelines on constipation. Gastroenterology, 119(6), 1761–1766.
9. Neurogenic bowel management in adults with spinal cord injury. (1998). Paralyzed Veterans of America, Consortium for Spinal Cord Medicine: Clinical Practice Guidelines. Washington (DC).
10. Doenges, M. E., Moorhouse, M. F., & Geissler-Murr, A. C. (2002). Nurse's Pocket Guide: Diagnoses, Interventions, and Rationales, ed 8. Philadelphia: F. A. Davis, p.151.

compromised family Coping

Definition: Usually supportive primary person (family member or close friend [SO]) provides insufficient, ineffective, or compromised support, comfort, assistance, or encouragement that may be needed by the client to manage or master adaptive tasks related to his/her health challenge

RELATED FACTORS

Inadequate or incorrect information or understanding by a primary person

Temporary preoccupation by a significant person who is trying to manage emotional conflicts and personal suffering and is unable to perceive or act effectively in regard to client's needs

Temporary family disorganization and role changes

Other situational or developmental crises or situations the significant person may be facing

Little support provided by client, in turn, for primary person

Prolonged disease or disability progression that exhausts the supportive capacity of SO(s)

[Unrealistic expectations of client/SOs or each other]

[Lack of mutual decision-making skills]

[Diverse coalitions of family members]

DEFINING CHARACTERISTICS

Subjective

Client expresses or confirms a concern or complaint about SO's response to his or her health problem

SO describes preoccupation with personal reaction (e.g., fear, anticipatory grief, guilt, anxiety) to client's illness/disability, or other situational or developmental crises

SO describes or confirms an inadequate understanding or knowledge base that interferes with effective assistive or supportive behaviors

Objective

SO attempts assistive or supportive behaviors with less than satisfactory results

SO withdraws or enters into limited or temporary personal communication with the client at the time of need

SO displays protective behavior disproportionate (too little or too much) to the client's abilities or need for autonomy

[SO displays sudden outbursts of emotions/shows emotional lability or interferes with necessary nursing/medical interventions]

SAMPLE CLINICAL APPLICATIONS: chronic conditions (e.g., COPD, AIDS, Alzheimer's disease, pain, renal failure), substance abuse, cancer, depression, hypochondriasis

DESIRED OUTCOMES/EVALUATION CRITERIA

Sample NOC linkages:

Family Coping: Family actions to manage stressors that tax family resources

Family Normalization: Ability of the family to develop and maintain routines and management strategies that contribute to optimal functioning when a member has a chronic illness or disability

Family Environment: Internal: Social climate as characterized by family member relationships and goals

Family Will

- Identify/verbalize resources within themselves to deal with the situation.
- Interact appropriately with the client, providing support and assistance as indicated.
- Provide opportunity for client to deal with situation in own way.
- Verbalize knowledge and understanding of illness/disability/disease.
- Express feelings honestly.
- Identify need for outside support and seek such.

ACTIONS/INTERVENTIONS

Sample NIC linkages:

Family Involvement Promotion: Facilitating family participation in the emotional and physical care of the patient

Family Support: Promotion of family values, interests, and goals

Family Mobilization: Utilization of family strengths to influence patient's health in a positive direction

NURSING PRIORITY NO. 1. To assess causative/contributing factors:

- Identify underlying situation(s) that may contribute to the inability of family to provide needed assistance to the client. *Circumstances may have preceded the illness and now have a significant effect (e.g., client had a heart attack during sexual activity, mate is afraid of repeating).*[1]
- Note the length of illness such as cancer, multiple sclerosis, and/or other long-term situations that may exist. *Chronic/unresolved illness, accompanied by changes in role performance/responsibility, often exhausts supportive capacity and coping abilities of SO/family.*[1]

 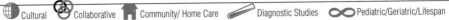

- Assess information available to and understood by the family/SO(s). *Access to and understanding of information regarding the specific illness/condition, treatment and prognosis is essential to family cooperation and care of the client.*[2]
- Discuss family perceptions of situation. *Expectations of client and family members may/may not be realistic and may interfere with ability to cope with situation.*[1]
- Identify role of the client in family and how illness has changed the family organization. *Illness affects how client performs usual functions in the family and affects how others in the family take over those responsibilities. These changes may result in dysfunctional behaviors, anger, hostility and hopelessness.*[1]
- Note other factors besides the client's illness that are affecting abilities of family members to provide needed support. *Individual members' preoccupation with own needs/concerns can interfere with providing needed care/support for stresses of long-term illness. Additionally, caregivers may incur decrease or loss of income/risk of losing own health insurance if they alter their work hours to care for client.*[1]

NURSING PRIORITY NO. 2. To assist family to reactivate/develop skills to deal with current situation:

- Listen to client's/SO's comments, remarks, and expression of concern(s). Note nonverbal behaviors and/or responses and congruency. *Provides information and promotes understanding of client's view of the illness and needs related to current situation.*[1]
- Encourage family members to verbalize feelings openly/clearly. *Promotes understanding of feelings in relationship to current events and helps them to hear what other person is saying, leading to more appropriate interactions.*[5]
- Discuss underlying reasons for client's behavior. *Helps family/SO understand and accept/deal with client behaviors that may be triggered by emotional or physical effects of illness.*[4]
- Assist the family and client to understand "who owns the problem" and who is responsible for resolution. Avoid placing blame or guilt. *When these boundaries are defined, each individual can begin to take care of own self and stop taking care of others in inappropriate ways.*[4]
- Encourage client and family to develop problem-solving skills to deal with the situation. *Use of these skills enables each member of the family to identify what he or she sees as the problem to be dealt with and contribute ideas for solutions that are acceptable to them, promoting more effective interactions among the family members.*[4]

NURSING PRIORITY NO. 3. To promote wellness (Teaching/Discharge Considerations):

- Provide information for family/SO(s) about specific illness/condition. *Promotes better understanding of need for following therapeutic regimen to provide maximum benefit.*[9]
- Involve client and family in planning care as often as possible. *When family members are knowledgeable and understand needs, commitment to plan is enhanced.*[9]
- Promote assistance of family in providing client care as appropriate. *Identifies ways of demonstrating support while maintaining client's independence (e.g., providing favorite foods, engaging in diversional activities).*[5]
- Note cultural factors related to family relationships which may be involved in problems of caring for member who is ill. *Family composition and structure, methods of decision making, gender issues and expectations will affect how family deals with stress of illness, negative prognosis.*[6]

- Refer to appropriate resources for assistance as indicated (e.g., counseling, psychotherapy, financial, spiritual). *May need additional help and getting to the appropriate resource provides accurate help for individual situation (e.g., family counseling, financial planning).*[9]
- Refer to NDs: Fear, Anxiety/death Anxiety, ineffective Coping, readiness for enhanced family Coping, disabled family Coping, anticipatory Grieving as appropriate.

DOCUMENTATION FOCUS

Assessment/Reassessment
- Assessment findings, including current/past coping behaviors, emotional response to situation/stressors, support systems available.

Planning
- Plan of care, who is involved in planning and areas of responsibility.
- Teaching plan.

Implementation/Evaluation
- Responses of family members/client to interventions/teaching and actions performed.
- Attainment/progress toward desired outcome(s).
- Modifications to plan of care.

Discharge Planning
- Long-range plan and who is responsible for actions.
- Specific referrals made.

References

1. Doenges, M., Moorhouse, M., & Geissler-Murr, A. (2002). Nursing Care Plans Guidelines for Individualizing Patient Care, ed 6. Philadelphia: F. A. Davis.
2. Bluman, I. G., et al. (1999). Attitudes, knowledge, and risk perceptions of women with breast and/ovarian cancer considering testing for BRCA1 and BRCA2. J Clin Oncol, 17(3), 1040–1046.
3. Doenges, M., Townsend, M., & Moorhouse, M. (1998). Psychiatric Care Plans: Guidelines for Individualizing Care, ed 3. Philadelphia: F. A. Davis.
4. Townsend, M. (2003). Psychiatric Mental Health Nursing: Concepts of Care, ed 4. Philadelphia: F. A. Davis.
5. Cox, H., Hinz, M., Lubno, M. A., Newfield, S., Ridenour, N., Slater, M., & Sridaromont, K. (2002). Clinical Applications of Nursing Diagnosis: Adult, Child, Women's, Psychiatric, Gerontic and Home Health Considerations, ed 4. Philadelphia: F. A. Davis.
6. Lipson, J. G., Dibble, S. L., & Minarik, P. A. (1996). Culture & Nursing Care: A Pocket Guide. San Francisco: School of Nursing, UCSF Nursing Press.
7. Townsend, M. (2001). Nursing diagnoses in Psychiatric Nursing: Care Plans and Psychotropic Medications, ed 5. Philadelphia: F. A. Davis.
8. Haeven, T. K., & Adams, K. J. (eds). (1982). Aging and life course transitions: An interdisciplinary perspective. New York: Guilford.
9. Ammon, S. (2001). Managing patients with heart failure. AJN, 101(12), 34–40.

defensive Coping

Definition: Repeated projection of falsely positive self-evaluation based on a self-protective pattern that defends against underlying perceived threats to positive self-regard.

 Cultural   Collaborative   Community/ Home Care   Diagnostic Studies   Pediatric/Geriatric/Lifespan   Medications

RELATED FACTORS

To be developed by nurse researchers and submitted to NANDA
[Refer to ND ineffective Coping]

DEFINING CHARACTERISTICS

Subjective

Denial of obvious problems/weaknesses
Projection of blame/responsibility
Hypersensitive to slight/criticism
Grandiosity
Rationalizes failures
[Refuses or rejects assistance]

Objective

Superior attitude toward others
Difficulty establishing/maintaining relationships, [avoidance of intimacy]
Hostile laughter or ridicule of others [aggressive behavior]
Difficulty in reality testing perceptions
Lack of follow-through or participation in treatment or therapy
[Attention-seeking behavior]

SAMPLE CLINICAL APPLICATIONS: eating disorders, substance abuse, chronic illness, bipolar/adjustment/dissociative disorders

DESIRED OUTCOMES/EVALUATION CRITERIA

Sample NOC linkages:
Self-Esteem: Personal judgment of self-worth
Coping: Actions to manage stressors that tax an individual's resources
Social Interaction Skills: An individual's use of effective interaction behaviors

Client Will (Include Specific Time Frame)

- Verbalize understanding of own problems/stressors.
- Identify areas of concern/problems.
- Demonstrate acceptance of responsibility for own actions, successes, and failures.
- Participate in treatment program/therapy.
- Maintain involvement in relationships.

ACTIONS/INTERVENTIONS

Sample NIC linkages:
Self-Awareness Enhancement: Assisting a patient to explore and understand his/her thoughts, feelings, motivations, and behaviors
Coping Enhancement: Assisting a patient to adapt to perceived stressors, changes, or threats that interfere with meeting life demands and roles
Counseling: Use of an interactive helping process focusing on the needs, problems, or feelings of the patient and significant others to enhance or support coping, problem-solving, and interpersonal relationships

NURSING PRIORITY NO. 1. To determine degree of impairment:

- Assess ability to comprehend current situation, developmental level of functioning. *Crucial to planning care for this individual. Client will have difficulty functioning in these circumstances.*[1]

- Determine level of anxiety and effectiveness of current coping mechanisms. *Severe anxiety will interfere with ability to cope, and client will need to assess what is working and develop new ways to deal with current situation.*[2]
- Determine coping mechanisms used (e.g., projection, avoidance, rationalization) and purpose of coping strategy (e.g., may mask low self-esteem). *Provides information about how these behaviors affect current situation.*[3]
- Assist client to identify/consider need to address problem differently. *Until client is willing to consider different approaches to dealing with situation, little progress can be expected.*[1]
- Describe all aspects of the problem through the use of therapeutic communication skills such as Active-listening. *Provides an opportunity for the client to clarify the situation and begin to look at options for problem-solving.*[2]
- Observe interactions with others. *Noting difficulties/ability to establish satisfactory relationships can provide clues to client behaviors that interfere with interactions with others.*[2]
- Note expressions of grandiosity in the face of contrary evidence (e.g., "I'm going to buy a new car" when the individual has no job or available finances). *Evidence of distorted thinking and possibility of mental illness.*[3]

NURSING PRIORITY NO. 2. To assist client to deal with current situation:

 - Provide explanation of the rules of the treatment program and discuss consequences of lack of cooperation. Encourage client participation in setting of consequences and agreement to them. *Promotes understanding and possibility of cooperation on the part of the client, especially when they have been involved in the decisions.*[2]
 - Set limits on manipulative behavior; be consistent in enforcing consequences when rules are broken and limits tested. *Providing clear information and following through on identified consequences reduce the ability to manipulate staff and environment.*[3]
 - Develop therapeutic relationship to enable client to test new behaviors in a safe environment. Use positive, nonjudgmental approach and "I" language. *Promotes sense of self-esteem and enhances sense of control.*[1]
 - Encourage control in all situations possible; include client in decisions and planning. *Preserves autonomy enabling realization of sense of self-worth.*[1]
 - Acknowledge individual strengths and incorporate awareness of personal assets/strengths in plan. *Promotes use of positive coping behaviors and progress toward effective solutions.*[4]
 - Convey attitude of acceptance and respect (unconditional positive regard). *Avoids threatening client's self-concept, preserving existing self-esteem.*[2]
 - Encourage identification and expression of feelings. *Provides opportunity for client to learn about and accept self and feelings as normal.*[2]
 - Provide/encourage use of healthy outlets for release of hostile feelings (e.g., punching bags, pounding boards). Involve in outdoor recreation program when available. *Promotes acceptable expression of these feelings which when unexpressed can lead to development of undesirable behaviors and make situation worse.*[4]
 - Provide opportunities for client to interact with others in a positive manner. *Promotes self-esteem and encourages client to learn how to develop/enhance relationships.*[4]
 - Assist client with problem-solving process. Identify and discuss responses to situation, maladaptive coping skills. Suggest alternative responses to situation. *Helps client select more adaptive strategies for coping.*[2]
 - Use confrontation judiciously *to help client begin to identify defense mechanisms (e.g., denial/projection) that are hindering development of satisfying relationships.*[2]

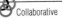 Cultural   Collaborative   Community/ Home Care   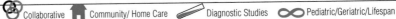 Diagnostic Studies   Pediatric/Geriatric/Lifespan   Medications

NURSING PRIORITY NO. 3. To promote wellness (Teaching/Discharge Considerations):

- Encourage client to learn relaxation techniques, use of guided imagery, and positive affirmation of self. *Enables client to incorporate and practice new behaviors to deal with stressors and view/respond to situation in a more realistic and positive manner.*[4]
- Promote involvement in activities/classes. *Client can practice new skills, develop new relationships, and learn new and positive ways of interacting with others.*[1]
- Refer to additional resources (e.g., substance rehabilitation, family/marital therapy) as indicated. *Can be useful in making desired changes and developing new coping skills.*[2]
- Refer to ND ineffective Coping for additional interventions.

DOCUMENTATION FOCUS

Assessment/Reassessment
- Assessment findings/presenting behaviors.
- Client perception of the present situation and usual coping methods/degree of impairment.

Planning
- Plan of care and interventions and who is involved in development of the plan.
- Teaching plan.

Implementation/Evaluation
- Response to interventions/teaching and actions performed.
- Attainment/progress toward desired outcome(s).
- Modifications to plan of care.

Discharge Planning
- Referrals and follow-up programing.

References

1. Doenges, M., Moorhouse, M., Murr, A. (2002). Nursing Care Plans, Guidelines for Individualizing Patient Care, ed 6. Philadelphia: F. A. Davis.
2. Doenges, M., Townsend, M., & Moorhouse, M. (1998). Psychiatric Care Plans: Guidelines for Individualizing Care, ed 3. Philadelphia: F. A. Davis.
3. Townsend, M. (2003). Psychiatric Mental Health Nursing: Concepts of Care, ed 4. Philadelphia: F. A. Davis.
4. Cox, H., Hinz, M., Lubno, M. A., Newfield, S., Ridenour, N., Slater, M., Sridaromont, K. (2002). Clinical Applications of Nursing Diagnosis Adult, Child, Women's Psychiatric, Gerontic and Home Health Considerations, ed 4. Philadelphia: F. A. Davis.

disabled family Coping

Definition: Behavior of SO (family member or other primary person) that disables his/her capacities and the client's capacity to effectively address tasks essential to either person's adaptation to the health challenge

RELATED FACTORS

Significant person with chronically unexpressed feelings of guilt, anxiety, hostility, despair, and so forth

Dissonant discrepancy of coping styles for dealing with adaptive tasks by the significant person and client or among significant people

Highly ambivalent family relationships

Arbitrary handling of a family's resistance to treatment that tends to solidify defensiveness as it fails to deal adequately with underlying anxiety

[High-risk family situations, such as single or adolescent parent, abusive relationship, substance abuse, acute/chronic disabilities, member with terminal illness]

DEFINING CHARACTERISTICS

Subjective
[Expresses despair regarding family reactions/lack of involvement]

Objective
Intolerance, rejection, abandonment, desertion

Psychosomaticism

Agitation, depression, aggression, hostility

Taking on illness signs of client

Neglectful relationships with other family members

Carrying on usual routines, disregarding client's needs

Neglectful care of the client in regard to basic human needs and/or illness treatment

Distortion of reality regarding the client's health problem, including extreme denial about its existence or severity

Decisions and actions by family that are detrimental to economic or social well-being

Impaired restructuring of a meaningful life for self, impaired individualization, prolonged overconcern for client

Client's development of helpless, inactive dependence

SAMPLE CLINICAL APPLICATIONS: chronic conditions (e.g., COPD, AIDS, Alzheimer's disease, chronic pain, renal failure, brain/spinal cord injury), substance abuse, cancer, genetic conditions (e.g., Down syndrome, sickle cell disease, Huntington's disease), depression, hypochondriasis

DESIRED OUTCOMES/EVALUATION CRITERIA

Sample NOC linkages:

Family Normalization: Ability of the family to develop and maintain routines and management strategies that contribute to optimal functioning when a member has a chronic illness or disability

Family Coping: Family actions to manage stressors that tax family resources

Family Environment: Internal: Social climate as characterized by family member relationships and goals

Family Will (Include Specific Time Frame)
- Verbalize more realistic understanding and expectations of the client.
- Visit/contact client regularly.
- Participate positively in care of client, within limits of family's abilities and client's needs.
- Express feelings and expectations openly and honestly as appropriate.

ACTIONS/INTERVENTIONS

Sample NIC linkages:

Family Therapy: Assisting family members to move their family toward a more productive way of living

 Cultural   Collaborative   Community/ Home Care   Diagnostic Studies 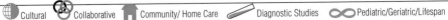 Pediatric/Geriatric/Lifespan   Medications

Family Support: Promotion of family values, interests, and goals
Family Involvement Promotion: Facilitating family participation in the emotional and physical care of the patient

NURSING PRIORITY NO. 1. To assess causative/contributing factors:

- Ascertain preillness behaviors/interactions of the family. *Provides comparative baseline for developing plan of care and determining interventions needed.*[4]
- Identify current behaviors of the family members (e.g., withdrawal—not visiting, brief visits, and/or ignoring client when visiting; anger and hostility toward client and others; ways of touching between family members, expressions of guilt). *Indicators of extent of problems existing in family. Relationships among family members before and after current illness affect ability to deal with problems of caretaking and lengthy illness.*[1]
- Discuss family perceptions of situation. *Expectations of client and family members may/may not be realistic and interfere with ability to deal with situation.*[6]
- Note cultural factors related to family relationships which may be involved in problems of caring for member who is ill. *Family composition and structure, methods of decision making, gender issues, and expectations will affect how family deals with stress of illness, negative prognosis.*[7]
- Note other factors that may be stressful for the family (e.g., financial difficulties or lack of community support, as when illness occurs when out of town). *Appropriate referrals can be made to provide information and assistance as needed. These problems can lead to caregiver burnout and compassion fatigue.*[6]
- Determine readiness of family members to be involved with care of the client. *Family members are involved in their lives, jobs, and families and may find it difficult to manage tasks necessary for helping with care of the client.*[6]

NURSING PRIORITY NO. 2. To provide assistance to enable family to deal with the current situation:

- Establish rapport with family members who are available. *Promotes therapeutic relationship and support for problem-solving solutions.*[1]
- Acknowledge difficulty of the situation for the family. *Communicates understanding of family's feelings and can reduce blaming and guilt feelings.*[2]
- Active-listen concerns, note both overconcern/lack of concern. *Identifies accuracy of client's information and measure of concern, which may interfere with ability to resolve situation.*[2]
- Allow free expression of feelings, including frustration, anger, hostility, and hopelessness while placing limits on acting-out/inappropriate behaviors. *Provides opportunity to identify accuracy and validate appropriateness of feelings. Limits minimize risk of violent behavior.*[4]
- Give accurate information to SO(s) from the beginning. *Establishes trust and promotes opportunity for clarification and correction of misunderstandings.*[4]
- Act as liaison between family and healthcare providers. *Provides single contact to provide explanations and clarify treatment plan, enhancing reliability of information.*[4]
- Provide brief, simple explanations about use and alarms when equipment (such as a ventilator) is involved. Identify appropriate professional(s) for continued support/problem solving. *Having information and ready access to appropriate resources can reduce feelings of helplessness and promote sense of control.*[1]
- Provide time for private interaction between client and family/significant other(s). *Individuals need to talk about what is happening and process new and frightening information to learn to deal with situation/diagnosis within family relationships.*[3]

- Include SO(s) in the plan of care. Provide instruction/demonstrate necessary skills. *Promotes family's ability to provide care and develop a sense of control over difficult situation.*[3]
- Accompany family when they visit client. *Being available for questions, concerns, and support promotes trusting relationship in which family feels free to learn all they can about situation/diagnosis.*[3]
- Assist SO(s) to initiate therapeutic communication with client. *Learning to use new methods of communication (Active-listening and I-messages) can enhance relationships and promote effective problem-solving for the family.*[3]
- Refer client to protective services as necessitated by risk of physical harm/neglect. *Removing client from home enhances individual safety. May reduce stress on family to allow opportunity for therapeutic intervention.*[3]

NURSING PRIORITY NO. 3. To promote wellness (Teaching/Discharge Considerations):

- Assist family to identify coping skills being used and how these skills are/are not helping them deal with situation. *When family members know this information, they can begin to enhance those skills that are more effective in promoting healthy family functioning in difficult times.*[3]
- Answer family's questions patiently and honestly. Reinforce information provided by other providers. *Continues trusting relationship with family members and promotes understanding of the situation/prognosis so family members can deal more effectively with what is happening.*[1]
- Reframe negative expressions into positive whenever possible. *A positive frame contributes to supportive interactions and can lead to better outcomes.*[3]
- Respect family needs for withdrawal and intervene judiciously. *Situation may be overwhelming and time away can be beneficial to continued participation. A brief respite can refresh family members who are serving as caregivers and permit renewed ability to manage situation.*[1]
- Encourage family to deal with the situation in small increments rather than trying to deal with the whole picture. *Reduces likelihood of individual being overwhelmed by possibilities that may face them in potentially disabling or fatal outcomes.*[1]
- Assist the family to identify familiar things that would be helpful to the client (e.g., a family picture on the wall), especially when hospitalized for long time, such as in hospice or long-term care. *Reinforces/maintains orientation and provides a sense of home and family for client.*[1]
- Refer family to appropriate resources as needed (e.g., family therapy, financial counseling, spiritual advisor). *May need additional help to deal with difficult situation/illness.*[6]
- Refer to ND anticipatory Grieving as appropriate.

DOCUMENTATION FOCUS

Assessment/Reassessment
- Assessment findings, current/past behaviors including family members who are directly involved and support systems available.
- Emotional response(s) to situation/stressors.

Planning
- Plan of care/interventions and who is involved in planning.
- Teaching plan.

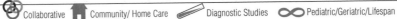 Cultural Collaborative Community/ Home Care Diagnostic Studies Pediatric/Geriatric/Lifespan Medications

Implementation/Evaluation
- Responses of individuals to interventions/teaching and actions performed.
- Attainment/progress toward desired outcome(s).
- Modifications to plan of care.

Discharge Planning
- Ongoing needs/resources/other follow-up recommendations and who is responsible for actions.
- Specific referrals made.

References

1. Doenges, M., Moorhouse, M., & Murr, A. (2002). Nursing Care Plans, Guidelines for Individualizing Patient Care, ed 6. Philadelphia: F. A. Davis.
2. Doenges, M., Townsend, M., & Moorhouse, M. (1998). Psychiatric Care Plans: Guidelines for Individualizing Care, ed 3. Philadelphia: F. A. Davis.
3. Townsend, M. (2003). Psychiatric Mental Health Nursing: Concepts of Care, ed 4. Philadelphia: F. A. Davis.
4. Cox, H., Hinz, M., Lubno, M. A., Newfield, S., Ridenour, N., Slater, M., & Sridaromont, K. (2002). Clinical Applications of Nursing Diagnosis Adult, Child, Women's Psychiatric, Gerontic and Home Health Considerations, ed 4. Philadelphia: F. A. Davis.
5. Hareven, T. K., & Adams, K. J. (eds). (1982). Aging and life course transitions. An interdisciplinary perspective. New York: Guilford.
6. Sims, D.D. (1993). If I Could Just See Hope, Finding Your Way Through Grief. Louisville, KY: Grief Inc.
7. Lipson, J. G., Dibble, S. L., & Minarik, P. A. (1996). Culture & Nursing Care: A Pocket Guide. San Francisco: School of Nursing, UCSF Nursing Press.

ineffective Coping

Definition: Inability to form a valid appraisal of the stressors, inadequate choices of practiced responses, and/or inability to use available resources

RELATED FACTORS
Situational/maturational crises

High degree of threat

Inadequate opportunity to prepare for stressor; disturbance in pattern of appraisal of threat

Inadequate level of confidence in ability to cope/perception of control; uncertainty

Inadequate resources available; inadequate social support created by characteristics of relationships

Disturbance in pattern of tension release; inability to conserve adaptive energies

Gender differences in coping strategies

[Work overload, no vacations, too many deadlines; little or no exercise]

[Impairment of nervous system; cognitive/sensory/perceptual impairment, memory loss]

[Severe/chronic pain]

DEFINING CHARACTERISTICS

Subjective
Verbalization of inability to cope or inability to ask for help

Sleep disturbance; fatigue

Abuse of chemical agents

[Reports of muscular/emotional tension, lack of appetite]

Objective

Lack of goal-directed behavior/resolution of problem, including inability to attend to and difficulty with organizing information; [lack of assertive behavior]

Use of forms of coping that impede adaptive behavior [including inappropriate use of defense mechanisms, verbal manipulation]

Inadequate problem solving

Inability to meet role expectations/basic needs

Decreased use of social supports

Poor concentration

Change in usual communication patterns

High illness rate [including high blood pressure, ulcers, irritable bowel, frequent headaches/neckaches]

Risk-taking

Destructive behavior toward self or others [including overeating, excessive smoking/drinking, overuse of prescribed/OTC medications, illicit drug use]

[Behavioral changes (e.g., impatience, frustration, irritability, discouragement)]

SAMPLE CLINICAL APPLICATIONS: new diagnosis of major illness, chronic conditions, major depression, substance abuse, eating disorders, bipolar disorder, social anxiety disorder, pregnancy/parenting

DESIRED OUTCOMES/EVALUATION CRITERIA

Sample NOC linkages:

Coping: Actions to manage stressors that tax an individual's resources

Impulse Control: Self-restraint of compulsive or impulsive behaviors

Decision Making: Ability to choose between two or more alternatives

Client Will (Include Specific Time Frame)

- Assess the current situation accurately.
- Identify ineffective coping behaviors and consequences.
- Verbalize awareness of own coping abilities.
- Verbalize feelings congruent with behavior.
- Meet psychological needs as evidenced by appropriate expression of feelings, identification of options, and use of resources.

ACTIONS/INTERVENTIONS

Sample NIC linkages:

Coping Enhancement: Assisting a patient to adapt to perceived stressors, changes, or threats that interfere with meeting life demands and roles

Decision-Making Support: Providing information and support for a person who is making a decision regarding healthcare

Impulse Control Training: Assisting the patient to mediate impulsive behavior through application of problem-solving strategies to social and interpersonal situations

NURSING PRIORITY NO. **1.** To determine degree of impairment:

- Evaluate ability to understand events, provide realistic appraisal of situation. *Necessary information for developing workable plan of care.*[2]
- Identify developmental level of functioning. *People tend to regress to a lower developmental stage during illness/crisis and recognition of client's level enables more appropriate interventions to be implemented.*[2]

 Cultural   Collaborative   Community/ Home Care 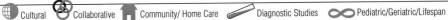 Diagnostic Studies   Pediatric/Geriatric/Lifespan   Medications

- Assess current functional capacity and note how it is affecting the individual's coping ability. *Promotes identification of strategies that will be helpful in current situation.*[4]
- Determine alcohol intake, drug use, smoking habits, sleeping and eating patterns. *Substance abuse impairs ability to deal with what is happening in current situation. Identification of impaired sleeping and eating patterns provides clues to extent of anxiety and impaired coping.*[2]
- Ascertain impact of illness on sexual needs/relationship. *Illnesses, medications and many treatment regimens can affect sexual functioning, and identification of individual problems can lead to appropriate interventions.*[2]
- Assess level of anxiety and coping on an ongoing basis. *Identifies changes in ability to cope and worsening of ability to understand at an early stage where intervention can be most effective.*[4]
- Note speech and communication patterns. *Identifies existing problems and assesses ability to understand situation/communicate needs.*[7]
- Observe and describe behavior in objective terms. Validate observations. *Promotes accuracy and assures correctness of conclusions to arrive at the best possible solutions.*[7]

NURSING PRIORITY NO. 2. To assess coping abilities and skills:

- Ascertain client's understanding of current situation and its impact. *Client may not understand situation and knowing these factors are necessary to planning care and identifying appropriate interventions.*[8]
- Active-listen and identify client's perceptions of what is happening. *Reflecting client's thoughts can provide a forum for understanding perceptions in relation to reality for planning care and determining accuracy of interventions needed.*[2]
- Evaluate client's decision-making ability. *When ability to make decisions is impaired by illness or treatment regimen, it is important to take this into consideration when planning care to maximize participation and positive outcomes.*[9]
- Determine previous methods of dealing with life problems. *Identifies successful techniques that can be used in current situation. Often client is preoccupied by current concerns and does not think about previous successful skills.*[8]

NURSING PRIORITY NO. 3. To assist client to deal with current situation:

- Call client by name. Ascertain how client prefers to be addressed. *Using client's name enhances sense of self and promotes individuality/self-esteem.*[2]
- Encourage communication with staff/SOs. *Developing positive interactions between staff, SO(s) and client ensures that everyone has the same understanding.*[8]
- Use reality orientation (e.g., clocks, calendars, bulletin boards) and make frequent references to time, place as indicated. Place needed/familiar objects within sight for visual cues. *Often client can be disoriented by changes in routine, anxiety about illness and treatment regimens, and these measures help the client maintain orientation and a sense of reality.*[9]
- Provide for continuity of care with same personnel taking care of the client as often as possible. *Developing relationships with same caregivers promotes trust and enables client to discuss concerns and fears freely.*[9]
- Explain disease process/procedures/events in a simple, concise manner. *Devoting time for listening may help client to express emotions, grasp situation, and feel more in control.*[10]
- Provide for a quiet environment/position equipment out of view as much as possible. *Anxiety is increased by noisy surroundings.*[8]
- Schedule activities so periods of rest alternate with nursing care. Increase activity slowly. *Client is weakened by illness and ensuring rest can promote ability to cope.*[8]

- 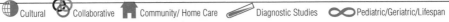 Assist client in use of diversion, recreation, relaxation techniques. *Learning new skills not only can be helpful for reducing stress, but will be useful in the future as the client learns to cope more successfully.*[8]
- Stress positive body responses to medical conditions, but do not negate the seriousness of the situation (e.g., stable blood pressure during gastric bleed or improved body posture in depressed client). *Acknowledging the reality of the illness while accurately stating the facts can provide hope and encouragement.*[8]
- Encourage client to try new coping behaviors and gradually master situation. *Practicing new ways of dealing with what is happening leads to being more comfortable and can promote a positive outcome as client relaxes and handles illness and treatment regimen more successfully.*[9]
- Confront client when behavior is inappropriate, pointing out difference between words and actions. *Provides external locus of control, enhancing safety while client learns self-control.*[2]
- Assist in dealing with change in concept of body image as appropriate. (Refer to ND disturbed Body Image.) *New view of self may be negative and client needs to incorporate change in a positive manner to enhance self-image.*[11]

NURSING PRIORITY NO. 4. To provide for meeting psychological needs:

- Treat the client with courtesy and respect. Converse at client's level, providing meaningful conversation while performing care. *Enhances therapeutic relationship.*[2]
- Take advantage of teachable moments. *Individuals learn best and are open to new information when they feel accepted and are in a comfortable environment.*[11]
- Allow client to react in own way without judgment by staff/caregivers. *Provide support and diversion as indicated. Unconditional positive regard and support promotes acceptance, enabling client to deal with difficult situation in a positive way.*[8]
- Encourage verbalization of fears and anxieties and expression of feelings of denial, depression, and anger. *Free expression allows for dealing with these feelings and when the client knows that these are normal reactions, he or she can deal with them better.*[11]
- Provide opportunity for expression of sexual concerns. *Important aspect of person that may be difficult to express. Providing an opening for discussion by asking sensitive questions can allow client to talk about concerns.*[11]
- Help client to set limits on acting-out behaviors and learn ways to express emotions in an acceptable manner. *Enables client to gain sense of self-esteem, promoting internal locus of control.*[2]

NURSING PRIORITY NO. 5. To promote wellness (Teaching/Discharge Considerations):

- Give updated/additional information needed about events, cause (if known), and potential course of illness as soon as possible. *Knowledge helps reduce anxiety/fear, allows client to deal with reality.*[8]
- Provide and encourage an atmosphere of realistic hope. *Promotes optimistic outlook energizing client to address situation. Client needs to hear positive things while undergoing difficult circumstances.*[8]
- Give information about purposes and side effects of medications/treatments. *Client feels included, promotes sense of control enabling client to cope with situation in a more positive manner.*[8]

- Stress importance of follow-up care. *Checkups to make sure regimen is being followed accurately and that healing is progressing promotes a satisfactory outcome.*[8]
- Encourage and support client in evaluating lifestyle, occupation, and leisure activities. *Helps client to look at difficult areas that may contribute to anxiety and to make changes gradually without undue/debilitating anxiety.*[8]
- Assess effects of stressors (e.g., family, social, work environment, or nursing/healthcare management) and discuss ways to deal with them. *Identifying these factors will enable client to develop strategies to make changes needed to promote wellness.*[8]
- Provide for gradual implementation and continuation of necessary behavior/lifestyle changes. *Change is difficult and beginning slowly enhances commitment to plan.*[8]
- Discuss/review anticipated procedures and client concerns, as well as postoperative expectations when surgery is recommended. *Knowledge allays fears and helps client to understand procedures and treatments and expected results. When client has prior information about what to expect during postoperative course, he or she will remain calm and anxiety is reduced.*[11]
- Refer to outside resources and/or professional therapy as indicated/ordered. *May be necessary to assist with long-term improvement.*[11]
- Determine need/desire for religious representative/spiritual counselor and make arrangements for visit. *Spiritual needs are an integral part of being human and determining and meeting individual preferences helps client deal with concerns/desires for discussion/assistance in this area.*[12]
- Provide information/consultation as indicated for sexual concerns. Provide privacy when client not in home. *Individuals are sexual beings and concerns about role in family/relationship, ability to function are often not readily expressed. Discussion opens opportunity for clarification and understanding and helps to meet need for intimacy.*[11]
- Refer to other NDs as indicated (e.g., Pain; Anxiety, impaired verbal Communication, [actual/] risk for self- or other-directed Violence). *Provides further assistance in area of identified need.*[13]

DOCUMENTATION FOCUS

Assessment/Reassessment
- Baseline findings, degree of impairment, and client's perceptions of situation.
- Coping abilities and previous ways of dealing with life problems.

Planning
- Plan of care/interventions and who is involved in planning.
- Teaching plan.

Implementation/Evaluation
- Client's responses to interventions/teaching and actions performed.
- Medication dose, time, and client's response.
- Attainment/progress toward desired outcome(s).
- Modifications to plan of care.

Discharge Planning
- Long-term needs and actions to be taken.
- Support systems available, specific referrals made, and who is responsible for actions to be taken.

References

1. Doenges, M., Moorhouse, M., & Murr, A.(2002). Nursing Care Plans, Guidelines for Individualizing Patient Care, ed 6. Philadelphia: F. A. Davis.
2. Doenges, M., Townsend, M., & Moorhouse, M. (1998). Psychiatric Care Plans: Guidelines for Individualizing Care, ed 3. Philadelphia: F. A. Davis.
3. Townsend, M. (2003). Psychiatric Mental Health Nursing: Concepts of Care, ed 4. Philadelphia: F. A. Davis.
4. Cox, H., Hinz, M., Lubno, M. A., Newfield, S., Ridenour, N., Slater, M., & Sridaromont, K. (2002). Clinical Applications of Nursing Diagnosis Adult, Child, Women's Psychiatric, Gerontic and Home Health Considerations, ed 3. Philadelphia: F. A. Davis.
5. Lipson, J. G. Dibble, S. L., & Minarik, P. A. (1996). Culture & Nursing Care: A Pocket Guide. San Francisco: School of Nursing, UCSF Nursing Press.
6. Townsend, M. (2001). Nursing diagnoses in Psychiatric Nursing: Care Plans and Psychotropic Medications, ed 5. Philadelphia: F. A. Davis.
7. Haeven, T. K., & Adams, K. J. (eds). (1982). Aging and Life Course Transitions: An Interdisciplinary Perspective. New York: Guilford.
8. Cherif, M., & Younis, E.I. (2000). Liver transplantation. Clin Fam Prac, 2(1), 117.
9. Liken, M. A. (2001b). Caregivers in crisis: Moving a relative with Alzheimer's to assisted living. Clin Nurs Res, 10(1), 53–69.
10. HIV/AIDS Treatment Information Service. (2001). Guidelines for the use of antiretroviral agents in HIV-infected adults and adolescents. Available at: www.hivatis.org/ guidelines/adult/aug13_01/pdf/aaaug 13s.pdf (9Nov. 2001).
11. Tan, G., Waldman, K., & Bostick, R. (Winter, 2002). Psychosocial issues, sexuality, and Cancer. Sexuality Disabil, 20(4), 297–318.
12. Geiter, H. (2002). The spiritual side of nursing. RN, 65(5), 43–44.
13. Doenges, M., Moorhouse, M., & Murr, A. (2004). Nurse's Pocket Guide diagnoses, Interventions, and Rationales, ed 9. Philadelphia: F. A. Davis.

ineffective community Coping

Definition: Pattern of community activities (for adaptation and problem solving) that is unsatisfactory for meeting the demands or needs of the community

RELATED FACTORS
Deficits in social support services and resources
Inadequate resources for problem solving
Ineffective or nonexistent community systems (e.g., lack of emergency medical system, transportation system, or disaster planning systems)
Natural or human-made disasters

DEFINING CHARACTERISTICS

Subjective
Community does not meet its own expectations
Expressed vulnerability; community powerlessness
Stressors perceived as excessive

Objective
Deficits of community participation
Excessive community conflicts
High illness rates

 Cultural Collaborative Community/ Home Care Diagnostic Studies 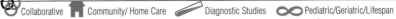 Pediatric/Geriatric/Lifespan Medications

Increased social problems (e.g., homicide, vandalism, arson, terrorism, robbery, infanticide, abuse, divorce, unemployment, poverty, militance, mental illness)

SAMPLE CLINICAL APPLICATIONS: high rate of illness/injury/violence

DESIRED OUTCOMES/EVALUATION CRITERIA

Sample NOC linkages:

Community Competence: The ability of a community to collectively problem solve to achieve goals

Community Health Status: The general state of well-being of a community or population

Community Will (Include Specific Time Frame)

- Recognize negative and positive factors affecting community's ability to meet its demands or needs.
- Identify alternatives to inappropriate activities for adaptation/problem solving.
- Report a measurable increase in necessary/desired activities to improve community functioning.

ACTIONS/INTERVENTIONS

Sample NIC linkages:

Community Health Development: Facilitating members of a community to identify a community's health concerns, mobilize resources, and implement solutions

Environmental Management: Community: Monitoring and influencing of the physical, social, cultural, economic, and political conditions that affect the health of groups and communities

Community Disaster Preparedness: Preparing for an effective response to a large-scale disaster

NURSING PRIORITY NO. 1. To identify causative or precipitating factors:

- Evaluate community activities as related to meeting collective needs within the community itself and between the community and the larger society. *Determining what activities are currently available and what needs are not being met, either by the local or county/state entities. Provide information on which to base the steps needed to begin planning for desired changes.*[1]
- Note community reports of community functioning including areas of weakness or conflict. *Community is responsible for identifying needed changes for possible action.*[1]
- Identify effects of Related Factors on community activities. Note immediate needs (e.g., healthcare, food, shelter, funds). *Provides a baseline to determine community needs and identifying factors that are pertinent to the community allows community to deal with current concerns.*[1,5]
- Plan for the possibility of a disaster when determined by current circumstances. *In relation to threats, terrorist activities, and natural disasters, actions need to be coordinated between the local and the larger community.*[5]
- Determine availability and use of resources. *Helpful to begin planning to correct deficiencies that have been identified. Sometimes even though resources are available, they are not being used appropriately or fully.*[2]
- Identify unmet demands or needs of the community. *Determining where the deficiencies are is a crucial step to beginning to make an accurate plan for correction. Sometimes elected bodies see the problems differently from the general population and conflict can arise, therefore it is important for communication to resolve the issues that are in question.*[2]

NURSING PRIORITY NO. 2. To assist the community to reactivate/develop skills to deal with needs:

 • Determine community *strengths. Promotes understanding of ways in which community is already meeting identified needs and once identified, they can be built on to develop plan to improve community.*[1]

 • Identify and prioritize community goals. *Goals enable the identification of actions to direct the changes that are needed to improve the community. Prioritizing enables actions to be taken in order of importance.*[1]

 • Encourage community members/groups to engage in problem-solving activities. *Individuals who are involved in the problem-solving process and make a commitment to the solutions have an investment and are more apt to follow through on their commitments.*[3]

 • Develop a plan jointly with community to deal with deficits in support. *Working together will enhance efforts and help to meet identified goals.*[3]

NURSING PRIORITY NO. 3. To promote wellness as related to community health:

 • Create plans managing interactions within the community itself and between the community and the larger society. *These activities will meet collective needs.*[1]

 • Assist the community to form partnerships within the community and between the community and the larger society. *Promotes long-term development of the community to deal with current and future problems.*[1]

 • Provide channels for dissemination of information to the community as a whole, for example, print media; radio/television reports and community bulletin boards; speakers' bureau; reports to committees, councils, advisory boards on file and accessible to the public. *Having information readily available for everyone provides opportunity for all members of the community to know what is being planned and have input into the planning. Keeping community informed promotes understanding of needs and plans and probability of follow-through to successful outcomes.*[1]

 • Make information available in different modalities and geared to differing educational levels/cultures of the community. *Assures understanding by all members of the community and promotes cooperation with planning and follow-through.*[1]

 • Seek out and evaluate underserved populations. *These members of the community deserve to be helped to become productive citizens and be involved in the changes that are occurring.*[3]

 • Work with community members to identify lifestyle changes that can be made to meet the goals identified to improve the community deficits. *Changing lifestyles can promote a sense of power and encourage members to become involved in improving their community.*[4]

DOCUMENTATION FOCUS

Assessment/Reassessment
• Assessment findings, including perception of community members regarding problems.

Planning
• Plan of care and who is involved in planning.
• Teaching plan.

Implementation/Evaluation
• Response of community entities to plan/interventions and actions performed.
• Attainment/progress toward desired outcome(s).
• Modifications to plan of care.

 Cultural Collaborative 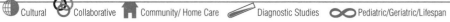 Community/ Home Care Diagnostic Studies Pediatric/Geriatric/Lifespan Medications

Discharge Planning
- Long-range plans and who is responsible for actions to be taken.

References

1. Higgs, Z.R., & Gustafson, D. (1985). Community as a Client: Assessment and Diagnosis. Philadelphia: F. A. Davis.
2. Hunt. R. (1998). Community-based nursing. AJN, 98(10), 44.
3. Schaeder, C, et al. (1997). Community nursing organizations: A new frontier. AJN, 97(1), 63.
4. Lai, S.C., & Cohen, M.N. (1999). Promoting lifestyle changes. AJN, 99(4), 63.
5. Doenges, M., Moorhouse, M., & Geissler-Murr, A. (2002). Nursing Care Plans Guidelines for Individualizing Patient Care, ed 6. Philadelphia: F. A. Davis.

readiness for enhanced Coping

Definition: A pattern of cognitive and behavioral efforts to manage demands that is sufficient for well-being and can be strengthened

RELATED FACTORS

To be developed by nurse researchers and submitted to NANDA

DEFINING CHARACTERISTICS

Subjective
Defines stressors as manageable
Seeks social support
Seeks knowledge of new strategies
Acknowledges power
Is aware of possible environmental changes

Objective
Uses a broad range of problem-oriented strategies
Uses spiritual resources

SAMPLE CLINICAL APPLICATIONS: chronic health conditions (e.g., asthma, diabetes mellitus, arthritis, systemic lupus, multiple sclerosis, AIDS), mental health concerns (e.g., seasonal affective disorder, attention deficit disorder, Down syndrome)

DESIRED OUTCOMES/EVALUATION CRITERIA
Sample NOC linkages:
Coping: Actions to manage stressors that tax an individual's resources
Quality of Life: An individual's expressed satisfaction with current life circumstances
Hope: Presence of internal state of optimism that is personally satisfying and life-supporting

Client Will (Include Specific Time Frame)
- Assess current situation accurately.
- Identify effective coping behaviors currently being used.
- Verbalize feelings congruent with behavior.
- Meet psychological needs as evidenced by appropriate expression of feelings, identification of options, and use of resources.

ACTIONS/INTERVENTIONS

Sample NIC linkages:

Coping Enhancement: Assisting a patient to adapt to perceived stressors, changes, or threats that interfere with meeting life demands and roles

Self-Awareness Enhancement: assisting a patient to explore and understand his/her thoughts, feelings, motivations, and behaviors

Teaching: Individual: Planning, implementation, and evaluation of a teaching program designed to address a patient's particular needs

NURSING PRIORITY NO. 1. To determine needs and desire for improvement:

- Evaluate client's understanding of situation, ability to provide realistic appraisal of situation. *Provides information about client's perception, cognitive ability, and whether the client is aware of the facts of the situation, providing essential information for planning care.*[1]

 • Determine stressors that may be affecting client. *Accurate identification of situation that client is dealing with provides information for planning interventions to enhance coping abilities.*[1]

 • Identify social supports available to client. *Available support systems, such as family/friends, can provide client with ability to handle current stressful events and often 'talking it out' with an empathic listener will help client move forward to enhance coping skills.*[1]

- Review coping strategies client is aware of and using. *The desire to improve one's coping ability is based on an awareness of the current status of the stressful situation.*[1]

- Determine use of alcohol/other drugs and smoking habits during times of stress. *Recognition of potential for substituting these actions or old habits to deal with anxiety increases individual's awareness of opportunity to choose new ways to cope with life stressors.*[2]

- Assess level of anxiety and coping on an ongoing basis. *Provides baseline to develop plan of care to improve coping abilities.*[2]

- Note speech and communication patterns. *Assesses ability to understand and provides information necessary to help client make progress in desire to enhance coping abilities.*[2]

 • Evaluate client's decision-making ability. *Understanding client's ability provides a starting point for developing plan and determining what information client needs to develop more effective coping skills.*[1]

NURSING PRIORITY NO. 2. To assist client to develop enhanced coping skills:

 • Active-listen and identify client's perceptions of current status. *Reflecting client's statements and thoughts can provide a forum for understanding perceptions in relation to reality for planning care and determining accuracy of interventions needed.*[3]

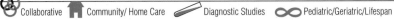 • Determine previous methods of dealing with life problems. *Enables client to identify successful techniques used in the past, promoting feelings of confidence in own ability.*[2]

- Discuss desire to improve ability to manage stressors of life. *Understanding motivation behind decision to seek new information to enhance life will help client know what is needed to learn new skills of coping.*[1]

- Discuss understanding of concept of knowing what can and cannot be changed. *Acceptance of reality that some things cannot be changed allows client to focus energies on dealing with things that can be changed.*[1]

Cultural   Collaborative   Community/ Home Care   Diagnostic Studies   Pediatric/Geriatric/Lifespan   Medications

NURSING PRIORITY NO. 3. To promote wellness (Teaching/Learning Considerations):

- Discuss predisposing factors related to any individual's response to stress. *Understanding that genetic influences, past experiences, and existing conditions determine whether a person's response is adaptive or maladaptive will give client a base on which to continue to learn what is needed to improve life.*[1]
- Assist client to develop a stress management program. *An individualized program of relaxation, meditation, involvement with caring for others/pets, etc., enhances sense of balance in life and strengthens client's ability to manage challenging situations.*[1]
- Help client develop problem-solving skills. *Learning the process for problem solving will promote successful resolution of potentially stressful situations that arise.*[4]
- Encourage involvement in activities of interest, such as exercise/sports, music, and art. *Individuals must decide for themselves what coping strategies are adaptive for them. Most people find enjoyment and relaxation in these kinds of activities.*[1]
- Discuss possibility of doing volunteer work in an area of the client's choosing. *Many individuals report satisfaction in giving of themselves and client may find sense of fulfillment in service to others.*[1]
- Refer to classes and/or reading material as appropriate. *May be helpful to further learning and pursuing goal of enhanced coping ability.*[1]

DOCUMENTATION FOCUS

Assessment/Reassessment
- Baseline information, client's perception of need.
- Coping abilities and previous ways of dealing with life problems.

Planning
- Plan of care/interventions and who is involved in planning.
- Teaching plan.

Implementation/Evaluation
- Client's responses to interventions/teaching and actions performed.
- Attainment/progress toward desired outcome(s).
- Modifications to plan of care.

Discharge Planning
- Long-term needs and actions to be taken
- Support systems available, specific referrals made, and who is responsible for actions to be taken.

References

1. Townsend, M. (2003). Psychiatric Mental Health Nursing Concepts of Care, ed 4. Philadelphia: F. A. Davis.
2. Doenges, M. E., Moorhouse, M. F., & Murr, A. C. (2004). Nurse's Pocket Guide Diagnoses, Interventions, and Rationales, ed 9. Philadelphia: F. A. Davis.
3. Doenges, M., Townsend, M., & Moorhouse, M. (1998). Psychiatric Care Plans: Guidelines for Individualizing Care, ed 3. Philadelphia: F. A. Davis.
4. Gordon, T. (2000). Parent Effectiveness Training, updated edition. New York: Three Rivers Press.

Definition: Pattern of community activities for adaptation and problem solving that is satisfactory for meeting the demands or needs of the community but can be improved for management of current and future problems/stressors

RELATED FACTORS

Social supports available
Resources available for problem solving
Community has a sense of power to manage stressors

DEFINING CHARACTERISTICS

Subjective
Agreement that community is responsible for stress management

Objective
Deficits in one or more characteristics that indicate effective coping
Active planning by community for predicted stressors
Active problem solving by community when faced with issues
Positive communication among community members
Positive communication between community/aggregates and larger community
Programs available for recreation and relaxation
Resources sufficient for managing stressors

Sample Clinical Applications: reducing rates of illness/injury/violence

DESIRED OUTCOMES/EVALUATION CRITERIA

Sample NOC linkages:

Community Competence: The ability of a community to collectively problem solve to achieve goals

Community Health Status: The general state of well-being of a community or population

Community Will (Include Specific Time Frame)
- Identify positive and negative factors affecting management of current and future problems/stressors.
- Have an established plan in place to deal with problems/stressors.
- Describe management of deficits in characteristics that indicate effective coping.
- Report a measurable increase in ability to deal with problems/stressors.

ACTIONS/INTERVENTIONS

Sample NIC linkages:

Program Development: Planning, implementating, and evaluating a coordinated set of activities designed to enhance wellness, or to prevent, reduce, or eliminate one or more health problems of a group or community

Environmental Management: Community: Monitoring and influencing of the physical, social, cultural, economic, and political conditions that affect the health of groups and communities

Health Policy Monitoring: Surveillance and influence of government and organization regulations, rules, and standards that affect nursing systems and practices to ensure quality care of patients

 Cultural Collaborative Community/ Home Care  Diagnostic Studies 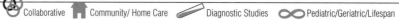 Pediatric/Geriatric/Lifespan Medications

NURSING PRIORITY NO. 1. To determine existence of and deficits or weaknesses in management of current and future problems/stressors:

- Review community plan for dealing with problems/stressors, untoward events such as natural disaster/terrorist activity. *Provides a baseline for comparision of preparedness with other communities and develops plan to address concerns.*[5]
- Assess effects of Related Factors on management of problems/stressors. *Identifying social supports available and awareness of the power of the community can enhance the plans needed to improve the community.*[1]
- Determine community's strengths. *Plan can build on strengths to address areas of weakness.*[2]
- Identify limitations in current pattern of community activities. *Recognition of the factors that can be improved through adaptation and problem solving will make it easier for the community to proceed with planning to make improvements that have been identified as necessary.*[4]
- Evaluate community activities as related to management of problems/stressors within the community itself and between the community and the larger society. *Disasters occurring in the community or in the country affect the local community and need to be recognized and addressed.*[5]

NURSING PRIORITY NO. 2. To assist the community in adaptation and problem solving for management of current and future needs/stressors:

- Define and discuss current needs and anticipated or projected concerns. *Agreement on scope/parameters of needs is essential for effective planning.*[2]
- Identify and prioritize goals to facilitate accomplishment. *Helps to bring the community together to meet a common concern/threat, maintain focus and facilitating accomplishment.*[5]
- Identify and interact with available resources (e.g., persons, groups, financial, governmental, as well as other communities). *Promotes cooperation. Major catastrophes, such as earthquakes, floods, terrorist activity, affect more than local community, and communities need to work together to deal with and accomplish reconstruction and future growth.*[6]
- Make a joint plan with the community and the larger community to deal with adaptation and problem solving. *Promotes management of problems/stressors to enable most effective solution for identified concern.*[3]
- Seek out and involve underserved/at-risk groups within the community. *Supports communication and commitment of community as a whole.*[3]

NURSING PRIORITY NO. 3. To enhance well-being of community:

- Assist the community to form partnerships within the community and between the community and the larger society. *Promotes long-term developmental growth of the community.*[5]
- Support development of plans for maintaining these interactions.
- Establish mechanism for self-monitoring of community needs and evaluation of efforts. *Facilitates proactive rather than reactive responses by the community.*
- Use multiple formats, for example, TV, radio, print media, billboards and computer bulletin boards, speakers' bureau, reports to community leaders/groups on file and accessible to the public. *Keeps community informed regarding plans, needs, outcomes to encourage continued understanding and participation.*[6]

Assessment/Reassessment

- Assessment findings and community's perception of situation.
- Identified areas of concern, community strengths/weaknesses.

Planning

- Plan and who is involved and responsible for each action.
- Teaching plan.

Implementation/Evaluation

- Response of community entities to the actions performed.
- Attainment/progress toward desired outcomes.
- Modifications to plan.

Discharge Planning

- Short-range and long-range plans to deal with current, anticipated, and potential problems and who is responsible for follow-through.
- Specific referrals made, coalitions formed.

References

1. Higgs, Z.R., & Gustafson, D. (1985). Community as a Client: Assessment and Diagnosis. Philadelphia: F. A. Davis.
2. Hunt. R. (1998). Community-based nursing. AJN, 98(10), 44.
3. Schaeder, C. et al. (1997). Community nursing organizations: A new frontier. AJN, 97(1), 63.
4. Lai, S.C., & Cohen, M.N. (1999). Promoting lifestyle changes. AJN, 99(4), 63.
5. Doenges, M., Moorhouse, M., & Geissler-Murr, A. (2002). Nursing Care Plans Guidelines for Individualizing Patient Care, ed 6. Philadelphia: F. A. Davis.
6. Stanhope, M., & Lancaster, J. (2000). Community and Public Health Nursing, ed 5. St. Louis, MO: Mosby.

readiness for enhanced family Coping

Definition: Effective managing of adaptive tasks by family member involved with the client's health challenge, who now exhibits desire and readiness for enhanced health and growth in regard to self and in relation to the client

RELATED FACTORS

Needs sufficiently gratified and adaptive tasks effectively addressed to enable goals of self-actualization to surface

[Developmental stage, situational crises/supports]

DEFINING CHARACTERISTICS

Subjective

Family member attempting to describe growth impact of crisis on his or her own values, priorities, goals, or relationships

Individual expressing interest in making contact on a one-to-one basis or on a mutual-aid group basis with another person who has experienced a similar situation

 Cultural Collaborative Community/ Home Care  Diagnostic Studies Pediatric/Geriatric/Lifespan Medications

Objective

Family member moving in direction of health-promoting and enriching lifestyle that supports and monitors maturational processes, audits and negotiates treatment programs, and generally chooses experiences that optimize wellness

SAMPLE CLINICAL APPLICATIONS: genetic disorders (e.g., Down syndrome, cystic fibrosis, neural tube defects), traumatic injury (e.g., amputation, spinal cord), chronic conditions (e.g., asthma, AIDS, Alzheimer's disease)

DESIRED OUTCOMES/EVALUATION CRITERIA

Sample NOC linkages:

Family Participation in Professional Care: Family involvement in decision making, delivery, and evaluation of care provided by health care professionals

Family Coping: Family actions to manage stressors that tax family resources

Family Functioning: Ability of the family to meet the needs of its members through developmental transitions

Family Will (Include Specific Time Frame)

- Express willingness to look at own role in the family's growth.
- Verbalize desire to undertake tasks leading to change.
- Report feelings of self-confidence and satisfaction with progress being made.

ACTIONS/INTERVENTIONS

Sample NIC linkages:

Normalization Promotion: Assisting parents and other family members of children with chronic diseases or disabilities in providing normal life experiences for their children and families

Family Support: Promotion of family values, interests, and goals

Family Involvement Promotion: Facilitating family participation in the emotional and physical care of the patient

NURSING PRIORITY NO. 1. To assess situation and adaptive skills being used by the family members:

- Determine individual situation and stage of growth family is experiencing/demonstrating. *Essential elements needed to identify family needs and develop plan of care for improving communication and interactions.*[1]
- Observe communication patterns of family. Listen to family's expressions of hope, planning, effect on relationships/life. *Provides clues to difficulties that individuals may have in expressing themselves effectively to others. Beginning to plan for the future with hope promotes changes in relationships that can enhance living for those involved.*[3]
- Note expressions such as "Life has more meaning for me since this has occurred." *Such statements identify change in values that may occur with the diagnosis/stress of a serious/potentially fatal illness.*[1]
- Identify cultural/religious health beliefs and expectations. *Beliefs about causes of illness may affect how family interacts with client (e.g., African-Americans may believe the illness is punishment for improper behavior, and may result in anger and statements of condemnation).*[6]

NURSING PRIORITY NO. 2. To assist family to develop/strengthen potential for growth:

- Provide time to talk with family to discuss their view of the situation. *Provides an opportunity to hear family's understanding and determine how realistic their ideas are for planning how they are going to deal with situation in the most positive manner.*[3]

- Establish a relationship with family/client. *Therapeutic relationships foster growth and enable family to identify skills needed for coping with difficult situation/illness.*[3]

- Provide a role model with which the family may identify. *Setting a positive example can be a powerful influence in changing behavior and as family members learn more effective communication skills, consideration for others, warmth and understanding, family relationships will be enhanced.*[2]

- Discuss importance of open communication and of not having secrets. *Functional communication is clear, direct, open and honest, with congruence between verbal and nonverbal. Dysfunctional communication is indirect, vague, controlled, with many double-bind messages. Awareness of this information can enhance relationships among family members.*[3]

- Demonstrate techniques such as Active-listening, I-messages, and problem solving. *Learning these skills can facilitate effective communication and improve interactions within the family.*[2]

NURSING PRIORITY NO. 3. To promote optimum wellness (Teaching/Discharge Considerations):

- Assist family to support the client in meeting own needs within ability and/or constraints of the illness/situation. *Family members may do too much for client or may not do enough, believing client 'wants to be babied.' With information and support they can learn to allow client to take the lead in doing what he or she is able to do.*[3]

- Provide experiences for the family to help them learn ways of assisting/supporting client. *Learning is enhanced when individual participates in hands-on opportunities to try out new activities.*[4]

- Discuss cultural beliefs and practices that may impact family members' interaction with client and dealing with condition. *Preconceived biases may interfere with efforts toward positive growth.*[6]

- Identify other clients/groups with similar conditions and assist client/family to make contact (groups such as Reach for Recovery, CanSurmount, Al-Anon, and so on). *Provides ongoing support for sharing common experiences, problem solving, and learning new behaviors.*[5]

- Assist family members to learn new, effective ways of dealing with feelings/reactions. *Awareness of ineffective methods that have been used and developing new and effective methods is essential to reach the goal of enhancing the family relationships.*[3]

DOCUMENTATION FOCUS

Assessment/Reassessment
- Adaptive skills being used, stage of growth.
- Family communication patterns.

Planning
- Plan of care/interventions and who is involved in planning.
- Teaching plan.

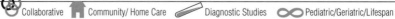 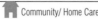

Implementation/Evaluation
- Client's responses to interventions/teaching and actions performed.
- Attainment/progress toward desired outcome(s).
- Modifications to plan of care.

Discharge Planning
- Identified needs/referrals for follow-up care, support systems.
- Specific referral.

References

1. Doenges, M., Moorhouse, M., Murr, A. (2002). Nursing Care Plans, Guidelines for Individualizing Patient Care, ed 6. Philadelphia: F. A. Davis.
2. Doenges, M., Townsend, M., & Moorhouse, M. (1998). Psychiatric Care Plans: Guidelines for Individualizing Care, ed 3. Philadelphia: F. A. Davis.
3. Townsend, M. (2003). Psychiatric Mental Health Nursing: Concepts of Care, ed 4. Philadelphia: F. A. Davis.
4. Cox, H., Hinz, M., Lubno, M. A., Newfield, S., Ridenour, N., Slater, M., Sridaromont, K. (2002). Clinical Applications of Nursing Diagnosis Adult, Child, Women's Psychiatric, Gerontic and Home Health Considerations, ed 4. Philadelphia: F. A. Davis.
5. Sims, D. (1993). If I Could Just See Hope. Louisville, KY: Grief Inc. Available at: www.griefinc.com.
6. Lipson, J. G., Dibble. S. L., Minarik, P. A. (1996). Culture & Nursing Care: A Pocket Guide. San Francisco: School of Nursing, UCSF Nursing Press, 1996.

risk for sudden infant Death Syndrome

Definition: Presence of risk factors for sudden death of an infant under 1 year of age

RISK FACTORS

Modifiable
Delayed or nonattendance of prenatal care
Infants placed to sleep in the prone or side-lying position
Soft underlayment/loose articles in the sleep environment
Infant overheating/overwrapping
Prenatal and postnatal smoke exposure

Potentially Modifiable
Young maternal age
Low birth weight; prematurity

Nonmodifiable
Male gender
Ethnicity (e.g., African American, Native American race of mother)
Seasonality of SIDS deaths (higher in winter and fall months)
SIDS mortality peaks between infant aged 2 to 4 months
SAMPLE CLINICAL APPLICATIONS: any child during first year of life
NOTE: A risk diagnosis is not evidenced by signs and symptoms, as the problem has not occurred and nursing interventions are directed at prevention.

DESIRED OUTCOMES/EVALUATION CRITERIA

Sample NOC linkages:

Risk Detection: Activities taken to identify personal health threats

Risk Control: Actions to eliminate or reduce actual, personal, and modifiable health threats

Knowledge: Infant Care: Extent of understanding conveyed about caring for a baby up to 12 months

Parent Will (Include Specific Time Frame)

- Verbalize knowledge of modifiable factors that can be addressed.
- Make changes in environment to prevent death occurring from other factors.
- Follows medically recommended prenatal and post-natal care.

ACTIONS/INTERVENTIONS

Sample NIC linkages:

Risk Identification: Analysis of potential risk factors, determination of health risks, and prioritization of risk reduction strategies for an individual or group

Parent Education: Infant: Instruction on nurturing and physical care during the first year of life

Teaching: Infant Safety: Instruction on safety during first year of life

NURSING PRIORITY NO. 1. To assess causative/contributing factors:

- Identify individual risk factors pertaining to situation. *Determines modifiable or potentially modifiable factors that can be addressed and treated. SIDS is the most common cause of death between 2 weeks and 1 year of age, with peak incidence occurring between the second and fourth month.*[1]
- Determine ethnicity, cultural background of family. *While distribution is worldwide, African-American babies are twice as likely to die of SIDS and American-Indian babies are nearly three times more likely to die than white babies.*[1,2]
- Note whether mother smoked during pregnancy or is currently smoking. *Many risk factors for SIDS also apply to non-SIDS deaths as well and smoking is known to negatively affect the fetus prenatally as well as after birth.*[1,2] *Some reports indicate an increased risk of SIDS in babies of smoking mothers.*[3]
- Assess extent of prenatal care, how early begun, extent to which mother followed recommended care measures. *Prenatal care is important for all pregnancies to afford the optimal opportunity for all infants to have a healthy start to life.*[4]
- Provide information about signs of premature labor and actions to be taken in the event they occur. *Prompt action can prevent early delivery and the complications of prematurity.*[4]
- Note use of alcohol/determine use of other drugs (including prescribed medications) during and after pregnancy. *Avoiding the use of alcohol and evaluating use of medications that may have an impact on the developing fetus enables management to minimize any damaging effects. While these are not known to affect the occurrence of SIDS, a healthy baby will be less apt to have problems.*[1]
- Evaluate the use of alcohol in American-Indian mother. *Infants whose mothers drank any amount of alcohol 3 months before conception through the first trimester had six times the risk of SIDS as those whose mothers did not drink. Mothers who consumed five or more drinks at one sitting during the first trimester had eight times the risk as those whose mothers did not binge drink.*[5]

 Cultural Collaborative 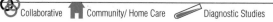 Community/ Home Care  Diagnostic Studies 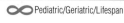 Pediatric/Geriatric/Lifespan Medications

NURSING PRIORITY NO. 2. Promote use of activities to minimize risk of SIDS:

- Stress importance of placing baby on his or her back to sleep, both at nighttime and naptime. *Research shows that fewer babies die of SIDS when they sleep on their backs. More than 5000 babies in the United States died of SIDS yearly until the Back to Sleep campaign began. Now the number of babies who die of SIDS is less than 3000 per year.*[6]

- Be sure that formal child care providers as well as grandparents, babysitters, neighbors or anyone who will have responsibility for the care of the child during sleep are aware of correct sleeping position. *The recommendation is to always place the child on his or her back until they roll over on their own; then repositioning is not required.*[1]

- Encourage parents to schedule awake tummy time. *This activity promotes strengthening of back and neck muscles while parents are close and baby is not sleeping.*[1]

- Encourage early and medically recommended prenatal care and continue with well-baby check-ups and immunizations after birth. *Prematurity presents many problems for the newborn and keeping babies healthy prevents problems that could put the infant at risk for SIDS. Immunizing infants prevent many illnesses that can be life-threatening.*[1,4]

- Encourage breastfeeding, if possible. *Breastfeeding has many advantages (immunological, nutritional, and psychosocial) promoting a healthy infant. While this does not preclude the occurrence of SIDS, healthy babies are less prone to many illnesses/problems.*[1,4]

- Discuss issues of bedsharing/co-sleeping and the concerns regarding sudden unexpected infant deaths from accidental entrapment under a sleeping adult or suffocation by becoming wedged in a couch or cushioned chair. *While co-sleeping is controversial, there are concerns about problems of accidental death from suffocation. Bedsharing or putting infant to sleep in an unsafe situation results in dangerous sleep environments that place infants at substantial risk for sudden unexpected death in infancy (SUDI).*[6]

- Note cultural beliefs about bedsharing. *Bedsharing is more common among breastfed infants, young, unmarried, low income, or those from a minority group. Additional study is needed to better understand bedsharing practices and its associated risks and benefits.*[6]

NURSING PRIORITY NO. 3. To promote wellness (Teaching/Discharge Considerations):

- Discuss known facts about SIDS with parents. *SIDS cannot be predicted or prevented. The cause while not known is not suffocation, aspiration, or regurgitation. A minor illness may be present but most victims are entirely healthy before death and many have recently been seen by their physician. It is not contagious or hereditary and is not an unusual disease (approximately 3000 babies die every year in the United States). Of every 1000 babies that are born, 999 survive, for a survival rate of 99.9%.*[1]

- Avoid overdressing or overheating infants during sleep. *Babies should be kept warm, but not too warm. Too many layers of clothing or blankets can overheat the infant. Room temperature that is comfortable for an adult will be comfortable for the baby. Infants who were dressed in two or more layers of clothes as they slept had six times the risk of SIDS as those dressed in fewer layers.*[1,4]

- Place the baby on a firm mattress in an approved crib. *Avoiding soft mattresses, sofas, cushions, waterbeds, other soft surfaces, while not known to prevent SIDS, will minimize chance of suffocation.*[1]

- Remove fluffy and loose bedding from sleep area, making sure baby's head and face are not covered during sleep. *Using only sleep clothing without a blanket, or if a blanket is used, making sure it is below baby's face and tucked in at the foot of the bed minimizes possibility of suffocation.*[1]

- Discuss the use of apnea monitors. *Apnea monitors are not recommended to prevent SIDS, but may be used to monitor other medical problems. Only a small percentage of infants who died of SIDS were known to have prolonged apnea episodes and monitors are also not medically recommended for subsequent siblings.*[1,2]

- Discourage frequent checking of the infant. *Since there is nothing that can be done to prevent the occurrence of SIDS, frequent checking only tires the parents and creates an atmosphere of tension and anxiety.*[1,2]
- Recommend public health nurse visit new mothers at least once or twice following discharge. *Researchers found that American-Indian infants whose mothers received such visits were 80% less likely to die from SIDS than those who were never visited.*[4]
- Refer parents to local SIDS programs and encourage consultation with health care provider if baby shows any signs of illness or behaviors that concern them. *Provides information to assure parents and/or correct treatable problems.*[1]

DOCUMENTATION FOCUS

Assessment/Reassessment
- Baseline findings, degree of parental anxiety/concern.

Planning
- Plan of care/interventions and who is involved in planning.
- Teaching plan.

Implementation/Evaluation
- Parent's responses to interventions/teaching and actions performed.
- Attainment/progress toward desired outcome(s)
- Modifications to plan of care.

Discharge Planning
- Long-term needs and actions to be taken.
- Support systems available, specific referrals made, and who is responsible for actions to be taken.

References

1. The Colorado SIDS Program, Inc, 6825 East Tennessee Ave, Suite 300, Denver, CO 80224–1631.
2. Beers, M.H., & Berkow, R. (1999). The Merck Manual of Diagnosis and Therapy, ed 17. Whitehouse Station, NJ: Merck Research Laboratories.
3. Phillips, C.R. (1996). Family-Centered Maternity and Newborn Care, ed 4. St. Louis, MO: Mosby.
4. London, M., Ladewig, P., Ball, J., Bindler, R. (2003). Maternal-Newborn & Child Nursing; Family-Centered Care. Upper Saddle River, NJ: Prentice Hall.
5. Iyasu, S., Randall, L.L., et al (2002). Risk factors for sudden infant death syndrome among Northern Plains Indians. JAMA, 288(21), 2717.
6. American Academy of Pediatrics, Task Force on Sleep Position and SIDS. (2000). Changing concepts of sudden infant death syndrome: Implications for infant sleep environment and position. Pediatrics, 105, 650–656.

ineffective Denial

Definition: Conscious or unconscious attempt to disavow the knowledge or meaning of an event to reduce anxiety/fear, but leading to the detriment of health

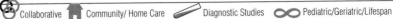
 Cultural Collaborative Community/ Home Care Diagnostic Studies 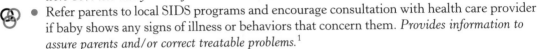 Pediatric/Geriatric/Lifespan Medications

To be developed by nurse researchers and submitted to NANDA

[Personal vulnerability; unmet self-needs]

[Presence of overwhelming anxiety-producing feelings/situation; reality factors that are consciously intolerable]

[Fear of consequences, negative past experiences]

[Learned response patterns, e.g., avoidance]

[Cultural factors, personal/family value systems]

DEFINING CHARACTERISTICS

Subjective

Minimizes symptoms; displaces source of symptoms to other organs

Unable to admit impact of disease on life pattern

Displaces fear of impact of the condition

Does not admit fear of death or invalidism

Objective

Delays seeking or refuses healthcare attention to the detriment of health

Does not perceive personal relevance of symptoms or danger

Makes dismissive gestures or comments when speaking of distressing events

Displays inappropriate affect

Uses home remedies (self-treatment) to relieve symptoms

SAMPLE CLINICAL APPLICATIONS: chronic illnesses, eating disorders, substance abuse, Alzheimer's disease, terminal conditions, bipolar disorder, body dysmorphic disorder

DESIRED OUTCOMES/EVALUATION CRITERIA

Sample NOC linkages:

Acceptance: Health Status: Reconciliation to health circumstances

Health Beliefs: Perceived Threat: Personal conviction that a health problem is serious and has potential negative consequences for lifestyle

Psychosocial Adjustment: Life Change: Psychosocial adaptation of an individual to a life change

Client Will (Include Specific Time Frame)

- Acknowledge reality of situation/illness.
- Express realistic concern/feelings about symptoms/illness.
- Seek appropriate assistance for presenting problem.
- Display appropriate affect.

ACTIONS/INTERVENTIONS

Sample NIC linkages:

Anxiety Reduction: Minimizing apprehension, dread, foreboding, or uneasiness related to an unidentified source or anticipated danger

Counseling: Use of an interactive helping process focusing on the needs, problems, or feelings of the patient and significant others to enhance or support coping, problem-solving, and interpersonal relationships

Coping Enhancement: Assisting a patient to adapt to perceived stressors, changes, or threats that interfere with meeting life demands and roles

NURSING PRIORITY NO. 1. To assess causative/contributing factors:

- Identify situational crisis/problem and client's perception of the situation. *Identification of both reality and client's perception, which may not be the same as the reality, are necessary for planning care accurately.*[1]
- Determine stage and degree of denial. *These factors will help identify whether the client is in early stages of denial and may be more amenable to intervention than those who are well entrenched in their beliefs. Treatment needs to begin where the client is and progress from there.*[1]
- Compare client's description of symptoms/conditions to reality of clinical picture and impact of illness/problem on lifestyle. *Identifies extent of discrepancy between the two and where treatment needs to start to help client accept reality.*[1]

NURSING PRIORITY NO. 2. To assist client to deal appropriately with situation:

- Develop nurse-client relationship by using therapeutic communication skills of Active-listening and I-messages. *Promotes trust in which client can begin to look at reality of situation and deal with it in a positive manner.*[2]
- Provide safe, nonthreatening environment. *Allows client to feel comfortable enough to deal with issues realistically.*[2]
- Encourage expressions of feelings, accepting client's view of the situation without confrontation. Set limits on maladaptive behavior *to promote safety. Allows client to work through and understand feelings. Unacceptable behavior is counterproductive to making progress as client will view self negatively.*[2]
- Present accurate information as appropriate, without insisting that the client accept what has been presented. *Avoids confrontation, which may further entrench client in denial. Open manner allows client to begin to accept reality.*[2]
- Discuss client's behaviors in relation to illness (e.g., diabetes mellitus, alcoholism, terminal cancer) and point out the results of these behaviors. *Information can help client accept reality and opt to change behaviors.*[3]
- Encourage client to talk with SO(s)/friends. *May clarify concerns and reduce isolation and withdrawal. Feedback from others facilitates understanding.*[4]
- Involve in group sessions. *Promotes discussion and feedback to enhance learning. Client can hear other views of reality and test own perceptions.*[4]
- Avoid agreeing with inaccurate statements/perceptions. *Prevents perpetuating false reality.*[2]
- Provide positive feedback for constructive moves toward independence. *Promotes repetition of desired behavior.*[4]

NURSING PRIORITY NO. 3. To promote wellness (Teaching/Discharge Considerations):

- Provide written information about illness/situation for client and family. *Can refer to for reminders as they consider options.*[1]
- Involve family members/SO(s) in long-range planning. *Helps to identify and meet individual needs for the future.*[4]
- Refer to appropriate community resources (e.g., Diabetes Association, Multiple Sclerosis Society, Alcoholics Anonymous). *May be needed to help client with long-term adjustment.*[2]
- Refer to ND ineffective Coping.

Assessment/Reassessment

- Assessment findings, degree of personal vulnerability/denial.
- Impact of illness/problem on lifestyle.

Planning

- Plan of care and who is involved in the planning.
- Teaching plan.

Implementation/Evaluation

- Client's response to interventions/teaching and actions performed.
- Use of resources.
- Attainment/progress toward desired outcome(s).
- Modifications to plan of care.

Discharge Planning

- Long-term needs and who is responsible for actions taken.
- Specific referrals made.

References

1. Doenges, M. E., Moorhouse, M. F., & Geissler-Murr, A. (2002). Nursing Care Plans Guidelines for Individualizing Patient Care, ed 6. Philadelphia: F. A. Davis.
2. Doenges, M. E., Townsend, M. C., Moorhouse, M. F. (1998). Psychiatric Care Plans, ed 3. Philadelphia: F. A. Davis.
3. Burgess, E. (1994). Denial and terminal illness. Am J Hospice Palliative Care, 11(2), 46–48.
4. Robinson, A.W. (1999). Getting to the heart of denial. AJN, 99(5), 38–42.
5. Townsend, M. C. (2003). Psychiatric Mental Health Nursing Concepts of Care, ed 4. Philadelphia: F. A. Davis.

impaired Dentition

Definition: Disruption in tooth development/eruption patterns or structural integrity of individual teeth

RELATED FACTORS

Dietary habits; nutritional deficits

Selected prescription medications; chronic use of tobacco, coffee or tea, red wine

Ineffective oral hygiene, sensitivity to heat or cold, chronic vomiting

Lack of knowledge regarding dental health, excessive use of abrasive cleaning agents/intake of fluorides

Barriers to self-care, access or economic barriers to professional care

Genetic predisposition, premature loss of primary teeth, bruxism

[Traumatic injury/surgical intervention]

DEFINING CHARACTERISTICS

Subjective
Toothache

Objective

Halitosis

Tooth enamel discoloration, erosion of enamel, excessive plaque

Worn down or abraded teeth, crown or root caries, tooth fracture(s)/ [pits/fissures]

Loose teeth, missing teeth or complete absence

Premature loss of primary teeth; incomplete eruption for age (may be primary or permanent teeth)

Excessive calculus

Malocclusion or tooth misalignment; asymmetrical facial expression

SAMPLE CLINICAL APPLICATIONS: facial trauma/surgery, malnutrition, eating disorders, head/neck cancer, seizure disorder

DESIRED OUTCOMES/EVALUATION CRITERIA

Sample NOC linkages:

Oral Health: Condition of the mouth, teeth, gums, and tongue

Self-Care: Oral Hygiene: Ability to care for own mouth and teeth

Knowledge: Health Behaviors: Extent of understanding conveyed about the promotion and protection of health

Client/SO Will (Include Specific Time Frame)

- Display clean teeth, pink healthy gums and mucous membranes.
- Verbalize and demonstrate effective dental hygiene skills.
- Engage in behaviors that improve oral/dental health.

ACTION/INTERVENTIONS

Sample NIC linkages:

Oral Health Maintenance: Maintenance and promotion of oral hygiene and dental health for the patient at risk for developing oral or dental lesions

Oral Health Restoration: Promotion of healing for a patient who has an oral mucosa or dental lesion

Referral: Arrangement for services by another care provider or agency

NURSING PRIORITY NO. 1. To assess causative/contributing factors:

- Inspect oral cavity. Note presence/absence and intactness of teeth or dentures and appearance of gums. *Provides baseline for planning and interventions in terms of safety, nutritional needs and aesthetics.*[1]
- Evaluate current status of dental hygiene and oral health *to determine need for teaching, assistive devices, and/or referral to dentist or periodontist.*[1]
- Note presence of halitosis. *Bad breath may be result of numerous local or systemic conditions, including smoking, periodontal disease, dehydration, malnutrition, ketoacidosis, infections, or some anti-seizure medications. Management can include simple mouth care or treatment of underlying conditions.*[2]
- Document age/developmental and cognitive status; manual dexterity. Evaluate nutritional and health state, noting presence of conditions such as bulimia/chronic vomiting; musculoskeletal impairments; or problems with mouth (e.g., bleeding disorders, cancer lesions/abscesses, facial trauma). *Factors affecting client's dental health and ability to provide own dental care.*[1]
- Note current situation that will affect dental health (e.g., presence of airway/ET intuba-

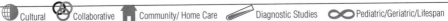

tion, facial fractures, jaw surgery, new braces, and use of anticoagulants or chemotherapy) *that require special mouth care activities.*[1]

- Document (photograph) facial injuries before treatment *to provide "pictorial baseline" for future comparison/evaluation.*

NURSING PRIORITY NO. 2. To treat/manage dental care needs:

- Ascertain client's usual method of oral care *to provide continuity of care or to build on client's existing knowledge base and current practices in developing plan of care.*[1]
- Remind client to brush teeth if indicated. *Cues may be needed if client is young, elderly or cognitively or emotionally impaired.*[1]
- Assist with/provide oral care, as indicated[1]:
  Offer/provide tap water or saline rinses, diluted alcohol-free mouthwashes. Provide gentle gum massage and tongue cleaning with soft toothbrush.
  Assist with brushing and flossing when client is unable to do self-care.
  Use foam sticks to swab gums and oral cavity.[8]
  Provide/assist with battery-powered mouth care devices (e.g., toothbrush, plaque remover etc) if indicated.
  Assist with/provide denture care when indicated (e.g., remove and clean after meals and at bedtime).
- Reposition endotracheal tubes and airway adjuncts routinely, carefully padding/protecting teeth/prosthetics.
- Suction as needed *(if client is unable to manage secretions).*
- Provide appropriate diet for optimal nutrition, considering client's ability to chew (e.g., liquids or soft foods), and offering low sugar, low starch foods and snacks *to minimize tooth decay.*
- Avoid thermal stimuli when teeth are sensitive. Recommend use of specific designed toothpastes *to reduce sensitivity of teeth.*
- Maintain good jaw/facial alignment when fractures are present.
- Administer antibiotics as needed *to treat oral/gum infections that may be present and/or to prevent nosocomial infection in critically ill client whose teeth may be colonized by significant bacteria.*[3]
- Recommend use of analgesics and topical analgesics as needed *when dental pain is present.*
- Administer antibiotic therapy prior to dental procedures in susceptible individuals (e.g., prosthetic heart valve clients) and/or ascertain that bleeding disorders or coagulation deficits are not present to prevent excess bleeding.
- Refer to appropriate care providers (e.g., dental hygienists, dentists, periodontist, oral surgeon).

NURSING PRIORITY NO. 3. To promote wellness (Teaching/Discharge Considerations):

- Instruct client/caregiver to inspect oral cavity and in home-care interventions *to provide good oral care, and/or prevent tooth decay and periodontal disease.*
- Review/demonstrate proper toothbrushing techniques (i.e., brushing with bristles perpendicular to teeth surfaces) after meals and flossing daily. Suggest brushing with floride-containing toothpaste if client able to swallow/manage oral secretions. *This is the most effective way of reducing plaque formation and preventing periodontal disease.*[8]

• Discuss dental and oral health needs, both as client perceives needs and according to professional standards. *Client's perceptions are shaped by self-image, family and cultural expectations and/or conditions created by disease or trauma. Current healthcare practices and education are geared toward practices that improve client's appearance and health including reduced consumption of refined sugars, optimal fluoridation, access to preventative and restorative dental care, prevention of oral cancers and prevention of craniofacial injuries.*[4]

 • Recommend that clients of all ages decrease sugary/high carbohydrate foods in diet and snacks *to reduce buildup of plaque and risk of cavities caused by acids associated with the breakdown of sugar and starch.*[4]

 ∞ • Instruct older clients and caregivers concerning their special needs and importance of regular dental care. *Elderly are prone to 1) experience decay around older fillings (also have more fillings in mouth); 2) receding gums exposing root surfaces, which decay easily; 3) have reduced production of saliva and use multiple medications that can cause dry mouth with loss of tooth and gum protection; and 4) loosening of teeth or poorly fitting dentures associated with gum bone loss. These factors (often compounded by disease conditions and lack of funds) affect nutrient intake, chewing, swallowing, and oral cavity health.*[5]

 ∞ • Advise mother regarding age-appropriate concerns[1,4-6]:

Instruct mother to refrain from allowing baby to fall asleep with bottle containing formula, milk or sweetened beverages. Suggest use of water and pacifier during night *to prevent bottle tooth decay.*

Determine pattern of tooth appearance and tooth loss and compare to norms for primary and secondary teeth.

Discuss tooth discoloration and needed follow-up, *e.g., brown or black spots on teeth usually indicates decay, gray tooth color may indicate nerve injury, multiple cavities in adolescent could be caused from vomiting/bulimia.*

Discuss pit and fissure sealants. *Painted-on tooth surface sealants are becoming widely available to reduce number of cavities, and sometimes are available through community dental programs.*

Determine if children have school dental health programs available and/or recommend regular professional dental examinations as child grows.

Discuss with children/parents problems associated with oral piercing, if individual is contemplating piercing, or needs to know what to watch for after piercing. *Common symptoms that occur with piercing of lips, gums, and tongue include pain, swelling, infection, increased flow of saliva and chipped or cracked teeth requiring diligent oral care and/or more frequent dental examination to prevent complications.*

Discuss use of/need for safety devices (e.g., helmets, facemask, mouth guards) *to prevent/limit severity of sports-related facial injuries and tooth damage/loss.*

 • Discuss with pregnant women special needs and regular dental care. *Pregnant women need additional calcium and phosphorus to maintain good dental health and provide for strong teeth and bones in fetal development. Many women avoid dental care during pregnancy whether because of concerns for fetal health or other reasons (including lack of financial resources). However, one research study of 400 women suggests that pregnant women who receive treatment for periodontal disease can reduce their risk of giving birth to low birth-weight or preterm baby.*[4]

 • Review resources that are needed/available for the client to perform adequate dental hygiene care (e.g., toothbrush/paste, clean water, referral to dental care providers, access to financial assistance, personal care assistant).

 • Encourage cessation of tobacco (especially smokeless) and enrolling in smoking cessation classes *to reduce risk of oral cancers and other health problems.*

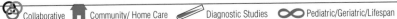 Cultural   Collaborative Community/ Home Care Diagnostic Studies   Pediatric/Geriatric/Lifespan   Medications

● Discuss advisability of dental checkup and/or care prior to instituting chemotherapy or radiation *to minimize oral/dental/tissue damage.*

DOCUMENTATION FOCUS

Assessment/Reassessment
● Individual findings, including individual factors influencing dentition problems.
● Baseline photos/description of oral cavity/structures.

Planning
● Plan of care and who is involved in planning.
● Teaching plan.

Implementation/Evaluation
● Responses to interventions/teaching and actions performed.
● Attainment/progress toward desired outcome(s).
● Modifications to plan of care.

Discharge Planning
● Individual long-term needs, noting who is responsible for actions to be taken.
● Specific referrals made.

References

1. Doenges, M. E., Moorhouse, M. F., & Murr, A. C. (2004). Nurse's Pocket Guide: Diagnoses, Interventions, and Rationales, ed 9. Philadelphia: F. A. Davis.
2. Ayers, K.M., & Colquhoun, A. N. (1998). NZ Dent J, 94(418), 156–160.
3. Scannapieco, F. A., Stewart, E. M., & Mylotte, J. M. (1992). Colonization of dental plaque by respiratory pathogens in medical intensive care patients. Crit Care Med, 20, 740.
4. Public education pamphlets from the American Dental Association: Your diet and dental health; Oral changes with age; Sealants; Oral piercing; National Academy of Sciences panel reaffirms effectiveness of fluoride; Periodontal treatment can reduce risk of some pregnancy complications: study. (Original study from the University of Chile was published in J Periodontology, August 2002.) Pamphlets published at various times on the ADA.org Web site and accessed July 2003. Available at: www.ada.org/public/media.
5. Diagnosis and management of dental caries throughout life. (2001). Office of Medical Applications of Research (OMAR). Bethesda, MD, March 2001. Retrieved through the National Guideline Clearinghouse Website, July 2003. Available at: www.guideline.gov.
6. Engel, J. (2002). Moby's Pocket Guide to Pediatric Assessment, ed 4. St Louis: Mosby.
7. Truman, B. I., Gooch, B. F., Sulemana, I., et al. (July, 2002). Recommendations on selected interventions to prevent dental caries, oral and pharyngeal cancers, and sports-related craniofacial injuries. Am J Prev Med, 23(1 suppl), 21–54.
8. Stiefel, K. A., et al. (2000). Improving oral hygiene for the seriously ill patient: Implementing research-based practice. Medsurg Nurs, 9(1), 40.

risk for delayed Development

Definition: At risk for delay of 25% or more in one or more of the areas of social or self-regulatory behavior, or cognitive, language, gross or fine motor skills

RISK FACTORS

Prenatal
Maternal age younger than 15 years or older than 35 years

Unplanned or unwanted pregnancy; lack of, late, or poor prenatal care

Inadequate nutrition; poverty; illiteracy

Genetic or endocrine disorders; infections; substance abuse

Individual

Prematurity; congenital or genetic disorders

Vision/hearing impairment or frequent otitis media

Failure to thrive, inadequate nutrition; chronic illness

Brain damage (e.g., hemorrhage in postnatal period, shaken baby, abuse, accident); seizures

Positive drug screening test; substance abuse

Lead poisoning; chemotherapy; radiation therapy

Foster or adopted child

Behavior disorders

Technology-dependent

Natural disaster

Environmental

Poverty

Violence

Caregiver

Mental retardation or severe learning disability

Abuse

Mental illness

NOTE: A risk diagnosis is not evidenced by signs and symptoms, as the problem has not occurred and nursing interventions are directed at prevention.

SAMPLE CLINICAL APPLICATIONS: congenital/genetic disorders, prematurity, infection, nutritional problems (malnutrition, anorexia, failure to thrive), toxic exposures (e.g., lead), substance abuse, endocrine disorders, abuse/neglect, developmental delay

DESIRED OUTCOMES/EVALUATION CRITERIA

Sample NOC linkage:

Child Development: [specify age]: Milestones of physical, cognitive, and psychosocial progression by [specify] months/years of age

Client Will (Include Specific Time Frame)

- Perform motor, social, self-regulatory behavior, cognitive and language skills appropriate for age or within scope of present capabilities.

Sample NOC linkages:

Knowledge: Infant Care: Extent of understanding conveyed about caring for a baby up to 12 months

Parenting: Provision of an environment that promotes optimum growth and development of dependent children

Caregiver Will (Include Specific Time Frame)

- Verbalize understanding of age-appropriate development/expectations

 Cultural Collaborative Community/ Home Care  Diagnostic Studies Pediatric/Geriatric/Lifespan Medications

- Identify individual risk factors for developmental delay/deviation and plan(s) for prevention.

ACTIONS/INTERVENTIONS

Sample NIC linkages:

Developmental Enhancement: Child or Adolescent: Facilitating or teaching parents/caregivers to facilitate the optimal gross motor, fine motor, language, cognitive, social, and emotional growth of preschool and school-age children/during the transition from childhood to adulthood

Risk Identification: Analysis of potential risk factors, determination of health risks, and prioritization of risk reduction strategies for an individual or group

NURSING PRIORITY NO. 1. To assess causative/contributing factors:

- Identify condition(s) that could contribute to developmental deviations as listed in Risk Factors, for example, extremes of maternal age, prenatal substance abuse/fetal alcohol syndrome, brain injury/damage, especially that occurring before or at time of birth, prematurity, family history of developmental disorders, chronic severe illness, brain infections, mental illness or retardation, shaken baby syndrome abuse, family violence, failure to thrive, poverty, inadequate nutrition. *Developmental delay occurs when a child fails to achieve one or more developmental milestones and may be the result of one or multiple factors. Delays may affect speech and language, fine and gross motor skills and/or personal and social skills.*[1]

- Obtain information from variety of sources. *Parents are often the first ones to think that there is a problem with their baby's development and should be encouraged to have routine well-baby checkups and screening for developmental delays. Teachers, family members, physicians, and others interacting with a client (older than infant) may have valuable input regarding behaviors that may indicate problems/developmental issues.*[1,2]

- Identify cultural beliefs, norms and values as they may impact parent/caregiver view of situation. *What is considered normal or abnormal development may be based on cultural beliefs/expectations.*[3]

- Ascertain nature of required caregiver activities and evaluate caregiver's abilities to perform needed activities.

- Note severity/pervasiveness of situation (e.g., potential for long-term stress leading to abuse/neglect, versus situational disruption during period of crisis or transition that may eventually level out). *Situations require different interventions in terms of the intensity and length of time that assistance and support may be critical to the caregiver. A crisis can produce great change within a family, some of which can be detrimental to the individual or family unit.*[4–6]

- Evaluate environment in which long-term care will be provided. *The physical, emotional, financial, and social needs of a family are impacted and intertwined with the needs of the ill person. Changes may be needed in the physical structure of the home and/or family roles, resulting in disruption and stress, placing everyone at risk.*[4,6]

NURSING PRIORITY NO. 2. To assist in preventing and/or limiting developmental delays:

- Note chronological *age to help determine developmental expectations (e.g., when child should roll over, sit up alone, speak first words, attain a certain weight/height, etc.), and how the expectations may be altered by child's condition. Pediatrition may screen with a motor quotient (MQ, which is child's age calculated by milestones met divided by chronological age and multiplied by 100). MQ between 50 and 70 requires further evaluation.*[1,7]

- Review expected skills/activities, using authoritative text (e.g., Gesell, Musen/Congor), reports of neurological exams, and/or assessment tools (e.g., Draw-a-Person, Denver Developmental Screening Test, Bender's Visual Motor Gestalt test, Early Language Milestone [ELM] Scale 2 and developmental language disorders [DLD]). *Provides guide for evaluation of growth and development, and for comparative measurement of individual's progress.*[2,4]

- Describe realistic, age-appropriate patterns of development to parent/caregiver and promote activities and interactions that support developmental tasks where client is at this time. *Important in planning interventions in keeping with the individual's current status and potential. Each child will have own unique strengths and difficulties.*[1–3]

- Collaborate with related professional resources (e.g., pediatritic specialists, occupational/rehabilitation/speech therapists, special education teacher, job counselor, professional counseling). *Multidisciplinary team care increases likelihood of developing a well-rounded plan of care that meets client/family's specialized and varied needs.*[4]

NURSING PRIORITY NO. 3. To promote wellness (Teaching/Discharge Considerations)[4]:

- Engage in/encourage prevention strategies (e.g., abstinence from drugs, alcohol and tobacco for pregnant women/child, referral for treatment programs, referral for violence prevention counseling, anticipatory guidance for potential handicaps [vision, hearing, failure to thrive]). *Promoting wellness starts with preventing complications and/or limiting severity of anticipated problems. Such strategies can often be initiated by nurses where the potential is first identified, in the community setting.*[1,4]

- Evaluate client's progress on continual basis. Identify target symptoms requiring intervention *to make referrals in a timely manner and/or to make adjustments in plan of care, as indicated.*[2]

- Provide/assist with follow-up appointments as indicated *to promote ongoing evaluation, support, or management of situation.*[2]

- Discuss proactive actions to take (e.g., periodic laboratory studies *to monitor nutritional status,* or getting immunizations on schedule *to prevent serious infections) to avoid preventable complications.*[2]

- Maintain positive, hopeful attitude. Encourage setting of short-term realistic goals for achieving developmental potential. *Small incremental steps are often easier to deal with, and successes enhance hopefulness and well-being.*[6]

- Provide information as appropriate, including pertinent reference materials. *Bibliotherapy provides opportunity to review data at own pace, enhancing likelihood of retention.*[1,2]

- Encourage attendance at educational programs (e.g., parenting classes, infant stimulation sessions, food buying/cooking/nutrition, home and family safety, anger management, seminars on life stresses, aging process) *to address specific learning need/desires and interact with others with similar life challenges.*[2]

- Identify available community and national resources as appropriate (e.g., early intervention programs, gifted and talented programs, sheltered workshop, crippled children's services, medical equipment/supplier, caregiver support and respite services). *Provides additional assistance to support family efforts and can help identify community responsibilities, (e.g., services required to be provided to school-age child).*[1]

  Cultural Collaborative Community/ Home Care 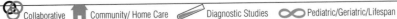 Diagnostic Studies Pediatric/Geriatric/Lifespan Medications

Assessment/Reassessment
- Assessment findings/individual needs including developmental level.
- Caregiver's understanding of situation and individual role.

Planning
- Plan of care and who is involved in the planning.
- Teaching plan.

Implementation/Evaluation
- Client's response to interventions/teaching and actions performed.
- Caregiver response to teaching.
- Attainment/progress toward desired outcome(s).
- Modifications to plan of care.

Discharge Planning
- Identified long-range needs and who is responsible for actions to be taken.
- Specific referrals made, sources for assistive devices, educational tools.

References

1. Developmental Delays: A Pediatrician's Guide to your Children's Health and Safety. Available at: www.keepkidshealthy.com. Accessed July 2003.
2. Practice parameters for the assessment and treatment of children, adolescents, and adults with autism and other pervasive developmental disorders. (1999). American Academy of Child and Adolescent Psychiatry Working Group on Quality Issues. J Am Acad Child Adolesc Psychiatry, 38 (12 Suppl):55s-76S. Available at: National Guideline Clearinghouse www.guideline.gov. Accessed July 2003.
3. Leininger, M.M. (1996). Transcultural Nursing: Theories, Research and Practices, ed 2. Hilliard., OH: McGraw-Hill.
4. Doenges, M. E., Moorhouse, M. F., & Geissler Murr, A. C. (2004). ND: Growth and Development, delayed. In Nurse's Pocket Guide: Diagnoses, Interventions, and Rationales, ed 9. Philadelphia: F. A. Davis.
5. Engel, J. (2002). Mosby's Pocket Guide to Pediatric Assessment. St Louis: Mosby.
6. Cox, H. C. et al. (2002). Clinical Applications of Nursing Diagnosis: Adult, Child, Women's Psychiatric, Gerontic, and Home Health Considerations, ed 4. Philadelphia: F. A. Davis.
7. Educating parents of extra-special children: Developmental delays. Available at: www.epeconline.com/DeveolpmentalDelays.html. Accessed January 2004.

Diarrhea

Definition: Passage of loose, unformed stools

RELATED FACTORS

Psychological
High stress levels and anxiety

Situational
Laxative/alcohol abuse, toxins, contaminants
Adverse effects of medications, radiation
Tube feedings
Travel

Physiologic
Inflammation, irritation
Infectious processes, parasites
Malabsorption

DEFINING CHARACTERISTICS

Subjective
Abdominal pain
Urgency, cramping

Objective
Hyperactive bowel sounds
At least three loose liquid stools per day

SAMPLE CLINICAL APPLICATIONS: inflammatory bowel disease, gastritis, enteral feedings, alcohol abuse, antibiotic use, food allergies/contamination, AIDS, radiation, parasites

DESIRED OUTCOMES/EVALUATION CRITERIA

Sample NOC linkages:

Bowel Elimination: Ability of the gastrointestinal tract to form and evacuate stool effectively

Symptom Severity: Extent of perceived adverse changes in physical, emotional, and social functioning

Hydration: Amount of water in the intracellular and extracellular compartments of the body

Client Will (Include Specific Time Frame)
- Reestablish and maintain normal pattern of bowel functioning.
- Verbalize understanding of causative factors and rationale for treatment regimen.
- Demonstrate appropriate behavior to assist with resolution of causative factors (e.g., proper food preparation or avoidance of irritating foods).

ACTIONS/INTERVENTIONS

Sample NIC linkages:

Diarrhea Management: Management and alleviation of diarrhea

Fluid Monitoring: Collection and analysis of patient data to regulate fluid balance

Perineal Care: Maintenance of perineal skin integrity and relief of perineal discomfort

NURSING PRIORITY NO. 1. To assess causative factors/etiology:

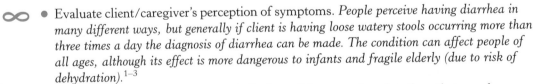

- Evaluate client/caregiver's perception of symptoms. *People perceive having diarrhea in many different ways, but generally if client is having loose watery stools occurring more than three times a day the diagnosis of diarrhea can be made. The condition can affect people of all ages, although its effect is more dangerous to infants and fragile elderly (due to risk of dehydration).*[1–3]
- Determine presence of systemic medical conditions or other situations that may be contributing to diarrhea. *Diarrhea may be a temporary problem (e.g., infections, reaction to food or medicine, after intestinal surgery) or it may be a long-term situation (e.g., celiac*

 Cultural Collaborative Community/ Home Care Diagnostic Studies 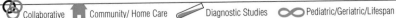 Pediatric/Geriatric/Lifespan Medications disease, inflammatory bowel disease, hyperthyroidism, tumor syndromes, AIDS, food intolerance/allergies, radiation or other cancer treatments; frequent use of magnesium-containing antacids; eating disorders with surreptitious laxative use).[2-5]

- Determine recent travel to developing countries/foreign environments; change in drinking water/food intake, consumption of unsafe food; swimming in untreated surface water, similar illness of family members/others close to client *that may help identify causative environmental factors.*[2,4-6]

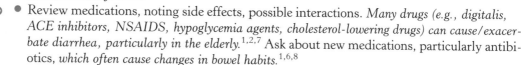

- Review medications, noting side effects, possible interactions. *Many drugs (e.g., digitalis, ACE inhibitors, NSAIDS, hypoglycemia agents, cholesterol-lowering drugs) can cause/exacerbate diarrhea, particularly in the elderly.*[1,2,7] Ask about new medications, particularly antibiotics, *which often cause changes in bowel habits.*[1,6,8]

- Obtain comprehensive history of symptoms *to help in identifying cause and treatment needs*[1,2,4-6]:

  Ascertain onset and pattern, noting whether onset was abrupt or gradual and whether the condition is acute or chronic.

  Determine frequency of stools and whether continuous or intermittent.

  Observe and record characteristics (e.g., watery, bloody, greasy), amount (e.g. small or copious), time of day (e.g., just after meals).

  Identify any associated factors (e.g., fever/chills, abdominal cramping, emotional upset, weight loss), aggravating factors (e.g., stress, foods), or mitigating factors (e.g., changes in diet, use of prescription or OTC medications).

  Note reports of pain. *Pain is often present with inflammatory bowel disease, irritable bowel syndrome, and mesenteric ischemia.*

- Assess for/remove fecal impaction, particularly in elderly where impaction may be accompanied by diarrhea.[3]

- Auscultate abdomen for presence, location, and characteristics of bowel sounds. *High-pitched, rapidly occurring, loud or tinkling bowel sounds often accompany diarrhea.*[9]

- Review results of laboratory testing on stool specimens. *Can reveal presence of bacterial infections, viral infections, parasites, blood, fat, offending drugs, inflammation, allergy, metabolic disorders, malabsorption syndromes, gastroenteritis or colitis, etc.*[1,2,4-6]

- Assist with, prepare for additional evaluation as indicated. *Tests may include upper and/or lower GI radiographs, ultrasound, endoscopic evaluations, biopsy, etc.*[12]

NURSING PRIORITY NO. 2. To alleviate/limit condition[1-6,8,10]:

- Assist with treatment of underlying cause: *Treatments are varied, and may be as simple as allowing time for recovery from a self-limiting gastroenteritis, or may require complex treatments including antimicrobials and rehydration, or community health interventions for contaminated food/water sources.*

- Provide/encourage bedrest during acute episode. *Rest decreases intestinal motility and reduces metabolic rate when infection or hemorrhage is a complication.*

- Restrict solid food intake, if indicated. *May help on short term to allow for bowel rest/ reduced intestinal workload, especially if cause of diarrhea is under investigation, or vomiting is present. Note: Child's preferred/usual diet may be continued to prevent or limit dehydration, with the possible limitation of fruit, fruit juices, or milk, if these factors are exacerbating the diarrhea.*[5,9]

- Limit caffeine and high-fat (e.g., butter, fried foods) or high-protein (e.g., meats) and foods known to cause/aggravate diarrhea (e.g., extremely hot/cold foods, chili), and milk and fruits/fruit juices as appropriate.

- Adjust strength/rate of enteral tube feedings; change formula as indicated *when diarrhea is associated with tube feedings.*
- Consider change in infant formula. *Diarrhea may be result of/aggravated by intolerance to specific formula.*
- Change medications as appropriate *(e.g., stopping magnesium-containing antacid or antibiotic causing diarrhea).*
- Promote the use of relaxation techniques (e.g., progressive relaxation exercise, visualization techniques) *to decrease stress/anxiety.*
- Administer medications to treat or limit diarrhea, as indicated, dependent on cause. *May include use of antidiarrheals (e.g., diphenoxylate [Lomotil]), anti-infectives (metronidazole [Flagyl]), antispasmodics (dicyclomine [Bentyl]), etc.*
- Assist client to manage situation[12]:
  Respond to call for assistance promptly.
  Place bedpan in bed with client (if desired) or commode chair near bed *to provide quick access/reduce need to wait for assistance of others.*
  Provide privacy; remove stool promptly; use room deodorizers *to reduce noxious odors, limit embarrassment.*
  Use incontinence pads depending on the severity of the problem.
  Provide emotional/psychological support. *Diarrhea can be source of great embarrassment and can lead to social isolation and feeling of powerlessness. Intimate relationship and sexual activity may be affected and need specific interventions to resolve.*
- Maintain skin integrity[12]:
  Assist as needed with pericare after each bowel movement *to prevent skin excoriation and breakdown.*
  Provide prompt diaper change and gentle cleansing *because skin breakdown can occur quickly when diarrhea occurs.*
  Apply lotion/ointment skin barrier as needed.
  Provide dry linen as necessary.
  Expose perineum/buttocks to air/use heat lamp with caution if needed *to keep area dry.*
  Refer to ND impaired Skin Integrity.

NURSING PRIORITY NO. 3. To restore/maintain hydration/electrolyte balance[1–3,5,6,10]:

- Note reports of thirst, less frequent or absent urination, dry mouth and skin, weakness, light-headedness, headache. *Signs/symptoms of dehydration and need for rehydration.*
- Observe for/question parents about young child crying with no tears, fever, decreased urination or no wet diapers for 6 to 8 hours, listlessness or irritability, sunken eyes, dry mouth and tongue and suspected or documented weight loss. *Child needs immediate facility treatment for dehydration if these signs are present and child is not taking fluids.*
- Note presence of low blood pressure/postural hypotension, tachycardia, poor skin hydration/turgor. *Presence of these factors indicates severe dehydration and electrolyte imbalance. The fragile elderly can progress quickly to this point, especially when vomiting is present, or client's normal food and fluid intake is below requirements.*
- Monitor total intake and output including stool output as possible. *Provides estimation of fluid needs.*
- Weigh infant's diapers *to determine output.*
- Offer/encourage water, plus broth or soups that contain sodium, and fruit juices/soft fruits or vegetables that contain potassium *to replace water and electrolytes.*

 Cultural Collaborative Community/ Home Care Diagnostic Studies 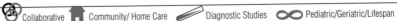 Pediatric/Geriatric/Lifespan Medications

• Recommend oral intake of beverages such as Gatorade, Pedialyte, Infalyte, bouillon. *Commercial rehydration solutions containing electrolytes may prevent/correct imbalances .*

• Administer enteral/parenteral feedings and IV/electrolyte fluids as indicated. *Intravenous fluids may be needed either short term to restore hydration status (e.g., acute gastroenteritis) or long term (severe osmotic diarrhea). Enteral/parenteral nutrition is reserved for clients unable to maintain adequate nutritional status because of long-term diarrhea (e.g., wasting syndrome, malnutrition states).*

NURSING PRIORITY NO. 4. To promote return to normal bowel function-ing[1,2,4–6,10]:

 • Increase oral fluid intake and gradually return to normal diet as tolerated.

• Encourage intake of nonirritating liquids.[11]

• Recommend products such as natural fiber, plain natural yogurt, Lactinex *to restore normal bowel flora.*[11]

 • Give medications as ordered *to treat infectious process, decrease motility, and/or absorb water.*

NURSING PRIORITY NO. 5. To promote wellness (Teaching/Discharge Considerations):

 • Review individual's causative factors and appropriate interventions to prevent recurrence.

• Discuss medication regimen, including prescription and OTC drugs, *especially when client has multiple medications with potential for diarrhea as side effect or interaction.*[12]

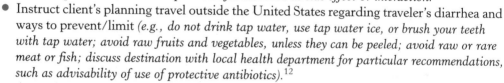 • Instruct client's planning travel outside the United States regarding traveler's diarrhea and ways to prevent/limit (*e.g., do not drink tap water, use tap water ice, or brush your teeth with tap water; avoid raw fruits and vegetables, unless they can be peeled; avoid raw or rare meat or fish; discuss destination with local health department for particular recommendations, such as advisability of use of protective antibiotics).*[12]

• Assess home/living environment, if indicated. *Discussion with client/caregivers may be needed regarding 1) sanitation and hygiene (e.g., handwashing and laundry practices), 2) safe food storage and preparation (to reduce risk of foodborne infections); and 3) particular risks in select populations (e.g., persons with chronic liver disease should avoid shellfish, persons with impaired immune defenses are at increased risk for diarrhea associated with raw dairy products or unheated deli meats; pregnant women should avoid undercooked meats [infectious diarrhea]).*[12]

• Teach parent/caregiver signs of dehydration, and instruct in the importance of fluid and electrolyte replacement, as well as simple food/fluids to provide rehydration.

• Instruct in perirectal skin care, if indicated. *Chronic diarrhea can result in skin excoriation and breakdown with potential for infection, itching and pain, and relationship/sexual difficulties.*[12]

DOCUMENTATION FOCUS

Assessment/Reassessment
• Assessment findings, including characteristics/pattern of elimination.

Planning
• Plan of care and who is involved in planning.
• Teaching plan.

Implementation/Evaluation
- Client's response to treatment/teaching and actions performed.
- Attainment/progress toward desired outcome(s).
- Modifications to plan of care.

Discharge Planning
- Recommendations for follow-up care.

References

1. Hogan, C. M. (1998). The nurse's role in diarrhea management. Oncol Nurs Forum, 25(5), 879–885.
2. Diarrhea. National Digestive Diseases Information Clearinghouse. (NDDIC). National Institutes of Health Publication No. 01–2749 January 2001.
3. Carnaveli, D. L., & Patrick, M. (1993). Nursing Management for the Elderly, ed 3. Philadelphia: JB Lippincott.
4. Evidence based clinical practice guideline for children with acute gastroenteritis (AGE). (2001). Cincinnati (OH) Children's Hospital Medical Center. Available at: the National Guideline Clearinghouse, www.guideline.gov. Accessed July 2003.
5. American Gastroenterological Association medical position statement: Guidelines for the evaluation of chronic diarrhea. (1999). Available at: the National Guideline Clearinghouse, www.guideline.gov. Accessed July 2003.
6. Guerrant, R. L., et al. (2001). Practice guidelines for the management of infectious diarrhea. Clin Infect Dis, 32(3), 331–351.
7. Ratnaike, R. N. (2000). Drug-induced diarrhea in older persons. Clin Geriatr, 8(1), 67–76.
8. Vogel, L. C. (1995). Antibiotic-induced diarrhea. Orthop Nurs, 14, 38–41.
9. Engel, J. (2002). Mosby's Pocket Guide to Pediatric Assessment, ed 4. St Louis: Mosby.
10. Larson, C. E. (2000). Evidence-based practice: Safety and efficacy of oral rehydration therapy for the treatment of diarrhea and gastroenteritis in pediatrics. Pediatr Nurs, 26(2), 177–179.
11. Peikin, S. R. (1999). Diarrhea in Gastrointestinal Health. New York: HarperCollins.
12. Doenges, M. E., Moorhouse, M. F., & Geissler-Murr, A. C. (2002). ND Diarrhea, risk for in Gastrointestinal Disorders. In Nursing Care Plans: Guidelines for Individualizing Patient Care, ed 6. Philadelphia: F. A. Davis.

risk for Disuse Syndrome

Definition: At risk for deterioration of body systems as the result of prescribed or unavoidable musculoskeletal inactivity

RISK FACTORS
Severe pain [chronic pain]
Paralysis [other neuromuscular impairment]
Mechanical or prescribed immobilization
Altered level of consciousness
[Chronic physical or mental illness]
[Adverse effects of aging]
NOTE: A risk diagnosis is not evidenced by signs and symptoms, as the problem has not occurred and nursing interventions are directed at prevention.

SAMPLE CLINICAL APPLICATIONS: multiple sclerosis, cerebral palsy, muscular dystrophy, post-polio syndrome, brain injury/stroke, spinal cord injury, arthritis, osteoporosis, fractures, amputation, dementia

DESIRED OUTCOMES/EVALUATION CRITERIA
Sample NOC linkages:
Immobility Consequences: Physiologic: Extent of compromise to physiologic functioning due to impaired physical mobility

 Cultural Collaborative 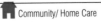 Community/ Home Care 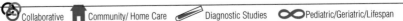 Diagnostic Studies Pediatric/Geriatric/Lifespan Medications

Risk Control: Actions to eliminate or reduce actual, personal, and modifiable health threats

Immobility Consequences: Psycho-Cognitive: Extent of compromise to psychcognitive functioning due to impaired physical mobility

Client Will (Include Specific Time Frame)

- Display intact skin/tissues or achieve timely wound healing.
- Maintain/reestablish effective elimination patterns.
- Be free of signs/symptoms of infectious processes.
- Demonstrate adequate peripheral perfusion with stable vital signs, skin warm and dry, palpable peripheral pulses.
- Maintain usual reality orientation.
- Maintain/regain optimal level of cognitive, neurosensory, and musculoskeletal functioning.
- Express sense of control over the present situation and potential outcome.
- Recognize and incorporate change into self-concept in accurate manner without negative self-esteem.

ACTIONS/INTERVENTIONS

Sample NIC linkages:

Energy Management: Regulating energy use to treat or prevent fatigue and optimize function

Environmental Management: Manipulation of the patient's surroundings for therapeutic benefit

Exercise Promotion: Facilitation of regular physical exercise to maintain or advance to a higher level of fitness and health

NURSING PRIORITY NO. 1. To evaluate probability of developing complications:

- Identify underlying conditions/pathology (e.g., cancer, lupus, diabetes mellitus, trauma, fractures with casting, immobilization devices; surgery; chronic disease conditions; malnutrition; neuromuscular diseases [e.g., stroke, post-polio, MS], spinal cord or brain injury, chronic pain, etc.) *that have potential for causing problems associated with inactivity and immobility.*
- Identify specific and potential concerns including client's age, cognition, mobility and exercise status. *Disuse syndrome can be a complication of and cause for bedridden state. The syndrome can include muscle and bone atrophy, stiffening of joints, brittle bones, reduction of cardiopulmonary function, loss of red blood cells, decreased sex hormones, decreased resistance to infections, increased proportion of body fat in relation to muscle mass and chemical changes in the brain which adversely impact client's activities of daily living, social life and quality of life.[1,2] Age-related physiological changes accompanied by chronic illness predispose older adults to functional decline related to inactivity and immobility.[3]*
- Determine if client's condition is acute/short-term or whether it may be a long-term/permanent condition. *Relatively short-term conditions (e.g., simple fracture treated with cast) may respond quickly to rehabilitative efforts. Long-term conditions (e.g., after stroke, aged person with dementia, cancers, demyelinating or degenerative diseases, SCI, and psychological problems such as depression or learned helplessness) have a higher risk of complications for the client and caregiver.*
- Evaluate client's risk for injury. *Risk is greater in client with cognitive problems, lack of safe or stimulating environment, inadequate mobility aids, and/or sensory-perception problems.[3]*

- Ascertain attitudes of individual/SO about condition (e.g., cultural values, stigma). Note misconceptions. Evaluate clients/family's understanding and ability to manage care for long period. Ascertain availability and use of support systems. *The client may be influenced (positively or negatively) by peer group and family role expectations. Caregivers may be influenced by their own physical/emotional limitations, degree of commitment to assisting the client toward optimal independence, and/or available time.*[3]
- Obtain psychological assessment of client's emotional status. *Potential problems that may arise from presence of condition need to be identified and dealt with to avoid further debilitation.*[3]

NURSING PRIORITY NO. 2. To identify/provide individually appropriate preventive or corrective interventions:

Skin[6,7]:

- Inspect skin on a frequent basis, noting changes. Monitor skin over bony prominences.
- Reposition frequently as individually indicated *to relieve pressure.*
- Provide skin care daily and PRN, drying well and using gentle massage and lotion *to stimulate circulation.*
- Keep skin, clothing and area clean/dry *to prevent/limit skin irritation and breakdown.*
- Initiate use of padding devices (e.g., sheepskin, egg-crate/gel/water/air mattress or cushions) *to reduce pressure on/enhance circulation to compromised tissues.*
- Review nutritional status and promote diet with adequate protein, calorie and vitamin/mineral intake *to aid in healing and promote general good health of skin/tissues.*
- Refer to ND impaired Skin Integrity, impaired Tissue Integrity for additional interventions.

Elimination[6,7]:

- Observe elimination patterns, noting changes and potential problems.
- Encourage balanced diet, including fruits and vegetables high in fiber and with adequate fluids *for optimal stool consistency and to facilitate passage through colon.*
- Provide/encourage adequate fluid intake, include water and cranberry juice *to reduce risk of urinary infections.*
- Maximize mobility at earliest opportunity.
- Evaluate need for stool softeners, bulk-forming laxatives.
- Implement consistent bowel management/bladder training programs, as indicated.
- Monitor urinary output/characteristics *to identify changes associated with infection.*
- Refer to NDs Constipation, Diarrhea, Bowel Incontinence, impaired Urinary Elimination, Urinary Retention for additional interventions.

Respiration[6,7]:

- Monitor breath sounds and characteristics of secretions *for early detection of complications (e.g., pneumonia).*
- Encourage ambulation and upright position. Reposition, cough, deep-breathe on a regular schedule *to facilitate clearing of secretions/prevent atelectasis.*
- Encourage use of incentive spirometry. Suction as indicated *to clear airways.*
- Demonstrate techniques/assist with postural drainage when indicated *for long-term airway clearance difficulties.*
- Assist with/instruct family and caregivers in quad coughing techniques/diaphragmatic weight training *to maximize ventilation in presence of SCI.*
- Discourage smoking. Refer for smoking cessation program as indicated.

 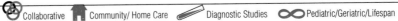

- Refer to NDs ineffective Airway Clearance, ineffective Breathing Pattern, impaired Gas Exchange, impaired spontaneous Ventilation for additional interventions.

Vascular (tissue perfusion)[6,7]:
- Assess cognition and mental status (ongoing). *Changes can reflect state of cardiac health, cerebral oxygenation impairment, or be indicative of a mental/emotional state that could adversely affect safety and self-care.*
- Determine core and skin temperature. Investigate development of cyanosis, changes in mentation *to identify changes in oxygenation status.*
- Routinely evaluate circulation/nerve function of affected body parts. *Changes in temperature, color, sensation, and movement can be the effect of immobility, disease, aging, or injury.*
- Encourage/provide adequate fluid *to prevent dehydration and circulatory stasis.*
- Monitor blood pressure before, during, and after activity— sitting, standing, and lying if possible *to ascertain response to/tolerance of activity.*
- Encourage being out of bed and ambulation, whenever possible. *Upright position and weight bearing helps maintain bone strength, increases circulation and prevents postural hypotension.*[4]
- Assist with position changes as needed. Raise head gradually. Institute use of tilt table/sitting upright on side of bed and arising slowly where appropriate *to reduce incidence of injury that may occur as a result of orthostatic hypotension.*
- Maintain proper body position; avoid use of constricting garments/restraints *to prevent vascular congestion.*
- Provide range of motion exercise. Refer for/assist with physical therapy *for strengthening, restoration of optimal range of motion and prevention of circulatory problems related to disuse.*
- Institute peripheral vascular support measures (e.g., elastic hose, Ace wraps, sequential compression devices—SCDs) *to enhance venous return and reduce incidence of thrombophlebitis.*
- Refer to NDs risk for Activity Intolerance; decreased Cardiac Output; ineffective Tissue Perfusion; risk for Peripheral Neurovascular Dysfunction for additional interventions.

Musculoskeletal (mobility/range of motion, strength/endurance)[6,7]:
- Perform/assist with range of motion exercises and involve client in active exercises with physical/occupational therapy *to promote bone health, muscle strengthening, flexibility optimal conditioning and functional ability.*
- Have client do exercises in bed if not contraindicated. *In-bed exercises help maintain muscle strength and tone.*[5]
- Maximize involvement in self-care *to restore/maintain strength and functional abilities.*
- Intersperse activity with rest periods. Pace activities as possible *to increase strength and endurance in a gradual manner and reduce failure of planned exercise because of exhaustion or overuse of weak muscles/injured area.*
- Identify needs/use supportive devices (e.g., cane/walker/functional positioning splints) as appropriate *to assist with safe mobility and functional independence.*
- Evaluate role of pain in mobility problem. Implement pain management program as individually indicated.
- Limit/monitor closely the use of restraints, and immobilize client as little as possible *to reduce possibility of agitation and injury.*
- Refer to NDs Activity Intolerance; impaired physical Mobility; acute Pain; chronic Pain; impaired Walking for additional interventions.

Sensory-perception[6,7]:

- Orient client as necessary to time, place, person, and situation. Provide cues for orientation (e.g., clock, calendar). *Disturbances of sensory interpretation and thought processes are associated with immobility as well as aging, being ill, disease processes/treatments and medication effects.*
- Provide appropriate level of environmental stimulation (e.g., music, television/radio, clock, calendar, personal possessions, and visitors). *Needs vary depending on the client, the nature of the current problem, and whether client is at home or in a healthcare facility. Having normal life cues can help with mental stimulation and restoration of health.*
- Encourage participation in recreational/diversional activities and regular exercise program (as tolerated) *to decrease the sensory deprivation associated with immobility and/or isolation.*
- Promote regular sleep hours, use of sleep aids, and usual presleep rituals *to promote normal sleep/rest cycle.*
- Refer to NDs disturbed Sensory Perception, disturbed Sleep Pattern, Social Isolation, deficient Diversional Activity for additional interventions.

Self-esteem, powerlessness, hopelessness, social isolation[6,7]:
- Determine factors that may contribute to impairment of client's self-esteem and social interactions. *Many things can be involved here, including the client's age, relationship status, usual health state; presence of disabilities including pain, or financial, environmental and physical problems; current situation causing immobility and client's state of mind concerning the importance of the current situation in regard to the rest of client's life and desired lifestyle.*
- Ascertain if changes in client's situation are likely to be short term/temporary or long-term/permanent. *Can affect both the client and care provider's coping abilities and willingness to engage in activities that prevent/limit effects of immobility.*
- Assess living situation (e.g. lives with spouse, parents, alone, etc.) and determine factors that may positively or adversely affect client's progress, roles, and/or safety.
- Explain/review all care procedures and plans. *Improves knowledge and facilitates decision-making. Involves client in own care, enhances sense of control and promotes independence.*
- Encourage questions and verbalization of feelings. *Aids in reducing anxiety and promotes learning about condition/specific needs.*
- Acknowledge concerns; provide presence and encouragement.
- Refer for mental/psychological/spiritual services as indicated *to provide counseling, support, and medications.*
- Provide for/assist with mutual goal setting, involving SO(s). *Promotes sense of control and enhances commitment to goals.*
- Ascertain that client can communicate needs adequately (e.g., call light, writing tablet, picture/letter board, interpreter).
- Refer to NDs impaired Adjustment, Hopelessness, Powerlessness, impaired verbal Communication, Self-Esteem [specify], ineffective Role Performance, impaired Social Interaction for additional interventions.

Body image[6,7]:
- Evaluate for presence/potential for emotional, mental and behavioral conditions that may contribute to isolation and degeneration. *Disuse syndrome often affects those individuals who are already isolated for one reason or another, e.g., serious illness/injury with disfigurement, frail elderly living alone, individual with severe depression, person with unacceptable behavior or without support system.*
- Orient to body changes through discussion and written information *to promote acceptance and understanding of needs.*

 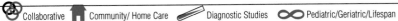

- Promote interactions with peers and normalization of activities within individual abilities.
- Refer to NDs disturbed Body Image, situational low Self-Esteem, Social Isolation, disturbed Personal Identity for additional interventions.

NURSING PRIORITY NO. 3. To promote wellness (Teaching/Discharge Considerations):

- Provide/review information about individual needs/areas of concern. *Treatment may be required for underlying condition(s), stress management, medications, therapies, and needed lifestyle changes.*
- Assist client/caregivers in development of individualized plan of care to best meet the client's potential. *Information can help client and care providers to understand what long-term goals could be attained, what barriers may need to be overcome, and what constitutes progress or lack of progress requiring further evaluation/intervention.*[6]
- Encourage involvement in regular exercise program including isometric/isotonic activities, active or assistive range of motion *to limit consequences of disuse and maximize level of function.*[2]
- Encourage/recommend suitable balanced nutrition as well as use of supplements if needed. Refer to appropriate community health providers and resources *to provide necessary assistance (e.g., help with meal preparation, financial help for groceries, dietitian/nutritionist, etc.).*[7]
- Review signs/symptoms requiring medical evaluation/follow-up *to promote timely interventions and limit adverse affects of situation.*[6]
- Identify community support services (e.g., financial, home maintenance, respite care, transportation).
- Refer to appropriate rehabilitation/home-care and support group resources to help client/care providers learn more about their condition, and acquire needed assistance.
- Provide sources for assistive devices/necessary equipment.

DOCUMENTATION FOCUS

Assessment/Reassessment
- Assessment findings, noting individual areas of concern, functional level, degree of independence, support systems/available resources.

Planning
- Plan of care and who is involved in planning.
- Teaching plan.

Implementation/Evaluation
- Client's response to interventions/teaching and actions performed.
- Changes in level of functioning.
- Attainment/progress toward desired outcome(s).
- Modifications to plan of care.

Discharge Planning
- Long-term needs and who is responsible for actions to be taken.
- Specific referrals made, resources for specific equipment needs.

References

1. Disuse Syndrome. (1999). Department for the Care of the Aged: Laboratory of Rehabilitation Research National Institute for Longevity Sciences Website. Available at: http://www.nils.go.jp/organ/dca/lrr/reh-e.html. Accessed August 2003.
2. Hanson, R. W. (2000). Physical Exercise, in Self-Management of Chronic Pain. Patient Handbook. Available at: http://www.aboutarachnoiditis.org. Accessed July 2003.
3. Blair, K. A. (1999). Immobility and activity intolerance in older adults. In Stanley, M. & Beare, P. G. (eds): Gerontological Nursing: A Health Promotion/Protection Approach, ed 2. Philadelphia: F. A. Davis.
4. Jiricka, M. K. (1994). Alterations in activity intolerance. In Port, C. M. (ed). Pathophysiology: Concepts of Altered Health States. Philadelphia: JB Lippincott.
5. Metzlar, D. J., & Harr, J. (1996). Positioning your patient properly. Am J Nurs, 96, 33–37.
6. Doenges, M. E., Moorhouse, M. F., & Geissler-Murr, A. C. (2004). Nurse's Pocket Guide: Diagnoses, Interventions, and Rationales, ed 9. Philadelphia: F. A. Davis.
7. Cox, H. C., et al. (2002). Clinical Applications of Nursing Diagnosis: Adult, Child, Women's, Psychiatric, Gerontic, and Home Health Considerations, ed 4. Philadelphia: F. A. Davis.

deficient Diversional Activity

Definition: Decreased stimulation from (or interest or engagement in) recreational or leisure activities [Note: Internal/external factors may or may not be beyond the individual's control.]

RELATED FACTORS

Environmental lack of diversional activity as in long-term hospitalization; frequent, lengthy treatments, [home-bound]

[Physical limitations, bedridden, fatigue, pain]

[Situational, developmental problem, lack of sources]

[Psychological condition, such as depression]

DEFINING CHARACTERISTICS

Subjective

Client's statement regarding the following:

Boredom; wish there were something to do, to read, and so on

Usual hobbies cannot be undertaken in hospital [home or other care setting]

[Changes in abilities/physical limitations]

Objective

[Flat affect, disinterest, inattentiveness]

[Restlessness, crying, yawning, sighing]

[Lethargy, withdrawal]

[Hostility]

[Overeating or lack of interest in eating, weight loss or gain]

SAMPLE CLINICAL APPLICATIONS: traumatic injuries, chronic pain, prolonged recovery (e.g., postoperative, complicated fractures), cancer therapy, chronic/debilitating conditions (e.g., congestive heart failure, COPD, renal failure, multiple sclerosis), awaiting organ transplantation

DESIRED OUTCOMES/EVALUATION CRITERIA

Sample NOC linkages:

 Cultural Collaborative Community/ Home Care 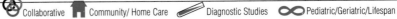 Diagnostic Studies Pediatric/Geriatric/Lifespan 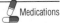 Medications

Leisure Participation: Use of restful or relaxing activities as needed to promote well-being

Social Involvement: Frequency of an individual's social interactions with persons, groups, or organizations

Health-Promoting Behavior: Actions to sustain or increase wellness

---

Client Will (Include Specific Time Frame)
- Recognize own psychological response (e.g., hopelessness and helplessness, anger, depression) and initiate appropriate coping actions.
- Engage in satisfying activities within personal limitations.

ACTIONS/INTERVENTIONS
Sample NIC linkages:

Recreation Therapy: Purposeful use of recreation to promote relaxation and enhancement of social skills

Activity Therapy: Prescription of and assistance with specific physical, cognitive, social, and spiritual activities to increase the range, frequency, or duration of an individual's (or group's) activity

Exercise Promotion: Facilitation of regular physical exercise to maintain or advance to a higher level of fitness and health

NURSING PRIORITY NO. 1. To assess precipitating/etiologic factors:

- Assess/review client's physical, cognitive, emotional, and environmental status. *Validates reality of diversional deprivation when it exists, or identifies the potential for loss of desired diversional activity, in order to plan for prevention or early intervention where possible.*
- Observe for restlessness, flat facial expression, withdrawal, hostility, yawning and/or statements of boredom as noted above, especially in individual likely to be confined either temporarily or long-term. *May be indicative of need for diversional interventions.*[1]
- Note potential impact of current disability/illness on lifestyle (e.g. young child with leukemia, elderly person with fractured hip, individual with severe depression). *Provides comparative baseline for assessments and interventions.*[9]
- Be aware of age/developmental level, gender and cultural factors, and the importance of a given activity in client's life. *When illness interferes with individual's ability to engage in usual activities, such as a lifelong dancer with incapacitating osteoporosis, a Mexican-American woman who is unable to take care of her family, the person may have difficulty engaging in meaningful substitute activities.*
- Determine client's actual ability to participate in available activities, noting attention span, physical limitations and tolerance, level of interest/desire, and safety needs. *Presence of depression/disinterest in life, problems of immobility, protective isolation, and lack of stimulation, developmental delay, or sensory deprivation may interfere with desired activity. However, lack of involvement may not reflect client's actual abilities, but may rather be a matter of misperception about abilities.*[9]

NURSING PRIORITY NO. 2. To motivate and stimulate client involvement in solutions:

- Institute/continue appropriate actions to deal with concomitant conditions such as anxiety, depression, grief, dementia, physical injury, isolation and immobility, malnutrition, acute or chronic pain, etc. *These conditions interfere with the individual's ability to engage in meaningful activities that will stimulate his or her interest.*

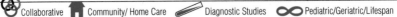 • Introduce activities at client's current level of functioning, progressing to more complex activities, as tolerated. *Provides opportunity for client to experience successes, reaffirming capabilities and enhancing self-esteem.*[8]

• Acknowledge reality of situation and feelings of the client *to establish therapeutic relationship in a situation where client may be feeling sense of loss when unable to participate in usual activities or to interact socially as desired.*[8]

• Accept hostile expressions while limiting aggressive acting-out behavior. *Permission to express feelings of anger, hopelessness allows for beginning resolution. However, destructive behavior is counterproductive to self-esteem and problem solving.*[8]

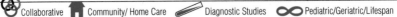 • Involve client, caregiver, and parent/SO in determining client's needs, desires and available resources. *Helps insure that plan is attentive to client's interests and resources, increasing likelihood of client participation.*[2]

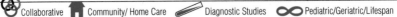 • Encourage parent/caregiver of young child to engage in play with confined child. *Reduces child's boredom, and play is essential to young child's development.*[3]

• Review history of lifelong activities and hobbies client has enjoyed. Discuss reasons client is not doing these activities now, and whether client can/would like to resume these activities. *Diversional activities can provide positive and productive avenues into which client can channel thoughts and time.*[4]

• Assist client/caregiver to set realistic goals for diversional activities, communicating hope and patience. *Can help client realize that this situation is not hopeless, that there are choices for improving the current situation, and that the future can hold the promise for improvement.*

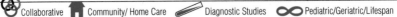 • Encourage/instruct in relaxation techniques (e.g., meditation, sharing experiences, reminiscence, soft music, guided visualization) *to enhance coping skills.*[8]

• Participate in decisions about timing and spacing of visitors, leisure and care activities *to promote relaxation/reduce sense of boredom as well as prevent overstimulation and exhaustion.*[8]

• Encourage client to assist in scheduling required and optional activity choices. *For example, client may want to watch favorite television show at bath time; if bath can be rescheduled later, client's sense of control is enhanced.*[8]

• Provide mix of desired activities/stimuli (e.g., music; news programs; educational presentations, personal interest TV/tapes (e.g., cooking, sports, religion, art); reading materials (e.g., books, papers, magazines, joke books); writing (e.g., journalizing, letters, taping experiences); games (e.g., board, card, video, computer); crafts and hobbies. *Activities need to be age/gender appropriate, personally meaningful and interspersed with rest/quiet periods for client to derive the most enjoyment.*[4]

• Refrain from making changes in schedule without discussing with client. *It is important for staff to be sensitive and responsible in making and following through on commitments to client.*[8]

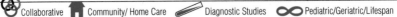 • Provide change of scenery (indoors and out where possible). Provide for periodic changes in the personal environment when client is confined inside, eliciting the client's input for likes and desires. *Change (e.g., new pictures on the wall, seasonal colors/flowers, altering room furniture, or outdoor light and air) can provide positive sensory stimulation, reduce client's boredom, improve sense of normalcy and control.*[5]

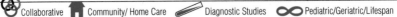 • Suggest activities such as bird feeders/baths for bird-watching, a garden in a window box/terrarium, or a fish bowl/aquarium *to stimulate observation as well as involvement and participation in activity (e.g., bird identification, picking out feeders and seeds).*[8]

 • Involve recreational/occupational/play/music/movement therapists as appropriate *to help identify fun things for individual to do within current situation, to procure assistive*

devices/make adaptations, to assist client to express needs/feelings, share experiences, escape healthcare routines and participate in self-healing.[1,6,7]

NURSING PRIORITY NO. 3. To promote wellness (Teaching/Discharge Considerations):

- Explore options for useful activities using the person's strengths/abilities and interests to engage the client/SO.
- Make appropriate referrals to available resources (e.g., exercise groups, senior activities, hobby clubs, volunteering, companion and service organizations) *to introduce or continue diversional activities in community/home settings.*
- Refer to NDs Powerlessness; Social Isolation; ineffective Coping; Hopelessness for additional interventions.

DOCUMENTATION FOCUS

Assessment/Reassessment
- Specific assessment findings, including blocks to desired activities.
- Individual choices for activities.

Planning
- Plan of care/interventions and who is involved in planning.

Implementation/Evaluation
- Client's responses to interventions/teaching and actions performed.
- Attainment/progress toward desired outcome(s).
- Modifications to plan of care.

Discharge Planning
- Long-term needs and who is responsible for actions to be taken.
- Referrals/community resources.

References

1. Radziewicz, R. M. (1992). Using diversional activities to enhance coping. Cancer Nurs, 15(4), 293.
2. Cox, H. C., et al. (2002). Adult, Child, Women's, Psychiatric, Gerontic, and Home Health Considerations, ed 4. Philadelphia: F. A. Davis, pp 275–278.
3. Engel, J. (2002). Mosby's Pocket Guide to Pediatric Assessment, ed 4. St. Louis: Mosby.
4. Harley, K., et al. (2002). Making each moment count: Developing a diversional therapies program for patients with hematologic malignancies. Abstract from Oncology Nursing Society Convention.
5. Dossey, B. M. (1998). Holistic modalities & healing moments. AJN, 98(6), 44.
6. Williams, M. A. (1988). The physical environment and patient care. Am Rev Nurs Res, 6, 61.
7. Coaten, R. (2002). Movement matters. National Healthcare J, (5), 53.
8. Psychosocial aspects of care. (2002). In Doenges, M. E., Moorhouse, M. F., & Geissler-Murr, A. C. Nursing Care Plans: Guidelines for Individualizing Patient Care, ed 6. Philadelphia: F. A. Davis.
9. Heriot, C. S. (1999). Developmental tasks and development in the later years of life. In Stanley, M. & Bear, P. G. (eds): Gerontological Nursing: A Health Promotion/Protection Approach, ed 2. Philadelphia: F. A. Davis.

Helpful Resource (guidelines for rationales not specifically cited)

Dossey, B. M. & Dossey, L. (1998). Body-mind-spirit: Attending to holistic care. AJN, 98(8), 35.

disturbed Energy Field

Definition: Disruption of the flow of energy [aura] surrounding a person's being that results in a disharmony of the body, mind and/or spirit

RELATED FACTORS

To be developed by nurse researchers and submitted to NANDA
[Block in energy field]
[Depression]
[Increased state anxiety]
[Impaired immune system]
[Pain]

DEFINING CHARACTERISTICS

Objective
Temperature change (warmth/coolness)
Visual changes (image/color)
Disruption of the field (vacant/hold/spike/bulge)
Movement (wave/spike/tingling/dense/flowing)
Sounds (tone/words)

SAMPLE CLINICAL APPLICATIONS: illness, trauma, cancer, pain, impaired immune system, fatigue, surgical procedures

DESIRED OUTCOMES/EVALUATION CRITERIA

Sample **NOC** linkages:
Well-Being: An individual's expressed satisfaction with health status
Spiritual Well-Being: Personal expression of connectedness with self, others, higher power, all life, nature, and the universe that transcends and empowers the self
Coping: Actions to manage stressors that tax an individual's resources

Client Will (Include Specific Time Frame)
- Acknowledge feelings of anxiety and distress.
- Verbalize sense of relaxation/well-being.
- Display reduction in severity/frequency of symptoms.

ACTIONS/INTERVENTIONS

Sample **NIC** linkages:
Therapeutic Touch: Attuning to the universal healing field, seeking to act as an instrument for healing influence, and using the natural sensitivity of the hands to gently focus and direct the intervention process
Meditation Facilitation: Facilitating a person to alter his/her level of awareness by focusing specifically on an image or thought
Pain Management: Alleviation of pain or a reduction in pain to a level of comfort that is acceptable to the patient

NURSING PRIORITY NO. **1.** To determine causative/contributing factors:

 • Develop therapeutic nurse-client relationship, initially accepting role of healer/guide as client desires. *This relationship is one in which both participants recognize each other as*

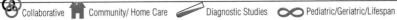 Cultural   Collaborative   Community/ Home Care   Diagnostic Studies   Pediatric/Geriatric/Lifespan   Medications

unique and important human beings and in which mutual learning occurs. The role of the nurse and the use of self as a therapeutic tool is recognized.[3]

- Provide opportunity for client to talk about illness, concerns, history, emotional state, or other relevant information. Note body gestures, tone of voice, words chosen to express feelings/issues. *In the safety of the nurse-client relationship, client can talk readily, identifying fears and concerns, nurse can identify meaning of other elements of communication.*[1]
- Determine client's motivation/desire for treatment. *Following explanation of Therapeutic Touch process and expected results, client may have unrealistic expectations or may understand purpose and believe process will be helpful.*[2]
- Note use of medications, other drug use (e.g., alcohol). *May affect client's ability to relax and take full advantage of the TT process.*[4]
- Use testing as indicated, such as the State-Trait Anxiety Inventory (STAI) or the Affect Balance Scale. *Provides measure of the client's anxiety to evaluate need for treatment/intervention.*[3]

NURSING PRIORITY NO. 2. To evaluate energy field:

- Place client in sitting or supine position with legs/arms uncrossed. Place pillows or other supports *to enhance comfort. Promotes relaxation and feelings of peace, calm and security, preparing the client to derive the most benefit from the procedure.*[1]
- Center self physically and psychologically. *A quiet mind and focused attention turns to the healing intent.*[6]
- Move hands slowly over the client at level of 2 to 3 inches above skin. *Assesses state of energy field and flow of energy within the system. The feelings that may be noted are tingling, warmth, coolness, comfort, peace, calm, and security.*[5]
- Identify areas of imbalance or obstruction in the field. *Areas of asymmetry; feelings of heat/cold, tingling, congestion or pressure, decreased or disrupted energy flow, pulsation, congestion, heaviness, decreased flow may be identified.*[7]

NURSING PRIORITY NO. 3. To provide therapeutic intervention:

- Explain the process of Therapeutic Touch (TT) and answer questions as indicated *to prevent unrealistic expectation. TT is the knowledgeable and purposeful patterning of the client environmental energy field and can relieve discomfort and anxiety. Providing information that the fundamental focus of TT is on healing and wholeness, not curing signs/symptoms of disease helps the client to understand the process.*[6]
- Discuss findings of evaluation with client. *Including the client in the process by sharing the findings of the nurse combined with sensations the client experienced provides the best opportunity to derive benefit from the procedure.*[2]
- Assist client with exercises to promote "centering." *Deep breathing, guided imagery, and the process of centering increase the potential to self-heal, enhance comfort, reduce anxiety.*[2]
- Perform unruffling process, keeping hands 2 to 3 inches from client's body and sweeping them downward and out of the field from head to toe, concentrating on areas of congestion. *Dissipates impediments to free flow of energy within the system and between nurse and client promoting the reception of healing energy and allowing the client to use own resources for self-healing.*[6]
- Focus on areas of disturbance identified, holding hands over or on skin, and/or place one hand in back of body with other hand in front. At the same time, concentrate on the intent to help the client heal. *This move allows the client's body to pull/repattern energy as needed and corrects energy imbalances.*[1]

• Shorten duration of treatment as appropriate. *Children and elderly individuals are generally more sensitive to therapeutic intervention.*[1,2]

• Make coaching suggestions in a soft voice. *Pleasant images/other visualizations, deep breathing enhance feelings of relaxation and help to relieve anxiety.*[1,2]

• Use hands-on massage/apply pressure to acupressure points as appropriate during process. *The addition of these methods can enhance the relaxation and benefit client receives from TT.*[6]

• Pay attention to changes in energy sensations as session progresses. Stop when the energy field is symmetrical and there is a change to feelings of peaceful calm. *Signifies energy is balanced, further intervention is not necessary and client is ready to rest.*[1,2]

• Hold client's feet for a few minutes at end of session. *Assists in "grounding" the body energy, completing the session.*[1]

• Provide client time for a period of peaceful rest following procedure. *TT promotes feelings of peace and comfort, relieving anxiety and promoting self-healing.*[1]

NURSING PRIORITY NO. 4. To promote wellness (Teaching/Discharge Considerations):

• Allow period of client dependency, as appropriate. *Period of dependency permits clients to strengthen own inner resources at their own pace.*[1]

• Encourage ongoing practice of the therapeutic process. *Helping client and family members to learn skill of TT will promote feelings of control of illness and health. It can be used anytime, anywhere, and with friends as well as family.*[4]

• Instruct in use of stress-reduction activities (e.g., centering/meditation, relaxation exercises, guided imagery). *Continuous use of these activities can promote harmony between mind-body-spirit.*[2]

• Discuss importance of integrating techniques into daily activity plan, for sustaining/enhancing sense of well-being. *Helping client to understand that making these a way of life will help them in dealing with challenges of illness and promote a healthy lifestyle.*[1]

• Have client practice each step and demonstrate the complete TT process following the session. *Client displays readiness to assume responsibilities for self-healing as he or she learns the TT process.*[1,2]

• Promote attendance at a support group where members can help each other practice and learn the techniques of TT. *The support of others helps the client to become proficient in the skill of TT.*[2]

 • Refer to other resources as identified (e.g., psychotherapy, clergy, medical treatment of disease processes, hospice). *Encourages the individual to address total well-being/facilitate peaceful death.*[6]

DOCUMENTATION FOCUS

Assessment/Reassessment
• Assessment findings, including characteristics and differences in the energy field.
• Client's perception of problem/need for treatment.

Planning
• Plan of care and who is involved in planning.
• Teaching plan.

 Cultural   Collaborative   Community/ Home Care   Diagnostic Studies   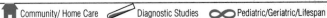 Pediatric/Geriatric/Lifespan   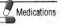 Medications

Implementation/Evaluation
- Changes in energy field.
- Client's response to interventions/teaching and actions performed.
- Attainment/progress toward desired outcomes.
- Modifications to plan of care.

Discharge Planning
- Long-term needs and who is responsible for actions to be taken.
- Specific referrals made.

Resources

1. Krieger, D. (1979). The Therapeutic Touch: How to Use Your Hands to Heal. Englewood Cliffs, NJ: Prentice Hall.
2. Buguslawski, M. (1980). Therapeutic touch: A facilitator of pain relief. Top Clin Nurs 2(27).
3. Townsend, M. C. (2003). Psychiatric Mental Health Nursing Concepts of Care, ed 4. Philadelphia: F. A. Davis.
4. Daglish, S. (1999). Therapeutic touch in an acute care community hospital. Can Nurse 95(3), 57–58.
5. Hayes, J., & Cox, C. (1999). The experience of therapeutic touch from a nusing perspective. Br JNurs 8(18), 1249.
6. Meehan, T. (1998). Therapeutic touch as a nursing intervention. J Adv Nurs 28(1), 117.
7. Marnhinweg, G. (1996). Energy field disturbance validation study. Healing Touch Newsletter 6(11).

impaired Environmental Interpretation Syndrome

Definition: Consistent lack of orientation to person, place, time, or circumstances over more than 3 to 6 months, necessitating a protective environment

RELATED FACTORS
Dementia (Alzheimer's disease, multi-infarct, Pick's disease, AIDS, alcoholism, Parkinson's disease)
Huntington's disease
Depression

DEFINING CHARACTERISTICS

Subjective
[Loss of occupation or social functioning from memory decline]

Objective
Consistent disorientation in known and unknown environments
Chronic confusional states; [loss of self-monitoring]
Inability to follow simple directions, instructions
Inability to reason; to concentrate; slow in responding to questions
Loss of occupation or social functioning from memory decline

SAMPLE CLINICAL APPLICATIONS: dementia (e.g., Alzheimer's, AIDS, alcoholism), depression, Huntington's disease

DESIRED OUTCOMES/EVALUATION CRITERIA
Sample **NOC** linkage:
Safety Status: Physical Injury: Severity of injuries from accidents and trauma

Cognitive Ability: Ability to execute complex mental processes

Safety Behavior: Home Physical Environment: Individual or caregiver actions to minimize environmental factors that might cause physical harm or injury in the home

---

Client Will (Include Specific Time Frame)
- Be free of harm.

Caregiver Will (Include Specific Time Frame)
- Identify individual client safety concerns/needs.
- Modify activities/environment to provide for safety.

ACTIONS/INTERVENTIONS

Sample **NIC** linkages:

Environment Management: Manipulation of the patient's surroundings for therapeutic benefit

Reality Orientation: Promotions of patient's awareness of personal identity, time, and environment

Surveillance: Purposeful and ongoing acquisition, interpretation, and synthesis of patient data for clinical decision making

NURSING PRIORITY NO. **1.** To assess causative/precipitating factors:

- Determine presence of conditions and/or behaviors leading to client's current problem. (Note: It is possible there is no identifiable event.) *Can provide clues for likelihood for improvement, as well as helping to identify potentially useful interventions and therapies.*[1]
- Note presence/reports of client's misinterpretation of environmental information (e.g., sensory, cognitive or social cues).
- Talk with SO(s) regarding baseline behaviors, length of time since onset/progression of problem, their perception of prognosis, and other pertinent information and concerns for client. *The client's SO/primary caregiver is an invaluable and essential source of information regarding past history and current situation, as both cognitive and behavioral symptoms tend to change over time, and are often variable from day to day.*[1]
- Obtain information regarding recent changes or disruptions in client's health or routine. *Decline in physical health or disruption in daily living situation (e.g., hospitalization, change in medications, or moving to new home) can exacerbate symptoms causing agitation or delirium.*[1]
- Identify potential environmental dangers and evaluate client's level of awareness (if any) of threat. Review client's physical conditions/limitations (e.g., decreased agility, reduced ROM of joints, loss of balance, and decline in visual acuity). *To note difficulties/problems that may impact client care and safety, or add to client's difficulties in interpretation of sensory input.*
- Review/evaluate responses of collaborative diagnostic examinations (e.g., cognition, functional capacity, and behavior, degree of memory impairments, reality orientation, general physical health and quality of life). *A combination of tests is often needed to complete an evaluation of client's overall condition relating to chronic/irreversible condition. These tests include (but are not limited to) MRI/brain scan; Mini-Mental State Examination (MMSE); Alzheimer's Disease Assessment Scale, cognitive subsection (ADAS-cog); Functional Assessment Questionnaire (FAQ); Clinical Global Impression of Change (CGIC); Neuropsychiatric Inventory (NPI).*[2]

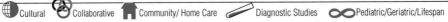 Cultural   Collaborative   Community/ Home Care   Diagnostic Studies   Pediatric/Geriatric/Lifespan   Medications

- Evaluate client's response to primary care providers as well as receptiveness to interventions. *Awareness of these dynamics is helpful for evaluation of ongoing needs for both client and caregiver, as client becomes increasingly dependent on caregivers and/or resistant to interventions.*[3]

NURSING PRIORITY NO. 2. To provide/promote safe environment:

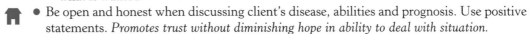
- Include SO(s)/caregivers in planning process. Identify previous/usual patterns for activities, such as sleeping, eating, self-care, etc. *to incorporate into plan of care to the extent possible and lessen confusion.*

- Implement behavioral and environmental management interventions, *to promote orientation, provide opportunity for client interaction using current cognitive skills, preserve client's dignity and safety*[1–6]:
  Provide calm environment, eliminate extraneous noise/stimuli
  Introduce yourself at each contact if needed. Call client by preferred name.
  Keep communication/questions simple. Use concrete terms. Use symbols instead of words when hearing/other impaired *to improve communication.*
  Avoid speaking in loud voice, crowding, restraining, shaming, demanding, or condescending actions toward client.
  Use touch judiciously. Tell client what is being done before touching.
  Simplify client's tasks and routines, limit number of decisions/choices client needs to make at one time, offer guided choices between two options
  Promote and structure activities and rest periods, allow adequate rest between stimulating events
  Recommend limiting number of visitors client interacts with at one time.
  Avoid challenging illogical thinking *because defensive reactions may result*
  Distract/redirect client's attention when behavior is agitated or dangerous. Set limits on acting-out behavior
  Remove from stressors and agitation triggers or danger; move client to quieter place; offer privacy
  Use lighting and visual aides to reduce confusion about surroundings.
  Maintain continuity of caregivers, care routines, and surroundings as much as possible
  Provide simple orientation measures, such as one-number calendar, personal items, seasonal decorations, etc.
  Be supportive and sensitive to fears, misperceived threats and frustration with expressing what is wanted

- Be open and honest when discussing client's disease, abilities and prognosis. Use positive statements. *Promotes trust without diminishing hope in ability to deal with situation.*

- Provide safety measures (e.g., close supervision, identification bracelet, alarms on exits, toxic substances and medication lockup, supervision of outdoor activities and wandering, locked unit areas, removal of car/car keys; lowered temperature on hot water tank); discourage/supervise smoking, monitor ADLs (e.g., use of stove/sharp knives, choice of clothing in relation to environment/season). *Impaired judgment and inattention to detail place client at increased risk for injury to self and others as well.*

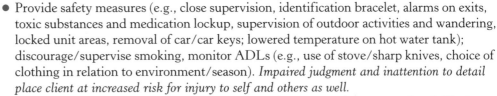
- Administer medications *to manage symptoms and maximize abilities* as ordered. Use lowest possible therapeutic dose and monitor for expected and/or adverse responses, side effects, and interactions.

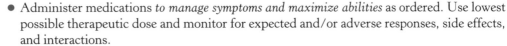
- Implement complimentary therapies as indicated/desired, e.g., music therapy, hand massage, Therapeutic Touch (if touch is tolerated), aromatherapy, bright-light treatment. *May help client relax, refocus attention, stimulate memories.*[7]

- Refer to NDs impaired verbal Communication; chronic Confusion; impaired Memory; disturbed Sensory Perception (specify); disturbed Thought Processes; risk for Trauma; Wandering as appropriate for additional interventions.

NURSING PRIORITY NO. 3. To assist caregiver to deal with situation:

 - Determine family dynamics, cultural values, resources, availability and willingness to participate in meeting client's needs.

- Evaluate SO's attention to own needs including health status, grieving process and respite. *Primary caregiver and other members of family will suffer from the stress that accompanies care giving and require information and support.*[2–6,9,10]

- Involve SO(s) in care and discharge planning. Maintain frequent interactions with SOs *to relay information, to change care strategies, try different responses, or implement other problem-solving solutions.*

- Review safety measures regarding client's environmental impairments. *Client can not only lose items, but also can get lost in familiar places, requiring special attention to client's possessions, as well as to physical safety in the home and community. The client may believe that caregivers are stealing the "lost" items; or the client may leave home and be unable to get back.*[8]

- Avoid leaving client alone in home. Consider use of home security system/motion detectors. Register client with Safe Return program of Alzheimer's Association. Talk with neighbors and police if client is prone to wander. *If the general public is on alert for a person with dementia who may need help, the chances of finding that person are greatly enhanced.*[8]

- Provide educational materials reflecting SO/family needs and learning styles and lists of available resources, such as newsletters, books, Web sites, telephone help lines, etc. *Reduces sense of overload, allows individuals to review/refer to resources as needed on their own time frame.*

- Identify appropriate community resources (e.g., Alzheimer's Disease and Related Disorders Association [ADRDA]; stroke or other brain injury support groups; senior support groups, respite care, clergy, social services, therapists, attorney services for advance directives and durable power of attorney) *to provide support for client and SOs, and assist with problem solving.*

- Discuss need for time for self away from client. (Refer to ND risk for Caregiver Role Strain.)

NURSING PRIORITY NO. 4. To promote wellness (Teaching/Discharge Considerations):

- Discuss how client's condition may progress, ongoing treatment needs and appropriate follow-up. *Intermittent evaluations are needed to determine client's general health, any deterioration in cognitive function, requiring adjustment in medication regimen, etc., to maintain the client at the highest possible level of functioning.*

- Develop plan of care with family to meet client's and SO(s') individual needs. *The individual plan is dependent on cultural and belief patterns, as well as family (personal, emotional, and financial) resources.*

- Instruct SO/caregivers to share information about client's condition, functional status and medications whenever encountering new providers. *Clients often have multiple doctors, each of whom may prescribe medications, with potential for adverse effects and overmedication.*[3,7]

 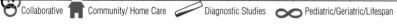

● Investigate local resources; provide appropriate referrals (e.g., Case managers, counselors, support groups, financial services, Meals on Wheels, adult day care, adult foster care, respite care for family, home care agency, nursing home placement). *Individuals are generally not capable of carrying alone the heavy burdens of caring for a relative with this problem. Caregivers need help and support (whether or not they are trying to provide total care) to deal with exhaustion and unresolved feelings.*[9,10]

 ● Discuss need for/appropriateness of genetic testing/counseling for family members. *Diagnosis of dementias such as early onset Alzheimer's or Huntington's disease necessitate additional support for family members who may be at risk themselves.*

DOCUMENTATION FOCUS

Assessment/Reassessment
● Assessment findings, including degree of impairment.

Planning
● Plan of care and who is involved in planning.
● Teaching plan.

Implementation/Evaluation
● Response to treatment plan/interventions and actions performed.
● Attainment/progress toward desired outcomes.
● Modifications to plan of care.

Discharge Planning
● Long-range needs, who is responsible for actions to be taken.
● Specific referrals made

References

1. Bostwick, J. M. (2000). The many faces of confusion: Timing and collateral history often holds the key to diagnosis. Postgrad Med, 108 (6), 60–72.
2. About Alzheimer's. (2003). Physicians and Care Professionals, Various Educational Materials. Alzheimer's Disease and Related Disorders Association (ADRDA). Available at: www.alz.org. Accessed 2003.
3. Doenges, M. E., Moorhouse, M. F., & Geissler-Murr, A. C. (2002). Nurse's Pocket Guide: Diagnoses, Interventions, and Rationales, ed 8. Philadelphia: F. A. Davis, pp 145–147.
4. Expert Consensus Guideline Series: Agitation in older persons with dementia: A guide for families and caregivers. (1998). Expert Knowledge Systems, LLC. Ross Editorial Services. Available at: www.psychguides.com. Accessed 2003.
5. Sommers, M. S., & Johnson, S. A. (1997). Alzheimer's disease and delirium/dementia. In Davis' Manual of Nursing Therapeutics for Diseases and Disorders. Philadelphia: F. A. Davis.
6. Kovach, C. R., & Wilson, S. A. (1999). Dementia in older adults. In Stanley, M., & Beare P. G. Gerontologic Nursing: A Health Promotion/Protection Approach, ed 2. Philadelphia: F. A. Davis.
7. Burns, A., Byrne, J., & Ballard, C. (2002). Sensory stimulation in dementia: An effective option for managing behavioral problems. BMJ, 325, 1312–1313. Summarized on Dementia Center Health and Age Website. Available at: www.healthandage.com.
8. Rowe, M. A. (2003). People with dementia who become lost. AJN 103(7), 32.
9. Brynes, G. (2000). Dealing with dementia: Help for relatives, friends and caregivers. Information brochure. Baltimore: Northern County Psychiatric Associates.
10. The mid stage of Alzheimer's disease: Tips for dealing with dementia sufferers. Available at: http://www.dementia.com. Accessed August 13, 2003.

Definition: Progressive functional deterioration of a physical and cognitive nature. The individual's ability to live with multisystem diseases, cope with ensuing problems, and manage his or her care are remarkably diminished

RELATED FACTORS

Depression; apathy

Fatigue

[Major disease/degenerative condition]

[Aging process]

DEFINING CHARACTERISTICS

Subjective

States does not have an appetite, not hungry, or "I don't want to eat"

Expresses loss of interest in pleasurable outlets, such as food, sex, work, friends, family, hobbies, or entertainment

Difficulty performing simple self-care tasks

Altered mood state—expresses feelings of sadness, being low in spirit

Verbalizes desire for death

Objective

Inadequate nutritional intake—eating less than body requirements; consumes minimal to none of food at most meals (i.e., consumes less than 75% of normal requirements at each or most meals); anorexia—does not eat meals when offered

Weight loss (decreased body mass from baseline weight)—5% unintentional weight loss in 1 month, 10% unintentional weight loss in 6 months

Physical decline (decline in bodily function)—evidence of fatigue, dehydration, incontinence of bowel and bladder

Cognitive decline (decline in mental processing)—as evidenced by problems with responding appropriately to environmental stimuli; demonstrates difficulty in reasoning, decision making, judgment, memory, concentration; decreased perception

Apathy as evidenced by lack of observable feeling or emotion in terms of normal ADLs and environment

Decreased participation in ADLs that the older person once enjoyed; self-care deficit—no longer looks after or takes charge of physical cleanliness or appearance; neglects home environment and/or financial responsibilities

Decreased social skills/social withdrawal—noticeable decrease from usual past behavior in attempts to form or participate in cooperative and interdependent relationships (e.g., decreased verbal communication with staff, family, friends)

Frequent exacerbations of chronic health problems such as pneumonia or urinary tract infections (UTIs)

SAMPLE CLINICAL APPLICATIONS: chronic debilitating conditions (e.g., AIDS, Alzheimer's disease, multiple sclerosis), cancer/terminal illnesses, major depression

DESIRED OUTCOMES/EVALUATION CRITERIA

Sample **NOC** linkages:

Will to Live: Desire, determination, and effort to survive

 Cultural Collaborative Community/ Home Care Diagnostic Studies Pediatric/Geriatric/Lifespan Medications

Psychosocial Adjustment: Life Change: Psychosocial adaptation of an individual to a life change

Physical Aging Status: Physical changes that commonly occur with adult aging

---

Client/ Caregiver Will (Include Specific Time Frame)
- Acknowledge presence of factors affecting well-being.
- Identify corrective/adaptive measures for individual situation.
- Demonstrate behaviors/lifestyle changes necessary to promote improved status.

ACTIONS/INTERVENTIONS
Sample **NIC** linkages:

Mood Management: Providing for safety, stabilization, recovery, and maintenance of a patient who is dysfunctionally depressed or elevated mood

Hope Instillation: Facilitation of the development of a positive outlook in a given situation

Self-Care Assistance: Assisting another to perform activities of daily living

NURSING PRIORITY NO. **1.** To identify causative/contributing factors:

- Assess client's/SO's perception of factors leading to present condition, noting onset, duration of decline. *Adult failure to thrive (FTT) is characterized by malnutrition associated with consistent weight loss, loss of physical, cognitive and social functioning, impaired immune function, and depression.*[1] *This condition may be identified when client is hospitalized for problems such as urinary tract infection, decubitus ulcers, falls, and mental confusion. Although it can occur as a result of an acute health problem or elder abuse, failure to thrive is most often associated with chronic health conditions, social isolation and budgetary constraints.*[2]

- Assist with testing as indicated (e.g., urea breath test, endoscopy; psychiatric evaluation). *Aversion to eating and decline in mental function with absence of usual symptoms associated with gastric disease may actually reflect gastric infection with* Helicobacter pylori.[9]

- Note presence/absence of physical complaints (e.g., fatigue, weight loss, others as noted in Defining Characteristics) and presence of conditions (e.g., heart disease, undetected diabetes mellitus, dementia, CVA, renal failure, terminal conditions). *These factors leading to failure to thrive may/may not be recognized by the client or SOs.*

- Assess for cultural beliefs, norms and values that are influencing client/caregiver understanding. *Although many cultures have their own distinct theories of nutritional practices for health promotion and disease prevention, the need for nutritional balance of a diet is almost universally recognized as essential for healing, general health and sustaining a quality life.*[3]

- Review with client/SO previous and current life situations, including role changes, multiple losses, and social isolation, grieving, *to identify stressors affecting current situation.*

- Determine nutritional status. *Poor nutrition (with weight loss, laboratory abnormalities) and factors contributing to failure to eat (e.g., chronic nausea, loss of appetite, no access to food or cooking, multiple medications, financial problems) greatly impact the health status and quality of life for the elderly individual.*[4–6]

- Determine client's cognitive and perceptual status and effect on self-care ability. *Various functional scales may be used, in addition to reports from client/caregiver regarding losses. Note: Failure to thrive is a recognized diagnosis for admission to hospice care.*[7]

- Evaluate client level of adaptive behavior, and client/caregiver knowledge, and skills about health maintenance, environment, and safety *in order to instruct, intervene, and refer appropriately.*

- Ascertain safety and effectiveness of home environment, and persons providing care *to identify potential for/presence of neglectful/abusive situations and/or need for referrals.*

NURSING PRIORITY NO. 2. To assess degree of impairment:

 ● Collaborate with multidisciplinary team to perform physical, psychological, nutritional and/or psychosocial assessment *to determine the extent of limitations, to intervene in treatment plan, and to make appropriate referrals.*

 ● Active-listen to client's/caregiver's perception of problem. *Conveys sense of confidence in client's ability to identify and solve current problems.*[8]

● Survey past and present availability/use of support systems. *Identification of sources of support can provide help for client to begin to accept help and improve situation.*[8]

NURSING PRIORITY NO. 3. To assist client to achieve/maintain general well-being:

 ● Develop plan of action with client/caregiver to meet immediate needs (physical safety, hygiene, nutrition, emotional support) and assist in implementation of plan.

 ● Refer to dietitian *to assist in planning nutritional meals to meet client's specific needs, taste, and abilities.* (Refer to ND imbalanced Nutrition: less than body needs for additional interventions.)

 ● Monitor caloric intake and weigh weekly. *Provides data to evaluate effectiveness of interventions.*

 ● Explore previously used successful coping skills and application to current situation. *Feelings of hopelessness and powerlessness interfere with ability to use coping skills and bringing them to mind can reinforce possibility of current use.*[8]

 ● Refine/develop new strategies as appropriate. (Refer to ND ineffective Coping for additional interventions.)

 ● Assist client to develop goals for dealing with life/illness situation. Involve SO in long-range planning. *Promotes commitment to goals and plan, maximizing outcomes.*

NURSING PRIORITY NO. 4. To promote wellness (Teaching/Discharge Considerations):

 ● Review medication regimen including potential side effects/adverse reactions. *Mood elevators, antibiotics, hydrogen-ion proton inhibitors, vitamin/mineral supplements, appetite stimulants, etc., may be ordered based on individual need.*

 ● Refer to other resources (e.g., social worker, occupational therapy, home care, assistive care, placement services, spiritual advisor). *Enhances coping, assists with problem solving, and may reduce risks to client and caregiver.*

 ● Promote socialization within individual limitations to *provide additional stimulation, reduce sense of isolation.*

 ● Help client find a reason for living or begin to deal with end-of-life issues and provide support for grieving. *Enhances sense of control, providing opportunity for client to take charge of own future.*[8]

DOCUMENTATION FOCUS

Assessment/Reassessment
● Individual findings, including current weight, dietary pattern, perceptions of self, food and eating, motivation for loss, support/feedback from SOs.
● Ability to perform ADLs/participate in care, meet own needs.

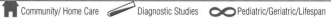 Cultural Collaborative Community/ Home Care Diagnostic Studies Pediatric/Geriatric/Lifespan Medications

Planning
- Plan of care/interventions and who is involved in planning.
- Teaching plan.

Implementation/Evaluation
- Responses to interventions and actions performed, general well-being, weekly weight.
- Attainment/progress toward desired outcome(s).
- Modifications to plan of care.

Discharge Planning
- Long-term needs and who is responsible for actions to be taken.
- Community resources/support groups.
- Specific referrals made.

References

1. Groom, D. D. (1993). Elder care: A diagnostic model for failure to thrive. J Gerontol Nurs 19,6.
2. Stanley, M. (1999). The aging gastrointestinal system, with nutritional considerations. In Stanley, M., & Beare, P. G. (eds): Gerontological Nursing: A Health Promotion/Protection Approach, ed 2. Philadelphia: F. A. Davis.
3. Purnell's Model for Cultural Competence. (1998). In Purnell, L. D., & Paulanka, B. J. (eds): Transcultural Health care: A Culturally Competent Approach. Philadelphia: F. A. Davis, p 34.
4. Wallace, J. I., & Schwartz, R. S. (1997). Involuntary weight loss in elderly outpatients. Clin Geriatr Med 13, 717.
5. Scott, D. D., & Chase, M. (2003). Nutritional management in the rehabilitation setting. Available at: www.emedicine.com. Accessed August 2003.
6. Karnofsky Performance Status Scale Rating Criteria. (1993). Oxford Textbook of Palliative Medicine. Oxford University Press.
7. Adult Failure to Thrive/Debility, Unspecified. (1993). Medicare worksheet for determining prognosis. Hospice of Southern Illinois, Inc.
8. Townsend, M. C. (2003). Psychiatric Mental Health Nursing Concepts of Care, (4th ed). Philadelphia: F. A. Davis.
9. Portnoi, V. A. (1997). *Helicobacter pylori* infection and anorexia of aging. Arch Intern Med, 157, 269.

risk for Falls

Definition: Increased susceptibility to falling that may cause physical harm

RISK FACTORS

Adults
History of falls
Wheelchair use; use of assistive devices (e.g., walker, cane)
Age 65 or over; female (if elderly)
Lives alone
Lower limb prosthesis

Physiological
Presence of acute illness; postoperative conditions
Visual/hearing difficulties
Impaired physical mobility; foot problems; decreased lower extremity strength; arthritis
Impaired balance; difficulty with gait;
Proprioceptive deficits (e.g., unilateral neglect); neuropathies
[Cardio and neuro] vascular disease; anemias; endoplasms (i.e., fatigue/limited mobility)

Orthostatic hypotension; [dehydration/blood loss]
Faintness when turning or extending neck
Sleeplessness/ [sleep disturbances]
Urgency and/or incontinence; diarrhea
Postprandial blood sugar changes/ [hypoglycemia]

Cognitive
Diminished mental status (e.g., confusion, [agitation]/delirium, dementia, impaired reality testing)
Medications; antihypertensive agents; ACE inhibitors; diuretics; tricyclic antidepressants; antianxiety agents; hypnotics or tranquilizers [polypharmacy (multiple medications)]
Alcohol use; narcotics

Environment
Restraints
Weather conditions (e.g., wet floors/ice)
Cluttered environment; throw/scatter rugs; no antislip material in bath and/or shower
Unfamiliar, dimly lit room

Children
2 years of age; male gender when <1 year of age
Lack of gate on stairs; window guards; auto restraints
Unattended infant on bed/changing table/sofa; bed located near window
Lack of parental supervision
NOTE: A risk diagnosis is not evidenced by signs and symptoms, as the problem has not occurred and nursing interventions are directed at prevention.
SAMPLE CLINICAL APPLICATIONS: osteoporosis, seizure disorder, cerebrovascular disease, cataracts, dementia, paralysis, hypotension, cardiac dysrhythmias, amputation, inner ear infection, alcohol abuse/intoxication

DESIRED OUTCOMES/EVALUATION CRITERIA
Sample **NOC** linkages:
Safety Behavior: Fall Prevention: Individual or caregiver actions to minimize risk factors that might precipitate falls
Risk Control: Actions to eliminate or reduce actual, personal, and modifiable health threats
Safety Status: Physical Injury: Severity of injuries from accidents and trauma

Client/Caregivers Will (Include Specific Time Frame)
- Verbalize understanding of individual risk factors that contribute to possibility of falls and take steps to correct situation(s).
- Demonstrate behaviors, lifestyle changes to reduce risk factors and protect self from injury.
- Modify environment as indicated to enhance safety.
- Be free of injury.

ACTIONS/INTERVENTIONS
Sample **NIC** linkages:
Fall Prevention: Instituting special precautions with patient at risk for injury from falling

 Cultural Collaborative Community/ Home Care Diagnostic Studies 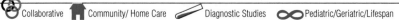 Pediatric/Geriatric/Lifespan Medications

Environment Management: Safety: Manipulation of the patient's surroundings for therapeutic benefit

Risk Identification: Analysis of potential risk factors, determination of health risks, and prioritization of risk reduction strategies for an individual or group

NURSING PRIORITY NO. 1. To evaluate source/degree of risk:

- Assess and document client's fall risk using a fall scale [e.g. Morse Fall Scale (MFS)] upon admission, change in status, transfer and discharge. *The MFS is widely used in acute care and long term settings and includes numbered rating scale for 1) history of falls, 2) secondary diagnosis, 3) use of ambulatory aid, 4) presence of IV, 5) gait/transfer abilities and 6) mental status. A MFS score of 25–50 places the client in low risk category and requires standard fall-prevention interventions. An MFS score of >51 indicates the client is at high risk for falls and requires high fall-prevention interventions.*[1,2]
- Note age, developmental level, decision-making ability, level of cognition and competence. *Infants, young children, young adult males, and elderly are at greatest risk because of developmental issues, inability to recognize danger, sensory impairments, or frailty.*
- Assess client for **significant** risk for injury. *Factors associated with increased risk for injury include current use of anticoagulants, significant vision, cognitive or mobility impairments; osteoporosis; or loss of muscle, fat and subcutaneous tissue.*[2]
- Assess mood, coping abilities, personality styles. *Individual's temperament, typical behavior, stressors, and level of self-esteem can affect attitude toward safety issues, resulting in carelessness or increased risk-taking without consideration of consequences.*
- Ascertain knowledge of safety needs/injury prevention and motivation to prevent injury. *Client/caregivers may not be aware of proper precautions or may not have the knowledge, desire, or resources to attend to safety issues in all settings.*[3]
- Discuss with caregivers importance of monitoring conditions that contribute to occurrence of injury (e.g., fatigue, objects that block traffic patterns, lack of sufficient light, attempting tasks that are too difficult for present level of functioning, lack of ability to contact someone when help is needed, etc.).
- Determine caregiver's expectations of children, cognitively impaired and/or elderly family members and compare with actual abilities. *Reality of client's abilities and needs may be different than perception or desires of caregivers.*
- Note socioeconomic status/availability and use of resources in other circumstances. *Can affect current coping abilities.*

NURSING PRIORITY NO. 2. To assist client/caregiver to reduce or correct individual risk factors:

- Review consequences of previously determined risk factors and client/SO response (e.g., previous falls caused by failure to make provisions for client's impairments related to physical, cognitive or environmental factors). *These factors are many and various and might include such things as an acute change in mental status and strength caused by a urinary infection, or a defective walker, or new room in a facility.*[3]
- Provide information regarding client's current disease/condition(s) (e.g., acute illness, dementia, incontinence, neurological or musculoskeletal conditions) *that may result in increased risk of falls.*
- Implement needed interventions and safety devices *to manage various conditions that could contribute to falling, and to promote safe environment for individual and others*[1–6]:
  Situate bed to enable client to exit toward his/her stronger side whenever possible.

Place bed in lowest possible position, use raised edge mattress, pad floor at side of bed, or place mattress on floor as appropriate

Use half side rail for repositioning in bed or upright pole to assist individual in arising from bed instead of full side rails. *Reduces risk of entrapment or falls from climbing over rails.*

Provide chairs with firm, high seats and lifting mechanisms when indicated

Provide adequate day/night lighting; evaluate vision/encourage use of prescription eyewear

Assist with transfers and ambulation; show client/SO ways to move safely

Provide/instruct in use of mobility devices and safety devices, like grab bars and call lights/personal assistance systems

Clear environment of hazards (e.g., obstructing furniture, small items on the floor, electrical cords, throw rugs)

Lock wheels on movable equipment (e.g., wheelchairs, beds)

Encourage use of treaded slippers, socks and shoes, and maintain non-skid floors and floor mats.

Provide foot and nail care

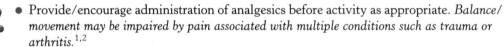 ● Provide/encourage administration of analgesics before activity as appropriate. *Balance/movement may be impaired by pain associated with multiple conditions such as trauma or arthritis.*[1,2]

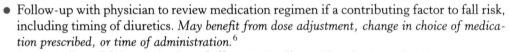 ● Follow-up with physician to review medication regimen if a contributing factor to fall risk, including timing of diuretics. *May benefit from dose adjustment, change in choice of medication prescribed, or time of administration.*[6]

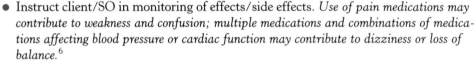 ● Instruct client/SO in monitoring of effects/side effects. *Use of pain medications may contribute to weakness and confusion; multiple medications and combinations of medications affecting blood pressure or cardiac function may contribute to dizziness or loss of balance.*[6]

● Refer to physical medicine specialist, physical or occupational therapist, recreation therapist as appropriate. *May require testing (e.g., balance, muscle strength) and exercises to improve strength or mobility, improve/relearn ambulation, or identify and obtain appropriate assistive devices for mobility, bathroom safety, or home modification.*

● Plan for home visit when appropriate. Determine that home safety issues are addressed, including supervision, access to emergency assistance, and client's ability to manage self-care in the home. *May be needed to adequately evaluate client's needs and available resources.*

NURSING PRIORITY NO. 3. To promote wellness (Teaching/Discharge Considerations)[1-6]:

● Educate client/SO/caregivers in fall prevention, address the need for exercise balanced with need for client/care provider safety. *While fall prevention is necessary, the need to protect the client from harm must be balanced with preserving client's independence. If the client is overly afraid of falling the lack of activity will result in deconditioning and even greater risk of falling.*[3]

● Discuss need for and sources of supervision (*e.g., babysitters, before and after school programs, elderly day care, personal companions, etc.*).

● Promote education geared to increasing individual's awareness of safety measures and available resources.

● Address individual environmental factors associated with falling and create/instruct in safe

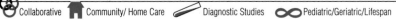

physical environment such as bed height, room lighting, inappropriate footwear/inadequate assistive devices, loose carpet or throw rugs, uneven flooring, grab bars in bathrooms.

- Refer to community resources as indicated. Provide written resources for later review/reinforcement of learning. *Client/caregivers may need/desire information (now or later) about financial assistance, home modifications, referrals for counseling, homecare, sources for safety equipment, or placement in extended care facility.*
- Connect client/family with community sources of assistance (e.g., neighbors, friends) *to check on client on regular basis, to assist elderly/handicapped individuals in providing such things as structural maintenance, clearing of snow, gravel or ice from walks and steps, etc.*
- Promote community awareness about the problems of design of buildings, equipment, transportation, and work-place accidents that contribute to falls.

DOCUMENTATION FOCUS

Assessment/Reassessment
- Individual risk factors noting current physical findings (e.g., bruises, cuts, anemia, and use of alcohol, drugs, and prescription medications).
- Client's/caregiver's understanding of individual risks/safety concerns.

Planning
- Plan of care and who is involved in planning.
- Teaching plan.

Implementation/Evaluation
- Individual responses to interventions/teaching and actions performed.
- Specific actions and changes that are made.
- Attainment/progress toward desired outcomes.
- Modifications to plan of care.

Discharge Planning
- Long-range plans for discharge needs, lifestyle, home setting and community changes, and who is responsible for actions to be taken.
- Specific referrals made.

References

1. Falls and fall risk. (1999) Clinical practice guideline. American Medical Directors Association (AMDA). Columbia MD. Available at: http://www.amda.com/. Accessed August 2003.
2. VA National Center for Patient Safety (NCPS) Fall Prevention and Management (updated 2002). Includes articles on Morse Fall Scale, standard and high risk fall prevention measures and safety education. Available at: http://www.patientsafety.gov. Accessed August 2003.
3. Henkel, G. (2002) Beyond the MDS. Team approach to falls assessment, prevention & management. Caring for the Aged, 3(4), 15–20.
4. Nursing Care Plan: Extended care, falls, risk for. (2002). In Doenges, M. E., Moorhouse, M. F., & Geissler-Murr, A. C. (eds): Nursing Care Plans: Guidelines for Individualizing Patient Care, ed 6, (CD-ROM). Philadelphia: F. A. Davis.
5. Daus, C. (1999). Maintaining mobility: Assistive equipment helps the geriatric population stay active and independent. Rehab Management, 12(5), 58–61.
6. Horn, L. B. (2000). Reducing the risk of falls in the elderly. Rehab Management, 13(3), 36–38.

dysfunctional Family Processes: alcoholism

Definition: Psychosocial, spiritual, and physiologic functions of the family unit are chronically disorganized, which leads to conflict, denial of problems, resistance to change, ineffective problem solving, and a series of self-perpetuating crises

RELATED FACTORS

Abuse of alcohol; resistance to treatment
Family history of alcoholism
Inadequate coping skills; addictive personality; lack of problem-solving skills
Biochemical influences; genetic predisposition

DEFINING CHARACTERISTICS

Subjective

Feelings

Anxiety/tension/distress, decreased self-esteem/worthlessness, lingering resentment
Anger/suppressed rage, frustration, shame/embarrassment, hurt, unhappiness, guilt
Emotional isolation/loneliness, powerlessness, insecurity, hopelessness, rejection
Responsibility for alcoholic's behavior, vulnerability, mistrust
Depression, hostility, fear, confusion, dissatisfaction, loss, repressed emotions
Being different from other people, misunderstood
Emotional control by others, being unloved, lack of identity
Abandonment, confused love and pity, moodiness, failure

Roles and Relationships

Family denial, deterioration in family relationships/disturbed family dynamics, ineffective spouse communication/marital problems, intimacy dysfunction
Altered role function/disruption of family roles, inconsistent parenting/low perception of parental support, chronic family problems
Lack of skills necessary for relationships, lack of cohesiveness, disrupted family rituals
Family unable to meet security needs of its members
Pattern of rejection, economic problems, neglected obligations

Objective

Roles and Relationships

Closed communication systems
Triangulating family relationships, reduced ability of family members to relate to each other for mutual growth and maturation
Family does not demonstrate respect for individuality and autonomy of its members

Behaviors

Expression of anger inappropriately, difficulty with intimate relationships, impaired communication, ineffective problem-solving skills, inability to meet emotional needs of its members, manipulation, dependency, criticizing, broken promises, rationalization/denial of problems
Refusal to get help/inability to accept and receive help appropriately, blaming

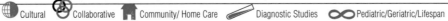 Cultural   Collaborative   Community/ Home Care   Diagnostic Studies   Pediatric/Geriatric/Lifespan   Medications

Loss of control of drinking, enabling to maintain drinking [substance use], alcohol [substance] abuse, inadequate understanding or knowledge of alcoholism [substance abuse]

Inability to meet spiritual needs of its members

Inability to express or accept wide range of feelings, orientation toward tension relief rather than achievement of goals, escalating conflict

Lying, contradictory, paradoxical communication, lack of dealing with conflict, harsh self-judgment, isolation, difficulty having fun, self-blaming, unresolved grief

Controlling communication/power struggles, seeking approval and affirmation

Lack of reliability, disturbances in academic performance in children, disturbances in concentration, chaos, failure to accomplish current or past developmental tasks/difficulty with life-cycle transitions

Verbal abuse of spouse or parent, agitation, diminished physical contact

Family special occasions are alcohol-centered, nicotine addiction, inability to adapt to change, immaturity, stress-related physical illnesses, inability to deal with traumatic experiences constructively, substance abuse other than alcohol

SAMPLE CLINICAL APPLICATIONS: alcohol abuse/withdrawal, prescription/illicit drug abuse

DESIRED OUTCOMES/EVALUATION CRITERIA

Sample **NOC** linkages:

Family Functioning: Ability of the family to meet the needs of its members through developmental transitions

Family Environment: Internal: Social climate as characterized by family member relationships and goals

Substance Addiction: Consequences: Compromise in health status and social functioning due to substance addiction

Family Will (Include Specific Time Frame)
- Verbalize understanding of dynamics of codependence.
- Participate in individual/family treatment programs.
- Identify ineffective coping behaviors/consequences.
- Demonstrate/plan for necessary lifestyle changes.
- Take action to change self-destructive behaviors/alter behaviors that contribute to client's drinking/substance use.

ACTIONS/INTERVENTIONS

Sample **NIC** linkages:

Substance Use Treatment: Supportive care of patient/family members with physical and psychosocial problems associated with the use of alcohol or drugs

Family Process Maintenance: Minimization of family process disruption effects

Counseling: Use of an interactive helping process focusing on the needs, problems, or feelings of the patient and SOs to enhance or support coping, problem solving, and interpersonal relationships

NURSING PRIORITY NO. 1. To assess contributing factors/underlying problem(s):

- Assess current level of functioning of family members. *Information necessary for planning care, determines areas for focus, potential for change.*[2]
- Ascertain family's understanding of current situation; note results of previous involvement

in treatment. *Family with a member who is addicted to alcohol has often had frequent hospitalizations in the past. Knowing what has brought about the current situation will determine a starting place for this treatment plan.*[2]

• Review family history, explore roles of family members and circumstances involving substance use. *Although one member may be identified as the client, all of the family members are participants in the problem and need to be involved in the solution.*[5]

• Determine history of accidents/violent behaviors within family and current safety issues. *Identifies level of concern needed to understand what actions can be taken to prevent further violence.*[2]

• Discuss current/past methods of coping. *Family members have developed coping skills to deal with behaviors of client which may or may not be useful to changing the situation. Skills identified as useful can help to change the present situation. Those identified as not helpful (enabling behaviors) can be targeted for intervention to bring about desired changes and improve family functioning.*[2,5]

• Determine extent of enabling behaviors being evidenced by family members. *Family members may have developed behaviors that support the client continuing the pattern of addiction. Awareness, identification, and knowledge of these behaviors provide opportunity for individuals to begin the process of change.*[2,5]

• Identify sabotage behaviors of family members. *Issues of secondary gain (conscious or unconscious) may impede recovery. Even though family member(s) may verbalize a desire for the individual to become substance-free, the reality of interactive dynamics is that they may unconsciously not want the individual to recover because this would affect the family member(s) own role in the relationship.*[2]

• Note presence/extent of behaviors of family, client, and self that might be "too helpful," such as frequent requests for help, excuses for not following through on agreed-on behaviors, feelings of anger/irritation with others. *Identification of specific behaviors (enabling) can help family members see what they do that complicates acceptance and helps with resolution of current problems.*[5]

NURSING PRIORITY NO. 2. To assist family to change destructive behaviors:

• Mutually agree on behaviors/responsibilities for nurse and client/family members. *Maximizes understanding of what is expected of each person and minimizes opportunity for manipulation.*[5]

• Confront and examine denial and sabotage behaviors used by family members. *Identifies specific behaviors that individuals can be aware of and begin to change so they can move beyond what can be blocks to recovery.*[6]

• Discuss use of anger, rationalization and/or projection and ways in which these interfere with problem resolution. *Awareness of own feelings can lead to a decision to change, client then has to face the consequences of his or her own actions and may choose to get well.*[6]

• Encourage family to identify and deal with anger. Solve concerns and develop solutions. *Understanding what leads to anger and violence can lead to new behaviors and changes in the family for healthier relationships.*[3]

• Determine family strengths, areas for growth, individual/family successes. *Family members may not have realized they have strengths and as they identify these areas, they can choose to learn and develop new strategies for a more effective family structure.*[2]

• Remain nonjudgmental in approach to family members and to member who uses alcohol/drugs. *Individual already sees self as unworthy and judgment on the part of caregivers to family will interfere with ability to be a change agent.*[5]

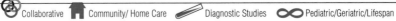 Cultural Collaborative Community/ Home Care Diagnostic Studies Pediatric/Geriatric/Lifespan Medications

- Provide information regarding effects of addiction on mood/personality of the involved person. *Family members have been dealing with client's behavior for a time and information can help them to understand and cope with negative behaviors without being judgmental or reacting angrily.*[2]
- Distinguish between destructive aspects of enabling behavior and genuine motivation to aid the user. *Family members often want to help but need to identify behavior that is helpful and that which is not, to begin to solve problems of addiction.*[6]
- Identify use of manipulative behaviors and discuss ways to avoid/prevent these situations. *The client often manipulates the people around him or her to maintain the status quo. When family begins to interact in a straightforward, honest manner, manipulation is not possible and healing can begin.*[2]

NURSING PRIORITY NO. 3. To promote wellness (Teaching/Discharge Considerations):

- Provide factual information to client/family about the effects of addictive behaviors on the family and what to expect after discharge. *Family may have unrealistic expectations about changes that have occurred in therapy and having information will help them deal more effectively with the difficulties of continuing the changes as they return to their new life without alcohol/substance.*[5]
- Provide information about enabling behavior, addictive disease characteristics for both user and nonuser who is codependent. *Education is a prime ingredient in treatment of addiction and can enable family members to deal realistically with these issues.*[6]
- Discuss importance of restructuring life activities, work/leisure relationships. *Previous lifestyle/relationships supported substance use requiring change to prevent relapse.*[7]
- Encourage family to refocus celebrations to exclude alcohol use. *Because celebrations often include the use of alcohol, this is one area where change can be made that can reduce the risk of relapse.*[7]
- Provide support for family members; encourage participation in group work. *Support is essential to changing client and family behaviors. Participating in group provides an opportunity to practice new skills of communication and behavior.*[5]
- Encourage involvement with/refer to self-help groups, Al-Anon, AlaTeen, Narcotics Anonymous, family therapy groups. *Regular attendance at a group can provide support; help client see how others are dealing with similar problems; and learn new skills, such as problem solving, for handling family disagreements.*[7]
- Provide bibliotherapy as appropriate. *Reading provides helpful information for making desired changes, especially when client/family members are dedicated to making change and willing to learn new ways of interacting within the family.*[7]
- Refer to NDs interrupted Family Processes; compromised/disabled family Coping as appropriate for additional interventions.

DOCUMENTATION FOCUS

Assessment/Reassessment
- Assessment findings, including history of substance(s) that have been used, and family risk factors/safety concerns.
- Family composition and involvement.
- Results of previous treatment involvement.

Planning
- Plan of care and who is involved in planning.
- Teaching plan.

Implementation/Evaluation
- Responses of family members to treatment/teaching and actions performed.
- Attainment/progress toward desired outcome(s).
- Modifications to plan of care.

Discharge Planning
- Long-term needs, who is responsible for actions to be taken.
- Specific referrals made.

References

1. Doenges, M. E., Moorhouse, M. F., & Geissler-Murr, A. C. (2004). Nurse's Pocket Guide: Diagnoses, Interventions, and Rationales, ed 9. Philadelphia: F. A. Davis.
2. Townsend, M. C. (2003). Psychiatric Mental Health Nursing Concepts of Care, ed 4. Philadelphia: F. A. Davis.
3. Gordon, T. (2000). Parent Effectiveness Training, updated edition. NY: Three Rivers Press.
4. Agency for Healthcare Research and Quality (AHRQ). (January, 1999). Evidence Report/ Technology Assessment Number 3: Pharmacotherapy for Alcohol Dependence. AHCPR Publication No. 99-E004a.
5. American Nurses Association (1987). Task Force on Substance Abuse Nursing Practice: The care of clients with addictions; dimensions of nursing practice. Kansas City, MO. American Nurses Association.
6. Nye, C. L., Zucker, R. A., & Fitzgerald H. E. (1999). Early family-based intervention in the path to alcohol problems, rationale and relationship between treatment process characteristics and child and parenting outcomes. J. Stud Alcohol Suppl, 13, 10–21.
7. Sielhamer, R. A., Jacob, T., & Dunn N. J. (1993). The impact of alcohol consumption on parent-child relationships in families of alcoholics. J Stud Alcohol. 54, 189.

interrupted Family Processes

Definition: Change in family relationships and/or functioning

RELATED FACTORS

Situational transition and/or crises (e.g., economic, change in roles, illness, trauma, disabling/expensive treatments)

Developmental transition and/or crises (e.g., loss or gain of a family member, adolescence, leaving home for college)

Shift in health status of a family member

Family roles shift; power shift of family members

Modification in family finances, family social status

Informal or formal interaction with community

DEFINING CHARACTERISTICS

Subjective

Changes in power alliances, satisfaction with family, expressions of conflict within family, effectiveness in completing assigned tasks, stress-reduction behaviors, expressions of conflict with and/or isolation from community resources, somatic complaints

[Family expresses confusion about what to do, verbalizes they are having difficulty responding to change]

 Cultural   Collaborative   Community/ Home Care   Diagnostic Studies   Pediatric/Geriatric/Lifespan   Medications

Objective

Changes in assigned tasks, participation in problem solving/decision making, communication patterns, mutual support, availability for emotional support/affective responsiveness and intimacy, patterns and rituals

SAMPLE CLINICAL APPLICATIONS: chronic illness, cancer, surgical procedures, traumatic injury, substance abuse, pregnancy

DESIRED OUTCOMES/EVALUATION CRITERIA

Sample **NOC** linkages:

Family Functioning: Ability of the family to meet the needs of its members through developmental transitions

Family Normalization: Ability of the family to develop and maintain routines and management strategies that contribute to optimal functioning when a member has a chronic illness or disability

Family Environment: Internal: Social climate as characterized by family member relationships and goals

Family Will (Include Specific Time Frame)

- Express feelings freely and appropriately.
- Demonstrate individual involvement in problem-solving processes directed at appropriate solutions for the situation/crisis.
- Direct energies in a purposeful manner to plan for resolution of the crisis.
- Verbalize understanding of illness/trauma, treatment regimen, and prognosis.
- Encourage and allow member who is ill to handle situation in own way, progressing toward independence.

ACTIONS/INTERVENTIONS

Sample **NIC** linkages:

Family Process Maintenance: Minimization of family process disruption effects

Family Integrity Promotion: Facilitating family participation in the emotional and physical care of the patient

Normalization Promotion: Assisting parents and other family members of children with chronic diseases or disabilities in providing normal life experiences for their children and families

NURSING PRIORITY NO. 1. To assess individual situation for causative/contributing factors:

- Determine pathophysiology, illness/trauma, developmental crisis present. *Identifies areas of need for planning care for this family.*[2]
- Identify family developmental stage (e.g., marriage, birth of a child, children leaving home, death of a spouse). *Developmental stage will affect family functioning, for instance, a couple who are newly married will be dealing with issues of learning how to live with each other; children leaving home may result in problems of "empty-nest syndrome"; or death of a spouse radically changes life for the survivor.*[2]
- Note components of family: parent(s), children, male/female, extended family available. *Affects how individuals deal with current stressors. Relationships among members may be supportive or strained.*[6]
- Observe patterns of communication in this family. Are feelings expressed? Freely? Who

talks to whom? Who makes decisions? For whom? Who visits? When? What is the interaction between family members? *Not only identifies weakness/areas of concern to be addressed, but also strengths that can be used for resolution of problem(s).*[6]

 ● Assess boundaries of family members. Do members share family identity and have little sense of individuality? Do they seem emotionally distant, not connected with one another? *These factors are critical to understanding individual family dynamics and developing strategies for change. Boundaries need to be clear so individual family members are free to be responsible for themselves.*[6]

 ● Ascertain role expectations of family members. Who is the ill member (e.g., nurturer, provider)? How does the illness affect the roles of others? *Each person may see the situation in own individual manner, and clear identification and sharing of these expectations promote understanding. Family members may expect client to continue to perform usual role or may not allow them to do anything. Either action can create problems for the ill member and realistic planning can provide positive sense of self for the client.*[2]

 ● Determine "Family Rules." For example, adult concerns (finances, illness, and so on) are kept from the children. *Rules may be imposed by adults rather than through a democratic process involving all family members, leading to conflict and angry confrontations. Setting positive family rules with all family members participating can promote a functional family.*[2,3]

 ● Identify parenting skills and expectations. *Ineffective parenting and unrealistic expectations may contribute to abuse. Understanding normal responses, progression of developmental milestones may help parent cope with changes necessitated by current crisis.*[2,3]

 ● Note energy direction. Are efforts at resolution/problem solving purposeful or scattered? *Provides clues about interventions that may be appropriate to assist client and family in directing energies in a more effective manner.*[2]

 ● Listen for expressions of despair/helplessness (e.g., "I don't know what to do") to note degree of distress. *Such feelings may contribute to difficulty adjusting to diagnosis and cooperating with treatment regimen required.*[4]

 ● Note cultural and/or religious *factors affecting perceptions/expectations of family members. Beliefs may affect client/SO reactions and adjustment to diagnosis, treatment and outcome of current problem/situation. For example, Arab-American family relationships include nuclear and extended family, make collective decisions, men are expected to be responsible for carrying out decisions, and women are usually delegated care for daily needs of the family.*[7]

 ● Assess support systems available outside of the family. *Having these resources can help the family begin to pull together and deal with current situation and problems they are facing.*[2]

NURSING PRIORITY NO. 2. To assist family to deal with situation/crisis:

● Deal with family members in warm, caring, respectful way. *Provides feelings of empathy and promotes individual's sense of worth and competence in ability to handle current situation.*[2]

● Acknowledge difficulties and realities of the situation. *Communicates message of understanding and reinforces that some degree of conflict is to be expected and can be used to promote growth.*[3]

 ● Encourage expressions of anger. Avoid taking them personally. *Feelings of anger are to be expected when individuals are dealing with difficult situation. Appropriate expression enables progress toward resolution of the stages of the grieving process when indicated. Not taking their anger personally maintains boundaries between nurse and family.*[2]

 ● Stress importance of continuous, open dialogue between family members to facilitate ongoing problem solving. *Promotes understanding and assists family members to maintain clear communication and resolve problems effectively.*[6]

 Cultural   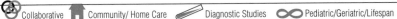 Collaborative   Community/ Home Care   Diagnostic Studies   Pediatric/Geriatric/Lifespan   Medications

- Provide information, verbal and written, and reinforce as necessary. *Promotes understanding and opportunity to review as needed.*[2]
- Assist family to identify and encourage their use of previously successful coping behaviors. *Most people have developed effective coping skills that when identified can be useful in current situation.*[6]
- Recommend contact by family members on a regular, frequent basis. *Promotes feelings of warmth and caring and brings family closer to one another enabling them to manage current difficult situation.*[2]
- Arrange for/encourage family participation in multidisciplinary team conference/group therapy as appropriate. *Participation in family and group therapy for an extended period increases likelihood of success as interactional issues (e.g., marital conflict, scapegoating of children) can be addressed and dealt with. Involvement with others can help family members to experience new ways of interacting and gain insight into their behavior, providing opportunity for change.*[2]
- Involve family in social support and community activities of their interest and choice. *Involvement with others outside of family constellation provides opportunity to observe how others handle problems and deal with conflict.*[2]

NURSING PRIORITY NO. 3. To promote wellness (Teaching/Discharge Considerations):

- Encourage use of stress-management techniques (e.g., appropriate expression of feelings, relaxation exercises). *The relaxation response helps members think more clearly, deal more effectively with conflict and promote more effective relationships to enhance family interactions.*[4]
- Provide educational materials and information. *Learning about the problems they are facing can assist family members in resolution of current crisis.*[2]
- Refer to classes (e.g., Parent Effectiveness, specific disease/disability support groups, self-help groups, clergy, psychological counseling/family therapy as indicated). *Can assist family to effect positive change/enhance conflict resolution skills. Presence of substance abuse problems requires all family members to seek support/assistance in dealing with situation to promote a healthy outcome.*[2,3]
- Assist family to identify situations that may lead to fear/anxiety. (Refer to NDs Fear; Anxiety.) *Promotes opportunity to provide anticipatory guidance.*[1]
- Involve family in mutual goal setting to plan for the future. *When all members of the family are involved, commitment to goals/continuation of plan are more likely to be maintained.*[3]
- Identify community agencies (e.g., Meals on Wheels, visiting nurse, trauma support group, American Cancer Society, Veterans Administration). *Provides both immediate and long-term support.*[6]

DOCUMENTATION FOCUS

Assessment/Reassessment
- Assessment findings including family composition, developmental stage of family, and role expectations.
- Family communication patterns.

Planning
- Plan of care/interventions and who is involved in planning.
- Teaching plan.

Implementation/Evaluation
- Each individual's response to interventions/teaching and actions performed.
- Attainment/progress toward desired outcome(s).
- Modifications to plan of care.

Discharge Planning
- Long-range needs, noting who is responsible for actions to be taken.
- Specific referrals made.

References
1. Doenges, M. E., Moorhouse, M. F., & Geissler-Murr, A. C. (2004). Nurse's Pocket Guide: Diagnoses, Interventions, and Rationales, ed 9. Philadelphia: F. A. Davis.
2. Townsend, M. C. (2003). Psychiatric Mental Health Nursing Concepts of Care, ed 4. Philadelphia: F. A. Davis.
3. Gordon, T. (2000). Parent Effectiveness Training, updated edition. New York: Three Rivers Press.
4. Cox, H. C., et al. (2002). Clinical Applications of Nursing Diagnosis: Adult, Child, Women's, Psychiatric, Gerontic, and Home Health Considerations, ed 4. Philadelphia: F. A. Davis.
5. Amato, P.R. & Booth, A. (1997). A generation at risk: Growing up in an era of family upheaval. Cambridge, MA: Harvard University Press.
6. Wright, L., & Leahey, M. (2000). Nurses and Families: A Guide to Assessment and Intervention, ed 3. Philadelphia: F. A. Davis.
7. Lipson, J. G., Dibble, S. L., & Minarik, P. A. (1996). Culture & Nursing Care: A Pocket Guide. San Francisco: UCSF Nursing Press.

readiness for enhanced Family Processes

Definition: A pattern of family functioning that is sufficient to support the well-being of family members and can be strengthened

RELATED FACTORS
To be developed by nurse researchers and submitted to NANDA

DEFINING CHARACTERISTICS

Subjective
Expresses willingness to enhance family dynamics
Communication is adequate
Relationships are generally positive; interdependent with community; family tasks are accomplished
Family adapts to change
Energy level of family supports activities of daily living

Objective
Family functioning meets physical, social and psychological needs of family members
Activities support the safety and growth of family members
Family roles are flexible and appropriate for developmental stages
Respect for family members is evident; boundaries of family members are maintained
Family resilience is efficient
Balance exists between autonomy and cohesiveness

SAMPLE CLINICAL APPLICATIONS: chronic health conditions (e.g., asthma, diabetes mellitus, arthritis, systemic lupus, multiple sclerosis, AIDS), mental health concerns (e.g., seasonal affective disorder, attention deficit disorder, Down syndrome)

 Cultural Collaborative Community/ Home Care Diagnostic Studies 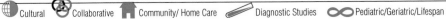 Pediatric/Geriatric/Lifespan Medications

Sample **NOC** linkages:

Family Social Climate: Supportive milieu as characterized by family member relationships and goals

Family Health Status: Overall health and social competence of family unit

Family Resiliency: Capacity of the family system to successfully adapt and function competently following significant adversity or crises

---

Client Will (Include Specific Time Frame)

- Express feelings freely and appropriately.
- Verbalizes understanding of desire for enhanced family dynamics.
- Demonstrate individual involvement in problem solving to improve family communications.
- Acknowledges awareness of boundaries of family members.

ACTIONS/INTERVENTIONS

Sample **NIC** linkages:

Family Support: Promotion of family values, interests and goals

Parent Education: Childrearing Family: Assisting parents to understand and promote the physical, psychological, and social growth and development of their toddler, preschool, or school-age child/children

Normalization Promotion: Assisting parents and other family members of children with chronic illnesses or disabilities in providing normal life experiences for their children and families

NURSING PRIORITY NO. **1.** To determine current status of family:

- Assess family composition: parent(s), children, male/female, extended family involved. *Many family forms exist in society today, such as biological, nuclear, single-parent, stepfamily, communal, and homosexual couple or family. A better way to determine a family may be to determine the attribute of affection, strong emotional ties, a sense of belonging and durability of membership.*[1]
- Note participating members of family: parent(s), children, male/female, extended family. *Identifies members of family who need to be involved and taken into consideration in developing plan of care to improve family functioning.*[1]
- Note stage of family development. *While the North American middle-class family stages may be described as single, young adult, newly married, family with young children, family with adolescents, grown children, later life, these developmental tasks may vary greatly among cultural groups. This information provides a framework for developing plan to enhance family processes.*[1]
- Observe patterns of communication in the family. Are feelings expressed: Freely? Who talks to whom? Who makes decisions? For whom? Who visits? When? What is the interaction between family members? *Not only identifies weakness/areas of concern to be addressed, but also strengths that can be used for planning improvement in family communication. Effective communication is that in which verbal and non-verbal messages are clear, direct, and congruent.*[1,2]
- Assess boundaries of family members. Do members share family identity and have little sense of individuality? Do they seem emotionally connected with one another? *Individuals need to respect one another and boundaries need to be clear so family members are free to be responsible for themselves.*[1,3]

• Identify "family rules" that are accepted in the family. *Families interact in certain ways over time and develop patterns of behavior that are accepted as the way "we behave" in this family. Functional families rules are constructive and promote the needs of all family members.*[1]

 • Note energy direction. *Efforts at problem solving, resolution of different opinions, growth may be purposeful or may be scattered and ineffective.*[3]

• Determine cultural and/or religious factors influencing family interactions. *Expectations related to socioeconomic beliefs may be different in various cultures, for instance, traditional views of marriage and family life may be strongly influenced by Roman Catholicism in Italian-American and Latino-American families. In some cultures, the father is considered the authority figure and the mother is the homemaker. These beliefs may be functional or dysfunctional in any given family and may change with stressors/circumstances (e.g., financial, loss/gain of a family member, personal growth).*[1,3]

NURSING PRIORITY NO. **2.** Assist the family to improve family interactions:

• Establish nurse-family relationship. *Promotes a warm, caring atmosphere in which family members can share thoughts, ideas, and feelings openly and nonjudgmentally.*[3]

• Acknowledge difficulties and realities of individual situation. *Reinforces that some degree of conflict is to be expected in family interactions that can be used to promote growth.*[1,3]

 • Stress importance of continuous, open dialogue between family members. *Facilitates ongoing expression of open, honest feelings and opinions and effective problem solving.*[1,4]

 • Assist family to identify and encourage use of previously successful coping behaviors. *Promotes recognition of previous successes and confidence in own abilities to learn and improve family interactions.*[2,4]

 • Acknowledge differences among family members with open dialogue about how these differences have occurred. *Conveys an acceptance of these differences among individuals and helps to look at how they can be used to facilitate the family process.*[3]

 • Identify effective parenting skills already being used and suggest new ways of handling difficult behaviors that may develop. *Allows the individual family members to realize that some of what has been done already has been helpful and helps them to learn new skills to manage family interactions in a more effective manner.*[3]

NURSING PRIORITY NO. **3.** To promote wellness (Teaching/Discharge Considerations):

 • Discuss and encourage use and participation in stress-management techniques. *Relaxation exercises, visualization, and similar skills can be useful for promoting reduction of anxiety and ability to manage stress that occurs in their lives.*[1]

 • Encourage participation in learning role-reversal activities. *Helps individuals to gain insight and understanding of other person's feelings and point of view.*[3]

 • Provide educational materials and information. *Enhances learning to assist in developing positive relationships among family members.*[4]

 • Assist family members to identify situations that may create problems and lead to fear/anxiety. *Thinking ahead can help individuals anticipate helpful actions to prevent conflict and untoward consequences.*[4]

 • Refer to classes/community resources as appropriate. *Family Effectiveness, self-help, psychology, religious affiliations can provide new information to assist family members to learn and apply to enhancing family interactions.*[4]

 • Involve family members in setting goals and planning for the future. *When individuals are involved in the decision making, they are more committed to carrying through plan to enhance family interactions as life goes on.*[2]

 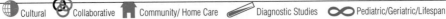

Assessment/Reassessment

- Assessment findings, including family composition, developmental stage of family and role expectations.
- Family communication patterns.

Planning

- Plan of care/interventions and who is involved in planning.
- Educational plan.

Implementation/Evaluation

- Each individual's response to interventions/teaching and actions performed.
- Attainment/progress toward desired outcome(s).
- Modifications to lifestyle/treatment plan.

Discharge Planning

- Long-range needs, noting who is responsible for actions to be taken.
- Specific referrals made.

References

1. Townsend, M. (2003). Psychiatric Mental Health Nursing Concepts of Care, ed 4. Philadelphia: F. A. Davis.
2. Gordon, T. (2000). Parent Effectiveness Training. New York: Three Rivers Press.
3. Doenges, M. E., Townsend, M. C., & Moorhouse, M. F. (1998). Psychiatric Care Plans Guidelines for Individualizing Care, ed 3. Philadelphia: F. A. Davis.
4. Doenges, M. E., Moorhouse, M. F., & Geissler-Murr, A. C. (2004). Nurse's Pocket Guide Diagnoses, Interventions, and Rationales, ed 9. Philadelphia: F. A. Davis.

Fatigue

Definition: An overwhelming sustained sense of exhaustion and decreased capacity for physical and mental work at usual level

RELATED FACTORS

Psychological

Stress, anxiety, boring lifestyle, depression

Environmental

Noise, lights, humidity, temperature

Situational

Occupation, negative life events

Physiologic

Increased physical exertion, sleep deprivation
Pregnancy, disease states, malnutrition, anemia
Poor physical condition
[Altered body chemistry (e.g., medications, drug withdrawal, chemotherapy)]

Subjective

Verbalization of an unremitting and overwhelming lack of energy, inability to maintain usual routines/level of physical activity

Perceived need for additional energy to accomplish routine tasks, increase in rest requirements

Tired, inability to restore energy even after sleep

Feelings of guilt for not keeping up with responsibilities

Compromised libido

Increase in physical complaints

Objective

Lethargic or listless, drowsy

Compromised concentration

Disinterest in surroundings/introspection

Decreased performance [accident-prone]

SAMPLE CLINICAL APPLICATIONS: anemia, hypothyroidism, cancer, multiple sclerosis, post-polio syndrome, AIDS, chronic renal failure, chronic fatigue syndrome, depression

DESIRED OUTCOMES/EVALUATION CRITERIA

Sample **NOC** linkages:

Endurance: Extent that energy enables a person to sustain activity

Energy Conservation: Extent of active management of energy to initiate and sustain activity

Activity Tolerance: Responses to energy-conserving body movements involved in required or desired daily activities

Client Will (Include Specific Time Frame)

- Report improved sense of energy.
- Identify basis of fatigue and individual areas of control.
- Perform ADLs and participate in desired activities at level of ability.
- Participate in recommended treatment program.

ACTIONS/INTERVENTIONS

Sample **NIC** linkages:

Energy Management: Regulating energy use to treat or prevent fatigue and optimize function

Exercise Promotion: Facilitation of regular physical exercise to maintain or advance to a higher level of fitness and health

Nutrition Management: Assisting with or providing a balanced dietary intake of foods and fluids

NURSING PRIORITY NO. 1. To assess causative/contributing factors:

- Identify presence of physical and/or psychological disease states (e.g., cancer and cancer therapies, severe/chronic pain, hepatitis, AIDS, MS/other neuromuscular disorders, major depressive disorder, anxiety states). *Important information can be obtained from knowing if fatigue is a result of an underlying condition or disease process (acute or chronic); whether an exacerbating/remitting condition is in exacerbation; and/or whether fatigue has been present over a longtime without any identifiable cause.*

 Cultural Collaborative Community/ Home Care 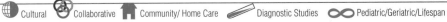 Diagnostic Studies Pediatric/Geriatric/Lifespan Medications

- Ascertain if client has a diagnosis of chronic fatigue syndrome (CFS). *This condition has recently been defined as a distinct disorder (affecting children and adults) characterized by chronic (often relapsing but always debilitating) fatigue, lasting for at least 6 months (often for much longer), causing impairments in overall physical and mental functioning and without an apparent etiology. Treatment is largely supportive.*[1]
- Assess cardiovascular and respiratory status, musculoskeletal strength, emotional health, and nutritional/fluid status. *Treatment of underlying conditions may resolve fatigue.*
- Note changes in life (e.g. relationship problems, family illness/injury/death, expanded responsibilities/demands of others, job-related conflicts) that can be causing or exacerbating level of fatigue. *Stress may be the result of dealing with disease or situational crises, dealing with the "unknowns" or trying to meet expectations of others.*[2] *Also, grief and depression can sap energy, and cause avoidance of social and/or physical interactions that could stimulate the mind and body. Persons with AIDS and the elderly are especially prone to this fatigue because they experience significant losses, often on a regular/recurring basis.*[3,4]
- Assess for sleep disturbances. *Sleep disturbance is both a contributor to and a manifestation of fatigue, (e.g., a client with chronic pain or depression may be sleeping long periods, but not experience refreshing sleep).*
- Test for/determine ability to participate in activities/level of mobility. *While many illness conditions negatively affect client's energy and activity tolerance, if the client is not engaged in light to moderate exercise, he/she may simply adjust to more sedentary activities, which can in turn exacerbate deconditioning and debilitation (chronic fatigue syndrome, cancer). However there are certain conditions (e.g., multiple sclerosis [MS] and post-polio syndrome) where the client's ability to do things reduces as he/she does them (e.g., at the beginning of a walk the client feels okay, but fatigue sets in [out of proportion to the activity] and the client is exhausted as if running a marathon).*[5,6]
- Review medication regimen/use. *Many medications have the potential side effect of causing/exacerbating fatigue (e.g., beta-blockers, chemotherapy agents, narcotics, sedatives, muscle relaxants, antiemetics, antidepressants, antiepileptics, diuretics, cholesterol-lowering drugs, HIV treatment agents).*
- Assess psychological and personality factors that may affect reports of fatigue level. *Client with severe/chronic fatigue may have issues affecting desire to be active (or work) resulting in secondary gain from exaggerating fatigue reports.*
- Evaluate aspect of "learned helplessness" that may be manifested by giving up. *Can perpetuate a cycle of fatigue, impaired functioning, increased anxiety and fatigue.*

NURSING PRIORITY NO. 2. To determine degree of fatigue/impact on life:

- Ask client to describe fatigue. *Individuals use different phrases (e.g. drained, exhausted, lousy, weak, lazy, worn out, whole-body tiredness, etc.).*
- Note client's belief about what is causing the fatigue and what relieves it. Note daily energy peaks/valleys. *Helpful in clarifying client's expressions for symptoms, pattern/timing of fatigue, which varies over time and may also vary in duration, unpleasantness and intensity from person to person.*[7]
- Assess severity of fatigue, using a 0–10 scale, noting frequency/pervasiveness of fatigue episodes, activities associated with increased fatigue, restfulness of sleep, ability to perform ADLs or desired activities, ability to concentrate/work, and mood. Use a fatigue assessment tool (e.g., Piper Fatigue Self-Report Scale, Multidimensional Fatigue Inventory, and Nail's General Fatigue Scale) as appropriate. *In initial evaluations, these scales can help determine manifestation, intensity, duration, and emotional meaning of fatigue. The scales can*

be used in ongoing evaluations to determine current status and estimate response to treatment strategies.[2,7–9]

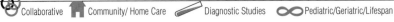 • Measure physiological response to activity (e.g., changes in blood pressure or heart/respiratory rate). *May indicate need for interventions to improve cardiovascular health, pulmonary status and conditioning.* (Refer to risk for Activity Intolerance for additional interventions.)

• Review availability and current use of assistance with daily activities, support systems and resources.

• Evaluate need for individual assistance/assistive devices. *Certain conditions causing fatigue (e.g., post-polio syndrome) worsen with overuse of weakened muscles. Client benefits from protection provided by braces, canes, power chairs, etc.*[6,7]

NURSING PRIORITY NO. 3. To assist client to cope with fatigue and manage with individual limits of ability:

• Accept reality of client reports of fatigue and avoid underestimating effect on quality of life the client experiences. *Fatigue is subjective and often debilitating, e.g., clients with cancer, AIDS, or MS are prone to more frequent episodes of severe fatigue following minimal energy expenditure and require longer recovery period; post-polio clients often display a cumulative effect if they fail to pace themselves and rest when early signs of fatigue are encountered.*[5,7,10]

• Treat underlying conditions where possible (e.g., manage pain, depression, or anemia; treat infections, reduce numbers of interacting medications, etc.), *to reduce fatigue caused by treatable conditions.*

• Involve client/SO/caregivers(s) in planning care *to incorporate their input, choices, and assistance.*

• Encourage client to do whatever activity possible (e.g., self-care, sit up in chair, walk for 5 minutes), pacing self, increasing activity level gradually. Schedule activities *for periods when client has the most energy, to maximize participation.*

• Structure daily routines and establish realistic activity goals with client, especially when depression is a factor in fatigue. *May enhance client's commitment to efforts and promote sense of self-esteem in accomplishing goals.*

• Instruct client/caregivers in alternate ways of doing familiar activities, and methods to conserve energy[2,3,7–10]:
    Sit instead of standing during daily care or kitchen activities
    Adjust the level/height of work surface *for ergonomic benefit/to prevent bending over*
    Carry several small loads instead of one large load
    Use assistive devices, e.g., adaptive eating utensils, wheeled walkers/chairs, electrically raised chairs, stair climbers
    Plan steps of activity before beginning *so that all needed materials are at hand*
    Delegate tasks/duties
    Combine and simplify activities

• Avoid temperature and humidity extremes. Provide environment conducive to relief of fatigue. *Temperature and level of humidity are known to affect exhaustion (especially in clients with MS).*[5]

• Encourage nutritional foods/refer to dietitian as indicated. *Nutritionally balanced diet with proteins, complex carbohydrates, vitamins, and minerals may boost energy. Frequent, small meals and simple-to-digest foods are beneficial when combating fatigue. Reduced amounts of caffeine and sugar can improve sleep and energy.*[3,7,10]

 Cultural  Collaborative   Community/ Home Care Diagnostic Studies 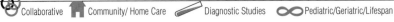 Pediatric/Geriatric/Lifespan   Medications

- Provide supplemental oxygen as indicated. *Presence of anemia/hypoxemia reduces oxygen available for cellular uptake and contributes to fatigue. If fatigue is related to oxygenation/perfusion problems, oxygen may improve energy level and ability to be active.* Refer to ND Activity Intolerance for additional interventions.
- Provide diversional activities, e.g., visiting with friends, family, doing hobbies or schoolwork *to reduce boredom, improve outlook and accomplish goals for activity.*
- Avoid over/understimulation (cognitive and sensory). *Impaired concentration can limit ability to block competing stimuli/distractions.* Refer to deficient Diversional Activity, for additional interventions.
- Recommend/implement routines and/or treatments that promote restful sleep, e.g.:
  Regular sleep hours at nights with beneficial nighttime rituals
  Short naps during day hours
  Quiet activities in the evening
  Warm baths
  Massage treatments and other therapies (e.g., meditation, visualization, acupuncture, osteopathic/chiropractic manipulations, mild exercise, yoga, T'ai chi)
  Refer to ND disturbed Sleep Pattern for additional interventions.
- Active-listen, provide support. Instruct in/refer for stress-management skills of visualization, deep breathing, relaxation, and biofeedback *to deal with situation, aid in relaxation, and to reduce boredom, pain, and sense of fatigue.*
- Implement physical therapy/exercise program in conjunction with the client and other team members such as physical and/or occupational therapist, exercise or rehabilitation physiologist. *Collaborative program with short-term achievable goals enhances likelihood of success and may motivate client to adopt a lifestyle of physical exercise for enhancement of health.*[2,7,8]

NURSING PRIORITY NO. 4. To promote wellness (Teaching/Discharge Considerations):

- Discuss therapy regimen relating to individual causative factors (e.g., physical and/or psychological illnesses) and help client/SO(s) to understand relationship of fatigue to illness.
- Assist client/SO(s) to develop plan for activity and exercise within individual ability.
- Stress necessity of allowing sufficient time to finish activities.
- Instruct client in ways to monitor responses to activity and significant signs/symptoms that indicate the need to modify activity level.
- Promote overall health measures (e.g., good nutrition, adequate fluid intake, appropriate vitamin/iron supplementation).
- Encourage client to develop assertiveness skills, prioritizing goals/activities, learning to say "No."
- Discuss burnout syndrome when appropriate and actions client can take to change individual situation.
- Assist client to identify appropriate coping behaviors. *Promotes sense of control and improves self-esteem.*
- Identify support groups/community resources (e.g., condition specific groups, transportation options).
- Refer to counseling/psychotherapy as indicated.
- Refer for resources to assist with routine needs (e.g., Meals on Wheels, homemaker/housekeeper services, yard care).

Assessment/Reassessment
- Manifestations of fatigue and other assessment findings.
- Degree of impairment/effect on lifestyle.
- Expectations of client/SO relative to individual abilities/specific condition.

Planning
- Plan of care/interventions and who is involved in the planning.
- Teaching plan.

Implementation/Evaluation
- Client's response to interventions/teaching and actions performed.
- Attainment/progress toward desired outcome(s).
- Modifications to plan of care.

Discharge Planning
- Discharge needs/plan, actions to be taken, and who is responsible.
- Specific referrals made.

References

1. Fukuda, K., Straus, S. D., Hickie, I., et al. (1994). The chronic fatigue syndrome: A comprehensive approach to its definition and study. International Chronic Fatigue Syndrome Study Group. Ann Intern Med, 121(12), 953–9 [Medline].
2. Vogin, G. (2001). Coping with fatigue. The Cleveland Clinic Condition Center. Available at: http://www.webmd.aol.com.
3. Zimmerman, J. (2002). Nutrition for health and healing in HIV. ACRIA Update, 11(2). Available at: http://www.thebody.comcria. Accessed August 2003.
4. Ackley, B. J. (2002). Fatigue. In Ackley, B. J., & Ladwig, G. B. (eds). Nursing Diagnosis Handbook: A Guide to Planning Care, ed 5. St. Louis: Mosby.
5. Understanding the unique role of fatigue in multiple sclerosis. (Updated 9/7/02). Multiple Sclerosis Encyclopaedia Website. Available at: http://www.mult-sclerosis.org/fatigue.html.
6. Perlman, S. (1999). Coping with fatigue of post-polio syndrome. Rancho Los Amigos Post Polio Support Group Newsletter.
7. Wells, J. N., & Fedric, T. (2001). Helping patients manage cancer-related fatigue. Home Healthcare Nurse, 19(8), 486.
8. VHA/DoD. (2001). Clinical practice guidelines for the management of medically unexplained symptoms: chronic pain and fatigue. Veterans Health Administration, Department of Defense. Washington, D.C. Available at: http://www.guideline.gov. Accessed August 2003.
9. Stewart, J. M., et al. (2001). Chronic Fatigue Syndrome. Available at: http://www.emedicine.com/ped/topic2795.htm. Accessed August 2003.
10. Common sense about AIDS: Fighting fatigue requires battle on many fronts. (1996). Article by American Health Consultants.

Fear [specify focus]

Definition: Response to perceived threat [real or imagined] that is consciously recognized as a danger

RELATED FACTORS

Natural/innate origin (e.g., sudden noise, height, pain, loss of physical support); innate releasers (neurotransmitters); phobic stimulus

 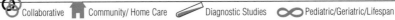

Learned response (e.g., conditioning, modeling from identification with others)

Unfamiliarity with environmental experiences

Separation from support system in potentially stressful situation (e.g., hospitalization, hospital procedures [/treatments])

Language barrier, sensory impairment

DEFINING CHARACTERISTICS

Subjective

Cognitive

Identifies object of fear; stimulus believed to be a threat

Physiologic

Anorexia, nausea, fatigue, dry mouth, [palpitations]

Apprehension, excitement, being scared, alarm, panic, terror, dread

Decreased self-assurance

Increased tension, jitteriness

Objective

Cognitive

Diminished productivity, learning ability, problem solving

Behaviors

Increased alertness, avoidance[/flight] or attack behaviors, impulsiveness, narrowed focus on "it" (e.g., the focus of the fear)

Physiologic

Increased pulse, vomiting, diarrhea, muscle tightness, increased respiratory rate and shortness of breath, increased systolic blood pressure, pallor, increased perspiration, pupil dilation

SAMPLE CLINICAL APPLICATIONS: phobias, hospitalization/diagnostic procedures, diagnosis of chronic/life-threatening condition

DESIRED OUTCOMES/EVALUATION CRITERIA

Sample **NOC** linkages:

Fear Control: Personal actions to eliminate or reduce disabling feelings of alarm aroused by an identifiable source

Coping: Actions to manage stressors that tax an individual's resources

Client Will (Include Specific Time Frame)

- Acknowledge and discuss fears, recognizing healthy versus unhealthy fears.
- Verbalize accurate knowledge of/sense of safety related to current situation.
- Demonstrate understanding through use of effective coping behaviors (e.g., problem solving) and resources.
- Display appropriate range of feelings and lessened fear.

ACTIONS/INTERVENTIONS

Sample **NIC** linkages:

Anxiety Reduction: Minimizing apprehension, dread, foreboding, or uneasiness related to an unidentified source or anticipated danger

Security Enhancement: Intensifying a patient's sense of physical and psychological safety

Coping Enhancement: Assisting a patient to adapt to perceived stressors, changes, or threats that interfere with meeting life demands and roles

NURSING PRIORITY NO. 1. To assess degree of fear and reality of threat perceived by the client:

 • Ascertain client/SO(s) perception of what is occurring and how this affects life. *Fear is a natural reaction to frightening events and how client views the event will determine how he or she will react.*[1]

 • Note degree of incapacitation (e.g., "frozen with fear," inability to engage in necessary activities). *Indicative of severe state (phobia), which determines type of actions needed.*[1]

 • Compare verbal/nonverbal responses. *Noting congruencies or incongruencies can help to identify client's misperceptions of situation and what actions may be helpful.*[1]

 • Be alert to signs of denial/depression. *Indicates need for specific interventions to identify and deal with problems. Client may deny problems until unable to deal with situation. Depression may accompany problems associated with fear that interfere with daily activities.*[2]

 • Identify sensory deficits that may be present, such as hearing impairment. *Affects reception and interpretation and inabilty to correctly sense and perceive stimuli leads to misunderstanding, increasing fear.*[4]

 • Note degree of concentration, focus of attention. *Indicative of extent of anxiety/fear related to what is happening and need for specific interventions to reduce physiologic reactions.*[4]

 • Investigate client's reports of subjective experiences. *May reflect delusions/hallucinations. It is important to understand how the client views the situation and need for reality orientation and further evaluation.*[4]

 • Be alert to and evaluate potential for violence. *Determines physiological changes due to fear. Client who is fearful may feel need to protect himself or herself and strike out at closest person. Proactive planning can avert or manage violent behaviors.*[5]

 • Measure vital signs/physiological responses to situation. *Provides baseline information of extent of response for comparison as needed at a later date. Stabilization can indicate effectiveness of interventions by lessening of response to identified fear.*[6]

 • Assess family dynamics. (Refer to other NDs such as interrupted Family Processes, readiness for enhanced family Coping, compromised/disabled family Coping, Anxiety.) *Actions and responses of family members may exacerbate or soothe fears of client.*[1]

NURSING PRIORITY NO. 2. To assist client/SOs in dealing with fear/situation:

• Stay with the client or make arrangements to have someone else be there. *Provides nonthreatening environment in which the presence of a calm, caring person can provide reassurance that individual will be safe. Sense of abandonment can exacerbate fear.*[6]

• Listen to, Active-listen client concerns. *Conveys message of belief in competence and ability of client, promoting understanding and clarify issues when client feels listened to so problem-solving can begin.*[2]

 • Provide information in verbal and written form. Speak in simple sentences and concrete terms. *Intense state of fear interferes with reception and interpretation of verbal information and supplementing it with written information facilitates understanding and retention of information.*[4]

 • Acknowledge normalcy of fear, pain, despair, and give "permission" to express feelings appropriately/freely. *Feelings are real, and it is helpful to bring them out in the open so they can be discussed and dealt with.*[6]

 Cultural Collaborative Community/ Home Care Diagnostic Studies 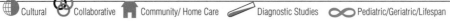 Pediatric/Geriatric/Lifespan Medications

- Provide opportunity for questions, answering honestly and providing information as appropriate. *Enhances sense of trust and enhances positive nurse-client relationship in which individual can verbalize fears and begin to problem-solve solutions.*[1]
- Present objective information when available and allow client to use it freely. Avoid arguing about client's perceptions of the situation. *Limits conflicts when fear response may impair rational thinking.*[6]
- Promote client control where possible and help client identify and accept those things over which control is not possible. *Life change and stressful events are viewed differently by individual. Providing opportunity to make own decision when possible strengthens internal locus of control. Individual with external locus of control may attribute feelings of anxiety and fear to an external source and may perceive it as beyond his or her control.*[1]
- Provide touch, Therapeutic Touch, massage, and other adjunctive therapies as indicated. *Aids in meeting basic human need, decreasing sense of isolation and assisting client to feel less anxious. Note: Therapeutic Touch requires the nurse to have specific knowledge and experience to use the hands to correct energy field disturbances by redirecting human energies to help or heal. Refer to ND: disturbed Energy Field.*[2,7]
- Encourage contact with a peer who has successfully dealt with a similarly fearful situation. *Provides a role model which can enhance sense of optimism. Client is more likely to believe others who have had similar experience(s).*[1]

NURSING PRIORITY NO. 3. To assist client in learning to use own responses for problem solving:

- Acknowledge usefulness of fear for taking care of self. *Provides new idea that can be a motivator to focus on dealing appropriately with situation.*[1]
- Identify client's responsibility for the solutions. Reinforce that the nurse will be available for help. *Enhances sense of control, self-worth, and confidence in own ability diminishing fear.*[8]
- Determine internal/external resources for help (e.g., awareness/use of effective coping skills in the past; SOs who are available for support). *Provides opportunity to recognize and build on resources client/SO may have used successfully in the past.*[1]
- Explain actions/procedures within level of client's ability to understand and handle. (Be aware of how much information client wants *to prevent confusion/overload.) Complex and/or anxiety-producing information can be given in manageable amounts over an extended period as opportunities arise and facts are given, individual will accept what he or she is ready for.*[8]
- Explain relationship between disease and symptoms if appropriate. *Lack of information can create anxiety and fear. Providing accurate information promotes understanding of why the symptoms occur, allaying anxiety about them.*[1]
- Review use of antianxiety medications and reinforce use as prescribed. *Anti-anxiety agents may be useful for brief periods to assist client to reduce anxiety to managable levels, providing opportunity for initation of client's own coping skills.*[1]

NURSING PRIORITY NO. 4. To promote wellness (Teaching/Discharge Considerations):

- Support planning for dealing with reality. *Assists in identifying areas in which control can be exercised and those in which control is not possible, enabling client to handle fearful situation/feelings.*[1]
- Assist client to learn relaxation/visualization and guided imagery skills (e.g., imagining a

pleasant place, use of music/tapes, deep-breathing, meditation, and mindfulness.) *Promotes release of endorphins and aids in developing internal locus of control, reducing fear/anxiety. May enhance coping skills, allowing body to go about its work of healing. Note: Mindfulness is a method of being in the here and now, concentrating on what is happening in the moment.*[7,8]

 • Encourage and assist client to develop exercise program (within limits of ability). *Provides a healthy outlet for energy generated by feelings and promotes relaxation. Has been shown to raise endorphin levels to enhance sense of well-being.*[2]

 • Provide for/deal with sensory deficits in appropriate manner (e.g., speak clearly and distinctly, use touch carefully as indicated by situation). *Hearing or visual impairments, other deficits can contribute to feelings of fear. Recognizing and providing for appropriate contact enhance communication promoting understanding.*[4]

• Refer to support groups, community agencies/organizations as indicated. *Provides information, ongoing assistance to meet individual needs, and opportunity for discussing concerns.*[2]

DOCUMENTATION FOCUS

Assessment/Reassessment
• Assessment findings, noting individual factors contributing to current situation.
• Manifestations of fear.

Planning
• Plan of care and who is involved in the planning.
• Teaching plan.

Implementation/Evaluation
• Client's responses to treatment plan/interventions and actions performed.
• Attainment/progress toward desired outcome(s).
• Modifications to plan of care.

Discharge Planning
• Long-term needs and who is responsible for actions to be taken.
• Specific referrals made.

References

1. Townsend, M. C. (2003). Psychiatric Mental Health Nursing Concepts of Care, ed 4. Philadelphia: F. A. Davis.
2. Doenges, M. E., Moorhouse, M. F., & Geissler-Murr, A. C. (2004). Nurse's Pocket Guide: Diagnoses, Interventions, and Rationales, ed 9. Philadelphia: F. A. Davis.
3. Gordon, T. (2000). Parent Effectiveness Training, updated edition. New York: Three Rivers Press.
4. Cox, H. C., et al. (2002). Clinical Applications of Nursing Diagnosis: Adult, Child, Women's, Psychiatric, Gerontic, and Home Health Considerations, ed 4. Philadelphia: F. A. Davis.
5. Lewis, M. I., & Dehn, D. S. (1999). Violence against nurses in outpatient mental health settings. J. Psychosoc Nurs, 37(6), 28.
6. Bay, E. J., & Algase, D. L. (1999). Fear and anxiety. A simultaneous concept analysis, Nurs Diagn, 10, 103.
7. Olson, M., & Sneed N. (1995). Anxiety and therapeutic touch. Issues Ment Health Nurs, 16(2), 97.
8. Kabat-Zinn, J. (1994). Wherever You Go There You Are, Mindfulness Meditation in Everyday Life. New York: Hyperion.

readiness for enhanced Fluid Balance

Definition: A pattern of equilibrium between fluid volume and chemical composition of body fluids that is sufficient for meeting physical needs and can be strengthened

 Cultural Collaborative Community/ Home Care Diagnostic Studies Pediatric/Geriatric/Lifespan Medications

To be developed by nurse researchers and submitted to NANDA

DEFINING CHARACTERISTICS

Subjective
Expresses willingness to enhance fluid balance
No excessive thirst

Objective
Stable weight
Moist mucous membranes
Food and fluid intake adequate for daily needs
Straw-colored urine with specific gravity within normal limits
Good tissue turgor
Urine output appropriate for intake
No evidence of edema or dehydration

SAMPLE CLINICAL APPLICATIONS: heart failure, irritable bowel syndrome, Addison's disease, enteral/parenteral feeding

DESIRED OUTCOME/EVALUATION CRITERIA
Sample **NOC** Linkages:
Hydration: Amount of water in the intracellular and extracellular compartments of the body
Fluid Balance: Balance of water in the intracellular compartments of the body
Risk Control: Actions to eliminate or reduce actual, personal, and modifiable health threats

Client Will (Include Specific Time Frame)
- Maintain fluid volume at a functional level as indicated by adequate urinary output, stable vital signs, moist mucous membranes, good skin turgor.
- Demonstrate behaviors to monitor fluid balance.
- Be free of thirst.
- Be free of evidence of fluid deficit or fluid overload.

ACTIONS/INTERVENTIONS
Sample **NIC** Linkages:
Fluid Management: Promotion of fluid balance and prevention of complications resulting from abnormal or undesired fluid levels
Fluid Monitoring: Collection and analysis of patient data to regulate fluid balance
Surveillance: Purposeful and ongoing acquisition, interpretation, and synthesis of patient data for clinical decision making

NURSING PRIORITY NO. 1. To assess potential for fluid imbalance, ways that client is managing:

 • Note presence of medical diagnoses with potential for fluid imbalance: 1) conditions/disease processes that may lead to deficits (e.g., diuretic therapy, hyperglycemia, ulcerative colitis, COPD, burns, cirrhosis of the liver, vomiting, diarrhea, hemorrhage, hot/humid climate, prolonged exercise, fever, excessive caffeine/alcohol intake); 2) risk factors that may lead to fluid excess (e.g., renal failure, heart failure, stroke, cerebral lesions, renal/adrenal insufficiency, psychogenic polydipsia, acute stress, surgical/anesthetic procedures, excessive or rapid infusion of IV fluids). *Body fluid balance is regulated by intake (food and fluid) output (kidney, gastrointestinal tract, skin, and lungs) and regulatory hormonal mechanisms. Balance is maintained within relatively narrow margin and can be easily disrupted by multiple factors.*[4]

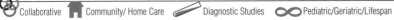

- Determine potential effects of age and developmental stage. *Elderly individuals have less body water than younger adults, decreased thirst response, and reduced effectiveness of compensatory mechanisms (e.g., kidneys are less efficient in conserving sodium and water). Infants and children have a relatively higher percentage of total body water and metabolic rate, and are often less able than adults to control their fluid intake.*[1,2,5]
- Evaluate environmental factors that could impact fluid balance. *Persons with impaired mobility, diminished vision or confined to bed cannot as easily meet their own needs and may be reluctant to ask for assistance. Persons whose work environment is restrictive or outside may also have greater challenges in meeting fluid needs.*[3]
- Assess vital signs (e.g., temperature, blood pressure, heart rate), skin/mucous membrane moisture, and urine output. Weigh as indicated. *Predictors of fluid balance that should be in client's usual range in a healthy state.*[4]

NURSING PRIORITY NO. 2. To prevent occurrence of imbalance:

- Monitor I/O balance being aware of insensible losses *to ensure accurate picture of fluid status.*[4]
- Weigh client regularly and compare with recent weight history. *Useful in early recognition of water retention/unexplained losses.*[1,4]
- Establish/review individual fluid needs and replacement schedule with client. Distribute fluids over 24-hour period. *Enhances likelihood of cooperation with meeting therapeutic goals while avoiding periods of thirst if fluids are restricted.*[1]
- Encourage regular oral intake of fluids (e.g., between meals, additional fluids during hot weather or when exercising) interspersed with high-fluid-content foods of client's choice. *Adds variety to maximize intake while maintaining fluid balance.*[1]
- Provide adequate free water with enteral feedings.
- Administer/discuss judicious use of medications as indicated (e.g., antiemetics, antidiarrheals, antipyretics, and diuretics). *Medications may be indicated to prevent fluid imbalance if individual becomes ill.*[1]

NURSING PRIORITY NO. 3. To enhance wellness (Teaching/Discharge Considerations):

- Discuss client's individual conditions/factors that could cause occurrence of fluid imbalance as appropriate, paying special attention to environmental factors such as hot/humid climate, lack of air conditioning, outdoor work setting *so that client/SO can take corrective action.*[1,3,6,7]
- Identify and instruct in ways to meet specific fluid needs (e.g., keep fluids near at hand/carry water bottle when leaving home, or measure specific 24-hour fluid portions if restrictions apply) *to manage fluid intake over time.*[1,3]
- Instruct client/SO(s) in how to measure and record I/O, including weighing diapers/continence pads when used, *if data needed for home management.*
- Identify actions (if any) client may take to correct imbalance (e.g., limiting caffeine intake, as needed use of diuretics, tight control of blood sugar).

 Cultural Collaborative Community/ Home Care   Diagnostic Studies   Pediatric/Geriatric/Lifespan Medications

- Review/instruct in medication regimen and administration and discuss potential for interactions/side effects that could disrupt fluid balance.[1,4,5]
- Instruct in signs and symptoms indicating need for immediate/further evaluation and follow-up *to prevent complications and/or allow for early intervention.*[1,4,5]

Assessment/Reassessment
- Individual findings, including factors affecting ability to manage (regulate) body fluids.
- I/O, fluid balance, changes in weight, and vital signs.
- Results of diagnostic testing/laboratory studies.

Planning
- Plan of care and who is involved in the planning.
- Teaching plan.

Implementation/Evaluation
- Client's responses to treatment/teaching and actions performed.
- Attainment/progress toward desired outcome(s).
- Modifications to plan of care.

Discharge Planning
- Long-term needs, noting who is responsible for actions to be taken.
- Specific referrals made.

References

1. Cox, H. C., et al. (2002). Clinical Applications of Nursing Diagnosis: Adult, Child, Women's Psychiatric, Gerontic, and Home Health Considerations, ed 4. Philadelphia: F. A. Davis.
2. Miller-Huey, R. Hydration in Elders: More than just a glass of water. Caregiver.com. Today's Caregiver Magazine. Available at: http://www.caregiver911.com. Accessed June 8, 2003.
3. Curtis, R. (1997). Guide to Heat Related Illnesses & Fluid Balance. Outdoor Action. Princeton University.
4. Metheny, N. (2000). Fluid and Electrolyte Balance: Nursing Considerations, ed 4. Philadelphia: J. B. Lippincott.
5. Engle, J. (2002). Pocket Guide to Pediatric Assessment, ed 4. St. Louis, MO: Mosby.
6. Curtis, R. (1997). Guide to Heat Related Illnesses & Fluid Balance. Outdoor Action. Princeton University.
7. Bennett, J. A. (2000). Dehydration: hazards and benefits. Geriatr Nurs, 21(2), 84–88.

[deficient Fluid Volume: hyper/hypotonic]

[**NOTE:** NANDA has restricted Fluid Volume, Deficient to address only isotonic dehydration. For client needs related to dehydration associated with alterations in sodium, the authors have provided this second diagnostic category.]

Definition: [Decreased intravascular, interstitial, and/or intracellular fluid. This refers to dehydration with changes in sodium.]

[**Hypertonic/hypernatremic dehydration:** uncontrolled diabetes mellitus/insipidus, diabetic ketoacidosis, diabetes insipidus, HHNC; prolonged NPO increased intake of hypertonic fluids/IV therapy, inability to respond to thirst reflex/inadequate free water

---

Information that appears in brackets has been added by the authors to clarify and enhance the use of nursing diagnoses.

supplementation (high-osmolarity enteral feeding formulas), hyperventilation, pure water loss with high fever and watery diarrhea, and renal insufficiency/failure]

[Hypotonic/hyponatremic dehydration: chronic illness/malnutrition, heat exhaustion and heat stroke, excessive use of hypotonic IV solutions (e.g., D_5W), renal insufficiency]

DEFINING CHARACTERISTICS

Subjective
[Reports of fatigue, nervousness, exhaustion]
[Thirst]

Objective
[Increased urine output, dilute urine (initially) and/or decreased output/oliguria]
[Weight loss]
[Decreased venous filling]
[Hypotension (postural); increased pulse rate; decreased pulse volume and pressure]
[Decreased skin turgor, dry skin/mucous membranes]
[Change in mental status (e.g., confusion)]
[Increased body temperature]
[Hemoconcentration; altered serum sodium]

SAMPLE CLINICAL APPLICATIONS: diabetes mellitus, diabetic ketoacidosis, renal failure, conditions requiring IV therapy or enteral feeding, heat exhaustion/stroke, presence of draining wounds/fistulas

DESIRED OUTCOMES/EVALUATION CRITERIA
Sample **NOC** linkages:
Fluid Balance: Balance of water in the intracellular compartments of the body
Hydration: Amount of water in the intracellular and extracellular compartments of the body
Electrolyte and Acid/Base Balance: Balance of electrolytes and non-electrolytes in the intracellular and extracellular compartments of the body

Client Will (Include Specific Time Frame)
- Maintain fluid volume at a functional level as evidenced by individually adequate urinary output, stable vital signs, moist mucous membranes, good skin turgor.
- Verbalize understanding of causative factors and purpose of individual therapeutic interventions and medications.
- Demonstrate behaviors to monitor and correct deficit as indicated when condition is chronic.

ACTIONS/INTERVENTIONS
Sample **NIC** linkages:
Fluid Management: Promotion of fluid balance and prevention of complications resulting from abnormal or undesired fluid levels
Hypovolemia Management: Reduction in extracellular and/or intracellular fluid volume and prevention of complications in a patient who is fluid overloaded
Shock Management: Volume: Promotion of adequate tissue perfusion for a patient with severely compromised intravascular volume.

 Cultural   Collaborative   Community/ Home Care 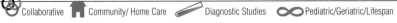 Diagnostic Studies  Pediatric/Geriatric/Lifespan   Medications

NURSING PRIORITY NO. 1. To assess causative/precipitating factors:

- Note possible medical diagnoses/disease processes that may lead to fluid deficits: 1) fluid loss (e.g., diarrhea/vomiting; fever; excessive sweating; heat stroke; diabetic ketoacidosis; burns, other draining wounds; gastrointestinal obstruction; salt-wasting diuretics; rapid breathing/mechanical ventilation, surgical drains); 2) limited intake (e.g., sore throat or mouth; client dependent on others for eating and drinking; vomiting); 3) fluid shifts (e.g., ascites, effusions, burns, sepsis); and 4) environmental factors (e.g., isolation, restraints, malfunctioning air conditioning, exposure to extreme heat).
- Determine effects of age, gender. Obtain weight and measure subcutaneous fat/muscle mass. *Factors that affect ratio of lean body mass to body fat, which influences total body water (TBW), which is approximately 60% of an adult's weight and 75% of an infant's weight.[1] In general, men have higher TBW than women, and the elderly's TBW is less than that of a youth. Elderly individuals are often at risk for underhydration because of a decreased thirst reflex, repeated infections, and chronic conditions. They may not be aware of water or nutritional needs, may be depressed or cognitively impaired, incontinent, and taking many medications.[2] Worldwide, dehydration (secondary to diarrheal illness) is the leading cause of infant and child mortality.[3]*
- Evaluate nutritional status, noting current intake, weight changes, problems with oral intake, use of supplements/tube feedings.

NURSING PRIORITY NO. 2. To evaluate degree of fluid deficit:

- Obtain history of usual pattern of fluid intake and recent alterations. *Intake may be reduced because of current physical or environmental issues (e.g., swallowing problems, vomiting; severe heat wave with inadequate fluid replacement); or a behavior pattern (e.g. elderly person refuses to drink water trying to control incontinence).[8]*
- Assess vital signs: including temperature (often elevated), pulse (elevated), respirations and blood pressure (may be low). Measure blood pressure *(lying/sitting/standing to evaluate orthostatic blood pressure)*, and monitor invasive hemodynamic parameters as indicated (e.g., central venous pressure [CVP]) to *determine degree of intravascular deficit and replacement needs.[7,8]*
- Note presence of dry mucous membranes, poor skin turgor, delayed capillary refill, flat neck veins, reports of thirst or weakness, child crying without tears, sunken eyeballs, fever, weight loss, little or no urine output. *Assessment signs of dehydration that client/SO may notice.[8]*
- Note change in usual mentation/behavior/functional abilities (e.g., confusion, falling, loss of ability to carry out usual activities, lethargy, dizziness). *These signs indicate sufficient dehydration to cause poor cerebral perfusion and/or electrolyte imbalance.*
- Observe/measure urinary output hourly or for 24 hours as indicated. Note color *(may be dark because of concentration)*, and specific gravity *(high number associated with dehydration with usual range being 1.010 to 1.025).[4]*
- Estimate or measure other fluid losses, (e.g., gastric, respiratory, and wound losses) *to more accurately determine fluid replacement needs.[8]*
- Review laboratory data (e.g., Hb/Hct, electrolytes [sodium, potassium, chloride, bicarbonate]; blood urea nitrogen [BUN], creatinine) *to evaluate body's response to fluid loss and to determine replacement needs.[4]*
- Collaborate with physician to identify/characterize the nature of fluid/electrolyte imbalance(s). *Dehydration is often categorized according to serum sodium concentration. Isonatremic*

(i.e., isotonic) dehydration is the most common type of dehydration. However, hypernatremic (also called hypertonic dehydration when relatively less sodium than water is lost) and hyponatremic (or hypotonic dehydration when relatively less water than sodium is lost) can both cause neurologic complications, and thus may be more dangerous.[3] *More than one cause may exist at a given time (e.g., increased loss of salt and water caused by diuretics that leads to decreased fluid intake as a result of lethargy and confusion).*[5]

NURSING PRIORITY NO. **3.** To correct/replace fluid losses to reverse pathophysiologic mechanisms:

 • Assist with treatment of underlying conditions causing or contributing to dehydration and electrolyte imbalances (e.g., change antibiotics causing diarrhea, treat fever/infection, malnutrition or severe depression; discontinue medications contributing to dehydration).

• Administer fluids and electrolytes as indicated. *Fluid used for replacement depends on the 1) type of dehydration present (e.g., hypertonic/ hypotonic), and 2) degree of deficit determined by age, weight and type of trauma/condition causing the fluid deficit. Multiple fluid resuscitation formulas (e.g., Parkland, Evans, Brooke burn formulas) exist with variations in both the volumes per weight suggested and the type or types of crystalloid or crystalloid-colloid combinations. Regardless of the formula or strategy used, the first 24 to 48 hours of fluid resuscitation require constant evaluation of the client's response, as well as frequent adjustments in fluid rates/solutions, to prevent complications (e.g. under/overhydration).*[2,6]

• Establish 24-hour replacement needs and routes to be used (e.g., IV/PO/tube feeding). *Entire fluid replacement may be done by IV or tube feeding if client is NPO, acutely ill or severely dehydrated. However, if client is be rehydrated orally, fluid replacement may be calculated to replace certain amount with meals (e.g., 75% to 80%) with the remainder offered during non-meal times. Steady rehydration rate reduces thirst, helps to balance electrolytes, and prevents peaks/valleys in fluid level. Managing oral rehydration in this manner can replace fluids, without resorting to IV therapy. These interventions should also be in place to prevent dehydration.*[2,3,5,6]

• Spread fluid intake throughout the day *to prevent periods of uncomfortable thirst.*[8]

 • Encourage increased intake of water and other fluids based on individual needs (up to 2.5 L/day or amount determined by physician for client's age, weight, and condition).

• Provide a variety of fluids in small frequent offerings, attempting to incorporate client's preferred beverage and temperature (e.g., iced or hot) *to enhance cooperation with regimen.*[8]

• Suggest intake of high-water content foods (e.g., popsicles, gelatin, soup, eggnog, watermelon) and/or electrolyte replacement drinks (e.g., Gatorade, Pedialyte) as appropriate. *Variety may stimulate intake.*

• Limit intake of alcohol/caffeinated beverages *that tend to exert a diuretic effect.*

• Engage client, family, and all caregivers in fluid management plan. *Everyone is responsible for the prevention or treatment of dehydration and should be involved in the planning and provision of adequate fluid on a daily basis.*

• Review diet orders to remove any nonessential fluid and salt restrictions. *As client's condition changes/new problems surface, old orders may contribute to dehydration.*

• Provide nutritionally balanced diet and/or enteral feedings (avoiding use of hyperosmolar to excessively high protein formulas) and provide adequate amount of free water with feedings.

• Maintain accurate intake and output (I/O), calculate 24-hour fluid balance, and weigh regularly (daily, in unstable client) *in order to monitor/document trends. Note: a 1-pound weight loss reflects fluid loss of about 500 mL in an adult.*[7]

 Cultural Collaborative Community/ Home Care Diagnostic Studies 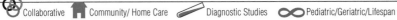 Pediatric/Geriatric/Lifespan Medications

NURSING PRIORITY NO. 4. To promote comfort and safety:

- Change position frequently. Bathe infrequently, using mild cleanser/soap and provide optimal skin care with suitable emollients *to maintain skin integrity and prevent excessive dryness caused by dehydration.*
- Provide frequent oral care and eye protection *to prevent injury from dryness.*
- Provide for safety measures when client is confused. (Refer to NDs acute Confusion, chronic Confusion for additional interventions.)
- Administer medications (e.g., antipyretics, insulin, antidiuretic hormone—ADH, vasopressin—Pitressin therapy) as indicated by contributing disease process.
- Adjust or discontinue medications (e.g., diuretics, laxatives, steroids, psychotropics, ACE inhibitors, etc.) that *may be contributing to dehydration.*[2,5]
- Observe for sudden/marked elevation of blood pressure, restlessness, moist cough, dyspnea, basilar crackles, and frothy sputum. *Too rapid a correction of fluid deficit may compromise the cardiopulmonary system, causing fluid overload and edema, especially if colloids are used in initial fluid resuscitation.*[8]

NURSING PRIORITY NO. 5. To promote wellness (Teaching/Discharge Considerations):

- Discuss factors related to occurrence of deficit as individually appropriate. *Early identification of risk factors can decrease occurrence and severity of complications associated with deficit fluid volumes.*[7]
- Recommend drinking more water when exercising/engaged in physical exertion, or during hot weather. Suggest carrying water bottle when away from home as appropriate.
- Identify and instruct in ways to meet specific fluid and nutritional needs.
- Discuss importance of not waiting to feel thirsty before injesting fluids. *Infants and the elderly may not sense/report thirst in timely fashion to prevent dehydration.*
- Review other actions (if any) that may be taken to prevent dehydration or correct deficiencies.
- Instruct client/SO(s) in how to monitor color of urine *(dark urine equates with concentration/dehydration)* and/or how to measure and record I/O (may include weighing or counting diapers in infant/toddler).
- Review/instruct in medication regimen and administration. Stress interactions/side effects to be reported to healthcare provider. *Facilitates timely intervention to prevent/lessen complications.*[8]
- Instruct in signs and symptoms indicating need for immediate/further evaluation and follow-up.

DOCUMENTATION FOCUS

Assessment/Reassessment
- Individual findings, including factors affecting ability to manage (regulate) body fluids and degree of deficit.
- I/O, fluid balance, changes in weight, urine-specific gravity, and vital signs.
- Results of diagnostic testing/laboratory studies.

Planning
- Plan of care and who is involved in the planning.
- Teaching plan.

Implementation/Evaluation

- Client's responses to treatment/teaching and actions performed.
- Attainment/progress toward desired outcome(s).
- Modifications to plan of care.

Discharge Planning

- Long-term needs, noting who is responsible for actions to be taken.
- Specific referrals made.

References

1. Cox, H. C., et al. (2002). Clinical Applications of Nursing Diagnosis: Adult, Child, Women's, Psychiatric, Gerontic, and Home Health Considerations, ed 4. Philadelphia: F. A. Davis, p 88.
2. Mentes, J. C. (1998). Hydration management. The Iowa Veterans Affairs Nursing Research Consortium. Iowa City, IA: University Iowa Gerontological Nursing Interventions Research Center, Research Dissemination Core.
3. Ellsbury, D. L., & Cantwell, G. P. Dehydration (Article last updated January 2003). Available at: http://www.emedicine.com. Accessed August 2003.
4. Cavanaugh, B. M. (1999). Nurse's Manual of Laboratory and Diagnostic Tests, ed 3. Philadelphia: F. A. Davis.
5. Dehydration and fluid maintenance. (2001). American Medical Directors Association (AMDA). Columbia, MD. Available at: http://www.guideline.gob. Accessed August 2003.
6. Oliver, R. I., Spain, D., & Stadelman, W. Burns, resuscitation and early management. Available at: http://www.emedicine.com. Accessed May 2003.
7. Matheny, N. (2000). Fluid and Electrolyte Balance: Nursing Considerations, ed 4. Philadelphia: J. B. Lippincott.
8. Fluid and Electrolyte Imbalances. In Doenges, M. E., Moorhouse, M. F., & Geissler-Murr, A. C. (2002). Nursing Care Plans: Guidelines for Individualizing Patient Care, ed 6. CD ROM. Philadelphia: F. A. Davis.

deficient Fluid Volume: [isotonic]

[NOTE: This diagnosis has been structured to address isotonic dehydration (hypovolemia) when fluids and electrolytes are lost in even amounts and excluding states in which changes in sodium occur. For client needs related to dehydration associated with alterations in sodium, refer to *[deficient Fluid Volume: hyper/hypotonic]*.]

Definition: Decreased intravascular, interstitial and/or intracellular fluid. This refers to dehydration, water loss alone without change in sodium.

RELATED FACTORS

Active fluid volume loss [e.g., hemorrhage, gastric intubation, diarrhea, wounds; abdominal cancer; burns, fistulas, ascites (third spacing); use of hyperosmotic radiopaque contrast agents]

Failure of regulatory mechanisms [e.g., fever/thermoregulatory response, renal tubule damage]

DEFINING CHARACTERISTICS

Subjective
Thirst

Weakness

Objective
Decreased urine output, increased urine concentration

Decreased venous filling, decreased pulse volume/pressure

 Cultural Collaborative Community/ Home Care Diagnostic Studies 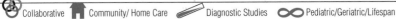 Pediatric/Geriatric/Lifespan Medications

Decreased BP, increased pulse rate
Sudden weight loss (except in third spacing)
Decreased skin/tongue turgor, dry skin/mucous membranes
Increased body temperature
Change in mental state
Elevated hematocrit

SAMPLE CLINICAL APPLICATIONS: hemorrhage, severe burns, gastroenteritis (with vomiting and diarrhea), malnutrition

DESIRED OUTCOMES/EVALUATION CRITERIA
Sample **NOC** linkages:
Hydration: Amount of water in the intracellular and extracellular compartments of the body
Fluid Balance: Balance of water in the intracellular compartments of the body
Coagulation Status: Extent to which blood clots within expected period of time

Client Will (Include Specific Time Frames)
- Maintain fluid volume at a functional level as evidenced by individually adequate urinary output with normal specific gravity, stable vital signs, moist mucous membranes, good skin turgor, and prompt capillary refill, resolution of edema.
- Verbalize understanding of causative factors and purpose of individual therapeutic interventions and medications.
- Demonstrate behaviors to monitor and correct deficit as indicated.

ACTIONS/INTERVENTIONS
Sample **NIC** linkages:
Hypovolemia Management: Reduction in extracellular and/or intracellular fluid volume and prevention of complications in a patient who is fluid overloaded
Shock Management: Volume: Promotion of adequate tissue perfusion for a patient with severely compromised intravascular volume
Bleeding Precautions: Reduction of stimuli that may induce bleeding or hemorrhage in at-risk patients

NURSING PRIORITY NO. 1. To assess causative/precipitating factors:
- Identify relevant diagnoses *that may create a fluid volume depletion (decreased intravascular plasma volume, such as might occur with rapid blood loss/hemorrhage from trauma, and vascular, pregnancy-related, or GI bleeding disorders; significant fluid (other than blood loss) such as might occur with severe gastroenteritis with vomiting and diarrhea, or extensive burns.*[1]
- Note presence of other factors (e.g., laryngectomy/tracheostomy tubes, drainage from wounds/fistulas or suction devices; water deprivation/fluid restrictions; decreased level of consciousness; dialysis; hot/humid climate, prolonged exercise; increased metabolic rate secondary to fever; increased caffeine/alcohol) *that may contribute to lack of fluid intake or loss of fluid by various routes.*
- Prepare for/assist with diagnostic evaluations (e.g., imaging studies, x-rays, etc.) *to locate source of bleeding/cause for hypovolemia.*

- Determine effects of age, gender. Obtain weight and measure subcutaneous fat/muscle mass. *These factors affect ratio of lean body mass to body fat, which influences total body water (TBW), and is approximately 60% of an adult's weight and 75% of an infant's weight.*[2] *In general, males have higher TBW than women, and the elderly's TBW is less than that of a*

youth. Elderly individuals are often at risk for underhydration because of a decreased thirst reflex, decreased effectiveness of compensatory mechanisms, repeated infections, and chronic conditions.[3] *Infants and children are less able to control their fluid intake. Worldwide, dehydration secondary to diarrheal illness is the leading cause of infant and child mortality.*[4]

NURSING PRIORITY NO. 2. To evaluate degree of fluid deficit:

- Estimate/measure traumatic or procedural fluid losses. Note possible routes of insensible fluid losses. Determine customary and current weight. *These factors are used to determine degree of dehydration and method of fluid replacement. The body surface area (BSA) method states that dehydration is related to deficit of TBW and assumes that loss of weight is loss of water. The caloric method states that the degree of dehydration is related to body weight (e.g., loss of 10% of usual body weight is considered "10% dry").*[5]
- Assess vital signs, including temperature (often elevated), pulse and respirations (elevated), and blood pressure (may be low). Measure blood pressure *(lying/sitting/standing to evaluate orthostatic blood pressure)*, and monitor invasive hemodynamic parameters as indicated (e.g., central venous pressure [CVP]) to *determine degree of intravascular deficit and replacement needs.*[8]
- Note presence of dry mucous membranes, poor skin turgor, delayed capillary refill, flat neck veins, and reports of thirst or weakness, child crying without tears, sunken eyeballs (or fontanels in infant), fever, weight loss, little or no urine output. *Assessment signs of dehydration that client/SO may notice. In an acute, life-threatening hemorrhage state, cold, pale, moist skin may be noted reflecting body compensatory mechanisms to profound hypovolemia.*[1]
- Note change in usual mentation/behavior/functional abilities (e.g. confusion, falling, loss of ability to carry out usual activities, lethargy, and dizziness). *These signs indicate sufficient dehydration to cause poor cerebral perfusion and/or electrolyte imbalance. In hypovolemic shock state, mentation changes rapidly and client may present in coma.*
- Observe/measure urinary output (hourly/24 hour totals). Note color *(may be dark because of concentration)* and specific gravity *(high number associated with dehydration with usual range being 1.010 to 1.025).*[6]
- Review laboratory data (e.g., Hb/Hct, electrolytes [sodium, potassium, chloride, bicarbonate]; blood urea nitrogen [BUN], creatinine) *to evaluate body's response to fluid loss and to determine replacement needs.*[6] *In isotonic dehydration, electrolyte levels may be lower, but concentrations remain near normal.*[5]

NURSING PRIORITY NO. 3. To correct/replace losses to reverse pathophysiological mechanisms:

- Stop blood loss (e.g., gastric lavage with room temperature or cool saline solution, drug administration, prepare for surgical intervention).
- Stop fluid loss (e.g., administer medication to stop vomiting/diarrhea, fever).[8]
- Administer fluids and electrolytes (e.g., blood, isotonic sodium chloride solution, lactated Ringer solution, fresh frozen plasma, dextran, hetastarch).[8]
- Establish/continually reevaluate 24-hour fluid replacement needs and routes to be used *to prevent peaks/valleys in fluid level and to prevent fluid overload.*[8]
- Control humidity and ambient air temperature as appropriate, especially when major burns are present, or in presence of fever *to reduce insensible losses.*
- Reduce bedding/clothes, provide tepid sponge bath.

 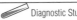

- Assist with hypothermia therapy as indicated *to decrease severe fever and elevated metabolic rate*. (Refer to ND Hyperthermia.)
- Maintain accurate I/O and weigh daily. Monitor urine specific gravity. Monitor vital signs (lying/sitting/standing) and invasive hemodynamic parameters as indicated (e.g., CVP, PAP/PCWP) *to evaluate effectiveness of resuscitation measures.*[8]

NURSING PRIORITY NO. 4. To promote comfort and safety:

- Change position frequently. Bathe infrequently, using mild cleanser/soap, and provide optimal skin care with emollients *to maintain skin integrity and prevent excessive dryness caused by dehydration.*
- Provide frequent oral care and eye care *to prevent injury from dryness.*
- Change dressings frequently/use adjunct appliances as indicated for draining wounds *to protect skin and to monitor/replace losses.*
- Administer medications (e.g., antiemetics, antidiarrheals to limit gastric/intestinal losses; antipyretics to reduce fever). Refer to NDs Diarrhea, Hyperthermia.
- Observe for sudden/marked elevation of blood pressure, restlessness, moist cough, dyspnea, basilar crackles, and frothy sputum. *Too rapid a correction of fluid deficit may compromise the cardiopulmonary system, causing fluid overload and edema, especially if colloids are used in initial fluid resuscitation.*[8]

NURSING PRIORITY NO. 5. To promote wellness (Teaching/Discharge Considerations):

- Discuss factors related to occurrence of fluid deficit as individually appropriate (e.g., reason for hemorrhage, potential for dehydration in children with fever/diarrhea, inadequate fluid replacement when performing strenuous work/exercise, living in hot climate, improper use of diuretics) *to reduce risk of recurrence.*[7]
- Identify actions (if any) client may take to prevent/correct deficiencies. *Carrying water bottle when away from home aids in maintaining fluid volume. Dressing in weather appropriate clothing, staying in shade during heat of day, engaging in exercise during early morning or evening hours, and installation of room cooler or electric fan for hot climates helps reduce risk of heat stress/hyperthermia. In cases of mild-to-moderate dehydration, use of oral solutions (e.g., Gatorade, Rehydralyte), soft drinks, breast milk, or formula can provide adequate rehydration.*[7]
- Instruct client/SO(s) in how to monitor color of urine *(dark urine equates with concentration/dehydration)* and/or how to measure and record I/O (may include weighing or counting diapers in infant/toddler).
- Review medications and interactions/side effects *especially as relates to medications that cause or exacerbate fluid loss (e.g., diuretics, laxatives), and those indicated to prevent fluid loss (e.g., antidiarrheals or anticoagulants).*
- Discuss signs/symptoms indicating need for emergent/further evaluation and follow-up. *Promotes timely intervention.*

DOCUMENTATION FOCUS

Assessment/Reassessment
- Assessment findings, including degree of deficit and current sources of fluid intake.
- I/O, fluid balance, changes in weight/edema, urine-specific gravity, and vital signs.

Planning
- Plan of care and who is involved in planning.
- Teaching plan.

Implementation/Evaluation
- Client's responses to interventions/teaching and actions performed.
- Attainment/progress toward desired outcome(s).
- Modifications to plan of care.

Discharge Planning
- Long-term needs, plan for correction, and who is responsible for actions to be taken.
- Specific referrals made.

References

1. Kolecki, P., & Meckhoff, C. R. (2001). Shock, hypovolemic. Article from Emedicine.com. Available at: http://www.emedicine.com. Accessed August 2003.
2. Cox, H. C., et al. (2002). Clinical Applications of Nursing Diagnosis: Adult, Child, Women's, Psychiatric, Gerontic, and Home Health Considerations, ed 4. Philadelphia: F. A. Davis, p. 88.
3. Mentes, J. C. (1998). Hydration management. The Iowa Veterans Affairs Nursing Research Consortium. Iowa City, IA: University Iowa Gerontological Nursing Interventions Research Center, Research Dissemination Core.
4. Ellsbury, D. L., & Cantwell, G. P. Dehydration. (Article last updated January 2003).Available at: http://www.emedicine.com. Accessed January 2003.
5. Welch, J. (1998). Isotonic dehydration. Available at: http://gucfm.georgetown.edu/welchjj/netscut/fen/isotonic_dehydration.html. Accessed August 2003.
6. Cavanaugh, B. M. (1999). Nurse's Manual of Laboratory and Diagnostic Tests, ed 3. Philadelphia: F. A. Davis.
7. Koch, H., & Graber, M. A. Pediatrics: Vomiting, Diarrhea, and Dehydration. University of Iowa Family Practice Handbook, ed 4 Available at: http://www.vh.org. Accessed August 2003.
8. Fluid and Electrolyte Imbalances. In Doenges, M. E., Moorhouse, M. F., & Geissler-Murr, A. C. (2002). Nursing Care Plans: Guidelines for Individualizing Patient Care, ed 6. C-D ROM. Philadelphia: F. A. Davis.

excess Fluid Volume

Definition: Increased isotonic fluid retention

RELATED FACTORS
Compromised regulatory mechanism [e.g., syndrome of inappropriate antidiuretic hormone—SIADH—or decreased plasma proteins as found in conditions such as malnutrition, draining fistulas, burns, organ failure]

Excess fluid intake

Excess sodium intake

[Drug therapies such as chlorpropamide, tolbutamide, vincristine, triptylines, carbamazepine]

DEFINING CHARACTERISTICS

Subjective
Shortness of breath, orthopnea

Anxiety

 Cultural   Collaborative   Community/ Home Care   Diagnostic Studies   Pediatric/Geriatric/Lifespan   Medications

Objective

Edema, may progress to anasarca; weight gain over short time

Intake exceeds output; oliguria

Abnormal breath sounds (rales or crackles), changes in respiratory pattern, dyspnea

Increased CVP; jugular vein distention; positive hepatojugular reflex

S_3 heart sound

Pulmonary congestion, pleural effusion, pulmonary artery pressure changes; BP changes

Change in mental status; restlessness

Specific gravity changes

Decreased Hb/Hct; azotemia, altered electrolytes

SAMPLE CLINICAL APPLICATIONS: congestive heart failure, renal failure, cirrhosis of liver, cancer, toxemia of pregnancy, conditions associated with SIADH (e.g., meningitis, encephalitis, Guillain-Barré syndrome), schizophrenia (where polydipsia is a prominent feature)

DESIRED OUTCOMES/EVALUATION CRITERIA

Sample **NOC** linkages:

Fluid Balance: Balance of water in the intracellular compartments of the body

Electrolyte & Acid/Base Balance: Balance of electrolytes and non-electrolytes in the intracellular and extracellular compartments of the body

Cardiac Pump Effectiveness: Extent to which blood is ejected from the left ventricle per minute to support systemic perfusion pressure

Client Will (Include Specific Time Frame)

- Stabilize fluid volume as evidenced by balanced I/O, vital signs within client's normal limits, stable weight, and free of signs of edema.
- Verbalize understanding of individual dietary/fluid restrictions.
- Demonstrate behaviors to monitor fluid status and reduce recurrence of fluid excess.
- List signs that require further evaluation.

ACTIONS/INTERVENTIONS

Sample **NIC** linkages:

Hypervolemia Management: Reduction in extracellular and/or intracellular fluid volume and prevention of complications in a patient who is fluid overloaded

Electrolyte Management: Promotion of electrolyte balance and prevention of complications resulting from abnormal or undesired serum electrolyte levels

Peritoneal Dialysis/Hemodialysis Therapy: Administration and monitoring of dialysis solution into and out of the peritoneal cavity/**or** Management of extracorporeal passage of the patient's blood through a dialyzer

NURSING PRIORITY NO. 1. To assess causative/precipitating factors:

- Be aware of conditions or risk factors associated with fluid excess (e.g., heart failure, chronic kidney disease, renal/adrenal insufficiency, excessive or rapid infusion of IV fluids, cerebral lesions, psychogenic polydipsia, acute stress, surgical/anesthetic procedures, decreased/loss of serum proteins) *that can contribute to excess fluid intake or retention.*[1]
- Determine/ estimate amount of fluid intake from all sources: PO, IV, ventilator, etc.
- Review nutritional issues, e.g., intake of sodium, potassium, and protein. *Imbalances in these areas are associated with fluid imbalances.*

NURSING PRIORITY NO. 2. To evaluate degree of excess:

- Note presence and location of edema (e.g., puffy eyelids, dependent swelling ankles/feet if ambulatory or up in chair; sacrum and posterior thighs when recumbent). Determine whether lower extremity edema is new or increasing. *Heart failure and renal failure are associated with dependent edema because of hydrostatic pressures, with dependent edema being a defining characteristic for excess fluid. Generalized edema (e.g., upper extremities and eyelids) is associated with nephrotic syndrome.*[2]

- Note presence of tachycardia, irregular rhythms. Auscultate heart tones for S_3, ventricular gallop. *Signs suggestive of heart failure, which results in decreased cardiac output and tissue hypoxia.*[7]

- Auscultate breath sounds for presence of crackles/congestion. Record occurrence of exertional breathlessness, dyspnea at rest, or paroxysmal nocturnal dyspnea. *Indication of pulmonary congestion and potential developing pulmonary edema that can interfere with oxygen-carbon dioxide exchange at the capillary level.*[3]

- Assess for presence of neck vein distention/hepatojugular reflux with head of bed elevated 30 to 45 degrees. *Signs of increased intravascular volume.*[6]

- Measure vital signs and invasive hemodynamic parameters (e.g., CVP, PAP/PCWP) if available. *Blood pressures may be high because of excess fluid volume, or be low if cardiac failure is occurring.*

- Measure abdominal girth *to evaluate changes that may indicate increasing fluid retention/edema.*[7]

- Measure/record intake and output accurately. Include "hidden" fluids (e.g., IV antibiotic additives, liquid medications, ice chips). Calculate fluid balance (plus/minus). Note patterns, times, and amount of urination (e.g., nocturia, oliguria).[6]

- Weigh daily or on a regular schedule, as indicated. Compare current weight with admission and/or previously stated weight. Assess lean body mass and total body water as indicated. *Provides a comparative baseline and is used to determine total body water, either by percentage or body surface area. Note: Volume overload can occur over weeks to months in patients with unrecognized renal failure where lean muscle mass is lost and fluid overload occurs with relatively little change in weight.*[4]

- Evaluate mentation for restlessness, anxiety, confusion, and personality changes. *Signs of decreased cerebral oxygenation may indicate electrolyte imbalance (e.g. hyponatremia) or cerebral edema.*[1]

- Assess appetite; note presence of nausea/vomiting. Assess neuromuscular reflexes *to determine presence of problems associated with imbalance of electrolytes (e.g., glucose, sodium, potassium, calcium).*

- Observe skin and mucous membranes. *Edematous tissues are prone to ischemia and breakdown/ulceration.*[5]

- Review laboratory data (e.g., BUN/Cr, Hb/Hct, serum albumin, proteins, and electrolytes; urine specific gravity/osmolality/sodium excretion) and chest radiograph. *These tests may be repeated to ascertain baseline imbalances and to monitor response to therapy.*

NURSING PRIORITY NO. 3. To promote mobilization/elimination of excess fluid:

- Restrict fluid intake as indicated *(especially when sodium retention is less than water retention and/or when fluid retention is related to renal failure).*[6]

- Provide for sodium restrictions if needed (as might occur in sodium retention in excess of water retention). *Restricting sodium favors renal excretion of excess fluid and may be more useful than fluid restriction.*[1]

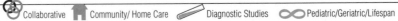

Cultural Collaborative Community/ Home Care Diagnostic Studies Pediatric/Geriatric/Lifespan Medications

- Set an appropriate rate of fluid intake/infusion throughout 24-hour period. Maintain steady rate of all IV infusions *to prevent exacerbation of excess fluid volume and to prevent peaks/valleys in fluid level.*[6]
- Administer medications (e.g., diuretics, cardiotonics, plasma or albumin volume expanders) *in order to improve cardiac output and kidney function thereby reducing congestion and edema.*
- Encourage bedrest when ascites is present. *May promote recumbency-induced diuresis.*
- Prepare for/assist with procedures as indicated (e.g., peritoneal or hemodialysis, mechanical ventilation). *May be done to correct volume overload, electrolyte and acid-base imbalances or to support individual during shock state.*[7]

NURSING PRIORITY NO. 4. To maintain integrity of skin and tissues:

- Promote early ambulation *to mobilize fluids and prevent/limit damage from venous stasis complications.*
- Evaluate edematous extremities, change position frequently *to reduce tissue pressure and risk of skin breakdown.*[7]
- Offer frequent mouth care when fluids are restricted using non-drying mouthwash and hard candies, etc., *to promote comfort of dry mucous membranes and prevent oral complications.*[7]
- Place in semi-Fowler's position as appropriate *to facilitate respiratory effort, especially when ascites is present or when breathing is impaired because of lung congestion.*
- Use safety precautions if client is confused/debilitated *as may occur with cerebral edema, electrolyte imbalance, heart failure, etc.*[7]
- Refer to NDs impaired/risk for impaired Skin Integrity, impaired Oral Mucous Membrane, risk for Activity Intolerance, and disturbed Thought Processes for additional interventions.

NURSING PRIORITY NO. 5. To promote wellness (Teaching/Discharge Considerations):

- Consult dietitian as needed *to develop dietary plan/identify foods to be limited or omitted.*
- Review dietary restrictions and safe substitutes for salt (e.g., lemon juice or spices such as oregano).
- Discuss fluid restrictions and "hidden sources" of fluids (e.g., foods high in water content such as fruits, ice cream, sauces, custard, etc.). Use small drinking cup or glass.
- Avoid salty or spicy foods *as they increase thirst or fluid retention.* Suck ice chips, hard candy, or slices of lemon *to help allay thirst.*[7]
- Suggest chewing gum, use of lip balm *to reduce discomforts of fluid restrictions.*[7]
- Instruct client/family in ways to keep track of intake. *For example, some may benefit from using a liter jug. Start each day with it empty and for every drink taken, pour the equivalent amount of water into the jug to check fluid intake through the day.*[6]
- Measure output, encourage use of voiding record when it is appropriate or weigh daily and report gain of more than 2 pounds/day (or as indicated by individual physician order). *If weight is higher than target weight, fluid is likely being retained.*[6]
- Discuss importance of/establish regular schedule for weighing. *Prompt reporting of changes facilitates timely intervention. Weight gain of 2.2 pounds can indicate one liter of retained fluid.*[7]

• Review drug regimen/side effects. *Many drugs have an impact on kidney function and fluid balance, especially in the elderly or those with cardiac and kidney impairments.*

• Stress need for mobility and/or frequent position changes *to prevent stasis and reduce risk of tissue injury.*[7]

• Identify "danger" signs requiring notification of healthcare provider *to ensure timely evaluation/intervention.*[6]

DOCUMENTATION FOCUS

Assessment/Reassessment
• Assessment findings, noting existing conditions contributing to and degree of fluid retention (vital signs, amount, presence and location of edema, and weight changes).
• I/O, fluid balance.

Planning
• Plan of care and who is involved in the planning.
• Teaching plan.

Implementation/Evaluation
• Response to interventions and teaching and actions performed.
• Attainment/progress toward desired outcome(s).
• Modifications to plan of care.

Discharge Planning
• Long-range needs, noting who is responsible for actions to be taken.

References

1. Fauci, A. S., et al. (eds). (1998). Harrison's Principles of Internal Medicine, ed 14. New York: McGraw-Hill, pp 268–269, 1292–1293.
2. Rios, H., et al. (1991). Validation of defining characteristics of four nursing diagnoses using a computerized data base. J Prof Nurs, 7, 293–299.
3. Matheny, N. (2000). Fluid and Electrolyte Balance: Nursing Considerations, ed 4. Philadelphia: J. B. Lippincott.
4. Veterans Health Administration, Department of Defense. VHA/DoD clinical practice guideline for the management of chronic kidney disease and pre-ERSD in the primary care setting. Department of Veterans Affairs (U.S.), Veterans Health Administration (2001), various pages. Available at: www.guideline.gov. Accessed August 2003.
5. Cullen, L. (1992). Interventions related to fluid and electrolyte imbalance. Nurs Clin North Am, 27, 569–597.
6. Hydration management. (2001). American Medical Directors Association (AMDA). Columbia, MD: National Guideline Clearinghouse. Available at: http://www.guideline.gov. Accessed August 2003.
7. Fluid and Electrolyte Imbalances. In Doenges, M. E., Moorhouse, M. F., & Geissler-Murr, A. C. (2002). Nursing Care Plans: Guidelines for Individualizing Patient Care, ed 6. CD ROM. Philadelphia: F. A. Davis.

risk for deficient Fluid Volume

Definition: At risk for experiencing vascular, cellular, or intracellular dehydration

RISK FACTORS
Extremes of age and weight
Loss of fluid through abnormal routes (e.g., indwelling tubes)
Knowledge deficiency related to fluid volume
Factors influencing fluid needs (e.g., hypermetabolic states)
Medications (e.g., diuretics)

 Cultural Collaborative Community/ Home Care Diagnostic Studies 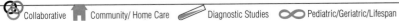 Pediatric/Geriatric/Lifespan Medications

Excessive losses through normal routes (e.g., diarrhea)

Deviations affecting access, intake, or absorption of fluids (e.g., physical immobility)

NOTE: A risk diagnosis is not evidenced by signs and symptoms, as the problem has not occurred and nursing interventions are directed at prevention.

SAMPLE CLINICAL APPLICATIONS: conditions with fever, diarrhea, nausea/vomiting; irritable bowel syndrome, draining wounds, dementia, depression, eating disorders

DESIRED OUTCOMES/EVALUATION CRITERIA

Sample **NOC** linkages:

Fluid Balance: Balance of water in the intracellular compartments of the body

Risk Control: Actions to eliminate or reduce actual, personal, and modifiable health threats

Knowledge: Disease Process: Extent of understanding conveyed about a specific disease process

---

Client Will (Include Specific Time Frame)

- Identify individual risk factors and appropriate interventions.
- Demonstrate behaviors or lifestyle changes to prevent development of fluid volume deficit.

ACTIONS/INTERVENTIONS

Sample **NIC** linkages:

Fluid Monitoring: Collection and analysis of patient data to regulate fluid balance

Hemodynamic Regulation: Optimization of heart rate, preload, afterload, and contractility

Bleeding Precautions: Reduction of stimuli that may indicate bleeding or hemorrhage in at-risk patients

NURSING PRIORITY NO. 1. To assess causative/contributing factors:

- Note possible medical diagnoses/disease processes that may lead to fluid deficits: 1) fluid loss (e.g., indwelling tubes, diarrhea/vomiting, fever, excessive sweating, diabetic ketoacidosis; burns, other draining wounds; gastrointestinal obstruction; use of diuretics); 2) limited intake (e.g., extremes of age, immobility, client dependent on others for eating and drinking; lack of knowledge related to fluid intake; heat exhaustion/stroke); 3) fluid shifts (e.g., ascites, effusions, burns, sepsis); or 4) environmental factors (e.g., isolation, restraints, very high ambient temperatures, malfunctioning air conditioning).[4]
- Determine effects of age, gender. Obtain weight and measure subcutaneous fat/muscle mass. *Factors that affect ratio of lean body mass to body fat, which influences total body water (TBW), which is approximately 60% of an adult's weight and 75% of an infant's weight.[1] In general, men have higher TBW than women, and the elderly's TBW is less than that of a youth. Elderly individuals are often at risk for underhydration because of a decreased thirst reflex, repeated infections, and chronic conditions. They may not be aware of water or nutritional needs, may be depressed or cognitively impaired, incontinent, and taking many medications.[2] Worldwide, dehydration (secondary to diarrheal illness) is the leading cause of infant and child mortality.[3]*
- Evaluate nutritional status, noting current food intake, type of diet (e.g., client is NPO or is on a restricted/pureed diet). Note problems (e.g., impaired mentation, nausea, wired jaws, immobility, insufficient time for meals, lack of finances restricting availability of food) *that can negatively affect fluid intake.*
- Refer to NDs [deficient Fluid Volume, hyper/hypotonic] or [isotonic] for additional interventions.

NURSING PRIORITY NO. 2. To prevent occurrence of deficit:

- Monitor I/O balance being aware of altered intake or output, as well as insensible losses *to ensure accurate picture of fluid status.*[4]
- Weigh client and compare with recent weight history. Perform serial weights *to determine trends.*[5]
- Note changes in vital signs (e.g., orthostatic hypotension, tachycardia, fever) *that may indicate or cause/exacerbate dehydration.*[4]
- Assess skin turgor/oral mucous membranes for signs of dehydration.
- Review laboratory data (e.g., Hb/Hct, electrolytes, BUN/Cr) *to evaluate fluid and electrolyte status.*[4]
- Administer medications as indicated (e.g., antiemetics, antidiarrheals, antipyretics) *to stop/limit fluid losses.*[4,5]
- Establish individual fluid needs/replacement schedule. Distribute fluids over 24-hours *to prevent periods of thirst.*[5]
- Provide supplemental fluids (tube feed, IV) as indicated.
- Encourage oral intake[4–6]:
  Provide water and other fluids to a minimum amount daily (up to 2.5 L/day or amount determined by physician for client's age, weight, and condition)
  Offer fluids between meals and regularly throughout the day
  Allow adequate time for eating and drinking at meals
  Provide fluids with manageable cup, bottle, or drinking straw
  Ensure that immobile/restrained client is assisted
  Encourage a variety of fluids in small frequent offerings, attempting to incorporate client's preferred beverage and temperature (e.g., iced or hot)
  Limit fluids that tend to exert a diuretic effect (e.g., caffeine, alcohol)
  Promote intake of high-water content foods (e.g., popsicles, gelatin, soup, eggnog, watermelon) and/or electrolyte replacement drinks (e.g., Gatorade, Pedialyte) as appropriate
  Encourage client to drink more fluids when exercising/ physical exertion, or during hot weather
  Review diet orders to remove any nonessential fluid and salt restrictions
  Provide nutritionally balanced diet and/or enteral feedings (avoiding use of hyperosmolar or excessively high protein formulas) and provide adequate amount of free water with feedings

NURSING PRIORITY NO. 3. To promote wellness (Teaching/Discharge Considerations):

- Discuss individual risk factors/potential problems and specific interventions *(e.g., proper clothing/bedding for infants and elderly during hot weather, use of room cooler/fan for comfortable ambient environment).*[7]
- Review appropriate use of medications and inform of side effects of medications *that have potential for causing/exacerbating dehydration.*
- Encourage client/caregiver to maintain diary of food/fluid intake, number and amount of voidings, and estimate of other fluid losses (e.g., wounds, liquid stools) *to determine replacement needs.*
- Engage client, family and all caregivers in fluid management plan. *Enhances cooperation with regimen and achievement of goals.*[5]

 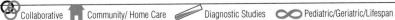

Assessment/Reassessment
- Individual findings, including individual factors influencing fluid needs/requirements.
- Baseline weight, vital signs.
- Specific client preferences for fluids.

Planning
- Plan of care and who is involved in planning.
- Teaching plan.

Implementation/Evaluation
- Responses to interventions/teaching and actions performed.
- Attainment/progress toward desired outcome(s).
- Modifications to plan of care.

Discharge Planning
- Individual long-term needs, noting who is responsible for actions to be taken.
- Specific referrals made.

References

1. Cox, H. C., et al. (2002). Clinical Applications of Nursing Diagnosis: Adult, Child, Women's, Psychiatric, Gerontic, and Home Health Considerations, ed 4. Philadelphia: F. A. Davis, p 88.
2. Mentes, J. C. (1998). Hydration management. The Iowa Veterans Affairs Nursing Research Consortium. Iowa City, IA: University Iowa Gerontological Nursing Interventions Research Center, Research Dissemination Core.
3. Ellsbury, D. L., & Cantwell, G. P. Dehydration. Available at: http://www.emedicine.com. Accessed August 2003.
4. Dehydration and fluid maintenance. (2001). American Medical Directors Association (AMDA). Columbia, MD: National Guideline Clearinghouse. Available at: http://www.guideline.gov. Accessed August 2003.
5. Fluid and Electrolyte Imbalances. In Doenges, M. E., Moorhouse, M. F., & Geissler-Murr, A. C. (2002). Nursing Care Plans: Guidelines for Individualizing Patient Care, ed 6. CD-ROM. Philadelphia: F. A. Davis.
6. Matheny, N. (2000). Fluid and Electrolyte Balance: Nursing Considerations, ed 4. Philadelphia: J. B. Lippincott.
7. Curtis, R. (1997). OA guide to heat related illnesses & fluid balance. Article for Princeton University Outdoor Action website. Available at: http://www.princeton.edu/~oa/safety/heatill.html. Accessed September 2003.

risk for imbalanced Fluid Volume

Definition: At risk for a decrease, an increase, or a rapid shift from one to the other of intravascular, interstitial, and/or intracellular fluid. This refers to body fluid loss, gain, or both.

RISK FACTORS

Scheduled for major invasive procedures

[Rapid/sustained loss, e.g., hemorrhage, burns, fistulas]

[Rapid fluid replacement]

Other risk factors to be determined

NOTE: A risk diagnosis is not evidenced by signs and symptoms, as the problem has not occurred and nursing interventions are directed at prevention.

SAMPLE CLINICAL APPLICATION: major surgical procedures, renal dialysis, conditions requiring IV therapy or parenteral/enteral nutrition, heart failure with use of diuretic therapy

Sample **NOC** linkages:

Fluid Balance: Balance of water in the intracellular compartments of the body

Risk Control: Actions to eliminate or reduce actual, personal, and modifiable health threats

Cardiac Pump Effectiveness: Extent to which blood is ejected from the left ventricle per minute to support systemic perfusion pressure

Client Will (Include Specific Time Frame)

- Demonstrate adequate fluid balance as evidenced by stable vital signs, palpable pulses/good quality, normal skin turgor, moist mucous membranes, individual appropriate urinary output, lack of excessive weight fluctuation (loss/gain), and no edema present.

ACTIONS/INTERVENTIONS

Sample **NIC** linkages:

Fluid Monitoring: Collection and analysis of patient data to regulate fluid balance

Intravenous [IV] Therapy: Administration and monitoring of intravenous fluids and medication

Bleeding Precautions: Reduction of stimuli that may induce bleeding or hemorrhage in at-risk patients

NURSING PRIORITY NO. 1. To determine causative/contributing factors:

- Note potential sources of fluid imbalances (e.g., presence of conditions such as diabetes insipidus, hyperosmolar nonketotic syndrome, bowel obstruction, heart/kidney/liver failure), major invasive procedures [e.g., surgery], use of anesthesia, preoperative vomiting and dehydration, draining wounds, use/overuse of certain medications [e.g., anticoagulants, diuretics, laxatives], use of IV fluids and delivery device, administration of total parenteral nutrition [TPN]).
- Note client's age, current level of hydration, and mentation. *Provides information regarding ability to tolerate fluctuations in fluid level and risk for creating or failing to respond to a problem (e.g., confused client may have inadequate intake, disconnect tubings, or readjust IV flow rate; infant or child unable to self-monitor or manage).*

NURSING PRIORITY NO. 2. To prevent fluctuations/imbalances in fluid levels:

- Measure and record intake:
  Include all sources (e.g., PO, IV, antibiotic additives, liquids with medications).
  Maintain IVs on volumetric infusion pumps, rapid infusion devices, as indicated *to deliver fluids accurately at desired rates to prevent either under or overinfusion.*[5]
- Measure and record output:
  Monitor urine output (hourly, or as often as needed). Report urine output <30 mL/hr or 0.5 mL/kg/hr *because it may indicate deficient fluid volume or cardiac or kidney failure.*
  Observe color of all excretions *to evaluate for bleeding.*
  Estimate volume/measure emesis when vomiting.
  Measure/estimate amount of liquid stool; weigh diapers/continence pads when indicated
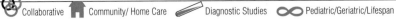 Inspect dressing(s), weigh dressings, estimate blood loss in surgical sponges, count

dressings/pads saturated per hour. *Note: Small losses can be life-threatening to pediatric clients.*[2]

Measure output from drainage devices.

Estimate/calculate insensible fluid losses *to include losses in replacement calculations. Note: Losses from diffusion through skin and via respiratory tract, are estimated at about 700 mL/24 hours in adult at ambient temperature,*[3] *while a diaphoretic episode requiring a full linen change may represent a fluid loss of as much as 1 L.*[5]

Calculate 24-hour fluid balance (noting intake > output, or output > intake).

- Weigh daily or as indicated, using same scale and clothing and evaluate changes as they relate to fluid status. *Provides for early detection and prompt intervention as needed.*[5]

- Monitor vital signs:

Evaluate vital signs at rest and with activities. *Blood pressure, heart and respiratory rate often increase when either volume deficit or fluid excess is present.*[5]

Calculate pulse pressure. *Pulse pressure often widens before systolic BP drops in response to fluid loss.*

Evaluate hemodynamic pressures when available. *Central venous pressure (CVP) and pulmonary artery wedge pressures (PAWP) may be used in critically ill to determine fluid balance and guide administration of vasoactive IV drips.*[2]

Note presence of hypotension, dry skin/mucous membranes, and delayed capillary refill. *Clinical signs of dehydration.*[4,5]

- Assess for peripheral/dependent edema, adventitious breath sounds, and distended neck veins; *clinical signs of fluid excess. Note that intravascular volume depletion can be present at the same time as extravascular fluid excess (seen as edema) is present, so hypertension or hypotension could be found.*[4,5]

- Note increased lethargy or reports of dizziness, weakness, muscle cramping. *Electrolyte imbalances (e.g., sodium, potassium, magnesium, calcium) may be present.*[5]

- Review laboratory data (e.g., electrolytes, Hgb/Hct, chest radiograph *to determine changes indicative of electrolyte and/or fluid imbalance.*[5]

- If fluid volume deficit is possible:

Anticipate fluid replacement needs (*e.g., need for blood/plasma transfusion in client with major trauma, planned surgery where blood and fluid loss can be expected, inability to take fluids voluntarily, major burn injury, person with heat stroke).*[5]

Establish/promote oral intake, incorporating beverage preferences when possible *to enhance cooperation with regimen.*[5] (Refer to NDs deficient Fluid Volume: [hypertonic/hypotonic], deficient Fluid Volume: [isotonic], and risk for deficient Fluid Volume for additional interventions.)

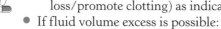

Administer IV fluids (e.g., crystalloids, colloids, blood/blood components) as prescribed using infusion pumps *to promote fluid management.*[4,5]

Tape tubing connections longitudinally *to reduce risk of disconnection and loss of fluids.*[5]

Administer medications (e.g., antidiarrheals, antiemetics, agents to reduce blood loss/promote clotting) as indicated *to reduce fluid loss.*[4,5]

- If fluid volume excess is possible:

Maintain fluid/sodium restrictions when needed. Offer small amounts of fluid over 24 hours. (Refer to ND excess Fluid Volume for additional interventions.)

Use IV volumetric pumps to deliver accurate amounts of fluid.

Administer medications (e.g., diuretics, cardiotonics) *to assist in management of fluid excess/edema.*[4,5]

Assist with/prepare for rotating tourniquets, phlebotomy, dialysis or ultrafiltration *to correct fluid overload situation.*[5]

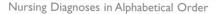

NURSING PRIORITY NO. 3. To promote wellness (Teaching/Discharge Considerations):

- Discuss individual risk factors/potential problems and specific interventions *to prevent/limit complications.*
- Instruct client/SO in how to measure and record I/O as appropriate.
- Review/instruct in medications or nutritionals (e.g., enteral/parenteral) regimen *to alert to potential complications and ways to manage.*
- Identify signs and symptoms indicating need for prompt evaluation/follow-up *to promote timely intervention/correction.*[5]
- Refer to NDs [deficient Fluid Volume: hypertonic/hypotonic], deficient Fluid Volume: [isotonic], excess Fluid Volume, risk for deficient Fluid Volume for additional interventions.

DOCUMENTATION FOCUS

Assessment/Reassessment
- Individual findings, including individual factors influencing fluid needs/requirements.
- Baseline weight, vital signs.
- Specific client preferences for fluids.

Planning
- Plan of care and who is involved in planning.
- Teaching plan.

Implementation/Evaluation
- Responses to interventions/teaching and actions performed.
- Attainment/progress toward desired outcome(s).
- Modifications to plan of care.

Discharge Planning
- Individual long-term needs, noting who is responsible for actions to be taken.
- Specific referrals made.

References

1. Cox, H. C., et al. (2002). Clinical Applications of Nursing Diagnosis: Adult, Child, Women's, Psychiatric, Gerontic, and Home Health Considerations, ed 4. Philadelphia: F. A. Davis, p 136.
2. Ackley, B. J. & Ladwig, G. B. Nursing Diagnosis Handbook: A Guide to Planning Care, ed 5. St Louis: Mosby, pp 359–360.
3. Guyton, A. C., & Hall, J. E. (1996). Textbook of Medical Physiology, ed 9. Philadelphia: W. B. Saunders.
4. Matheny, N. (2000). Fluid and Electrolyte Balance: Nursing Considerations, ed 4. Philadelphia: J. B. Lippincott.
5. Fluid and Electrolyte Imbalances, and Surgical Interventions. In Doenges, M. E., Moorhouse, M. F., & Geissler-Murr, A. C. (2002). Nursing Care Plans: Guidelines for Individualizing Patient Care, ed 6. CD-ROM. Philadelphia: F. A. Davis.

impaired Gas Exchange

Definition: Excess or deficit in oxygenation and/or carbon dioxide elimination at the alveoli-capillary membrane [This may be an entity of its own but also may be an end result of other pathology with an interrelatedness between airway clearance and/or breathing pattern problems.]

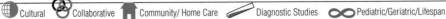
 Cultural Collaborative Community/ Home Care 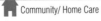 Diagnostic Studies Pediatric/Geriatric/Lifespan Medications

Ventilation perfusion imbalance [as in the following: altered blood flow (e.g., pulmonary embolus, increased vascular resistance), vasospasm, heart failure, hypovolemic shock]

Alveolar-capillary membrane changes [(e.g., acute respiratory distress syndrome); chronic conditions such as restrictive/obstructive lung disease, pneumoconiosis, respiratory depressant drugs, brain injury, asbestosis/silicosis]

[Altered oxygen supply (e.g., altitude sickness)]

[Altered oxygen-carrying capacity of blood (e.g., sickle cell/other anemia, carbon monoxide poisoning)]

DEFINING CHARACTERISTICS

Subjective
Dyspnea
Visual disturbances
Headache upon awakening
[Sense of impending doom]

Objective
Confusion [decreased mental acuity]
Restlessness, irritability [agitation]
Somnolence [lethargy]
Abnormal ABGs/arterial pH, hypoxia/hypoxemia, hypercapnia, hypercarbia, decreased carbon dioxide
Cyanosis (in neonates only), abnormal skin color (pale, dusky)
Abnormal rate, rhythm, depth of breathing; nasal flaring
Tachycardia [dysrhythmias]
Diaphoresis
[Anemia, polycythemia]

SAMPLE CLINICAL APPLICATIONS: COPD, asthma, pneumonia, tuberculosis, heart failure, respiratory distress syndrome, high altitude pulmonary edema, carbon monoxide poisoning

DESIRED OUTCOMES/EVALUATION CRITERIA

Sample **NOC** linkages:

Respiratory Status: Gas Exchange: Alveolar exchange of CO_2 or O_2 to maintain blood gas concentration

Tissue Perfusion: Pulmonary: Extent to which blood flows through intact pulmonary vasculature with appropriate pressure and volume, perfusing alveoli/capillary

Respiratory Status: Ventilation: Movement of air in and out of the lungs

Client Will (Include Specific Time Frame)
- Demonstrate improved ventilation and adequate oxygenation of tissues by ABGs within client's normal limits and absence of symptoms of respiratory distress (as noted in Defining Characteristics).
- Verbalize understanding of causative factors and appropriate interventions.
- Participate in treatment regimen (e.g., breathing exercises, effective coughing, and use of oxygen) within level of ability/situation.

ACTIONS/INTERVENTIONS

Sample **NIC** linkages:

Respiratory Monitoring: Collection and analysis of patient data to ensure airway patency and adequate gas exchange

Oxygen Therapy: Administration of oxygen and monitoring of its effectiveness

Airway Management: Facilitation of patency of air passages

NURSING PRIORITY NO. 1. To assess causative/contributing factors:

- Note presence of factors listed in Related Factors. *Gas exchange problems can be related to multiple factors, including anemias, anesthesia/surgical procedures, high altitude, allergic response, altered level of consciousness, anxiety/fear, aspiration, decreased lung compliance, excessive or thick secretions, immobility, infection, medication and drug toxicity/overdose, neuromuscular impairment of breathing pattern, pain, smoking.*
- Refer to NDs ineffective Airway Clearance, ineffective Breathing Pattern for additional nursing interventions and rationale as appropriate.

NURSING PRIORITY NO. 2. To evaluate degree of compromise:

- Evaluate respirations:
  Note respiratory rate, depth. *Increasing both rate and depth of respirations increases alveolar ventilation and occurs normally in response to exercise and stressors. Tachypnea is usually present to some degree, and can progress to hyperventilation with shallow respirations, dyspnea, and respiratory depression.*[1]
  Note client's reports/perceptions of breathing ease. *Client may report a range of symptoms (e.g., air hunger, shortness of breath with speaking, activity or at rest).*
  Observe for dyspnea on exertion, gasping; changing positions frequently to ease breathing; tendency to assume three-point position (bending forward while supporting self by placing one hand on each knee) *to maximize respiratory effort.*
  Note use of accessory muscles (e.g., scalene muscles, pectoralis minor, sternocleidomastoids and external intercostal muscles) *to assist diaphragm in increasing volume of thoracic cavity, which aids in inspiration.*[2]
  Observe infants/young children for nasal flaring and sternal retractions *indicating increased work of breathing/progressing respiratory distress.*
  Note use of abdominal muscles during expiration (normally a passive process) *to reduce thoracic dimensions and overcome airway resistance to expiration.*[2]
- Evaluate lungs:
  Auscultate and percuss chest, describing presence/absence of breath sounds, note adventitious breath sounds. *Although air may be heard moving through the lung fields, breath sounds may be faint because of decreased airflow or areas of consolidation. In this nursing diagnosis, ventilatory effort is insufficient to deliver enough oxygen, or to get rid of sufficient amounts of carbon dioxide. Abnormal breath sounds are indicative of numerous problems (e.g., hypoventilation such as might occur with chest or spinal cord injury, atelectasis or presence of secretions, improper endotracheal tube placement, collapsed lung) and must be evaluated for further intervention.*[3,4]
- Evaluate skin/mucous membrane color noting areas of pallor/cyanosis, for example, peripheral (nailbeds) versus central (around lips or earlobes) or general duskiness. *Duskiness and central cyanosis are indicative of advanced hypoxemia.*[4]
- Evaluate behavior:
  Assess level of consciousness and mentation changes. *Decreased level of consciousness*

 Cultural Collaborative Community/ Home Care Diagnostic Studies 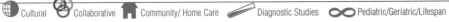 Pediatric/Geriatric/Lifespan Medications *impairs one's ability to protect the airway potentially adversely affecting oxygenation that in turn further impairs mentation.*

Note somnolence, restlessness, reports of headache on arising.

Assess energy level and activity tolerance, noting reports/evidence of fatigue, weakness, problems with sleep *that are associated with decreased oxygenation.*

- Monitor vital signs:

  Measure temperature. *High fever greatly increases metabolic demands and oxygen consumption.*

  Tachycardia and dysrhythmias may be noted *as heart reacts to ischemia, especially during activity.* Blood pressures can be variable, depending on underlying condition and cardiopulmonary response.

  Note increased pulmonary artery/right ventricular wedge pressures in critically ill client with central lines. *Indicative of increased pulmonary vascular resistance.*

- Review pertinent diagnostic data (e.g., ABGs, Hgb, red blood cells, electrolytes); chest radiography. Evaluate pulse oximetry (can be typical measurement along with vital signs in many facilities) and pulmonary function studies (e.g., lung volumes and capacities) *to determine presence/degree of lung function, and/or respiratory insufficiency and acid-base status; also used to monitor response to therapies. Client in respiratory failure typically shows hypoxemia and metabolic acidosis and is high risk for developing respiratory acidosis.*[5]

NURSING PRIORITY NO. 3. To correct/improve existing deficiencies:

- Elevate head of bed/position client appropriately. *Elevation/upright position facilitates respiratory function by gravity; however, client in severe distress will seek position of comfort. In ventilated client prone position may be indicated to improve pulmonary perfusion and increase oxygen diffusion.*[4]
- Provide airway adjuncts and suction as indicated *to clear/maintain airway and improve gas diffusion when client is unable to clear secretions or is showing desaturation of oxygen by oximetry or ABGs.*[4,6,7]
- Encourage frequent position changes, deep-breathing/directed coughing exercises, use of incentive spirometer, chest physiotherapy as indicated. *Promotes optimal chest expansion, mobilization of secretions, and oxygen diffusion.*[4]
- 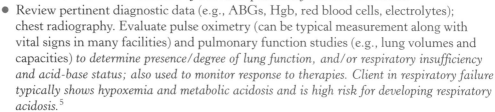 Provide supplemental oxygen (via cannula, mask) using lowest concentration possible *dictated by pulse oximetry, ABGs, and client symptoms/underlying condition.*
- Ensure availability of proper emergency equipment including ET/trach set and suction catheters appropriate for age and size of infant/child/adult. Avoid use of face mask in elderly emaciated client.
- Prepare for/assist with intubation and mechanical ventilation. *The decision to intubate and ventilate is made on a clinical diagnosis of increased work of breathing, hypoventilation, impaired mental status, or presence of a moribund state.*[5]
- Monitor/adjust ventilator settings (e.g., FIo_2, tidal volume, inspiratory/expiratory ratio, sigh, positive end-expiratory pressure—PEEP) as indicated when mechanical support is being used.
- Monitor for carbon dioxide narcosis (e.g., change in level of consciousness, changes in O_2 and CO_2 blood gas levels, flushing, decreased respiratory rate and headaches), *which may occur in clients receiving long-term oxygen therapy.*
- Maintain adequate I/O *for mobilization of secretions,* but avoid fluid overload *that may increase pulmonary congestion.*
- Provide psychological support, listening to questions/concerns. Deal with fear/anxiety

that may be present. Maintain calm attitude while working with client/SOs. *Anxiety is contagious and associated agitation can increase oxygen consumption/dyspnea.*

- Encourage adequate rest and limit activities to within client tolerance. Promote calm/restful environment. *Helps limit oxygen needs/consumption.*[4]
- Administer medications as indicated (e.g., corticosteroids, antibiotics, bronchodilators, expectorants, heparin) *to treat underlying conditions. Medications may be aerosolized/nebulized for enhanced response and limitation of side effects.*[4]
- Monitor therapeutic and adverse effects/interactions of drug therapy *to determine efficacy and need for change.*
- Use sedation judiciously *to avoid depressant effects on respiratory functioning.*[4]
- Minimize blood loss from procedures (e.g., blood draws—especially in neonates/infants, hemodialysis) *to limit effects of anemia and related gas diffusion impairment.*
- Assist with procedures as individually indicated (e.g., transfusion, phlebotomy, bronchoscopy) *to improve respiratory function/oxygen-carrying capacity.*
- Keep environment allergen/pollutant free *to reduce irritant effect on airways.*

NURSING PRIORITY NO. 4. To promote wellness (Teaching/Discharge Considerations)[4]:

- Review risk factors, particularly genetic/environmental/employment-related conditions (e.g., sickle-cell anemia, altitude sickness, exposure to toxins) *to help client/SO prevent complications or manage risk factors.*
- Discuss implications of smoking related to the illness/condition. Encourage client and SO(s) to stop smoking, attend cessation programs as necessary *to improve lung function.*
- Review oxygen-conserving techniques (e.g., organizing tasks before beginning, sitting instead of standing to perform tasks, eating small meals, performing slower-purposeful movements) *to reduce oxygen demands.*[4]
- Reinforce need for adequate rest, while encouraging activity within client's limitations.
- Instruct in the use of relaxation, stress-reduction techniques as appropriate.
- Review job description/work activities *to identify need for job modifications/vocational rehabilitation.*
- Discuss home oxygen therapy and instruct in safety concerns as indicated *to ensure client's safety, especially when used in the very young, fragile elderly, or when cognitive or neuromuscular impairment is present.*
- Identify specific supplier for supplemental oxygen/necessary respiratory devices, as well as other individually appropriate resources, such as home-care agencies, Meals on Wheels, etc., *to facilitate independence.*[4]

DOCUMENTATION FOCUS

Assessment/Reassessment
- Assessment findings, including respiratory rate, character of breath sounds; frequency, amount, and appearance of secretions; presence of cyanosis; laboratory findings; and mentation level.
- Conditions that may interfere with oxygen supply.

Planning
- Plan of care/interventions and who is involved in the planning.
- Ventilator settings, liters of supplemental oxygen.
- Teaching plan.

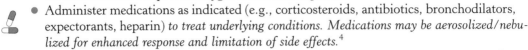

 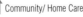

Implementation/Evaluation
- Client's responses to treatment/teaching and actions performed.
- Attainment/progress toward desired outcome(s).
- Modifications to plan of care.

Discharge Planning
- Long-range needs, identifying who is responsible for actions to be taken.
- Community resources for equipment/supplies postdischarge.
- Specific referrals made.

References

1. Seay, S. J., Gay, S. L., & Strauss, M. (2002). Tracheostomy emergencies. AJN, 102(3), 59.
2. Waldorf, A. (2003). Online course: Physiology of Exercise and Health. Pulmonary structure and function and gas exchange and transport. Cal State San Marcus. iLearn (Internet Learning Environments and Resource Network), available at: http://courses.csusm.edu/resources/biol325aw/chapter12_13.
3. Cox, H. C., et al. (2002) Clinical Applications of Nursing Diagnosis: Adult, Child, Women's Gerontic, and Home Health Considerations, ed 4. Philadelphia: F. A. Davis, pp 256–261.
4. Doenges, M. E., Moorhouse, M. F., & Geissler, Murr, A. C. (2002). Nursing Care Plans: Guidelines for Individualizing Patient Care, ed 6. Philadelphia: F. A. Davis, pp 112, 118–120, 130–131, 167.
5. Carcillo, J. A., & Fields A.I. (2002). Clinical practice parameters for hemodynamic support of pediatric and neonatal patients in septic shock. Crit Care Med, 30(6), 1365–78.
6. Fink, J. B., & Hess, D.R. (2002). Secretion clearance techniques. In Hess, D. R., et al. (eds): Respiratory Care: Principles and Practices. Philadelphia: W. B. Saunders.
7. Blair, K.A. (1999). The aging pulmonary system. In Stanley, M., & Beare, P. G. (eds): Gerontological Nursing: A Health Promotion/Protection Approach, ed 2. Philadelphia: F. A. Davis.
8. Argyle, B. (1996). Blood Gases Computer Program. Retrieved from Mad Scientist Software's Blood Gas tutorial. Available at: http://www.madsci.com/manu/indexgas.htm. Accessed August 2003.

anticipatory Grieving

Definition: Intellectual and emotional responses and behaviors by which individuals, families, communities work through the process of modifying self-concept based on the perception of potential loss [Note: May be a healthy response requiring interventions of support and information giving.]

RELATED FACTORS
To be developed by nurse researchers and submitted to NANDA

[Perceived potential loss of SO, physiological/psychosocial well-being (body part/function, social role), lifestyle/personal possessions]

DEFINING CHARACTERISTICS

Subjective
Sorrow, guilt, anger, [choked feelings]

Denial of potential loss; denial of the significance of the loss

Expression of distress at potential loss [ambivalence, sense of unreality]; bargaining

Alteration in activity level, sleep/dream patterns, eating habits, libido

Objective
Potential loss of significant object (e.g., people, job, status, home, ideals, part and processes of the body)

Altered communication patterns

Difficulty taking on new or different roles

Resolution of grief prior to the reality of loss

[Altered affect]

[Crying]

[Social isolation, withdrawal]

SAMPLE CLINICAL APPLICATIONS: cancer, traumatic injuries (e.g., brain/spinal cord), amputation, chronic/debilitating conditions (e.g., renal failure, COPD, MS, ALS), genetic/birth defects

DESIRED OUTCOMES/EVALUATION CRITERIA

Sample **NOC** linkages:

Grief Resolution: Adjustment to actual or impending loss

Caregiver Emotional Health: Feelings, attitudes, and emotions of a family care provider while caring for a family member or significant other over an extended period of time

Family Coping: Family actions to manage stressors that tax family resources

---

Client Will (Include Specific Time Frame)

- Identify and express feelings (e.g., sadness, guilt, fear) freely/effectively.
- Acknowledge impact/effect of the grieving process (e.g., physical problems of eating, sleeping) and seek appropriate help.
- Look toward/plan for future, one day at a time.

ACTIONS/INTERVENTIONS

Sample **NIC** linkages:

Grief Work Facilitation: Assistance with the resolution of a significant loss

Grief Work Facilitation: Perinatal Death: Assistance with the resolution of a perinatal loss

Dying Care: Promotion of physical comfort and psychological peace in the final phase of life

NURSING PRIORITY NO. 1. To assess causative/contributing factors:

- Determine client's perception of anticipated loss and meaning to him or her. "What are your concerns?" "What are your fears? Your greatest fear?" "How do you see this affecting you/your lifestyle?" *Identifying the needs to be addressed, acknowledging the client's responses are integral to planning care.*[9]
- Ascertain response of family/SO(s) to client's situation/concerns. *Family concerns affect client and need to be listened to and appropriate interventions taken. Problems may arise if family completes grieving prematurely and disengages from the dying member, who then feels abandoned at a time when the support is needed.*[2]
- Determine length of anticipatory grief process. *Some individuals may use the grieving as a defense against the inevitable loss. While some people may find this helpful when the loss occurs, many people find that intense feelings occur regardless of the period of anticipation.*[2]

NURSING PRIORITY NO. 2. To determine current response to anticipated loss:

- Note emotional responses, such as withdrawal, angry behavior, crying. Provide information about normal stages of grieving. *Awareness allows for appropriate choice of interventions because individuals handle grief in different ways. Knowledge promotes understanding of emotional responses.*[4]

 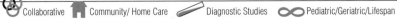

- Observe client's body language and check out meaning with the client. Note congruency of body language with verbalizations. *Body language is open to interpretation and needs to be validated so misinterpretation does not occur. Client may be saying one thing, but often body language is saying something else and identifying incongruencies can provide opportunity for individual to understand self in relation to grieving process.*[2]

- Note cultural factors/expectations that may impact client's responses to situation. *Cultural beliefs, such as Arab-Americans may want to pray in silence or private; African Americans may use faith and root healers in conjunction with biomedical resources; often beliefs vary with the individual and will affect how the client is responding to the situation.*[5]

- Identify problems with eating, activity level, sexual desire, role performance (e.g., work, parenting). *Indicators of severity of feelings client is experiencing and need for specific interventions to resolve these issues.*[5]

- Note family communication/interaction patterns. *Dysfunctional patterns of communication such as avoidance, preaching, giving advice can block effective communication and isolate family members.*[3]

- Discuss with client and family/SO's, and others as appropriate, plans that need to be made as well as anticipated adjustments/role changes related to the situation. Encourage/answer questions as needed. *This type of discussion will bring concerns out in the open and help with adaptation to the loss.*[5]

- Determine use/availability of community resources/support groups. *Appropriate use of support can help the individual feel less isolated and can promote feelings of inclusion and comfort.*[6]

NURSING PRIORITY NO. 3. To assist client/others to deal with situation:

- Provide open environment and trusting relationship. *Promotes a free discussion of feelings and concerns in a safe enviroment where client can reveal innermost fears and beliefs about anticipated loss.*[2]

- Use therapeutic communication skills of Active-listening, silence, acknowledgment. Respect client desire/request not to talk. *These skills convey belief in ability of client to deal with situation and develop a sense of competence. Client may not be ready to discuss feelings and situation and respecting client's own timeline conveys confidence.*[2,3]

- Inform children about the anticipated death/loss in age appropriate language. *Providing accurate information about impending loss or change in life situation will help the child begin the mourning process.*[10]

- Give permission to child to express feelings about situation and ask questions, being careful to provide honest answers within child's understanding. *Adults may be uncomfortable or upset talking about impending death/loss and children may be excluded from adult conversation about what is happening.*[10]

- Provide puppets or play therapy for toddlers/young children. Young children do not have the capacity to express their feelings and the use of play *may help them express grief and help deal with loss in ways that are appropriate to the age.*[2]

- Permit appropriate expressions of anger, fear. Note hostility toward/feelings of abandonment by spiritual power. (Refer to appropriate NDs.) *Anger is a normal part of the grieving process and talking about these feelings allows individual to think about them and move on, coming to some resolution regarding the anticipated loss.*[6]

- Provide information about normalcy of individual grief reaction. *Many people are not familiar with grief and are concerned that what they are experiencing is not normal. Letting them know that grief takes many forms and what they are feeling is alright, helps them deal with what is happening.*[9]

- Be honest when answering questions, providing information. *Enhances nurse-client relationship promoting trust and confidence.*[2]
- Provide assurance to child that cause for situation is not client's own doing, bearing in mind age and developmental level. *May lessen sense of guilt and affirm there is no need to assign blame to any family member.*[2]
- Provide hope within parameters of individual situation. Do not give false reassurance. *Something positive can be found in most situations. Helping client find the positives will help with management of current situation. Comments such as 'everything will be all right', or 'don't worry' are not helpful and convey lack of understanding to the client.*[2]
- Review life experiences/previous loss(es), role changes, and coping skills, noting strengths/successes. *Useful in dealing with current situation and problem solving existing needs.*[4]
- Discuss control issues, such as what is in the power of the individual to change and what is beyond control. *Recognition of these factors helps client focus energy for maximal benefit/outcome on what can be done.*[4]
- Incorporate family/SO(s) in problem solving. *Encourages family to support/assist client to deal with situation while meeting needs of family members.*[6]
- Determine client's status and role in family (e.g., parent, sibling, child), and address loss of family member role. *Client's illness affects their usual activities in the role he or she has in the family and inevitably affects all the other family members as responsibilities are taken over by them.*[6]
- Instruct in use of visualization and relaxation techniques. *These skills can be helpful to reduce anxiety and stress and help client and family members manage grief more effectively.*[7]
- Mobilize resources when client is the community. *When anticipated loss affects community as a whole, such as closing of manufacturing plant, impending disaster (e.g., wildfire, terrorist concerns), multiple supports will be required to deal with size and complexity of situation. When more people are directly or indirectly involved in the anticipated loss, emotions/anxiety tend to be amplified and transmitted, complicating the situation.*
- Use sedatives/tranquilizers with caution. *While the use of these medications may be helpful in the short term, too much dependence on them may retard passage through the grief process.*[2]

NURSING PRIORITY NO. 4. To promote wellness (Teaching/Discharge Considerations):

- Give information that feelings are OK and are to be expressed appropriately. *Talking about feelings can facilitate the grieving process, but destructive behavior can be damaging to the self-esteem.*[2]
- Encourage continuation of usual activities/schedule and involvement in appropriate exercise program as appropriate and able. *Promotes sense of control and self-worth, enabling client to feel more positive about ability to handle situation.*[6]
- Identify/promote involvement of family and social support systems. *A supportive environment enhances the effectiveness of interventions and promotes a successful grieving process.*[4]
- Discuss and assist with planning for future/funeral as appropriate. *Involving family members in this discussion assures that everyone knows what is desired and what is planned, avoiding unexpected disagreements.*[4]
- Refer to additional resources such as pastoral care, counseling/psychotherapy, community/organized support groups as indicated for both client and family/SO. *Useful for ongoing needs and facilitation of grieving process.*[6]

 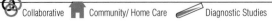

• Identfy resources/develop community plan to address anticipated large-scale losses. *Preparation for complex challenges facilitates prompt response as needs occur.*

DOCUMENTATION FOCUS

Assessment/Reassessment
- Assessment findings, including client's perception of anticipated loss and signs/symptoms that are being exhibited.
- Responses of family/SOs.
- Availability/use of resources.

Planning
- Plan of care and who is involved in planning.
- Teaching plan.

Implementation/Evaluation
- Client's response to interventions/teaching and actions performed.
- Attainment/progress toward desired outcome(s).
- Modifications to plan of care.

Discharge Planning
- Long-range needs and who is responsible for actions to be taken.
- Specific referrals made.

References

1. Doenges, M. E., Moorhouse, M. F., & Geissler-Murr, A. C. (2004). Nurse's Pocket Guide: Diagnoses, Interventions, and Rationales, ed 9. Philadelphia: F. A. Davis.
2. Townsend, M. C. (2003). Psychiatric Mental Health Nursing Concepts of Care, ed 4. Philadelphia: F. A. Davis.
3. Gordon, T. (2000). Parent Effectiveness Training, updated edition. New York: Three Rivers Press.
4. Cox, H. C., et al: (2002). Clinical Applications of Nursing Diagnosis: Adult, Child, Women's, Psychiatric, Gerontic, and Home Health Considerations, ed 4. Philadelphia: F. A. Davis.
5. Lipson, J. G., Dibble, S. L., & Minarik, P. A. (1996). Culture & Nursing Care: A Pocket Guide. San Francisco: UCSF Nursing Press.
6. Doenges, M. E., Townsend, M. C., & Moorhouse, M. F. (1998). Psychiatric Care Plans Guidelines for Individualizing Care, ed 3. Philadelphia: F. A. Davis.
7. Pearce, J. C. (2002). The Biology of Trancendence a Blueprint of the Human Spirit. Rochester, VT: Park St Press.
8. Matzo M., et al. (2002). Teaching cultural consideration at the end of life. End of Life Nursing Education Consortium program recommendations. J Contin Edu Nurs, 33(6), 270–278.
9. Neeld, E. H. (2003). Seven Choices, ed 4. Austin, TX: Centerpoint Press.
10. Riely, M. (2003). Facilitating Children's Grief. J School Nurs, 19(4), 212–218.

dysfunctional Grieving

Definition: Extended, unsuccessful use of intellectual and emotional responses by which individuals, families, and communities attempt to work through the process of modifying self-concept based on the perception of loss

RELATED FACTORS
Actual or perceived object loss (e.g., people, possessions, job, status, home, ideals, parts and processes of the body [e.g., amputation, paralysis, chronic/terminal illness])

[Thwarted grieving response to a loss, lack of resolution of previous grieving response]
[Absence of anticipatory grieving]

DEFINING CHARACTERISTICS

Subjective
Expression of distress at loss; denial of loss

Expression of guilt; anger; sadness; unresolved issues; [hopelessness]

Idealization of lost object (e.g., people, possessions, job, status, home, ideals, parts and processes of the body)

Reliving of experiences with little or no reduction (diminishment) of intensity of the grief

Alterations in eating habits, sleep/dream patterns, activity level, libido, concentration and/or pursuit of tasks

Objective
Onset or exacerbation of somatic or psychosomatic responses

Crying; labile affect

Difficulty in expressing loss

Prolonged interference with life functioning; developmental regression

Repetitive use of ineffectual behaviors associated with attempts to reinvest in relationships

[Withdrawal; isolation]

SAMPLE CLINICAL APPLICATIONS: cancer, traumatic injuries (e.g., brain/spinal cord), amputation, chronic/debilitating conditions (e.g., renal failure, COPD, ALS), genetic/birth defects, fetal demise, SIDS/other sudden unexpected deaths (e.g., suicide), infertility

DESIRED OUTCOMES/EVALUATION CRITERIA

Sample **NOC** linkages:

Grief Resolution: Adjustment to actual or impending loss

Family Coping: Family actions to manage stressors that tax family resources

Psychosocial Adjustment: Life Change: Psychosocial adaptation of an individual to a life change

Client Will (Include Specific Time Frame)
- Acknowledge presence/impact of dysfunctional situation.
- Demonstrate progress in dealing with stages of grief at own pace.
- Participate in work and self-care/ADLs as able.
- Verbalize a sense of progress toward resolution of the grief and hope for the future.

ACTIONS/INTERVENTIONS

Sample **NIC** linkages:

Grief Work Facilitation: Assistance with the resolution of a significant loss

Grief Work Facilitation: Perinatal Death: Assistance with the resolution of a perinatal loss

Coping Enhancement: Assisting a patient to adapt to perceived stressors, changes, or threats that interfere with meeting life demands and roles

NURSING PRIORITY NO. 1. To assess causative/contributing factors:

 • Identify loss that is present. Look for cues of sadness (e.g., sighing, faraway look, unkempt appearance, inattention to conversation). *Indicators of extent of grief and how individual is dealing with situation.*[6]

 Cultural Collaborative Community/ Home Care  Diagnostic Studies 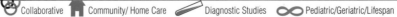 Pediatric/Geriatric/Lifespan Medications

- Identify stage of grief being expressed: denial, isolation, anger, bargaining, depression, acceptance. *Helps to establish how client is dealing with grieving and degree of difficulty client is having adjusting to the death/loss.*[10]
- Determine level of functioning, ability to care for self. *Individual may be incapacitated by depth of loss and be unable to manage day-to-day activities adequately, necessitating intervention/assistance.*[6]
- Be aware of avoidance behaviors (e.g., anger, withdrawal, long periods of sleeping or refusing to interact with family). *Additional indicators of depth of grieving being experienced and need for more intensive support/monitoring to help client deal effectively with death/loss.*[10]
- Note availability/use of support systems and community resources. *Identification of these supports can be helpful for the client to access the assistance they can provide. Client may be so distraught, it is difficult to reach out and avail self of this help.*[9]
- Identify cultural factors and ways individual(s) has dealt with previous loss(es). *Way of expressing self may reflect cultural background and religious beliefs. Understanding cultural expectations will help to determine the nature/degree of dysfunction.*[8]
- Ascertain response of family/SO(s) to situation. Assess needs of SO(s). *Response of family members will affect how client is dealing with situation and this information is important for planning care to enable all members to effectively cope with events.*[9]
- Perform/refer for psychological testing, as indicated (e.g., Beck's Depression Scale). *Determines degree of depression and indication of need for medication.*[2]
- Refer to ND anticipatory Grieving as appropriate.

NURSING PRIORITY NO. 2. To assist client/others to deal appropriately with loss:

- Encourage verbalization without confrontation about realities. *It is helpful to listen without correcting misperceptions in the beginning, allowing free flow of expression. Provides opportunity for reflection aiding resolution and acceptance.*[6]
- Encourage client to choose topics of conversation and refrain from forcing client to "face the facts." *Talking freely about concerns can help client identify what is important to deal with and how to cope with situation.*[9]
- Active-listen feelings and be available for support/assistance. Speak in soft, caring voice. *Communicates acceptance and caring, enabling client to seek own answers to current situation.*[3]
- Encourage expression of anger/fear, guilt, and anxiety. Refer to appropriate NDs. *These feelings are part of the grieving process and to accomplish the work of grieving, they need to be expressed and accepted.*[9]
- Permit verbalization of anger with acknowledgment of feelings and setting of limits regarding destructive behavior. *Enhances client safety, promotes resolution of grief process by encouraging expression of feelings that are not usually accepted, and supports self-esteem.*[2]
- Acknowledge reality of feelings of guilt/blame, including hostility toward spiritual power. (Refer to ND Spiritual Distress.) *Assists client to take steps toward resolution by being available to listen to ideas client expresses.*[7]
- Respect the client's needs and wishes for quiet, privacy, talking, or silence. *Individual may not be ready to talk about or share grief and needs to be allowed to make own timeline.*[6]
- Give "permission" to be at this point when the client is depressed. *Assures client that feelings are normal and can be a starting point to deal with loss/death that has occurred in a positive manner.*[9]
- Provide comfort and availability as well as caring for physical needs. *Client needs to know that they will be supported and helped when not able to care for self.*[6]

● Reinforce use of previously effective coping skills. Instruct in/encourage use of visualization and relaxation techniques. *Identifying and discussing how client has dealt with loss in the past can provide opportunity to use them in current situation. Use of these techniques helps client to learn to relax and consider options for dealing with loss/death.*[2]

 ● Assist SOs to cope with client's response. Include age-specific interventions. *Family/SO(s) may not be dysfunctional but may be intolerant, not recognizing needs of the client. Family members, including children may express their feelings in anger, resulting in punishment for behavior that is deemed unacceptable, rather than recognizing the basis in grief.*[10]

 ● Include family/SO(s) in setting realistic goals for meeting needs of client and family members. *Involving all members enhances the probability that each member will express their needs and hear what the needs of others are, ensuring a more effective outcome.*[2]

● Use sedatives/tranquilizers with caution. *While the use of these medications may be helpful in the short term, too much dependence on them may retard passage through the grief process.*[2]

NURSING PRIORITY NO. 3. To promote wellness (Teaching/Discharge Considerations):

 ● Discuss healthy ways of dealing with difficult situations. *Identifying ways individual(s) has dealt with losses in the past will help him or her to look at what has been helpful in the past and what might be useful in the current situation.*[2]

● Have individual(s) identify familial, religious, and cultural factors that have meaning. *One's family of origin has a major impact on what the individuals learn about these issues and how to deal with losses. Identifying and discussing how they affect the current situation may help bring loss into perspective and promote grief resolution.*[8]

 ● Encourage involvement in usual activities, exercise, and socialization within limits of physical ability, and psychological state. *Keeping life to a somewhat normal routine can provide individual(s) with some sense of control over events that are not controllable.*[8]

 ● Suggest client keep a journal of experiences and feelings. *As client writes about what is happening, new insights may occur. Reading over what has been written can help individual see progress that has been made and begin to have hope for the future.*[9]

 ● Discuss and assist with planning for future/funeral as appropriate. *Provides a sense of control and involvement in these activities and ensures that own wishes will be heard and respected.*[10]

 ● Identify volunteer opportunities, e.g., community reorganization/cleanup; investigating new employment/relocation opportunities. *Exercising control in a productive manner empowers individuals and promotes rebuilding of community.*

● Refer to other resources (e.g., pastoral care, counseling, psychotherapy, organized support groups). *Provides additional help when needed to resolve situation, continue grief work.*[8]

DOCUMENTATION FOCUS

Assessment/Reassessment
● Assessment findings, including meaning of loss to the client, current stage of the grieving process, and responses of family/ SOs.
● Availability/use of resources.

Planning
● Plan of care and who is involved in the planning.
● Teaching plan.

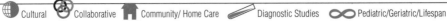   Cultural   Collaborative   Community/ Home Care   Diagnostic Studies   Pediatric/Geriatric/Lifespan   Medications

Implementation/Evaluation
- Client's response to interventions/teaching and actions performed.
- Attainment/progress toward desired outcome(s).
- Modifications to plan of care.

Discharge Planning
- Long-term needs and who is responsible for actions to be taken.
- Specific referrals made.

References

1. Doenges, M. E., Moorhouse, M. F., & Geissler-Murr, A. C. (2004). Nurse's Pocket Guide: Diagnoses, Interventions, and Rationales, ed 9. Philadelphia: F. A. Davis.
2. Townsend, M. C. (2003). Psychiatric Mental Health Nursing Concepts of Care, ed 4. Philadelphia: F. A. Davis.
3. Gordon, T. (2000). Parent Effectiveness Training, updated edition. New York: Three Rivers Press.
4. Cox, H. C., et al. (2002). Clinical Applications of Nursing Diagnosis: Adult, Child, Women's, Psychiatric, Gerontic, and Home Health Considerations, ed 4. Philadelphia: F. A. Davis.
5. Lipson, J. G., Dibble, S. L., & Minarik, P. A. (1996). Culture & Nursing Care: A Pocket Guide. San Francisco: UCSF Nursing Press.
6. Doenges, M. E., Townsend, M. C., & Moorhouse, M. F. (1998). Psychiatric Care Plans Guidelines for Individualizing Care, ed 3. Philadelphia: F. A. Davis.
7. Pearce, J. C. (2002). The Biology of Trancendence a Blueprint of the Human Spirit. Rochester, VT: Park St Press.
8. Matzo M., et al. (2002). Teaching cultural consideration at the end of life. End of Life Nursing Education Consortium program recommendations. J Contin Edu Nurs, 33(6), 270–278.
9. Neeld, E. H. (2003). Seven Choices, ed 4. Austin, TX: Centerpoint Press.
10. Riely, M. (2003). Facilitating children's grief. J School Nurs, 19(4), 212–218.

risk for disproportionate Growth

Definition: At risk for growth above the 97th percentile or below the third percentile for age, crossing two percentile channels; disproportionate growth

RISK FACTORS

Prenatal
Maternal nutrition, multiple gestation
Substance use/abuse, teratogen exposure
Congenital/genetic disorders [e.g., dysfunction of endocrine gland, tumors]

Individual
Organic (e.g., pituitary tumors) and inorganic factors
Prematurity
Malnutrition; caregiver and/or individual maladaptive feeding behaviors; insatiable appetite; anorexia; [impaired metabolism, greater-than-normal energy requirements]
Infection; chronic illness [e.g., chronic inflammatory diseases]
Substance [use]/abuse [including anabolic steroids]

Environmental
Deprivation, poverty
Violence, natural disasters
Teratogen, lead poisoning

Caregiver

Abuse

Mental illness/retardation, severe learning disability

NOTE: A risk diagnosis is not evidenced by signs and symptoms, as the problem has not occurred and nursing interventions are directed at prevention.

SAMPLE CLINICAL APPLICATIONS: congenital/genetic disorders, prematurity, infection, nutritional problems (malnutrition, anorexia, failure to thrive, excessive intake), toxic exposures (e.g., lead), abuse/neglect, endocrine disorders, pituitary tumor

DESIRED OUTCOMES/EVALUATION CRITERIA

Sample **NOC** linkages:

Growth: A normal increase in body size and weight

Nutritional Status: Body Mass: Congruence of body weight, muscle, and fat to height, frame, and gender

Client Will (Include Specific Time Frame)

- Receive appropriate nutrition as indicated by individual needs.
- Demonstrate weight/growth stabilizing or progress toward age-appropriate size.
- Participate in plan of care as appropriate for age/ability.

Sample **NOC** linkages:

Child Development: [specify age group]: Milestones of physical, cognitive, and psychosocial progression by [specify] months/years of age

Caregiver Will (Include Specific Time Frame)

- Verbalize understanding of growth delay/deviation and plans for intervention

ACTIONS/INTERVENTIONS

Sample **NIC** linkages:

Nutritional Monitoring: Collection and analysis of patient data to prevent or minimize malnourishment

Teaching: Infant/Toddler Nutrition: Instruction on nutrition and feeding practices during the first/second and third years of life

Weight Management: Facilitating maintenance of optimal body weight and percent body fat

NURSING PRIORITY NO. 1. To assess causative/contributing factors:

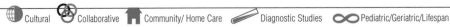

- Determine factors/condition(s) existing that could contribute to growth deviation as listed in Risk Factors, including familial history of pituitary tumors, Marfan's syndrome, genetic anomalies; prematurity; family living conditions of poverty, malnutrition, drug abuse, etc. *Information essential to developing plan of care.*[1]
- Identify nature and effectiveness of parenting/caregiving activities. *Inadequate, inconsistent caregiving, unrealistic/insufficient expectations, lack of stimulation, inadequate limit setting, lack of responsiveness indicate problems in parent-child relationship.*[4]
- Note severity/pervasiveness of situation (e.g., individual/SO showing effects of long-term physical/emotional abuse/neglect versus individual experiencing recent onset situational disruption or inadequate resources during period of crisis or transition).
- Assess significant stressful events, losses, separation and environmental changes (e.g., abandonment, divorce, death of parent/sibling, aging, move).

Cultural   Collaborative   Community/ Home Care   Diagnostic Studies   Pediatric/Geriatric/Lifespan   Medications

- Assess cognition, awareness, orientation, behavior of the client/caregiver. *Actions such as withdrawal/aggression, reactions to environment and stimuli provide information for identifying needs and planning care.*[1]
- Active-listen concerns about body size, ability to perform competitively (e.g., sports, body building) *to ascertain the potential for use of anabolic steroids/other drugs.*

NURSING PRIORITY NO. 2. To prevent/limit deviation from growth norms:

- Note chronological age, familial factors (body build/stature) *to determine growth expectations.* Note reported losses/alterations in functional level. *Provides comparative baseline.*
- Identify present growth age/stage. *Measurements are compared to "standard" or normal range for children of same gender and age.*
- Review expectations for current height/weight percentiles and degree of deviation. Plan for periodic evaluations. *Growth rates are measured in terms of how much a child grows within a specified time. These rates vary dramatically as a child grows (normal growth is a discontinuous process) and must be evaluated periodically over time to ascertain that child has definite growth disturbance. Accelerated or slowed growth rates are rarely normal and warrant further evaluation.*[1]
- Investigate deviations in height/weight/head size. *Deviations may include weight only (increased or decreased) or height (increased or decreased) and head size (disproportionate to rest of body). These deviations may be seen alone or in combination, all requiring additional testing over time to determine cause and effect on child's growth and development. Some are more urgent than others (e.g., small head size is evaluated further/treated as soon as identified, whereas short stature may require a longer evaluation period to determine if developmental problem exists).*[1]
- Determine if child's growth is above 97th percentile (very tall and large) for age. *Child should be further evaluated for endocrine disorders/pituitary tumor (could result in gigantism). Other disorders may be characterized by excessive weight for height (e.g., hypothyroidism, Cushing syndrome), abnormal sexual maturation or abnormal body/limb proportions.*[2]
- Determine if child's growth is below third percentile (very short and small) for age. *Child should have further evaluations for failure to thrive related to intrauterine growth retardation, prematurity/very low birth weight, small parents, poor nutrition, stress/trauma, or medical condition (e.g., intestinal disorders with malabsorption, diseases of heart, kidneys, diabetes mellitus). Treatment of underlying condition may alter/improve child's growth pattern.*[3]
- Perform nutritional assessment. *Overfeeding and malnutrition (protein and other basic nutrients) on a constant basis prevents children from reaching healthy growth potential, even if no disease/disorder is present. A well-balanced diet will help prevent or overcome this disorder.* Refer to ND imbalanced Nutrition: [specify].
- Review results of radiographs *(to determine bone age/extent of bone and soft-tissue growth),* laboratory studies *(to measure endocrine/hormone levels),* and diagnostic scans *(to identify tumors).*
- Assist with therapy to treat/correct underlying conditions (e.g., Crohn's disease, cardiac problems, or renal disease); endocrine problems (e.g., hypothyroidism, type 1 diabetes mellitus, growth hormone abnormalities); genetic/intrauterine growth retardation; infant feeding problems, nutritional deficits.
- Include nutritionist and other specialists as indicated (e.g., physical/occupational therapist) in developing plan of care. *Helpful in determining specific dietary needs for growth/weight reduction,*[6] *assistive devices to facilitate intake, or appropriate exercise programs.*
- Determine need for medications (e.g., appetite stimulants, antidepressants, growth hormones, etc.).

NURSING PRIORITY NO. 3. To promote wellness (Teaching/Discharge Considerations):

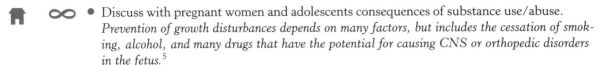 • Discuss with pregnant women and adolescents consequences of substance use/abuse. *Prevention of growth disturbances depends on many factors, but includes the cessation of smoking, alcohol, and many drugs that have the potential for causing CNS or orthopedic disorders in the fetus.*[5]

• Refer for genetic screening as appropriate. *There are many reasons for referral including (and not limited to) positive family history of a genetic disorder (e.g., fragile X syndrome, muscular dystrophy), woman with exposure to toxins/potential teratogenic agents, women older than 35 years at delivery, previous child born with congenital anomalies, history of intrauterine growth retardation, etc.*

• Provide information regarding normal growth as appropriate, including pertinent reference materials. *Bibliotherapy provides opportunity to review data at own pace, enhancing likelihood of retention.*

• Discuss appropriateness of appearance, grooming, touching, language, and other associated developmental issues. Refer to NDs delayed Growth and Development, risk for delayed Development, Self-Care Deficit [specify].

• Recommend involvement in regular monitored exercise/sports program *to enhance muscle tone/strength and appropriate body building.*

• Discuss actions to take to prevent/limit complications associated with stature/size.

• Review prescribed medications (e.g., growth hormone, thyroid replacement) noting potential side effects/adverse reactions *to promote adherence to regimen and reduce risk of untoward responses.*

• Identify available community resources as appropriate (e.g., public health programs such as WIC, medical equipment suppliers, nutritionist, substance abuse programs, specialists in endocrine problems/genetics).

• Stress importance of regular follow-up *to monitor progress of growth/weight changes.*

DOCUMENTATION FOCUS

Assessment/Reassessment
- Assessment findings/individual needs, including current growth status, and trends.
- Caregiver's understanding of situation and individual role.

Planning
- Plan of care and who is involved in the planning.
- Teaching plan.

Implementation/Evaluation
- Client's responses to interventions/teaching and actions performed.
- Caregiver response to teaching.
- Attainment/progress toward desired outcome(s).
- Modifications to plan of care.

Discharge Planning
- Identified long-range needs and who is responsible for actions to be taken.
- Specific referrals made, sources for assistive devices, educational tools.

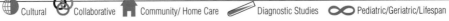 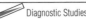

References

1. Leglar, J. D. and Rose, L. C. (1998). Assessment of abnormal growth curves, Article for "Problem-Oriented Diagnoses" series for Department of Family Practice, University of Texas Health Science Center, San Antonio, TX. American Academy of Family Physicians website. Available at: http://www.aafp.org. Accessed September 2003.
2. Gigantism. (2003) Fact sheet: University of Pennsylvania Health System website. Available at: http://www.pennhealth.com.
3. Endocrinology and short stature. (2001). Patient Fact Sheets. The Endocrine Society website. Available at: http://www.endo society.org.
4. Gordon, T. (2000). Parent Effectiveness Training, updated edition. New York: Three Rivers Press.
5. Maloni J. A., et al. (2003). Implementing evidence-based practice: reducing risk for low birth weight through pregnancy smoking cessation. J Obstet Gynecol Neonatal Nurs, 32(5), 676–682.
6. American Dietetic Association: Nutrition in comprehensive program planning for persons with developmental disabilities (1996–1999). Available at: www.eatright.org/adap0297b.html. Accessed March 29, 1990.

delayed Growth and Development

Definition: Deviations from age-group norms

RELATED FACTORS

Inadequate caretaking, [physical/emotional neglect or abuse]

Indifference, inconsistent responsiveness, multiple caretakers

Separation from SOs

Environmental and stimulation deficiencies

Effects of physical disability [handicapping condition]

Prescribed dependence [insufficient expectations for self-care]

[Physical/emotional illness (chronic, traumatic), e.g., chronic inflammatory disease, pituitary tumors, impaired nutrition/metabolism, greater-than-normal energy requirements; prolonged/painful treatments; prolonged/repeated hospitalizations]

[Sexual abuse]

[Substance use/abuse]

DEFINING CHARACTERISTICS

Subjective

Inability to perform self-care or self-control activities appropriate for age

Objective

Delay or difficulty in performing skills (motor, social, or expressive) typical of age group; [loss of previously acquired skills, precocious or accelerated skill attainment]

Altered physical growth

Flat affect, listlessness, decreased responses

[Sleep disturbances, negative mood/response]

SAMPLE CLINICAL APPLICATIONS: congenital/genetic disorders, prematurity, infection, nutritional problems (malnutrition, anorexia, failure to thrive), toxic exposures (e.g., lead), substance abuse, endocrine disorders, abuse/neglect, developmental delay

DESIRED OUTCOMES/EVALUATION CRITERIA

Sample **NOC** linkages:

Child Development: [specify age group]: Milestones of physical, cognitive, and psychosocial progression by [specify] months/years of age

Physical Maturation: Female/Male: Normal physical changes in the female/male that occur with the transition from childhood to adulthood

---

Client Will (Include Specific Time Frame)
- Perform motor, social, and/or expressive skills typical of age group within scope of present capabilities.
- Perform self-care and self-control activities appropriate for age.
- Demonstrate weight/growth stabilization or progress toward age-appropriate size.

Sample **NOC** linkages:

Child Development: [specify age group]: Milestones of physical, cognitive, and psychosocial progression by [specify] months/years of age

Growth: A normal increase in body size and weight

Parents/Caregivers Will (Include Specific Time Frame)
- Verbalize understanding of growth/developmental delay/deviation and plan(s) for intervention.

ACTIONS/INTERVENTIONS

Sample **NIC** linkages:

Developmental Enhancement: Child/Adolescent [specify]: Facilitating or teaching parents/caregivers to facilitate the optimal gross motor, fine motor, language, cognitive, social, and emotional growth of preschool and school-age children/of individuals during the transition from childhood to adulthood

Nutritional Monitoring: Collection and analysis of patient data to prevent or minimize malnourishment

Developmental Care: Structuring the environment and providing care in response to the behavioral cues and states of the preterm infant

NURSING PRIORITY NO. **1.** To assess causative/contributing factors:

 • Determine existing condition(s) (e.g., limited intellectual capacity, physical disabilities, accelerated physical growth, early or delayed puberty, chronic illness, tumors, genetic anomalies, substance use/abuse, violence, poverty; multiple birth [twins]/minimal length of time between pregnancies). *These conditions contribute to growth/developmental deviation, necessitating specific evaluation and interventions depending on the situation.*[6]

- Identify child with developmental delays using standard screening tests. *Developmental surveillance is a flexible, ongoing process that involves the use of both skilled observation of the child and concerns of parents, health professionals, teachers and others to identify children with variations in normal growth and development.*[1]

• Determine nature of parenting/caretaking activities. *Presence of conflict and negative interaction between parent/caregiver and child (e.g., inadequate, inconsistent parenting, unrealistic/insufficient expectations; lack of stimulation, limit setting, and responsiveness) interferes with the development of age appropriate skills and maturation.*[1,3]

• Note severity/pervasiveness of situation (e.g., long-term physical/emotional abuse versus situational disruption or inadequate assistance during period of crisis or transition). *Problems existing over a long period may have more severe effects and require longer course of treatment to reverse.*

• Assess occurrence/frequency of significant stressful events, losses, separation and environmental changes (e.g., loss, separation, abandonment, divorce; death of parent/sibling; aging; unemployment, new job; moves; new baby/sibling, marriage, new stepparent). *Lack*

 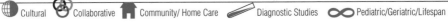

of resolution or repetition of stressor can have a cumulative effect over time and result in regression in/or deterioration of functional level.

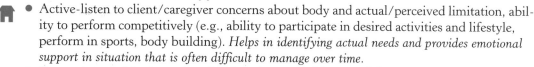

- Active-listen to client/caregiver concerns about body and actual/perceived limitation, ability to perform competitively (e.g., ability to participate in desired activities and lifestyle, perform in sports, body building). *Helps in identifying actual needs and provides emotional support in situation that is often difficult to manage over time.*

- Determine need for/use of medications (e.g., steroids, growth hormones), *which can affect body growth and development. Potential for good and for harm exists in the use of these agents.*

- Evaluate home/daycare/hospital/institutional environment *to determine adequacy of care provision, including nourishing meals, healthy sleep/rest time, stimulation, diversional or play activities.*

NURSING PRIORITY NO. 2. To determine degree of deviation from growth/developmental norms:

- Identify present growth age/stage. *Provides baseline for identification of needs and effectiveness of therapy.*[2]

- Review expectations for current height/weight percentiles. *Measurements are compared to "standard" or normal range for children of same gender and age to determine degree of deviation.*[2]

- Note chronological age, familial factors (body build/stature) *to help determine developmental expectations, (e.g., when child should roll over, sit up alone, speak first words, attain a certain weight/height, etc.), and how the expectations may be altered by child's condition. Pediatrician may screen with a motor quotient (MQ, which is child's age calculated by milestones met divided by chronological age and multiplied by 100). MQ between 50 and 70 requires further evaluation.*[3,9]

- Review expected skills/activities, using authoritative text (e.g., Gesell, Musen/Congor), reports of neurologic examinations, and/or assessment tools (e.g., Draw-a-Person, Denver Developmental Screening Test, Bender's Visual Motor Gestalt test. Early Language Milestone [ELM] Scale 2 and developmental language disorders [DLD]). *Provides guide for evaluation of growth and development, and for comparative measurement of individual's progress.*[4]

- Assess client/family for influence of cultural beliefs, norms, and values. *What is considered normal and abnormal development may be based on familial and cultural perceptions.*[5]

- Note signs of sexual maturation in child (e.g., development of pubic/axillary hair, breast enlargement, presence of body odor, acne, rapid linear growth, and adolescent-type behavior, with or without maturation of gonads). *Precocious puberty in females before age 8 or males before age 10 may occur because of lesions of hypothalamus/intracranial tumors.*

- Evaluate sexual behavior, as indicated. Investigate sexual acting-out behaviors inappropriate for age. *May indicate sexual abuse.*

- Note findings of psychological evaluation of client and family *to determine factors that can cause or exacerbate growth or development of client, or impair the psychological health of the family.*

NURSING PRIORITY NO. 3. To correct/minimize growth deviations and associated complications:

- Assist with therapies to treat/correct underlying conditions (e.g., intestinal malabsorption conditions, cardiac or kidney disease); endocrine problems (e.g., hypothyroidism, diabetes, growth hormone abnormalities); infant feeding problems, nutritional deficits. *May facilitate return to previous developmental levels or growth patterns.*

- Collaborate with physician, nutritionist, and other specialists (e.g., physical/occupational therapists) in developing plan of care. *Multidisciplinary team care increases likelihood of developing a well-rounded plan of care that meets client/family's specialized and varied needs.*

- Describe realistic, age-appropriate patterns of development to parent/caregiver, whether child's deviation is likely to be temporary or permanent (set-back or delay versus permanent brain injury); and promote activities and interactions that support developmental tasks where client is at this time. *Increases likelihood of commitment to interventions in keeping with the child's current status and potential. Each child will have own unique strengths and difficulties. Some children will catch up with other children in early childhood; some will have problems into adulthood.* [1,5,6]

- Recommend involvement in regular exercise/sports program *to enhance muscle tone/strength and appropriate body building.*

- Administer/monitor responses to medications. *May be given to stimulate growth as appropriate, or possibly to shrink tumor when present.* Stress necessity of not stopping medications without approval of healthcare provider *in order to maximize benefit and limit adverse side effects.*

- Prepare child for surgical interventions/radiation therapy when indicated to treat pituitary tumor. Discuss appropriateness and potential complications of bone-lengthening procedures.

- Plan for/stress importance of periodic evaluations. *Growth rates are measured in terms of how much a child grows within a specified time. These rates vary dramatically as a child grows (normal growth is a discontinuous process) and must be evaluated periodically over time to ascertain that child has definite growth disturbance. Accelerated or slowed growth rates are rarely normal and warrant further evaluation.* [2]

NURSING PRIORITY NO. 4. To assist clients (and/or caregivers) to prevent, minimize, or overcome delay/regressed or precocious development:

- Provide anticipatory guidance for parents/care providers regarding expectations for client's development *to clarify misconceptions, and assist them in dealing with reality of situation. May help in providing nurturing care.* [7]

- Communicate with client at appropriate cognitive level of development. Give client tasks and responsibilities appropriate to age or functional level *to model age and cognitively appropriate caregiver skills.* [8]

- Encourage client to perform activities of daily living (ADLs) as indicated. Discuss appropriateness of appearance, grooming, touching, language, play, safety, and other associated developmental issues. *Promotes independence and helps client develop sense of what is appropriate for age.*

- Involve client in opportunities to practice progress in activities of life, or to try new behaviors (e.g., role play, group activities). *Facilitates learning process/retention of new skills.*

- Encourage setting of short-term, realistic goals *for achieving developmental potential.* Evaluate progress on continual basis *to increase complexity of tasks/goals* as indicated.

- Consult additional professional resources (e.g., occupational/rehabilitation/speech therapists, special education teacher, job counselor) *to address specific individual needs.*

- Encourage recognition that certain deviations/behaviors are appropriate for a specific developmental age level (e.g., 14-year-old child functioning at level of 6-year-old child is

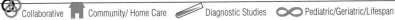

not able to anticipate the consequences of his or her actions) or chronological age (e.g., 9-year-old is displaying pubertal changes). *Promotes acceptance of client as presented and helps shape expectations reflecting actual situation.*

- Avoid blame when discussing contributing factors. *Parent/caregivers usually feel inadequate and blame themselves for being "a poor parent/care provider." Adding blame further diverts the individual's focus from learning new/changing behaviors to achieve the desired outcomes.*

- Maintain positive, hopeful attitude. Support self-actualizing nature of the individual and attempts to maintain or return to optimal level of self-control or self-care activities.

- Provide positive feedback for efforts/successes and adaptation while minimizing failures. *Encourages continuation of efforts, improving outcome.*

- Identify equipment needs/refer to suppliers (e.g., adaptive/growth-stimulating computer programs, communication devices) *to provide client/caregivers access to assistive devices that could improve involvement in/quality of life.*

- Assist client/caregivers to accept and adjust to irreversible developmental deviations (e.g., Down syndrome is not currently correctable). *Helps refocus attention and energy to areas that can be changed/improved.*

- Assist client/family to identify lifestyle changes that may be required (e.g., care for handicaps [blindness, musculoskeletal or cognitive deficits], proper use of assistive devices, learning new skills, development of routines and support systems).

- Provide support for caregiver during transitional crises (e.g., residential schooling, institutionalization).

- Refer family/client for counseling/psychotherapy *to deal with issues of grief and loss, time and stress management, lifestyle changes, abuse/neglect and other needs as indicated.*

NURSING PRIORITY NO. 5. To promote wellness (Teaching/Discharge Considerations):

- Provide information regarding normal growth and development process as appropriate. *Individuals need to know about normal process so deviations can be recognized when necessary.*

- Suggest genetic testing/counseling for family/client dependent on causative factors. *May be necessary for planning for future pregnancies.*

- Discuss consequences of substance use/abuse. *May be involved in the problems of growth/development that individual is experiencing.*

- Discuss actions to take *to avoid preventable complications* (e.g., periodic laboratory studies *to monitor hormone levels/nutritional status*).

- Recommend wearing medical alert bracelet when taking replacement hormones. *Provides information in case of an emergency.*

- Encourage attendance at appropriate educational programs. *Parenting classes, infant stimulation sessions, seminars on life stresses, aging process can provide information for client/family to learn to manage current situation and future changes.*

- Provide information regarding normal growth/development as appropriate, including pertinent reference materials. *Bibliotherapy provides opportunity to review data at own pace, enhancing likelihood of retention.*

- Discuss community responsibilities (e.g., services required to be provided to school-age child). Include social worker/special education team in process *to plan for meeting educational, physical, psychological, and monitoring needs of child.*

- Identify community resources as appropriate: public health programs such as Women, Infants, and Children (WIC), nutritionist, substance abuse programs; early intervention programs, seniors' activity/support groups, gifted and talented programs, Sheltered

Workshop, crippled children's services, medical equipment/supplier. *Provides additional assistance to support family efforts in treatment program.*

- Evaluate/refer to social services to determine safety of client and consideration of placement in foster care.
- Refer to the NDs impaired Parenting, interrupted Family Processes for additional interventions.

DOCUMENTATION FOCUS

Assessment/Reassessment
- Assessment findings/individual needs including current growth status/trends and developmental level/evidence of regression.
- Caregiver's understanding of situation and individual role.
- Safety of individual/need for placement.

Planning
- Plan of care and who is involved in the planning.
- Teaching plan.

Implementation/Evaluation
- Client's responses to interventions/teaching and actions performed.
- Caregiver response to teaching.
- Attainment/progress toward desired outcome(s).
- Modifications to plan of care.

Discharge Planning
- Identified long-range needs and who is responsible for actions to be taken.
- Specific referrals made; sources for assistive devices, educational tools.

References

1. Curry, D. M., & Duby, J. C. (1994). Developmental surveillance by pediatric nurses. Pediatr Nurs, 20, 40–44.
2. Leglar, J. D., & Rose, L. C. (1998). Assessment of abnormal growth curves, Article for "Problem-Oriented Diagnoses" series for Department of Family Practice, San Antonio, TX: University of Texas Health Science Center. Available at: http://www.aafp.org. Accessed September 2003.
3. Developmental Delays: A Pediatrician's Guide to your Children's Health and Safety. Available at: www.keepkidshealthy.com. Accessed July 2003.
4. American Academy of Child and Adolescent Psychiatry Working Group on Quality Issues. (1999). J Am Acad Child Adolesc Psychiatry, 38 (12 Suppl), 55S–76S. Available at: www.guideline.gov. Accessed July 2003.
5. Leininger, M. M. (1996). Transcultural Nursing: Theories, Research and Practices, ed 2. Hilliard, OH: McGraw-Hill.
6. Engel, J. (2002). Mosby's Pocket Guide to Pediatric Assessment. St Louis: Mosby.
7. Denehy, J. A. (1990). Anticipatory guidance. In Craft, M. J., Denehy, J. A. (eds): Nursing Interventions for Infants and Children. Philadelphia: WB Saunders.
8. McCloskey, J. C., & Bulechek, G. M. (eds). (1992). Nursing Interventions Classification (NIC). St. Louis: Mosby.
9. Educating parents of extra-special children: Developmental delays. Available at: www.epeconline.com/DevelopmentalDelays.html. Accessed January 2004.

Helpful Resource

Pediatric considerations. (2002). In Doenges, M. E., Moorhouse, M. F. & Geissler, A. C. Nursing Care Plans: Guidelines for Individualizing Patient Care, ed 6. CD-ROM. Philadelphia: F. A. Davis.

 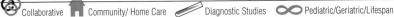

ineffective Health Maintenance

Definition: Inability to identify, manage, and/or seek out help to maintain health [This diagnosis contains components of other NDs. We recommend subsuming health maintenance interventions under the "basic" nursing diagnosis when a single causative factor is identified (e.g., deficient Knowledge (specify); ineffective Therapeutic Regimen Management, chronic Confusion, impaired verbal Communication, disturbed Thought Process, ineffective Coping, compromised family Coping, delayed Growth and Development).]

RELATED FACTORS

Lack of or significant alteration in communication skills (written, verbal, and/or gestural)
Unachieved developmental tasks
Lack of ability to make deliberate and thoughtful judgments
Perceptual or cognitive impairment (complete or partial lack of gross and/or fine motor skills)
Ineffective individual coping; dysfunctional grieving; disabling spiritual distress
Ineffective family coping
Lack of material resource; [lack of psychosocial supports]

DEFINING CHARACTERISTICS

Subjective

Expressed interest in improving health behaviors
Reported lack of equipment, financial and/or other resources; impairment of personal support systems
Reported inability to take the responsibility for meeting basic health practices in any or all functional pattern areas
[Reported compulsive behaviors]

Objective

Demonstrated lack of knowledge regarding basic health practices
Observed inability to take the responsibility for meeting basic health practices in any or all functional pattern areas; history of lack of health-seeking behavior
Demonstrated lack of adaptive behaviors to internal/external environmental changes
Observed impairment of personal support system; lack of equipment, financial and/or other resources
[Observed compulsive behaviors]

SAMPLE CLINICAL APPLICATIONS: chronic conditions (e.g., MS, rheumatoid arthritis, chronic pain), brain injury/stroke, spinal cord injury/paralysis, laryngectomy, dementia/Alzheimer's disease, developmental delay

DESIRED OUTCOMES/EVALUATION CRITERIA

Sample **NOC** linkages:

Health Promoting Behaviors: Actions to sustain or increase wellness
Knowledge: Health Behaviors: Extent of understanding conveyed about the promotion and protection of health
Participation: Health Care Decisions: Personal involvement in selecting and evaluating health care options

Client Will (Include Specific Time Frame)

- Identify necessary health maintenance activities.
- Verbalize understanding of factors contributing to current situation.
- Assume responsibility for own healthcare needs within level of ability.
- Adopt lifestyle changes supporting individual healthcare goals.

Sample **NOC** linkages: **Risk Detection**, Social Support: Perceived availability and actual provision of reliable assistance from others: Personal actions to identify personal health threats

SO/Caregiver Will (Include Specific Time Frame)

- Verbalize ability to cope adequately with existing situation, provide support/monitoring as indicated.

ACTIONS/INTERVENTIONS

Sample **NIC** linkages:

Health System Guidance: Facilitating a patient's location and use of appropriate health services

Support System Enhancement: Facilitation of support to patient by family, friends, and community

Health Education: Developing and providing instruction and learning experiences to facilitate voluntary adaptation of behavior conducive to health in individuals, families, groups, or communities

NURSING PRIORITY NO. 1. To assess causative/contributing factors:

 ● Determine level of dependence/independence and type/presence of developmental disabilities. *May range from complete dependence (dysfunctional) to partial or relative independence and determines type of interventions needed.*[1]

● Ascertain client's ability and desire to learn. Determine barriers to learning (e.g., can't read, speaks/understands different language, is overcome with stress or grief). *May not be physically, emotionally or mentally capable now because of current situation or may need information in small, manageable increments.*[1]

● Assess communication skills/ability/need for interpreter. Identify support person requiring/willing to accept information. *Ability to understand is essential to identification of needs and planning care. May need to provide the information to another individual if client is unable to comprehend.*[9]

● Note whether impairment is related to an acute/sudden onset situation, or a progressive illness/long-term health problem. *May require more intensive/long-lasting support.*[4]

● Evaluate for substance use/abuse (e.g., alcohol, narcotics). *Affects client's desire/ability to help self.*[6]

● Note desire/level of ability to meet health maintenance needs, as well as self-care ADLs. *Care may need to begin with helping client make a decision to improve ability as well as noting factors that are interfering with meeting needs.*[3]

● Note setting where client lives (e.g., long-term care facility, homebound, or homeless). *May contribute to inability/desire to meet healthcare needs.*[10]

● Ascertain recent changes in lifestyle. *For instance, a man whose wife dies and who has no skills for taking care of his own/family's health needs may need assistance to learn how to manage new situation.*[8]

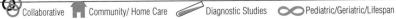 Cultural Collaborative Community/ Home Care Diagnostic Studies Pediatric/Geriatric/Lifespan Medications

- Determine level of adaptive behavior, knowledge, and skills about health maintenance, environment, and safety. *Will determine beginning point for planning and intervening to help client learn necessary skills to maintain health in a positive manner.*[7]
- Evaluate environment *to note individual adaptation* needs *(e.g., supplemental humidity, air purifier, change in heating system).*[1]
- Note client's use of professional services and resources (e.g., appropriate or inappropriate/nonexistent).[9]

NURSING PRIORITY NO. 2. To assist client/caregiver(s) to maintain and manage desired health practices:

- Develop plan with client/SO(s) for self-care. *Allows for incorporating existing disabilities, adapting and organizing care as necessary.*[1]
- Provide time to listen to concerns of client/SO(s). *Provides opportunity to clarify expectations/misconceptions.*
- Provide anticipatory guidance *to maintain and manage effective health practices during periods of wellness, and identify ways client can adapt when progressive illness/long-term health problems occur.*[9]
- Encourage socialization, "buddy system" and personal involvement *to enhance support system, provide pleasant stimuli, and limit permanent regression.*[2]
- Provide for communication and coordination between healthcare facility teams and community healthcare providers *to promote continuation of care/maximize outcomes.*[2]
- Involve comprehensive specialty health teams when available/indicated (e.g., pulmonary, psychiatric, enterostomal, IV therapy, nutritional support, substance abuse counselors).[9]
- Monitor adherence to prescribed medical regimen *to problem solve difficulties in adherence and alter the plan of care as needed.*[1]

NURSING PRIORITY NO. 3. To promote wellness (Teaching/Discharge Considerations):

- Provide information about individual healthcare needs, using client's preferred learning style (e.g., pictures, words, video, Internet). *Use of methods which help client to understand own situation can enhance cooperation with the plan of care.*[8]
- Limit amount of information presented at one time, especially when dealing with elderly client. Present new material through self-paced instruction when possible. *Allows client time to process and store new information.*[8]
- Help client/SO(s) develop realistic healthcare goals. Provide a written copy to those involved in planning process for future reference/revision as appropriate. *Promotes planning to enable the client to maintain a healthy/productive lifestyle.*[10]
- Assist client/SO(s) to develop stress management skills. *Knowing ways to manage stress helps individual to develop and maintain a healthy lifestyle.*[3]
- Identify ways to adapt exercise program *to meet client's changing needs/abilities and environmental concerns.*[5]
- Identify signs and symptoms requiring further evaluation and follow-up. *Essential to identify developing problems that could interfere with maintaining a healthy lifestyle.*[10]
- Make referral as needed for community support services (e.g., homemaker/home attendant, Meals on Wheels, skilled nursing care, Well-Baby Clinic, senior citizen healthcare activities). *May need additional assistance to maintain self-sufficiency.*[9]
- Refer to social services as indicated. *May need assistance with financial, housing, or legal concerns (e.g., conservatorship).*[2]

● Refer to support groups as appropriate (e.g., senior citizens, Red Cross, Salvation Army, Alcoholics or Narcotics Anonymous). *Provides information and help for specific needs.*[9]

 ● Arrange for hospice service for client with terminal illness. *Will help client and family deal with end-of-life issues in a positive manner.*[3,4]

DOCUMENTATION FOCUS

Assessment/Reassessment

● Assessment findings, including individual abilities, family involvement, and support factors/availability of resources.

Planning

● Plan of care and who is involved in planning.
● Teaching plan.

Implementation/Evaluation

● Responses of client/SO(s) to plan/interventions/teaching and actions performed.
● Attainment/progress toward desired outcome(s).
● Modifications to plan of care.

Discharge Planning

● Long-range needs and who is responsible for actions to be taken.
● Specific referrals made.

References

1. Bohny, B. (1997). A time for self-care: Role of the home healthcare nurse. Home Healthcare Nurs, 15(4), 281–286.
2. Callaghan, P., & Morrissey, G. (1993). Social support and health: A review. J Adv Nurs, 203, 18.
3. Dossey, B. M., & Dossey, L. (1998). Body-Mind-Spirit: Attending to holistic care. AJN, 998(6), 44.
4. Gregory, C. M. (1997). Caring for caregivers: Proactive planning eases burden on caregivers. Lifelines, 1(2), 51.
5. Lai, S. C., & Cohen, M. N. (1999). Promoting lifestyle changes. AJN, 99(4), 63.
6. Larsen, L. S. (1998). Effectiveness of counseling intervention to assist family caregivers of chronically ill relatives. J Psychosoc Nurs, 36(8), 26.
7. MacNeill, D., & Weis, T. (1998). Case study: Coordinating care. Continuing Care, 17(4), 78.
8. Pocinki, K. (1990). Writing for an older audience: Ways to maximize understanding and acceptance. AMWA, 3(5), 6.
9. Stuifbergen, A. (1997). Health promotion: An essential component of rehabilitation for persons with chronic disabling conditions. Adv Nurs Sci, 19(4), 138–147.
10. Healthy People 2010 Toolkit: A Field Guide for Health Planning. Washington, DC: Public Health Foundation. Available at: http://www.phf.org/HPtools/state.htm. Accessed February 2002.

Health-Seeking Behaviors (specify)

Definition: Active seeking (by a person in stable health) of ways to alter personal health habits and/or the environment in order to move toward a higher level of health (Note: Stable health is defined as achievement of age-appropriate illness-prevention measures; client reports good or excellent health, and signs and symptoms of disease, if present, are controlled.)

RELATED FACTORS

To be developed by nurse researchers and submitted to NANDA
[Situational/maturational occurrence precipitating concern about current health status]

 Cultural   Collaborative   Community/ Home Care   Diagnostic Studies   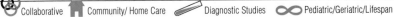 Pediatric/Geriatric/Lifespan   Medications

Subjective

Expressed desire to seek a higher level of wellness

Expressed desire for increased control of health practice

Expression of concern about current environmental conditions on health status

Stated unfamiliarity with wellness community resources

[Expressed desire to modify codependent behaviors]

Objective

Observed desire to seek a higher level of wellness

Observed desire for increased control of health practice

Demonstrated or observed lack of knowledge in health promotion behaviors, unfamiliarity with wellness community resources

SAMPLE CLINICAL APPLICATIONS: seasonal allergies/episodic asthma, familial risk factors for major disease conditions (e.g., myocardial infarction, breast cancer, hypertension), well-controlled chronic diseases (e.g., diabetes, MS, Crohn's)

DESIRED OUTCOMES/EVALUATION CRITERIA

Sample **NOC** linkages:

Health-Seeking Behavior: Actions to promote optimal wellness, recovery, and rehabilitation

Health-Promoting Behavior: Actions to sustain or increase wellness

Hope: Presence of internal state of optimism that is personally satisfying and life-supporting

Knowledge: Health Promotion: Extent of understanding of information needed to obtain and maintain optimal health

Client Will (Include Specific Time Frame)

- Express desire to change specific habit/lifestyle patterns to achieve/maintain optimal health.
- Participate in planning for change.
- Seek community resources to assist with desired change.

ACTIONS/INTERVENTIONS

Sample **NIC** linkages:

Self-Modification Assistance: Reinforcement of self-directed change initiated by the patient to achieve personally important goals

Health Education: Developing and providing instruction and learning experiences to facilitate voluntary adaptation of behavior conducive to health in individuals, families, groups, or communities

Health System Guidance: Facilitating a patient's location and use of appropriate health services

NURSING PRIORITY NO. 1. To assess specific concerns/habits/issues client desires to change:

- Ascertain client's belief about health and his/her ability to maintain health. *Belief in ability to accomplish desired action is predictive of performance.*[7]

Nursing Diagnoses in Alphabetical Order

- Discuss concerns with client and Active-listen to identify underlying issues (e.g., physical and/or emotional stressors; and/or external factors such as environmental pollutants or other hazards). *Helps to determine client's level of satisfaction with current health issues and readiness for change.*

- Review knowledge base and note coping skills that have been used previously to change behavior/habits. *Brings these to client's awareness and promotes use in current situation.*[1]

- Determine family and cultural perspectives, values, concerns and behaviors about health, well-being, and illness. *Influences client/SO and healthcare provider's perception of health and needs, which are not necessarily congruent. Also affects healthcare delivery systems and client's desire for/access to services.*[8]

- Use testing such as Myers-Briggs or other psychological tests, as indicated and review results with client/SO(s). *Can identify client strengths and help with development of plan of action. May also help client make decisions for the future.*[1]

- Identify behaviors that tend to promote or compromise health. *Identifies strengths and/or areas client may need to change, especially in long-term illnesses such as asthma, diabetes mellitus, or habits such as smoking or substance abuse.*[3]

NURSING PRIORITY NO. 2. To assist client to develop plan for improving health:

- Discuss risk-taking behaviors with client (e.g., smoking, drinking, self-medicating, lack of healthy food or exercise). Explore with client/SO(s) areas of health over which each individual has control and discuss barriers (e.g., lack of time, access to convenient facilities or safe environment in which to exercise). *Identifies actions individual can take to plan for improving health practices.*[5]

- Address barriers to health care (e.g., transportation services, lack of insurance, costs of services, unavailability of child/elder care, communication barriers, fear of/actual criticism from peers, etc.). *Nurse/other professionals can help reduce some of these barriers by advocating for the client and encouraging client's efforts in self-health.*[6]

- Problem-solve options for change. *Helps identify actions to be taken to achieve desired improvement.*[6]

- Provide information about conditions/health risk factors or concerns in desired format (e.g., pictures, TV programs, articles, handouts, audio/video tape, classes, group discussions, Internet, and other databases) as appropriate. *Use of multiple modalities enhances acquisition/retention of information and gives client choices for accessing and applying information.*

- Discuss assertive behaviors and provide opportunity for client to practice new behaviors. *Promotes positive change to improve lifetime healthcare practices for the individual.*[6]

- Use therapeutic communication skills. *Promotes effective interactions within the family and with helping resources to provide support for desired changes.*[1]

NURSING PRIORITY NO. 3. To promote wellness (Teaching/Discharge Considerations):

- Acknowledge client's strengths in present health management and build on in planning for future. *Promotes feelings of self-esteem and recognition of current positive actions can help client progress in own care.*[5]

 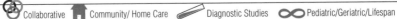 Cultural   Collaborative   Community/ Home Care   Diagnostic Studies   Pediatric/Geriatric/Lifespan   Medications

- Encourage use of exercise, relaxation skills, yoga, medication, visualization, and guided imagery *to assist in management of stress and promote general health/well being.*[2]
- Instruct in individually appropriate wellness behaviors. Regular scheduling of breast self-examination/mammogram, testicular self-examination/prostate examination; flu shots, immunizations, regular medical and dental examinations, healthy diet, exercise program. *Helps client efficiently manage health care practices.*[6]
- Identify and refer child/family member to health resources for immunizations, basic health services, and to learn health promotion/monitoring skills (e.g., monitoring hydration, measuring fever). *May facilitate long-term attention to health issues.*
- Refer to community resources (e.g., dietitian/weight control program, smoking cessation groups, Alcoholics Anonymous, codependency support groups, assertiveness training/Parent Effectiveness classes, clinical nurse specialists/psychiatrists) *to address specific concerns and apply health promotion skills.*[6]
- Refer to other wellness NDs such as readiness for enhanced Therapeutic Regimen Management, Knowledge, Nutrition, or Parenting for additional interventions as appropriate.

DOCUMENTATION FOCUS

Assessment/Reassessment
- Assessment findings including individual concerns/risk factors.
- Client's request for change.

Planning
- Plan of care and who is involved in planning.
- Teaching plan.

Implementation/Evaluation
- Responses to wellness plan, interventions/teaching and actions performed.
- Attainment/progress toward desired outcome(s).
- Modifications to plan of care.

Discharge Planning
- Long-range needs and who is responsible for actions to be taken.
- Specific referrals.

References

1. Townsend, M. C. (2003). Psychiatric Mental Health Nursing Concepts of Care, ed 4. Philadelphia: F. A. Davis.
2. Herrick, C. M., & Ainsworth, A. F. (2000). Invest in yourself: Yoga as a self-care strategy. Nurs Forum, 35(2), 32–36.
3. Patel, A. M. (2001). Using the Internet in the management of asthma. Curr Opin Pulm Med, 7(1), 39–42.
4. Rich, J. S., & Black, W. C. (2000). When should we stop screening. Eff Clin Pract, 3(2), 78–84.
5. U.S. Department of Health and Human Services: Healthy People 2000 national health promotion and disease prevention objectives. DHHS No (PHS) 91–50212, Washington, DC, 1991, U.S. Government Printing Office.
6. Healthy People 2010 Toolkit A Field Guide to Health Planning, February 2002. Available at: http://www.phf.org/HPtools/state.htm.
7. Fenn, M. (1998). Health promotion: Theoretical perspectives and clinical applications. Holis Nurs Pract, 19(2), 1–7.
8. Purnell, L. D., & Paulanka, B. J. (1998). Transcultural Health Care: A Culturally Competent Approach. Philadelphia: F. A. Davis.

Definition: Inability to independently maintain a safe growth-promoting immediate environment

RELATED FACTORS

Individual/family member disease or injury
Insufficient family organization or planning
Insufficient finances
Impaired cognitive or emotional functioning
Lack of role modeling
Unfamiliarity with neighborhood resources
Lack of knowledge
Inadequate support systems

DEFINING CHARACTERISTICS

Subjective

Household members express difficulty in maintaining their home in a comfortable [safe] fashion
Household requests assistance with home maintenance
Household members describe outstanding debts or financial crises

Objective

Accumulation of dirt, food, or hygienic wastes
Unwashed or unavailable cooking equipment, clothes, or linen
Overtaxed family members (e.g., exhausted, anxious)
Repeated hygienic disorders, infestations, or infections
Disorderly surroundings, offensive odors
Inappropriate household temperature
Lack of necessary equipment or aids
Presence of vermin or rodents

SAMPLE CLINICAL APPLICATIONS: chronic conditions (e.g., AIDS, MS, rheumatoid arthritis), depression, dementia, developmental delay

DESIRED OUTCOMES/EVALUATION CRITERIA

Sample **NOC** linkages:

Self-Care: Instrumental Activities of Daily Living [IADL]: Ability to perform activities needed to function in the home or community

Family Functioning: Ability of the family to meet the needs of its members through developmental transitions

Safety Behavior: Home Physical Environment: Individual or caregiver actions to minimize environmental factors that might cause physical harm or injury in the home

Client/Caregiver Will (Include Specific Time Frame)

- Identify individual factors related to difficulty in maintaining a safe environment.
- Verbalize plan to eliminate health and safety hazards.
- Adopt behaviors reflecting lifestyle changes to create and sustain a healthy/growth-promoting environment.
- Demonstrate appropriate, effective use of resources.

 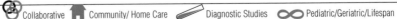

ACTIONS/INTERVENTIONS

Sample **NIC** linkages:

Home Maintenance Assistance: Helping the patient/family to maintain the home as a clean, pleasant place to live

Environmental Management: Manipulation of the patient's surroundings for therapeutic benefit

Support System Enhancement: Facilitation of support to patient by family, friends, and community

NURSING PRIORITY NO. 1. To assess causative/contributing factors:

- Identify presence of/potential for conditions such as diabetes, fractures/spinal cord injury; amputation, multiple sclerosis, arthritis, stroke, Parkinson's disease, mental illness (schizophrenia) *that can compromise client/SO's functional abilities in taking care of home.*[3]

- Note presence of personal and/or environmental factors (e.g., severe depression, memory lapses/dementia; high-risk newborn or family member with multiple care tasks; substance abuse; absence of family or support systems) *that may overwhelm caregiver with responsibilities.*[2]

- Determine reason for problem in the household and degree of discomfort and unsafe conditions noted by client/SO. *Some safety problems may be immediately obvious (e.g., lack of heat, water) while other problems may be more subtle and difficult to manage (e.g., lack of sufficient finances for home repairs, or lack of knowledge about food storage or rodent control). Client and/or SO may need assistance or teaching regarding safety of their environment if it is negatively impacting their health.*[2]

- Assess level of cognitive/emotional/physical functioning *to ascertain client's needs and caregiver's capabilities when developing plan of care for preventive, supportive, and therapeutic care.*[1]

- Identify lack of knowledge/misinformation *to determine need for health education/home safety program.*

- Discuss home environment/perform home visit as indicated *to determine client's ability to care for self, to identify potential health and safety hazards, and to determine adaptations that may be needed (e.g., wheelchair accessible doors/hallways, safety bars in bathroom, safe place for child play, clean water available, working cook stove/microwave, screens on windows).*[2]

- Identify support systems available to client/SO(s) *to determine needs and initiate referrals (e.g., companionship, daily care, respite care, homemaking, running errands, meal preparation or meal-service program, financial assistance, etc.).*[1]

- Determine financial resources to meet needs of individual situation. *May need referral to social services for funds, necessary equipment, home repairs, transportation, etc.*[2]

NURSING PRIORITY NO. 2. To help client/SO(s) to create/maintain a safe, growth-promoting environment:

- Coordinate planning with multidisciplinary team and client/SO. *Coordination and cooperation of team improves motivation and maximizes outcomes.*

- Assist client/SO(s) to develop plan for maintaining a clean, healthful environment. *Activities such as sharing of household tasks/repairs between family members, contract services, exterminators, trash removal can promote ongoing maintenance.*

- Assist client/SO(s) to identify and acquire necessary equipment and services (e.g., chair/stair lifts, commode chair, safety grab bar, structural adaptations, service animals, aids for hearing/seeing, mobility; trash removal, cleaning supplies) *to meet individual needs.*[3]

 • Identify resources available for appropriate assistance (e.g., visiting nurse, budget counseling, homemaker, Meals on Wheels, physical/occupational therapy, social services).[2]

 • Identify options for financial assistance with housing needs. *Client may be able to stay in home with minimal assistance, or may need significant assistance over a wide range of possibilities, including removal from the home.*[2]

NURSING PRIORITY NO. 3. To promote wellness (Teaching/Discharge Considerations):

 • Evaluate client at each community contact or before facility discharge *to determine if home maintenance needs are ongoing in order to initiate appropriate referrals.*[3]

 • Identify environmental hazards that may negatively affect health. Discuss long-term plan for taking care of environmental needs.

 • Provide information necessary for the individual situation. *Helps client/family decide what can be done to improve situation.*[3]

 • Identify community resources and support systems (e.g., extended family, neighbors, church group, seniors program).

• Refer to NDs deficient Knowledge (specify), Self-Care deficit [specify], Caregiver Role Strain, ineffective Coping, compromised family Coping, risk for Injury for additional interventions as appropriate.

DOCUMENTATION FOCUS

Assessment/Reassessment
• Assessment findings include individual/environmental factors, presence and use of support systems.

Planning
• Plan of care and who is involved in planning; support systems and community resources identified.
• Teaching plan.

Implementation/Evaluation
• Client's/SO's responses to interventions/teaching and actions performed.
• Attainment/progress toward desired outcome(s).
• Modifications to plan of care.

Discharge Planning
• Long-term needs and who is responsible for actions to be taken.
• Specific referrals made, equipment needs/resources.

References

1. Townsend, M. C. (2003). Psychiatric Mental Health Nursing Concepts of Care, ed 4. Philadelphia: F. A. Davis.
2. Available at: http://www.msue.msu.edu/msue/imp/mod02/master02.html Accessed 2003.
3. Fenn, M. (1998). Health promotion: Theoretical perspectives and clinical application. Holis Nurs Pract, 19(2), 1–7.
4. Purnell, L. D., & Paulanka, B. J. (1998). Transcultural Health Care: A Culturally Competent Approach. Philadelphia: F. A. Davis.

 Cultural Collaborative Community/ Home Care Diagnostic Studies 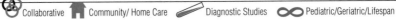 Pediatric/Geriatric/Lifespan Medications

Hopelessness

Definition: Subjective state in which an individual sees limited or no alternatives or personal choices available and is unable to mobilize energy on own behalf

RELATED FACTORS
Prolonged activity restriction creating isolation
Failing or deteriorating physiologic condition
Long-term stress; abandonment
Lost belief in transcendent values/God

DEFINING CHARACTERISTICS

Subjective
Verbal cues (despondent content, "I can't," sighing); [believes things will not change/problems will always be there]

Objective
Passivity, decreased verbalization
Decreased affect
Lack of initiative
Decreased response to stimuli, [depressed cognitive functions, problems with decisions, thought processes; regression]
Turning away from speaker; closing eyes; shrugging in response to speaker
Decreased appetite, increased/decreased sleep
Lack of involvement in care/passively allowing care
[Withdrawal from environs]
[Lack of involvement/interest in SOs (children, spouse)]
[Angry outbursts]

SAMPLE CLINICAL APPLICATIONS: chronic conditions, terminal diagnoses, infertility

DESIRED OUTCOMES/EVALUATION CRITERIA
Sample **NOC** linkages:
Depression Control: Personal actions to minimize melancholy and maintain interest in life events
Hope: Presence of internal state of optimism that is personally satisfying and life-supporting
Quality of Life: An individual's expressed satisfaction with current life circumstances

Client Will (Include Specific Time Frame)
- Recognize and verbalize feelings.
- Identify and use coping mechanisms to counteract feelings of hopelessness.
- Involve self in and control (within limits of the individual situation) own self-care and ADLs.
- Set progressive short-term goals to develop/foster/sustain behavioral changes/outlook.
- Participate in diversional activities of own choice.

ACTIONS/INTERVENTIONS
Sample **NIC** linkages:
Hope Instillation: Facilitation of the development of a positive outlook in a given situation

---

Emotional Support: Provision of reassurance, acceptance, and encouragement during times of stress

Mood Management: Providing for safety, stabilization, recovery, and maintenance of a patient who is experiencing dysfunctionally depressed or elevated mood

NURSING PRIORITY NO. 1. To identify causative/contributing factors:

 • Review familial/social history and physiologic history contributing to current problems. *History of poor coping abilities, disorder of familial relating patterns, emotional problems, language/cultural barriers (leading to feelings of isolation), recent or long-term illness of client or family member, multiple social and/or physiologic traumas to individual or family members can all affect client's feelings of hopelessness.*[2]

 • Note current familial/social/physical situation of client. *Issues such as the newly diagnosed chronic/terminal disease, language/cultural barriers, lack of support system, recent job loss, loss of spiritual/religious faith, recent multiple traumas can result in an individual giving up. Identification of the issues involved in each person's situation are necessary to appropriately plan for care.*[2]

 • Determine coping behaviors and defense mechanisms displayed previously and in current situation as well as client's perception of effectiveness then and now. *It is important to identify client's strengths and encourage their use as client begins to deal with what is currently happening.*[2]

 • Have client describe events that lead to feeling inadequate or having no control. *Identifies sources of frustration and defines problem areas so action can be taken to learn how to deal with them in more positive ways.*[6]

 • Determine presence of suicidal ideation, availability of plan, and means to follow through with plan. *Hopelessness is identified as a central underlying factor in the predisposition to suicide, and the client sees no other way out of a hopeless situation.*[7] Refer to ND risk for suicide

NURSING PRIORITY NO. 2. To assess level of hopelessness:

 • Note behaviors indicative of hopelessness. (Refer to Defining Characteristics.) *Provides information to develop effective plan of care and suggests possible resources needed.*[6]

 • Evaluate/discuss use of defense mechanisms (useful or not). *Identifying behaviors such as increased sleeping, use of drugs, illness behaviors, eating disorders, denial, forgetfulness, daydreaming, ineffectual organizational efforts, exploiting own goal setting, and regression can provide accurate information for client to begin changing behavior/inaccurate beliefs.*[6]

 • Discuss client's feelings about life not being worth living and other signs of hopelessness and worthlessness. Evaluate degree of hopelessness using psychological testing. *Identifying the degree of hopelessness and suicidal ideation is crucial to instituting treatment to prevent the client from carrying out the plan.*[10]

NURSING PRIORITY NO. 3. To assist client to identify feelings and to begin to cope with problems as perceived by the client:

 • Establish a therapeutic/facilitative relationship showing positive regard for the client. *Client may then feel safe to disclose feelings and feel understood and listened to.*[3]

 • Explain all tests/procedures thoroughly. Involve client in planning schedule for care. Answer questions truthfully. *Promotes understanding and sense of control to enhance trust and therapeutic relationship.*[2]

 • Encourage client to verbalize and explore feelings and perceptions of what is happening. *Talking about feelings of anger, helplessness, powerlessness, confusion, despondency, isolation,*

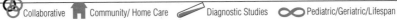 Cultural   Collaborative   Community/ Home Care   Diagnostic Studies   Pediatric/Geriatric/Lifespan   Medications

and grief (which can lead to a sense of hopelessness and the belief that nothing can be done) provides opportunity for reflection and enables client to begin to understand self and that there are actions that can be helpful.[3]

- Provide opportunity for children to "play out" feelings (e.g., puppets or art for preschooler, peer discussions for adolescents). *Provides insight into perceptions and can give direction for developing coping strategies.*[2]

- Express hope to client and encourage SOs and other health-team members to also do so. Avoid expressions of false hope. *Client may not identify positives in own situation and may find it difficult to accept them from others, but will hear them. False reassurances will undermine sense of security.*[2]

- Assist client to identify short-term goals. Promote activities to achieve goals, and facilitate contingency planning. *Dealing with situation in manageable steps, enhances chances for success, promotes sense of control, and encourages belief that there is hope for resolution of situation.*[6]

- Discuss current options and list actions, in conjunction with the client, that can be taken. Correct misconceptions expressed by the client. *Encourages use of own actions, validates reality and promotes sense of control of the situation.*[2]

- Endeavor to prevent situations that might lead to feelings of isolation or lack of control in client's perception. *Client will interpret these occurrences as further proof that there is no hope.*[6]

- Promote client control in establishing time, place, and frequency of treatment/therapy sessions. *Involve family members in the appointments as appropriate. Allows individual to assume control over own situation, engendering positive feelings of ability to manage what is happening. Involvement of family members provides support and encouragement for client.*[2]

- Help client recognize areas in which he or she has control versus those that are not within his or her control. *Often the individual who is feeling hopeless is focusing on issues that cannot be changed. When the client begins to focus on things that are within control, a sense of hope can be nurtured.*[6]

- Encourage risk-taking in situations in which the client can succeed. *Succeeding in new ventures can improve self-esteem and hope for more successful actions.*[2]

- Help client begin to develop new coping mechanisms. *These can be learned and used effectively to counteract hopelessness.*[3]

- Encourage structured/controlled increase in physical activity as tolerated. *Promotes the release of endorphins, enhancing sense of well-being.*[2]

- Demonstrate and encourage use of relaxation exercises, guided imagery. *Anxious feelings create tension and learning to relax can help client begin to look at possibilities of feeling more hopeful.*[9]

NURSING PRIORITY NO. 4. To promote wellness (Teaching/Discharge Considerations):

- Provide positive feedback for actions taken to deal with and overcome feelings of hopelessness. *Encourages changes in thinking patterns and continuation of desired behaviors.*[10,12]

- Assist client/family to become aware of factors/situations leading to feelings of hopelessness. *Helps individuals to identify precipitating events and provides opportunities to avoid/modify situation, promoting sense of control over life.*[8]

- Discuss initial signs of hopelessness. *Helps client to identify behaviors such as procrastination, increased need for sleep, decreased physical activity, and withdrawal from social/familial activities and how they have affected thinking and ability to deal with current situation. Awareness provides the opportunity to begin to change.*[9]

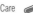

- Facilitate client's incorporation of personal loss. *Often losses in individual's life result in feelings of hopelessness and lack of control in current events that are happening. Enhancing grief work and promoting resolution of feelings helps client to begin to feel hope again and look forward to life.*[9]
- Encourage client/family to develop support systems in the immediate community. *Having support close at hand provides individuals with assistance, advocacy for moving forward enabling them to look toward future with hope.*[6]
- Help client to become aware of, nurture, and expand spiritual self. (Refer to ND Spiritual Distress.) *Acknowledging and learning about spiritual aspect of self can help client look toward the future with hope for improved sense of well-being.*[11]
- Introduce the client into a support group before the individual therapy is terminated for continuation of therapeutic process. *Provides for a smooth transition so client feels accepted and comfortable in the presence of others.*[6]
- Refer to other resources for assistance as indicated (e.g., clinical nurse specialist, psychiatrist, social services, spiritual advisor). *May need additional help to develop hope for the future, sustain efforts for change.*[2]

DOCUMENTATION FOCUS

Assessment/Reassessment
- Assessment findings, including degree of impairment, use of coping skills and support systems.

Planning
- Plan of care and who is involved in planning.
- Teaching plan.

Implementation/Evaluation
- Responses to interventions/teaching and actions performed.
- Attainment/progress toward desired outcome(s).
- Modifications to plan of care.

Discharge Planning
- Identified long-range needs/client's goals for change and who is responsible for actions to be taken.
- Specific referrals made.

References

1. Doenges, M. E., Moorhouse, M. F., & Geissler-Murr, A. C. (2002). Nurse's Pocket Guide: Diagnoses, Interventions, and Rationales, ed 8. Philadelphia: F. A. Davis.
2. Townsend, M. C. (2003). Psychiatric Mental Health Nursing Concepts of Care, ed 4. Philadelphia: F. A. Davis.
3. Gordon, T. (2000). Parent Effectiveness Training, updated edition. New York: Three Rivers Press.
4. Cox, H. C., et al (2002). Clinical Applications of Nursing Diagnosis: Adult, Child, Women's, Psychiatric, Gerontic, and Home Health Considerations, ed 4. Philadelphia: F. A. Davis.
5. Lipson, J. G., Dibble, S. L., & Minarik, P. A. (1996). Culture & Nursing Care: A Pocket Guide. San Francisco: UCSF Nursing Press.
6. Doenges, M. E., Townsend, M. C., & Moorhouse, M. (1998). Psychiatric Care Plans Guidelines for Individualizing Care, ed 3. Philadelphia: F. A. Davis.
7. Ghosh, T. B., & Victor, B. S. (1994). Suicide. In Hales, R. R., Yudofsky, S. C., & Talbott, J. A. (eds): The American Psychiatric Press Textbook of Psychiatry, ed 2. Washington, DC: American Psychiatric Press.
8. Drew, B. (1990). Differentiation of hopelessness, helplessness, and powerlessness using Erik Erikson's "Roots of Virtue". Arch Psychiatr Nurs, 4, 332.

 Cultural Collaborative Community/ Home Care Diagnostic Studies 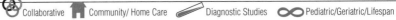 Pediatric/Geriatric/Lifespan Medications

9. Miller, J. F. (2000). Coping with Chronic illness: Overcoming Powerlessness. Philadelphia: F. A.Davis.
10. Beck, A. T., Brown, G., & Berchick, R. J. (1990). Relationship between hopelessness and ulimate suicide: A replication with psychiatric out-patients. Am J Psychiatry 147, 190–195.
11. Pearce, J. C. (2000). The Biology of Trancendence a Blueprint of the Human Spirit. Rochester, VT: Park St Presss.
12. Seligman, M. E. P. (1998). Learned Optimism: How to Change Your Mind & Your Life. New York Pocket Books/Simon & Schuster.

Hyperthermia

Definition: Body temperature elevated above normal range

RELATED FACTORS

Exposure to hot environment; inappropriate clothing
Vigorous activity; dehydration
Inability or decreased ability to perspire
Medications or anesthesia
Increased metabolic rate; illness or trauma

DEFINING CHARACTERISTICS

Subjective
[Headache]
[Weakness, faintness]
[Thirst/absence of thirst]
[Nausea]

Objective
Increase in body temperature above normal range
[Dry], flushed skin; warm to touch
Increased respiratory rate, tachycardia; [unstable BP]
Seizures or convulsions; [muscle rigidity/fasciculation]
[Confusion, combativeness, delirium, coma]

SAMPLE CLINICAL APPLICATIONS: infectious diseases, head trauma, hyperthyroidism, heat exhaustion/stroke, surgical procedure/anesthesia

DESIRED OUTCOMES/EVALUATION CRITERIA

Sample **NOC** linkages:

Thermoregulation: Balance among heat production, heat gain, and heat loss

Thermoregulation: Neonate: Balance among heat production, heat gain, and heat loss during the neonatal period

Safety Behavior: Personal: Individual or caregiver efforts to control behaviors that might cause physical injury

Client Will (Include Specific Time Frame)
- Maintain core temperature within normal range.
- Be free of complications such as irreversible brain/neurological damage, and acute renal failure.
- Identify underlying cause/contributing factors and importance of treatment, as well as signs/symptoms requiring further evaluation or intervention.
- Demonstrate behaviors to monitor and promote normothermia.
- Be free of seizure activity.

ACTIONS/INTERVENTIONS

Sample **NIC** linkages:

Temperature Regulation: Attaining and/or maintaining body temperature within a normal range

Fever Treatment: Management of a patient with hyperpyrexia caused by nonenvironmental factors

Malignant Hyperthermia Precautions: Prevention or reduction of hypermetabolic response to pharmacological agents used during surgery

NURSING PRIORITY NO. 1. To assess causative/contributing factors:

- Identify underlying cause *(e.g., **excessive heat production** such as occurs with strenuous exercise, fever, shivering, tremors, convulsions, hyperthyroid state, infection/sepsis; malignant hyperpyrexia/heat stroke, sympathomimetic drugs; **impaired heat dissipation** such as occurs with heatstroke, dermatologic diseases, burns, inability to perspire such as occurs with spinal cord injury and certain medications [e.g., diuretics, sedatives, certain heart and blood pressure medications]; **hypothalamic dysfunction causing loss of thermoregulation** such as may occur in infections, brain lesions, drug overdose).*[1]

- Note chronological and developmental age of client. *Infants, young children, and elderly persons are most susceptible to damaging hyperthermia. Environmental factors and relatively minor infections can produce a much higher temperature in infants and young children than older children and adults. Infants, children, or impaired individuals are not able to protect themselves, and cannot recognize and/or act on symptoms of hyperthermia. Elderly persons have age-related risk factors (e.g. poor circulation, inefficient sweat glands, skin changes caused by normal aging, chronic diseases).*[1–4]

NURSING PRIORITY NO. 2. To evaluate effects/degree of hyperthermia[1–3,5,6]:

- Monitor core temperature by appropriate route (e.g., tympanic, rectal). Note presence of temperature elevation (>98.6 °F [37 °C]) or fever (100.4 °F [38 °C]). *Rectal and tympanic temperatures most closely approximate core temperature; however, shell temperatures (oral, axillary, touch) are often measured at home and are predictive of fever. Rectal temperature measurement may be the most accurate, but is not always expedient (e.g., client declines, is agitated, has rectal lesions or surgery, etc.). Abdominal temperature monitoring may be done in the premature neonate.*

- Assess whether body temperature reflects heatstroke. *Defined as body temperature higher than 106 °F (41.1 °C) that is associated with neurological dysfunction and is potentially life-threatening.*[1]

- Assess neurologic response, noting level of consciousness and orientation, reaction to stimuli, reaction of pupils, presence of posturing or seizures. *High fever accompanied by changes in mentation may indicate septic state or heatstroke.*

- Monitor blood pressure and invasive hemodynamic parameters if available (e.g., cardiac output, arterial pressures). *Hypodynamic state can occur, especially in person with preexisting cardiovascular disease if heat-related illness (e.g., heat stroke or malignant hyperthermia reaction to anesthesia) has rendered the client critically ill.*

- Monitor heart rate and rhythm. *Tachycardia, dysrhythmias and ECG changes are common due to electrolyte and acid-base imbalance, dehydration, specific action of catecholamines, and direct effects of hyperthermia on blood and cardiac tissue.*

- Monitor respirations. *Hyperventilation may initially be present, but ventilatory effort may eventually be impaired by seizures, hypermetabolic state (shock and acidosis).*

 Cultural Collaborative Community/ Home Care 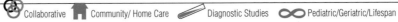 Diagnostic Studies Pediatric/Geriatric/Lifespan Medications

- Auscultate breath sounds *to note presence/progression of adventitious sounds such as crackles (rales) especially when heart failure or pneumonia is present.*
- Monitor/record all sources of fluid loss such as urine *(oliguria and/or renal failure may occur due to hypotension, dehydration, shock, and tissue necrosis)*; vomiting and diarrhea, wounds/fistulas, and insensible losses *(potentiates fluid and electrolyte losses).*
- Note presence/absence of sweating. *The body attempts to increase heat loss by evaporation, conduction, and diffusion. Evaporation is decreased by environmental factors of high humidity and high ambient temperature as well as body factors producing loss of ability to sweat or sweat gland dysfunction (e.g., spinal cord transection, cystic fibrosis, dehydration, and vasoconstriction).*

- Monitor laboratory studies such as ABGs, electrolytes, cardiac and liver enzymes *(may reveal tissue degeneration)*; glucose *(hypoglycemia)*; BUN/Cr *(acute renal failure)*; urinalysis *(myoglobinuria, proteinuria, and hemoglobinuria can occur as products of tissue necrosis).*[1]

NURSING PRIORITY NO. 3. To assist with measures to reduce body temperature/restore normal body/organ function[1–,3,5,6]:

- Administer antipyretics, orally/rectally (e.g., aspirin, acetaminophen), as ordered.
  Promote cooling by means of:
  Limiting clothing/dressing in lightweight, loose-fitting clothes. *Encourages heat loss by radiation and conduction.*
  Cool the environment with air-conditioning or fans. *Promotes heat loss by convection.*
  Provide cool/tepid sponge baths or immersion if temperature is >104 °F *for heat loss by evaporation and conduction,* or local ice packs, especially in groin and axillae (Note: In pediatric clients especially, room temperature [tepid] water is preferred *as cold-water sponges/immersion can increase shivering, producing heat and increasing fever.*)

  Lavage body cavities with cold water in presence of malignant hyperthermia *to promote core cooling.*
  Keep clothing and linens dry *to reduce shivering.*

  Use hypothermia blanket wrapping extremities with bath towels *to minimize shivering.*
    Turn off hypothermia blanket when core temperature is within 1° to 3° of desired temperature *to allow for downward drift.*

  Administer medications (e.g., dantrolene, chlorpromazine, or diazepam) as ordered, *to manage hyperthermia, control shivering and seizures.*

- Provide hydration:
  Offer/force plenty of fluids, by appropriate route (e.g., oral, IV) even if client is not thirsty to *replace fluids lost through perspiration and respiration.*
  Avoid alcohol and caffeinated beverages *(increases fluid loss by diuresis).*
  Administer replacement IV fluids and electrolytes *to support circulating volume and tissue perfusion and treat acid-base imbalance.*
- Promote client safety (e.g., maintain patent airway, padded side rails, quiet environment; mouth care for dry mucous membranes, skin protection from cold when hypothermia blanket is used, observation of equipment safety measures).
- Maintain bedrest *to reduce metabolic demands/oxygen consumption.*

- Provide supplemental oxygen *to offset increased oxygen demands and consumption.*
- Administer medications as indicated *to treat underlying cause, such as antibiotics (for infection), dantrolene (for malignant hyperthermia), β-blockers (for thyroid storm).*

- Provide high-calorie diet, tube feedings, or parenteral nutrition *to meet increased metabolic demands.*

NURSING PRIORITY NO. 4. To promote wellness (Teaching/Discharge Considerations):

- Teach parents how to measure child's temperature, at what body temperature to give antipyretic medications, and what symptoms to report to physician. *Low-grade fever enhances immune system functioning in presence of infection and is not harmful as long as individual is not dehydrated or susceptible to febrile seizures.*[3,7] *Fever may be treated at home because of the general discomfort and lethargy associated with fever. Fever is reportable, however, especially if it is unresponsive to antipyretics and fluids, because it often accompanies a treatable infection (viral or bacterial).*[5]
- Instruct families/caregivers (of young children, persons who are outdoors in very hot climate, elderly living alone) in dangers of heat exhaustion and heat stroke and ways to manage hot environments. *Heat injuries can be immediately life-threatening. Being aware of environmental hazards and hydration levels can save one's life.*[8]
- Review client's specific cause such as underlying disease process (thyroid storm); environmental factors (heatstroke); reaction to anesthesia (malignant hyperthermia); loss of ability to perspire. *Helps to identify those factors that client can control (if any), such as correction of underlying disease process (e.g., thyroid suppression medication); ways to protect oneself from excessive exposure to environmental heat (e.g., proper clothing, restriction of activity, scheduling outings during cooler part of day); and understanding of family traits (e.g., malignant hyperthermia reaction to anesthesia is often familial).*[9]
- Discuss importance of adequate fluid intake at all times and ways to improve hydration status when ill, or when under stress (e.g., exercise, hot environment).
- Recommend avoidance of hot tubs/saunas as appropriate *(e.g., clients with cardiac conditions compromised by decreased cardiac output associated with peripheral vasodilation, pregnancy that may affect fetal development or increase maternal cardiac workload).*

DOCUMENTATION FOCUS

Assessment/Reassessment
- Temperature and other assessment findings, including vital signs and state of mentation.

Planning
- Plan of care/interventions and who is involved in the planning.
- Teaching plan.

Implementation/Evaluation
- Responses to interventions/teaching and actions performed.
- Attainment/progress toward desired outcome(s).
- Modifications to plan of care.

Discharge Planning
- Referrals that are made, those responsible for actions to be taken.

References

1. Helman, R. S. (2002). Heatstroke. Emedicine article. Available at http://www.emedicine.com. Accessed September 2003.
2. Evidence-based clinical practice guideline of fever of uncertain source: Outpatient evaluation and management for children 2 months to 36 months of age. (2002). Cincinnati, OH: Cincinnati Children's Hospital Medical Center. Available at: www.guideline.gov. Accessed September 2003.
3. Engel, J. (2002). Mosby's Pocket Guide to Pediatric Assessment, ed 4. St Louis: Mosby.
4. Brody, G. M. (1994). Hyperthermia and hypothermia in the elderly. Clin Geriatr Med, 10, 213.

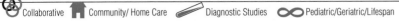 Cultural Collaborative Community/ Home Care Diagnostic Studies Pediatric/Geriatric/Lifespan Medications

5. Doenges, M. E., Moorhouse, M. F., & Geissler-Murr, A. C. (2004). Nurse's Pocket Guide: Diagnoses, Interventions, and Rationales, ed 9. Philadelphia: F. A. Davis.
6. Sepsis/Septicemia. (2002). In Doenges, M. E., Moorhouse, M. F., and Geissler-Murr, A. C. Nursing Care Plans: Guidelines for Individualizing Patient Care, ed 6. Philadelphia: F. A. Davis, pp 676–677.
7. Roberts, N. J. (1991). The immunological consequences of fever. In Mackowiak, P. A. (ed): Fever: Basic Mechanisms and Management. New York: Raven.
8. Curtis, R. (1997). Outdoor Action guide to heat related illnesses & fluid balance. Article for Princeton University Outdoor Action website. Available at: http://www.princeton.edu/~oa/safety/heatill.html. Accessed September 2003.
9. Malignant Hyperthermia. (1989). Dantrolene-Medstudents-Anesthesiology. Fact Sheet. National Institute on Aging. U.S. Dept Health and Human Services.

Hypothermia

Definition: Body temperature below normal range

RELATED FACTORS

Exposure to cool or cold environment [prolonged exposure, e.g., homeless, immersion in cold water/near drowning; induced hypothermia/cardiopulmonary bypass]

Inadequate clothing

Evaporation from skin in cool environment

Inability or decreased ability to shiver

Aging [or very young]

[Debilitating] illness or trauma, damage to hypothalamus

Malnutrition; decreased metabolic rate, inactivity

Consumption of alcohol; medications [/drug overdose] causing vasodilation

DEFINING CHARACTERISTICS

Objective

Reduction in body temperature below normal range

Shivering; piloerection

Cool skin

Pallor

Slow capillary refill; cyanotic nailbeds

Hypertension; tachycardia

[Core temperature 95 °F/35 °C: increased respirations, poor judgment, shivering]

[Core temperature 95 °F to 93.2 °F/35 ° to 34 °C: bradycardia or tachycardia, myocardial irritability/dysrhythmias, muscle rigidity, shivering, lethargic/confused, decreased coordination]

[Core temperature 93.2 °F to 86 °F/34 °C to 30 °C: hypoventilation, bradycardia, generalized rigidity, metabolic acidosis, coma]

[Core temperature below 86 °F/30 °C: no apparent vital signs, heart rate unresponsive to drug therapy, comatose, cyanotic, dilated pupils, apneic, areflexic, no shivering (appears dead)]

SAMPLE CLINICAL APPLICATIONS: dementia, malnutrition/anorexia nervosa, brain trauma/ stroke, some surgical procedures (e.g., craniotomy), alcohol intoxication, abuse/neglect, prematurity, near drowning/cold water immersion

DESIRED OUTCOMES/EVALUATION CRITERIA

Sample **NOC** linkages:

Thermoregulation: Individual or caregiver efforts to control behaviors that might cause physical injury

Thermoregulation: Neonate: Balance among heat production, heat gain, and heat loss during the neonatal period

Safety Behavior: Personal: Individual or caregiver efforts to control behaviors that might cause physical injury

Client Will (Include Specific Time Frame)
- Display core temperature within normal range.
- Be free of complications such as cardiac failure, respiratory infection/failure, thromboembolic phenomena.
- Identify underlying cause/contributing factors that are within client control.
- Verbalize understanding of specific interventions to prevent hypothermia.
- Demonstrate behaviors to monitor and promote normothermia.

ACTIONS/INTERVENTIONS
Sample **NIC** linkages:

Hypothermia Treatment: Rewarming and surveillance of a patient whose core body temperature is below 35 °C

Temperature Regulation: Attaining and/or maintaining body temperature within a normal range

Temperature Regulation: Intraoperative: Attaining and/or maintaining desired intraoperative body temperature

NURSING PRIORITY NO. **1.** To assess causative/contributing factors:

- Note underlying cause, e.g., 1) **decreased heat production** *such as occurs with hypopituitary, hypoadrenal and hypothyroid conditions, hypoglycemia and neuromuscular inefficiencies seen in extremes of age)*; 2) **increased heat loss** *(e.g., exposure to cold weather/cold wind; cold water drenching or immersion, improper clothing/shelter/food for conditions; vasodilation from medications, drugs or poisons; skin surface problems such as burns or psoriasis; fluid losses/dehydration; surgery, open wounds/exposed skin/viscera; multiple rapid infusions of cold solutions or transfusions of banked blood; over-treatment of hyperthermia)*; 3) **impaired thermoregulation** *(e.g., hypothalamus failure such as might occur with CNS trauma or tumor; intracranial bleeding/stroke; toxicologic and metabolic disorders; Parkinson's disease, multiple sclerosis).*[1,2]
- Note contributing factors: age of client (e.g., premature neonate, child, elderly person); concurrent/coexisting medical problems (e.g., brainstem injury, near drowning, sepsis, hypothyroidism, alcohol intoxication); nutrition status (e.g., thin tall person loses heat easier than short stature, fat person); living condition/relationship status (e.g., aged/cognitive impaired client living alone).

NURSING PRIORITY NO. **2.** To prevent further decrease in body temperature:

- Treat mild-to-moderate hypothermia[1–4]:
  Add layers of clothing. Remove wet clothing/bedding. Wrap in warm blankets.
  Increase physical activity if possible.
  Provide warm liquids after shivering stops if client is alert and can swallow.
  Provide warm nutrient-dense food (carbohydrates, proteins, and fats) and fluids (hot sweet liquids are easily digestible and absorbable).
  Avoid alcohol, caffeine, and tobacco *(to prevent vasodilation, diuresis, or vasoconstriction, respectively)*

 Cultural Collaborative Community/ Home Care 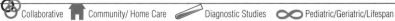 Diagnostic Studies Pediatric/Geriatric/Lifespan Medications

Place in warm ambient temperature environment, provide external heat sources.

Prevent pooling of antiseptic/irrigating solutions under client in operating room; cover skin areas outside of operative field; wrap in warmed blankets.

Provide stockinet hat, open radiant warmer, isolette, or heating blanket for newborn infant.

Treat severe hypothermia[1-4]:

Remove client from causative/contributing factors

Dry the skin, cover with blankets, provide shelter with warm ambient temperature; use radiant lights

Provide heat to trunk, not to extremities, initially. Avoid use of heat lamps or hot water bottles. *Surface rewarming can result in rewarming shock due to surface vasodilation.*

Keep individual lying down. Avoid jarring *(can trigger an abnormal heart rhythm).*

NURSING PRIORITY NO. 3. To evaluate effects of hypothermia[1-4]:

- Measure core temperature with low register thermometer (measuring below 94°F/34°C).
- Assess respiratory effort *(rate and tidal volume are reduced when metabolic rate decreases and respiratory acidosis occurs).*
- Auscultate lungs, noting adventitious sounds. *Pulmonary edema, respiratory infection, and pulmonary embolus are potential complications of hypothermia.*
- Monitor heart rate and rhythm. *Cold stress reduces pacemaker function, and bradycardia (unresponsive to atropine), atrial fibrillation, atrioventricular blocks, and ventricular tachycardia can occur. Ventricular fibrillation occurs most frequently when core temperature is 82°F/28°C or below.*
- Monitor BP, noting hypotension. *Can occur due to vasoconstriction, and shunting of fluids as a result of cold injury effect on capillary permeability.*
- Measure urine output. *Oliguria/renal failure can occur due to low flow state and/or following hypothermic osmotic diuresis.*
- Note CNS effects (e.g., mood changes, sluggish thinking, amnesia, complete obtundation); and peripheral CNS effects (e.g., paralysis—87.7°F/31°C, dilated pupils—below 86°F/30°C, flat EEG—68°F/20°C).
 - Monitor laboratory studies such as ABGs *(respiratory and metabolic acidosis)*; electrolytes; CBC *(increased hematocrit, decreased white blood cell count)*; cardiac enzymes *(myocardial infarct may occur owing to electrolyte imbalance, cold stress catecholamine release, hypoxia, or acidosis)*; coagulation profile; glucose; pharmacologic profile *(for possible cumulative drug effects).*

NURSING PRIORITY NO. 4. To restore normal body temperature/organ function[1-4]:

- Assist with surface warming by means of warmed blankets, warm environment/radiant heater, and electronic warming devices. Cover head/neck and thorax, leaving extremities uncovered as appropriate to maintain peripheral vasoconstriction. Note: Do not institute surface rewarming prior to core rewarming in severe hypothermia *(causes afterdrop of temperature by shunting cold blood back to heart in addition to rewarming shock as a result of surface vasodilation).*
- Assist with core rewarming measures, such as warmed IV solutions, and warm-solution lavage of body cavities (gastric, peritoneal, bladder) or cardiopulmonary bypass if indicated *to normalize core temperature.* Rewarm no faster than 1°F to 2°F per hour *to avoid sudden vasodilation, increased metabolic demands on heart, and hypotension (rewarming shock).*

- Protect skin/tissues by repositioning, applying lotion/lubricants, and avoiding direct contact with heating appliance/blanket. *Impaired circulation can result in severe tissue damage.*
- Keep client quiet; handle gently *to reduce potential for fibrillation in cold heart.*
- Provide CPR as necessary, with compressions initially at one-half normal heart rate. *Severe hypothermia causes slowed conduction, and cold heart may be unresponsive to medications, pacing, and defibrillation.*
- Maintain patent airway. Assist with intubation if indicated. Provide heated, humidified oxygen when used.
- Turn off warming blanket when temperature is within 1°F to 3°F of desired temperature *to avoid hyperthermia situation.*
- Administer IV fluids with caution to prevent overload as the vascular bed expands. *Cold heart is slow to compensate for increased volume.*
- Avoid vigorous use of pharmacologic therapy *to prevent overdose. As rewarming occurs, organ function returns, correcting endocrine abnormalities, and tissues become more receptive to the effects of drugs previously administered.*
- Perform range-of-motion exercises, provide support hose, reposition, encourage coughing/deep-breathing exercises, avoid restrictive clothing/restraints *to reduce effects of circulatory stasis.*
- Provide well-balanced, high-calorie diet/feedings *to replenish glycogen stores and nutritional balance.*

NURSING PRIORITY NO. 5. To promote wellness (Teaching/Discharge Considerations):

- Review client's specific cause of hypothermia. Inform client/SO(s) of procedures being used to rewarm client.
- Identify factors that client can control (if any), such as protection from environment, appropriate clothing/layering when outdoors; potential risk for future hypersensitivity to cold; drugs/alcohol/medications that predispose to hypothermia, and so forth.
- Discuss signs/symptoms of early hypothermia (e.g., changes in mentation, somnolence, impaired coordination, slurred speech) *to facilitate recognition of problem and timely intervention. Information may be especially important if client works or plays outdoors (e.g., camping, skiing, hiking).*
- Identify assistive community resources, as indicated (social services, emergency shelters, clothing suppliers, food bank, public service company, financial resources, etc.). *Individual/SO may be in need of numerous resources if hypothermia was caused by inadequate housing, homelessness, malnutrition.*

DOCUMENTATION FOCUS

Assessment/Reassessment
- Findings, noting degree of system involvement, respiratory rate, ECG pattern, capillary refill, and level of mentation.
- Graph temperature.

Planning
- Plan of care and who is involved in planning.
- Teaching plan.

 Cultural   Collaborative   Community/ Home Care   Diagnostic Studies 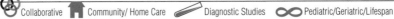 Pediatric/Geriatric/Lifespan   Medications

Implementation/Evaluation
- Responses to interventions/teaching, actions performed.
- Attainment/progress toward desired outcome(s).
- Modifications to plan of care.

Discharge Planning
- Long-term needs, identifying who is responsible for each action.

References

1. Curtis, R. (2002). Outdoor Action guide to hypothermia and cold weather injuries. Princeton University Outdoor Action website. Available at: http://www.princeton.edu/~oa/safety/hypocold.html. Accessed August 2003.
2. Decker, W., et al. (2001). Hypothermia. Article for Emedicine website. Available at: http://www.emedicine.com. Accessed August 2003.
3. Surgical Intervention. (2002). In Doenges, M. E., Moorhouse, M. F., & Geissler-Murr, A. C. Nursing Care Plans: Guidelines for Individualizing Patient Care, ed 6. Philadelphia: F. A. Davis, pp 771–772.
4. State of Alaska cold injuries and cold water near drowning guidelines. (Revised 01/96). Available at: www.hypothermia.org/protocol.htm. Accessed January 2004.

disturbed personal Identity

Definition: Inability to distinguish between self and nonself

RELATED FACTORS

To be developed by nurse researchers and submitted to NANDA
[Organic brain syndrome]
[Poor ego differentiation, as in schizophrenia]
[Panic/dissociative states]
[Biochemical body change]

DEFINING CHARACTERISTICS

To be developed by nurse researchers and submitted to NANDA

Subjective
[Confusion about sense of self, purpose or direction in life, sexual identification/preference]

Objective
[Difficulty in making decisions]
[Poorly differentiated ego boundaries]
[See ND Anxiety for additional characteristics]

SAMPLE CLINICAL APPLICATIONS: schizophrenia, dissociative disorders, borderline personality disorder, developmental delay, autism, gender identity conflict, dementia, traumatic injury (e.g., amputation, spinal cord injury, brain injury)

DESIRED OUTCOMES/EVALUATION CRITERIA

Sample **NOC** linkages:

Identity: Ability to distinguish between self and non-self and to characterize one's essence

Distorted Thought Control: Self-restraint of disruption in perception, thought processes, and thought content

Anxiety Control: Personal actions to eliminate or reduce feelings of apprehension and tension from an unidentifiable source

Client Will (Include Specific Time Frame)

- Acknowledge threat to personal identity.
- Integrate threat in a healthy, positive manner (e.g., state anxiety is reduced, make plans for the future).
- Verbalize acceptance of changes that have occurred.
- State ability to identify and accept self (long-term outcome).

ACTIONS/INTERVENTIONS

Sample **NIC** linkages:

Self-Esteem Enhancement: Assisting a patient to increase his/her personal judgment of self-worth

Self-Awareness Enhancement: Assisting a patient to explore and understand his/her thoughts, feelings, motivations, and behaviors

Decision-Making Support: Providing information and support for a person who is making a decision regarding healthcare

NURSING PRIORITY NO. 1. To assess causative/contributing factors:

- Ascertain client's perception of the extent of the threat to self and how client is handling the situation. *Many factors can affect an individual's self-image, illness (chronic or terminal), injuries, changes in body structure (amputation, spinal cord damage), and client's view of what has happened will affect development of plan of care and interventions to be used.*[1]
- Determine speed of occurrence of threat. *An event, such as an accident or sudden diagnosis of diabetes, cancer, that has happened quickly may be more threatening.*[7]
- Define disturbed body image. *Body image is the basis of personal identity and changes that prevent individual from achieving ideals and expectancies can have a negative impact.*[1]
- Be aware of physical signs of panic state. (Refer to ND Anxiety.)
- Note age of client. *An adolescent may struggle with the developmental task of personal/sexual identity, whereas an older person may have more difficulty accepting/dealing with a threat to identity, such as progressive loss of memory, or aging body changes.*[3]
- Assess availability and use of support systems. Note response of family/SO(s). *During stressful situations, support is essential for client to cope with changes that are occurring and response of family will need to be noted and interventions developed to help client and family members deal with situation/illness.*[3]
- Note withdrawn/automatic behavior, regression to earlier developmental stage, general behavioral disorganization, or display of self-mutilation behaviors in adolescent or adult; delayed development, preference for solitary play, display of self-stimulation in child. *Indicators of poor coping skills and need for specific interventions to help client develop sense of self and identity. Inability to identify self interferes with interactions with others.*[3]
- Determine presence of hallucinations/delusions, distortions of reality. *Indicators of presence of psychosis and need for interventions to deal with inability to distinguish between self and nonself.*[3]

NURSING PRIORITY NO. 2. To assist client to manage/deal with threat:

- Make time to listen/Active-listen to client, encouraging appropriate expression of feelings, including anger and hostility. *Conveys a sense of confidence in client's ability to identify extent of threat, how it is affecting sense of identity, and how to deal with feelings in acceptable ways.*[7,8]

 Cultural Collaborative 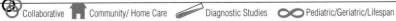 Community/ Home Care Diagnostic Studies Pediatric/Geriatric/Lifespan Medications

- **⌂** ● Provide calm environment. *Feelings of anxiety are contagious and calm surroundings can help client to quiet down and be able to think more clearly about how illness/situation can be managed effectively.*[9]
- **⌂** ● Use crisis-intervention principles when indicated. *May be necessary to help client restore equilibrium when situation escalates.*[1]
- **⌂** ● Assist client to develop strategies to cope with threat to identity. *Reduces anxiety, promotes self-awareness and enhances self-esteem enabling client to deal with threat more realistically.*[10]
- **⌂** ● Engage client in activities appropriate to individual situation. *Using activities such as a mirror for visual feedback, tactile stimulation to reconnect with parts of the body (amputation, unilateral neglect), can help to identify self as an individual.*[2]
- **⌂** ● Provide for simple decisions, concrete tasks, calming activities. *Promotes sense of control and positive expectations to enable client to regain sense of self.*[3]
- **⌂** ● Allow client to deal with situation in small steps. *May have difficulty coping with larger picture when in stress overload. Taking small steps promotes feelings of success and abililty to manage illness/situation.*[9]
- **⌂** ● Assist client in developing/participating in an individualized exercise program. *Walking is an excellent beginning program. It is helpful to choose activities that client enjoys. Exercise releases endorphins thereby reducing stress and anxiety.*[1]
- **⌂** ● Provide concrete assistance as needed. *Until basic-level needs, such as ADLs and food, are met, individual is unable to deal with higher level needs. Once these needs are met, client can begin to deal with threat to identity.*[1]
- **⌂** ● Take advantage of opportunities to promote growth. Realize that client will have difficulty learning while in a dissociative state. *Alterations in mental status can interfere with ability to process information and new information can increase confusion and disorientation.*[3]
- **⌂** ● Maintain reality orientation without confronting client's irrational beliefs. *Client may become defensive, blocking opportunity to look at other possibilities. Arguing does not change the perceptions and can interfere with nurse/client relationship.*[1]
- **⌂** ● Use humor judiciously when appropriate. *While humor can lift spirits and provide a moment of levity, it is important to note the mood/receptiveness of the client before using it.*[3]
- **⌂** ● Discuss options for dealing with issues of gender identity. *Identification of client's concerns about role dysfunction/conflicting feelings about sexual identity will indicate need for therapy, possible gender-change surgery when client is a transsexual, or other available choices.*[2]
- ● Refer to NDs disturbed Body Image, Self-Esteem [specify], Spiritual Distress.

NURSING PRIORITY NO. 3. To promote wellness (Teaching/Discharge Considerations):

- **⌂** ● Provide accurate information about threat to and potential consequences for individual in current situation. *Fear and anxiety regarding the threat represented by the illness/situation can be potentiated by lack of knowledge, unknown consequences and inaccurate beliefs. Accurate information can help client incorporate new knowledge into changed self-concept.*[7]
- **⌂** ● Assist client and SO(s) to acknowledge and integrate threat into future planning. *A diagnosis, accident, etc., can require major life changes, such as wearing identification bracelet when prone to mental confusion; a new lifestyle to accommodate change of gender for transsexual client; diet and medication routine with the diagnosis of diabetes mellitus. Planning can help the client to make the changes required to move forward with new life.*[4]
- **⊕** ● Refer to appropriate support groups. *May need additional assistance, such as day-care program, counseling/psychotherapy, gender identity, family/marriage counseling, parenting.*[2]

Assessment/Reassessment
- Findings, noting degree of impairment.
- Nature of and client's perception of the threat.

Planning
- Plan of care and who is involved in the planning.
- Teaching plan.

Implementation/Evaluation
- Client's response to interventions/teaching and actions performed.
- Attainment/progress toward desired outcome(s).
- Modifications to plan of care.

Discharge Planning
- Long-term needs and who is responsible for actions to be taken.
- Specific referrals made.

References

1. Townsend, M. (2003). Psychiatric Mental Health Nursing: Concepts of Care, ed 4. Philadelphia: F. A. Davis.
2. Doenges, M., Moorhouse, M., & Murr, A. (2002). Nursing Care Plans, Guidelines for Individualizing Patient Care, ed 6. Philadelphia: F. A. Davis.
3. Doenges, M., Townsend, M., & Moorhouse, M. (1998). Psychiatric Care Plans: Guidelines for Individualizing Care, ed 3. Philadelphia: F. A. Davis.
4. Pinhas-Hamiel, O., Dolan, L. M., et al. (1996). Increased incidence of non-insulin-dependent diabetes mellitus among adolescents. J Pediatr, 128(8), 608.
5. Deckelbaum, R. J., Williams, C. L. (2001). Childhood obesity: The health issue. Obesity Res, 9(5), 239s.
6. Badger, J. M. (2001). Burns: the psychological aspect. AJN, 101(11), 38–41.
7. Bartol, T. (2002). Putting a patient with diabetes in the driver's seat. Nursing, 32(2), 53–55.
8. Bruera, E., et al. (1995). The frequency of alcoholism among patients with pain due to terminal cancer. J Pain Symptom Management, 10(8), 599–603.
9. Paice, J. (2002). Managing psychological conditions in palliative care. AJN, 102(11), 36–43.
10. Cox, H., Hinz, M., Lubno, M. A., Newfield, S., Ridenour, N., Slater, M., & Sridaromont, K. (2002). Clinical Applications of Nursing Diagnosis Adult, Child, Women's Psychiatric, Gerontic and Home Health Considerations, ed 4. Philadelphia: F. A. Davis.
11. Lipson, J. G., Dibble, S. L., & Minarik, P. A. (1996). Culture & Nursing Care: A Pocket Guide. San Francisco: School of Nursing, UCSF Nursing Press.
12. Townsend, M. (2001). Nursing diagnoses in Psychiatric Nursing: Care Plans and Psychotropic Medications, ed 5. Philadelphia: F. A. Davis.

disorganized Infant Behavior

Definition: Disintegrated physiological and neuro-behavioral responses to the environment

RELATED FACTORS

Prenatal
Congenital or genetic disorders; teratogenic exposure; [exposure to drugs]

Postnatal
Prematurity; oral/motor problems; feeding intolerance; malnutrition
Invasive/painful procedures; pain

 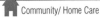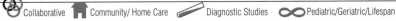

Individual
Gestational/postconceptual age; immature neurological system
Illness; [infection]; [hypoxia/birth asphyxia]

Environmental
Physical environment inappropriateness
Sensory inappropriateness/overstimulation/deprivation
[Lack of containment/boundaries]

Caregiver
Cue misreading/cue knowledge deficit
Environmental stimulation contribution

DEFINING CHARACTERISTICS

Objective
Regulatory Problems
Inability to inhibit [e.g., "locking in"-inability to look away from stimulus]; irritability

State-Organization System
Active-awake (fussy, worried gaze); quiet-awake (staring, gaze aversion)
Diffuse/unclear sleep, state-oscillation
Irritable or panicky crying

Attention-Interaction System
Abnormal response to sensory stimuli (e.g., difficult to soothe, inability to sustain alert
status)

Motor System
Increased, decreased, or limp tone
Finger splay, fisting or hands to face; hyperextension of arms and legs
Tremors, startles, twitches; jittery, jerky, uncoordinated movement
Altered primitive reflexes

Physiologic
Bradycardia, tachycardia, or arrhythmias; bradypnea, tachypnea, apnea
Pale, cyanotic, mottled, or flushed color
"Time-out signals" (e.g., gaze, grasp, hiccough, cough, sneeze, sigh, slack jaw, open mouth,
tongue thrust)
Oximeter desaturation
Feeding intolerances (aspiration or emesis)

SAMPLE CLINICAL APPLICATIONS: prematurity, congenital/genetic disorders, meconium
aspiration, respiratory distress syndrome, small for gestational age

DESIRED OUTCOMES/EVALUATION CRITERIA
Sample **NOC** linkage:
Neurologic Status: Extent to which the peripheral and central nervous system receive,
process, and respond to internal and external stimuli

Infant Will (Include Specific Time Frame)

- Exhibit organized behaviors that allow the achievement of optimal potential for growth and development as evidenced by modulation of physiological, motor, state, and attentional-interactive functioning.

Sample **NOC** linkages:

Child Development: [specify age group]: Milestones of physical, cognitive, and psychosocial progression by [specify] months of age

Growth: A normal increase in body size and weight

Parent/Caregiver Will (Include Specific Time Frame)

- Recognize individual infant cues.
- Identify appropriate responses (including environmental modifications) to infant's cues.
- Verbalize readiness to assume caregiving independently.

ACTIONS/INTERVENTIONS

Sample **NIC** linkages:

Environmental Management: Manipulation of the patient's surroundings for therapeutic benefit

Developmental Care: Structuring the environment and providing care in response to the behavioral cues and states of the preterm infant

Newborn Care: Management of neonate during the transition to extrauterine life and subsequent period of stabilization

NURSING PRIORITY NO. 1. To assess causative/contributing factors:

- Determine infant's chronological and developmental age; note length of gestation. *These factors (prematurity, infant maturity and stages of development) help to determine plan of care.*[1,2,5]
- Observe for cues suggesting presence of situations that may result in pain/discomfort. *Some behavior that appears to be disorganized may be caused by a pain source that once identified may be alleviated.*[1]
- Determine adequacy of physiological support. *Identifies areas of additional need.*[1]
- Evaluate level/appropriateness of environmental stimuli. *Infant behavior is affected by a wide range of stimuli. Careful assessment narrows focus of concerns.*[2]
- Ascertain parents' understanding of infant's needs/abilities. *Identifies knowledge base and areas of learning need.*[2–4]
- Listen to parent's concerns about their capabilities to meet infant's needs. *Active-listening can reassure parents, pinpoint areas to be addressed, as well as provide opportunity to correct misconceptions.*[2,3]

NURSING PRIORITY NO. 2. To assist parents in providing co-regulation to the infant:

- Provide a calm, nurturant physical and emotional environment. *Provides optimal infant comfort. Models behavior for parent(s) and optimizes learning.*[2,3]
- Encourage parents to hold infant, including skin-to-skin contact as appropriate. *Touch enhances parent-infant bonding, as well as provides means of calming.*[3]
- Model gentle handling of baby and appropriate responses to infant behavior. *Provides cues to parent.*[3]

 Cultural Collaborative Community/ Home Care Diagnostic Studies 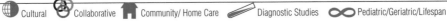 Pediatric/Geriatric/Lifespan Medications

- Support and encourage parents to be with infant and participate actively in all aspects of care. *Situation may seem overwhelming to new parents. Emotional and physical support enhances coping. Parents that are able to help in the care of their infant express lower levels of helplessness and powerlessness.*[1,2]
- Discuss infant growth/development, pointing out current status and progressive expectations as appropriate. *Augments parent knowledge of co-regulation.*[2]
- Incorporate the parents' observations and suggestions into plan of care. *Demonstrates valuing of parents' input and encourages continued involvement.*[2,4]

NURSING PRIORITY NO. 3. To deliver care within the infant's stress threshold:

- Provide a consistent caregiver. *Facilitates recognition of infant cues/changes in behavior. Communication is optimized if family is familiar with caregiver.*[2]
- Identify infant's individual self-regulatory behaviors (e.g., sucking, mouthing; grasp, hand-to-mouth, face behaviors; foot clasp, brace; limb flexion, trunk tuck; boundary seeking).
- Support hands to mouth and face; offer pacifier or non-nutritive sucking at the breast with gavage feedings. *Provides opportunities for infant to self-regulate.*[2]
- Avoid aversive oral stimulation, such as routine oral suctioning; suction ET tube only when clinically indicated. *Maximizes infant comfort, preventing undue/noxious stimulation.*[1,2]
- Use oxy-hood large enough to cover the infant's chest so arms will be inside the hood. *Allows for hand-to-mouth self-calming activities during this therapy.*[2]
- Provide opportunities for infant to grasp. *Helps with development of motor function skills.*[2]
- Provide boundaries and/or containment during all activities. Use swaddling, nesting, bunting, caregiver's hands as indicated. *Enhances infant's feelings of security and safeness. Avoids startle reflex and accompanying distress.*[2,3]
- Allow adequate time/opportunities to hold infant. Handle infant very gently, move infant smoothly, slowly and contained, avoiding sudden/abrupt movements. *Provides comfort to infant and models behavior to parent(s).*[3]
- Maintain normal alignment, position infant with limbs softly flexed, shoulders and hips adducted slightly. Use appropriate-sized diapers. *Avoids unnecessary discomfort.*[2]
- Evaluate chest for adequate expansion, placing rolls under trunk if prone position indicated. *Provides for ease of respirations.*[2]
- Avoid restraints, including at IV sites. If IV board is necessary, secure to limb positioned in normal alignment. *Optimizes comfort and movement.*[1,2]
- Provide a sheepskin, egg-crate mattress, water bed, and/or gel pillow/mattress for infant who does not tolerate frequent position changes. *Minimizes tissue pressure and risk of tissue injury.*[2]
- Visually assess color, respirations, activity, invasive lines without disturbing infant. Assess with "hands on" every 4 hours as indicated and PRN. *Allows for undisturbed rest/quiet periods.*[2,3]
- Schedule daily activities, time for rest, and organization of sleep/wake states to maximize tolerance of infant. Defer routine care when infant in quiet sleep. *Gives infant a sense of routine and also provides for undisturbed rest/quiet periods.*[2,3]
- Provide care with baby in side-lying position. Begin by talking softly to the baby, then placing hands in containing hold on baby, allow baby to prepare. Proceed with least invasive manipulations first. *Gradual build from comforting touch, to nursing care, to invasive interventions decreases overall stress of infant. Shortens perception of "being bothered" time and facilitates more rapid calming phase.*[3]

- Respond promptly to infant's agitation or restlessness. Provide "time out" when infant shows early cues of overstimulation. Comfort and support the infant after stressful interventions. *Decreases stress for both infant and family. Facilitates calming phase.*[3]
- Remain at infant's bedside for several minutes after procedures/caregiving to monitor infant's response and provide necessary support. *Allows for more rapid intervention(s) if infant becomes overstressed.*[3]

- Administer analgesics as individually appropriate. *Maintains optimal comfort.*[1–4,]

NURSING PRIORITY NO. 4. To modify the environment to provide appropriate stimulation:

- Introduce stimulation as a single mode and assess individual tolerance.

Light/Vision
- Reduce lighting perceived by infant, introduce diurnal lighting (and activity) when infant achieves physiological stability. (Day light levels of 20 to 30 candles and night light levels of less than 10 candles are suggested.) Change light levels gradually to allow infant time to adjust. *Lowering light levels reduces visual stimulation, provides comforting environment. Diurnal lighting allows the stable infant to begin perception of day and night cycles and to establish circadian rhythms.*[1]
- Protect the infant's eyes from bright illumination during examinations/procedures, as well as from indirect sources such as neighboring phototherapy treatments. *Prevents retinal damage and reduces visual stressors.*[2]
- Deliver phototherapy (when required) with Biliblanket devices if available. *Alleviates need for eye patches to protect vision.*[2]
- Provide caregiver face (preferably parent's) as visual stimulus when infant shows readiness (awake, attentive). *Begins process of visual recognition.*[1]

Sound
- Identify sources of noise in environment and eliminate/reduce *to minimize auditory stimulus, reduces startle response in infant, provides comforting environment*[2]:
  Speak in a low voice.
  Reduce volume on alarms/telephones to safe but not excessive volume.
  Pad metal trash can lids.
  Open paper packages such as IV tubing and suction catheters slowly and at a distance from bedside.
  Conduct rounds/report away from bedside.
  Place soft/thick fabric such as blanket rolls and toys near infant's head *to absorb sound.*
  Keep all incubator portholes closed, closing with two hands *to avoid loud snap with closure and associated startle response.*
- Do not play musical toys or tape players inside incubator. *Even very soft sounds echo in an enclosed space. What an adult may find soothing is likely to overstimulate an infant.*[2,3]
- Avoid placing items on top of incubator; if necessary to do so, pad surface well. *Contact with the external parts of the incubator causes reverberation inside the chamber.*
- Conduct regular decibel checks of interior noise level in incubator (recommended not to exceed 60 dB). *Verifies that decibel levels are within acceptable range.*[2]
- Provide auditory stimulation to console, support infant before and through handling or to reinforce restfulness. *Provides modeling of behavior for family and increased comfort for infant.*[3]

 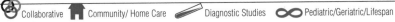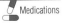

Olfactory

- Be cautious in exposing infant to strong odors (such as alcohol, Betadine, perfumes). *Olfactory capability of the infant is very sensitive.*[1]
- Place a cloth or gauze pad scented with milk near the infant's face during gavage feeding. *Enhances association of milk with act of feeding/gastric fullness.*[2]
- Invite parents to leave a handkerchief that they have scented by wearing close to their body near infant. *Strengthens infant recognition of parents.*[2]

Vestibular

- Move and handle the infant slowly and gently. Do not restrict spontaneous movement. *Maintains comfort while at the same time encouraging motor function skill.*[2]
- Provide vestibular stimulation *to console, stabilize breathing/heart rate, or enhance growth.* Use a waterbed (with or without oscillation), a motorized/moving bed or cradle, or rocking in the arms of a caregiver.

Gustatory

- Dip pacifier in milk and offer to infant for sucking and tasting during gavage feeding. *Further enhances feeding recognition with touch and taste cues.*[2]

Tactile

- Maintain skin integrity and monitor closely. Limit frequency of invasive procedures. *Decreases chance of infections. Decreases infant discomfort.*[1]
- Minimize use of chemicals on skin (e.g., alcohol, povidone-iodine, solvents) and remove afterward with warm water. *Chemical compounds remove the natural protective mechanisms of skin, and infants are often very sensitive to integumentary injury.*[1]
- Limit use of tape and adhesives directly on skin. Use DuoDerm under tape. *Helps prevent dermal injury/allergic reactions.*[1]
- Touch infant with a firm containing touch, avoid light stroking. Provide a sheepskin, soft linen. Note: Tactile experience is the primary sensory mode of the infant. *Light stroking can cause tickle sensations that are irritating rather than pleasurable. Firm touch is reassuring.*[2]
- Encourage frequent parental holding of infant (including skin-to-skin). Supplement activity with extended family, staff, volunteers. *For family members touch enhances bonding. If family is not readily available, infant needs regular skin-to-skin contact from caregivers for comfort and reassurance.*[3]

NURSING PRIORITY NO. 5. To promote wellness (Teaching/Discharge Considerations):

- Evaluate home environment to identify appropriate modifications. *Helps the family identify needs and begin to mentally prepare for infant homecoming.*[3]

- Identify community resources (e.g., early stimulation program, qualified child-care facilities/respite care, visiting nurse, home-care support, specialty organizations). *Begins process of resource utilization.*[2–4]

- Determine sources for equipment/therapy needs. *Facilitates transition to at-home care.*[3]

- Refer to support/therapy groups as indicated. *Provides role models, facilitates adjustment to new roles/responsibilities, and enhances coping.*[2,3]

- Provide contact number, as appropriate (e.g., primary nurse). *Supports adjustment to home setting, enhances problem solving.*[3]
- Refer to additional NDs such as risk for impaired parent/infant/child Attachment, compromised/disabled/readiness for enhanced family Coping, delayed Growth and Development, risk for Caregiver Role Strain.

Assessment/Reassessment

- Findings, including infant's cues of stress, self-regulation, and readiness for stimulation; chronological/developmental age.
- Parent's concerns, level of knowledge.

Planning

- Plan of care and who is involved in the planning.
- Teaching plan.

Implementation/Evaluation

- Infant's responses to interventions/actions performed.
- Parents' participation and response to interactions/teaching.
- Attainment/progress toward desired outcome(s).
- Modifications of plan of care.

Discharge Planning

- Long-term needs and who is responsible for actions to be taken.
- Specific referrals made.

References

1. Creasy, R., & Resnik, R. (1999). Maternal-Fetal Medicine, ed 4. Philadelphia: W. B. Saunders.
2. London, M., Ladewig, P., Ball, J., & Bindler, R. (2003). Maternal-Newborn & Child Nursing; Family-Centered Care. Upper Saddle River, NJ: Prentice Hall.
3. Ladewig, P., London, M., Moberly, S., & Olds, S. (2002). Contemporary Maternal-Newborn Nursing Care, ed 5. Upper Saddle River, NJ: Prentice Hall.
4. Lowdermilk, D., Perry, S., & Bobak, I. (2001). Maternity & Women's Health Care, ed 6. St. Louis: Mosby.
5. Mandeville, L., & Troiano, N. (1999). High-Risk & Critical Care; Intrapartum Nursing, ed 2. Philadelphia: Lippincott.

risk for disorganized Infant Behavior

Definition: Risk for alteration in integration and modulation of the physiological and behavioral systems of functioning (i.e., autonomic, motor, state, organizational, self-regulatory, and attentional-interactional systems)

RISK FACTORS

Pain

Oral/motor problems

Environmental overstimulation

Lack of containment/boundaries

Invasive/painful procedures

Prematurity; [immaturity of the CNS; genetic problems that alter neurological and/or physiological functioning, conditions resulting in hypoxia and/or birth asphyxia]

[Malnutrition; infection; drug addiction]

[Environmental events or conditions such as separation from parents, exposure to loud noise, excessive handling, bright lights]

 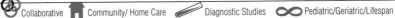

NOTE: A risk diagnosis is not evidenced by signs and symptoms, as the problem has not occurred and nursing interventions are directed at prevention.

SAMPLE CLINICAL APPLICATIONS: prematurity, congenital/genetic disorders, meconium aspiration, respiratory distress syndrome, small for gestational age

DESIRED OUTCOMES/EVALUATION CRITERIA

Sample **NOC** linkage:

Neurologic Status: Extent to which the peripheral and central nervous system receive, process, and respond to internal and external stimuli

Infant Will (Include Specific Time Frame)
- Exhibit organized behaviors that allow the achievement of optimal potential for growth and development as evidenced by modulation of physiologic, motor, state, and attentional-interactive functioning.

Sample **NOC** linkages:

Child Development: [specify age group 2/4/6/12 months]: Milestones of physical, cognitive, and psychosocial progression by [specify] months of age

Risk Detection: Activities taken to identify personal health threats

Parent/Caregiver Will (Include Specific Time Frame)
- Identify cues reflecting infant's stress threshold and current status.
- Develop/modify responses (including environment) to promote infant adaptation and development.

ACTIONS/INTERVENTIONS AND DOCUMENTATION FOCUS

Refer to ND *disorganized Infant Behavior* for Actions/Interventions and Documentation Focus.

readiness for enhanced organized Infant Behavior

Definition: A pattern of modulation of the physiological and behavioral systems of functioning (i.e., autonomic, motor, state-organizational, self-regulators, and attentional-interactional systems) in an infant that is satisfactory but that can be improved resulting in higher levels of integration in response to environmental stimuli

RELATED FACTORS
Prematurity
Pain

DEFINING CHARACTERISTICS

Objective
Stable physiologic measures
Definite sleep-wake states
Use of some self-regulatory behaviors
Response to visual/auditory stimuli

SAMPLE CLINICAL APPLICATIONS: prematurity, congenital/genetic disorders, meconium aspiration, respiratory distress syndrome, small for gestational age

Sample **NOC** linkage:

Neurologic Status: Extent to which the peripheral and central nervous system receive, process, and respond to internal and external stimuli

---

Infant Will (Include Specific Time Frame)
- Continue to modulate physiologic and behavioral systems of functioning.
- Achieve higher levels of integration in response to environmental stimuli.

Sample **NOC** linkages:

Child Development: [specify age group 2/4/6/12 months]: Milestones of physical, cognitive, and psychosocial progression by [specify] months of age

Knowledge: Infant Care: Extent of understanding conveyed about caring for a baby up to 12 months

---

Parent/Caregiver Will (Include Specific Time Frame)
- Identify cues reflecting infant's stress threshold and current status.
- Develop/modify responses (including environment) to promote infant adaptation and development.

ACTIONS/INTERVENTIONS

Sample **NIC** linkages:

Developmental Care: Structuring the environment and providing care in response to the behavioral cues and states of the preterm infant

Environmental Management: Manipulation of the patient's surroundings for therapeutic benefit

NURSING PRIORITY NO. 1. To assess infant status and parental skill level:

- Determine infant's chronological and developmental age; note length of gestation. *These factors (prematurity, infant maturity and stages of development) help to determine plan of care.*[1,2,5]
- Identify infant's individual self-regulatory behaviors: suck, mouth; grasp, hand-to-mouth, face behaviors; foot clasp, brace; limb flexion, trunk tuck; boundary seeking. *Assessing the infant's own regulatory coping tools alerts family and caregiver when infant is entering a stress cycle, and helps determine if the infant needs assistance coping. This knowledge also helps development of a care plan if situation warrants.*[1,2,4]
- 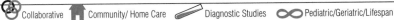 Observe for cues suggesting presence of situations that may result in pain/discomfort. *Some behavior that appears to be disorganized may be caused by a pain source that once identified may be alleviated.*[1]
- Evaluate level/appropriateness of environmental stimuli. *Infant behavior is affected by a wide range of stimuli. Careful assessment narrows focus of concerns.*[2]
- Ascertain parents' understanding of infant's needs/abilities. *Identifies knowledge base and areas of additional learning need.*[2–4]
- Listen to parents' perceptions of their capabilities to promote infant's development. *Active listening can reassure parents as well as pinpoint areas amenable to improvement.*[2,3]

NURSING PRIORITY NO. 2. To assist parents to enhance infant's integration:

- Review infant growth/development, pointing out current status and progressive expectations. Identify cues reflecting infant stress. *Increases parental knowledge base and*

  Cultural  Collaborative Community/ Home Care Diagnostic Studies Pediatric/Geriatric/Lifespan Medications

level of confidence. Attention to cues allow for early intervention in case of problem development.[2–4]

 • Discuss parent's perceptions of needs/provide recommendations for modifications of environmental stimuli/activity schedule, sleep and pain control needs. *While care provided is satisfactory, some modifications may enhance infant's integration/development.*[1,4]

 • Incorporate parents' observations and suggestions into plan of care. *Demonstrates valuing of parents' input and encourages continued involvement.*[2,4]

NURSING PRIORITY NO. 3. To promote wellness (Teaching/Learning Considerations):

• Identify community resources (e.g., visiting nurse, home care support, child care). *Begins process of resource utilization.*[2–4]

• Refer to support group/individual role model *to facilitate ongoing adjustment to new roles/responsibilities and problem solving.*[2,3]

• Refer to additional NDs, for example, readiness for enhanced family Coping.

DOCUMENTATION FOCUS

Assessment/Reassessment
• Findings, including infant's self-regulation and readiness for stimulation; chronological/developmental age.
• Parents' concerns, level of knowledge.

Planning
• Plan of care and who is involved in the planning.
• Teaching plan.

Implementation/Evaluation
• Infant's responses to interventions/actions performed.
• Parents' participation and response to interactions/teaching.
• Attainment/progress toward desired outcome(s).
• Modifications of plan of care.

Discharge Planning
• Long-term needs and who is responsible for actions to be taken.
• Specific referrals made.

References

1. Creasy, R., & Resnik, R. (1999). Maternal-Fetal Medicine, ed 4. Philadelphia: W. B. Saunders.
2. London, M., Ladewig, P., Ball, J., & Bindler, R. (2003). Maternal-Newborn & Child Nursing; Family-Centered Care. Upper Saddle River, NJ: Prentice Hall.
3. Ladewig, P., London, M., Moberly, S., & Olds, S. (2002). Contemporary Maternal-Newborn Nursing Care, ed 5. Upper Saddle River, NJ: Prentice Hall.
4. Lowdermilk, D., Perry, S., & Bobak, I. (2001). Maternity & Women's Health Care, ed 6. St. Louis: Mosby.
5. Mandeville, L., & Troiano, N. (1999). High-Risk & Critical Care; Intrapartum Nursing, ed 2. Philadelphia: Lippincott.

Definition: Impaired ability to suck or coordinate the suck-swallow response

RELATED FACTORS
Prematurity
Neurologic impairment/delay
Oral hypersensitivity
Prolonged NPO
Anatomic abnormality

DEFINING CHARACTERISTICS

Subjective
[Caregiver reports infant is unable to initiate or sustain an effective suck]

Objective
Inability to initiate or sustain an effective suck
Inability to coordinate sucking, swallowing, and breathing

SAMPLE CLINICAL APPLICATIONS: prematurity, cleft lip/palate, thrush, hydrocephalus, cerebral palsy, fetal alcohol syndrome, respiratory distress, severe developmental delay

DESIRED OUTCOMES/EVALUATION CRITERIA
Sample **NOC** linkages:
Swallowing Status: Oral Phase: Adequacy of preparation, containment, and posterior movement of fluids and/or solids in the mouth for swallowing
Breastfeeding Establishment: Infant: Proper attachment of an infant to and sucking from the mother's breast for nourishment during the first 2 to 3 weeks
Hydration: Amount of water in the intracellular and extracellular compartments of the body

Infant Will (Include Specific Time Frame)
● Display adequate output as measured by sufficient number of wet diapers daily.
● Demonstrate appropriate weight gain.
● Be free of aspiration.

ACTIONS/INTERVENTIONS
Sample **NIC** linkages:
Lactation Counseling: Use of an interactive helping process to assist in maintenance of successful breastfeeding
Swallowing Therapy: Facilitating swallowing and preventing complications of impaired swallowing
Nutrition Monitoring: Collection and analysis of patient data to prevent or minimize malnourishment

NURSING PRIORITY NO. 1. To identify contributing factors/degree of impaired function:

● Assess developmental age, structural abnormalities (e.g., cleft lip/palate), mechanical barriers (e.g., ET tube, ventilator). *These factors (infant maturity and structural/mechanical barriers to infant feeding) help to determine plan of care.*[1,2,5]

  Cultural Collaborative Community/ Home Care 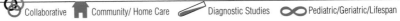 Diagnostic Studies Pediatric/Geriatric/Lifespan Medications

- Determine level of consciousness, neurological damage, seizure activity, presence of pain. *Provides baseline information and identifies areas of special need.*[1,2]
- Note type/scheduling of medications. *May cause sedative effect/impair feeding activity.*[2]
- Compare birth and current weight/length measurements. *Monitors effectiveness of infant feeding technique.*[1,2,4]
- Assess signs of stress when feeding (e.g., tachypnea, cyanosis, fatigue/lethargy). *Detects areas of increased need for alternate feeding methods and/or rest periods.*[1]
- Note presence of behaviors indicating continued hunger after feeding. *Determines if infant is receiving adequate amount during feeding.*[2,4]

NURSING PRIORITY NO. 2. To promote adequate infant intake:

- Determine appropriate method for feeding (e.g., special nipple/feeding device, gavage/enteral tube feeding) and choice of formula/breast milk to meet infant needs. *Individualizes care and maintains infant health status.*[1]
- Demonstrate techniques/procedures for feeding. Note proper positioning of infant, "latching-on" techniques, rate of delivery of feeding, frequency of burping. *Models appropriate feeding methods, increases parental knowledge base and confidence.*[2–4,]
- Monitor caregiver's efforts. Provide feedback and assistance as indicated. *Enhances learning, encourages continuation of efforts.*[2,3]
- Refer mother to lactation specialist for assistance and support in dealing with unresolved issues (e.g., teaching infant to suck). *Provides resource for future needs and problem solving. Begins pattern of resource utilization.*[2–4,]
- Emphasize importance of calm/relaxed environment during feeding.
- Adjust frequency and amount of feeding according to infant's response. *Prevents infant's frustration associated with under/overfeeding.*
- Advance diet, adding solids or thickening agent as appropriate for age and infant needs. *Provides for infant's nutrition and health needs.*[2,4]
- Alternate feeding techniques (e.g., nipple and gavage) according to infant's ability and level of fatigue. *Individualizes plan of care to enhance successful feeding.*[1]
- Alter medication/feeding schedules as indicated to minimize sedative effects. *Altered states of function and consciousness interfere with feeding and may lead to choking or aspirating.*[1]

NURSING PRIORITY NO. 3. To promote wellness (Teaching/Discharge Considerations):

- Instruct caregiver in techniques to prevent/alleviate aspiration. *Helps parent/caregiver feel more confident, promotes infant safety.*[1,4]
- Discuss anticipated growth and development goals for infant, corresponding caloric needs. *Accommodating infant maturity and development help to individualize and update plan of care.*[1,2,5]
- Suggest recording infant's weight and nutrient intake periodically. *Monitors effectiveness of infant feeding technique by providing measurable data. Provides positive reinforcement to implementation of care plan.*[1,2,4]
- Recommend participation in classes as indicated (e.g., first aid, infant cardiopulmonary resuscitation). *Increases knowledge base for infant safety and caregiver confidence.*[2–4,]

Assessment/Reassessment
- Type and route of feeding, interferences to feeding and reactions.
- Infant's measurements.

Planning
- Plan of care/interventions and who is involved in planning.
- Teaching plan.

Implementation/Evaluation
- Infant's response to interventions (e.g., amount of intake, weight gain, response to feeding) and actions performed.
- Caregiver's involvement in infant care, participation in activities, response to teaching.
- Attainment of/progress toward desired outcome(s).
- Modifications to plan of care.

Discharge Planning
- Long-term needs/referrals and who is responsible for follow-up actions.

References

1. Creasy, R., & Resnik, R. (1999). Maternal-Fetal Medicine, ed 4. Philadelphia: W. B. Saunders.
2. London, M., Ladewig, P., Ball, J., & Bindler, R. (2003). Maternal-Newborn & Child Nursing; Family-Centered Care. Upper Saddle River, NJ: Prentice Hall.
3. Ladewig, P., London, M., Moberly, S., & Olds, S. (2002). Contemporary Maternal-Newborn Nursing Care, ed 5. Upper Saddle River, NJ: Prentice Hall.
4. Lowdermilk, D., Perry, S., & Bobak, I. (2001). Maternity & Women's Health Care, ed 6. St. Louis: Mosby.

risk for Infection

Definition: At increased risk for being invaded by pathogenic organisms

RISK FACTORS

Inadequate primary defenses (broken skin, traumatized tissue, decrease in ciliary action, stasis of body fluids, change in pH secretions, altered peristalsis)

Inadequate secondary defenses (e.g., decreased hemoglobin, leukopenia, suppressed inflammatory response) and immunosuppression

Inadequate acquired immunity; tissue destruction and increased environmental exposure; invasive procedures

Chronic disease, malnutrition, trauma

Pharmaceutical agents [including antibiotic therapy]

Rupture of amniotic membranes

Insufficient knowledge to avoid exposure to pathogens

NOTE: A risk diagnosis is not evidenced by signs and symptoms, as the problem has not occurred and nursing interventions are directed at prevention.

SAMPLE CLINICAL APPLICATIONS: immune suppressed conditions (e.g., HIV positive/AIDS, cancer), COPD, long-term use of steroids (e.g., asthma, rheumatoid arthritis, SLE), diabetes mellitus, malnutrition, surgical/invasive procedures, substance abuse, burns, premature rupture of membranes

 Cultural Collaborative Community/ Home Care Diagnostic Studies 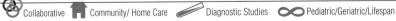 Pediatric/Geriatric/Lifespan Medications

Sample **NOC** linkages:

Immune Status: Adequacy of natural and acquired appropriately targeted resistance to internal and external antigens

Knowledge: Infection Control: Extent of understanding conveyed about prevention and control of infection

Risk Control: Actions to eliminate or reduce actual, personal, and modifiable health threats

---

Client Will (Include Specific Time Frame)

- Verbalize understanding of individual causative/risk factor(s).
- Identify interventions to prevent/reduce risk of infection.
- Demonstrate techniques, lifestyle changes to promote safe environment.
- Achieve timely wound healing; be free of purulent drainage or erythema; be afebrile.

ACTIONS/INTERVENTIONS

Sample **NIC** linkages:

Infection Protection: Prevention and early detection of infection in a patient at risk

Infection Control: Minimizing the acquisition and transmission of infectious agents

Surveillance: Purposeful and ongoing acquisition, interpretation, and synthesis of patient data for clinical decision making

NURSING PRIORITY NO. 1. To assess causative/contributing factors:

- Assess for host-specific factors that affect immunity[1]:

    Extremes of age. *Newborns and the elderly are more susceptible to disease/infection than general population.*

    Presence of underlying disease: *Client may have disease that directly impacts immune system (e.g., cancer, AIDS, autoimmune disorder) or may be weakened by any disease condition.*

    Lifestyle: *Personal habits may make person more or less susceptible (e.g., alcoholics are more susceptible to certain pneumonias; or individual with regular exercise may have more resistance to infections).*

    Nutritional status: *Malnutrition weakens the immune system, making the individual more susceptible.*

    Trauma (with loss of skin or mucous membrane integrity) or invasive procedures (e.g., urinary catheterizations, oral intubation, parenteral injection, sharps/needle sticks) *are common paths of pathogen entry.*

     Certain medications: *Steroids, chemotherapeutic agents directly affect immune system. Long-term or improper antibiotic treatment can disrupt body's normal flora and result in increased susceptibility to antibiotic-resistant organisms.*

    Presence or absence of immunity: *Natural immunity may be acquired as a result of development of antibodies to a specific agent following infection, preventing recurrence of specific disease (e.g., chickenpox). Active immunization (via vaccination, e.g., measles, polio) and passive immunization (e.g., antitoxin or immune globulin administration) can prevent certain communicable diseases.*

- Observe for redness, warmth, swelling, pain, red streaks surrounding acquired injuries (e.g., knife cuts, toe injuries, insect bites); also inspect in the same manner: insertion sites of invasive lines, sutures, surgical incisions/wounds. *Signs of localized infection that may have systemic implications if treatment is delayed.*[9,10]

- Assess and document skin conditions around insertions of orthopedic pins, wires, and

---

tongs, noting inflammation and drainage. *Local infections in bone sites can lead to osteomyelitis and long-term delays of healing, or bone loss.*[9,10]

- Note onset of fever, chills, diaphoresis, and altered level of consciousness. *Signs and symptoms of sepsis (systemic infection), requiring intensive medical treatment and acquisition of appropriate tissue/fluid specimens for observation and culture and sensitivities.*[1,11]

- Note and report laboratory values (e.g., white blood cell count and differential, blood/urine/wound cultures).

NURSING PRIORITY NO. 2. To reduce/correct existing risk factors:

- Stress proper handwashing techniques (using antibacterial soap and running water) before and after all care contacts, and after contact with items likely to be contaminated. Wash hands after glove removal. Instruct client/SO/visitors to wash hands, as indicated. *A first-line defense against nosocomial infections/cross-contamination.*[1,3]
- Provide clean, well-ventilated environment. *May require turning off central air-conditioning and opening window for good ventilation; room with negative air pressure, etc.*[6]
- Recommend individuals/staff isolate self at home when ill *to prevent spread of infection to others, including co-workers.*[11]
- Monitor visitors/caregivers for signs of infection, restrict access and traffic flow. *Prevents transmission to and/or from client and may reveal additional cases.*[1,8,11]
- Provide for appropriate isolation as indicated (e.g., total/wound/skin/reverse; single room with own bathroom and door closed, etc.) *to prevent transmission to other clients/staff.*[6,8]
- Group/cohort individuals with same diagnosis/exposure as resources require. *Limited resources (as may occur with an outbreak/epidemic) may dictate a ward-like environment but need for regular precautions to control spread of infection still exists.*[11]
- Use appropriate isolation coverings, as indicated for particular exposure risk (e.g., airborne, droplet, splash risk) including mask/respiratory filter of appropriate particulate regulator, gowns, aprons, head covers, face shields, protective eyewear.[1,4,6,8,11]
- Use disposable equipment whenever possible. Sterilize reusable equipment and surfaces according to manufacturer recommendations.[1,8]
- Dispose of needles and sharps in approved containers *to reduce risk of needle stick/sharps injury.*[1,8]
- Handle and properly package tissue/fluid specimens.[1,7]
- Perform/instruct in preoperative body shower/scrubs when indicated (e.g., orthopedic, plastic surgery).
- Maintain sterile technique for invasive procedures (e.g., IV, urinary catheter, tracheostomy care, pulmonary suctioning).[1]
- Maintain the cleanliness of all irrigation and cleansing solutions.
- Maintain appropriate hang times for parenteral solutions (IVs, additives, nutritional solutions) *to reduce opportunity for contamination/bacterial growth.*[2]
- Cleanse incisions/insertion sites daily and as needed with povidone-iodine or other appropriate solution *to prevent growth of bacteria.*[9]
- Cover dressings/casts with plastic when using bedpan *to prevent contamination when wound is in perineal/pelvic region.*
- Change dressings as needed/indicated. Handle and properly dispose of soiled dressings using barriers and bags *to contain fluids in dressings.*[8,9]
- Separate touching surfaces of excoriated skin (e.g., in herpes zoster or weeping dermatitis)

and apply appropriate skin barriers. Use gloves when caring for open lesions *to minimize autoinoculation/transmission of viral diseases.*[9]

- Encourage early ambulation, deep breathing, coughing, and position change *for mobilization of respiratory secretions.* Monitor/assist with use of adjuncts (e.g., respiratory aids such as incentive spirometry) *to reduce atelectasis/prevent pneumonia.*
- Maintain adequate hydration, stand/sit to void, and catheterize if necessary *to avoid bladder distention.* Provide regular catheter/perineal care. *Reduces risk of ascending urinary tract infection.*
- Maintain fluid and electrolyte balance *to prevent imbalances that would predispose to infection.*
- Provide/encourage balanced diet, emphasizing proteins to feed the immune system. *Immune function is affected by protein intake, the balance between omega-6 and omega-3 fatty acid intake, and adequate amounts of vitamins A, C, and E and the minerals zinc and iron. A deficiency of these nutrients puts the client at an increased risk of infection.*[2]
- Administer/monitor medication regimen (e.g., antimicrobials, drip infusion into osteomyelitis, subeschar clysis, and topical antibiotics) and note client's response *to determine effectiveness of therapy/presence of side effects.*
- Administer prophylactic antibiotics and immunizations as indicated.
- Alert infection control officer/proper authorities to presence of specific infectious agents and number of cases as required. *Provides for case finding and helps curtail outbreak.*[11]

NURSING PRIORITY NO. 3. To promote wellness (Teaching/Discharge Considerations):

- Review individual nutritional needs, appropriate exercise program, and need for rest *to enhance immune system function and healing.*[2,10,11]
- Instruct client/SO(s) in techniques to protect the integrity of skin, care for lesions, temperature measurement, and prevention of spread of infection in the home setting. *Provides basic knowledge for self-help and self-protection.*[7,10]
- Emphasize necessity of taking antibiotics as directed (e.g., dosage and length of therapy). *Premature discontinuation of treatment may result in return of infection with resistance to antibiotic therapies.*[10,11]
- Discuss importance of not taking antibiotics/using "leftover" drugs unless specifically instructed by healthcare provider. *Inappropriate use can lead to development of drug-resistant strains/secondary infections.*[10]
- Discuss the role of smoking and second-hand smoke in respiratory infections. Refer to smoking cessation programs as indicated.
- Promote safe-sex practices and reporting sexual contacts of infected individuals *to prevent the spread of sexually transmitted disease.*[1,10]
- Involve individuals/community in education programs *to increase awareness of spread/prevention of communicable diseases.*[1,10,11]
- Promote childhood immunization program. Encourage adults to update immunizations as appropriate.
- Encourage high-risk persons, including healthcare workers to have influenza and pneumonia vaccinations *to help prevent flu and viral pneumonias.*[1,11]
- Provide preoperative teaching *to reduce potential for postoperative infection (e.g., respiratory measures to prevent pneumonia, wound/dressing care, avoidance of others with infection).*[5,9]
- Review use of prophylactic antibiotics if appropriate *(e.g., before dental work for clients with history of rheumatic fever, heart valve replacements, etc.).*[10]

- Identify resources available to the individual (e.g., substance abuse/rehabilitation or needle exchange program as appropriate; available/free condoms, and so on).
- Refer to NDs risk for imbalanced Body Temperature, ineffective Health Maintenance, Hyperthermia, impaired/risk for impaired Skin Integrity for additional interventions.

DOCUMENTATION FOCUS

Assessment/Reassessment
- Individual risk factors that are present including recent/current antibiotic therapy.
- Wound and/or insertion sites, character of drainage/body secretions.
- Signs/symptoms of infectious process

Planning
- Plan of care/interventions and who is involved in planning.
- Teaching plan.

Implementation/Evaluation
- Responses to interventions/teaching and actions performed.
- Attainment/progress toward desired outcome(s).
- Modifications to plan of care.

Discharge Planning
- Discharge needs/referrals and who is responsible for actions to be taken.
- Specific referrals made.

References

1. Mechanisms of transmission and pathogenic organisms in the health care setting and strategies for prevention and control. (2001). Elements One and Two of online course of Infection Control Learning Institute. Available at: http://www.proceo.com. Accessed September 2003.
2. Lehmann, S. (1991). Immune function and nutrition: The clinical role of the intravenous nurse. J Intraven Nurs, 14, 406.
3. Garner, J., & Favero, M. (1986). CDC Guideline for handwashing and hospital environmental control. Am J Infection Control, 16, 28–40.
4. Borton, D. (1997). Isolation precautions: Clearing up the confusion. Nursing97, 21(1), 49.
5. Emori, L., Culver, D., & Horan, T. (1995). National Nosocomial Infections Surveillance System (NNIS): Description of surveillance methods. Am J Infection Control, 19, 259–267.
6. Garner, J. S. (1996). Guideline for isolation precautions in hospitals. Infection Control and Hospital Epidemiology, 17(1), 53–80.
7. Friedman, M. M. (2002). Improving infection control in home care: From ritual to science-based practice. Home Healthcare Nurse, 18(2), 99.
8. Hospital infection control guidance: Communicable Disease Surveillance & Response (CSR). World Health Organization (WHO) website. Available at: http://www.who.int/csr/en.
9. Thompson, J. (2000). A practical guide to wound care. RN, 63(1), 48–52.
10. Androwich, I., Burkhart, L., & Gettrust, K.V. (1996). Community and Home Health Nursing. Albany, NY: Delmar.
11. Care Plan: Disaster Considerations; and ND Infection, risk for, in numerous care plans. In Doenges, M. E., Moorhouse, M. F., & Geissler-Murr, A. C. (2002). Nursing Care Plans: Guidelines for Individualizing Patient Care, ed 6. Philadelphia: F. A. Davis.

risk for Injury

Definition: At risk of injury as a result of environmental conditions interacting with the individual's adaptive and defensive resources

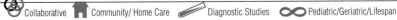 Cultural Collaborative  Community/ Home Care Diagnostic Studies Pediatric/Geriatric/Lifespan Medications

Internal

Biochemical, regulatory function (e.g., sensory dysfunction)

Integrative or effector dysfunction; tissue hypoxia; immune/autoimmune dysfunction; malnutrition; abnormal blood profile (e.g., leukocytosis/leukopenia, altered clotting factors, thrombocytopenia, sickle cell, thalassemia, decreased hemoglobin)

Physical (e.g., broken skin, altered mobility); developmental age (physiological, psychosocial)

Psychological (affective, orientation)

External

Biologic (e.g., immunization level of community, microorganism)

Chemical (e.g., pollutants, poisons, drugs, pharmaceutical agents, alcohol, caffeine, nicotine, preservatives, cosmetics, dyes); nutrients (e.g., vitamins, food types)

Physical (e.g., design, structure, and arrangement of community, building, and/or equipment), mode of transport or transportation

People/provider (e.g., nosocomial agent, staffing patterns; cognitive, affective, and psychomotor factors).

NOTE: A risk diagnosis is not evidenced by signs and symptoms, as the problem has not occurred and nursing interventions are directed at prevention.

SAMPLE CLINICAL APPLICATIONS: seizure disorder, dementia/AIDS, cataracts, glaucoma, substance abuse, malnutrition

DESIRED OUTCOMES/EVALUATION CRITERIA

Sample **NOC** linkages:

Safety Behavior: Personal: Individual or caregiver efforts to control behaviors that might cause physical injury

Risk Control [specify]: Actions to eliminate or reduce actual, personal, and modifiable health threats [such as alcohol/drug use, altered visual function]

Safety Status: Physical Injury: Severity of injuries from accidents and trauma

Client/Caregivers Will (Include Specific Time Frame)

- Verbalize understanding of individual factors that contribute to possibility of injury and take steps to correct situation(s).
- Demonstrate behaviors, lifestyle changes to reduce risk factors and protect self from injury.
- Modify environment as indicated to enhance safety.
- Be free of injury.

ACTIONS/INTERVENTIONS

In reviewing this ND, it is apparent there is much overlap with other diagnoses. We have chosen to present generalized interventions. Although there are commonalities to injury situations, we suggest that the reader refer to other primary diagnoses as indicated, such as risk for Poisoning, Suffocation, Trauma, and Falls; Activity Intolerance; Wandering, impaired physical Mobility, disturbed Thought Processes, acute/chronic Confusion, disturbed Sensory Perception, ineffective Health Maintenance, impaired Home Maintenance, imbalanced Nutrition: less/more than body requirements; impaired/risk for impaired Skin Integrity, impaired Gas Exchange, ineffective Tissue Perfusion, decreased Cardiac Output, risk for Infection, risk for other-directed/self-directed Violence, impaired/risk for impaired Parenting.

Sample **NIC** linkages:

Surveillance: Safety: Purposeful and ongoing collection and analysis of information about the patient and the environment for use in promoting and maintaining patient safety

Risk Identification: Analysis of potential risk factors, determination of health risks, and prioritization of risk reduction strategies for an individual or group

Environmental Management: Safety: Manipulation of the patient's surroundings for therapeutic benefit

NURSING PRIORITY NO. 1. To evaluate degree/source of risk inherent in the individual situation:

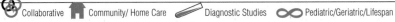
- Perform thorough assessments regarding safety issues when planning for client care/discharge. *Failure to accurately assess and intervene or refer regarding these issues can place the client at needless risk and creates negligence issues for the healthcare practitioner.*
- Note age and gender (children, young adults, elderly persons, and men are at greater risk). *Affects client's ability to protect self and/or others.*
- Evaluate developmental level, decision-making ability, level of cognition, competence and independence. *Determines client/SO's ability to attend to safety issues.*
- Assess mood, coping abilities, personality styles (i.e., temperament, aggression, impulsive behavior, level of self-esteem). *May result in careless/increased risk taking without consideration of consequences.*[1,2]
- Evaluate individual's response to violence in surroundings (e.g., neighborhood, television, peer group). *May affect client's regard for own/others' safety.*[1,2]
- Determine presence of firearms in home, how they are stored, and ease of access.[3,12]
- Ascertain knowledge of safety needs/injury prevention and motivation to prevent injury in home, community, and work setting. *Information may reveal areas of misinformation, lack of knowledge, need for teaching.*[4]
- Note socioeconomic status/availability and use of resources.
- Assess muscle strength, gross and fine motor coordination.
- Determine potential for abusive behavior by family members/SO(s)/peers. Observe client for signs of injury and age (e.g., old/new bruises, history of fractures, frequent absences from school/work). *Client or care providers may require further evaluation/investigation for abuse.*[5]

NURSING PRIORITY NO. 2. To assist client/caregiver to reduce or correct individual risk factors:

- Provide information regarding client's specific disease/condition (e.g., weakness, dementia, osteoporosis, head injury) *to enhance decision making, clarify expectations and individual needs.*
- Orient/reorient client to environment as needed. Remove hazards from environment as needed (e.g., razors, medications, lighter, high beds without rails; unsafe oxygen equipment, extraneous furniture, throw rugs, etc.).
- Place confused client or young children near nurses' station *to provide for frequent observation.*[6]
- Identify interventions/safety devices to promote safe physical environment and individual safety. *This can include a wide variety of interventions, including (and not limited to) stand assist/repositioning/lifting devices, back safety classes and injury-prevention devices/exercises; seat raisers for chairs; ergonomic beds, chairs, workstations; safety lock exit/stairwell doors when client can wander away, adequate lighting; electrical and fire safety devices, extinguish-*

 Cultural Collaborative Community/ Home Care Diagnostic Studies 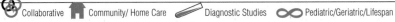 Pediatric/Geriatric/Lifespan Medications *ers, and alarms; storage/disposal of volatile liquids; appropriate use of car restraints, bicycle and other helmets; installation of proper ventilation for use when mixing/using toxic substances; use of safety glasses/goggles; electrical outlet covers/lockouts; care of old appliances to prevent suffocation; window locks, obtaining visual aids, communication devices (telephone, computer, hearing aid, medical alert devices, etc); mobility devices (canes, wheelchair, crutches, walkers, etc); installing handrails, ramps, bathtub safety tapes; oxygen safety rules; swimming pool fencing and supervision; childproof cabinets and medication/toxic substance containers* [1-13].

- Review client's level of physical activity in his/her lifestyle *to determine changes/adaptations that may be required by current situation.*
- Determine if reckless behavior is occurring/likely to occur *to initiate appropriate wellness counseling/referrals.*
- Refer to physical or occupational therapist as appropriate *to identify high-risk tasks, conduct site visits, select/create/modify equipment and provide education about body mechanics and musculoskeletal injuries, as well as provide therapies as indicated.*[6]
- Explore behaviors related to use of alcohol, tobacco and recreational drugs and other substances.
- Review with client/SO consequences of previously determined risk factors (e.g., increase in oral cancer among teenagers using smokeless tobacco; potential consequences of illegal activities; person needing surgery who is smoking and has heart disease; occurrence of spontaneous abortion, fetal alcohol syndrome/neonatal addiction in prenatal women using tobacco, alcohol, and other drugs).
- Demonstrate/encourage use of techniques to reduce/manage stress and vent emotions such as anger, hostility. *Identifying and dealing with emotions appropriately enables individual to maintain control of behavior and avoid possibility of violent outbursts.*[2,5,7]
- Discuss importance of self-monitoring of factors that can contribute to occurrence of injury (e.g., fatigue, anger, irritability). *Client/SO may be able to modify risk through monitoring of actions, or postponement of certain actions, especially during times when client is likely to be highly stressed.*
- Encourage participation in self-help programs, such as assertiveness training, positive self-image *to enhance self-esteem*; smoking cessation; weight management.
- Review expectations caregivers have of children, cognitively impaired, and/or elderly family members.[13]
- Discuss need for and sources of supervision (e.g., before and after school programs, elderly day care).
- Discuss concerns about childcare, discipline practices.
- Administer all medications safely. *Requires diligence in prescribing, preparing, dispensing, storing and administering to prevent errors that may result in harm, adverse side effects or toxic interactions.*[8]

NURSING PRIORITY NO. 3. To promote wellness (Teaching/Discharge Considerations):

- Identify individual needs/resources for safety education such as first aid/CPR classes, babysitter class, water or gun safety.[3,10,11]
- Refer to other resources as indicated (e.g., counseling/psychotherapy, budget counseling, and parenting classes).
- Provide telephone numbers and other contact numbers as individually indicated (e.g., doctor, 911, poison control, police).
- Provide bibliotherapy/written resource lists *for later review and self-paced learning.*

- Refer to/assist with community education programs *to increase awareness of safety measures and resources available to the individual.*[4]
- Promote community awareness about the problems of design of buildings, equipment, transportation, and workplace practices that contribute to accidents.[4]
- Identify community resources/neighbors/friends to assist elderly/handicapped individuals in providing such things as structural maintenance, snow and ice removal from walks and steps, etc.
- Identify emergency escape plans/routes for home and community *to be prepared in the event of natural or man-made disaster (e.g., fire, hurricane, earthquake, toxic chemical release).*[4]
- Refer to NDs risk for Poisoning, Suffocation, Trauma, and Falls; and Wandering for additional interventions as appropriate.

DOCUMENTATION FOCUS

Assessment/Reassessment
- Individual risk factors, noting current physical findings (e.g., bruises, cuts).
- Client's/caregiver's understanding of individual risks/safety concerns.

Planning
- Plan of care and who is involved in planning.
- Teaching plan.

Implementation/Evaluation
- Individual responses to interventions/teaching and actions performed.
- Specific actions and changes that are made.
- Attainment/progress toward desired outcome(s).
- Modifications to plan of care.

Discharge Planning
- Long-range plans for discharge needs, lifestyle and community changes, and who is responsible for actions to be taken.
- Specific referrals made.

References

1. Gorman-Smith, D., & Tolan, P. (1998). The role of exposure to community violence and developmental problems among inner city youth. Dev Psychopathol, 10(1), 101.
2. Youth Violence in the United States. National Center for Injury Prevention and Control. Available at: www.cdc.gov/ncipc/factsheet. Accessed January 2004.
3. Gun Safety. Available at: www.ena.org. Accessed January 2004.
4. Care Plan: Disaster Considerations; and ND Infection, risk for, in numerous care plans. In Doenges, M. E., Moorhouse, M. F., & Geissler-Murr, A. C. (2002). Nursing Care Plans: Guidelines for Individualizing Patient Care, ed 6. Philadelphia: F. A. Davis.
5. Intimate Partner Violence. National Center for Injury Prevention and Control. Retrieved from www.cdc.gov/ncipc/factsheet. Accessed January 2004.
6. Nelson, A, et al. (2003). Safe patient handling & movement. AJN 103(3):32–43.
7. Sexual Violence. National Center for Injury Prevention and Control. Available at: www.cdc.gov/ncipc/factsheet. Accessed January 2004.
8. Cohen, M. (2000). Medication Errors: Causes, Prevention and Risk Management. Boston: Jones and Bartlett.
9. Bicycle/Helmet Safety. Available at: www.ena.org. Accessed January 2004.
10. Water Safety. Emergency Nurses Association. Available at: www.ena.org. Accessed January 2004.
11. Drowning Prevention. National Center for Injury Prevention and Control. Available at: www.cdc.gov/ncipc/factsheet. Accessed January 2004.

 Cultural   Collaborative   Community/ Home Care   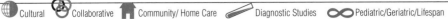 Diagnostic Studies    Pediatric/Geriatric/Lifespan   Medications

12. Suicide in the United States. National Center for Injury Prevention and Control. Available at: www.cdc.gov/ncipc/factsheet. Accessed January 2004.
13. Safety for older consumers' home safety checklist. Consumer Product Safety Commission (CPSC) document no. 701. Available at: http://www.cpsc.gov. Accessed September 2003.

risk for perioperative positioning Injury

Definition: At risk for injury as a result of the environmental conditions found in the perioperative setting

RISK FACTORS

Disorientation; sensory/perceptual disturbances due to anesthesia
Immobilization, muscle weakness; [preexisting musculoskeletal conditions]
Obesity; emaciation; edema
[Elderly]
NOTE: A risk diagnosis is not evidenced by signs and symptoms, as the problem has not occurred and nursing interventions are directed at prevention.
SAMPLE CLINICAL APPLICATIONS: operative procedures, arthritis, obesity, malnutrition, peripheral vascular disease

DESIRED OUTCOMES/EVALUATION CRITERIA

Sample **NOC** linkages:
Risk Detection: Activities taken to identify personal health threats
Risk Control: Actions to eliminate or reduce actual, personal, and modifiable health threats
Circulation Status: Extent to which blood flows unobstructed, unidirectionally, and at an appropriate pressure through large vessels of the systemic and pulmonary circuits

Client Will (Include Specific Time Frame)
- Be free of injury related to perioperative disorientation.
- Be free of untoward skin and tissue injury or changes lasting beyond 24 to 48 hours postprocedure.
- Report resolution of localized numbness, tingling, or changes in sensation related to positioning within 24 to 48 hours as appropriate.

ACTIONS/INTERVENTIONS

Sample **NIC** linkages:
Positioning: Intraoperative: Moving the patient or body part to promote surgical exposure while reducing the risk of discomfort and complications
Skin Surveillance: Collection and analysis of patient data to maintain skin and mucous membrane integrity
Circulatory Precautions: Protection of a localized area with limited perfusion

NURSING PRIORITY NO. 1. To identify individual risk factors/needs:

- Consider anticipated type and length of procedure, type of anesthesia to be used, and customary required position (e.g., supine, lithotomy, prone, lateral, sitting) *to increase awareness of potential complications (e.g., supine position may cause low back pain and skin pressure at heels/elbows/sacrum, lateral chest position can cause shoulder and neck pain plus eye and ear injury on the client's downside. Also normal defense mechanisms are altered due to anesthetic agents and medications as well as forced prolonged immobility during the procedure).*[1,2]

- Review client's history, noting age, weight, height, nutritional status, physical limitations (e.g., prostheses, implants, and range-of-motion restrictions) and preexisting conditions (vascular, respiratory, circulatory, neurologic, immunocompromise). *These factors affect choice of position for the procedure (e.g., elderly person with no subcutaneous padding or severe arthritis). Presence of certain conditions can cause the risk of skin/tissue integrity problems during surgery (e.g., diabetes mellitus, obesity, presence of peripheral vascular disease, level of hydration, temperature of extremities).*[1,2]

- Assess the individual's responses to preoperative sedation/medication, noting level of sedation and/or adverse effects (e.g., drop in blood pressure) and report to surgeon as indicated. *Hypotension is a common factor associated with nerve ischemia.*[3]
- Evaluate environmental conditions/safety issues surrounding the sedated client (e.g., client alone in holding area, siderails up on bed/cart, use of tourniquets/armloads, need for local injections, etc.) *that predispose client to potential tissue injury.*[1,3]

NURSING PRIORITY NO. 2. To position client to provide protection for anatomic structures and to prevent client injury:

- Stabilize both transport cart and operating room bed when transferring client to and from operating room table. Provide body and limb support for client during transfers, using adequate numbers of personnel *to prevent client fall or compromise of any body system, and/or to prevent injury to personnel.*[4]
- Position client, using appropriate positioning equipment/devices, *to provide optimal exposure of surgical site*[1,2]:

  Keep head in neutral position (when client in supine position) and arm boards at less than 90-degree angle and level with floor *to prevent neural injuries.*

  Maintain cervical neck alignment, and provide protection/padding for forehead, eyes, nose, chin, breasts, genitalia, knees, and feet *when client in prone position.*

  Protect bony prominences and pressure points on dependent side (e.g., axillary roll for dependent axilla, lower leg flexed at hip, upper leg straight padding between knees, ankles, and feet) *when client in lateral position.*

  Place legs in stirrups simultaneously, adjusting stirrup height to client's legs, maintaining symmetrical position, pad popliteal space as indicated *to reduce risk of peroneal and tibial nerve damage, prevent muscle strain, and reduce risk of hip dislocation when lithotomy position used.*

- Check that positioning equipment is correct size for client, is firm and stable, and is adjusted accordingly.[2,4]
- Use gel pads or similar devices over the operating room bed. *Decreases pressure at any given point by redistributing overall pressures across a larger surface area.*[2]
- Limit use of pillows, blankets, molded foam devices, towels, and sheet rolls, *which may produce only a minimum of pressure reduction, or contribute to friction injuries.*[2]
- Place safety straps strategically *to secure client for specific procedure.* Avoid pressure on extremities when securing straps *to limit possibility of pressure injuries.*[4]
- Realign/maintain body alignment during procedure as needed. *Changes in position may expose or damage otherwise protected body tissue. The position change may be planned, or imperceptible, and may result from adding or deleting positioning devices, adjusting the procedure bed in some manner, or moving the client on the procedure bed.*[2]
- Apply and periodically reposition padding of pressure points/bony prominences (e.g., arms, shoulders, ankles) and neurovascular pressure points (e.g., breasts, knees, ears) *to maintain position of safety and prevent injury from prolonged pressure.*

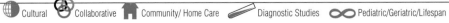

- Protect body from contact with metal parts of the operating table, *which could produce electrical injury/burns.*[1,5]
- Position extremities to facilitate periodic evaluation of hands, fingers, and toes. *Prevents accidental trauma from moving table attachments, allows for repositioning of extremities to prevent neurovascular injuries from prolonged pressure. Extremities should not extend beyond the end of operating table to reduce risk of compression or stretch injury.*[6]
- Check peripheral pulses and skin color/temperature periodically *to monitor circulation.*
- Ascertain that eyelids are closed and secured *to prevent corneal abrasions.*[6]
- Prevent pooling of prep and irrigating solutions, and body fluids. *Pooling of liquids in areas of high pressure under client increases risk of pressure ulcer development.*[7]
- Reposition slowly at transfer and in bed (especially halothane-anesthetized client) *to prevent severe drop in blood pressure, dizziness, or unsafe transfer.*
- Position client following extubation *to protect airway and facilitate respiratory effort.*
- Determine specific postoperative positioning guidelines (e.g., head of bed slightly elevated following spinal anesthesia *to prevent headache;* turn to unoperated side following pneumonectomy *to facilitate maximal respiratory effort).*[1]

NURSING PRIORITY NO. 3. To promote wellness (Teaching/Discharge Considerations):

- Maintain equipment in good working order *to identify potential hazards in the surgical suite and implement corrections as appropriate.*
- Provide perioperative teaching relative to client safety issues (including not crossing legs during procedures performed under local or light anesthesia, postoperative needs/limitations, and signs/symptoms requiring medical evaluation) *to reduce incidence of preventable complications.*
- Inform client and postoperative caregivers of expected/transient reactions (such as low backache, localized numbness, and reddening or skin indentations, which should quickly resolve), *to help them identify problems/concerns that require follow-up.*
- Assist with therapies/nursing actions including skin care measures, application of elastic stockings, early mobilization *to enhance circulation and venous return, and promote skin and tissue integrity.*
- Encourage/assist with frequent range-of-motion exercises *to prevent/reduce joint stiffness.*
- Refer to appropriate resources as needed.

DOCUMENTATION FOCUS

Assessment/Reassessment
- Findings, including individual risk factors for problems in the perioperative setting/need to modify routine activities or positions.
- Periodic evaluation of monitoring activities.

Planning
- Plan of care and who is involved in planning.
- Teaching plan.

Implementation/Evaluation
- Response to interventions and actions performed.
- Attainment/progress toward desired outcome(s).
- Modifications to plan of care.

Discharge Planning
- Long-term needs and who is responsible for actions to be taken.

References
1. Surgical Intervention. (2002). In Doenges, M. E., Moorhouse, M. F., & Geissler-Murr, A. C.: Nursing Care Plans: Guidelines for Individualizing Patient Care, ed 6. Philadelphia: F. A. Davis, pp 766–767.
2. AORN Standards and Recommended Practices for Perioperative Nursing (2001). Denver, CO: Association of Perioperative Registered Nurses, (AORN).
3. No author listed. Prevention of injuries in the anaesthetised patient. (1997–2004). Available at: www.surgical-tutor.org. Accessed February 2004.
4. Gruendemann, B. J., & Fernsebner, B. (1995). Comprehensive Perioperative Nursing, vol. 1. Boston: Jones & Bartlett.
5. Rothrock, J. (1996). Perioperative nursing care planning. St. Louis: Mosby.
6. Spry, C. (1997). Essentials of perioperative nursing. Gaithersburg, MD: Aspen.
7. Meeker, M., & Rothrock, J. (1999). Alexander's Care of the Patient in Surgery, ed 11. St. Louis: Mosby.

decreased adaptive capacity Intracranial

Definition: Intracranial fluid dynamic mechanisms that normally compensate for increases in intracranial volume are compromised, resulting in repeated disproportionate increases in intracranial pressure (ICP) in response to a variety of noxious and non-noxious stimuli

RELATED FACTORS
Brain injuries
Sustained increase in ICP = 10 to 15 mm Hg
Decreased cerebral perfusion pressure = 50 to 60 mmHg
Systemic hypotension with intracranial hypertension

DEFINING CHARACTERISTICS

Objective
Repeated increases in ICP of >10 mm Hg for more than 5 minutes following a variety of external stimuli
Disproportionate increase in ICP following single environmental or nursing maneuver stimulus
Elevated P_2 ICP waveform
Volume pressure response test variation (volume-pressure ratio 2, pressure-volume index <10)
Baseline ICP equal to or greater than 10 mm Hg
Wide amplitude ICP waveform
[Altered level of consciousness—coma]
[Changes in vital signs, cardiac rhythm]

SAMPLE CLINICAL APPLICATIONS: traumatic brain injury (TBI), cerebral edema, cranial tumors/hematomas, hydrocephalus

DESIRED OUTCOMES/EVALUATION CRITERIA
Sample **NOC** linkages:
Neurologic Status: Extent to which the peripheral and central nervous system receive, process, and respond to internal and external stimuli

 Cultural Collaborative Community/ Home Care Diagnostic Studies 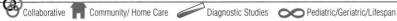 Pediatric/Geriatric/Lifespan Medications

Fluid Balance: Balance of water in the intracellular compartments of the body
Neurologic Status: Cranial Sensory/Motor Function: Extent to which cranial nerves convey sensory and motor information

Client Will (Include Specific Time Frame)
- Demonstrate stable ICP as evidenced by normalization of pressure waveforms/response to stimuli.
- Display improved neurological signs.

ACTIONS/INTERVENTIONS

Sample **NIC** linkages:
Cerebral Edema Management: Limitation of secondary cerebral injury resulting from swelling of brain tissue
Cerebral Perfusion Promotion: Promotion of adequate perfusion and limitation of complications for a patient experiencing or at risk for inadequate cerebral perfusion
Intracranial Pressure (ICP) Monitoring: Measurement and interpretation of patient data to regulate intracranial pressure

NURSING PRIORITY NO. 1. To assess causative/contributing factors:

- Determine factors related to individual situation (e.g., cause for coma/decreased cerebral perfusion and potential for increased ICP). *Deterioration in neurologic signs/symptoms or failure to improve after initial insult may reflect decreased adaptive capacity.*[1]

- Monitor/document changes in ICP waveform/pressure reading and corresponding event (e.g., suctioning, position change, monitor alarms, family visit). *Intracranial pressure monitoring may be done in client with severe head injury (hematomas, contusions, edema or compressed cranial fractures, Glasgow Coma Scale [GCS] <8 with abnormal computed tomography scan). Elevated pressure reading (>20–25) can be caused by the injury, and/or treatment modalities.*[1,2]

NURSING PRIORITY NO. 2. To note degree of impairment:

- Evaluate coma, using Glasgow Coma Scale, noting numbers less than 8. *Typically seen in clients with severe head injury and increased ICP with impaired cerebral perfusion pressure (CPP). Assesses eye opening (e.g., awake, opens only to painful movement, keeps eyes closed); and position/movement (e.g., spontaneous, purposeful, posturing); pupils (size, shape, equality, light reactivity), and consciousness/mental status (e.g., comatose, responds to pain, awake/confused, etc.). Determines level of dysfunction and influences choice of interventions.*[1–3]
- Note purposeful and nonpurposeful motor response (e.g., posturing), comparing right/left sides. *Posturing and abnormal flexion of extremities usually indicates diffuse cortical damage. Absence of spontaneous movement on one side indicates damage to the motor tracts in the opposite cerebral hemisphere.*[1]
- Test for presence/absence of reflexes (e.g., blink, cough, gag, Babinski's reflex), nuchal rigidity. *Helps identify location of injury (e.g., loss of blink reflex suggests damage to the pons and medulla, absence of cough and gag reflexes reflects damage to medulla, and presence of Babinski's reflex indicates injury along pyramidal pathways in the brain).*[1]
- Monitor vital signs and cardiac rhythm before/during/after activity. *Helps determine parameters for "safe" activity. Mean arterial blood pressure should be maintained above 90*

mm Hg to maintain CCP greater than 70 mm Hg, *which reflects adequate blood supply to the brain.*[1,3] *Fever in brain injury can be associated with injury to the hypothalamus or bleeding, systemic infection (e.g., pneumonia) or drugs. Hyperthermia exacerbates cerebral ischemia. Irregular respiration patterns can suggest location of cerebral insult. Cardiac dysrhythmias can be due to brainstem injury and stimulation of the sympathetic nervous system. Bradycardia may occur with high ICP.*[1,3]

 • Monitor urine output and serum sodium (Na). *Post-traumatic neuroendocrine dysfunction can result in a hyponatremic or hypernatremic state. When hyponatremia exists cerebral edema and/or syndrome of inappropriate antidiuretic hormone (SIADH) can occur requiring correction with fluid restriction and hypertonic IV solution. Hypernatremia can occur because of injury to the hypothalamus or pituitary stalk causing diabetes insipidus (DI) resulting in huge urine losses; or be the result of excessive diuresis due to use of mannitol or furosemide administered to reduce cerebral edema.*[3]

NURSING PRIORITY NO. 3. To minimize/correct causative factors/maximize perfusion:

• Elevate head of bed as individually appropriate. *Optimal head of bed position is determined by both ICP and CCP measurements, that is, which degree of elevation lowers ICP while maintaining adequate cerebral blood flow.*[4] *Studies show that in most cases, 30 degrees elevation significantly decreases ICP while maintaining cerebral blood flow.*[1]

• Maintain head/neck in neutral position, supporting with small towel rolls or pillows *to maximize venous return. Note: Lateral and rotational neck flexion has been shown to be the most consistent trigger of sustained increases in ICP.*[5]

• Avoid causing hip flexion of 90 degrees or more. *Hip flexion may trap venous blood in the intraabdominal space, increasing abdominal and intrathoracic pressure, and reducing venous outflow from the head, increasing cerebral pressure.*[6]

• Decrease extraneous stimuli/provide comfort measures (e.g., quiet environment, soft voice, tapes of familiar voices played through earphones, back massage, gentle touch as tolerated) *to reduce CNS stimulation and promote relaxation.*[1,5]

• Limit painful procedures (e.g., venipunctures, redundant neurologic evaluations) to those that are absolutely necessary *in order to minimize preventable elevations in ICP.*[1,3]

• Encourage family/SOs to talk to patient. *Familiar voices appear to have a relaxing effect on many comatose individuals (thereby reducing ICP).*[1]

• Provide rest periods between care activities and limit duration of procedures. Lower lighting/noise level, schedule and limit activities *to provide restful environment and limit spikes in ICP associated with noxious stimuli.*[1]

• Limit/prevent activities *that increase intrathoracic/abdominal pressures (e.g., coughing, vomiting, straining at stool).* Avoid/ limit use of restraints *(often increase agitation and markedly increase ICP).*[1]

• Suction with caution (only when needed and limit to two passes of 10 seconds each with negative pressure no more than 120 mm Hg). Suction just beyond end of endo/tracheal tube without touching tracheal wall or carina. Administer lidocaine intratracheally *to reduce cough reflex.* Hyperoxygenate before suctioning as appropriate *to minimize hypoxia. Note: Routine hyperventilation is to be avoided, but it can be used in acute neurologic deterioration to rapidly decrease catastrophic elevations in ICP.*[3]

• Maintain patency of urinary drainage system *to reduce risk of hypertension, increased ICP, associated dysreflexia if spinal cord injury is also present, and spinal cord shock is past.* (Refer to ND Autonomic Dysreflexia.)

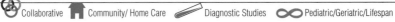

 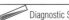

- Weigh as indicated. Calculate fluid balance every shift/daily *to determine fluid needs/maintain hydration and prevent fluid overload.*[1]
- Administer fluids as indicated via IV/enteral routes. *Fluid is needed to maintain adequate blood pressure for cerebral and body organ perfusion and to reduce potential for dehydration due to fluid loss, use of diuretics and insensible losses.*[3]
- Restrict fluid intake as necessary, administer IV fluids via pump/control device *to prevent inadvertent vascular overload, cerebral edema, and increased ICP.*[1]
- Regulate environmental temperature/bed linens, use cooling blanket as indicated *to decrease metabolic and oxygen needs when fever present. Lowering the body temperature has been shown to decrease ICP and improve outcomes for recovery.*[3]
- Investigate increased restlessness *to determine causative factors and initiate corrective measures as indicated.*
- Provide appropriate safety measures/initiate treatment for seizures *to prevent injury/increase of ICP/hypoxia.*
- Administer supplemental oxygen; hyperventilate as indicated when on mechanical ventilation. Monitor arterial blood gases (ABGs), particularly pH, CO_2 and Pao_2 levels. *$PaCO_2$ level of 28 to 30 mmHg decreases cerebral blood flow while maintaining adequate cerebral oxygenation, while a PaO_2 of less than 65 mm Hg may cause cerebral vascular dilation.*[1-,3]
- Administer enteral/parenteral nutrition *to achieve positive nitrogen balance reducing effects of post brain injury metabolic and catabolic states, which can lead to complications such as immunosuppression, infection, poor wound healing, loss of body mass, and multiple organ dysfunction.*[3]
- Administer medications (e.g., antihypertensives, diuretics, analgesics/sedatives, antipyretics, vasopressors, antiseizure drugs, neuromuscular blocking agents, and corticosteroids) as appropriate *to maintain homeostasis and treat/prevent complications.*
- Prepare client for surgery as indicated (e.g., evacuation of hematoma/space-occupying lesion) *to reduce ICP/enhance circulation.*

NURSING PRIORITY NO. 4. To promote wellness (Teaching/Discharge Considerations):

- Discuss with caregivers specific situations (e.g., if client choking or experiencing pain, needing to be repositioned, constipated, blocked urinary flow) and review appropriate interventions *to prevent/limit episodic increases in ICP.*
- Identify signs/symptoms suggesting increased ICP (in client at risk without an ICP monitor), for example, restlessness, deterioration in neurologic responses. Review appropriate interventions.

DOCUMENTATION FOCUS

Assessment/Reassessment
- Neurologic findings noting right/left sides separately (such as pupils, motor response, reflexes, restlessness, nuchal rigidity).
- Response to activities/events (e.g., changes in pressure waveforms/vital signs).
- Presence/characteristics of seizure activity.

Planning
- Plan of care and who is involved in planning.
- Teaching plan.

Implementation/Evaluation

- Response to interventions and actions performed.
- Attainment/progress toward desired outcome(s).
- Modifications to plan of care.

Discharge Planning

- Future needs, plan for meeting them, and determining who is responsible for actions.
- Referrals as identified.

References

1. Craniocerebral trauma (acute rehabilitative phase). In Doenges, M. E., Moorhouse, M. F., & Geissler-Murr, A. C. (2002): Nursing Care Plans: Guidelines for Individualizing Patient Care, ed 6. Philadelphia: F. A. Davis.
2. Part 1: Guidelines for the management of severe traumatic brain injury. (2000). Brain Trauma Foundation, Inc. New York: American Association of Neurological Surgeons. Available at: http://www.guideline.gov. Accessed November 2003.
3. Acute care management of severe traumatic brain injuries. (2001). Crit Care Nurse Q, 23(4), 1.
4. Simmons, B. J. (1997). Management of intracranial hemodynamics in the adult: A research analysis of head positioning and recommendations for clinical practice and future research. J Neurosci Nurs, 29, 44.
5. Mitchell, P. H., & Habermann, B. (1999). Rethinking physiological stability: Touch and intracranial pressure. Biol Res Nurs, 1(1), 12–19.
6. Vos, H. R. (1993). Making headway with intracranial hypertension. Am J Nurs, 93, 28.

deficient Knowledge [Learning Need] (specify)

Definition: Absence or deficiency of cognitive information related to specific topic [Lack of specific information necessary for clients/SO(s) to make informed choices regarding condition/treatment/lifestyle changes]

RELATED FACTORS

Lack of exposure
Information misinterpretation
Unfamiliarity with information resources
Lack of recall
Cognitive limitation
Lack of interest in learning
[Client's request for no information]
[Inaccurate/incomplete information presented]

DEFINING CHARACTERISTICS

Subjective

Verbalization of the problem
[Request for information]
[Statements reflecting misconceptions]

Objective

Inaccurate follow-through of instruction
Inadequate performance of test
Inappropriate or exaggerated behaviors (e.g., hysterical, hostile, agitated, apathetic)
[Development of preventable complication]

 Cultural Collaborative Community/ Home Care Diagnostic Studies Pediatric/Geriatric/Lifespan Medications

SAMPLE CLINICAL APPLICATIONS: any newly diagnosed disease or traumatic injury, progression of/deterioration in a chronic condition

DESIRED OUTCOMES/EVALUATION CRITERIA
Sample **NOC** linkages:
Knowledge: [specify—25 choices]: Extent of understanding conveyed about a specific disease process, the promotion and protection of health, maintaining optimal health, etc.
Information Processing: Ability to acquire, organize, and use information

Client Will (Include Specific Time Frame)
- Participate in learning process.
- Identify interferences to learning and specific action(s) to deal with them.
- Exhibit increased interest/assume responsibility for own learning and begin to look for information and ask questions.
- Verbalize understanding of condition/disease process and treatment.
- Identify relationship of signs/symptoms to the disease process and correlate symptoms with causative factors.
- Perform necessary procedures correctly and explain reasons for the actions.
- Initiate necessary lifestyle changes and participate in treatment regimen.

ACTIONS/INTERVENTIONS
Sample **NIC** linkages:
Teaching: Individual [or 13 other choices]: Planning, implementation, and evaluation of a teaching program designed to address a patient's particular needs
Learning Facilitation: Promoting the ability to process and comprehend information
Learning Readiness Enhancement: Improving the ability and willingness to receive information

NURSING PRIORITY NO. 1. To assess readiness to learn and individual learning needs:

- Ascertain level of knowledge, including anticipatory needs. *Learning needs can include many things (e.g., disease cause and process, factors contributing to symptoms, procedures for symptom control, needed alterations in lifestyle, ways to prevent complications). Client may or may not ask for information, or may express inaccurate perceptions of health status and needed behaviors to manage self-care.*[1]
- Engage in Active-listening. *Conveys expectation of confidence in client's ability to determine learning needs and best ways of meeting them.*[5]
- Determine client's ability to learn. *Client may not be physically, emotionally, or mentally capable at this time, and may need time to work through and express emotions before teaching.*[1]
- Be alert to signs of avoidance. *May need to allow client to suffer the consequences of lack of knowledge before client is ready to accept information.*[1]
- Identify SO(s)/family members requiring information. *Providing appropriate information to others can provide reinforcement for learning as everyone will understand what is to be expected.*[4]

NURSING PRIORITY NO. 2. To determine other factors pertinent to the learning process:

- Note personal factors (e.g., age and developmental level, sex, social/cultural influences, religion, life experiences, level of education, sense of powerlessness) *that affect ability and desire to learn/assimilate new information.*[2]

- Assess client/SO's preferred learning mode (e.g., auditory/visual, group classes, one-to one instruction). *Identifying how client learns facilitates learning, especially when faced with a stressful situation, illness/new treatment regimen.*[3]
- Determine blocks to learning including 1) language barriers (e.g., can't read or write, speaks/understands a different language than that spoken by teacher), 2) physical factors (e.g., sensory deficits, such as aphasia, dyslexia, hearing or vision impairment), 3) physical constraints (e.g., acute illness, activity intolerance; impaired thought processes), 4) complexity of material to be learned (e.g., caring for colostomy, giving own insulin injections), 5) forced change in lifestyle (e.g., stopping smoking), or 6) have stated no need/desire to learn. *Many factors affect the client's ability and desire to learn and his or her expectations of the learning process must be addressed if learning is to be successful.*[1]
- Assess the level of the client's capabilities and the possibilities of the situation. *May need to assist SO(s) and/or caregivers to learn by introducing one new idea, by building on previous information, or by finding pictures to demonstrate an idea, etc. to adapt teaching to client's specific needs.*[6]

NURSING PRIORITY NO. 3. To assess the client's/SO(s') motivation:

- Identify motivating factors for the individual. *Provides information that can direct plan of care and appropriate content specific to client's situation and motivations.*[3]
- Provide information relevant to the situation. *Narrowing the amount of information helps to keep the client focused and prevents client from feeling overwhelmed.*[4]
- Provide positive reinforcement rather than negative reinforcers (e.g., criticism and threats). *Enhances cooperation and encourages continuation of efforts.*[5]

NURSING PRIORITY NO. 4. To establish priorities in conjunction with client:

- Determine client's most urgent need from both client's and nurse's viewpoint. *Identifies whether client and nurse are together in their thinking and provides a starting point for teaching and outcome planning for optimal success.*[6]
- Discuss client's perception of need. *Takes into account the client's personal desires/needs and values/beliefs providing a basis for planning appropriate care.*[6]
- Differentiate "critical" content from "desirable" content. *Identifies information that must be learned now as well as content that could be addressed at a later time. Client's emotional state may preclude hearing much of what is presented and by only providing what is essential, client may hear it.*[3]

NURSING PRIORITY NO. 5. To determine the content to be included:

- Identify information that needs to be remembered (cognitive) at client's level of development and education. *Enhances possibility that information will be heard and understood.*[6]
- Identify information having to do with emotions, attitudes, and values (affective). *The affective learning domain addresses a learner's emotions towards learning experiences and attitudes, interest, attention, awareness, and values are demonstrated by affective behaviors. Knowing the client's affective state enhances learning possibilities.*[7]
- Identify psychomotor skills that are necessary for learning. *Psychomotor learning involves both cognitive learning and muscular movement. The phases for learning these skills are cognitive (what), associative (how), and autonomous (practice to automaticity). Learners need to know what, why, and how they will learn. For instance, papers need to be typed, so the psychomotor skill will be touch typing. The individual will learn touch typing finger placement and how to type smoothly and rhythmically.*[8]

 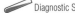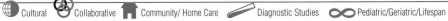

NURSING PRIORITY NO. 6. To develop learner's objectives:

- State objectives clearly in learner's terms *to meet learner's (not instructor's) needs. Understanding why the material is important to the learner provides motivation to learn.*[8]
- Identify outcomes (results) to be achieved. *Understanding what the outcomes will be helps the client realize the importance of learning the material, providing the motivation necessary to learning.*[8]
- Recognize level of achievement, time factors, and short-term and long-term goals. *Learning progresses in stages. Stage 1) Unconsciously unskilled where we don't know we don't know; stage 2) consciously unskilled, we know we don't know and start to learn; stage 3) consciously skilled, we know how to do it, but need to think and work hard to do it; and stage 4) we become unconsciously skilled, where the new skills are easier and even seem natural.*[9]
- Include the affective goals (e.g., reduction of stress). *The learner's emotional behaviors affect the learning experience and need to be actively addressed for maximum effectiveness.*[7]

NURSING PRIORITY NO. 7. To identify teaching methods to be used:

- Determine client's method of accessing information (e.g., visual, auditory, kinesthetic, gustatory/olfactory) and include in teaching plan. *Using multiple modes of instruction enhances retention.*[10]
- Involve the client/SO(s) by using interactive programmed books, questions/dialogue, and audio/visual materials. *Provides mental images to help individual learn more effectively.*[3]
- Involve with others who have same problems/needs/concerns. *Group presentations, support groups provide role models and opportunity for sharing of information to enhance learning.*
- Provide mutual goal setting and learning contracts. *Clarifies expectations of teacher and learner.*
- Use team and group teaching as appropriate.

NURSING PRIORITY NO. 8. To facilitate learning:

- Provide written information/guidelines at client's level of reading comprehension to refer to as necessary. *Reinforces learning process.*
- Pace and time learning sessions and learning activities to individual's needs. *Client statements, questions, comments indicating confusion or boredom provide feedback indicating client's ability to grasp information being presented.*
- Provide an environment that is conducive to learning *to limit distractions and allow client to focus on the material presented.*
- Be aware of factors related to teacher in the situation (e.g., vocabulary, dress, style, knowledge of the subject, and ability to impart information effectively) *that may affect client's reaction to teacher/ability to learn from this individual.*
- Begin with information the client already knows and move to what the client does not know, progressing from simple to complex. *Eases client into learning process and limits sense of being overwhelmed.*
- Deal with the client's anxiety. Present information out of sequence, if necessary, dealing first with material that is most anxiety-producing *when the anxiety is interfering with the client's learning process.*
- Provide active role for client in learning process, including questions and discussion. *Promotes sense of control over situation and identifies misconceptions that require clarification.*
- Have client paraphrase content in own words, perform return demonstration, and explain how learning can be applied in own situation *to enhance internalization of material and to evaluate learning.*[3]

- Provide for feedback (positive reinforcement) and evaluation of learning/acquisition of skills. *Validates current level of understanding and identifies areas requiring follow-up.*[5]

- Be aware of informal teaching and role modeling that takes place on an ongoing basis. *Answering specific questions/reinforcing previous teaching during routine care enhances learning on a regular basis.*[1]

- Assist client to use information in all applicable areas (e.g., situational, environmental, personal). *Enhances learning to promote better understanding of situation/illness.*[1]

NURSING PRIORITY NO. 9. To promote wellness (Teaching/Discharge Considerations):

- Provide telephone number of contact person *to answer questions/validate information after discharge.*[1]

- Identify available community resources/support groups *to assist with problem solving, provide role models, support personal growth/change.*[4]

- Provide bibliotherapy and additional learning resources (e.g., audio/visual media and Internet sites) as appropriate. *May assist with further learning/promote learning at own pace.*[7]

DOCUMENTATION FOCUS

Assessment/Reassessment
- Individual findings/learning style and identified needs, presence of learning blocks (e.g., hostility, inappropriate behavior).

Planning
- Plan for learning, methods to be used, and who is involved in the planning.
- Teaching plan.

Implementation/Evaluation
- Responses of the client/SO(s) to the learning plan and actions performed. How the learning is demonstrated.
- Attainment/progress toward desired outcome(s).
- Modifications to plan of care.

Discharge Planning
- Additional learning/referral needs.

References

1. Bohny, B. A. (1997). A time for self-care: Role of the home healthcare nurse. Home Health Nurse, 15(4), 281–286.
2. Purnell, L. D., & Paulanka, B. J. (1998). Purnell's model for cultural competence. In Purnell, L. D., & Paulanka, B. J. (eds): Transcultural Health Care: A culturally Competent Approach. Philadelphia: F. A. Davis.
3. Duffy, B. (1997). Using a creative teaching process with adult patients. Home Health Nurse, 15(2), 102–108.
4. Bartholomew L. K, et al. (2000). Watch, discover, think, and act: A model for patient education program development. Patient Educ Couns, 39(2–3), 269–280.
5. Gordon, T. (2000). Parent Effectiveness Training. New York: Three Rivers Press.
6. Townsend, M. C. (2003). Psychiatric Mental Health Nursing Concepts of Care, ed 4. Philadelphia: F. A. Davis.
7. Bloom B. Bloom's Learning Domains. From Encyclopedia of Educational Technology. Available at: http://coe.sdsu.edu/eet/Articles/BloomsLD. Accessed March 2004.

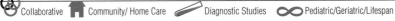
Cultural   Collaborative   Community/ Home Care   Diagnostic Studies   Pediatric/Geriatric/Lifespan   Medications

8. Cook, S. L. Strategies for Psychomotor Skills. From Instructional Strategies. Available at: http://www.signaleader.com/IDTPortfolio/IT800/psychomotor.html. Accessed March 2004.
9. Adams, L. (March, 2004). Learning a New Skill is Easier Said Than Done. Working Together (electronic newsletter). Gordon Training International.
10. Kolb, D. A. (1984). Experiential Learning: Experience as the Source of Learning and Development. New Jersey: Prentice Hall.

Helpful Resources

ND: Knowledge, deficient [Learning Needs] in multiple care plans. In Doenges, M. E., Moorhouse, M. F., & Geissler-Murr, A. C. (2002). Nursing Care Plans: Guidelines for Individualizing Patient Care, ed 6. Philadelphia: F. A. Davis.
ND: Knowledge, deficient. In Cox, H. C, et al. (2002). Clinical Applications of Nursing Diagnosis: Adult, Child, Women's, Psychiatric, Gerontic, and Home Health Considerations, ed 4. Philadelphia: F. A. Davis.

ready for enhanced Knowledge (specify)

Definition: The presence or acquisition of cognitive information related to a specific topic is sufficient for meeting health-related goals and can be strengthened

RELATED FACTORS

To be developed by nurse researchers and submitted to NANDA

DEFINING CHARACTERISTICS

Subjective
Expresses an interest in learning
Explains knowledge of the topic; describes previous experiences pertaining to the topic

Objective
Behaviors congruent with expressed knowledge
SAMPLE CLINICAL APPLICATIONS: as a health seeking behavior the client may be healthy or this diagnosis can occur in any clinical condition

DESIRED OUTCOMES/EVALUATION CRITERIA
Sample **NOC** linkages:
Knowledge: [specify—30 choices]: Extent of understanding conveyed about a specific disease process, the promotion and protection of health, maintaining optimal health, etc.
Information Processing: Ability to acquire, organize, and use information

Client Will (Include Specific Time Frame)
● Exhibit responsibility for own learning and seek answers to questions.
● Verify accuracy of informational resources.
● Verbalize understanding of information gained.
● Use information to develop individual plan to meet healthcare needs/goals.

ACTIONS/INTERVENTIONS
Sample **NIC** linkages:
Teaching: Individual [or 16 other choices]: Planning, implementation, and evaluation of a teaching program designed to address a patient's particular needs
Learning Facilitation: Promoting the ability to process and comprehend information
Learning Readiness Enhancement: Improving the ability and willingness to receive information

NURSING PRIORITY NO. 1. To develop plan for learning:

 • Verify client's level of knowledge about specific topic. *Provides opportunity to assure accuracy and completeness of knowledge base for future learning.*[4]

 • Determine motivation/expectation for learning. *Provides insight useful in developing goals and identifying information needs.*[4]

 • Assist client to identify learning goals. *Helps to frame or focus content to be learned and provides measure to evaluate learning process.*[10]

 • Ascertain preferred methods of learning (e.g., auditory, visual, interactive, or "hands-on"). *Identifies best approaches for the individual to facilitate learning process.*[10]

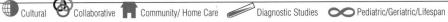 • Note personal factors (e.g., age, gender, social/cultural influences, religion, life experiences, level of education) *that may impact learning style, choice of informational resources.*[1]

 • Determine challenges to learning: language barriers (e.g., cannot read, speak/understand dominant language); physical factors (e.g., sensory deficits such as aphasia, dyslexia); physical stability (e.g., acute illness, activity intolerance); difficulty of material to be learned. *Identifies special needs to be addressed if learning is to be successful.*[6]

NURSING PRIORITY NO. 2. To facilitate learning:

• Identify/provide information in varied formats appropriate to client's learning style (e.g., audiotapes, print materials, videos, classes/seminars). *Use of multiple formats increases learning and retention of material.*[3]

• Provide information about additional/outside learning resources (e.g., bibliography, pertinent Web sites). *Promotes ongoing learning at own pace.*[7]

• Discuss ways to verify accuracy of informational resources. *Encourages independent search for learning opportunities while reducing likelihood of acting on erroneous or unproven data that could be detrimental to client's well-being.*[4]

• Identify available community resources/support groups. *Provides additional opportunities for role-modeling, skill training, anticipatory problem solving, and so forth.*[1]

• Be aware of/discuss informal teaching and role modeling that takes place on an ongoing basis. *Incongruencies in community/peer role models, support group feedback, print advertisements, popular music/videos may exist creating questions/potentially undermining learning process.*[4]

NURSING PRIORITY NO. 3. To enhance optimum wellness:

• Assist client to identify ways to integrate and use information in all applicable areas (e.g., situational, environmental, personal). *Ability to apply/use information increases desire to learn and retention of information.*[10]

• Encourage client to journal, keep a log or graph as appropriate. *Provides opportunity for self-evaluation of effects of learning, such as better management of chronic condition, reduction of risk factors, acquisition of new skills.*[6,9]

DOCUMENTATION FOCUS

Assessment/Reassessment
• Individual findings/learning style and identified needs, presence of challenges to learning.

Planning
- Plan for learning, methods to be used, and who is involved in the planning.
- Educational plan.

Implementation/Evaluation
- Responses of the client/SO(s) to the educational plan and actions performed.
- How the learning is demonstrated.
- Attainment/progress toward desired outcome(s).
- Modifications to lifestyle/treatment plan.

Discharge Planning
- Additional learning/referral needs.

References

1. Bohny, B.A. (1997). A time for self-care: Role of the home healthcare nurse. Home Health Nurse, 15(4), 281–286.
2. Purnell, L. D., & Paulanka, B. J. (1998). Purnell's model for cultural competence. In Purnell, L. D., & Paulanka, B. J. (eds): Transcultural Health Care: A Culturally Competent Approach. Philadelphia: F. A. Davis.
3. Duffy, B. (1997). Using a creative teaching process with adult patients. Home Health Nurse, 15(2), 102–108.
4. Bartholomew, L. K., et al. (2000). Watch, discover, think, and act: A model for patient education program development. Patient Educ Couns, 39(2–3), 269–280.
5. Gordon, T. (2000). Parent Effectiveness Training. New York: Three Rivers Press.
6. Townsend, M. C. (2003). Psychiatric Mental Health Nursing Concepts of Care, ed 4. Philadelphia: F. A. Davis.
7. Bloom, B. Bloom's Learning Domains. From Encyclopedia of Educational Technology. Available at: http://coe.sdsu.edu/eet/Articles/BloomsLD. Accessed March 2004.
8. Cook, S. L. Strategies for Psychomotor Skills. From Instructional Strategies. Available at: http://www.signaleader.com/IDTPortfolio/IT800/psychomotor.html. Accessed March 2004.
9. Adams, L. Learning a New Skill is Easier Said Than Done. From Gordon Training International. Available from: newsletter@gordontraining.com. Accessed March 2004.
10. Don Clark. (1999). Learning Styles, or How We Go From the Unknown To the Known. Available at: http://www.nwlink.com/~don clark/hrd/learning/styles.html. Accessed January 2004.

risk for Loneliness

Definition: At risk for experiencing vague dysphoria

RISK FACTORS
Affectional deprivation
Physical isolation
Cathectic deprivation
Social isolation
NOTE: A risk diagnosis is not evidenced by signs and symptoms, as the problem has not occurred and nursing interventions are directed at prevention.
SAMPLE CLINICAL APPLICATIONS: debilitating conditions (e.g., MS, COPD, renal failure), cancer, AIDS, major depression

DESIRED OUTCOMES/EVALUATION CRITERIA
Sample **NOC** linkages:
Loneliness: The extent of emotional, social, or existential isolation response

Social Involvement: Frequency of an individual's social interactions with persons, groups, or organizations

Immobility Consequences: Psycho-Cognitive: Extent of compromise in psycho-cognitive functioning due to impaired physical mobility

Client Will (Include Specific Time Frame)
- Identify individual difficulties and ways to address them.
- Engage in social activities.
- Report involvement in interactions/relationship client views as meaningful.

ACTIONS/INTERVENTIONS
Sample **NIC** linkages:

Socialization Enhancement: Facilitation of another person's ability to interact with others

Hope Instillation: Facilitation of the development of a positive outlook in a given situation

Emotional Support: Provision of reassurance, acceptance, and encouragement during times of stress

NURSING PRIORITY NO. 1. To identify causative/precipitating factors:

- Differentiate between ordinary loneliness and a state of constant sense of dysphoria. *Being alone is a different state than loneliness.*[3]
- Note client's age and duration of problem, that is, situational (such as leaving home for college) or chronic. *Elderly individuals incur multiple losses associated with aging, loss of spouse, decline in physical health, and changes in roles intensifying feelings of loneliness.*[3]
- Determine degree of distress, tension, anxiety, restlessness present. Note history of frequent illnesses, accidents, crises. *Identifies somatic complaints that can result from loneliness. Individuals under stress tend to have more illnesses and accidents related to inattention and anxiety.*[6]
- Note presence/proximity of family, SO(s). *Loneliness may not be related to being alone, but knowing that family is available can help with planning care. Client may be estranged from other family members or they may not be willing to be involved with client.*[6]
- Determine how individual perceives/deals with solitude. *Client may see being alone as positive, allowing time to pursue own interests, or may view solitude as sad and long for lost objects, such as spouse.*[6]
- Review issues of separation from parents as a child, loss of SO(s)/spouse. *Often early separation from parents affects the individual as other losses occur throughout life, leading to feelings of inadequacy and inability to deal with current situation.*[6]
- Assess sleep/appetite disturbances, ability to concentrate. *Feelings of loneliness often accompany depression and identifying whether client is adequately taking care of self is important to planning care.*[7]
- Note expressions of "yearning" for an emotional partnership. *Widows are particularly prone to feelings of loneliness. Going from being a "couple" to being alone is a difficult transition and these feelings are indicative of a desire to return to the "couple" state.*[7]

NURSING PRIORITY NO. 2. To assist client to identify feelings and situations in which he or she experiences loneliness:

- Establish therapeutic nurse-client relationship. Provides *a sense of connection with someone, enabling client to feel free to talk about feelings of loneliness and current situation that is related to these feelings.*[1]

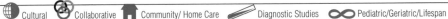

- Discuss individual concerns about feelings of loneliness and relationship between loneliness and lack of SOs. Note desire/willingness to change situation. *Motivation can impede—or facilitate—achieving desired outcomes. Often feelings of loneliness arise from underlying depression related to loss affecting individual's coping abilities.*[7]
- Support expression of negative perceptions of others and whether client believes they are true. *Provides opportunity for client to clarify reality of situation, recognize own denial. Individual's view of the world is colored by feelings of loneliness/depression.*[1]
- Accept client's expressions of loneliness as a primary condition and not necessarily as a symptom of some underlying condition. *Provides a beginning point which will allow the client to look at what loneliness means in life without having to search for deeper meaning.*[1]

NURSING PRIORITY NO. 3. To assist client to become involved:

- Discuss reality versus perceptions of situation. Have client identify people who he or she interacts with on a regular basis. *Provides opportunity for reality check and beginning to understand own feelings of loneliness related to what is happening in own life.*[2]
- Discuss importance of emotional bonding (attachment) between infants/young children, parents/caregivers as appropriate. *Understanding the importance of attachment provides parents with information that will help them take measures to be sure this bonding occurs.*[2]
- Involve in classes such as assertiveness, language/communication, social skills. *Addressing individual needs will enhance socialization and provide client with the skills to become involved in social activities, promoting self-confidence and alleviating feelings of loneliness.*[3]
- Role-play situations that are new or are anxiety-provoking for client. *Practicing new situations helps develop self-confidence and provides client with information about what to expect and how to deal with the unexpected in a positive manner.*[2]
- Discuss positive health habits, including personal hygiene, exercise activity of client's choosing. *Improves feelings of self-esteem, enabling client to feel more confident in social situations.*[7]
- Identify individual strengths, areas of interest that client identifies and is willing to pursue. *Provides opportunities for involvement with others to develop new social skills.*[7]
- Encourage attendance at support groups (e.g., therapy, separation/grief, religious). *Participating in these activities can meet individual needs and help client begin to deal with feelings of loneliness.*[7]
- Help client establish plan for progressive involvement, beginning with a simple activity such as calling an old friend, speaking to a neighbor, and leading to more complicated interactions/activities. *Taking small steps promotes success and confidence is gained as each step is taken, helping client to be more involved and to resolve feelings of loneliness.*[7]
- Provide opportunities for interactions in a supportive environment (e.g., have client accompanied as in a "buddy system") during initial attempts to socialize. *Helps reduce stress, provides positive reinforcement, and facilitates successful outcome.*[7]

NURSING PRIORITY NO. 4. To promote wellness (Teaching/Discharge Considerations):

- Encourage involvement in special-interest groups (computers, bird watchers); charitable services (serving in a soup kitchen, youth groups, animal shelter). *Becoming involved with others takes focus off of self and own concerns, promoting feelings of self-worth and encouraging client to again be an active part of society.*[7]
- Suggest volunteering for church committee or choir; attending community events with

friends and family; becoming involved in political issues/campaigns; enrolling in classes at local college/continuing education programs, as able. *When client is willing to become involved in these kinds of activities, perception of loneliness fades into the background and even though individual may still be lonely, the sense of loneliness is not so pervasive.*[7]

 • Refer to appropriate counselors for help with relationships, social skills or identified needs. *May provide additional assistance for specific needs to help client deal with feelings of loneliness and isolation.*[9]

• Refer to NDs Hopelessness, Anxiety, Social Isolation.

DOCUMENTATION FOCUS

Assessment/Reassessment
• Assessment findings, including client's perception of problem, availability of resources/support systems.
• Client's desire/commitment to change.

Planning
• Plan of care and who is involved in planning.
• Teaching plan.

Implementation/Evaluation
• Response to interventions/teaching and actions performed.
• Attainment/progress toward desired outcome(s).
• Modifications to plan of care.

Discharge Planning
• Long-term needs, plan for follow-up and who is responsible for actions to be taken.
• Specific referrals made.

References

1. Doenges, M. E., Townsend, M., & Moorhouse, M. F. (1998). Psychiatric Care Plans: Guidelines for Individualizing Care, ed 3. Philadelphia: F. A. Davis.
2. Townsend, M. (2003). Psychiatric Mental Health Nursing: Concepts of Care, ed 4. Philadelphia: F. A. Davis.
3. Lipson, J. G., Dibble, S. L., & Minarik, P. A. (1996). Culture & Nursing Care: A Pocket Guide. San Francisco: School of Nursing, UCSF Nursing Press.
4. Doenges, M. E., Moorhouse, M. F., & Geissler-Murr, A. C. (2004). Nurse's Pocket Guide Diagnoses, Interventions, and Rationales, ed 9. Philadelphia: F. A. Davis.
5. Paice, J. (2002) Managing psychological conditions in palliative care. AJN, 102(11), 36–43.
6. Killeen, C. (1998). Loneliness, an epidemic in modern society. J Adv Nurs, 28(4), 762–770.
7. McAuley, E., et al. (2000). Social relations, physical activity, and well-being in older adults. Prev Med, 31, 608–617.
8. Acorn, S., & Bampton, E. (1992). Patient's loneliness: A challenge for rehabilitation nurses. Rehabil Nurs, 17, 22.
9. Davidson, L., & Stayner, D. (1997). Loss, loneliness, and the desire for love: perspectives on the social lives of people with schizophrenia. Psychiatr Rehab J, 20, 3–12.

impaired Memory

Definition: Inability to remember or recall bits of information or behavioral skills (Impaired memory may be attributed to physiopathologic or situational causes that are either temporary or permanent)

 Cultural Collaborative Community/ Home Care Diagnostic Studies 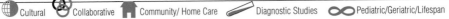 Pediatric/Geriatric/Lifespan Medications

RELATED FACTORS

Acute or chronic hypoxia; anemia
Decreased cardiac output
Fluid and electrolyte imbalance
Neurologic disturbances [e.g., brain injury/concussion]
Excessive environmental disturbances; [manic state, fugue, traumatic event]
[Chronic pain; stress overload]
[Substance use/abuse; effects of medications]
[Age]

DEFINING CHARACTERISTICS

Subjective
Reported experiences of forgetting
Inability to recall recent or past events, factual information, [or familiar persons, places, items]

Objective
Observed experiences of forgetting
Inability to determine if a behavior was performed
Inability to learn or retain new skills or information
Inability to perform a previously learned skill
Forget to perform a behavior at a scheduled time

SAMPLE CLINICAL APPLICATIONS: brain injury/stroke, dementia/Alzheimer's disease, hypoxia (e.g., COPD, anemia, altitude sickness), alcohol intoxication/substance abuse

DESIRED OUTCOMES/EVALUATION CRITERIA

Sample **NOC** linkages:
Memory: Ability to cognitively retrieve and report previously stored information
Cognitive Orientation: Ability to identify person, place, and time
Cognitive Ability: Ability to execute complex mental processes

Client Will (Include Specific Time Frame)
- Verbalize awareness of memory problems.
- Establish methods to help in remembering essential things when possible.
- Accept limitations of condition and use resources effectively.

ACTIONS/INTERVENTIONS

Sample **NIC** linkages:
Memory Training: Facilitation of memory
Reality Orientation: Promotions of patient's awareness of personal identity, time, and environment
Dementia Management: Provision of a safe and therapeutic environment for the patient who is experiencing an acute confusional state

NURSING PRIORITY NO. 1. To assess causative factor(s)/degree of impairment:

- Determine physical/biochemical factors (e.g., recent surgery, infections, brain injury; use of multiple medication, exposure to toxic substances, use/abuse of alcohol/other drugs; pain, depression, etc.) *that may be related to changes in memory.*

• Note client's age, and potential for depression symptoms in elderly. *Depressive disorders are particularly prevalent in older adults (approximately 15%) who report inability to concentrate and poor memory. Kuljis (2003) calls it a prevalent myth that substantial memory loss is a normal aspect of aging barring effects of illness or injury. However, it is known that memory is somehow altered in the aging process and that generally memory for past occurrences is superior to the retention and recall of more recent information.*[1,2]

• Note presence/degree of anxiety. *Can increase the client's confusion and disorganization and further interfere with attempts at recall.* Refer to ND Anxiety for additional interventions as indicated.

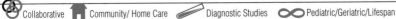 • Collaborate with medical and psychiatric providers *to evaluate extent of impairment to orientation, attention span, ability to follow directions, send/receive communication, appropriateness of response.*

• Assist with/review results of cognitive testing (e.g., Blessed Information-Memory-Concentration (BIMC) test, Clinical Dementia Rating (CDR) Scale, Mini-Mental State Examination (MMSE). *Although the etiology for some memory impairments may be obvious or established by client/SO/caregiver report, a combination of tests may be needed to complete evaluation of the client's overall condition and prognosis.*[3]

• Evaluate skill proficiency levels. *Evaluation may include many self-care activities (e.g., daily grooming, steps in preparing a meal, participating in a lifelong hobby, balancing a checkbook, and driving ability) to determine level of independence/needed assistance.*

• Ascertain how client/family view the problem (e.g., practical problems of forgetting to turn off the stove; or role and responsibility impairments related to loss of memory and concentration) *to determine significance/impact of problem and suggest direction of interventions.*

NURSING PRIORITY NO. 2. To maximize level of function:

 • Assist with treatment of underlying conditions (e.g., electrolyte imbalance, reaction to medications, drug intoxication) *where treatment can improve memory processes.*

 • Orient/reorient client as needed to environment. Introduce self with each client contact *to meet client's safety and comfort needs.* (Refer to ND chronic Confusion for additional interventions.)

• Implement appropriate memory retraining techniques (e.g., keeping calendars, writing lists, memory cue games, mnemonic devices, using computers, etc.) *to provide restorative or compensatory training for cognitive function.*[4]

• Assist in/instruct client and family in associate-learning tasks (e.g., practice sessions recalling personal information, reminiscing, locating a geographic location (Stimulation Therapy). *Practice may improve performance and integrate new behaviors into the client's coping strategies.*

• Support and reinforce client's efforts to remember information or behavioral skills. *Can decrease anxiety levels and perhaps help with further memory recovery.*

• Encourage ventilation of feelings of frustration, helplessness, etc. Refocus attention to areas of control and progress *to lessen feelings of powerlessness/hopelessness.*

• Provide for/emphasize importance of pacing learning activities and having appropriate rest *to avoid fatigue that may further impair cognitive abilities.*

• Monitor client's behavior and assist in use of stress-management techniques (e.g., music therapy, reading, television, games, socialization) *to reduce frustration and enhance enjoyment of life.*

• Structure teaching methods and interventions *to client's level of functioning and/or potential for improvement.*

- Determine client's response to/effects of medications prescribed to improve attention, concentration, memory processes and to lift spirits/modify emotional responses. *Medications used for cognitive enhancement can be effective, but benefits should be weighed against whether quality of life is improved when considering side effects/cost of drugs.*[3]

NURSING PRIORITY NO. 3. To promote wellness (Teaching/Discharge Considerations):

- Assist client/SO(s) to establish compensation strategies *to improve functional lifestyle and safety, such as menu planning with a shopping list; timely completion of tasks on a daily planner, checklists at the front door to ascertain that lights and stove are off before leaving.*

- Teach client and family/care providers memory involvement tasks, e.g., reminiscence and memory practice exercises *geared toward improving client's functional ability.*

- Refer to/encourage follow-up with counselors, rehabilitation programs, job coaches, social/financial support systems *to help deal with persistent/difficult problems.*

- Refer to rehabilitation services *that are matched to the needs, strengths, and capacities of individual and modified as needs change over time.*[4]

- Assist client to deal with functional limitations (e.g., inability to prepare meals, loss of driving privileges) and identify resources to meet individual needs (e.g., home care assistant, companion, Meals on Wheels, etc.), *maximizing independence and general well-being.*

DOCUMENTATION FOCUS

Assessment/Reassessment
- Individual findings, testing results, and perceptions of significance of problem.
- Actual impact on lifestyle and independence.

Planning
- Plan of care and who is involved in planning process.
- Teaching plan.

Implementation/Evaluation
- Responses to interventions/teaching and actions performed.
- Attainment/progress toward desired outcome(s).
- Modifications to plan of care.

Discharge Planning
- Long-term needs and who is responsible for actions to be taken.
- Specific referrals made.

References

1. Kuljis, R. O. Minimal cognitive impairment. (2003). Available at: http://www.emedicine.com.
2. Roussel, L. A. (1999). The aging neurological system. In Stanley, M., and Beare, P. G. (eds): Gerontological Nursing: A Health Promotion/Protection Approach, ed 2. Philadelphia: F. A. Davis.
3. About Alzheimer's. (2003). Physicians and care Professionals educational materials. Retrieved from Alzheimer's Disease and Related Disorders Association (AARDA) website. Available at: http://www.alz.org.
4. Rehabilitation of persons with traumatic brain injury. (1999). NIH Consensus Panel, JAMA, 8(10), 974–983.

Definition: Limitation of independent movement from one bed position to another

RELATED FACTORS

To be developed by nurse researchers and submitted to NANDA
[Neuromuscular impairment]
[Pain/discomfort]

DEFINING CHARACTERISTICS

Subjective
[Reported difficulty performing activities]

Objective
Impaired ability to: turn side to side, move from supine to sitting or sitting to supine, "scoot" or reposition self in bed, move from supine to prone or prone to supine, from supine to long-sitting or long-sitting to supine

SAMPLE CLINICAL APPLICATIONS: paralysis (e.g., spinal cord injury, stroke), traumatic brain injury, neuromuscular disorders (e.g., ALS), major chest/back surgery, severe depression, dementia, catatonic schizophrenia

DESIRED OUTCOMES/EVALUATION CRITERIA

Sample **NOC** linkages:

Body Positioning: Self-Initiated: Ability to change own body position

Muscle Function: Adequacy of muscle contraction needed for movement

Immobility Consequences: Physiological: Extent of compromise to physiological functioning due to impaired physical mobility

Client/Caregiver Will (Include Specific Time Frame)
- Verbalize willingness to/and participate in repositioning program.
- Verbalize understanding of situation/risk factors, individual therapeutic regimen, and safety measures.
- Demonstrate techniques/behaviors that enable safe repositioning.
- Maintain position of function and skin integrity as evidenced by absence of contractures, foot drop, decubitus, and other skin disorders.
- Maintain or increase strength and function of affected and/or compensatory body part.

ACTIONS/INTERVENTIONS

Sample **NIC** linkages:

Bed Rest Care: Promotion of comfort and safety and prevention of complications for a patient unable to get out of bed

Positioning: Deliberative placement of the patient or a body part to promote physiologic and/or psychological well-being

Teaching: Prescribed Activity/Exercise: Preparing a patient to achieve and/or maintain a prescribed level of activity

 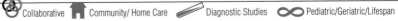

NURSING PRIORITY NO. 1. To identify causative/contributing factors:

- Determine diagnoses that contribute to immobility (e.g., MS, arthritis, parkinsonism, hemi/para/tetraplegia, fractures/multiple trauma, mental illness, severe depression) *to identify interventions specific to client's mobility impairment and needs.*
- Note individual risk factors related to current situation (e.g., surgery, casts, amputation, traction, pain, advanced age, weakness/debilitation, severe depression, head injury, dementia, burns, spinal cord injury) *to identify interventions related to client's specific problems related to bedrest and potential complications.*
- Determine degree of perceptual/cognitive impairment and/or ability to follow directions. *Impairments related to age, chronic or acute disease condition, trauma, surgery, or medications require alternative interventions and/or changes in plan of care.*

NURSING PRIORITY NO. 2. To assess functional ability:

- Determine functional level classification 1 to 4 *(level 1 requires use of equipment or device, level 2 requires help from another person for assistance, level 3 requires help from another person and equipment device, level 4 is totally dependent, does not participate in activity).*
- Note emotional/behavioral responses to problems of immobility. *Can negatively affect self-concept and self-esteem, autonomy and independence. Feelings of frustration and powerlessness may impede attainment of goals. Social, occupational and relationship roles can change, leading to isolation, depression, and economic consequences.*[4,5]
- Note presence of complications related to immobility. *Studies have shown that as much as 5.5% of muscle strength can be lost each day of rest and immobility.*[1] *Other complications include changes in circulation and impairments of organ function affecting the whole person (e.g., cognition, immune system function, emotional state, etc.).* Refer to ND risk for Disuse Syndrome.

NURSING PRIORITY NO. 3. To promote optimal level of function and prevent complications:

- Instruct client/caregivers in bed-mobility movements and set positions, encouraging client to participate as much as possible, even if only to move head, or run bed controls. *Promotes independence and prepares body for purposeful movement.*
- Provide/assist with daily range-of-motion interventions (active and passive) *to maintain joint mobility, improve circulation and prevent contractures.*
- Collaborate with rehabilitation team *to create exercise and adaptive program designed specifically for client,* identifying assistive devices (e.g., splints, braces, boots) and equipment (e.g., transfer board/sling, trapeze, hydraulic lift, specialty beds, etc.).
- Perform periodic assessment of equipment to verify good working order *and ensure safety for client and care provider.*
- Change client's position frequently, moving individual parts of the body (e.g., legs, arms, head) using appropriate support and proper body alignment. Encourage periodic changes in head of bed (if not contraindicated by conditions such as acute spinal cord injury), with client in supine and prone positions at intervals *to improve circulation, reduce tightening of muscles and joints, normalizing body tone and more closely simulating body positions individual would normally use.*[2]
- Instruct caregivers in methods of moving client relative to specific situations (e.g., turning side to side, or prone or sitting) *to provide support for the client's body and to prevent injury*

to the lifter. Note: Positioning instructions and detailed sketches are available (e.g., Therapist Guide: Adult Positions, Transitions and Transfers, Ossmand & Campbell, 1990) on proper positions for certain conditions (e.g., paralyzed client) as well as the safe movement and positioning of body parts (e.g., rolling, bridging, scooting, sitting, etc.), which should become well known to caregivers in order to prevent injury to both the client and the caregivers.

• Place in upright position at intervals, or out of bed into upright chair, if condition allows. *Being vertical has been shown to reduce the work of heart, improve circulation and lung ventilation, and may improve cognition and awareness.*[3]

• Perform/encourage regular skin examination and care *to reduce pressure on sensitive areas and prevent development of problems with skin integrity.*

• Provide egg-crate, alternating air pressure or water mattress. *Reduces tissue pressure and aids in maximizing cellular perfusion to prevent dermal injury.*

• Use padding and positioning devices (e.g., foam wedge, pillows, hand rolls, etc. for bony prominences, feet, hands, elbows, head) *to prevent stress on tissues and reduce potential for disuse complications.*

• Note change in strength to do more or less self-care (e.g., hygiene, feeding, toileting) *to promote psychological and physical benefits of self-care and to adjust level of assistance as indicated.*

• Assist on/off bedpan (with head of bed low) and then raise into sitting position (when condition allows), *to reduce skin shear and improve elimination, which can be impaired by immobility.*

• Administer medication before activity as needed for pain relief *to permit maximal effort/involvement in activity.*

• Provide diversional activities (e.g., television, books, music, games, visiting) as appropriate *to decrease boredom and potential for depression.*

• Ensure telephone/call bell is within reach. Provides individually appropriate methods for client to communicate needs for assistance.

• Refer to NDs, impaired physical Mobility, impaired wheelchair Mobility, Activity Intolerance, risk for Disuse Syndrome, impaired Transfer Ability, impaired Walking for additional interventions.

NURSING PRIORITY NO. 4. To promote wellness (Teaching/Discharge Considerations):

• Involve client/SO in determining activity schedule. *Promotes commitment to plan, maximizing outcomes.*

• Instruct all caregivers in safety concerns regarding body mechanics, as well as client's required positions and exercises *to prevent injury to both, and to minimize potential for preventable complications.*

• Encourage continuation of regular exercise program *to maintain/enhance gains in strength/muscle control.*

• Obtain/identify sources for assistive devices. Demonstrate safe use and proper maintenance. *Promotes independence and enhances safety.*

DOCUMENTATION FOCUS

Assessment/Reassessment
• Individual findings, including level of function/ability to participate in specific/desired activities.

 Cultural   Collaborative   Community/Home Care   Diagnostic Studies   Pediatric/Geriatric/Lifespan   Medications

Planning
- Plan of care and who is involved in the planning.

Implementation/Evaluation
- Responses to interventions/teaching and actions performed.
- Attainment/progress toward desired outcome(s).
- Modification to plan of care.

Discharge Planning
- Discharge/long-range needs, noting who is responsible for each action to be taken.
- Specific referrals made.
- Sources of/maintenance for assistive devices.

References

1. Pattillo, M. A. and Stanley, M. (1999). The aging musculoskeletal system. In Stanley, M. and Beare, P. G. (eds): Gerontological Nursing: A Health Promotion/Protection Approach, ed 2. Philadelphia: F. A. Davis.
2. Kumagai, K. A. S. (1998). Physical management of the neurologically involved client: techniques for bed mobility and transfers. In Chin, P. A., Finocchiaro, D., & Rosebrough, A. (eds.): Rehabilitation Nursing Practice. New York: McGraw-Hill.
3. Palmer, M., & Wyness, M. A. (1988). Positioning and handling: Important considerations in the care of the severely head-injured patient. J Neurosurg Nurs, 20(1), 42–49.
4. Mass, M. L. (1989). Impaired physical mobility. Unpublished manuscript. Cited in research article for National Institutes for Health.
5. Hogue, C. C. (1984). Falls and mobility late in life: An ecological model. J Am Geriatr Soc, 32, 858–861.

Helpful Resource

Doenges, M. E., Moorhouse, M. F., & Geissler-Murr, A. C. (2002), Nursing Care Plans: Guidelines for Individualizing Patient Care, ed 6. Philadelphia: F. A. Davis.

impaired physical Mobility

Definition: Limitation in independent, purposeful physical movement of the body or of one or more extremities

RELATED FACTORS
Sedentary lifestyle, disuse or deconditioning; limited cardiovascular endurance

Decreased muscle strength, control and/or mass; joint stiffness or contracture; loss of integrity of bone structures

Intolerance to activity/decreased strength and endurance

Pain/discomfort

Neuromuscular/musculoskeletal impairment

Sensoriperceptual/cognitive impairment; developmental delay

Depressive mood state or anxiety

Selective or generalized malnutrition; altered cellular metabolism; body mass index above 75th age-appropriate percentile

Lack of knowledge regarding value of physical activity; cultural beliefs regarding age-appropriate activity; lack of physical or social environmental supports

Prescribed movement restrictions; medications

Reluctance to initiate movement

Subjective
[Report of pain/discomfort on movement]

Objective
Limited range of motion; limited ability to perform gross fine/motor skills; difficulty turning

Slowed movement; uncoordinated or jerky movements, decreased [sic] reaction time

Gait changes (e.g., decreased walking speed; difficulty initiating gait, small steps, shuffles feet; exaggerated lateral postural sway)

Postural instability during performance of routine ADLs

Movement-induced shortness of breath/tremor

Engages in substitutions for movement (e.g., increased attention to other's activity, controlling behavior, focus on pre-illness/disability activity)

SAMPLE CLINICAL APPLICATIONS: neuromuscular disorders (e.g., MS, ALS), Parkinson's disease, traumatic injuries (e.g., fractures, spinal cord/brain injuries), rheumatoid arthritis, severe depression

SUGGESTED FUNCTIONAL LEVEL CLASSIFICATION:
- 0—Completely independent
- 1—Requires use of equipment or device
- 2—Requires help from another person for assistance, supervision, or teaching
- 3—Requires help from another person and equipment device
- 4—Dependent, does not participate in activity

DESIRED OUTCOMES/EVALUATION CRITERIA
Sample **NOC** linkages:

Mobility Level: Ability to move purposefully

Immobility Consequences: Physiologic: Extent of compromise to physiological functioning due to impaired physical mobility

Knowledge: Prescribed Activity: Extent of understanding conveyed about prescribed activity and exercise

Client Will (Include Specific Time Frame)
- Verbalize willingness to and demonstrate participation in activities.
- Verbalize understanding of situation/risk factors and individual treatment regimen and safety measures.
- Demonstrate techniques/behaviors that enable resumption of activities.
- Maintain position of function and skin integrity as evidenced by absence of contractures, footdrop, decubitus, and so forth.
- Maintain or increase strength and function of affected and/or compensatory body part.

ACTIONS/INTERVENTIONS
Sample **NIC** linkages:

Exercise Therapy: [specify]: Use of active or passive body movement to maintain or restore flexibility; use of specific activity or exercise protocols to enhance or restore controlled body movement, etc.

 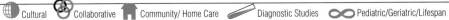

Pain Management: Alleviation of pain or a reduction in pain to a level of comfort acceptable to the patient

Traction/Immobilization Care: Management of a patient who has traction and/or a stabilizing device to immobilize and stabilize a body part

NURSING PRIORITY NO. 1. To identify causative/contributing factors:

- Determine diagnosis that contributes to immobility (e.g., MS, arthritis, parkinsonism, hemiplegia/paraplegia, depression, developmental delays, etc.). *These conditions can cause physiologic and psychological problems that can seriously impact physical, social, and economic well-being.*[1]
- Note factors affecting current situation (e.g., surgery, fractures, amputation, tubings (chest tube, Foley catheter, IVs, pumps, etc.) and potential time involved (e.g., few hours in bed after surgery vs. serious trauma requiring long-term bedrest/debilitating disease limiting movement). *Identifies potential impairments and determines type of interventions needed.*
- Assess client's developmental level, motor skills, ease and capability of movement, posture and gait to *determine presence of characteristics of client's unique impairment and to guide choice of interventions.*
- Note older client's general health status. *Hogue (1984) identified mobility as the most important functional ability that determines the degree of independence and healthcare needs among older persons.*[2] *While aging per se does not cause impaired mobility, several predisposing factors in addition to age-related changes can lead to immobility, e.g., diminished body reserves of musculoskeletal system, chronic diseases, sedentary lifestyle, decreased ability to quickly and adequately correct movements affecting center of gravity. Thus falls are a major source of morbidity and mortality for older persons.*[3]
- Assess degree of pain, listening to client's description. *Nurses must be willing to accept client's definition and self-rating of pain and believe their need for analgesics.*[4]
- Ascertain client's perception of activity/exercise needs and impact of current situation. *Helps to determine client's usual lifestyle as it relates to activity, and potential long-term effect of current immobility. Also identifies barriers that may be addressed (e.g., lack of safe place to exercise, focus on pre-illness/disability activity, controlling behavior, depression, cultural expectations, distorted body image, etc.).*[5]
- Assess nutritional status and energy level. *Deficiencies in nutrients and water, electrolytes and minerals can negatively affect energy and activity tolerance.*
- Determine history of falls and relatedness to current situation. *Client may be restricting activity because of actual injury or from psychological distress (i.e., fear and anxiety) that can persist after a fall.*[6]

NURSING PRIORITY NO. 2. To assess functional ability:

- Determine degree of immobility in relation to 0–4 scale, noting muscle strength and tone, joint mobility, cardiovascular status, balance and endurance. *Identifies strengths and deficits (e.g., ability to ambulate with/without assistive devices, or inability to transfer safely from bed to wheelchair) and may provide information regarding potential for recovery (e.g., client with severe brain injury may have permanent limitations because of impaired cognition affecting memory, judgment, problem solving and motor planning, requiring more intensive inpatient and long-term care).*
- Determine degree of perceptual/cognitive impairment and ability to follow directions.

Impairments related to age, chronic or acute disease condition, trauma, surgery, or medications require alternative interventions and/or changes in plan of care.

- Observe movement when client is unaware of observation *to note any incongruency with reports of abilities.*
- Note emotional/behavioral responses to problems of immobility. *Can negatively affect self-concept and self-esteem, autonomy and independence. Feelings of frustration and powerlessness may impede attainment of goals. Social, occupational, and relationship roles can change, leading to isolation, depression, and economic consequences.*[1,2]
- Determine presence of complications related to immobility (e.g., pneumonia, elimination problems, contractures, decubitus, anxiety). *Studies have shown that as much as 5.5% of muscle strength can be lost each day of rest and immobility.*[5] *Other complications include changes in circulation and impairments of organ function affecting the whole person (e.g., cognition, bone demineralization, venous pooling and thromboembolic pneumonia, weakened immune system function, muscle contractures, etc.)* See ND risk for Disuse Syndrome.

NURSING PRIORITY NO. 3. To promote optimal level of function and prevent complications:

- Assist with treatment of underlying condition causing pain and/or dysfunction *to maximize function.*
- Assist/have client reposition self on a regular schedule as dictated by individual situation (including frequent shifting of weight when client is wheelchair-bound) *to enhance circulation to tissues, reduce risk of tissue ischemia.*
- Demonstrate/assist with use of side rails, overhead trapeze, roller pads, hydraulic lifts/chairs *for position changes/transfers.* Instruct in safe use of walker/cane *for ambulation.*
- Review/encourage use of proper body mechanics *to prevent injury to client or caregiver.*
- Support affected body parts/joints using pillows/rolls, foot supports/shoes air mattress, waterbed, etc. *to maintain position of function and reduce risk of pressure ulcers.*
- Perform/encourage regular skin examination and care *to reduce pressure on sensitive areas and to prevent development of problems with skin integrity.*
- Provide/recommend egg-crate, alternating air pressure or water mattress. *Reduces tissue pressure and aids in maximizing cellular perfusion to prevent dermal injury.*
- Use padding and positioning devices (e.g., foam wedge, pillows, hand rolls, etc.) for bony prominences, feet, hands, elbows, head) *to prevent stress on tissues and reduce potential for disuse complications.*
- Collaborate with physical medicine specialist and occupational/physical therapists in providing range of motion exercise (active or passive), isotonic muscle contractions (e.g., flexion of ankles, push/pull exercises), assistive devices, and activities (e.g., early ambulation, transfers, stairs) *to limit/reduce effects and complications of immobility (e.g., contracture deformities, deep vein thromboses). Techniques such as gait training, strength training and exercise to improve balance and coordination can be helpful in rehabilitating client.*[7]
- Encourage client's participation in self-care activities, physical/occupational therapies as well as diversional/recreational activities. *Reduces sensory deprivation, enhances self-concept and sense of independence, and improves body strength and function.*
- Note change in strength to do more or less self-care (e.g., hygiene, feeding, toileting, therapies) *to promote psychological and physical benefits of self-care and to adjust level of assistance as indicated.*
- Discuss discrepancies in movement with client aware and unaware of observation and methods for dealing with identified problems. *May be necessary when client is using avoidance or controlling behavior, or is not aware of own abilities due to anxiety/fear.*[7]

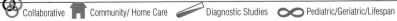

- Avoid routinely assisting or doing for client those activities that client can do for self. *Caregivers can contribute to impaired mobility by being overprotective or helping too much.*
- Administer medications before activity as needed for pain relief *to permit maximal effort/involvement in activity.*
- Provide client with ample time to perform mobility-related tasks. Schedule activities with adequate rest periods during the day *to reduce fatigue.*
- Identify/encourage energy-conserving techniques for ADLs. *Limits fatigue, maximizing participation.*
- Provide for safety measures as indicated by individual situation, including environmental management/fall prevention. Refer to ND risk for Falls.
- Encourage adequate intake of fluids/nutritious foods. *Promotes well-being and maximizes energy production.*
- Refer to NDs impaired bed Mobility, impaired wheelchair Mobility, Activity Intolerance, risk for Disuse Syndrome, impaired Transfer Ability, and impaired Walking for additional interventions.

NURSING PRIORITY NO. 4. To promote wellness (Teaching/Discharge Considerations):

- Encourage client's/SO's involvement in decision making as much as possible. *Enhances commitment to plan, optimizing outcomes.*
- Teach client/SO importance and purpose of exercise (e.g., increased cardiovascular and respiratory tolerance, improved flexibility, balance, and muscle strength/tone, enhanced sense of well-being).
- Discuss safe ways that client can exercise (e.g., walking around the block with companion or in a mall during bad air days, participating in a water aerobics class, attending regular rehab sessions).
- Assist client/SO to learn safety measures as individually indicated. *May need instruction and to give return demonstration (e.g., use of heating pads, locking wheelchair before transfers, removal or securing of scatter/area rugs, judicious and accurate use of medications, supervised exercise).*[7]
- Involve client and SO(s) in care, assisting them to learn ways of managing problems of immobility, especially when impairment is expected to be long-term. *May need referral for support and community services to provide care, supervision, companionship, respite services, nutritional and ADL assistance, adaptive devices or changes to living environment, financial assistance, etc.*[7]
- Demonstrate use of adjunctive devices (e.g., walkers, braces, prosthetics) and ascertain that client can safely use them. Identify appropriate resources for obtaining and maintaining appliances/equipment. *Promotes independence and enhances safety.*

DOCUMENTATION FOCUS

Assessment/Reassessment
- Individual findings, including level of function/ability to participate in specific/desired activities.

Planning
- Plan of care and who is involved in the planning.
- Teaching plan.

Implementation/Evaluation
- Responses to interventions/teaching and actions performed.
- Attainment/progress toward desired outcome(s).
- Modifications to plan of care.

Discharge Planning
- Discharge/long-range needs, noting who is responsible for each action to be taken.
- Specific referrals made.
- Sources of/maintenance for assistive devices.

References

1. Mass, M. L. (1989). Impaired physical mobility. Unpublished manuscript. Cited in research article for National Institutes for Health.
2. Hogue, C. C. (1984). Falls and mobility late in life: An ecological model. J Am Geriatr Soc, 32, 858–861.
3. Rowe, J. W., & Kahn, R. L. (1987). Human aging: Usual and successful. Science, 237, 143–149.
4. McCaffrey, M., & Pasero, C. (1999). Pain: Clinical Manual, ed 2. St. Louis: Mosby.
5. Pattillo, M. A., & Stanley, M. (1999). The aging musculoskeletal system. In Stanley, M. & Beare, P. G. Gerontological Nursing: A Health Promotion/Protection Approach, ed 2. Philadelphia: F. A. Davis.
6. Tinetti, M. E., Williams, T. F., & Mayewski, R. (1986). Fall risk index for elderly patients based on number of chronic disabilities. Am J Med, 80, 429–434.
7. Doenges, M. E., Moorhouse, M. F., & Geissler-Murr, A. C. (2002), Nursing Care Plans: Guidelines for Individualizing Patient Care, ed 6. Philadelphia: F. A. Davis.

impaired wheelchair Mobility

Definition: Limitation of independent operation of wheelchair within environment

RELATED FACTORS
To be developed by nurse researchers and submitted to NANDA

DEFINING CHARACTERISTICS
Impaired ability to operate manual or power wheelchair on even or uneven surface, on an incline or decline, on curbs

Note: Specify level of independence (Refer to ND impaired physical Mobility)

SAMPLE CLINICAL APPLICATIONS: neuromuscular disorders (e.g., MS, ALS), paralysis (e.g., brain injury/stroke, spinal cord injury), muscular dystrophy, cerebral palsy, fractures

DESIRED OUTCOMES/EVALUATION CRITERIA
Sample **NOC** linkage:
Ambulation: Wheelchair: Ability to move from place to place in a wheelchair

Client Will (Include Specific Time Frame)
- Be able to move safely within environment, maximizing independence.
- Identify and use resources appropriately.

Sample **NOC** linkages:
Risk Detection: Activities taken to identify personal health threats
Risk Control: Actions to eliminate or reduce actual, personal, and modifiable health threats

Caregiver Will (Include Specific Time Frame)
- Provide safe mobility within environment and community

 Cultural Collaborative Community/ Home Care Diagnostic Studies 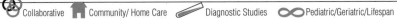 Pediatric/Geriatric/Lifespan Medications

ACTIONS/INTERVENTIONS

Sample **NIC** linkages:

Positioning: Wheelchair: Placement of a patient in a properly selected wheelchair to enhance comfort, promote skin integrity, and foster independence

Exercise Therapy: Muscle Control: Use of specific activity or exercise protocols to enhance or restore controlled body movement

Transport: Moving a patient from one location to another

NURSING PRIORITY NO. 1. To identify causative/contributing factors:

● Determine diagnosis that contributes to immobility (e.g., amyotrophic lateral sclerosis— ALS, spinal cord injury, spastic cerebral palsy, brain injury) and client's functional level/individual abilities (0–4 scale, see ND impaired physical Mobility).

● Identify factors in environments frequented by the client that contribute to inaccessibility (e.g., uneven floors/surfaces, lack of ramps, steep incline/decline, narrow doorways/spaces).

● Ascertain access to and appropriateness of public and/or private transportation.

NURSING PRIORITY NO. 2. To promote optimal level of function and prevent complications:

● Collaborate with physical medicine, physical, and occupational therapists in planning activities to improve client's ability to independently operate wheelchair within limits of tolerance and adjustment to various environments. *May require individual instruction and encouragement, strengthening exercises, assistance with various tasks and close supervision.*

● Ascertain that wheelchair provides the base mobility to maximize function. *Wheelchairs must be matched with client's age, size, developmental level and unique functional needs (e.g., proper seating and support for children in wheelchairs is critical to their ability to learn at school, to play and to interact with friends).[1] Correct seating is essential for prevention, correction, and compensation for postural changes in order to maintain client's comfort and function. Chair should provide for maximum reach, maneuverability, function and center of gravity positioning and propulsion; should recline to change back contours, hip angles and pelvic restrictions; should have back adjustment for changing trunk stability requirements and should tilt for reposition, pressure relief and comfort.[1,2]*

● Perform periodic assessments of client and wheelchair to monitor chair usage and function, as well as changes in client's postural, behavioral and functional status. *Helps to identify problems (e.g., abnormal wear patterns on the chair requiring mechanical adjustments/repair; or loss of client's strength where power add-ons to the chair would improve mobility, or alternate methods of mobility might be needed).[2]*

● Provide for/instruct client in safety while in a wheelchair (e.g., supports for all body parts, repositioning and transfer assistive devices, position and pressure relief products, feet and leg support, armrest choices, and back and height adjustment).

● Note evenness of surfaces client would need to negotiate and refer to appropriate sources for modifications (e.g., replacing carpet with tile, revising ramps that are too steep, narrow or slippery). Clear pathways of obstructions.

● Recommend/arrange for alterations to home/work or school/recreational settings frequented by client. *Although most public buildings have certain adaptations in rooms and accesses, they are not always well constructed or in good working order. The client may need assistance in these settings and with demanding that alterations be carried out.*

• Determine need for and capabilities of assistive persons. Provide training and support as indicated.

 • Monitor client's use of joystick, sip and puff, sensitive mechanical switches, etc., *to provide necessary equipment if condition/capabilities change.*

 • Monitor client for adverse effects of immobility (e.g., contractures, muscle atrophy, deep venous thrombosis, pressure ulcers).

NURSING PRIORITY NO. 3. To promote wellness (Teaching/Discharge Considerations):

 • Consult with therapist and identify/refer to medical equipment suppliers *to customize client's wheelchair for size, positioning aids, and electronics suited to client's ability (e.g., sip and puff, head movement, sensitive switches, etc.).*

 • Encourage client's/SO(s') involvement in decision making as much as possible. *Enhances commitment to plan, optimizing outcomes.*

 • Involve client/SO in care, assisting them in managing immobility problems. *Promotes independence in self-evaluation and self-care, including managing the type of wheelchair/other assistive devices best for client, how the user's needs and abilities change over time, modifications that might be made (e.g., number and placement of ramps around the home, modifications to rooms, doors and vehicles, etc.).*[3]

 • Demonstrate/provide information regarding individually appropriate safety, including wheelchair preventative maintenance measures (e.g., for wheelchair locks, tires, axels, casters, metal parts, batteries, etc.). *Wheelchair safety involves the maintenance of the chair and provision for obtaining relief when chair malfunctions. Many states have enacted so-called Wheelchair Lemon Laws that "mandate warranties to maintain assistive technology in proper working condition, to assure availability of appropriate loaner replacement chairs during repair time and to encourage manufacturers and dealers to cooperatively pool assistive technology resources for loaner purposes to assure availability without undue burden."*[4]

 • Refer to support groups relative to specific medical condition/disability and geared toward client's independence. *Provides role modeling, assistance with problem solving.*

 • Identify community resources to provide ongoing support. *The current societal view (that persons with disabilities have the right to be self-determining and to make their own choices about their lives and to achieve the quality of life each believes is personal best) places as much emphasis on community (re)integration as on physical rehabilitation and functional capabilities.*[5]

DOCUMENTATION FOCUS

Assessment/Reassessment
• Individual findings, including level of function/ability to participate in specific/desired activities.

Planning
• Plan of care and who is involved in the planning.
• Teaching plan.

Implementation/Evaluation
• Responses to interventions/teaching and actions performed.

 Cultural   Collaborative   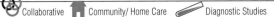 Community/ Home Care   Diagnostic Studies   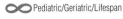 Pediatric/Geriatric/Lifespan   Medications

Discharge Planning

- Discharge/long-range needs, noting who is responsible for each action to be taken.
- Specific referrals made.
- Sources of/maintenance for assistive devices.

References

1. Taylor, S. J. Seating for children: What to consider. Article on wheelchairs, on SpinTips website. Available at: http://www.spinlife.com. Accessed November 2003.
2. Buck, S. (2001). Mobility and the aged: The importance of adjustability and consistent reassessment when treating mobility-impaired elderly clients. Article retrieved from Rehab Management, Interdisciplinary Journal of Rehabilitation International website. Available at: http://www.rehabinternationalpub.com/fall2001/7.asp.
3. Lathrop, D. (2000). Ramp the planet! Reprinted from New Mobility: Life on Wheels. Available at: http://www.spinlife.com.
4. Colorado House Bill 97–1194, *Concerning Self-Sufficiency for Persons with Disabilities by Assuring Reliable Assistive Technology*. Bill signed into law April 30, 1997. Denver, CO.
5. Scherer, M. (2002). The importance of assistive technology outcomes. Article for Institute for Matching Person & Technology, Washington DC.

Nausea

Definition: A subjective unpleasant, wavelike sensation in the back of the throat, epigastrium, or abdomen that may lead to the urge or need to vomit

RELATED FACTORS

Treatment Related

Gastric irritation: pharmaceutical agents (e.g., aspirin, nonsteroidal anti-inflammatory drugs, steroids, antibiotics), alcohol, iron, and blood

Gastric distention: delayed gastric emptying caused by pharmaceutical interventions (e.g., narcotics administration, anesthesia agents)

Pharmaceutical agents(e.g., analgesics, antiviral for HIV, aspirin, opioids, chemotherapeutic agents)

Toxins (e.g., radiation therapy)

Biophysical

Biochemical disorders (e.g., uremia, diabetic ketoacidosis, pregnancy)

Cardiac pain; cancer of stomach or intra-abdominal tumors (e.g., pelvic or colorectal cancers); local tumors (e.g., acoustic neuroma, primary or secondary brain tumors, bone metastases at base of skull)

Esophageal or pancreatic disease; liver or splenetic capsule stretch

Gastric distention due to delayed gastric emptying, pyloric intestinal obstruction, genitourinary and biliary distention, upper bowel stasis, external compression of the stomach, liver, spleen, or other organ enlargement that slows stomach functioning (squashed stomach syndrome)

Gastric irritation due to pharyngeal and peritoneal inflammation

Motion sickness, Meniere's disease, or labyrinthitis

Physical factors (e.g., increased intracranial pressure, meningitis)

Toxins (e.g., tumor-produced peptides, abdominal metabolites due to cancer)

Situational

Psychological factors (e.g., pain, fear, anxiety, noxious odors, taste, unpleasant visual stimulation)

DEFINING CHARACTERISTICS

Subjective

Reports "nausea" or "sick to stomach"

Objective

Usually precedes vomiting, but may be experienced after vomiting or when vomiting does not occur

Accompanied by swallowing movement affected by skeletal muscles; pallor, cold and clammy skin, increased salivation, tachycardia, gastric stasis, and diarrhea

SAMPLE CLINICAL APPLICATIONS: surgery/anesthesia, cancer, pregnancy, AIDS, gastritis, peptic ulcer disease, renal failure, brain injury, meningitis, panic disorders/phobias

DESIRED OUTCOMES/EVALUATION CRITERIA

Sample **NOC** linkages:

Symptom Severity: Extent of perceived adverse changes in physical, emotional, and social functioning

Hydration: Amount of water in the intracellular and extracellular compartments of the body

Nutritional Status: Food & Fluid Intake: Amount of food and fluid taken into the body over a 24-hour period

Client Will (Include Specific Time Frame)

- Be free of nausea.
- Manage chronic nausea, as evidenced by acceptable level of dietary intake.
- Maintain/regain weight as appropriate.

ACTIONS/INTERVENTIONS

Sample **NIC** linkages:

Nausea Management: Prevention and alleviation of nausea

Vomiting Management: Prevention and alleviation of vomiting

Fluid Management: Promotion of fluid balance and prevention of complications resulting from abnormal or undesired fluid levels

NURSING PRIORITY NO. 1. To determine causative/contributing factors:

- Assess for presence of conditions of the GI tract (e.g., peptic ulcer disease, cholecystitis, appendicitis, gastritis, intestinal blockage, ingestion of "problem" foods). *Dietary changes may be sufficient to decrease frequency of nausea in some situations.*
- Note systemic conditions that may result in nausea (e.g., pregnancy, cancer treatment, myocardial infarction, hepatitis, acid-base and metabolic disturbances, systemic infections, drug toxicity, migraine headache, presence of neurogenic causes-stimulation of the vestibular system, concussion, CNS trauma/tumor). *Helpful in determining appropriate interventions/need for treatment of underlying conditions.*[4]
- Identify situations that client perceives as anxiety-inducing, threatening, or distasteful

 Cultural Collaborative Community/ Home Care Diagnostic Studies Pediatric/Geriatric/Lifespan Medications

(e.g., "this is nauseating") such as might occur if client is having multiple diagnostic studies, facing surgery. *May be able to limit/control exposure to situations or take medication prophylactically.*

 • Note psychological factors, including those that are culturally determined (e.g., eating certain foods considered repulsive in one's culture).[4]

• Determine if nausea is potentially self-limiting and/or mild (e.g., first trimester of pregnancy, 24-hour GI tract viral infection) or is severe and prolonged (e.g., cancer treatment, hyperemesis gravidarum). *Indicates potential degree of effect on fluid/electrolyte balance and nutritional status.*[4]

• Record food intake and changes in symptoms *to help identify food intolerances when nausea is chronic.*

 • Assess vital signs, especially for older clients, and note signs of dehydration. *Nausea may occur in the presence of postural hypotension/fluid volume deficit, or in severe hypertension.*

NURSING PRIORITY NO. 2. To promote comfort and enhance intake:

 • Collaborate with physician *to treat underlying medical condition when cause of nausea is known (e.g., infection, adverse side effect of medications, food allergies, gastrointestinal reflux).*

 • Administer/monitor response to medications that prevent or relieve nausea. *Antiemetic agents may be administered prophylactically to prevent/limit severity of nausea and vomiting in some conditions (e.g., during chemotherapy or radiation or postoperative clients at high risk for vomiting).*[1]

 • Administer antiemetic on regular schedule before/during and after administration of antineoplastic agents.[1]

 • Administer analgesics *when postoperative pain is a factor in nausea/vomiting.* Observe for nausea *when opioids are used for pain management.*[2]

• Time chemotherapy doses *for least interference with food intake.*

• Review medications, especially in elderly client on multiple drugs. *Polypharmacy with drug interactions and side effects may cause/exacerbate nausea.*

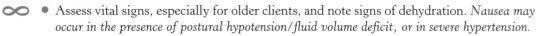 • Manage food and fluids:

Have client try dry foods such as toast, crackers, dry cereal before arising *when nausea occurs in the morning, or throughout the day* as appropriate.

Advise client to drink liquids before or after meals, instead of with meals. Sip fluids slowly and use cool, clear liquids (e.g., water, ginger ale/lemon-lime soda—if tolerated, electrolyte drinks).

Recommend avoiding milk and other dairy products during acute episodes.

Provide diet and snacks high in carbohydrates with substitutions of preferred foods (including bland/noncaffeinated beverages, gelatin, sherbet) when available *to reduce gastric acidity and improve nutrient intake.* Avoid overly sweet, fried and fatty foods *that may increase nausea/be more difficult to digest.*[4]

Instruct client to eat small meals spaced throughout the day rather than large meals *so stomach does not feel too full.*[4]

Instruct client to eat and drink slowly, chewing food well *for easier digestion.*

Advise client to suck on ice cubes, tart or hard candies, chew gum. *Keeps mucous membranes moist and can provide some fluid/nutrient intake.*

Monitor infusion rate of tube feeding, if present *to prevent rapid administration that can cause gastric distention/produce nausea.*

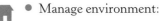 • Manage environment:

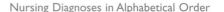

Elevate head of bed or have client sit upright after meals *to promote digestion by gravity and eliminate feeling of fullness when that is causing nausea.*
Avoid sudden changes in position.
Apply cool cloth to face and neck.
Provide clean, pleasant smelling, quiet environment.
Avoid offending odors (e.g., cooking smells, smoke, perfumes, mechanical emissions, etc.)

 ● Provide nonpharmacologic measures:
Encourage deep, slow breathing *to promote relaxation.*
Use distraction with music, guided imagery, music therapy, chatting with family/friends, watching television *to refocus attention away from unpleasant sensations.*
Provide frequent oral care *to cleanse mouth and minimize "bad tastes."*

● Investigate use of electrical nerve stimulation, or acupressure point therapy (e.g., elastic band worn around wrist with small, hard bump that presses against acupressure point). *Some individuals with chronic nausea report this to be helpful and without sedative effect of medication.*[3]

NURSING PRIORITY NO. 3. To promote wellness (Teaching/Discharge Considerations):

 ● Review individual factors causing nausea and ways to avoid problem (e.g., identifying offending medications or foods). *Provides necessary information for client to manage own care.*

● Instruct in proper use, side effects, and adverse reactions of antiemetic medications. *Enhances client safety and effective management of condition.*

 ● Advise client/SO to prepare and freeze meals in advance *for days when nausea is severe or cooking is impossible as with chemo/radiation therapy.*

● Discuss potential complications and possible need for medical follow-up or alternative therapies. *Timely recognition and intervention may limit severity of complications (e.g., dehydration).*

 ● Review signs of dehydration and stress importance of replacing fluids and/or electrolytes (with products such as Gatorade or Pedialyte) if vomiting occurs, especially in young children or frail elderly. *Increases likelihood of preventing potentially serious complications.*

DOCUMENTATION FOCUS

Assessment/Reassessment
● Individual findings, including individual factors causing nausea.
● Baseline weight, vital signs.
● Specific client preferences for nutritional intake.

Planning
● Plan of care and who is involved in planning.
● Teaching plan.

Implementation/Evaluation
● Response to interventions/teaching and actions performed.
● Attainment/progress toward desired outcome(s).
● Modifications to plan of care.

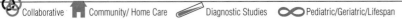 

Discharge Planning
- Individual long-term needs, noting who is responsible for actions to be taken.
- Specific referrals made.

References
1. American Society of Health System Pharmacists, (ASHP) therapeutic guidelines on the pharmacologic management of nausea and vomiting in adult and pediatric patients receiving chemotherapy or radiation therapy or undergoing surgery (1999). Am J Health Syst Pharm, 56(8), 729.
2. Thompson, H. J. (1999). The management of post-operative nausea and vomiting. J Adv Nurs, 29(5), 1130–1136.
3. Mann, E. (1999). Using acupuncture and acupressure to treat postoperative emesis. Prof Nurs, 14(10), 691–694.
4. The American Gastroenterological Association Medical Position Statement: Nausea and Vomiting. (2001). Gastroenterology, 120(1), 261–262. Available at: http://www.guideline.gov. Accessed January 2004.

unilateral Neglect

Definition: Lack of awareness and attention to one side of the body

RELATED FACTORS
Effects of disturbed perceptual abilities (e.g., [homonymous] hemianopsia, one-sided blindness; [or visual inattention])
Neurologic illness or trauma
[Impaired cerebral blood flow]

DEFINING CHARACTERISTICS

Subjective
[Reports feeling that part does not belong to own self]

Objective
Consistent inattention to stimuli on an affected side
Inadequate self-care [inability to satisfactorily perform ADLs]
[Lack of] positioning and/or safety precautions in regard to the affected side
Does not look toward affected side; [does not touch affected side]
Leaves food on plate on the affected side
[Failure to use the affected side of the body without being reminded to do so]
SAMPLE CLINICAL APPLICATIONS: traumatic brain injury, cerebrovascular accident/ruptured cerebral aneurysm, brain tumor, glaucoma

DESIRED OUTCOMES/EVALUATION CRITERIA
Sample **NOC** linkages:
Self-Care: Activities of Daily Living (ADL): Ability to perform the most basic physical tasks and personal care activities
Body Positioning: Self-Initiated: Ability to change own body position
Safety Behavior: Personal: Individual or caregiver efforts to control behaviors that might cause physical injury

Client Will (Include Specific Time Frame)
- Acknowledge presence of sensory-perceptual impairment.
- Verbalize positive realistic perception of self, incorporating the current dysfunction.

- Identify adaptive/protective measures for individual situation.
- Perform self-care within level of ability.
- Demonstrate behaviors, lifestyle changes necessary to promote physical safety.

ACTIONS/INTERVENTIONS

Sample **NIC** linkages:

Unilateral Neglect Management: Protecting and safely reintegrating the affected part of the body while helping the patient adapt to disturbed perceptual abilities

Positioning: Deliberative placement of the patient or a body part to promote physiologic and/or psychological well being

Environmental Management: Safety: Manipulation of the patient's surroundings for therapeutic benefit

NURSING PRIORTIY NO. **1.** To assess the extent of altered perception and the related degree of disability:

- Measure visual acuity and field of vision *to determine presence/degree of interference if problem is due to actual loss of visual field as can occur with some types of stroke, causing 1) failure to recognize an object, or 2) define where an object is located. However, the client can have intact visual fields and still experience spatial neglect.*[1]
- Assess ability to distinguish between right and left. *Unilateral spatial neglect is observed in stroke, brain tumor, or accident victims with damage to the right parietal or parietal-occipital lobe, resulting in misperceptions of space opposite to brain damage. The individual with this condition has information from the left hemispace, but no conscious awareness of the information; thus will pay no attention to the left space.*[1–4]
- Assess sensory awareness (e.g., response to stimulus of hot/cold, dull/sharp); note problems with awareness of motion and proprioception. *Disturbances in these areas may be result of spinal cord injury (where loss of sensation affects body awareness) or brain lesion (where sensation may be intact, but awareness is impaired).*
- Observe client's behavior *to determine the extent of impairment (e.g., failure to respond to stimuli, objects, or people on the contralesional side).*
- Note physical signs of neglect (e.g., disregard for position of affected limb(s), bumping into walls when ambulating, shaving only right side of face, skin irritation/injury, etc.).
- Observe ability to function within limits of impairment. Compare with client's perception of own abilities. *Client may or may not be able to learn from mistakes or from observing others, depending upon the location/severity of the brain lesion.*[5]
- Explore and encourage verbalization of feelings *to identify meaning of loss/dysfunction/change to the client and impact it may have on assuming ADLs.*

NURSING PRIORITY NO. **2.** To promote optimal comfort and safety for the client in the environment:

- Approach client, and instruct others to approach client, from the unaffected side (e.g., right side, or side where vision is not impaired) *to enhance client's awareness and potential for communication.*
- Orient/reorient to physical environment and persons interacting with client. *Client with unilateral neglect can also have numerous other cognitive defects affecting ability to think, remember, speak or understand language, and/or interpret environment.*[5]

 Cultural Collaborative Community/ Home Care Diagnostic Studies 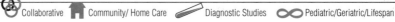 Pediatric/Geriatric/Lifespan Medications

- Provide vision and hearing aids if condition requires/client usually wears them *to improve sensory input and interpretation.*
- Remove excess stimuli from the environment *to decrease confusion and reactive stress.*
- Encourage client to turn head and eyes in full rotation and "scan" the environment *to compensate for visual field loss or if neglect therapies include scanning.*
- Position bedside table and objects (such as call bell, tissues) *within functional field of vision or awareness to facilitate self-care.*
- Monitor affected body part(s) for positioning/anatomic alignment, pressure points/skin irritation/injury, and dependent edema. *Increased risk of injury/ulcer formation necessitates close observation and timely intervention.*
- Describe where affected areas of body are *when moving/repositioning client.*
- Protect affected body part(s) from pressure/injury/burns, and help client/caregivers learn to assume this responsibility.
- Provide visual cues/assist client to position the affected extremity carefully and teach to routinely visualize placement of the extremity. When client completely ignores one side of the body, use of positioning *improves perception and awareness, and/or prevents injury.*
- Provide assistance with ADLs (e.g., feeding, bathing, dressing, grooming, toileting, etc.), *help client tend to affected side, or compensate for client's impairments.*
- Assist with ambulation/movement, using appropriate mobility and assistive devices *to promote safety of client and caregiver.*
- Protect from falls and/or collision with objects:
  Position furniture and equipment *so travel path is not obstructed.*
  Monitor environment, remove articles *that may create a safety hazard (e.g., footstool, throw rug).*
  Ensure adequate lighting in the environment.
  Keep doors wide open or completely closed.
- Refer to NDs impaired Environmental Interpretation Syndrome, risk for Falls/Injury, and Self-Care Deficit (specify) for additional interventions regarding comfort and safety.

NURSING PRIORITY NO. 3. To promote wellness (Teaching/Discharge Considerations):

- Collaborate with rehabilitation team *to identify strategies (e.g., sensory stimulation techniques such as tapping or stroking, active and passive range-of-motion exercises and temporary restraint of healthy limb while practicing motor skills) to assist client to compensate for deficits.*[5]
- Refer for/participate in neuropsychological therapies, as indicated. *Rehabilitation may address 1) visual attention deficits (e.g., scanning, training) or 2) spatial representation deficits (e.g., mental imagery training, eye patching, stimulation therapy, etc.).*[3]
- Reinforce to client the reality of the dysfunction and need to compensate. Avoid participating in the client's use of denial. *Delays dealing with reality of situation and limits progress towards goals.*
- Acknowledge and accept feelings of despondency, grief, and anger. *When feelings are openly expressed, client can deal with them and move forward.*
- Encourage family members/SO(s) to treat client normally, perform own care as able and include in family activities/outings. *Promotes sense of self-worth and encourages participation in life activities to limit withdrawal/depression.*
- Encourage client to accept affected limb/side as part of self even when it no longer feels like

it belongs. Have client look at and handle affected side *to stimulate awareness* and bring the affected limb across the midline *for client to visualize during care.*

 • Provide tactile stimuli to the affected side by touching/manipulating, stroking, and providing objects of various weight, texture, and size for the client to handle.

 • Suggest using a mirror to help client adjust position. *Allows client to visualize both sides of the body.*

 • Place nonessential items (e.g., television, pictures, hairbrush) on affected side during post acute phase once client begins to cross midline *to encourage continuation of retraining behaviors.*

 • Use descriptive terms to identify body parts rather than "left" and "right"; for example, "Lift this leg" (point to leg) or "Lift your affected leg."

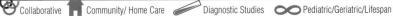 • Refer to/encourage client to continue rehabilitative services *to enhance independence in functioning.*

 • Identify additional resources to meet individual needs (e.g., Meals on Wheels, home-care rehabilitation services) *to maximize independence, allow client to return to/succeed in community setting.*

DOCUMENTATION FOCUS

Assessment/Reassessment
- Individual findings, including extent of altered perception, degree of disability, effect on independence/participation in ADLs.

Planning
- Plan of care and who is involved in the planning.
- Teaching plan.

Implementation/Evaluation
- Responses to intervention/teaching and actions performed.
- Attainment/progress toward desired outcome(s).
- Modifications to plan of care.

Discharge Planning
- Long-term needs and who is responsible for actions to be taken.
- Available resources, specific referrals made.

References

1. Walker, R. (1994). Unilateral Neglect: Clinical and experimental studies edited by Ian H. Robertson and John C. Marshall. Review for Psyche: An Interdisciplinary Journal of Research on Consciousness. Available at: http://psyche.cs.monash.edu.au/v1/psyche-1-08-walker.html. Accessed September 2003.
2. Mansoori, L. Hemispatial neglect syndrome. Student lecture for Brain, Thought and Action (MCDB 3650) University of Colorado, Boulder.
3. Ricci, R., Calhoun, J., & Chatterjee, A. (2000). Orientation bias in unilateral neglect: Representational contributions. (Research article). Philadelphia: Department of Neurology and the Center for Cognitive Neuroscience, University of Pennsylvania.
4. Sinclair, C. (2001). Brain organization as seen in unilateral special neglect. Available at: http://serendip.brynmawr.edu/bb/neuro/neuro01/web2/Sinclair.html. Accessed September 2003.
5. No author listed. Post-stroke rehabilitation fact sheet. Available at: National Institute for Neurological Disorders and Stroke (NINDS), http://www.ninds.gov. Accessed March 2004.

Noncompliance [ineffective Adherence] (specify)

Definition: Behavior of person and/or caregiver that fails to coincide with a health-promoting or therapeutic plan agreed on by the person (and/or family and/or community) and healthcare professional; in the presence of an agreed-on health-promoting or therapeutic plan, person's or caregiver's behavior is fully or partially adherent or nonadherent and may lead to clinically ineffective, partially ineffective outcomes

RELATED FACTORS

Healthcare plan
Duration
SOs; cost; intensity; complexity

Individual factors
Personal and developmental abilities; knowledge and skill relevant to the regimen behavior; motivational forces
Individual's value system; health beliefs, cultural influences, spiritual values
[Altered thought processes such as depression, paranoia]
[Difficulty changing behavior, as in addictions]
[Issues of secondary gain]

Health system
Individual health coverage; financial flexibility of plan
Credibility of provider; client-provider relationships; provider continuity and regular follow-up; provider reimbursement of teaching and follow-up; communication and teaching skills of the provider
Access and convenience of care; satisfaction with care

Network
Involvement of members in health plan; social value regarding plan
Perceived beliefs of SOs' communication and teaching skills

DEFINING CHARACTERISTICS

Subjective
Statements by client or SO(s) of failure to adhere; [does not perceive illness/risk to be serious, does not believe in efficacy of therapy, unwilling to follow treatment regimen or accept side effects/limitations]

Objective
Behavior indicative of failure to adhere (by direct observation)
Objective tests (e.g., physiologic measures, detection of physiologic markers)
Failure to progress
Evidence of development of complications/exacerbation of symptoms
Failure to keep appointments

[Inability to set or attain mutual goals]

[Denial]

SAMPLE CLINICAL APPLICATIONS: any new diagnosis, chronic conditions, or situations requiring lifestyle changes

DESIRED OUTCOMES/EVALUATION CRITERIA

Sample **NOC** linkages:

Compliance Behavior: Actions taken on the basis of professional advice to promote wellness, recovery, and rehabilitation

Health Beliefs: [specify]: Personal convictions that influence health behaviors

Caregiver-Patient Relationship: Positive interactions and connections between the caregiver and care recipient

---

Client Will (Include Specific Time Frame)

- Participate in the development of mutually agreeable goals and treatment plan.
- Verbalize accurate knowledge of condition and understanding of treatment regimen.
- Make choices at level of readiness based on accurate information.
- Access resources appropriately.
- Demonstrate progress toward desired outcomes/goals.

ACTIONS/INTERVENTIONS

Sample **NIC** linkages:

Mutual Goal Setting: Collaborating with patient to identify and prioritize care goals, then developing a plan for achieving those goals

Self-Modification Assistance: Reinforcement of self-directed change initiated by the patient to achieve personally important goals

Values Clarification: Assisting another to clarify her/his own values in order to facilitate effective decision making

NURSING PRIORITY NO. 1. To determine reason for alteration/disregard of therapeutic regimen/instructions:

- 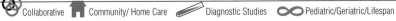 Discuss with client/SO(s) their perception/understanding of the situation (illness/treatment). *Basic information needed to understand client's/SO(s) position and develop plan of care.*[2]
- Listen to/Active-listen client's complaints, comments. *Conveys confidence in individual's ability to understand and manage own care.*[1]
- Note language spoken, read, and understood. *Lack of understanding of words that are used in explanations may result in client lack of cooperation with therapeutic regimen.*[2]
- Be aware of developmental level as well as chronological age of client. *Determines how to interact with client on appropriate level to enhance relationship and ability to discuss lack of cooperation with medical regimen.*[2]
- Assess level of anxiety, locus of control, sense of powerlessness, and so forth. *Presence of these factors will affect how client is managing illness/situation and therapeutic regimen.*[1]
- Note length of illness. *People tend to become passive and dependent in long-term, debilitating illnesses and find it difficult to expend energy to follow through with therapeutic regimen.*[6]
- Clarify value system: cultural/religious values, health/illness beliefs of the client/SO(s). *These factors will influence individual's view of the therapeutic regimen, for instance, Mexican Americans may believe the future is in God's hands, women may delay Pap smears and mammograms because of modesty.*[10]

- Determine social characteristics, demographic and educational factors, as well as personality of the client. *Educated individuals may be more oriented to health promotion and disease prevention, while lower socioeconomic individuals may be focused on the basics of living and may not pay attention to/follow healthcare recommendations. Personality characteristics such as suspiciousness, obsessive features may affect how client views medical regimen.*[9]

- Verify psychological meaning of the behavior (e.g., may be denial). Note issues of secondary gain. *Family dynamics, school/workplace issues, involvement in legal system may unconsciously affect client's decision regarding care and necessary follow-through.*[3]

- Assess availability/use of support systems and resources. *Failure to follow through with recommended therapies may be due to lack of/incorrect usage of support that is available.*[9]

- Be aware of nurses'/healthcare providers' attitudes and behaviors toward the client. Do they have an investment in the client's compliance/recovery? What is the behavior of the client and nurse when client is labeled "noncompliant"? *Some care providers may be enabling client whereas others' judgmental attitudes may impede treatment progress.*[1]

NURSING PRIORITY NO. 2. To assist client/SO(s) to develop strategies for dealing effectively with the situation:

- Develop therapeutic nurse-client relationship. *Promotes trust, provides atmosphere in which client/SO(s) can freely express views/concerns and explore reasons for lack of compliance with therapeutic regimen.*[1]

- Explore client involvement in or lack of mutual goal setting. *Client will be more likely to follow through on goals he or she participated in developing.*[7]

- Review treatment strategies. Identify which interventions in the plan of care are most important in meeting therapeutic goals and which are least amenable to cooperation. *Sets priorities and encourages problem solving areas of conflict, enabling client to make decisions related to choices of care.*[7]

- Contract with the client for participation in care. *Enhances commitment to follow-through.*[3]

- Encourage client to maintain self-care, providing for assistance when necessary. Accept client's evaluation of own strengths/limitations while working with client to improve abilities. *Promotes self-esteem enabling client to have a sense of control over illness and treatment regimen.*[7]

- Provide for continuity of care in and out of the hospital/care setting, including long-range plans. *Supports trust, facilitates progress toward goals as client illness is dealt with over time.*[6]

- Provide information and help client to know where and how to find it on own. *Promotes independence and encourages informed decision making and control over illness, enhancing compliance with therapeutic regimen.*

- Give information in manageable amounts, using verbal, written, and audiovisual modes at level of client's ability. *Individuals learn in many ways and using these different modes at client's own pace facilitates learning and enables assimilation of the information.*[3]

- Have client paraphrase instructions/information heard. *Validates client's understanding and reveals misconceptions so corrections can be made and appropriate questions can be asked and answered.*[4]

- Accept the client's choice/point of view, even if it appears to be self-destructive. Avoid confrontation regarding beliefs. *Maintaining open communication is important to continuing to provide correct information and therapeutic relationship with the client/SO(s). If illness is terminal, accept client's wishes regarding continued care or treatments, providing what is accepted.*[1]

• Establish graduated goals or modified regimen as necessary. *Client with COPD who smokes a pack of cigarettes a day may be willing to reduce that amount but not give up smoking altogether. This choice may improve quality of life and encourage progression to more advanced goals.*[3]

NURSING PRIORITY NO. 3. To promote wellness (Teaching/Discharge Considerations):

 • Stress importance of the client's knowledge and understanding of the need for treatment/medication, as well as consequences of actions/choices. *Client who is not adhering to the treatment regimen may not have full information or may not understand the reasons for the recommendations. With full understanding, client can make a more informed decision about care.*[1]

 • Develop a system for self-monitoring. *Provides a sense of control and enables the client to follow own progress and assist with making choices.*[7]

 • Provide support systems to reinforce negotiated behaviors. Encourage client to continue positive behaviors, especially if client is beginning to see benefit. *Individuals who feel alone and do not hear any positive reinforcement for changes that have been made will have difficulty maintaining the changes. When clients do hear positive comments and see the results for themselves, they are more apt to be willing to continue treatment regimen.*[7]

 • Refer to counseling/therapy and/or other appropriate resources. *May need additional assistance to resolve situation and enable client to progress as desired.*[1]

• Refer to NDs ineffective Coping, compromised family Coping, deficient Knowledge (specify); Anxiety.

DOCUMENTATION FOCUS

Assessment/Reassessment
• Individual findings/deviation from prescribed treatment plan and client's reasons in own words.
• Consequences of actions to date.

Planning
• Plan of care and who is involved in planning.
• Teaching plan.

Implementation/Evaluation
• Response to interventions/teaching and actions performed.
• Attainment/progress toward desired outcome(s).
• Modifications to plan of care.

Discharge Planning
• Long-term needs and who is responsible for actions to be taken.
• Specific referrals made.

References

1. Doenges, M., Townsend, M., & Moorhouse, M. (1998). Psychiatric Care Plans: Guidelines for Individualizing Care, ed 3. Philadelphia: F. A. Davis.
2. Locher, J., et al. (2002). Effects of age and casual attribution to aging on health-related behaviors associated with urinary incontinence in older women. Gerontologist, 42(4), 525.

 Cultural 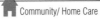 Collaborative Community/ Home Care Diagnostic Studies 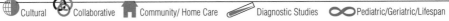 Pediatric/Geriatric/Lifespan Medications

3. Cox, H., et al. (2002). Clinical Applications of Nursing Diagnoses, ed 4. Philadelphia: F. A. Davis.
4. Pinhas-Hamiel, O., Dolan, L. M., et al. (1996). Increased incidence of non-insulin-dependent diabetes mellitus among adolescents. J Pediatr, 128(8), 608.
5. Deckelbaum, R. J., & Williams, C. L. (2001). Childhood obesity: The health issue. Obesity Research, 9(5), 239s.
6. Badger, J. M. (2001). Burns: The psychological aspect. AJN, 101(11), 38–41.
7. Bartol, T. (2002). Putting a patient with diabetes in the driver's seat. Nursing, 32(2), 53–55.
8. Doughty, D. B. (2001). The state of ostomy care, tremendous progress, continued challenges. J Wound Ostomy Continence Nurs, 28(1), 1–2.
9. American Society of Pain Management Nurses. (2002). Position paper on pain management in patients with addictive disease. Pensacola, FL.
10. Lipson, J. G., Dibble, S. L., & Minarik, P. A. (1996). Culture & Nursing Care A Pocket Guide. San Francisco: UCSF Nursing Press.

imbalanced Nutrition: less than body requirements

Definition: Intake of nutrients insufficient to meet metabolic needs

RELATED FACTORS

Inability to ingest or digest food or absorb nutrients because of biological, psychological, or economic factors

[Increased metabolic demands, e.g., burns]

[Lack of information, misinformation, misconceptions]

DEFINING CHARACTERISTICS

Subjective

Reported inadequate food intake less than recommended daily allowances (RDA)

Reported lack of food

Aversion to eating; reported altered taste sensation; satiety immediately after ingesting food

Abdominal pain with or without pathological condition; abdominal cramping

Lack of interest in food; perceived inability to digest food

Lack of information, misinformation, misconceptions [Note: The authors view this as a related factor rather than a defining characteristic.]

Objective

Body weight 20% or more under ideal [for height and frame]

Loss of weight with adequate food intake

Evidence of lack of [available] food

Weakness of muscles required for swallowing or mastication

Sore, inflamed buccal cavity

Poor muscle tone

Capillary fragility

Hyperactive bowel sounds; diarrhea and/or steatorrhea

Pale conjunctiva and mucous membranes

Excessive loss of hair [or increased growth of hair on body (lanugo)]

[Cessation of menses]

[Decreased subcutaneous fat/muscle mass]

[Abnormal laboratory studies (e.g., decreased albumin, total proteins; iron deficiency; electrolyte imbalances)]

SAMPLE CLINICAL APPLICATIONS: cancer, AIDS, anorexia/bulimia nervosa, burns, facial trauma, brain injury/coma, stroke, Parkinson's disease, cleft lip/palate, anemia, dementia/Alzheimer's disease, major depression, schizophrenia

DESIRED OUTCOMES/EVALUATION CRITERIA
Sample **NOC** linkages:
Nutritional Status: Extent to which nutrients are available to meet metabolic needs
Knowledge: Diet: Extent of understanding conveyed about diet
Weight Control: Personal actions resulting in achievement and maintenance of optimum body weight for health

Client Will (Include Specific Time Frame)
- Demonstrate progressive weight gain toward goal.
- Display normalization of laboratory values and be free of signs of malnutrition as reflected in Defining Characteristics.
- Verbalize understanding of causative factors when known and necessary interventions.
- Demonstrate behaviors, lifestyle changes to regain and/or maintain appropriate weight.

ACTIONS/INTERVENTIONS
Sample **NIC** linkages:
Nutrition Management: Assisting with or providing a balanced dietary intake of foods and fluids
Weight Gain Assistance: Facilitating gain of body weight
Eating Disorders Management: Prevention and treatment of severe diet restrictions and overexercising or binging and purging of foods and fluids

NURSING PRIORITY NO. **1.** To assess causative/contributing factors:

- Identify hospitalized clients at risk for inadequate quality/quantity of nutrients such as following intestinal surgery, hypermetabolic states (e.g., burns, trauma, severe infection), restricted oral intake/NPO for procedure.
- Obtain dietary history *to determine chronic problems/ongoing needs:*
  Increased caloric requirements with difficulty ingesting sufficient calories (e.g., cancer)
  Maturational/developmental issues (e.g., premature baby with sucking difficulties, child with lack of emotional stimulation; frail elderly living alone)
  Swallowing problems (e.g., stroke, Parkinson's disease, cerebral palsy/other neuromuscular disorders)[10]
  Decreased absorption (e.g., lactose intolerance, Crohn's disease)
  Decreased desire/refusal to eat (e.g., anorexia nervosa, cirrhosis, pancreatitis, alcoholism, bipolar disorder, chronic fatigue)[10]
  Treatment–related issues (e.g., chemotherapy, radiation, stomatitis, facial surgery/wired jaw)
  Personal/situational factors (e.g., inability to procure or prepare food; damaged or missing teeth, ill-fitting dentures, gum disease; social isolation, grief/loss).[10]
- Assess pediatric concerns, (e.g., changes in nutritional needs related to growth phase; congenital anomalies including tracheoesophageal fistula, cleft lip/palate; metabolic/malabsorption problems such as diabetes, phenylketonuria, cerebral palsy; chronic infections).[5]
- Determine weight change patterns and lifestyle factors that may affect weight.
  Socioeconomic resources, amount of money available for purchasing food, proximity of grocery

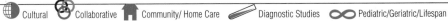

store, and available storage space for food are all factors that may impact food choices and intake.

- Evaluate impact of cultural, ethnic, and religious factors. *The nutritional balance of a diet is recognized by most cultures, with distinct theories of nutritional practices for health promotion and disease prevention. Foods are used for prevention or treatment of disease (e.g., client may believe in use of hot or cold foods to treat certain conditions; or use low-fat, low-sodium foods to prevent heart disease). Certain foods may be thought to cause a disease condition (e.g., upset stomach caused from eating too many cold foods). Special diets or food preparation may be cultural or religious based (e.g., kosher preparation for Jewish client; vegetarian eating no meat or meat byproducts).*[1]
- Explore specific eating habits, the meaning of food to client (e.g., never eats breakfast, snacks throughout entire day; fasts for weight control, no time to eat properly), and individual food preferences and intolerances/aversions. *Identifies poor eating practices to be corrected and provides insight into dietary interventions that may appeal to client.*
- Assess client's knowledge of nutritional needs and ways client is meeting these needs. *Identifies teaching needs and/or helps guide choice of interventions.*[10]
- Note availability/use of financial resources and support systems. *These factors affect/determine ability to acquire, prepare and store food. Lack of support or socialization may impact client's desire to eat.*
- Assess medication regimen, noting possible drug side effects/interactions, allergies, use of laxatives, diuretics. *These factors may be affecting appetite, food intake, or absorption.*[10,11]
- Note client's ability to feed self/presence of interfering factors. *Difficulties such as paralysis, tremor, or injury to hands/arms with inability to grasp or lift utensils to mouth; cognitive impairments affecting coordination or remembering to eat, age and/or developmental issues may require input of multiple providers/therapists to develop individualized plan of care.*[10]
- Determine psychological factors that may affect food choices. Perform psychological assessment as indicated, *to assess body image and congruency with reality, and/or to identify factors (e.g., dementia, severe depression) that may be interfering with client's appetite and food intake.*[10]
- Note occurrence of amenorrhea, tooth decay, swollen salivary glands, or report of constant sore throat. *May be signs of eating disorder, such as bulimia, affecting eating patterns and requiring additional evaluation.*[7,8]
- Review usual activities/exercise program noting repetitive activities (e.g., constant pacing) or inappropriate exercise (e.g., prolonged jogging). *Clients who have eating disorders, such as anorexia or bulimia, may use these obsessive activities as weight-control measures.*[8]

NURSING PRIORITY NO. 2. To evaluate degree of deficit:

- Weigh and measure on admission and periodically, using same scale, same time of day and same clothing, as much as possible *to provide for accurate comparison/evaluate effectiveness of therapeutic regimen.*[10]
- Compare current weight with client's usual weight, and norms for age and body size *to identify changes (e.g., sudden loss related to medical illness vs. ongoing chronic depression with anorexia and weight loss; or toddler with failure to meet growth expectations) that affect choice of intervention.*
- Measure/calculate body fat, body water and muscle mass (via anthropometric measurements); or calculate body mass index (BMI) *to establish baseline parameters and assist in determining therapeutic goals. Note: [BMI = weight (lbs)/height (inches squared) x 704]. Desirable BMI is 23–25, with <19 being severely underweight.*[2,10]

• Calculate growth percentiles in infants/children using growth chart *to identify deviations from the norm.*[5]

• Assess client's deficits relative to age, body build, strength, activity level, etc. *Provides comparative baseline and helps clarify expectations.*

• Obtain history and/or review diary of daily portion (or calorie) intake, patterns and times of eating *to reveal recent changes in client's weight or appetite; and identify strengths and weaknesses in client's dietary habits.*[10]

• Review laboratory studies (e.g., comprehensive metabolic panel, including liver enzymes, total protein and albumin, glucose, insulin levels, cholesterol/other lipids, calcium, phosphorus, and magnesium; thyroid stimulating hormone [TSH]; serum electrolytes, etc.) *to determine degree of nutritional deficits and effect on body function dictating specific dietary needs.*[6,10] *Note: Baseline screening may be done (e.g., albumin, cholesterol and CBC) to determine whether more in-depth evaluation is needed.*[2]

• Assist with/review results of diagnostic procedures (e.g., Schilling's test, D-xylose test, 72-hour stool fat, GI series, gastric reflux scanning).[2]

NURSING PRIORITY NO. 3. To establish a nutritional plan that meets individual needs:

• Collaborate with physician/dietitian/nutritional team *to implement interdisciplinary management and set nutritional goals, especially when malnutrition is profound, client has specific dietary needs; and or long-term feeding problems exist.*[9,10]

• Calculate basal energy expenditure (BEE) using Harris-Benedict formula and estimate energy and protein requirements *to aid in developing components of nutritional plan.*[8]

• Establish ongoing method of evaluating intake (e.g., calories/day, percent of food consumed at each feeding, etc.) *to assist in determining both amount of food taken and what food groups are consumed or left uneaten, to identify nutritional deficits.*[10]

• Discuss with client/SO aspects of diet that can remain unchanged *to preserve those that are valuable/meaningful.* Negotiate with client aspects of diet that need to be changed, especially if eating/psychiatric disorder is limiting food intake.

• Provide diet modifications as indicated:

Avoid/limit withholding of food (e.g., prolonged NPO for surgery) as much as possible and reinstitute oral feedings as early as possible *to reduce adverse effects of malnutrition.*

Increase specific nutrients (e.g., protein, carbohydrates, fats and calories) as needed, providing client with preferred food and seasoning choices where possible *to enhance intake.*

Determine when client prefers/tolerates largest meal of the day. Maintain flexibility in timing of food intake *to promote sense of control and give client opportunity to eat when feeling more rested, less pain or nausea, or family coming at mealtime, etc.*[11]

Provide numerous small feedings, as indicated; supplement with easily digested snacks *to reduce feeling of fullness that can accompany larger meals, and to improve chances of increasing the amount of nutrients taken over 24-hour period.*[3]

Promote adequate/timely fluid intake. *Fluid is essential to the digestive process and is often taken with meals. Fluids may need to be withheld before meals or with meals if interfering with food intake.*

Encourage variety in food choices, varying textures and taste sensations (e.g., sweet, salty, fresh, methods of cooking) *to enhance food satisfaction and stimulate appetite.*

Offer/keep available to client, finger foods and snacks *that are easy to self-feed.*

Use alternative flavoring agents (e.g., lemon and herbs) *to enhance taste of foods especially if salt is restricted.*

 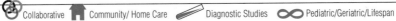

Add nonfat milk powder to foods with a high liquid content (e.g., gravy, puddings, cooked cereal) or sugar/honey in beverages if carbohydrates are tolerated *to increase caloric value.*[10]

Avoid foods that cause intolerances/increase gastric motility (e.g., gas-forming foods, hot/cold, spicy, caffeinated beverages, milk products, and the like) *to reduce postprandial discomfort that may discourage client from eating.*

Limit high-fat foods or fiber/bulk if indicated, *because they may lead to early satiety.*

Offer supplement drinks (or dispense in 2- to 4-oz portions several times/day). *Client may view this as a "medication" and thus will drink it, improving intake and energy level.*[10]

- Promote pleasant, relaxing environment, including socialization when possible. *Promotes focus on activity of eating, enhancing intake.*[11]
- Suggest use of glass of wine before meal *to stimulate appetite.*
- Administer pharmaceutical agents as indicated. *Appetite stimulants, dietary supplements; digestive drugs/enzymes, vitamins/minerals (e.g., iron); antacids, anticholinergics, antiemetics, or antidiarrheals, etc. may be used to enhance intake, improve digestion, and correct nutritional deficiencies.*[10]
- Address disease-specific condition or treatments[9–11]:

Assist in treatments to correct/control underlying causative factors (e.g., cancer, malabsorption syndrome, anorexia) *to improve intake and utilization of nutrients.*

Assess/monitor client's ability to chew, taste and swallow. *Impairments in these areas may be caused by neurological problems (e.g., stroke, ALS); lesions in the mouth (e.g., candidiasis, herpes); or treatments (e.g., intubation, chemotherapy) and limit client's ability and/or desire for food.*

Auscultate for presence/character of bowel sounds *to determine ability/readiness of intestinal tract to handle digestive processes (e.g., hypermotility accompanies vomiting/diarrhea, while absence of bowel sounds may indicate bowel obstruction).*

Medicate for pain or nausea, and manage drug side effects *to increase physical comfort and appetite.*

Prevent/minimize unpleasant odors/sights, or cooking odors. *Often have a negative effect on appetite or activate gag reflex.*

Provide oral care before/after meals. *Reduces discomfort associated with nausea, vomiting, oral lesions, mucosal dryness and halitosis, making eating easier/food more palatable.*

Encourage use of lozenges, gum, hard candy, beverages, etc., *to stimulate salivation when dryness is a factor.*

Provide blenderized foods, formula tube feedings or parenteral nutrition infusions when indicated by client's condition (e.g., wired jaws or paralysis following stroke) and degree of malnutrition. *Enteral route is preferred when oral feeding is not appropriate; however, parenteral nutrition is recommended if client not able to tolerate at least 50% of the goal rate of enteral feedings.*[9]

Consult occupational therapist *to identify appropriate assistive devices,* or speech therapist *to enhance swallowing ability. (Refer to ND impaired Swallowing.)*

Develop/refer client to structured (Behavioral Modification) program of nutrition therapy, which may include documenting time/length of eating period, putting food in a blender and tube-feeding food not eaten). *These programs are used to change the maladaptive eating behaviors of clients with anorexia and bulimia and ensure adequate caloric intake. Because "control" is central to the etiology of these disorders it is important to ensure that the client is perceived to be "in control."*[8]

Recommend/support hospitalization for controlled environment as indicated in severe malnutrition/life-threatening situations.

NURSING PRIORITY NO. 4. To promote wellness (Teaching/Discharge Considerations):

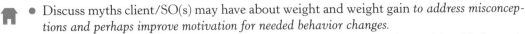

- 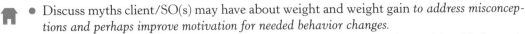 Discuss myths client/SO(s) may have about weight and weight gain *to address misconceptions and perhaps improve motivation for needed behavior changes.*
- Emphasize importance of well-balanced, nutritious intake. Provide nutritional information as indicated, balancing calorie intake and energy expenditure, taking into account client's age and developmental stage (e.g., toddler, teenager, pregnant woman, elderly person with chronic disease), physical health and activity tolerance, financial and socioeconomic factors, and client/SOs potential for management of underlying conditions. *For example, older adults need same nutrients as younger adults, but in smaller amounts, and with attention to certain components, such as calcium, fiber, vitamins, protein and water.*[4] *Infants/children require small meals and constant attention to needed nutrients for proper growth/development while dealing with child's food preferences and eating habits.*[5]
- Involve SO(s) in treatment plan as much as possible *to provide ongoing support and increase likelihood of accomplishing dietary goals.*
- Consult with dietitian/nutritional support team as necessary *for long-term needs.*[9,10]
- Involve client in developing behavior modification program appropriate to specific needs based on consistent, realistic weight gain goal. *Enhances commitment to change and likelihood of accomplishing desired outcomes.*[8]
- Provide positive regard, love, and acknowledgment of "voice within" guiding client with eating disorder. *These efforts encourage the client to recognize maladaptive eating patterns as defense mechanisms to ease the emotional pain and begin to resolve underlying issues and develop more adaptive coping strategies for dealing with stressful situations.*[8]
- Weigh weekly and document results *to monitor effectiveness of dietary plan.*[10]
- Develop regular exercise/stress reduction program. *Enhances general well-being, improves organ function/muscle tone, and increases appetite.*[10]
- Review medical regimen and provide information/assistance as necessary. Discuss drug regimen, side effects, and potential interactions with other medications/over-the-counter drugs.
- Assist client to identify/access community resources such as food stamps, budget counseling, Meals on Wheels, community food banks, and/or other appropriate assistance programs.
- Refer for dental hygiene/professional care, counseling/psychiatric care, family therapy as indicated.
- Provide/reinforce client teaching regarding preoperative/postoperative dietary needs when surgery is planned.
- Assist client/SO(s) to learn how to blenderize food and/or perform tube feeding. *Promotes independence/self-care and sense of some degree of control in a difficult situation.*
- Refer to home health resources *for initiation/supervision of home nutrition therapy when used.*

DOCUMENTATION FOCUS

Assessment/Reassessment
- Baseline and subsequent assessment findings to include signs/symptoms as noted in Defining Characteristics and laboratory diagnostic findings.
- Caloric intake.
- Individual cultural/religious restrictions, personal preferences.
- Availability/use of resources.
- Personal understanding/perception of problem.

 Cultural Collaborative Community/ Home Care Diagnostic Studies 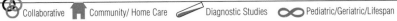 Pediatric/Geriatric/Lifespan Medications

Planning
- Plan of care and who is involved in planning.
- Teaching plan.

Implementation/Evaluation
- Client's responses to interventions/teaching and actions performed.
- Results of weekly weigh-in.
- Attainment/progress toward desired outcome(s).
- Modifications to plan of care.

Discharge Planning
- Long-term needs/who is responsible for actions to be taken.
- Specific referrals made.

References

1. Purnell, L. D., & Paulanka, B. J. (1998). Transcultural Health Care: A Culturally Competent Approach. Philadelphia: F. A. Davis, pp 33–35.
2. Lawhorne, L. S. (2001). Altered nutritional status: Guideline. Columbia, MD: American Medical Directors Association (AMDA). Available at: www.guideline.gov. Accessed January 2004.
3. Love, C. C., & Seaton, H. (1991). Eating disorders: Highlights of nursing assessment and therapeutics. Nurs Clin North Am, 26, 667–697.
4. Older Americans Month. Food & Nutrition Information. Available at: http://www.eatright.org/Public/Nutritioninformation. Accessed June 2003.
5. Engel, J. (2002). Pocket Guide to Pediatric Assessment, ed 4. St. Louis: Mosby.
6. Vogelzang, J. L. (2003). Making nutrition sense from OASIS. Home Healthcare Nurse, 21(9), 592–600.
7. Could You or Someone You Care about Have an Eating Disorder. Available at: http://www.eating-disorder.com. Accessed February 2004.
8. Townsend, M. C. (2003). Psychiatric Mental Health Nursing Concepts of Care, ed 4. Philadelphia: F. A. Davis.
9. Practice management guidelines for nutritional support of the trauma patient. (2001). Eastern Association for the Surgery of Trauma - Professional Association, 112 pp. NGC:002187. Available at: www.guideline.gov. Accessed February 2004.
10. Altered nutritional status. (2001). American Medical Directors Association - Professional Association, 32 pages. NGC:002530. Available at: www.guideline.gov. Accessed February 2004.
11. Mealtime difficulties for older persons: assessment and management. (2003). The John A. Hartford Foundation Institute for Geriatric Nursing - Academic Institution, 23 pages. NGC:002732. Available at: www.guideline.gov. Accessed February 2004.

imbalanced Nutrition: more than body requirements

Definition: Intake of nutrients that exceeds metabolic needs

RELATED FACTORS
Excessive intake in relationship to metabolic need

DEFINING CHARACTERISTICS

Subjective
Reported dysfunctional eating patterns:
Pairing food with other activities

Eating in response to external cues such as time of day, social situation
Concentrating food intake at end of day
Eating in response to internal cues other than hunger, for example, anxiety
Sedentary activity level

Objective
Weight 20% over ideal for height and frame [obese]
Triceps skin fold greater than 15 mm in men and 25 mm in women
Weight 10% over ideal for height and frame [overweight]
Observed dysfunctional eating patterns [as noted in subjective]
[Percentage of body fat greater than 22% for trim women and 15% for trim men]

SAMPLE CLINICAL APPLICATIONS: bulimia nervosa, morbid obesity, diseases requiring long-term steroid use (e.g., COPD), conditions associated with immobility (stroke/paralysis, MS, amputation), Alzheimer's disease, depression, developmental delay

DESIRED OUTCOMES/EVALUATION CRITERIA

Sample **NOC** linkages:

Weight Control: Personal actions resulting in achievement and maintenance of optimum body weight for health

Knowledge: Diet: Extent of understanding conveyed about diet

Nutritional Status: Extent to which nutrients are available to meet metabolic needs

Client Will (Include Specific Time Frame)
- Verbalize a more realistic self-concept/body image (congruent mental and physical picture of self).
- Demonstrate acceptance of self as is rather than an idealized image.
- Demonstrate appropriate changes in lifestyle and behaviors, including eating patterns, food quantity/quality, and exercise program.
- Attain desirable body weight with optimal maintenance of health.

ACTIONS/INTERVENTIONS
Sample **NIC** linkages:

Weight Reduction Assistance: Facilitating loss of weight and/or body fat

Nutrition Management: Assisting with or providing a balanced dietary intake of foods and fluids

Eating Disorders Management: Prevention and treatment of severe diet restrictions and overexercising or binging and purging of foods and fluids

NURSING PRIORITY NO. 1. To identify causative/contributing factors:

- Note presence of/potential for conditions (e.g., family influence, genetics [including client's basal metabolic rate]; pregnancy, menopause, hypothyroidism, depression, use of certain medications such as steroids, birth control pills; physical disabilities/limitations) *that can contribute to obesity.*
- Obtain weight history, noting if client has weight gain out of character for self or family, is/was obese child, or used to be much more physically active than is now *to identify trends. Note: Obesity is now the most prevalent nutritional disorder among children and adolescents in the United States.*[1]
- Assess client's knowledge of own body weight and nutritional needs, and determine cultural influences. *Although nutritional needs are not always understood, being overweight or having large body size may not be viewed negatively by individual, since it is considered within*

  Collaborative Community/ Home Care 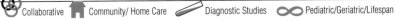 Diagnostic Studies Pediatric/Geriatric/Lifespan  Medications

relationship to family eating patterns, peer and cultural influences.[1] *African-American women's frame of reference for "normal body weight" was much larger than standard indicators.*[2] *And some cultures even place importance on large body size (e.g., Samoan people, or Cuban children).*[3]

- Identify familial and cultural influences. *Different cultures place high importance on food and food-related events (e.g., Greeks, Italians, and many other cultures), while some cultures routinely observe fasting days (e.g., Arab, Greek, Irish, Jewish) that may be done for health and/or religious purposes.*[3]
- Ascertain how client perceives food and the act of eating. *Individual beliefs, values and types of foods available influence what people eat, avoid or alter. Client may be eating to satisfy an emotional need rather than physiological hunger because food can offer security and acceptance, and often plays a significant role in socialization.*[3,4]
- Assess dietary practices, asking for recall of foods/fluids ingested, times and patterns of eating, activities/place, whether alone or with other(s); and feelings before, during, and after eating. *Provides opportunity for individual to focus on/internalize realistic picture of the amount of food ingested and corresponding eating habits/feeling. Identifies patterns requiring change and/or a base on which to tailor dietary program.*[5]
- Calculate total calorie intake, using client's 24-hour recall or weekly food diary. Evaluate usual intake of different food groups. *Helps identify strengths and weaknesses. For example, client may report normal or excessive intake of food, but calories and intake of certain food groups (e.g., sweets and fats) are often underestimated.*
- Ascertain previous dieting history. *Client may report experimentation with numerous types of diets ("yo-yo" dieting) with varying results, or may never have attempted a weight management program.*
- Discuss client's view of self, including what being fat does for the client. Note negative/positive monologues (self-talk) of the individual.
- Obtain body drawing. (Client draws self on wall with chalk, then stands against it and actual body is drawn to determine difference between the two). *Determines whether client's view of self-body image is congruent with reality.*
- Ascertain occurrence of negative feedback from SO(s). *May reveal control issues, impact motivation for change.*
- Review daily activity and exercise program *to identify areas for modification.*
- Measure/calculate body fat, body water and muscle mass (via anthropometric measurements); or calculate body mass index (BMI) *to establish baseline parameters.* [*BMI = weight (lbs)/height (inches squared) x704*] *Desirable BMI is 23–25, with >30 being obese and >40 being morbidly obese.*[6] *Children who are 120% or more of ideal body weight for height and age are considered obese.*[7]
- Calculate waist to hip ratio (WHR). *A WHR >8.2 in women and >1.0 in men (apple-shaped fat distribution in abdomen/around torso) is associated with increased risk of complications of obesity (e.g., cardiovascular disease).*[8–10]
- Review laboratory testing (e.g., total cholesterol/other blood lipids, fasting glucose, thyroid, hormones, etc.) *that may reveal medical conditions contributing to obesity, and/or identify problems that may be treated with alterations in diet.*[11]

NURSING PRIORITY NO. 2. To establish weight reduction program:

- Discuss client's motivation for weight loss (e.g., for own satisfaction/self-esteem, to improve health status, or to gain approval from another person). *Helps client determine realistic motivating factors for individual situation (e.g., acceptance of self "as is," improvement of health status).*

- Obtain commitment for weight loss. *Verbal agreement to goals or written contract formalizes the plan and may enhance efforts/maximize outcomes.*
- Calculate calorie requirements based on physical factors and activity. *Calories are usually counted according to three substances (e.g., carbohydrates = 4 calories/g, protein = 4 calories/g, fats = 9 calories/g). Note: Alcohol (a fourth separate group) = 7 calories/g). Decreasing calories by 500/day or expending 500 calories/day through exercise results in a weight loss of about 1 pound/week.[9]*

- Collaborate with physician, dietitian *to develop/implement comprehensive weight loss program that includes food, activity, behavior alteration, and support.*
- Provide information regarding specific nutritional needs. *Individual may be deficient in needed nutrients (e.g., proteins, vitamins, or minerals), or may eat too much of one food group (e.g., fats or carbohydrates). Depending on client's desires and needs, many weight management programs are available that focus on particular factors (e.g., low carbohydrates, low fat, low calories). Reducing portion size and following a balanced diet along with increasing exercise is often what is needed to improve health.[12]*

- Assist in/encourage periodic evaluation and alteration of nutritional program. *May be desired/needed for addressing special needs (e.g., diabetes mellitus, age considerations, very low calorie/fasting), incorporating client's culture and preferences, and ongoing monitoring in long-term weight management programs.*
- Set realistic goals for weekly weight loss. *Reasonable weight loss (1–2 lbs/week) has been shown to have more lasting effects than rapid weight loss, although sustaining motivation for small losses often makes it difficult for client to stick with a program. Note: A loss of 5–20% of total body weight can reduce many of the health risks associated with obesity in adults.[1]*
- Address need to give self permission to occasionally include desired/craved food items in eating plan. *Denying self often results in sense of deprivation and feelings of guilt/failure when individual "succumbs to temptation." These feelings can lead to binging that can sabotage weight loss and/or put a halt to weight management efforts.*

- Identify unhelpful eating behaviors (e.g., eating over sink, "gobbling, nibbling or grazing") and address kinds of activities associated with eating (e.g., watching television or reading, being unmindful of eating or food) *that results in taking in too many calories as well as eliminating the joy of food because of failure to notice flavors or sensation of fullness/satiety.*

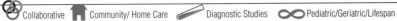

- Discuss necessary modifications/develop eating re-education plan (e.g., planning meals and what to eat at restaurants, eating small portions, limiting eating to one location in house, eating slowly and savoring food, drinking water before meals, viewing exercise as a means of controlling hunger; rewarding self for progress with something besides food) *to promote healthy eating patterns and support continuation of behavioral changes.[6]*

- Stress need for adequate fluid intake *to assist in digestive process and to slake thirst, which is often mistakenly identified as hunger.*
- Encourage involvement in planned activity program of client's choice and within physical abilities. *Moderately increased physical activity for 30–45 minutes 5 days/week can expend 1500–2000 calories/week, supporting both loss of pounds and maintenance of lower weight.[13]*
- Recommend reading labels of nonprescription diet aids if used. *Herbals containing diuretics or Ma-huang (product similar to ephedrine) may cause adverse side effects in vulnerable persons.*
- Monitor individual prescribed drug regimen (e.g., appetite suppressants, hormone therapy, vitamin/mineral supplements) *for benefits or adverse side effects/drug interactions.*
- Provide positive reinforcement/encouragement for efforts, as well as actual weight loss. *Enhances commitment to program and enhances person's sense of self-worth.*

- Refer to bariatric physician/surgeon when indicated. *Evaluation for special measures may be needed (e.g., supervised fasting or bariatric surgery) for morbidly obese persons with BMI >40.*[9]

NURSING PRIORITY NO. 3. To promote wellness (Teaching/Discharge Considerations):

- Discuss myths client/SO(s) may have about weight and weight loss *to address misconceptions and perhaps improve motivation for needed behavior changes.*
- Emphasize importance of avoiding fad diets *that may be harmful to health, and often do not produce long-term positive results.*
- Assist client to choose nutritious foods that reflect personal likes, meet individual needs, and are within financial budget.
- Identify ways to manage stress/tension during meals. *Promotes relaxation to permit focus on act of eating and awareness of satiety.*
- Review and discuss strategies to deal appropriately with feelings *to avoid overeating.*
- Encourage variety and moderation in dietary plan *to decrease boredom.*
- Advise to plan for special occasions (birthday/holidays) by reducing intake before event and/or eating "smart" *to redistribute/reduce calories and allow for participation.*
- Discuss importance of an occasional treat by planning for inclusion in diet, *to avoid feelings of deprivation arising from self-denial.*
- Recommend client weigh only once per week, same time/clothes, and graph on chart. Measure/monitor body fat when possible *(more accurate measure).*
- Discuss normalcy of ups and downs of weight loss: plateau, set point (at which weight is not being lost), hormonal influences, etc. *Prevents discouragement when progress stalls.*
- Encourage buying personal items/clothing *as a reward for weight loss or other accomplishments.* Suggest disposing of "fat clothes" *to encourage positive attitude of permanent change and remove "safety valve" of having wardrobe available "just in case" weight is regained.*
- Involve SO(s) in treatment plan as much as possible *to provide ongoing support and increase likelihood of success.*
- Refer to community support groups/psychotherapy as indicated *to provide role models, address issues of body image or self-worth.*
- Provide contact number for dietitian *to address ongoing nutrition needs/dietary changes.*
- Refer to NDs disturbed Body Image, ineffective Coping for additional interventions as appropriate.

DOCUMENTATION FOCUS

Assessment/Reassessment
- Individual findings, including current weight, dietary pattern; perceptions of self, food, and eating; motivation for loss, support/feedback from SO(s).

Planning
- Plan of care/interventions and who is involved in planning.
- Teaching plan.

Implementation/Evaluation
- Responses to interventions, weekly weight, and actions performed.
- Attainment/progress toward desired outcome(s).
- Modifications to plan of care.

Discharge Planning
- Long-term needs and who is responsible for actions to be taken.
- Specific referrals made.

References

1. Freemark, M. (2002). Obesity. Available at: http://www.emedicine.com. Accessed November 2003.
2. Gore, S. V. (1999). African-American women's perceptions of weight: Paradigm shift for advanced practice. Holist Nurs Pract, 13(4), 71–79.
3. Purnell, L. D., & Paulanka, B. J. (1998). Transcultural Health Care: A Culturally Competent Approach. Philadelphia: F. A. Davis, p 22.
4. Leininger, M. E. (1988). Transcultural eating patterns and nutrition: Transcultural nursing and anthropological perspectives. Holist Nurs Pract, 3(1), 16–25.
5. Fleury, J. (1991). Empowering potential: A theory of wellness motivation. Nurs Res, 40, 288.
6. Lawhorne, L. S. (2001). Altered nutritional status: Guideline. Columbia, MD: American Medical Directors Association (AMDA). Available at: www.guideline.gov. Accessed November 2003.
7. Dimensions of Nutritional Assessment. In Engel, J. (2002), Pocket Guide to Pediatric Assessment, ed 4. St. Louis: Mosby, p 58.
8. Stanley, M. (1999). The aging gastrointestinal system, with nutritional considerations. In Stanley, M., & Beare, P. G. Gerontological Nursing: A Health Promotion/Protection Approach, ed 2. Philadelphia: F. A. Davis.
9. Galletta, G. M. (2003). Obesity and weight control. Available at: http://www.emedicine.com. Accessed November 2003.
10. Lutz, CA, & Przytulski, KR. (2001). Nutrition and Diet Therapy, 3rd ed. Philadelphia: F. A. Davis.
11. Woods, A. (2003). X marks the spot: Understanding metabolic syndrome. Nursing Made Incredibly Easy! 1(1), 19–26.
12. Nonas, C. A. (1998). A model for chronic obesity through dietary treatment. J Am Diet Assoc, (suppl 2), S16.
13. Rippe, J. M., & Hess, S. (1998). The role of physical activity in the prevention and management of obesity. J Am Diet Assoc, (suppl 2), S9.

imbalanced Nutrition: risk for more than body requirements

Definition: At risk for an intake of nutrients that exceeds metabolic needs

RISK FACTORS

Reported/observed obesity in one or both parents [/spouse; hereditary predisposition]

Rapid transition across growth percentiles in infants or children [adolescents]

Reported use of solid food as major food source before 5 months of age

Reported/observed higher baseline weight at beginning of each pregnancy [frequent, closely spaced pregnancies]

Dysfunctional eating patterns; concentrating food intake at end of day; eating in response to external cues such as time of day, social situation/to internal cues other than hunger (such as anxiety); observed use of food as reward or comfort measure

Pairing food with other activities

[Frequent/repeated dieting]

[Socially/culturally isolated; lacking other outlets]

[Alteration in usual activity patterns/sedentary lifestyle]

[Alteration in usual coping patterns]

[Majority of foods consumed are concentrated, high-calorie/fat sources]

[Significant/sudden decline in financial resources, lower socioeconomic status]

NOTE: A risk diagnosis is not evidenced by signs and symptoms, as the problem has not occurred and nursing interventions are directed at prevention.

 Cultural Collaborative Community/ Home Care 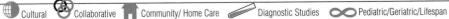 Diagnostic Studies Pediatric/Geriatric/Lifespan Medications

SAMPLE CLINICAL APPLICATIONS: bulimia nervosa, diseases requiring long-term steroid use (e.g., COPD), conditions associated with immobility (stroke/paralysis, MS, amputation), Alzheimer's disease, depression, developmental delay

DESIRED OUTCOMES/EVALUATION CRITERIA
Sample **NOC** linkages:

Weight Control: Personal actions resulting in achievement and maintenance of optimum body weight for health

Knowledge: Diet: Extent of understanding conveyed about diet

Nutritional Status: Nutrient Intake: Adequacy of nutrients taken into the body

Client Will (Include Specific Time Frame)
- Verbalize understanding of body and energy needs.
- Identify lifestyle/cultural factors that predispose to obesity.
- Demonstrate behaviors, lifestyle changes to reduce risk factors.
- Acknowledge responsibility for own actions and need to "act, not react" to stressful situations.
- Maintain weight at a satisfactory level for height, body build, age, and gender.

ACTIONS/INTERVENTIONS
Sample **NIC** linkages:

Weight Management: Facilitating maintenance of optimal body weight and percent body fat

Nutritional Counseling: Use of an interactive helping process focusing on the need for diet modification

Nutrition Management: Assisting with or providing a balanced dietary intake of foods and fluids

NURSING PRIORITY NO. 1. To assess potential factors for undesired weight gain:

- Note presence/number of risk factors *to help determine degree of risk. For example: A high correlation exists between obesity in parents and children, which may reflect (in part) family patterns of food intake, exercise, selection of leisure activity (e.g., amount of television watching), family and cultural patterns of food selection. Also family studies (e.g., twin and adoption) suggest genetic factors.*[1]
- Evaluate familial and cultural influences *that often place high importance on food and food-related events, or that place importance on large body size (e.g., Samoan people, or Cuban children).*[2]
- Determine age and activity level/exercise patterns *to note areas where changes might be useful to prevent obesity/promote health.*
- Calculate growth percentiles in infants/children using growth chart *to identify deviations from the norm.*
- Review laboratory data (e.g., growth hormones, thyroid, glucose and insulin levels, lipids, total protein) *to determine health status/presence of endocrine/metabolic disorders dictating specific dietary needs.*[6]
- Determine weight change patterns, lifestyle, and cultural factors that may predispose to weight gain. *Socioeconomic resources, amount of money available for purchasing food, proximity of grocery store, and available storage space for food are all factors that may impact food choices and intake.*

- Assess eating patterns in relation to risk factors. *Food choices and amounts of certain food groups are known to impact health and cause/exacerbate disease conditions (e.g., heart disease, diabetes, hypertension, gallstones, colon cancer).*[3]
- Determine patterns of hunger and satiety. *Eating patterns often differ in those who are predisposed to weight gain, and may include such factors as skipping meals (decreases the metabolic rate), fasting and binging (causes wide fluctuations in glucose and insulin), eating or overeating in response to emotions (e.g., loneliness, anger, happiness).*
- Note history of dieting/kinds of diets used. *Individual may have tried multiple diets with varying degrees of success; but often have history of regaining weight (yo-yo dieting) or finding that diets are not desirable. Repeated dieting is thought to promote obesity.*
- Determine whether bingeing/purging (bulimia) is a factor *to identify potential for eating disorder requiring in-depth intervention.*
- Identify personality characteristics (such as rigid thinking patterns, external locus of control, negative body image/self-concept, negative monologues [self-talk], and dissatisfaction with life) *that are often associated with obesity.*
- Determine psychological significance of food to the client.
- Listen to concerns and assess motivation to prevent weight gain. *If client's concern regarding weight control are motivated for reasons other than personal well-being (e.g., partner's expectations/demands), the likelihood of success is decreased.*

NURSING PRIORITY NO. 2. To assist client to develop preventive program to avoid weight gain:

- Assess client's knowledge of nutritional needs and ways client is meeting these needs. *Provides baseline for further teaching and/or interventions.*
- Provide information as indicated on nutrition, balancing calorie intake and energy expenditure, taking into account client's age and developmental stage (e.g., toddler, teenager, pregnant woman, elderly person with chronic disease), physical health and activity tolerance, financial and socioeconomic factors, and client's/SO's potential for management of risk factors. *For example, older adults need same nutrients as younger adults, but in smaller amounts, and with attention to certain components, such as calcium, fiber, vitamins, protein and water.*[4] *Infants/children require small meals and constant attention to needed nutrients for proper growth/development while dealing with child's food preferences and eating habits.*[5]
- Review healthy eating patterns/habits (e.g., eating slowly and only when hungry; stopping when full; avoiding skipping meals; eating foods from every food group; using smaller plates; chewing food thoroughly; making healthy food choices even when eating fast food, etc). *Most fast foods and packaged foods are highly processed or are high in sugar, fat, and calories.*
- Discuss importance/help client develop a program of exercise and relaxation techniques. *Promotes incorporation of healthy habits into lifestyle.*
- Assist client to develop strategies for reducing stressful thinking/actions. *Promotes relaxation, reduces likelihood of stress/comfort eating.*

NURSING PRIORITY NO. 3. To promote wellness (Teaching/Discharge Considerations):

- Provide information about individual risk factors *to enhance decision making and support motivation.*

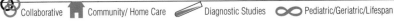

- Consult with dietitian *to address specific nutrition/dietary issues (e.g., food groups, liquid diets, dietary restrictions that might be needed for certain chronic diseases such as renal failure or diabetes mellitus).*
- Provide information to new mothers about nutrition for developing babies *to reduce potential for childhood obesity related to lack of knowledge.*
- Encourage the client to make a commitment to lead an active life and control food habits.
- Assist client in learning to be in touch with own body to identify feelings such as anger, anxiety, boredom, sadness *that may provoke "comfort eating."*
- Develop a system for self-monitoring *to provide a sense of control and enable the client to follow own progress and assist with making choices.*
- Refer to support groups and appropriate community resources for behavior modification as indicated. *Provides role models and assistance for making lifestyle changes.*

DOCUMENTATION FOCUS

Assessment/Reassessment
- Findings related to individual situation, risk factors, current caloric intake/dietary pattern.

Planning
- Plan of care and who is involved in the planning.
- Teaching plan.

Implementation/Evaluation
- Response to interventions/teaching and actions performed.
- Attainment/progress toward desired outcome(s).
- Modifications to plan of care.

Discharge Planning
- Long-range needs, noting who is responsible for actions to be taken.
- Specific referrals made.

References

1. Freemark, M. (2002). Obesity. Available at: http://www.emedicine.com. Accessed November 2003.
2. Purnell, L. D., & Paulanka, B. J. (1998). Transcultural Health Care: A Culturally Competent Approach. Philadelphia: F. A. Davis.
3. Galletta, G. M. (2003). Obesity and weight control. Available at: http://www.emedicine.com. Accessed November 2003.
4. Older Americans Month. Food & Nutrition Information. Available at: http://www.eatright.org/Public/Nutritioninformation. Accessed June 2003.
5. Engel, J. (2002). Pocket Guide to Pediatric Assessment, ed 4. St. Louis: Mosby.
6. Vogelzang, J. L. (2003). Making nutrition sense from OASIS. Home Healthcare Nurse, 21(9), 592–600.

readiness for enhanced Nutrition

Definition: A pattern of nutrient intake that is sufficient for meeting metabolic needs and can be strengthened

RELATED FACTORS
To be developed by nurse researchers and submitted to NANDA

Subjective

Expresses willingness to enhance nutrition

Eats regularly

Expresses knowledge of healthy food and fluid choices

Attitude toward eating and drinking is congruent with health goals

Objective

Consumes adequate food and fluid

Follows an appropriate standard for intake (e.g., the food pyramid or American Diabetic Association Guidelines)

Safe preparation and storage for food and fluids

SAMPLE CLINICAL APPLICATIONS: as a health-seeking behavior the client may be healthy or this diagnosis can occur in any clinical condition

DESIRED OUTCOMES/EVALUATION CRITERIA

Sample **NOC** linkages:

Nutritional Status: Extent to which nutrients are available to meet metabolic needs

Knowledge: Diet: Extent of understanding conveyed about diet

Health Promoting Behavior: Actions to sustain or increase wellness

Client Will (Include Specific Time Frame)

- Demonstrate behaviors to attain/maintain appropriate weight
- Be free of signs of malnutrition
- Be able to safely prepare and store foods

ACTIONS/INTERVENTIONS

Sample **NIC** linkages:

Nutrition Management: Assisting with or providing a balanced dietary intake of foods and fluids

Teaching: Prescribed Diet: Preparing a patient to correctly follow a prescribed diet

Weight Management: Facilitating maintenance of optimal body weight and percent body fat

NURSING PRIORITY NO. **1.** To determine current nutritional status and eating patterns:

- Assess client's knowledge of current nutritional needs and ways client is meeting these needs. *Provides baseline for further teaching and/or interventions.*
- Assess eating patterns and food/fluid choices in relation to any health-risk factors and health goals. *Helps to identify specific strengths and weaknesses that can be addressed.*
- Determine that age-related and developmental needs are met. *These factors are constantly present throughout the lifespan, although differing for each age group. For example, older adults need same nutrients as younger adults, but in smaller amounts, and with attention to certain components, such as calcium, fiber, vitamins, protein and water.[1] Infants/children require small meals and constant attention to needed nutrients for proper growth/development while dealing with child's food preferences and eating habits.[2]*
- Evaluate for influence of cultural factors *to determine what client considers to be normal dietary practices, as well as to identify food preferences and eating patterns that can be strengthened and/or altered, if indicated.[3]*

 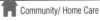Cultural 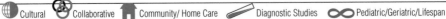Collaborative Community/ Home Care Diagnostic Studies Pediatric/Geriatric/Lifespan Medications

- Assess how client perceives food, food preparation, and the act of eating *to determine client's feeling and emotions regarding food and self-image.*
- Ascertain occurrence of/potential for negative feedback from SO(s). *May reveal control issues that could impact client's motivation for change.*
- Determine patterns of hunger and satiety. *Helps identify strengths and weaknesses in eating patterns and potential for change, e.g., person predisposed to weight gain may need a different time for a big meal than evening, or learn what foods reinforce feelings of satisfaction.*
- Assess client's ability to shop for, safely store, and/or prepare foods *to determine if health information or resources might be needed.*

NURSING PRIORITY NO. 2. To assist client/SO(s) to develop plan to meet individual needs:

- Assist in obtaining/review results of individual testing, e.g., weight/height, body fat percent, lipids, glucose, complete blood count, total protein, etc. *to determine that client is healthy and/or identify dietary changes that may be helpful in attaining health goals.*[5]
- Encourage client's new eating patterns/habits (e.g., controlling portion size, eating regular meals, reading product labels, reducing high-fat, high sugar, or fast-food intake, following specific dietary program, drinking water and healthy beverages). *Provides reinforcement/ supports client's efforts to incorporate changes into lifestyle habits and continue with new behaviors.*
- Provide instruction/reinforce information regarding special needs. *Client/SO may benefit from or desire assistance in learning new eating habits or following medically prescribed diets (e.g., very low calorie diet, tube-feedings, and diabetic or renal dialysis diet).*[4]
- Address reading of food labels, instructing in meaning of labeling as indicated, to assist client/SO in making healthful choices.
- Encourage safe preparation and storage of food *to avoid foodborne illnesses.*
- Consult/refer to dietitian or primary care provider as indicated. *Client/SO may benefit from advice regarding specific nutrition/dietary issues, or may require regular follow-up to determine that needs are being met when following a medically prescribed program.*
- Develop a system for self-monitoring *to provide a sense of control and enable the client to follow own progress, and assist in making choices.*

NURSING PRIORITY NO. 3. To enhance wellness (Teaching/Discharge Considerations):

- Review individual risk factors and provide additional information/response to concerns. *Assists the client with motivation and decision-making.*
- Provide bibliotherapy and help client/SO(s) identify and evaluate resources they can access on their own. *When referencing the Internet or nontraditional/unproven resources, the individual must exercise some restraint and determine the reliability of the source/information before acting on it.*
- Involve SO(s) in treatment plan as much as possible *to provide ongoing support and increase likelihood of success.*
- Encourage variety and moderation in dietary plan *to decrease boredom and encourage client in efforts to make healthy choices about eating and food.*
- Assist client to identify/access community resources when indicated. *May benefit from assistance such as food stamps, budget counseling, Meals on Wheels, community food banks, and/or other assistance programs.*

Assessment/Reassessment

- Baseline information, client's perception of need.
- Nutritional intake and metabolic needs.

Planning

- Plan of care/interventions and who is involved in planning.
- Teaching Plan.

Implementation/Evaluation

- Client's responses to interventions/teaching and actions performed.
- Attainment/progress toward desired outcome(s).
- Modifications to plan of care.

Discharge Planning

- Long-term needs and actions to be taken
- Support systems available, specific referrals made, and who is responsible for actions to be taken.

References

1. Older Americans Month. Food & Nutrition Information. Available at: http://www.eatright.org/Public/Nutritioninformation. Accessed June 2003.
2. Engel, J. (2002). Pocket Guide to Pediatric Assessment, ed 4. St. Louis: Mosby.
3. Purnell, L. D., & Paulanka, B. J. (1998) Transcultural Health Care: A Culturally Competent Approach. Philadelphia: F. A. Davis.
4. Pignone, MP, et al. (2003). Counseling to promote a healthy diet in adults: A summary of the evidence for the U. S. Preventive Services Task Force. Am J Prev Med, 24(1), 75–92.
5. Vogelzang, J. L. (2003). Making nutrition sense from OASIS. Home Healthcare Nurse, 21(9):592–600.

impaired Oral Mucous Membrane

Definition: Disruption of the lips and soft tissue of the oral cavity

RELATED FACTORS

Pathologic conditions—oral cavity (radiation to head or neck); cleft lip or palate; loss of supportive structures

Trauma

Mechanical (e.g., ill-fitting dentures; braces; tubes [ET, nasogastric], surgery in oral cavity)

Chemical (e.g., alcohol, tobacco, acidic foods, regular use of inhalers)

Chemotherapy; immunosuppression/compromised; decreased platelets; infection; radiation therapy

Dehydration, malnutrition or vitamin deficiency

NPO for more than 24 hours

Lack of/impaired or decreased salivation; mouth breathing

Ineffective oral hygiene; barriers to oral self-care/professional care

Medication side effects

Stress; depression

 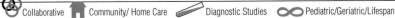

Diminished hormone levels (women); aging-related loss of connective, adipose, or bone tissue

Subjective
Xerostomia (dry mouth)
Oral pain/discomfort
Self-report of bad/diminished or absent taste; difficulty eating or swallowing

Objective
Coated tongue; smooth atrophic, sensitive tongue; geographic tongue
Gingival or mucosal pallor
Stomatitis; hyperemia; bleeding gingival hyperplasia; macroplasia; vesicles, nodules, or papules
White patches/plaques, spongy patches or white curdlike exudate, oral lesions or ulcers; fissures; cheilitis; desquamation; mucosal denudation
Edema
Halitosis [carious teeth]
Gingival recession, pockets deeper than 4 mm
Purulent drainage or exudates; presence of pathogens
Enlarged tonsils beyond what is developmentally appropriate
Red or bluish masses (e.g., hemangiomas)
Difficult speech

SAMPLE CLINICAL APPLICATIONS: oral trauma, cancer, chemo/radiation therapy, malnutrition, infection, oral surgery, cleft lip/palate, conditions requiring endotracheal intubation (e.g., brain or spinal cord injury/stroke, COPD, acute respiratory distress syndrome, ALS)

DESIRED OUTCOMES/EVALUATION CRITERIA
Sample **NOC** linkages:
Oral Health: Condition of the mouth, teeth, gums, and tongue
Self-Care: Oral Hygiene: Ability to care for own mouth and teeth
Tissue Integrity: Skin and Mucous Membrane: Structural intactness and normal physiologic function of skin and mucous membranes

Client Will (Include Specific Time Frame)
- Verbalize understanding of causative factors.
- Identify specific interventions to promote healthy oral mucosa.
- Demonstrate techniques to restore/maintain integrity of oral mucosa.
- Report/demonstrate a decrease in symptoms/complaints as noted in Defining Characteristics.

ACTIONS/INTERVENTIONS
Sample **NIC** linkages:
Oral Health Restoration: Promotion of healing for a patient who has an oral mucosa or dental lesion
Oral Health Maintenance: Maintenance and promotion of oral hygiene and dental health for the patient at risk for developing oral or dental lesions

Oral Health Promotion: Promotion of oral hygiene and dental care for a patient with normal oral and dental health

NURSING PRIORITY NO. 1. To identify causative/contributing factors to condition:

- Note presence of illness/disease/trauma (e.g., herpes simplex, gingivitis, facial fractures, cancer or cancer therapies, as well as generalized debilitating conditions).
- Determine presence/type of oral problem (e.g., stomatitis is an inflammation ranging from redness to severe ulceration and is a side effect of many cancer treatments; oral thrush presents as distinctive lesions of mouth, tongue and cheeks, caused by yeast; taste sensation may be altered by certain medications or CNS dysfunction) *to identify appropriate interventions or preventative measures.*
- Assess for presence, type, and location of oral pain, noting whether pain is caused by oral lesions, dry mouth, teeth or gum problems *to determine needed interventions and to reduce potential for complications (e.g., infection) associated with sore mouth.*[1]
- Determine nutrition/fluid intake and reported changes. *Malnutrition and dehydration predispose clients to problems with oral mucous membranes.*
- Note use of tobacco (including smokeless) and alcohol. *Associated with cancers of the oral cavity and with nutritional deficiencies affecting the oral mucosa.*
- Observe for chipped or sharp-edged teeth. Note fit of dentures or other prosthetic devices when used. *Factors that increase the risk of injury to delicate tissues.*
- Assess medication use and possibility of side effects. *For example, use of antihypertensives and anticholinergics impairs salivary function/promotes xerostomia.*[8]
- Determine allergies to food/drugs, other substances *that may result in irritation of oral mucosa.*
- 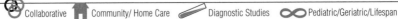 Assess mouth, tongue, gums and lips for color, moisture *to ascertain general health of oral mucous membranes.* Take note of abnormal lesions (e.g., inflammation, edema, white or red patches, ulcers, etc.). *White ulcerated spots may be canker sores, especially in children; white curd patches (thrush) are common in infants. Reddened, swollen bleeding gums may indicate infection, poor nutrition, or poor oral hygiene. A red tongue may be related to vitamin deficiencies.*[2] *Malignant lesions are more common in elderly than younger persons (especially if there is a history of smoking or alcohol use) and many elderly persons rarely visit a dentist.*[3]
- Evaluate client's ability to provide self-care and availability of necessary equipment/assistance. *Client's age (very young or elderly) impacts ability to provide self-care, as well as current health issues (e.g., disease condition or treatment, weakness), and client's habits and lifestyle.*
- Review oral hygiene practices, noting frequency and type (e.g., brushing/flossing/Water Pik); inquire about client's professional dental care, regularity and date of last dental examination.

NURSING PRIORITY NO. 2. To correct identified/developing problems:

- Routinely inspect oral cavity for sores, lesions, and/or bleeding. Recommend client establish regular schedule of self-inspection, when possible, such as when performing oral care activities. *Can help with early identification of oral disease; reveal symptoms of systemic disease, drug side effects, or trauma of the oral cavity.*[4]
- Encourage adequate fluids *to prevent dehydration/oral dryness and limit bacterial overgrowth.*[8]

 Cultural   Collaborative   Community/ Home Care   Diagnostic Studies   Pediatric/Geriatric/Lifespan   Medications

- Provide for increased humidity by vaporizer or room humidifier, *if client is mouth breather or ambient humidity is low.*
- Plan diet to avoid irritating foods/fluids, temperature extremes. Provide soft or pureed diet as required. *Abrasive foods may open healing lesions. Open lesions are painful and aggravated by salt, spice, acidic food/beverages. Extreme cold or hot can cause pain to sensitive membranes.*
- Recommend avoiding alcohol, smoking/chewing tobacco, *which may further dehydrate and irritate mucosa.*
- Provide/encourage regular oral care (including after meals/at bedtime, and frequently to critically ill client) using water, or mouthwash (especially before meals), avoiding those containing alcohol *(drying effect)* or hydrogen peroxide *(drying and foul tasting).*[5]
- Use soft-bristle brush or sponge/cotton-tip applicators to cleanse teeth and tongue. *Brushing the teeth is the most effective way of reducing plaque and managing periodontal disease.*[6]
- Floss gently/use WaterPik *to remove food particles that promote bacterial growth and gum disease.*
- Use foam sticks to swab mouth, tongue and gums (when client has no teeth). Use lemon/glycerin swabs with caution. *Can result in decreased salivary amylase and oral moisture, as well as erosion of tooth enamel.*[6]
- Suction oral cavity gently/frequently if client cannot swallow secretions. *Saliva contains digestive enzymes that may be erosive to exposed tissues (e.g., such as might occur because of heavy drooling following radical neck surgery). Suctioning can improve comfort and enhance oral hygiene.*
- Provide low-intensity suctioning during oral care *to reduce risk of aspiration in intubated clients or those with decreased gag/swallow reflexes.*[8]
- Provide/assist with denture care, as needed. *Evidence-based protocol for denture care states that dentures are to be removed and scrubbed at least once daily, removed and rinsed after every meal, and kept in an appropriate solution at night.*[7]
- Lubricate lips and provide commercially prepared oral lubricant solution, when indicated. Encourage use of chewing gum, hard candy, etc., *to stimulate flow of saliva to neutralize acids and limit bacterial growth.*
- Provide anesthetic lozenges or analgesics such as Stanford solution, viscous lidocaine (Xylocaine), hot pepper (capsaicin) candy, as indicated *to reduce oral discomfort/pain.*
- Administer medications, as ordered, (e.g., antibiotics, antifungal agents) including antimicrobial mouth rinse or spray (i.e., chlorhexidine) *to treat oral infections or reduce potential for bacterial overgrowth and risk of ventilator-associated pneumonia (VAP).*[8,9]
- Change position of ET tube/airway every 8 hours and as needed when client is on ventilator *to minimize pressure on fragile tissues and improve access to all areas of oral cavity.*
- Provide adequate nutritional intake *to prevent complications associated with nutritional deficiencies.*

NURSING PRIORITY NO. 3. To promote wellness (Teaching/Discharge Considerations):

- Review current oral hygiene patterns and provide information as required/desired *to correct deficiencies and encourage proper care.*
- Instruct parents in oral hygiene techniques and proper dental care for infants/children (e.g., safe use of pacifier, brushing of teeth and gums, avoidance of sweet drinks and candy, recognition and treatment of thrush). *Encourages early initiation of good oral health practices and timely intervention for treatable problems.*

• Discuss special mouth care required during and after illness/trauma, or following surgical repair (e.g., cleft lip/palate) *to facilitate healing.*

 • Identify need for/demonstrate use of special "appliances" to perform own oral care. *Enhances independence in self-care.*

 • Listen to concerns about appearance and provide accurate information about possible treatments/outcomes. Discuss effect of condition on self-esteem/body image, noting withdrawal from usual social activities/relationships, and/or expressions of powerlessness.

• Review information regarding drug regimen, use of local anesthetics *for safe use.*

 • Promote general health/mental health habits. *(Altered immune response can negatively affect the oral mucosa.)*

 • Provide nutritional information *to correct deficiencies, reduce irritation/gum disease, and prevent dental caries.*

• Stress importance of limiting nighttime regimen of bottle of milk for infant in bed. Suggest pacifier or use of water during night *to prevent bottle syndrome with decaying of teeth.*

• Recommend regular dental checkups/care and episodic evaluation of oral health prior to certain medical treatments (e.g., chemotherapy or heart valve replacement) *to maintain oral health/reduce risk of oropharyngeal colonization leading to bacterial growth on heart valves, endocarditis, etc.*[8]

• Identify community resources (e.g., low-cost dental clinics, Meals on Wheels/food stamps, home care aide) *to meet individual needs.*

DOCUMENTATION FOCUS

Assessment/Reassessment
• Condition of oral mucous membranes, routine oral care habits and interferences.

Planning
• Plan of care and who is involved in planning.
• Teaching plan.

Implementation/Evaluation
• Responses to interventions/teaching and actions performed.
• Attainment/progress toward desired outcome(s).
• Modifications to plan of care.

Discharge Planning
• Long-term needs and who is responsible for actions to be taken.
• Specific referrals made, resources for special appliances.

References

1. Carl, W., & Havens, J. (2000). The cancer patient with severe mucositis. Cur Rev Pain, 4(3), 197–202.
2. Engel, J. (2002) Pocket Guide to Pediatric Assessment, ed 4. St. Louis: Mosby, pp 155–156.
3. Aubertin, M. A. (1997). Oral cancer screening in the elderly: The home healthcare nurse's role. Home Health Nurs, 15(9), 594–604.
4. White, R. (2000). Nurse assessment of oral health: A review of practice and education. Br J Nurs, 9(5), 260–266.
5. Winslow, E. H. (1994). Don't use H_2O_2 for oral care. Am J Nurse, 94(3),19.
6. Stiefel, K. A., et al. (2000). Improving oral hygiene for the seriously ill patient: Implementing research-based practice. Medsurg Nurs, 9(1), 40–43, 46.
7. Curzio, J., & McCowan, M. (2000). Getting research into practice: Developing oral hygiene standards. Br J Nurs, 9(7), 434–438.

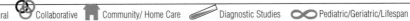 Cultural   Collaborative   Community/ Home Care   Diagnostic Studies   Pediatric/Geriatric/Lifespan   Medications

8. Trieger, N. (2004). Oral care in the intensive care unit. Am J Crit Care, 13(1), 24.
9. Munro, C., & Grap, M. J. (2004). Oral health and care in the intensive care unit: Stat of science. Am J Crit Care, 13(1), 25–33.

acute Pain

Definition: Unpleasant sensory and emotional experience arising from actual or potential tissue damage or described in terms of such damage (International Association for the Study of Pain); sudden or slow onset of any intensity from mild to severe with an anticipated or predictable end and a duration of less than 6 months

RELATED FACTORS

Injuring agents (biologic, chemical, physical, psychological)

DEFINING CHARACTERISTICS

Subjective

Verbal or coded report [may be less from clients younger than age 40, men, and some cultural groups]
Changes in appetite and eating
[Pain unrelieved and/or increased beyond tolerance]

Objective

Guarded/protective behavior; antalgic position/gestures
Facial mask; sleep disturbance (eyes lack luster, beaten look, fixed or scattered movement, grimace)
Expressive behavior (restlessness, moaning, crying, vigilance, irritability, sighing)
Distraction behavior (pacing, seeking out other people and/or activities, repetitive activities)
Autonomic alteration in muscle tone (may span from listless [flaccid] to rigid)
Autonomic responses (diaphoresis; blood pressure, respiration, pulse change; pupillary dilation)
Self-focusing
Narrowed focus (altered time perception, impaired thought process, reduced interaction with people and environment)
[Fear/panic]

SAMPLE CLINICAL APPLICATIONS: traumatic injuries, surgical procedures, infections, cancer, burns, skin lesions, gangrene, thrombophlebitis/pulmonary embolus, neuralgia

DESIRED OUTCOMES/EVALUATION CRITERIA

Sample **NOC** linkages:

Pain Level: Severity of reported or demonstrated pain

Pain Control: Personal actions to control pain

Pain: Disruptive Effects: Observed or reported disruptive effects of pain on emotions and behavior

Client Will (Include Specific Time Frame)

- Report pain is relieved/controlled.
- Follow prescribed pharmacologic regimen.
- Verbalize methods that provide relief.
- Demonstrate use of relaxation skills and diversional activities as indicated for individual situation.

ACTIONS/INTERVENTIONS

Sample **NIC** linkages:

Pain Management: Alleviation of pain or a reduction in pain to a level of comfort that is acceptable to the patient

Analgesic Administration: Use of pharmacologic agents to reduce or eliminate pain

Environmental Management: Comfort: Manipulation of the patient's surroundings for promotion of optimal comfort

NURSING PRIORITY NO. 1. To assess etiology/precipitating contributory factors:

- Perform a comprehensive assessment of pain including location, characteristics, onset/duration, frequency, quality, severity (using numeric, pain thermometer, adolescent pediatric pain tool [APPT] or Wong-Baker faces pain scale).[1,2] Note precipitating/aggravating factors.
- Determine possible pathophysiological/psychological causes of pain (e.g., inflammation, fractures, neuralgia, surgery, influenza, pleurisy, angina/acute MI, cholecystitis, burns, headache, herniated disc, grief, fear/anxiety, and concurrent medical conditions). *Acute pain is that which follows a surgical procedure, or trauma, or occurs suddenly with the onset of a painful condition (e.g., heart attack, migraine headache, pancreatitis).*[3]
- Note anatomical location of surgical incisions/procedures. *This can influence the amount of postoperative pain experienced, for example, vertical/diagonal incisions are more painful than transverse or S-shaped. Presence of known/unknown complication(s) may make the pain more severe than anticipated.*[4,5,10]
- Determine history/presence of chronic conditions (e.g., multiple sclerosis, stroke, mental distortions, trauma) *that may also cause pain and interfere with accurate assessment of acute pain.*[2]
- Assess client's perceptions of pain, along with behavioral (e.g., agitation, withdrawal) and physiologic (e.g., hypertension, tachycardia, tachypnea) responses, and cultural expectations regarding pain. *Client's perception of pain is influenced by age and developmental stage, underlying problem causing pain, cognitive, behavioral and sociocultural factors.*[2]
- Note client's attitude toward pain and use of specific pain medications, including any history of substance abuse. *Client may have beliefs restricting use of medications, or may have a high tolerance for drugs because of recent/current use; or may not be able to take pain medications at all if participating in a substance abuse recovery program.*
- Note client's locus of control (internal/external). *Individuals with external locus of control may take little or no responsibility for pain management.*
- Determine medications currently being used (e.g., anticoagulants) and any medication allergies *that may affect choice of analgesics.*[4,5]
- Assist in thorough diagnosis, including neurologic and psychological factors (pain inventory, psychological interview) as appropriate when pain persists.
- Refer for/review results of diagnostic studies (e.g., laboratory studies, radiographs, scans, etc) depending on results of history and physical examination.
- Refer for specialty consults (e.g., surgical, orthopedic, anesthesiologist) *for treatment of underlying problem causing pain or to provide modalities to treat the pain.*

NURSING PRIORITY NO. 2. To evaluate client's response to pain:

- Perform pain assessment each time pain occurs, using flow sheet or pain diary, as indicated. Document and investigate changes from previous reports and evaluate results of pain inter-

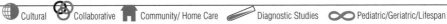

ventions *to demonstrate improvement in status or to identify worsening of underlying condition/development of complications.*[6]

- Be aware of client's "Right to Treatment" *that includes prevention of or adequate relief from pain*[7] *and that failure to meet the standard of assessing for pain can be considered negligence.*[8]

- Accept client's description of pain (e.g., quality, intensity, duration, onset, location). Be aware of the terminology client uses for pain experience (e.g., young child may say "owie"; elderly may say "it aches so bad"). *Pain is a subjective experience and cannot be felt by others.*[2] Note: Some elderly clients experience a reduction in perception of pain or have difficulty localizing/describing pain and pain may be manifested as a change in behavior (e.g., restlessness, increased confusion/wandering, acting out).

- Note cultural and developmental influences affecting pain response. *These factors affect client's and caregiver's attitudes and beliefs regarding the pain experience, expressions of pain, and expectations regarding pain management.*[2,9]

- Observe nonverbal cues (e.g., how client walks, holds body, guarding behaviors; sleeplessness, grimacing facial expressions; distraction behaviors, narrowed focus; crying, poor feeding, lethargy in infants) especially in persons who cannot communicate verbally. *Cues not congruent with verbal reports indicate need for further evaluation.*[1-6,9]

- Assess for referred pain, as appropriate, *to help determine possibility of underlying condition or organ dysfunction causing pain to be perceived in area other than site of the problem.*

- Monitor vital signs during episodes of pain. *Blood pressure, respiratory and heart rate are usually altered in acute pain.*[1,2,4,5]

- Ascertain client's knowledge of and expectations about pain management. *Provides baseline for interventions and teaching, provides opportunity to allay common fears/misconceptions (e.g., fears about addiction to opiates, belief that complete pain relief is possible in every situation) or to address expected side effects of analgesics (e.g., constipation).*[2]

- Review client's previous experiences with pain and methods found either helpful or unhelpful for pain control in the past. *Helpful in determining appropriate interventions.*

NURSING PRIORITY NO. 3. To assist client to explore methods for alleviation/control of pain:

- Work with client *to prevent rather than "chase" pain.* Use flow sheet *to document pain, therapeutic interventions, response, and length of time before pain recurs.* Instruct client to report pain as soon as it begins *because timely intervention is more likely to be successful in alleviating pain.*[2,11]

- Determine client's acceptable level of pain on a 0 to 10 or faces scale. *Client may not be 100% pain-free, but may feel that a "3" is a manageable level of discomfort, or may require medication for pain level of "5," because the experience is subjective.*[1,2,4-6,9]

- Encourage verbalization of feelings about the pain *to evaluate coping abilities and to identify areas of additional concern.*[1,11]

- Review procedures/expectations and tell client when treatments will hurt. Discuss pain management methods that will be used *to reduce concerns of the unknown and muscle tension associated with anxiety/fear.*

- Use puppets/dolls for explanations/teaching when indicated, *to demonstrate procedures for child and enhance understanding to reduce level of anxiety/fear.*

- Provide/promote nonpharmacological pain management[1-12]:
  Quiet environment, calm activities.
  Comfort measures (e.g., back rub, change of position, use of heat/cold compresses)
  Use of relaxation exercises (e.g., focused breathing, visualization, guided imagery)

Diversional/distraction activities such as television/radio, socialization with others, commercial or individualized tapes (e.g., "white" noise, music, instructional). Involve client and family in pain management.

 Suggest parent be present during painful procedures *to comfort child.* Identify ways of avoiding/minimizing pain. *Splinting incision during cough, keeping body in good alignment and using proper body mechanics, resting between activities can reduce occurrence of muscle tension/spasms or undue stress on incision.*

- Establish collaborative approach for pain management based on client's understanding about, and acceptance of, available treatment options. *Pharmacologic management is based on client's symptomatology and mechanism of pain, as well as tolerance for pain and for the various analgesics. Pain medications may include pills, injections, intravenous dosing/patient-controlled analgesia (PCA), or regional analgesia (e.g., epidural and spinal blocking).*[2–5,11,12]

- Administer analgesics to maximal dosage as needed *to maintain "acceptable" level of pain. The type of medication(s) ordered depends on the type and severity of pain (e.g., acetaminophen and nonsteroidal anti-inflammatory medications [NSAIDs] are commonly used to treat mild-to-moderate pain, while opiates [e.g., morphine, oxycodone and fentanyl] are used to treat moderate to severe pain). Note: Combinations of medications may be used on prescribed intervals.*[5,12]

- Notify physician/healthcare provider if regimen is inadequate to meet pain control goal. Assist client to prevent (rather than treat pain) and alter drug regimen based on individual needs. *Once established, pain is more difficult to suppress. Increasing dosage, changing medication or using a stepped program (e.g., switching from injection to oral route, or lengthening time interval between doses) helps in self-management of pain.*[4,7]

- Address with client side effects of medication regimen (e.g., constipation caused by use of opiates) and planned interventions *to limit adverse effects and barriers to adequate use of analgesics.*[2]

- Evaluate for adverse medication effects (e.g., decrease in mental acuity, change in thought processes, confusion/delirium, urinary retention, severe nausea, vomiting, pruritus). *Intolerable symptoms that usually require change of medication(s).*[2,3,5,11,12]

- Demonstrate/monitor use of self-administration/patient-controlled analgesia (PCA) that involves client in plan *to administer own IV pain medication, or bolus additional dose when on continual basis drip.*[2–5,11,12]

- Provide information/monitor use of site-specific medications (e.g., spinal/epidural/regional anesthesia) *that might be used for certain procedures such as back surgery or amputation, labor/delivery).*[3,4,11,12]

- Instruct client in use of transcutaneous electrical stimulation (TENS) unit when ordered.

NURSING PRIORITY NO. 4. To promote wellness (Teaching/Discharge Considerations):

- Acknowledge the pain experience and convey acceptance of client's response to pain. *Reduces defensive responses, promotes trust and enhances cooperation with regimen.*

- Encourage adequate rest periods *to prevent fatigue that can impair ability to manage/cope with pain.*

- Review nonpharmacologic measures for lessening pain. *Relaxation skills and techniques such as self-hypnosis, biofeedback, and Therapeutic Touch (TT) have no detrimental side effects.*

- Provide information/discuss pain management before planned procedures. *The primary concern of most clients/families is pain and discomfort following surgery/invasive procedure.*

- Address impact of pain on lifestyle/independence. *Understanding that pain can be manage-*

  Cultural Collaborative 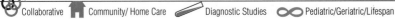 Community/ Home Care Diagnostic Studies Pediatric/Geriatric/Lifespan Medications *able and that there are ways to maximize level of functioning promotes hope and cooperation with regimen.*

 • Encourage performance of individualized physical therapy/exercise program. *Promotes active role in preventing muscle spasms/contractures.*

 • Discuss ways SO(s) can assist client with pain management. *Helping to reduce precipitating factors that may cause or exacerbate pain (e.g., need to walk distances or climb stairs, strenuous activity including household chores/yard work, noisy environment), supporting timely pain control, encouraging eating nutritious meals to enhance wellness, and providing gentle massage to reduce muscle tension facilitate recovery/pain control.*

 • Identify specific signs/symptoms and changes in pain *requiring medical follow-up.*

DOCUMENTATION FOCUS

Assessment/Reassessment
- Individual assessment findings, including client's description of response to pain, specifics of pain inventory, expectations of pain management, and acceptable level of pain.
- Prior medication use; substance abuse.

Planning
- Plan of care and who is involved in planning.
- Teaching plan.

Implementation/Evaluation
- Response to interventions/teaching and actions performed.
- Attainment/progress toward desired outcome(s).
- Modifications to plan of care.

Discharge Planning
Long-term needs, noting who is responsible for actions to be taken.
Specific referrals made.

References

1. Engel, J.(2002). Pocket Guide to Pediatric Assessment, ed 4. St Louis: Mosby, pp 249, 259.
2. Young, D. (1999). Acute pain management. Iowa City, IA: University of Iowa Gerontological Nursing Interventions Research Center. Research Dissemination Core.
3. Information about Acute Pain Management. Available at: http://www.sepaincare.com/pain_acute.htm. Accessed September 2003.
4. Clinical practice guideline for the management of postoperative pain. Version 1.2. (2002). Washington, DC: Department of Defense, Veterans Health Administration. Available at: http://www.guideline.gov. Accessed July 2004.
5. Ameres, M. J., & Yeh, B. (2001). Pain after surgery. Available at: http://www.emedicine.com. Accessed December 2003.
6. Smith, R., Curci, M., & Silverman, A. (2002). Pain management: The global connection. Nursing Management, 33(6), 26–29.
7. Acute pain management: Operative or medical procedures and trauma. (Clinical Practice Guideline). (1992). Pub No. AHCPR 92-0019. Rockville, MD: Agency for Health Care Policy and Research, Public Health Service, U.S. Dept of Health and Human Services.
8. Pain Standards for 2001. (2001). Joint Commission on Accreditation of Healthcare Organizations. Available at:www.jcaho.org/standards/stds2001_mpfrm.html. Accessed January 2004.
9. Purnell, L. D., & Paulanka, B. J. (1998). Transcultural Health Care: A Culturally Competent Approach. Philadelphia: F. A. Davis.

10. ND Pain, acute. In Doenges, M. E., Moorhouse, M. F., & Geissler-Murr, A. C. (2002). *Nurse's Pocket Guide: Diagnoses, Interventions and Rationales*, ed 8. Philadelphia: F. A. Davis.

11. Assessment and management of acute pain. (2002). Bloomington, MN: Institute for Clinical Systems Improvement (ICSI). Available at: http://www.guideline.gov.

12. Michael, J. A. (2002). Pain Medicine, Types. Available at: http://www.emedicine.com. Accessed December 2003.

chronic Pain

Definition: Unpleasant sensory and emotional experience arising from actual or potential tissue damage or described in terms of such damage (International Association for the Study of Pain); sudden or slow onset of any intensity from mild to severe, constant or recurring without an anticipated or predictable end and a duration of greater than 6 months

[Pain is a signal that something is amiss in the body. It may be associated with an incurable disease or it may be the result of nerve fibers transmitting painful impulses to the brain which become "trained" to deliver pain signals better (just as muscle function improves with training).[1] Chronic pain can be recurrent and periodically disabling (e.g., migraine headaches) or may be unremitting (e.g., pain associated with osteoporosis, bone cancer). While chronic pain syndrome includes various learned behaviors, psychological factors can become the primary contribution to impairment. This is a complex entity, combining elements from other NDs (e.g., Powerlessness, deficient Diversional Activity, interrupted Family Processes, Self-Care deficit, and risk for Disuse Syndrome.)]

RELATED FACTORS

Chronic physical/psychosocial disability

DEFINING CHARACTERISTICS

Subjective

Verbal or coded report

Fear of reinjury

Altered ability to continue previous activities

Changes in sleep patterns; fatigue

[Changes in appetite]

[Preoccupation with pain]

[Desperately seeks alternative solutions/therapies for relief/control of pain]

Objective

Observed evidence of: protective/guarding behavior; facial mask; irritability; self-focusing; restlessness; depression

Reduced interaction with people

Anorexia, weight changes

Atrophy of involved muscle group

Sympathetic mediated responses (temperature, cold, changes of body position, hypersensitivity)

SAMPLE CLINICAL APPLICATIONS: traumatic injuries, migraines, repetitive motion injury (carpal/cubital tunnel syndrome), rheumatoid arthritis, peripheral neuropathies in diabetes or AIDS, cancer, burns, endometriosis, neuralgia, gangrene

 Cultural Collaborative Community/ Home Care Diagnostic Studies 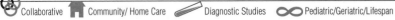 Pediatric/Geriatric/Lifespan Medications

Sample **NOC** linkages:

Pain Control: Personal actions to control pain

Pain: Disruptive Effects: Observed or reported disruptive effects of pain on emotions and behavior

Pain: Psychological Response: Cognitive and emotional responses to physical pain

---

Client Will (Include Specific Time Frame)

- Verbalize and demonstrate (nonverbal cues) relief and/or control of pain/discomfort.
- Verbalize recognition of interpersonal/family dynamics and reactions that affect the pain problem.
- Demonstrate/initiate behavioral modifications of lifestyle and appropriate use of therapeutic interventions.

Sample **NOC** linkage:

Family Coping: Family actions to manage stressors that tax family resources

---

Family/SO(s) Will (Include Specific Time Frame)

- Cooperate in pain management program. (Refer to ND readiness for enhanced family Coping.)

ACTIONS/INTERVENTIONS

Sample **NIC** linkages:

Pain Management: Alleviation of pain or a reduction in pain to a level of comfort that is acceptable to the patient

Medication Management: Facilitation of safe and effective use of prescription and over-the-counter drugs

Simple Relaxation Therapy: Use of techniques to encourage and elicit relaxation for the purpose of decreasing undesirable signs and symptoms such as pain, muscle tension, or anxiety

NURSING PRIORITY NO. 1. To assess etiology/precipitating factors:

- Identify contributing factors (e.g., musculoskeletal trauma with lasting effects, chronic pancreatitis, cancers, osteoporosis, peripheral neuropathies from conditions such as diabetes or AIDS, fibromyalgia, overuse syndromes such as tendonitis; mechanical low back pain, spinal stenosis, amputation, urologic disorders, ulcer disease, endometriosis, cardiovascular disease, poor circulation, arthritis, recurrent migraines, bipolar disorders, depression, personality disorders, etc.). *These conditions can cause/exacerbate pain that persists for longer than 6 months.*[2]
- Assist in diagnostic testing, including physical, neurological, psychological evaluation (e.g., Minnesota Multiphasic Personality Inventory—MMPI, pain inventory, psychological interview). *Chronic pain syndrome (CPS) is a common problem that presents a major challenge to healthcare providers because of its complex history, often unclear etiology, and poor response to therapy. The pathophysiology is multifactorial and some believe that CPS is a learned behavioral syndrome that begins with a noxious stimulus causing pain that is then somehow reinforced internally or externally.*[2]
- Evaluate emotional/physical components of individual situation. *Individuals with certain psychological syndromes (e.g., major depression, somatization disorder, hypochondriasis) are prone to develop CPS. Many painful conditions cause or exacerbate emotional responses (e.g.,*

depression, withdrawal, agitation, anger) that worsen over time. Persistent long-term pain (and/or pain medications) can unconsciously be used to avoid unpleasant situations, or to obtain relief from emotions or responsibilities (e.g., guilt, anger; fear of work, sex or relationships).[2]

 • Determine relevant cultural factors. *Pain is accepted and expressed in different ways (e.g., moaning aloud or enduring in stoic silence), some may magnify symptoms to convince others of reality of pain, or believe that suffering in silence helps atone for past wrongdoing.*[3]

 • Note gender and age of client. *There may be differences between women and men, as to how they perceive and/or respond to pain. Pain in children, ethnic minorities, or cognitively impaired persons is often underestimated and undertreated.*[4] *While the prevalence of chronically painful conditions (e.g., arthritis) and illnesses (e.g., cancers) is common in the elderly, they may be reluctant to report pain.*[5,6]

 • Evaluate current and past analgesic/narcotic drug use and nonprescription drug use (including alcohol). *Provides clues to options to try or avoid, identifies need for changes in medication regimen, as well as need for detoxification program.*

NURSING PRIORITY NO. 2. To determine client response to chronic pain situation:

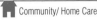 • Evaluate pain behavior, noting past and current pain experience, using pain rating scale or pain diary. *Pain behaviors can include the same ones present in acute pain (e.g., crying, grimacing, withdrawal, narrowed focus), but may also include other behaviors (e.g., dramatization of complaints, depression, drug misuse). Pain complaints may be exaggerated, because of client's perception that pain is not believed, or because client believes caregivers are discounting reports of pain.*[12]

• Provide comprehensive assessment of pain problem, noting its duration, who has been consulted, and what therapies (including alternative/complementary) have been used. *The pathophysiology of chronic pain is multifactorial. If the condition causing the persistent pain is physiological and noncurable (e.g., terminal cancer), all diagnostics and treatments may have been exhausted, and pain management becomes the primary goal. If medical treatments are ongoing for painful conditions (e.g., spinal stenosis, pancreatitis, endometriosis, arthritis), consultations with specialists may be helpful in finding curative or palliative treatments. If pain is present without a clear etiology and/or continues unabated, complex rehabilitation techniques may be required, incorporating physical, occupational, psychological, and recreational therapies.*[1,2]

• Note lifestyle effects of pain. *Major effects of chronic pain on the client's life can include depressed mood, fatigue, weight loss or gain, sleep disturbances, reduced activity and libido, excessive use of drugs and alcohol, dependent behavior and disability out of proportion to impairment.*[2,6]

• Assess degree of personal maladjustment of the client such as isolationism, anger, irritability, loss of work time/job/school. *Chronic pain reduces client's coping abilities and psychological well-being, often resulting in problems with relationships and life functioning.*[12]

• Determine issues of secondary gain for the client/SO(s) (e.g., financial/insurance compensation pending, marital/family concern, school or work issues) *which may be present if there is marked discrepancy between claimed distress and objective findings, or there is a lack of cooperation during evaluation and in complying with prescribed treatment.*[7]

• Note codependent components, enabling behaviors of caregivers/family members *that support continuation of the status quo, and may interfere with progress in pain management/resolution of situation.*

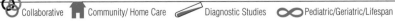 • Note availability/use of personal and community resources. *Client/SO may need many*

things (e.g., equipment, financial resources, vocational training, respite services or placement in rehabilitation facility) in order to manage painful conditions and/or concerns or disabilities associated with condition.[12]

- Make home visit when indicated, observing such factors as client's safety, equipment, adequate lighting, or family interactions *to note impact of home environment on the client and to determine changes that might be useful in improving client's life (e.g., grab bars in bathrooms and hallways, wider doors, ramps, assistance with activities of daily living, housekeeping, yard work).*

- Acknowledge and assess pain matter-of-factly, avoiding undue expressions of concern, as well as expressions of disbelief about client's suffering. *Conveying an attitude of empathic understanding of client's disabling distress can have a beneficial impact on client's perception of health.*[8]

NURSING PRIORITY NO. 3. To assist client to deal with pain:

- Encourage participation in multidisciplinary pain management plan. *Comprehensive team may include physical medicine specialist; physical, occupational, recreational and vocational therapists; and emotional/behavioral therapists to address complex issues of unresolved pain issues, to set goals for pain relief, and to develop an individualized treatment and evaluation plan. Treatments could involve surgery, nerve blocks, injections, massage and other hands-on therapies, as well as counseling and home exercise programs.*[12]

- Administer/encourage client use of analgesics, as indicated. *Different medications or combinations of drugs may be used such as opioids/narcotics, non-opioids (e.g., acetaminophen, Cox-2 inhibitors, and NSAIDs) and adjuvant medications (e.g., muscle relaxants, anticonvulsants, antidepressants) to manage persistent pain, so that client may find relief, and/or increase level of function.*[1,2]

- Provide consistent and sufficient medication for pain relief especially in individuals who tend to be undermedicated (e.g., elderly, cognitively impaired, person with life-long pain, those with terminal cancer). *Medications may need to be administered regularly (not as needed), doses titrated either up or down, and dose maximized to optimize pain relief while managing side effects.*

- Use nonpharmacological interventions (as found in ND acute Pain) as appropriate (e.g., heat/cold, splinting, exercises, hydrotherapy, electrical stimulation/TENS unit, visualization, guided imagery, Therapeutic Touch [TT], progressive muscle relaxation, biofeedback, massage) *to obtain comfort, improve healing, and decrease dependency on analgesics.*[12]

- Assist client to learn breathing techniques (e.g., diaphragmatic breathing) and exercise/body movement *to relieve muscle tension and enhance generalized relaxation.*

- Discuss pain management goals/review client expectations versus reality, *because it may be that while pain cannot be resolved, it can be significantly lessened or managed, improving quality of life.*[12]

- Address medication misuse with client/SO and refer for appropriate counseling/interventions *when addiction is known or suspected to be interfering with client's well being. Most people (if they don't already have a substance [drug or alcohol] abuse problem), don't become addicted to pain medications, even when used on a long-term basis. These individuals will take the pain medications in order to go about the business of their lives. Addicts lie about their pain levels and about their activities in order to obtain pain medications or progressively higher doses of medications; and require special evaluation and interventions.*[1,2]

- Include client and SO(s) in limiting or removing attention for pain behavior, when appropriate (e.g., discussing pain for only a specified time; or acknowledging "I'm sorry your pain returned today, but you need to go to school"; or actively practicing relaxation or coping skills). *Limits focusing on pain, especially if client is highly dependent on pain for secondary gain issues, or is addicted to medications.*[9]

 • Discuss the physiologic dynamics of tension/anxiety and how this affects the pain. *Increasing muscle tension/anxiety can escalate pain and reduce effectiveness of therapeutic interventions.*

 • Encourage client to use positive affirmations: "I am healing." "I am relaxed." "I love this life." Have client be aware of internal-external dialogue. Say "cancel" when negative thoughts develop. *Negative thinking can exacerbate feelings of hopelessness and replacing those thoughts with positive ones can be helpful to pain management.*[12]

• Use tranquilizers, narcotics, and analgesics sparingly. *These drugs are physically and psychologically addicting and promote sleep disturbances, especially interference with deep REM—rapid eye movement—sleep. Client may need to be detoxified if many medications are currently used.*

 • Encourage right-brain stimulation with activities such as love, laughter, and music. *These actions can release endorphins, enhancing sense of well-being.*[12]

 • Encourage use of subliminal tapes *to bypass logical part of the brain by reinforcing: "I am becoming a more relaxed person." "It is all right for me to relax."*

 • Assist family to develop an individualized approach for dealing with client's pain behavior. *Positive reinforcement, encouraging client to use own control, and diminishing attention given to pain behavior can aid in refocusing energies on more productive activities.*

 • Be alert to changes in pain *that may indicate a new physical problem/developing complication.*

NURSING PRIORITY NO. 4. To promote wellness (Teaching/Discharge Considerations):

 • Address client's preferences and wishes for incurable pain or end-of-life pain management via advance directives *in order to assist family/SO in attending to client's needs.*[10]

 • Incorporate folk healthcare practices and beliefs into care whenever possible. *Has been shown to increase compliance with pain management treatment plan.*[11]

 • Provide client/SO education and encouragement regarding client's individual painful condition and management plan *to promote hope, as well as maximize participation in efforts for reduction of pain and optimal level of function.*

 • Assist client and SO(s) *to learn how to heal by developing sense of internal control, by being responsible for own treatment, and by obtaining the information and tools to accomplish this.*

• Discuss potential for developmental delays in child with chronic pain. Identify current level of function *to establish a baseline and determine appropriate expectations for individual child.*

• Teach client/SO medication administration, including use of PCA pumps, as indicated. Review safe use of medications, side effects requiring home management (e.g., constipation) or medical evaluation (e.g., possible drug reactions). *Appropriate instruction in home management increases the accuracy and safety of medication administration.*[12]

 • Assist client to learn to change pain behavior. *Focusing on wellness behavior (e.g., "Act as if you are well and pain-free") enhances sense of control and refocuses attention away from pain."*[12]

 • Encourage and assist family member/SO(s) to learn home care interventions. *Massage and other nonpharmacologic pain management techniques benefit the client through reduction of pain level and sense that client is not alone/has support of SO.*

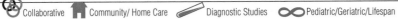 Cultural   Collaborative   Community/Home Care   Diagnostic Studies   Pediatric/Geriatric/Lifespan   Medications

- Recommend that client and SO(s) take time for themselves. *Provides opportunity to re-energize and refocus on tasks at hand.*
- Identify and discuss potential hazards of unproved and/or nonmedical therapies/remedies. *While some remedies may be harmless or even helpful for some individuals, others may have the potential for injury, negate therapeutic effect of prescribed therapies, or waste the client's money.*
- Identify community support groups/resources to meet individual needs (e.g., yard care, home maintenance, alternative transportation). *Proper use of resources may reduce negative pattern of "overdoing" heavy activities, then spending several days in bed recuperating.*
- Refer for counseling and/or marital therapy, Parent Effectiveness classes, and so forth as needed. *Presence of chronic pain affects all relationship/family dynamics.*[12]
- Refer to NDs ineffective Coping, compromised family Coping.

DOCUMENTATION FOCUS

Assessment/Reassessment

Individual findings, including duration of problem/specific contributing factors, previously/currently used interventions.

Perception of pain, effects on lifestyle, and expectations of therapeutic regimen.

Family's/SO's response to client, and support for change.

Planning

- Plan of care and who is involved in planning.
- Teaching plan.

Implementation/Evaluation

- Responses to interventions/teaching and actions performed.
- Attainment/progress toward desired outcome(s).
- Modifications to plan of care.

Discharge Planning

- Long-term needs and who is responsible for actions to be taken.
- Specific referrals made.

References

1. Farkas H. (2002). Chronic pain. Available at: http://www.emedicine.com. Accessed December 2003.
2. Singh, M. K., Patel, J., & Gallagher, R. M. (2002). Chronic pain syndrome. Available at: http://www.emedicine.com. Accessed September 2003.
3. Purnell, L. D., & Paulanka, B. J. (1998). Transcultural Health Care: A Culturally Competent Approach. Philadelphia: F. A. Davis, p 44.
4. Young, D. (1999). Acute pain management. Iowa City, IA: University of Iowa Gerontological Nursing Interventions Research Center. Research Dissemination Core.
5. McGuire, L. (1999). Pain management in older adults. In Stanley, M., & Beare, P. G. Gerontological Nursing: A Health Promotion/Prevention Approach, ed 2. Philadelphia: F. A. Davis.
6. The management of persistent pain in older persons. (2002). J Am Geriatr Soc, 50(6 Suppl):S205–24. Available at: http://www.guideline.gov. Accessed September 2003.
7. Bienenfeld, D. (2003). Malingering. Available at: http://www.emedicine.com. Accessed January 2004.
8. Smith, G. R., Rost, K., & Kashner, T. M. (1995). A trial of the effect of a standardized psychiatric consultation on health outcomes and costs in somatizing patients. Arch Gen Psychiatry, 52(3), 238–243.
9. Spratt, E. G., & DeMaso, D. (2002). Somatoform disorder: Somatization. Available at: http://www.emedicine.com. Accessed January 2004.

10. American Medical Directors Association (AMDA). (1999). Chronic pain management in the long-term care setting. Available at: http://www.guideline.gov. Accessed September 2003.
11. Juarez, G., Ferrell, B., & Borneman, T. (1998). Influence of culture on cancer pain management in Hispanic clients. Cancer Practice, 6(5), 262–269.
12. McCaffrey, M., & Pasero, C. (1999). Pain: Clinical Manual. St. Louis: Mosby.

impaired Parenting

Definition: Inability of the primary caretaker to create, maintain, or regain an environment that promotes the optimum growth and development of the child (Note: It is important to reaffirm that adjustment to parenting in general is a normal maturational process that elicits nursing behaviors to prevent potential problems and to promote health.)

RELATED FACTORS

Social
Presence of stress (e.g., financial, legal, recent crisis, cultural move [e.g., from another country/cultural group within same country]); unemployment or job problems; financial difficulties; relocations; poor home environments
Lack of family cohesiveness; marital conflict, declining satisfaction; change in family unit
Role strain or overload; single parents; father of child not involved
Unplanned or unwanted pregnancy; lack of, or poor, parental role model; low self-esteem
Low socioeconomic class; poverty; lack of resources, access to resources, social support networks, transportation
Inadequate child-care arrangements; lack of value of parenthood; inability to put child's needs before own
Poor problem-solving skills; maladaptive coping strategies
Social isolation
History of being abusive/being abused; legal difficulties

Knowledge
Lack of knowledge about child health maintenance, parenting skills, child development; inability to recognize and act on infant cues
Unrealistic expectation for self, infant, partner
Low educational level or attainment; limited cognitive functioning; lack of cognitive readiness for parenthood
Poor communication skills
Preference for physical punishment

Physiologic
Physical illness

Infant or child
Premature birth; multiple births; unplanned or unwanted child; not gender desired
Illness; prolonged separation from parent/separation at birth
Difficult temperament; lack of goodness of fit (temperament) with parental expectations
Handicapping condition or developmental delay; altered perceptual abilities; attention-deficit hyperactivity disorder

 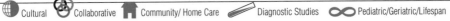

Psychologic

Young age, especially adolescent

Lack of, or late, prenatal care; difficult labor and/or delivery; multiple births; high number or closely spaced pregnancies

Sleep deprivation or disruption; depression

Separation from infant/child

History of substance abuse or dependencies

Disability; history of mental illness

DEFINING CHARACTERISTICS

Subjective

Parental

Statements of inability to meet child's needs; cannot control child

Negative statements about child

Verbalization of role inadequacy frustration

Objective

Infant or Child

Frequent accidents/illness; failure to thrive

Poor academic performance/cognitive development

Poor social competence; behavioral disorders

Incidence of physical and psychological trauma or abuse

Lack of attachment; separation anxiety

Runaway

Parental

Maternal-child interaction deficit; poor parent-child interaction; little cuddling; insecure or lack of attachment to infant

Inadequate child health maintenance; unsafe home environment; inappropriate child-care arrangements; inappropriate visual, tactile, auditory stimulation

Poor or inappropriate caretaking skills; inconsistent care/behavior management

Inflexibility to meet needs of child, situation

High punitiveness; rejection or hostility to child; child abuse; child neglect; abandonment

SAMPLE CLINICAL APPLICATIONS: prematurity, multiple births, genetic/congenital defects, chronic illness (parent/child), substance abuse, physical/psychological abuse, major depression, developmental delay, schizophrenia

DESIRED OUTCOMES/EVALUATION CRITERIA

Sample **NOC** linkages:

Role Performance: Congruence of an individual's role behavior with role expectations

Parenting: Provision of an environment that promotes optimum growth and development of dependent children

Child Development: [specify age group]: Milestones of physical, cognitive, and psychosocial progression by [specify] months/years of age

Parent Will (Include Specific Time Frame)

- Verbalize realistic information and expectations of parenting role.
- Verbalize acceptance of the individual situation.

- Identify own strengths, individual needs, and methods/resources to meet them.
- Demonstrate appropriate attachment/parenting behaviors.

ACTIONS/INTERVENTIONS

Sample **NIC** linkages:

Parenting Promotion: Providing parenting information, support, and coordination of comprehensive services to high-risk families

Family Integrity Promotion: Promotion of family cohesion and unity

Developmental Enhancement: Child/Adolescent: Facilitating or teaching parents/caregivers to facilitate the optimal gross motor, fine motor, language, cognitive, social, and emotional growth of preschool and school-age children. Facilitating optimal physical, cognitive, social, and emotional growth of individuals during the transition from childhood to adulthood

NURSING PRIORITY NO. **1.** To assess causative/contributing factors:

- Note family constellation; two-parent, single, extended family, or child living with other relative such as grandparent. *Helps identify problem areas/strengths to formulate plans to change situation that is currently creating problems for the parents.*[3]
- Review type, severity, duration of problem and contribution of, as well as impact on, individual family members. *Affects choice of interventions. When abuse is the problem, it is an act of commission, whereas neglect is considered an act of omission. These behaviors indicate the presence of problems with relationships and/or parenting skills and individual problems such as inability to deal with stressors, substance abuse, mental illness, cognitive limitations or criminality.*[1]
- Determine developmental stage of the family (e.g., new child, adolescent, child leaving/returning home). *Affects individual situation and provides direction for interventions after problem(s) are identified.*[1]
- Assess family relationships/boundaries and identify needs of individual members. *These factors are critical to understanding individual family dynamics and developing strategies for change.*[3]
- Report and take necessary actions as legally/professionally indicated if child's safety is a concern.. *Safety of child is paramount and needs to be dealt with immediately.*[5]
- Assess parenting skill level, taking into account the individual's intellectual, emotional, and physical strengths and weaknesses. *Parents with significant impairments may need more education/assistance. Ineffective parenting and unrealistic expectations contribute to problems of abuse and neglect. Understanding normal responses, progression of developmental milestones can help parents understand and cope with changes.*[1]
- Observe attachment behaviors between parental figure and child, recognizing cultural background. (Refer to ND risk for impaired parent/infant/child Attachment.) *Lack of eye contact and touching may indicate bonding problems. Failure to bond effectively is thought to affect subsequent parent-child interaction. Behaviors such as eye-to-eye contact, use of en face position, talking to the infant in a high-pitched voice are indicative of attachment behaviors in American culture but may not be appropriate in another culture.*[1,4]
- Note presence of factors in the child, e.g., birth defects, hyperactivity, which may be related to difficulties of parenting. *Unanticipated needs of the child may affect attachment and care-taking needs. Parents have an ideal of what is expected in a child and when circumstances dictate otherwise they may experience feelings of sadness and anger.*[1]Refer to dysfunctional Grieving.
- Evaluate physical challenges/limitations. *Might affect the parent's ability to care for a child*

 Cultural Collaborative 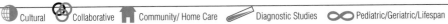 Community/ Home Care Diagnostic Studies Pediatric/Geriatric/Lifespan Medications *(e.g., visual/hearing impairment, quadriplegia, severe depression, mental illness) and indicated need for additional planning to assist the parents.*[1]

- Determine presence/effectiveness of support systems, role models, extended family, and community resources available to the parent(s). *Lack of/ineffective use of support systems increase risk of recidivism and continued inability to parent effectively.*[5]
- Note absence from home setting/lack of child supervision by parent. *Demands of working long hours/out of town, multiple responsibilities such as working and attending educational classes will affect relationship between parent and child and ability to provide the care and nurturing necessary for children to grow and prosper.*[7]

NURSING PRIORITY NO. 2. To foster development of parenting skills:

- Create an environment in which relationships can be developed and needs of each individual met. *Learning is more effective when individuals feel safe and free to express feelings and concerns without fear of judgment.*[6,7]
- Make time for listening to concerns of the parent(s). *Listening conveys respect and acceptance, enabling parent(s) to openly discuss needs and desires regarding the illness/situation and future plans.*[2]
- Emphasize positive aspects of the situation. *Maintaining a hopeful attitude toward the parent's capabilities and potential for improving the situation will help them to manage what is happening more effectively.*[1]
- Note staff attitudes toward parent/child and specific problem/disability. *The needs of disabled parent(s) to be seen as an individual and evaluated apart from a stereotype are crucial to helping individual to cope with difficult situation. Negative attitudes are detrimental to promoting positive outcomes.*[3]
- Encourage expression of feelings, such as helplessness, anger, frustration. Set limits on unacceptable behaviors. *When feelings are expressed openly, they can be acknowledged and dealt with, enabling parent(s) to move forward in dealing with illness/situation. Individual may express anger by acting-out behaviors which need to be restrained before damage is done to self, self-esteem, others or environment.*[5,6]
- Acknowledge difficulty of situation and normalcy of feelings. *Individuals feel validated when difficulty is recognized, enhancing feelings of acceptance.*[1]
- Recognize stages of grieving process when the child is disabled or other than anticipated. *Expectation of a "normal"/desired child (for instance, having a girl instead of boy, child with a misshapen head/prominent birthmark, or birth defect such as cleft palate) results in grieving for the loss of that expectation.*[1]
- Allow time for parents to express feelings and deal with the "loss." *Each person grieves at own pace and allowing this time facilitates the process.*[8]
- Encourage attendance at skill classes, such as Parent Effectiveness. *Helps parents to develop communication and problem-solving techniques that promote positive relationships between parent and child.*[6,7]
- Emphasize parenting functions rather than mothering/fathering skills. *By virtue of gender, each person brings something to the parenting role; however, nurturing tasks can be done by both parents.*[1]

NURSING PRIORITY NO. 3. To promote wellness (Teaching/Discharge Considerations):

- Involve all available members of the family in learning. *Promotes understanding and effective communication when each individual has the same information and is able to ask questions and clarify what has been heard.*[5]

• Provide information appropriate to the situation, including time management, limit setting, and stress-reduction techniques. *Facilitates satisfactory implementation of plan/new behaviors.*[5]

 • Develop support systems appropriate to the situation. *Extended family, friends, social worker, home care services may be needed to help parents cope positively with what is happening.*[3]

 • Assist parent to plan time and conserve energy in positive ways. *Enables individual to cope effectively with difficulties as they arise.*[3]

 • Encourage parents to identify positive outlets for meeting their own needs. *Going out for dinner, making time for their own interests and each other/dating promotes general well-being, helps reduce burnout.*[3]

 • Refer to appropriate support/therapy groups as indicated. *Underlying issues may interfere with adaptation to situation and additional support may help individuals to deal more effectively with them.*[5]

 • Identify community resources (e.g., child-care services). *Will assist with individual needs to provide respite and support.*[3]

• Refer to NDs such as ineffective Coping, compromised family Coping, risk for Violence [specify], Self-Esteem [specify], interrupted Family Processes.

DOCUMENTATION FOCUS

Assessment/Reassessment
• Individual findings, including parenting skill level, deviations from normal parenting expectations, family makeup and developmental stages.
• Availability/use of support systems and community resources.

Planning
• Plan of care and who is involved in planning.
• Teaching plan.

Implementation/Evaluation
• Parent(s')/child's responses to interventions/teaching and actions performed.
• Attainment/progress toward desired outcome(s).
• Modification to plan of care.

Discharge Planning
• Long-range needs and who is responsible for actions to be taken.
• Specific referrals made.

References

1. Townsend, M. C. (2003). Psychiatric Mental Health Nursing Concepts of Care, ed 4. Philadelphia: F. A. Davis.
2. Gordon, T. (2000). Parent Effectiveness Training, (updated ed). New York: Three Rivers Press.
3. Cox, H. C., et al. (2002). Clinical Applications of Nursing Diagnosis: Adult, Child, Women's, Psychiatric, Gerontic, and Home Health Considerations, ed 4. Philadelphia: F. A. Davis.
4. Lipson, J. G., Dibble, S. L., & Minarik, P. A. (1996). Culture & Nursing Care: A Pocket Guide. San Francisco: UCSF Nursing Press.
5. Doenges, M. E., Townsend, M. C., & Moorhouse, M. F. (1998). Psychiatric Care Plans Guidelines for Individualizing Care, ed 3. Philadelphia: F. A. Davis.
6. Gordon, T. (1989). Teaching Children Self-discipline: At Home and At School. New York: Random House.
7. Gordon, T. (2000). Family Effectiveness Training Video. Solana Beach, CA: Gordon Training Intnl.
8. Neeld, E. H. (1997). Seven Choices, ed 3. Austin, TX: Centerpoint Press.

 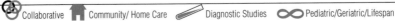

risk for impaired Parenting

Definition: Risk for inability of the primary caretaker to create, maintain, or regain an environment that promotes the optimum growth and development of the child. (Note: It is important to reaffirm that adjustment to parenting in general is a normal maturational process that elicits nursing behaviors to prevent potential problems and to promote health.)

RISK FACTORS

Lack of role identity; lack of available role model, ineffective role model

Social

Stress [e.g., financial, legal, recent crisis, cultural move (e.g., from another country/cultural group within same country)]; unemployment or job problems; financial difficulties; relocations; poor home environments

Lack of family cohesiveness; marital conflict, declining satisfaction; change in family unit

Role strain/overload; single parents; father of child not involved

Unplanned or unwanted pregnancy; lack of, or poor, parental role model; low self-esteem

Low socioeconomic class; poverty; lack of: [resources], access to resources, social support networks, transportation

Inadequate child-care arrangements; lack of value of parenthood; inability to put child's needs before own

Poor problem-solving skills; maladaptive coping strategies

Social isolation

History of being abusive/being abused; legal difficulties

Knowledge

Lack of knowledge about child health maintenance, parenting skills, child development; inability to recognize and act on infant cues

Unrealistic expectation of child

Low educational level or attainment; low cognitive functioning; lack of cognitive readiness for parenthood

Poor communication skills

Preference for physical punishment

Physiologic

Physical illness

Infant or Child

Premature birth; multiple births; unplanned or unwanted child; not gender desired

Illness; prolonged separation from parent/separation at birth

Difficult temperament; lack of goodness of fit (temperament) with parental expectations

Handicapping condition or developmental delay; altered perceptual abilities; attention-deficit hyperactivity disorder

Psychological

Young age, especially adolescent

Lack of, or late, prenatal care; difficult labor and/or delivery; multiple births; high number or closely spaced pregnancies

Sleep deprivation or disruption; depression

Separation from infant/child

History of substance abuse or dependencies

Disability; history of mental illness

NOTE: A risk diagnosis is not evidenced by signs and symptoms, as the problem has not occurred and nursing interventions are directed at prevention.

SAMPLE CLINICAL APPLICATIONS: prematurity, multiple births, genetic/congenital defects, chronic illness (parent/child), substance abuse, physical/psychological abuse, major depression, developmental delay, schizophrenia

DESIRED OUTCOMES/EVALUATION CRITERIA

Sample **NOC** linkages:

Parenting: Provision of an environment that promotes optimum growth and development of dependent children

Role Performance: Congruence of an individual's role behavior with role expectations

Social Support: Perceived availability and actual provision of reliable assistance from other persons

Client Will (Include Specific Time Frame)

- Verbalize awareness of individual risk factors.
- Identify own strengths, individual needs, and methods/resources to meet them.
- Demonstrate behavior/lifestyle changes to reduce potential for development of problem or reduce/eliminate effects of risk factors.
- Participate in activities, classes to promote growth.

ACTIONS/INTERVENTIONS AND DOCUMENTATION FOCUS

- Refer to impaired Parenting or risk for impaired parent/infant/child Attachment

Readiness For Enhanced Parenting

Definition: A pattern of providing an environment for children or other dependent person(s) that is sufficient to nurture growth and development and can be strengthened

RELATED FACTORS

To be developed by nurse researchers and submitted to NANDA

DEFINING CHARACTERISTICS

Subjective

Expresses willingness to enhance parenting

Children or other dependent person(s) express satisfaction with home environment

Objective

Emotional and tacit support of children or dependent person(s) is evident; bonding or attachment evident

Physical and emotional needs of children/dependent person(s) are met

Realistic expectations of children/dependent person(s) exhibited

SAMPLE CLINICAL APPLICATIONS: as a health-seeking behavior the client/family may be healthy or this diagnosis can be associated with any clinical condition

 Cultural   Collaborative  Community/ Home Care  Diagnostic Studies 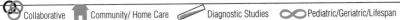 Pediatric/Geriatric/Lifespan   Medications

Sample **NOC** linkages:

Parenting: Provision of an environment that promotes optimum growth and development of dependent children

Parent-Infant Attachment: Behaviors which demonstrate an enduring affectionate bond between a parent and infant

Parenting: Social Safety: Parental actions to avoid social relationships that might cause harm or injury

Client Will (Include Specific Time Frame)
Verbalize realistic information and expectations of parenting role.
Identify own strengths, individual needs, and methods/resources to meet them.
Demonstrate appropriate attachment/parenting behaviors.

ACTIONS/INTERVENTIONS

Sample **NIC** linkages:

Parent Education: Childrearing Family: Assisting parents to understand and promote the physical, psychological, and social growth and development of their toddler, preschool, or school-age child/children

Parent Education: Infant: Instruction on nurturing and physical care needed during the first year of life

Parenting Promotion: Providing parenting information, support, and coordination of comprehensive services to high-risk families

NURSING PRIORITY NO. 1. To determine need/motivation for improvement:

- Note family constellation: two-parent, single, extended family, or child living with other relative, such as grandparent. *Understanding make-up of the family provides information about needs to assist them in improving their family connections.*[1]
- Determine developmental stage of the family (e.g., new child, adolescent, child leaving/returning home, retirement). *These maturational crises bring changes in the family that can provide opportunity for enhancing parenting skills and improving family interactions.*[1]
- Assess family relationships and identify needs of individual members, noting any special concerns that exist, such as birth defects, illness, hyperactivity. *The family is a system and when members make decisions to improve parenting skills, the changes affect all parts of the system. Identifying needs, special situations, and relationships can help to develop plans to bring about effective change.*[1]
- Assess parenting skill level, taking into account the individual's intellectual, emotional, and physical strengths and weaknesses. *Identifies areas of need for education, skill training, and information on which to base plan for enhancing parenting skills.*[2]
- Observe attachment behaviors between parent(s) and child(ren), recognizing cultural background, which may influence expected behaviors. *Behaviors such as eye-to-eye contact, use of enface position, talking to infant in high-pitched voice are indicative of attachment behaviors in American culture but may not be appropriate in another culture. Failure to bond is thought to affect subsequent parent-child interactions.*[3]
- Determine presence/effectiveness of support systems, role models, extended family, and community resources available to the parent(s). *Parents desiring to enhance abilities and improve family life can benefit by role models that help them strengthen own style of parenting.*[3]
- Note cultural/religious influences on parenting, expectations of self/child, sense of success

or failure. *Expectations may vary with different cultures, such as Arab Americans hold children to be sacred but childrearing is based on negative rather than positive reinforcements and parents are more strict with girls than boys. These beliefs may interfere with desire to improve parenting skills when there is conflict between the two.*[3,4]

NURSING PRIORITY NO. 2. To foster development of parenting skills:

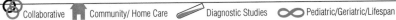 • Create an environment in which relationships can be developed and needs of each individual family member can be met. *A safe environment in which individuals can freely express their thoughts and feelings optimizes learning and positive interactions among family members enhancing relationships.*[2,5]

 • Make time for listening to concerns of the parent(s). *Promotes sense of importance and of being heard and identifies accurate information regarding needs of the family for enhancing relationships.*[2]

 • Encourage expression of feelings, such as helplessness, anger while setting limits on unacceptable behaviors. *Identification of feelings promotes understanding of self and enhances connections with others in the family. Unacceptable behaviors result in feelings of anger and diminished self-esteem and can lead to problems in the family relationships.*[3]

 • Emphasize parenting functions rather than mothering/fathering skills. *By virtue of gender, each person brings something to the parenting role; however, nurturing tasks can be done by both parents, enhancing family relationships.*[5]

 • Encourage attendance at skill classes, such as Parent Effectiveness Training. *Assists in developing communication skills of Active-listening, I-messages, and problem-solving techniques to improve family relationships and promote a win-win environment.*[2]

NURSING PRIORITY NO. 3. To promote optimum parenting skills:

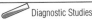 • Involve all members of the family in learning. *The family system benefits from all members participating in learning new skills to enhance family relationships.*[1]

• Encourage parents to identify positive outlets for meeting their own needs. *Activities such as going out for dinner, making time for their own interests and each other/dating promotes general well-being, enhances family relationships and improves family functioning.*[2]

• Provide information as indicated, including time management, stress-reduction techniques. *Learning about positive parenting skills, understanding growth and developmental expectations, and ways to reduce stress and anxiety promotes individual's ability to deal with problems that may arise in the course of family relationships.*[1]

• Discuss current "family rules," identifying areas of needed change. *Rules may be imposed by adults, rather than through a democratic process, involving all family members, leading to conflict and angry confrontations. Setting positive family rules with all family members participating can promote an effective, functional family.*[2]

• Discuss need for long-term planning and ways in which family can maintain desired positive relationships. *Each stage of life brings its own challenges, and understanding and preparing for each one enables family members to move through them in positive ways, promoting family unity and resolving inevitable conflicts with win-win solutions.*[6]

DOCUMENTATION FOCUS

Assessment/Reassessment
• Individual findings, including parenting skill level, parenting expectations, family makeup and developmental stages.
• Availability/use of support systems and community resources.

🌐 Cultural ☸ Collaborative 🏠 Community/ Home Care Diagnostic Studies ∞ Pediatric/Geriatric/Lifespan Medications

Planning
- Plan for enhancement, who is involved in planning.

Implementation/Evaluation
- Family members' responses to interventions/teaching and actions performed.
- Attainment/progress toward desired outcome(s).
- Modifications to plan.

Discharge Planning
- Long-range needs and who is responsible for actions to be taken.
- Modification to plan.

References
1. Townsend, M. C. (2003). Psychiatric Mental Health Nursing Concepts of Care, ed 4. Philadelphia: F. A. Davis.
2. Gordon, T. (2000). Parent Effectiveness Training (updated). New York: Three Rivers Press.
3. Doenges, M. E., Townsend, M. C., & Moorhouse, M. F. (1998). Psychiatric Care Plans Guidelines for Individualizing Care, ed 3. Philadelphia: F. A. Davis.
4. Lipson, J. G., Dibble, S. L. & Minarik, P. A. (1996). Culture & Nursing Care: A Pocket Guide. San Francisco: UCSF Nursing Press.
5. Doenges, M. E., Moorhouse, M. F., & Geissler-Murr, A. C. (2004). Nurses' Pocket Guide, Diagnoses, Interventions, and Rationales, ed 9. Philadelphia: F. A. Davis.
6. Gordon, T. (1989). Teaching Children Self-Discipline, At Home and At School. New York: Random House.

risk for Peripheral Neurovascular Dysfunction

Definition: At risk for disruption in circulation, sensation, or motion of an extremity

RISK FACTORS
Fractures
Mechanical compression (e.g., tourniquet, cast, brace, dressing, or restraint)
Orthopedic surgery; trauma
Immobilization
Burns
Vascular obstruction
NOTE: A risk diagnosis is not evidenced by signs and symptoms, as the problem has not occurred and nursing interventions are directed at prevention.
SAMPLE CLINICAL APPLICATIONS: atherosclerosis, traumatic injuries, burns, orthopedic surgery, Buerger's disease, Raynaud's disease, diabetes mellitus

DESIRED OUTCOMES/EVALUATION CRITERIA
Sample **NOC** linkages:
Tissue Perfusion: Peripheral: Extent to which blood flows through the small vessels of the extremities and maintains tissue function
Risk Detection: Activities taken to identify personal health threats
Risk Control: Actions to eliminate or reduce actual, personal, and modifiable health threats

Client Will (Include Specific Time Frame)
- Maintain function as evidenced by sensation/movement within normal range for the individual.

- Identify individual risk factors.
- Demonstrate/participate in behaviors and activities to prevent complications.
- Relate signs/symptoms that require medical reevaluation.

ACTIONS/INTERVENTIONS

Sample **NIC** linkages:

Peripheral Sensation Management: Prevention or minimization of injury or discomfort in the patient with altered sensation

Circulatory Care: Arterial/Venous Insufficiency: Promotion of arterial/venous circulation

NURSING PRIORITY NO. 1. To determine significance/degree of potential for compromise:

- Assess for individual risk factors: 1) trauma to extremity(ies) that cause internal tissue damage such as high-velocity and penetrating trauma; fractures (especially long-bone fractures) with hemorrhage; or external pressures from burn eschar; 2) immobility (e.g., long-term bedrest, tight dressings, splints or casting); 3) presence of conditions affecting peripheral circulation, such as atherosclerosis, Buerger's disease, Raynaud's disease, or diabetes mellitus; 4) women older than age 60; 5) smoking; 6); obese and sedentary individuals; 7) high levels of homocysteine and cholesterol; 8) use of anticoagulants; and 9) vigorous exercise *that potentiates risk of circulation insufficiency and occlusion.*[1–3]
- Note presence and degree (1+-4+ scale) of peripheral edema. Evaluate entire length of injured extremity. Measure both affected and unaffected extremity and compare *to determine degree of impairment and establish baseline to monitor improvement or progression of condition.*
- Monitor for tissue bleeding, and spread of hematoma formation *that can compress blood vessels and raise compartment pressures.*[1,2]
- Note position/location of casts, braces, and traction apparatus *to ascertain potential for pressure on tissues.*
- Assess skin for signs of ulceration *as can occur when circulation is impaired.*
- Review recent/current drug regimen, noting use of anticoagulants and vasoactive agents.

NURSING PRIORITY NO. 2. To prevent deterioration/maximize circulation of affected limb(s):

- Perform neurovascular assessments in person immobilized for any reason (e.g., surgery, prolonged bedrest, diabetic neuropathy, fractures) or individuals with suspected neurovascular problems, always noting differences in affected limb as compared with unaffected limb. Use five Ps of assessment[4]:

  NOTE: Some literature sources warn that the 5 Ps are not diagnostic of compartment syndrome, and that with the exception of pain and paresthesia, these traditional signs are not reliable (e.g., the 5 Ps assume a conscious patient, and not a young child).[2]

  1. Pain: Using 0–10 (or similar pain scale), assess for presence, location, severity, and duration of pain. *Pain may be intermittent (e.g., intermittent claudication) or more constant (e.g., compartment syndrome or arterial occlusion). Pain may range from muscle tension/tenderness and burning, to severe pain (out of proportion to chief complaint). Pain may be present with exertion, with passive movement, or at rest.*[2,5]
  2. Pulses: Monitor presence and quality of peripheral pulses (distal to injury or impairment) via palpation and/or Doppler. *Intact pulse usually indicates adequate circulation.*

 Cultural Collaborative Community/ Home Care 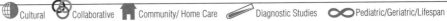 Diagnostic Studies Pediatric/Geriatric/Lifespan Medications

However, occasionally a pulse may be palpated even though circulation is blocked by a soft clot; or perfusion through larger arteries may continue after increased compartment pressure has collapsed the arteriole/venule circulation in the muscle.[1,2,5]

3. Pallor: Evaluate skin temperature, capillary refill and color changes *to assess perfusion. Pallor with shiny, taut skin and slow venous refill is indicative of circulatory impairment. Cold, pale, bluish color with purpura indicates arterial insufficiency.*[6]
4. Paresthesia: Assess sensation. *Changes may include feelings of tingling, numbness, "pins and needles" or diminished or absence of sensation. Note: Sensation may be normal early (in the presence of compartmental syndrome), because superficial circulation is usually not compromised.*[2]
5. Paralysis: Evaluate for range of motion below injury. *Movement may be limited or absent because of tissue edema and nerve compression.*[2]

- Prevent/limit potential for complications[1–3,5,6]:

(Refer to ND ineffective peripheral Tissue Perfusion for additional interventions.)

Position all extremities in proper alignment *to maximize circulation and maintain position of function.*

Provide nutritional support (with adequate calories and micronutrients) and fluids *to promote healing and reduce sluggishness of circulation, as indicated.*

Remove jewelry from affected limb *to limit injury caused by pressure on/edema of tissues.*

Elevate injured extremity(ies) to limit swelling unless contraindicated by confirmed presence of compartment syndrome *where elevation can actually impede arterial flow, decreasing perfusion.*

Apply ice bags around injury/fracture site as indicated *to limit tissue swelling/hematoma formation.*

Limit/avoid use of restraints. Use padding, and evaluate extremity circulation, movement and sensation frequently, when restraints are required.

Monitor corrective devices (e.g., cast, splint, traction equipment) frequently *for proper application and function.* Use repositioning/padding *to relieve pressure.*

Split/bivalve cast, reposition traction/restraints as appropriate *to release pressure/prevent permanent tissue damage.*

Inspect skin/tissues around cast edges and traction devices *for pressure points.* Investigate reports of "burning sensation" under cast.

Observe position/location of supporting ring of splints/sling. Readjust as indicated.

Provide/assist with range of motion exercises to all joints. Encourage client to routinely exercise digits/joints distal to injury *to enhance circulation.*

Assist with/encourage early ambulation *to help prevent thrombophlebitis formation.*

Evaluate bedfast client frequently for calf tenderness, redness, swelling, (or less frequently) pain on dorsiflexion of foot (positive Homans' sign).

 Apply antiembolic hose/sequential pressure device as indicated.

Use bed cradle to keep linens off affected extremity.

Provide pressure reduction devices for heels, toes and other bony prominences.

 Recommend/refer for professional nail and foot care.

Monitor Hgb/Hct, coagulation studies (e.g., prothrombin time) if either clotting or bleeding into tissues is known or suspected, or client is receiving anticoagulant therapy.

Administer IV fluids, blood products as needed *to maintain circulating volume and reduce potential for irreversible tissue injury associated with loss of perfusion.*

 Administer anticoagulants as indicated *for thrombotic vascular obstructions.*

- Investigate sudden changes (e.g., decreased skin temperature, pallor, reports of pain that are extreme for type of injury, increased pain at rest/on passive movement of extremity, development of burning/tingling sensations, muscle tension/tenderness with erythema, change in pulse quality distal to injury) *that are suggestive of compartment syndrome.*

- Place limb in neutral position, avoiding elevation *to maximize circulation.*
 • Report symptoms to physician at once *to provide for timely evaluation and intervention.*
- Assist with diagnostic studies (e.g., ultrasound, angiography/arteriography or measurements of ankle-brachial ratio, segmental arterial pressures, or intracompartmental pressures), as indicated. *Confirms diagnosis of circulatory occlusion (s)/evaluates effectiveness of therapeutic interventions.*[1,2,5–7]
 • Prepare for surgical intervention/other therapies (e.g., fibulectomy, fasciotomy, bypass surgery, hyperbaric oxygen therapy) as indicated *to relieve increasing pressure/restore circulation.*

NURSING PRIORITY NO. 3. To promote wellness (Teaching/Discharge Considerations)[1–3,5,6]:

- Instruct client/family in performance and reporting of neurovascular findings, when indicated (e.g., client with new fractures at home in cast, client at risk for DVT, etc.) *to limit preventable complications through early intervention.*
- Review proper body alignment of limbs (e.g., elevated, dependent or neutral), as appropriate for client's individual situation.
- Promote benefits of walking and smoking cessation *to improve circulation.*
- Discuss necessity of avoiding constrictive clothing, sharp angulation of legs, crossing legs, and thermal/chemical/mechanical trauma especially if client has known diabetes or at risk for DVT or peripheral vascular insufficiency.
- Demonstrate proper application and removal of antiembolic hose.
- Review safe use of heat/cold therapy as indicated, especially if client has poor sensation in extremities *to avoid thermal injury.*
- Instruct client/SO(s) in use of properly fitting footwear, and to wear clean, wrinkle-free socks *to reduce risk of skin breakdown on feet.*
- Demonstrate/recommend continuation of prescribed exercise program *to maintain function and circulation of limbs.*
- Recommend regular follow-up with healthcare provider to monitor status of condition, provide for timely intervention.

DOCUMENTATION FOCUS

Assessment/Reassessment
- Specific risk factors, nature of injury to limb.
- Assessment findings, including comparison of affected/unaffected limb, characteristics of pain in involved area.

Planning
- Plan of care and who is involved in the planning.
- Teaching plan.

Implementation/Evaluation
- Response to interventions/teaching and actions performed.
- Attainment/progress toward desired outcome(s).
- Modification of plan of care.

 Cultural Collaborative Community/ Home Care Diagnostic Studies Pediatric/Geriatric/Lifespan Medications

Discharge Planning
- Long-term needs, referrals and who is responsible for actions to be taken.
- Specific referrals made.

References

1. Fort, C. W. (2003). How to combat 3 deadly trauma complications. Nursing, 33(5), 58–63.
2. Paula, R. (2002). Compartment syndrome, extremity. Available at: http://www.emedicine.com. Accessed January 2004.
3. Peripheral vascular disease. Public information sheet. Available at: http://ivillagehealth.com. Accessed January 2004.
4. Ackley, B. J. (2002). ND Risk for peripheral neurovascular dysfunction. In Ackley, B. J., & Ladwig, G. B. Nursing Diagnosis Handbook: A Guide to Planning Care, ed 5. St. Louis: Mosby.
5. Peripheral Arterial Occlusive Disease. Fact sheet for Family Practice notebook.com, a Family Medicine Resource. Available at: http://www.fpnotebook.com. Accessed January 2004.
6. Guideline for management of wounds in patients with lower-extremity arterial disease. (2002). Wound Ostomy and Continence Nurses Society (WOCN), Clinical practice guideline series; No 1. Available at: http://www.guideline.gov. Accessed September 2003.
7. Carrington, A. L., et al. (2001). Peripheral vascular and nerve function associated with lower limb amputation in people with and without diabetes. Clin Sci, 101, 261–266.

risk for Poisoning

Definition: At accentuated risk of accidental exposure to or ingestion of drugs or dangerous products in doses sufficient to cause poisoning [or the adverse effects of prescribed medication/drug use]

RISK FACTORS

Internal (individual)
Reduced vision

Lack of safety or drug education

Lack of proper precaution; [unsafe habits, disregard for safety measures, lack of supervision]

Insufficient finances

Verbalization of occupational setting without adequate safeguards

Cognitive or emotional difficulties; [behavioral]

[Age (e.g., young child, elderly person)]

[Chronic disease state, disability]

[Cultural or religious beliefs/practices]

External (environmental)
Large supplies of drugs in house

Medicines stored in unlocked cabinets accessible to children or confused persons

Availability of illicit drugs potentially contaminated by poisonous additives

Flaking, peeling paint or plaster in presence of young children

Dangerous products placed or stored within the reach of children or confused persons

Unprotected contact with heavy metals or chemicals

Paint, lacquer, and so forth in poorly ventilated areas or without effective protection

Chemical contamination of food and water

Presence of poisonous vegetation

Presence of atmospheric pollutants, [proximity to industrial chemicals/pattern of prevailing winds]

[Therapeutic margin of safety of specific drugs (e.g., therapeutic versus toxic level, half-life, method of uptake and degradation in body, adequacy of organ function)]

[Use of multiple herbal supplements or megadosing]

NOTE: A risk diagnosis is not evidenced by signs and symptoms, as the problem has not occurred and nursing interventions are directed at prevention.

SAMPLE CLINICAL APPLICATIONS: dementia, cataracts/glaucoma, substance abuse, depression, developmental delay

DESIRED OUTCOMES/EVALUATION CRITERIA

Sample **NOC** linkages:

Risk Control: Drug Use: Actions to eliminate or reduce drug use that poses a threat to health

Knowledge: Medication: Extent of understanding conveyed about the safe use of medication

Safety Behavior: Home Physical Environment: Individual or caregiver actions to minimize environmental factors that might cause physical harm or injury in the home

---

Client/SO Will (Include Specific Time Frame)

- Verbalize understanding of dangers of poisoning.
- Identify hazards that could lead to accidental poisoning.
- Correct environmental hazards as identified.
- Demonstrate necessary actions/lifestyle changes to promote safe environment.

ACTIONS/INTERVENTIONS

Sample **NIC** linkages:

Environmental Management: Safety: Manipulation of the patient's surroundings for therapeutic benefit

Medication Management: Facilitation of safe and effective use of prescription and over-the-counter drugs

Surveillance: Safety: Purposeful and ongoing collection and analysis of information about the patient and the environment for use in promoting and maintaining patient safety

NURSING PRIORITY NO. 1. To assess causative/contributing factors:

 • Determine presence of internal/external risk factors in client's environment. *Deaths from poisoning are most commonly from drugs, medicines, gases and vapors, mushrooms and shellfish, as well as commonly recognized poisons (e.g., lead, mercury, arsenic, cleaning products and pesticides).*[1]

 • Determine client's allergies (e.g., medications, bee stings, foods) in order *to avoid exposure to substances causing potentially lethal reactions, or to provide preventative measures (e.g., client carries an epinephrine injector/inhaler).*

 • Note age and cognitive status of client and careproviders *to identify individuals that could be at higher risk for accidental poisoning. Babies, toddlers and preschoolers are at risk because they are curious, like to put things into their mouths, and aren't aware of what's safe to eat. While school age child can recognize danger and is at lower risk of unintentional poisoning, child is at risk for inadvertent overdose when taking medications without adequate supervision. The adolescent is at higher risk of suicide attempts (with overdose of medications, and/or from*

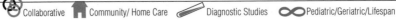

illicit drug overdose/adverse reactions or alcohol toxicity), due to natural inclination to take risks, peer pressure, and easy access to drugs. Infants, children and unborn babies are more vulnerable than healthy adults to other poisons, too (e.g., carbon monoxide [CO] due to their higher metabolic rates and oxygen requirements).[2–4] Elderly persons are at risk because of the higher number of prescription and OTC medications they consume, and because of visual and cognitive impairments, which can cause them to forget what medications have been consumed and in what amounts they are taken. Elderly persons are also likely to share medications. Also the presence of nutritional deficits and renal or hepatic degeneration can reduce ability to detoxify drugs.[5,6]

- Ascertain client's use of medications. *Some individuals (especially elderly) believe that medication offers the solution to every health problem, a belief bolstered by frequent television, radio and written advertising promising relief from a multitude of conditions from colds to sexual vitality. This often leads to multiple drug use (polypharmacy) and contributes to potential for overdose, adverse reactions (e.g., digitalis toxicity) and drug interactions.[5]*

- Evaluate client's/SO's knowledge/beliefs about poisoning *to determine baseline knowledge and potential for exposure.* Poison is anything that kills or injures through its chemical actions. Poisons come in four different forms (e.g., solids, liquids, sprays, and invisible vapors) and can enter the body through 1) ingestion, 2) inhalation, 3) absorption through the skin/mucous membranes/eye, and 4) via IV injection.[7,8]

- Identify drug hazards:
  Alcohol and other drugs. *These substances have potential for adverse reactions, and intentional and accidental overdose. Alcohol is found in many products (e.g., perfumes, aftershave, cough medications, mouthwash, flavoring extracts.) Note: As little as 1 ounce of alcohol can cause serious injury in a small child.[9]*
  Prescription, OTC medications and culturally-based home remedies. *These have potential for intentional and accidental overdose, as well as dangerous interactions. Drugs that are therapeutic in small doses may be deadly when taken in excess (e.g., beta-blockers, warfarin, digitalis). One of the most common problems is inadvertent overdosage of acetaminophen (Tylenol), either by increased dosing or by taking it with a combination product, also containing acetaminophen. In children, the most serious accidental poisonings occur with iron, methadone, and tricyclic antidepressants.[1,6,8]*
  Vitamins, mineral and herbal supplements. *Vitamins (especially A and D) are toxic in large doses and iron is especially harmful to children.[8] Herbal drugs can be a source of poisoning (usually when taken chronically), due to toxicity of individual ingredients or from contaminants (e.g., mercury, lead and arsenic).[1]*

- Look for environmental hazards:
  Household products (e.g., oven, toilet bowel or drain cleaners; fertilizers, rust remover; dishwasher products, bleach, hydrogen peroxide, essential oils, button batteries, fluoride preparations, antifreeze; furniture polish, lighter fluid, lamp oil, kerosene; paints, lubricant oils, turpentine; bug sprays and powders) *are readily available toxins in various forms that are often improperly stored.[1,7,8]*
  Gases (e.g., car exhaust fumes, gasoline/oil/wood/propane burning fumes [carbon monoxide], methane, radon). *Persons most at risk for carbon monoxide poisoning are those with heart/lung disease or anemia, infants and children (due to higher metabolic rates), elderly persons, and pregnant women.[1,4,6,10]*
  Foods/water (e.g., wild mushrooms, berries; food that has not been properly handled/stored; water contaminated by agricultural or industrial activities).[1,8]
  Heavy metals (lead and mercury). *Lead can be ingested or inhaled from multiple sources (e.g., paint chips; stained glass, welding, industrial machinery/equipment, battery manufac-*

turing/repair; construction sites; hazardous waste sites).[1,11] *Mercury is usually ingested via contaminated fish and seafood, but is also an environmental pollutant (e.g., emissions from plants burning fossil fuels or incinerated medical waste, and groundwater contamination).*[12]

 ● Review results of laboratory tests/toxicology screening as indicated. *Guides treatment when overdose or accidental poisoning is known or suspected.*

NURSING PRIORITY NO. 2. To assist in correcting factors that can lead to accidental poisoning:

 ● Determine use of prescribed medications, OTC medications and drugs (e.g., alcohol, marijuana, heroin) *to provide opportunity to discuss potential for client's/SO's accidental overdose, or accidental ingestion by children when drugs/drug paraphernalia are in the home, or when medications are carelessly stored.*

 ● Evaluate client/family risk for lead or mercury (other heavy metal) and refer for further evaluation/screening tests (e.g., public health, physician office). *Assessment of exposure risk and blood level testing are important preventative/corrective measures.*[13]

● Discuss poison prevention measures[4,5,7–10,12,14]:

Teach children about hazards of poisonous substances. Teach them to "ask first" before eating or drinking anything.

Use safety caps, labels, and/or lockup cabinets for all medicines, cleaning products, paint/solvents, and other toxic substances.

Don't leave child alone with household products or medications. *Many accidental poisonings occur when parent steps away for a moment and child gets into product that parent left out.*

Store foods separately from household chemicals. *Containers often look similar.*

Store cleaning solutions and other household/garage chemicals in original container/avoid pouring into drinking glasses or bottles. *Child may take a drink, thinking it is juice/soda. Also products are clearly labeled as to ingredients and safety needs if ingestion does occur. (This information is important for Poison Control Center to direct emergency care.)*

Do not mix different chemical products (e.g., bleach and ammonia) *that can create poisonous gases.*

Administer children's medications as drugs, not candy. *Prevent confusion for child.*

Recap medication containers immediately after obtaining current dosage. *Open containers increase risk of accidental ingestion.*

Stress importance of supervising infant/child or individuals with cognitive limitations.

Note: Children visiting elderly may be exposed to medications without child safety caps or medication boxes left on counter top.

Code medicines for the visually impaired.

Turn on light and put on glasses (if visually impaired) before taking or giving medications.

Do not share medications with anyone else, or take medications prescribed for another person.

Have responsible SO(s)/home health nurse supervise medication regimen/prepare medications for the cognitively or visually impaired, or obtain prefilled medication box from pharmacy.

Wear protective clothing and eye gear when using pesticides and other spray chemicals. Avoid areas that have recently been sprayed. *These chemicals are absorbed easily through skin and can be very poisonous.*

Discard outdated and unused products/drugs safely (disposing in hazardous waste collection areas, not down drain/toilet).

 Cultural   Collaborative   Community/ Home Care  Diagnostic Studies 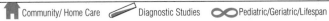 Pediatric/Geriatric/Lifespan   Medications

Monitor air quality in house. Place carbon monoxide and smoke detectors near bedrooms, and radon detectors in basement if indicated.

Have all fuel-burning appliances (e.g., gas, wood) professionally installed and annually inspected. Clean fireplace chimneys yearly.

Check house for, and remove, lead-based paint if living in an older home (built before 1950) or flaking plaster.

- Examine yard/remove plants for potentially harmful or poisonous (e.g., mushrooms, flowers, shrubs) *that can be ingested by children.*

- Refer identified health/safety violations to the appropriate resource (e.g., health department, Occupational Safety and Health Administration—OSHA) when workplace exposures are suspected.

NURSING PRIORITY NO. 3. To promote wellness (Teaching/Discharge Considerations)[4,5,7–10,12,14]:

- Institute community programs *to assist individuals to identify and correct risk factors in own environment.*

- Review proper food storage/canning techniques and appropriate preparation and serving *to reduce risk of food poisoning (e.g., salmonella,* Escherichia coli, *botulism).*

- Instruct family: in the event of poisoning, look for container and contact professional help. Keep list of emergency numbers (e.g., local or 1–800 Poison Control, EMS, physician, pharmacist, nurse) on or by telephone.

- Instruct in first aid measures or ascertain that client/SO has access to written literature *when potential exists for accidents/trauma.*

- Encourage emergency measures, awareness and education (e.g., CPR/first aid class, community safety programs, and ways to access emergency medical personnel).

- Instruct family to not try to induce vomiting if ingestion is suspected, and dispose of Ipecac if on hand. *Induced vomiting is unpleasant and can make things worse. Until recently, the American Academy of Pediatrics (AAP) advised parents to keep Ipecac syrup on hand at home in the event that a doctor/poison control center advised its use to induce vomiting. The AAP changed this recommendation in 2003 after concluding that Ipecac increases the risk of aspiration and is inadequate for removing poisons from the body.*[10]

- Review drug side effects/potential interactions with client/ SO(s). Discuss use of OTC drugs/herbal supplements and possibilities of misuse, drug interactions, and overdosing (e.g., vitamin or acetaminophen megadosing, etc). Avoid mixing alcohol with medications *(potentiates effects of many drugs).*

- Refer substance abuser to detoxification programs, inpatient/outpatient rehabilitation, counseling, support groups, and psychotherapy.

- Teach client/SO risk of injury to fetus when pregnant woman engages in substance abuse or is exposed to toxins (e.g., carbon monoxide, mercury).[11,12]

- Educate client to outdoor hazards, both locally and vacation sites (e.g., vegetation [poison ivy], insects [bees.] air pollutants). Encourage susceptible person to carry kit with a prefilled syringe of epinephrine and an epinephrine nebulizer *for immediate use when necessary.*

- Encourage periodic inspection of household well water/tap water *to identify possible contaminants.*

- Review community sources of possible water contamination (e.g., sewage disposal, agricultural/industrial runoff).

- Review pertinent job-related health department/OSHA regulations.

- Refer to resources that provide information about air quality (e.g., pollen index, "bad air days") *to promote informed decision making/limit exposure.*

- Refer for therapy/counseling as indicated *when individual is depressed and expressing suicidal ideation.*

DOCUMENTATION FOCUS

Assessment/Reassessment
- Identified risk factors noting internal/external concerns.

Planning
- Plan of care and who is involved in the planning.
- Teaching plan.

Implementation/Evaluation
- Response to interventions/teaching and actions performed.
- Attainment/progress toward desired outcome(s).
- Modification to plan of care.

Discharge Planning
- Long-term needs and who is responsible for actions to be taken.
- Specific referrals made.

References

1. What's your poison? Available at: http://www.dotpharmacy.co.uk/uppoison.html. Accessed January 2004.
2. Poisoning risk factors. (1997). Information sheet from Centers for Disease Control and Prevention, "What Affects a Child's Risk of Poisoning?" Adapted from recommendations in Injury Prevention and Injury Control for Children and Youth. Atlanta, GA: Committee on Injury and Poison Prevention of the American Academy of Pediatrics.
3. Barela, T. (2001). What affects a child's risk of poisoning? TORCH magazine. Available at: http://www.randolph.af.mil/se2/torch. Accessed September 2003.
4. Children are at greater risk for CO poisoning: Know how to protect your family. Available at: http://www.kidsource.com. Accessed September 2003.
5. Stoehr, G. P. (1999). Pharmacology and older adults: The problem of polypharmacy. In Stanley, M., & Beare, P. G. (eds): Gerontological Nursing: A Health Promotion/Protection Approach, ed 2. Philadelphia: F. A. Davis, pp 66–73.
6. Older adults are at risk for poisoning exposures. (2002). News release from Illinois Poison Control Center. Available at: http://www.mchc.org. Accessed September 2003.
7. Nathan, M. S. (2001). Poison proofing your home. Available at: http://www.emedicine.com. Accessed January 2004.
8. Cohen, J. S. Poisoning. Available at: http://www.emedince.com. Accessed January 2004.
9. Is my child at risk for poisoning during the holidays? (2003). Information sheet. Available at: http://www.phoenixchildrens.com. Accessed September 2003.
10. Keep your children safe: Prevent accidental poisoning. Available at: http://www.cnn.com/HEALTH/library. Accessed January 2004.
11. Lead Poisoning Risk Factors. (2001). Information sheet. Available at: http://www.keepkidshealthy.com. Accessed September 2003.
12. Fetuses at risk of mercury poisoning. (2000). Fact sheet for United Press. Available at: http://www.apples-forhealth.com. Accessed September 2003.
13. U.S. Department of Health and Human Services, U.S. Public Health Service. (1994). Put prevention into practice lead screening in children. J Am Acad Nurs Pract, 6, 379.
14. ND: Poisoning, risk for. In Doenges, M. E., Moorhouse, M. F., & Geissler-Murr, A. C. (2004). Nurse's Pocket Guide: Diagnoses, Interventions, and Rationales, ed 9. Philadelphia: F. A. Davis.

 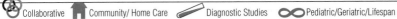

Post-Trauma Syndrome [specify stage]

Definition: Sustained maladaptive response to a traumatic, overwhelming event

RELATED FACTORS

Events outside the range of usual human experience

Serious threat or injury to self or loved ones; serious accidents; industrial and motor vehicle accidents

Physical and psychosocial abuse; rape

Witnessing mutilation, violent death, or other horrors; tragic occurrence involving multiple deaths

Natural and/or manmade disasters; sudden destruction of one's home or community; epidemics

Wars; military combat; being held prisoner of war or criminal victimization (torture)

DEFINING CHARACTERISTICS

Subjective

Intrusive thoughts/dreams; nightmares; flashbacks

Palpitations; headaches [loss of interest in usual activities, loss of feeling of intimacy/sexuality]

Hopelessness; shame

[Excessive verbalization of the traumatic event, verbalization of survival guilt or guilt about behavior required for survival]

Gastric irritability [changes in appetite; sleep disturbance/insomnia; chronic fatigue/easy fatigability]

Objective

Anxiety; fear

Hypervigilant; exaggerated startle response; neurosensory irritability; irritability

Grief; guilt

Difficulty in concentrating; depression

Anger and/or rage; aggression

Avoidance; repression; alienation; denial; detachment; psychogenic amnesia; numbing

Altered mood states; [poor impulse control/irritability and explosiveness]; panic attacks; horror

Substance abuse; compulsive behavior

Enuresis (in children)

[Difficulty with interpersonal relationships; dependence on others; work/school failure]

[Stages:

ACUTE SUBTYPE: Begins within 6 months and does not last longer than 6 months.

CHRONIC SUBTYPE: Lasts more than 6 months.

DELAYED SUBTYPE: Period of latency of 6 months or more before onset of symptoms.]

SAMPLE CLINICAL APPLICATIONS: traumatic injuries, physical/psychological abuse, dissociative disorder

DESIRED OUTCOMES/EVALUATION CRITERIA

Sample **NOC** linkages:

Fear Control: Personal actions to eliminate or reduce disabling feelings of alarm aroused by an identifiable source

Abuse Protection: Protection of self or dependent others from abuse

Abuse Recovery: [specify Emotional or Sexual]: Healing of psychologic injuries due to abuse/Healing following sexual abuse or exploitation

---

Client Will (Include Specific Time Frame)
- Express own feelings/reactions, avoiding projection.
- Verbalize a positive self-image.
- Report reduced anxiety/fear when memories occur.
- Demonstrate ability to deal with emotional reactions in an individually appropriate manner.
- Demonstrate appropriate changes in behavior/lifestyle (e.g., share experiences with others, seek/get support from SO(s) as needed, change in job/residence).
- Report absence of physical manifestations (such as pain, chronic fatigue).
- Refer to ND Rape-Trauma Syndrome for additional outcomes when trauma is the result of rape.

ACTIONS/INTERVENTIONS

Sample **NIC** linkages:

Support System Enhancement: Facilitation of support to patient by family, friends, and community

Counseling: Use of an interactive helping process focusing on the needs, problems, or feelings of the patient and significant others to enhance or support coping, problem-solving, and interpersonal relationships

Anxiety Reduction: Minimizing apprehension, dread, foreboding, or uneasiness related to an unidentified source or anticipated danger

NURSING PRIORITY NO. **1.** To assess causative factor(s) and individual reaction:

Acute phase
- Observe for/elicit information about physical or psychological injury and note associated stress-related symptoms such as "numbness," headache, tightness in chest, nausea, pounding heart, and so forth. *Anxiety is viewed as a normal reaction to a realistic danger or threat and noting these factors can identify the severity of the anxiety the client is experiencing in the circumstances.*[4]
- Identify psychological responses: anger, shock, acute anxiety, confusion, denial. Note laughter, crying; calm or agitated, excited (hysterical) behavior; expressions of disbelief and/or self-blame, lability of emotional changes. *Indicators of severe response to trauma that client has experienced and need for specific interventions.*[9]
- Assess client's knowledge of and anxiety related to the situation. Note ongoing threat to self, e.g., contact with perpetrator and/or associates, and/or perception of others as threatening. *Client may be aware but speak as though the incident related to someone else. Flashbacks may occur with the individual reliving the incident/event.*[9]
- Note occupation (e.g., police, fire, emergency department, etc.), as listed in Risk Factors. *These occupations carry a high risk for constantly being involved in traumatic events and the potential for exacerbation of stress response/block to recovery.*[1]
- Identify social aspects of trauma/incident. *May have been injured during incident/event with resultant disfigurement, chronic conditions/permanent disabilities which affect ability to return to normal involvement in activities/work.*[9]

 Cultural 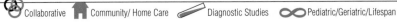 Collaborative   Community/ Home Care Diagnostic Studies Pediatric/Geriatric/Lifespan   Medications

- Ascertain ethnic background/cultural and religious perceptions and beliefs about the occurrence. *Client may believe occurrence is retribution from God, or result of some indiscretion on his or her part, or in some way blame themselves for the incident/occurrence. Individual's view of how he or she is coping may be influenced by cultural background, religious beliefs and family influence.*[5,9]
- Determine degree of disorganization. *Presence of persistent frightening thoughts and memories, reliving the event, feeling emotionally numb and unable to be close to friends and family members, sleep and eating problems interfere with ability to manage daily living, work and relationships with others.*[9]
- Identify whether incident has reactivated preexisting or coexisting situations (physical/psychological). *Traumas or difficulties in client's life and how they were dealt with will affect how the client views the current trauma.*[7]
- Determine disruptions in relationships (e.g., family, friends, coworkers, SOs). *Support persons may not know how to deal with client/situation and may be oversolicitous or withdraw and either of these actions will be counterproductive to client's ability to cope with situation.*[9]
- Note withdrawn behavior, use of denial, and use of chemical substances or impulsive behaviors (e.g., chain-smoking, overeating). *Indicators of severity of anxiety and client's difficulty dealing with post-traumatic stress disorder (PTSD) and need for interventions to address these behaviors.*[9]
- Be aware of signs of increasing anxiety (e.g., silence, stuttering, inability to sit still). *Increasing anxiety may indicate risk for violence, need for medication or other measures to decrease anxiety and help client manage feelings.*[9]
- Note verbal/nonverbal expressions of guilt or self-blame when client has survived trauma in which others died. *Sense of own responsibility (blame) and guilt about not having done something to prevent incident or not having been "good enough" to deserve surviving are strong beliefs, especially in individuals who are influenced by background, religious and cultural factors.*[2]
- Assess signs/stage of grieving for self and others. *Identification and understanding of stages of grief assist with choice of interventions, planning of care, and movement toward resolution.*[2]
- Identify development of phobic reactions to ordinary articles (e.g., knives); situations (e.g., walking in groups of people, strangers ringing doorbell). *These may trigger feelings from original trauma and need to be dealt with sensitively, accepting reality of feelings and stressing ability of client to deal with them.*[2]

Chronic phase (in addition to previous assessment)
- Evaluate continued somatic complaints. Investigate reports of new/changes in symptoms. *Reports of physical symptoms, such as gastric irritation, anorexia, insomnia, muscle tension, headache may accompany disorganization and need further evaluation and interventions.*[2]
- Note manifestations of chronic pain or pain symptoms in excess of degree of physical injury. *Psychological responses may magnify/exacerbate physical symptoms, indicating need for interventions to help client deal with pain.*[7]
- Be aware of signs of severe/prolonged depression; note presence of flashbacks, intrusive memories, and/or nightmares and stay with client during these episodes. *May calm fears and assure client that he or she is not "going crazy" but that these symptoms are not uncommon following a trauma of such magnitude.*[4]
- Assess degree of dysfunctional coping (including substance use/abuse) and consequences. *Identifies needs/depth of interventions required. Individuals display different levels of dysfunctional behavior in response to stress and often the choice of chemical substances/substance abuse is a way of deadening the psychic pain.*[2]

NURSING PRIORITY NO. 2. To assist client to deal with situation that exists:

Acute phase

- Provide a calm, safe environment. *Promotes sense of trust and safety and can help client maintain control when anxiety is at a panic level.*[12]
- Assist with documentation for police report, as indicated, and stay with the client. *Developing accurate chain of evidence (maintaining sequencing and collection of evidence), labeling each specimen and storing/packaging it properly provides important evidence for possibility of future prosecution.*[2]
- Listen to/investigate physical complaints. *Physical injuries may have occurred during incident/panic of recurrence, which may be masked by emotional reactions and limit client's ability to recognize them. These need to be identified and differentiated from anxiety symptoms so appropriate treatment may be instituted.*[2]
- Identify supportive persons for this individual. *Having unconditional support from loving/caring others can help the client cope with the situation, and move on to live more fully.*[2]
- Remain with client, listen as client recounts incident/concerns—possibly repeatedly. If client does not want to talk, accept silence. *Establishes trust providing psychological support and allowing client opportunity to vent emotions.*[4]
- Provide nonthreatening, consistent environment in which client can talk freely about feelings, fear (including concerns about relationship with/response of SO), and experiences/sensations (e.g., loss of control, "near-death experience"). *Minimizes stimuli, reducing anxiety and calming individual, helping to break the cycle of anxiety/fear and encouraging them to express feelings and relive event.*[2]
- ∞ Help child to express feelings about event using techniques appropriate to developmental level (e.g., play for young child, stories/puppets for preschooler, peer group for adolescent). *Children are more likely to express in play what they may not be able to verbalize directly. Adolescents may benefit from groups, gaining knowledge, support, decreased sense of isolation and improved coping skills.*[3]
- Assist with practical realities (e.g., temporary housing, money, notifications of family members, or other needs). *Dealing with these issues is necessary and helps client remain connected to reality and maintain sense of control over daily living concerns.*[2]
- Be aware of and assist client to use ego strengths in a positive way by acknowledging ability to handle what is happening. *Enhances self-concept, reduces sense of helplessness and powerlessness, enabling client to move on with life.*[3]
- Allow the client to work through own kind of adjustment. If the client is withdrawn or unwilling to talk, do not force the issue. *Each person is an individual and has own ways of coping. Being there, and allowing client to choose own path conveys sense of confidence in ability to deal with situation.*[10]
- Listen for expressions of fear of crowds and/or people. *May indicate continuing anxiety and difficulty re-entering normal activities.*[9]
- Encourage learning stress-management techniques, such as deep breathing, meditation, relaxation, exercise. *Reduces stress, enhancing coping skills and helping to resolve situation.*[11]
- 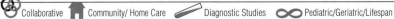 Identify employment, community resource groups. *Provides opportunity for ongoing support to deal with recurrent stressors as individual moves on with life.*[12]

Chronic phase

- Continue listening to expressions of concern. *May have recurring symptoms and need to continue to talk about the incident.*[9]
- Permit free expression of feelings (may continue from the crisis phase). Do not rush client

 Cultural   Collaborative   Community/ Home Care   Diagnostic Studies   ∞ Pediatric/Geriatric/Lifespan   Medications through expressions of feelings too quickly and do not reassure inappropriately. *Client may believe pain and/or anguish is misunderstood and may be depressed. Statements such as "You don't understand" or "You weren't there" are a defense, a way of pushing others away and need to be responded to with empathy and concern.*[10]

- Encourage client to talk out experience, expressing feelings of fear, anger, loss/grief. (Refer to ND dysfunctional Grieving). *Client may need to repeat story over and over and needs to be accepted and assured that feelings are normal for the unusual event that has been experienced.*[9]
- Note whether feelings expressed appear congruent with events the client experienced. *Expressing feelings helps client recognize and identify them to enhance coping. Incongruency may indicate deeper conflict and can impede resolution.*[11]
- Ascertain/monitor sleep pattern of children as well as adults. *Sleep disturbances/nightmares may develop, delaying resolution, impairing coping abilities and interferring with return to desired lifstyle.*[7]
- Encourage client to become aware and accepting of own feelings and reactions when they are identified. *There are no "bad" feelings and awareness and acceptance enables client to deal with feelings once identified and move forward in recovery from traumatic event.*[6]
- Acknowledge reality of loss of self which existed before the incident. Assist client to move toward an acceptance of the potential for growth that exists within client. *Recognition that individual can never go back to being the person he or she was before the incident allows progress toward life as a different person.*[11]
- Continue to allow client to progress at own pace. *Taking own time to talk about what has happened, allowing feelings to be fully expressed, aids in the healing process. If rushed, client may believe he or she is not accepted or understood.*[2]
- Give "permission" to express/deal with anger at the assailant/situation in acceptable ways. *Being free to express anger appropriately allows it to be dissipated so underlying feelings can be identified and dealt with, strengthening coping skills.*[2]
- Keep discussion on practical and emotional level rather than intellectualizing the experience. *When feelings (the experience) are intellectualized, uncomfortable insights and/or awareness are avoided by the use of rationalization, blocking resolution of feelings and impairing coping abilities.*[2]
- Assist in dealing with practical concerns and effects of the incident, such as court appearances, altered relationships with SO(s), employment problems. *In the period immediately following the traumatic incident, individual is in a state of numbness and shock. Thinking becomes difficult and assistance with practical matters will help manage necessary activities for the person to move through this time.*[10]
- Provide for sensitive, trained counselors/therapists and engage in therapies such as psychotherapy in conjunction with medications, Implosive Therapy (flooding), hypnosis, relaxation, Rolfing, memory work, cognitive restructuring, Eye Movement Desensitization and Reprocessing (EMDR), physical and occupational therapies. *Although it is not necessary for the helping person to have experienced the same kind of trauma as the client's, sensitivity and listening skills are important to helping the client confront fears and learn new ways to cope with what has happened. Therapeutic use of desensitization techniques (flooding, implosive therapy) provides for extinction through exposure to the fear. Body work can alleviate muscle tension. Some techniques (Rolfing) help to bring blocked emotions to awareness as sensations of the traumatic event are reexperienced.*[9]
- Discuss use of medication (e.g., antidepressants). *May be used to decrease anxiety, lift mood, aid in management of behavior, and ensure rest until client regains control of own self. Lithium may be used to reduce explosiveness; low-dose psychotropics may be used when loss of contact with reality is a problem.*[8]

NURSING PRIORITY NO. 3. To promote wellness (Teaching/Discharge Considerations):

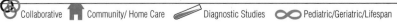 • Assist client to identify and monitor feelings while therapy is occurring. *Promotes awareness and helps client know that control of feelings as they arise will help move beyond traumatic episode.*[9]

 • Provide information about what reactions client may expect during each phase. Let client know these are common reactions. Be sure to phrase in neutral terms of "You may or you may not...." *Knowledge of what may be experienced helps reduce fear of the unknown, enabling client to manage reactions if they occur. Use of neutral terms lets client understand that not all reactions may occur in own situation.*[3]

 • Assist client to identify factors that may have created a vulnerable situation and that he or she may have power to change to protect self in the future. *While client is not responsible for event, may have unknowingly contributed to occurrence by their actions. Identifying those actions that are within their power to change provides sense of control over seemingly uncontrollable situations.*[9]

 • Avoid making value judgments. *Client may be judging self and caregiver needs to convey nonjudgmental stance to allow individual to deal with feelings of guilt and recrimination, accepting fact that he or she did the best they were capable of in the circumstances.*[3]

 • Discuss lifestyle changes client is contemplating and how they may contribute to recovery. *Client needs to evaluate appropriateness of plans and look at long-range consequences to make the best choice for the future.*[4]

 • Assist with learning stress-management techniques. *Deep breathing, counting to 10, reviewing the situation, reframing skills assist client in developing constructive ways to cope with feelings of powerlessness and to regain control of self. Reframing stressors/situation in other words or positive ideas can help client recognize and consider alternatives.*[4]

 • Discuss recognition of and ways to manage "anniversary reactions," letting client know normalcy of recurrence of thoughts and feelings at this time. *Understanding that these feelings are to be expected and planning for them helps client get through the anniversary of the event with the least difficulty.*[10]

• Suggest support group for SO(s). *Family members may not understand client's reactions and need help with understanding them and learning how to deal with client in the most helpful manner.*[2]

• Encourage psychiatric consultation. *May need additional therapy if client is unable to maintain control, is violent, inconsolable, or does not seem to be making an adjustment. Participation in a group may be helpful.*[2]

• Refer for family/marital counseling if indicated. *Additional/ongoing support and/or therapy may be needed to help family resolve family crisis and look at potential for growth. Client problems affect others in family/relationships, and further counseling may help resolve issues of enabling behavior/communication problems.*[12]

• Refer to NDs Powerlessness; ineffective Coping, anticipatory/dysfunctional Grieving.

DOCUMENTATION FOCUS

Assessment/Reassessment
• Individual findings, noting current dysfunction and behavioral/emotional responses to the incident.
• Specifics of traumatic event.
• Reactions of family/SO(s).

Cultural   Collaborative   Community/ Home Care   Diagnostic Studies   Pediatric/Geriatric/Lifespan   Medications

Planning

- Plan of care and who is involved in the planning.
- Teaching plan.

Implementation/Evaluation

- Responses to interventions/teaching and actions performed.
- Emotional changes.
- Attainment/progress toward desired outcome(s).
- Modifications to plan of care.

DischargePlanning

- Long-term needs and who is responsible for actions to be taken.
- Specific referrals made.

References

1. Doenges, M., Moorhouse, M., & Geissler-Murr, A. (2002). Nursing Care Plans, Guidelines for Individualizing Patient Care, ed 6. Philadelphia: F. A. Davis.
2. Doenges, M., Townsend, M., & Moorhouse, M. (1998). Psychiatric Care Plans: Guidelines for Individualizing Care, ed 3. Philadelphia: F. A. Davis.
3. Cox, H., et al. (2002). Clinical Applications of Nursing Diagnoses, ed 4. Philadelphia: F. A. Davis.
4. Townsend, M. (2003). Psychiatric Mental Health Nursing: Concepts of Care, ed 4. Philadelphia: F. A. Davis.
5. Lipson, J. G., Dibble, S. L., & Minarik, P. A. (1996). Culture & Nursing Care: A Pocket Guide. San Francisco: School of Nursing, UCSF Nursing Press.
6. Stuart, G. W. (2001). Anxiety responses and anxiety disorders. In Stuart, G. W., & Laraia, M. T. (eds): Principles and Practice of Psychiatric Nursing, ed 7. St. Louis: Mosby.
7. Kunert P. K. (2002). Stress and adaptation. In Porth, C. M. (ed): Pathophysiology: Concepts of Altered Health States. Philadelphia: J.B. Lippincott.
8. Townsend, M. (2001). Nursing Diagnoses in Psychiatric Nursing: Care Plans and Psychotropic Medications, ed 5. Philadelphia: F. A. Davis.
9. National Institute of Mental Health (2000). Anxiety Disorders, NIH Publication No. 00–3879. Rockville, MD: author. Available at: www.nimh.nih.gov.anxiety/anxiety.cfm. Accessed December 2003.
10. Harper, N. E. (1997). Seven Choices. Austin, TX: Centerpoint Press.
11. Harvard Mental Health Letter. (June, 1996). Posttraumatic stress disorder – Part I. Boston, MA: Harvard Medical School Health Publications Group.
12. Harvard Mental Health Letter. (July, 1996). Posttraumatic stress disorder – Part II. Boston, MA: Harvard Medical School Health Publications Group.

risk for Post-Trauma Syndrome

Definition: At risk for sustained maladaptive response to a traumatic, overwhelming event

RISK FACTORS

Occupation (e.g., police, fire, rescue, corrections, emergency room staff, mental health worker, [and their family members])

Perception of event; exaggerated sense of responsibility; diminished ego strength

Survivor's role in the event

Inadequate social support; nonsupportive environment; displacement from home

Duration of the event

NOTE: A risk diagnosis is not evidenced by signs and symptoms, as the problem has not occurred and nursing interventions are directed at prevention.

Sᴀᴍᴘʟᴇ Cʟɪɴɪᴄᴀʟ Aᴘᴘʟɪᴄᴀᴛɪᴏɴs: traumatic injuries, physical/psychological abuse, disssociative disorder

DESIRED OUTCOMES/EVALUATION CRITERIA
Sample **NOC** linkages:
Grief Resolution: Adjustment to actual or impending loss
Anxiety Control: Personal actions to eliminate or reduce feelings of apprehension and tension from an unidentifiable source
Social Support: Perceived availability and actual provision of reliable assistance from other persons

---

Client Will (Include Specific Time Frame)
- Be free of severe anxiety.
- Demonstrate ability to deal with emotional reactions in an individually appropriate manner.
- Report absence of physical manifestations (pain, nightmares/flashbacks, fatigue) associated with event.

ACTIONS/INTERVENTIONS
Sample **NIC** linkages:
Crisis Intervention: Use of short-term counseling to help the patient cope with a crisis and resume a state of functioning comparable to or better than the pre-crisis state
Coping Enhancement: Assisting a patient to adapt to perceived stressors, changes, or threats that interfere with meeting life demands and roles
Support System Enhancement: Facilitation of support to patient by family, friends, and community

NURSING PRIORITY NO. 1. To assess contributing factors and individual reaction:

- Note occupation (e.g., police, fire, emergency department, etc.), as listed in Risk Factors. *These occupations carry a high risk for constantly being involved in traumatic events and the potential for PTSD to develop.*[1]
- Assess client's knowledge of and anxiety related to potential or recurring situations. *Having information about these situations enables individuals to think about and plan for eventualities so anxiety can be dealt with in a positive manner.*[7]
- Ascertain ethnic background and cultural/religious perceptions and beliefs about the occurrence. *Client may believe occurrence is retribution from God, or result of some indiscretion on his or her part, or in some way blame themselves for the incident/occurrence. Individual's view of how he or she is coping may be influenced by cultural background, religious beliefs and family influence.*[7]
- Identify how client's experiences may affect current situation. *Individual who has had previous experiences with traumatic events, (i.e., fireman who deals with trauma on a regular basis, or person who has been involved in a trauma herself or himself) may be more susceptible to PTSD and ineffective coping abilities.*[2]
- Listen for comments of taking on responsibility (e.g., "I should have been more careful/gone back to get her"). *Expressing guilt for actions that individual might have taken can lead to ruminations about lack of responsible behavior, leading to anxiety and PTSD.*[9]
- Note verbal/nonverbal expressions of guilt or self-blame when client has survived trauma in which others died. *Sense of own responsibility (blame) and guilt about not having done*

 Cultural Collaborative Community/ Home Care 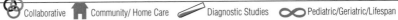 Diagnostic Studies Pediatric/Geriatric/Lifespan 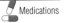 Medications

something to prevent incident or not having been "good enough" to deserve surviving are strong beliefs, especially in individuals who are influenced by background, religious and cultural factors.[2]

- Evaluate for life factors/stressors currently or recently occurring, such as displacement from home due to catastrophic event (e.g., illness/injury, fire/flood/violent storm/earthquake). *Such occurrences can put the individual at risk for developing PTSD and indicates need for preventive measures to be taken.*[4]

- Identify client's coping mechanisms. *Resolution of the posttrauma response is largely dependent on the coping skills the client has developed throughout own life and is able to bring to bear on current situation.*[4]

- Determine availability/usefulness of client's support systems, family, social, community, and so forth. (Note: Family members can also be at risk.) *Having an effective available support system and talking with them about what is happening can help client and family members resolve feelings and move on with life in a positive manner.*[10]

NURSING PRIORITY NO. 2. To assist client to deal with situation that exists:

- Educate high-risk persons/families about signs/symptoms of post-trauma response, especially if it is likely to occur in their occupation/life. *Debriefing following events can help client recognize own feelings and concerns and take appropriate steps to prevent development of PTSD.*[9]

- Help child to express feelings about event using techniques appropriate to developmental level (e.g., play for young child, stories/puppets for preschooler, peer group for adolescent). *Children are more likely to express in play what they may not be able to verbalize directly. Adolescents may benefit from groups, gaining knowledge, support, decreased sense of isolation and improved coping skills.*[3]

- Identify and discuss client's strengths (e.g., very supportive family, usually copes well with stress, etc.) as well as vulnerabilities (e.g., client tends toward alcohol/other drugs for coping, client has witnessed a murder, etc.). *Knowing one's strengths and weaknesses helps client know what actions to take to cope with and prevent anxiety from becoming overwhelming.*[9]

- Discuss how individual coping mechanisms have worked in past traumatic events. *Awareness of previous successful experiences can help client remember coping skills that can be used in current situation to deal with it in a positive manner.*[4]

- Evaluate client's perceptions of events and personal significance (e.g., policeman/parent investigating death of a child). *Individuals perceive events depending on their previous experiences, cultural and religious background and family of origin and will respond to any given trauma based on these factors. Incidents that touch a person's own life will be more difficult to deal with and may have a deeper effect.*[3]

- Provide emotional and physical presence to strengthen client's coping abilities. *Spending time with the client promotes trust and provides an opportunity for client to review coping mechanisms that have worked in previous situations and think about what will help in the current situation.*[4]

- Encourage expression of feelings. Note whether feelings expressed appear congruent with events the client experienced. *Expressing feelings helps client recognize and identify them to enhance coping. Incongruency may indicate deeper conflict and can impede resolution.*[7]

- Observe for signs and symptoms of stress responses, such as nightmares, reliving an incident, poor appetite, irritability, numbness and crying, family/relationship disruption. *These responses are normal in the early postincident time frame. If prolonged and persistent, the client may be experiencing post-traumatic stress disorder.*[9]

NURSING PRIORITY NO. 3. Promote wellness (Teaching/Discharge Considerations):

● Provide a calm, safe environment. *Client can deal with disruption of life more effectively when surrounded by quiet and by knowing he or she is safe.*[11]

● Encourage client to identify and monitor feelings on an ongoing basis. *Promotes awareness of changes in ability to deal with stressors, allowing prompt intervention when necessary.*[5]

● Encourage learning stress-management techniques, such as deep breathing, meditation, relaxation, exercise. *Reduces stress, enhancing coping skills and helping to resolve situation.*[6]

● Recommend participation in debriefing sessions that may be provided following major events. *Dealing with the stressor promptly may facilitate recovery from event/prevent exacerbation. Debriefing is being used by many organizations who regularly deal with traumatic events to prevent the development of PTSD.*[4]

● Encourage individual to develop a survivor mentality. *People often have it within their means to head off life-threatening situations and even survive the worst when they plan for emergencies and think ahead about ways to survive, such as taking food, water and protective gear on a day hike in case you get lost, fall and break a bone, or in other ways have to spend more time than anticipated.*[11]

● Identify employment, community resource groups. *Provides opportunity for ongoing support to deal with recurrent stressors as individual moves on with life.*[8]

● Refer for individual/family counseling as indicated. *May need additional assistance to prevent continuation of anxiety and the onset of PTSD.*[7]

DOCUMENTATION FOCUS

Assessment/Reassessment
● Identified risk factors noting internal/external concerns.
● Client's perception of event and personal significance.

Planning
● Plan of care and who is involved in the planning.
● Teaching plan.

Implementation/Evaluation
● Response to interventions/teaching and actions performed.
● Attainment/progress toward desired outcome(s).

Discharge Planning
● Long-term needs and who is responsible for actions to be taken.
● Specific referrals made.

References

1. Doenges, M. E., Moorhouse, M .F., & Geissler-Murr, A. C. (2002). Nursing Care Plans, Guidelines for Individualizing Patient Care, ed 6. Philadelphia: F. A. Davis.
2. Doenges, M., Townsend, M., & Moorhouse, M. (1998). Psychiatric Care Plans: Guidelines for Individualizing Care, ed 3. Philadelphia: F. A. Davis.
3. Cox, H., et al. (2002). Clinical Applications of Nursing Diagnoses, ed 4. Philadelphia: F. A. Davis.
4. Townsend, M. (2003). Psychiatric Mental Health Nursing: Concepts of Care, ed 4. Philadelphia: F. A. Davis.
5. Stuart, G. W. (2001). Anxiety responses and anxiety disorders. In Stuart, G. W., & Laraia, M. T. Principles and Practice of Psychiatric Nursing, ed 7. St. Louis: Mosby.

 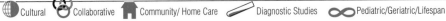

6. Kunert P. K. (2002). Stress and adaptation. In Porth, C. M. (ed): Pathophysiology: Concepts of Altered Health States. Philadelphia: J.B. Lippincott.
7. National Institute of Mental Health. (2000). Anxiety Disorders. NIH Publication No. 02–3879. Rockville, MD: author. Available at: www.nimh.nih.gov.anxiety/anxiety.cfm. Accessed January 2004.
8. Harper, N. E. (1997). Seven Choices, ed 5. Austin, TX: Centerpoint Press.
9. Harvard Mental Health Letter (June, 1996). Posttraumatic stress disorder—Part I. Boston, MA: Harvard Medical School Health Publications Group.
10. Harvard Mental Health Letter (July, 1996). Posttraumatic stress disorder—Part II. Boston, MA: Harvard Medical School Health Publications Group.
11. Kamier, K. (2004). Surviving the Extremes: A Doctor's Journey to the Limits of Human Endurance. Boston: St. Martin's.

Powerlessness [specify level]

Definition: Perception that one's own action will not significantly affect an outcome; a perceived lack of control over a current situation or immediate happening

RELATED FACTORS

Healthcare environment [e.g., loss of privacy, personal possessions, control over therapies]
Interpersonal interaction [e.g., misuse of power, force; abusive relationships]
Illness-related regimen [e.g., chronic/debilitating conditions]
Lifestyle of helplessness [e.g., repeated failures, dependency]

DEFINING CHARACTERISTICS

Subjective

Severe
Verbal expressions of having no control or influence over situation, outcome, or self-care
Depression over physical deterioration that occurs despite client compliance with regimens

Moderate
Expressions of dissatisfaction and frustration over inability to perform previous tasks and/or activities
Expression of doubt regarding role performance
Reluctance to express true feelings; fear of alienation from caregivers

Low
Expressions of uncertainty about fluctuating energy levels

Objective

Severe
Apathy [withdrawal, resignation, crying]
[Anger]

Moderate
Does not monitor progress
Nonparticipation in care or decision making when opportunities are provided
Dependence on others that may result in irritability, resentment, anger, and guilt
Inability to seek information regarding care

Does not defend self-care practices when challenged
Passivity

Low
Passivity

SAMPLE CLINICAL APPLICATIONS: chronic/debilitating conditions (e.g., COPD, MS), cancer, spinal cord injury, major depressive disorder, somatization disorders

DESIRED OUTCOMES/EVALUATION CRITERIA
Sample **NOC** linkages:

Health Beliefs: Perceived Control: Personal conviction that one can influence a health outcome

Participation: Health Care Decisions: Personal involvement in selecting and evaluating healthcare options

Family Participation in Professional Care: Family involvement in decision making, delivery, and evaluation of care provided by healthcare professionals

Client Will (Include Specific Time Frame)
- Express sense of control over the present situation and future outcome.
- Make choices related to and be involved in care.
- Identify areas over which individual has control.
- Acknowledge reality that some areas are beyond individual's control.

ACTIONS/INTERVENTIONS
Sample **NIC** linkages:

Self-Responsibility Facilitation: Encouraging a patient to assume more responsibility for own behavior

Health System Guidance: Facilitating a patient's location and use of appropriate health services

Decision-Making Support: Providing information and support for a person who is making a decision regarding healthcare

NURSING PRIORITY NO. **1.** To assess causative/contributing factors:

 - Identify situational circumstances (e.g., strange environment, immobility, diagnosis of terminal/chronic illness, lack of support system(s), lack of knowledge about situation) affecting the client at this time. *Knowing the specific situation of the client is essential to planning care and empowering the individual.*[4]

 - Determine client's perception/knowledge of condition and treatment plan. *Identifying how client views and understands what is happening and what the plan of care entails is essential to begin to help client feel empowered.*[2]

- Ascertain client response to treatment regimen. Does client see reason(s) for and understand it is in the client's interest or is client compliant and helpless? *The manner in which the individual responds to the treatment indicates the depth of feelings of powerlessness and may interfere with progress.*[4]

- Identify client locus of control and associated cultural factors impacting self-view. Internal control (expressions of responsibility for self and ability to control outcomes— "I didn't quit smoking") or external (expressions of lack of control over self and environment— "Nothing ever works out"; "What bad luck to get lung cancer"). *Locus of control is a term used in reference to an individual's sense of mastery or control over events, and one's culture*

 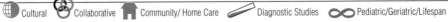

may dictate gender roles and the individual's expectations of control. These beliefs can influence a client's practice of health-related behaviors.[9,11]

- Assess degree of mastery client has exhibited in life. *How this individual has dealt with problems throughout life will help to understand feelings of powerlessness client is feeling during this crisis.*[4,5]
- Determine if there has been a change in relationships with SO(s). *Conflict in relationships may be contributing to sense of powerlessness. Domestic violence situations often leave the individuals involved feeling powerless to change what is happening.*[4]
- Note availability/use of resources. *Client who has few options for assistance or who is not knowledgeable about how to use resources needs to be given information and assistance to know how and where to seek help.*[3]
- Investigate caregiver practices. Do they support client control/responsibility? *Caregivers who do for the client what he or she is able to do for own self diminish sense of control. When client is given as much control as possible over self, sense of power is regained.*[3]

NURSING PRIORITY NO. 2. To assess degree of powerlessness experienced by the client/SO(s):

- Listen to statements client makes: "They don't care"; "It won't make any difference"; "Are you kidding?" *Indicators of sense of powerlessness and hopelessness and need for specific interventions to provide sense of control over what is happening.*[2]
- Note expressions that indicate "giving up," such as "It won't do any good." *May indicate suicidal intent, indicating need for immediate evaluation and intervention.*[6]
- Note behavioral responses (verbal and nonverbal) including expressions of fear, interest or apathy, agitation, withdrawal. *These responses can show depth of anxiety, feelings of powerlessness over what is happening and indicate need for intervention to help client begin to look at situation with some sense of hope.*[6]
- Note lack of communication, flat affect, and lack of eye contact. *May indicate more severe state of mind, such as psychotic episode, and need for immediate evaluation and treatment.*[4]
- Identify the use of manipulative behavior and reactions of client and caregivers. *Manipulation is used for management of powerlessness because of distrust of others, fear of intimacy, search for approval, and validation of sexuality.*[1]

NURSING PRIORITY NO. 3. To assist client to clarify needs relative to ability to meet them:

- Show concern for client as a person. *Communicates value of the individual, enhancing self-esteem.*[8]
- Make time to listen to client's perceptions and concerns and encourage questions. *Provides time for client to explore views and understand what is happening in order to come to some decisions about situation, enhancing sense of control.*[8]
- Accept expressions of feelings, including anger and hopelessness. *Communicates empathy and understanding of reality of those feelings and provides a point of discussion to move toward sense of control.*[4]
- Avoid arguing or using logic with hopeless client. *Client will not accept that anything can make a difference. Arguing denies client's reality and may impede client/nurse relationship.*[2]
- Express hope for the client. *Although client may not accept expressions of hope, there is always hope of something, and when options are explored, client may begin to see there is hope.*[8]

- Identify strengths/assets and past coping strategies that were successful. *Helps client to recognize own ability to deal with difficult situation, providing sense of power.*[5]
- Assist client to identify what he or she can do for self. Identify things the client can/cannot control. *Accomplishing something can provide a sense of control and helps client understand that there are things he or she can manage. Accepting that some things cannot be controlled helps client to stop using energy to try to control them.*[1]
- Encourage client to maintain a sense of perspective about the situation. *Discussing ways client can look at options and make decisions based on which ones will be best leads to the most effective solutions for situation.*[6]

NURSING PRIORITY NO. 4. To promote independence:

- Use client's locus of control to develop individual plan of care. *Tailoring care to the individual's ability will maximize effectiveness. For instance, client with internal control can take control of own care, and those with external control may need to begin with small tasks and add as tolerated, moving toward learning to take more control of care.*[6]
- Develop contract with client specifying goals agreed on. *When client is involved in planning commitment to plan is enhanced, optimizing outcomes.*[2]
- Treat expressed decisions and desires with respect. Avoid critical parenting behaviors. *Listening to client and accepting what is said, no matter what the content, helps client hear own words and begin to process information and feelings to make positive decisions to prevent development of PTSD. Comments that are heard as critical or condescending will block communication and growth.*[1]
- Provide client opportunities to control as many events as energy and restrictions of care permit. *Promotes sense of control over situation and helps client begin to feel more confident about own ability to manage what is happening.*[6]
- Discuss needs openly with client and set up agreed-on routines for meeting identified needs. *Minimizes use of manipulation. Manipulative behavior is often used to influence others to do what the person thinks he or she should do. Usually this results in defensiveness or outright rebellion against what is suggested, resulting in lack of trust and withdrawal on the part of the person being manipulated.*[10]
- Minimize rules and limit continuous observation to the degree that safety permits. *Provides sense of control for the client while maintaining a safe environment for the client.*[6]
- Support client efforts to develop realistic steps to put plan into action, reach goals, and maintain expectations. *Noting progress that is being made can provide a sense of control and diminish sense of powerlessness.*[6]
- Provide positive reinforcement for desired behaviors. *In Behavioral Therapy, the belief that when a behavior reinforces the probability that the behavior will recur, it is called a positive reinforcer and the function is called positive reinforcement. By providing this reinforcement, the desired behaviors are more likely to continue.*[4]
- Direct client's thoughts beyond present state to future when appropriate. *Focusing on possibilities in small steps can help the client see that there can be hope in small things each day.*[1]
- Schedule frequent contacts to check on client, deal with client needs, and let client know someone is available. *Communicates caring and concern for client and needs, reinforcing sense of worthiness.*[1]
- Involve SO(s) in client care as appropriate. *Personal involvement by supportive family members can help client see the possibilities for resolving problems related to feelings of powerlessness.*[6]

 Cultural Collaborative Community/ Home Care 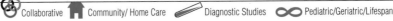 Diagnostic Studies ∞ Pediatric/Geriatric/Lifespan Medications

NURSING PRIORITY NO. 5. To promote wellness (Teaching/Discharge Considerations):

- Instruct in/encourage use of anxiety and stress-reduction techniques. *Most individuals react to stress in predictable physiological and psychological ways. Feelings of powerlessness related to client's situation can be relieved by use of these techniques.*[5]

- Provide accurate verbal and written information about what is happening and discuss with client/SO(s). Repeat as often as necessary. *Providing information in different modalities allows better access and opportunity for increased understanding. People don't always hear every piece of information the first time it is presented because of anxiety and inattention, so repetition helps to fill in the missed information.*[6]

- Assist client to set realistic goals for the future. *Provides opportunity for client to decide what direction is desired and to gain confidence from completion of each goal.*[10]

- Assist client to learn/use assertive communication skills. *Practicing a new way of expressing thoughts and requests provides the client with a skill to achieve desires and improve relationships.*[10]

- Facilitate return to a productive role in whatever capacity possible for the individual. Refer to occupational therapist/vocational counselor as indicated. *Feelings of powerlessness may result from inability to engage in or resume previous activities, and learning new ways to be productive enhances self-esteem and reduces feelings of powerlessness.*[6]

- Encourage client to think productively and positively and take responsibility for choosing own thoughts. *Negative thinking can result in feelings of powerlessness and learning to use positive thinking can reverse this pattern, promoting feelings of control and self-worth.*[6]

- Problem-solve with client/SO(s). *Learning a problem-solving method that results in a win-win solution improves family relationships and promotes feelings of self-worth in those involved.*[10]

- Suggest client periodically review own needs/goals. *It is easy to become discouraged as time goes on, and reviewing thinking about needs and how previously set goals are relevant in the present, helps to either renew those goals, or develop new goals to meet current situation.*[6]

- Refer to support groups, counseling/therapy, and so forth as indicated. *May need additional assistance to resolve current problems/feelings of powerlessness.*[4]

DOCUMENTATION FOCUS

Assessment/Reassessment
- Individual findings, noting degree of powerlessness, locus of control, individual's perception of the situation.

Planning
- Plan of care and who is involved in the planning.
- Teaching plan.

Implementation/Evaluation
- Responses to interventions/teaching and actions performed.
- Specific goals/expectations.
- Attainment/progress toward desired outcome(s).
- Modifications to plan of care.

Discharge Planning
- Long-term needs and who is responsible for actions to be taken.
- Specific referrals made.

References

1. Doenges, M., Moorhouse, M., & Geissler-Murr, A. (2002). Nursing Care Plans, Guidelines for Individualizing Patient Care, ed 6. Philadelphia: F. A. Davis.
2. Doenges, M., Townsend, M., & Moorhouse, M. (1998). Psychiatric Care Plans: Guidelines for Individualizing Care, ed 3. Philadelphia: F. A. Davis.
3. Cox, H., et al. (2002). Clinical Applications of Nursing Diagnoses, ed 4. Philadelphia: F. A. Davis.
4. Townsend, M. (2003). Psychiatric Mental Health Nursing: Concepts of Care, ed 4. Philadelphia: F. A. Davis.
5. Stuart, G. W. (2001). Anxiety responses and anxiety disorders. In Stuart, GW, & Laraia, MT. Principles and Practice of Psychiatric Nursing, ed 7. St. Louis: Mosby.
6. Kunert, P. K. (2002). Stress and adaptation. In Porth, C. M. (ed): Pathophysiology: Concepts of Altered Health States. Philadelphia: J.B. Lippincott.
7. National Institute of Mental Health (2000). Anxiety Disorders, NIH Publication No. 00–3879. Rockville, MD: author. Available at: www.nimh.nih.gov.anxiety/anxiety.cfm. Accessed December 2003.
8. Neeld, E. H. (1997). Seven Choices. Austin, TX: Centerpoint Press.
9. Venes, D. (ed) (1997). Taber's Cyclopedic Medical Dictionary, ed 18. Philadelphia: F. A. Davis.
10. Gordon, T. (2000). Parent Effectiveness Training, (updated ed). New York: Three Rivers Press.
11. Lipson, J. G., Dibble, S. L., & Minarik, P. A. (1996). Culture & Nursing Care: A Pocket Guide. San Francisco: School of Nursing, UCSF Nursing Press.

risk for Powerlessness

Definition: At risk for perceived lack of control over a situation and/or one's ability to significantly affect an outcome

RISK FACTORS

Physiologic
Chronic or acute illness (hospitalization, intubation, ventilator, suctioning); dying
Acute injury or progressive debilitating disease process (e.g., spinal cord injury, multiple sclerosis)
Aging (e.g., decreased physical strength, decreased mobility)

Psychosocial
Lack of knowledge of illness or healthcare system
Lifestyle of dependency with inadequate coping patterns
Absence of integrality (e.g., essence of power)
Decreased self-esteem; low or unstable body image
NOTE: A risk diagnosis is not evidenced by signs and symptoms, as the problem has not occurred and nursing interventions are directed at prevention.
SAMPLE CLINICAL APPLICATIONS: new/unexpected diagnoses, chronic/debilitating conditions (e.g., COPD, MS), cancer, spinal cord injury, major depressive disorder, somatization disorders

DESIRED OUTCOMES/EVALUATION CRITERIA
Sample **NOC** linkages:
Health Beliefs: Perceived Control: Personal conviction that one can influence a health outcome

 Cultural   Collaborative   Community/ Home Care  Diagnostic Studies 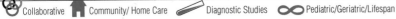 Pediatric/Geriatric/Lifespan   Medications

Participation: Health Care Decisions: Personal involvement in selecting and evaluating healthcare options

Family Participation in Professional Care: Family involvement in decision making, delivery, and evaluation of care provided by healthcare professionals

---

Client Will (Include Specific Time Frame)

- Express sense of control over the present situation and hopefulness about future outcomes.
- Make choices related to and be involved in care.
- Identify areas over which individual has control.
- Acknowledge reality that some areas are beyond individual's control.

ACTIONS/INTERVENTIONS

Sample **NIC** linkages:

Self-Responsibility Facilitation: Encouraging a patient to assume more responsibility for own behavior

Health System Guidance: Facilitating a patient's location and use of appropriate health services

Decision-Making Support: Providing information and support for a person who is making a decision regarding healthcare

NURSING PRIORITY NO. 1. To assess causative/contributing factors:

- Identify situational circumstances (e.g., acute illness, sudden hospitalization, diagnosis of terminal or debilitating/chronic illness, very young or aging with decreased physical strength and mobility, lack of knowledge about illness, healthcare system). *Necessary information to develop individualized plan of care for this client.*[1]
- Determine client's perception/knowledge of condition and proposed treatment plan. *Identifying how client views and understands what is happening and what the plan of care entails is essential to begin to help client feel empowered.*[7]
- Identify client locus of control and associated cultural factors impacting self-view. Internal control (expressions of responsibility for self and ability to control outcomes— "I didn't quit smoking") or external (expressions of lack of control over self and environment— "Nothing ever works out"; "What bad luck to get lung cancer"). *Locus of control is a term used in reference to an individual's sense of mastery or control over events and one's culture may dictate gender roles and the individual's expectations of control. These beliefs can influence a client's practice of health-related behaviors.*[9,11]
- Assess client's self-esteem and degree of mastery client has exhibited in life situations. *Provides clues to client's ability to see self as in control and deal with current situation.*[7]
- Note availability and use of resources. *Client who has few options for assistance or who is not knowledgeable about how to use resources needs to be given information and assistance to know how and where to seek help.*[3]
- Listen to statements client makes that might indicate feelings of loss of control (e.g., "They don't care," "It won't make a difference," "It won't do any good"). *Indicators of sense of powerlessness and hopelessness and need for specific interventions to provide sense of control over what is happening.*[4]
- Observe behavioral responses (verbal and nonverbal) for expressions of fear, disinterest or apathy, or withdrawal. *These responses can show depth of anxiety over what is happening and indicate need for intervention to help client begin to look at situation with some sense of hope.*[5]

• Be alert for signs of manipulative behavior and note reactions of client and caregivers. *Manipulation may be used for management of powerlessness because of fear and distrust.*[4]

NURSING PRIORITY NO. 2. To assist client to clarify needs and ability to meet them:

 • Show concern for client as a person. Encourage questions. *Communicates value of the individual, enhancing self-esteem. Questions may reveal lack of information or concerns client may have.*[8]

 • Make time to listen to client's perceptions of the situation as well as concerns. *Provides time for client to explore views and understand what is happening to come to some decisions about situation, enhancing sense of control.*[5]

 • Accept expressions of feelings, including anger and reluctance to try to work things out. *Communicates unconditional regard for the client and encourages individual to think about options even though situation may look hopeless.*[5]

 • Express hope for client and encourage review of past experiences with successful strategies. *Provides an opportunity for person to remember and accept that he or she has managed difficult situations before and can do the same in current difficulty.*[4]

 • Assist client to identify what he or she can do to help self and what situations can/cannot be controlled. *Accomplishing something can provide a sense of control and helps client understand that there are things he or she can manage. Accepting that some things cannot be controlled helps client to stop using energy to try to control them.*[1]

NURSING PRIORITY NO. 3. To promote wellness (Teaching/Discharge Considerations):

 • Encourage client to be active in own healthcare management and to take responsibility for choosing own actions and reactions. *Discussing ways client can look at options and make decisions based on which ones will be best leads to the most effective solutions for situation.*[6]

 • Plan and problem-solve with client and SOs. *Learning a problem-solving method that results in a win-win solution improves family relationships and promotes feelings of self-worth in those involved.*[10]

 • Support client efforts to develop realistic steps to put plan into action, reach goals, and maintain expectations. *Noting progress that is being made can provide a sense of control and prevent sense of powerlessness.*[6]

 • Provide accurate verbal and written instructions about what is happening and what realistically might happen. *Providing information in different modalities allows better access and opportunity for increased understanding.*[6]

 • Suggest client periodically review own needs/goals. *Reviewing needs and how previously set goals are relevant in the present helps to either renew those goals, or develop new goals to meet current situation.*[5]

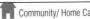 • Refer to support groups or counseling/therapy as appropriate. *May need additional assistance to manage difficulties of current situation.*[4]

DOCUMENTATION FOCUS

Assessment/Reassessment
• Individual findings, noting potential for powerlessness, locus of control, individual's perception of the situation.

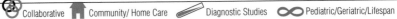 Cultural Collaborative Community/ Home Care  Diagnostic Studies ∞ Pediatric/Geriatric/Lifespan Medications

Planning
- Plan of care and who is involved in the planning.
- Teaching plan.

Implementation/Evaluation
- Responses to interventions/teaching and actions performed.
- Specific goals/expectations.
- Modifications to plan of care.

Discharge Planning
- Long-term needs and who is responsible for actions to be taken.
- Specific referrals made.

References

1. Doenges, M. E., Moorhouse, M. F., & Geissler-Murr, A. C. (2002). Nursing Care Plans, Guidelines for Individualizing Patient Care, ed 6. Philadelphia: F. A. Davis.
2. Doenges, M., Townsend, M., & Moorhouse, M. (1998). Psychiatric Care Plans: Guidelines for Individualizing Care, ed 3. Philadelphia: F. A. Davis.
3. Cox, H., et al. (2002). Clinical Applications of Nursing Diagnoses, ed 4. Philadelphia: F. A. Davis.
4. Townsend, M. (2003). Psychiatric Mental Health Nursing: Concepts of Care, ed 4. Philadelphia: F. A. Davis.
5. Stuart, G. W. (2001). Anxiety responses and anxiety disorders. In Stuart, G. W., & Laraia, M. T. Principles and Practice of Psychiatric Nursing, ed 7. St. Louis: Mosby.
6. Kunert, P. K. (2002). Stress and adaptation. In Porth, C. M. (ed): Pathophysiology: Concepts of Altered Health States. Philadelphia: J.B. Lippincott.
7. National Institute of Mental Health. (2000). Anxiety Disorders. NIH Publication No. 00–3879. Rockville, MD: author. Available at: www.nimh.nih.gov.anxiety/anxiety.cfm. Accessed January 2004.
8. Neeld, E. H. (1997). Seven Choices. Austin, TX: Centerpoint Press.
9. Venes, D. (ed.). (1997). Taber's Cyclopedic Medical Dictionary, ed 18. Philadelphia: F. A. Davis.
10. Gordon, T. (2000). Parent Effectiveness Training, (updated ed). New York: Three Rivers Press.
11. Lipson, J. G., Dibble, S. L., & Minarik, P. A. (1996). Culture & Nursing Care: A Pocket Guide. San Francisco: School of Nursing, UCSF Nursing Press.

ineffective Protection

Definition: Decrease in the ability to guard self from internal or external threats such as illness or injury

RELATED FACTORS
Extremes of age
Inadequate nutrition
Alcohol abuse
Abnormal blood profiles (e.g., leukopenia, thrombocytopenia, anemia, coagulation)
Drug therapies (e.g., antineoplastic, corticosteroid, immune, anticoagulant, thrombolytic)
Treatments (e.g., surgery, radiation)
Diseases, such as cancer and immune disorders

DEFINING CHARACTERISTICS

Subjective
Neurosensory alterations
Chilling

Itching
Insomnia; fatigue; weakness
Anorexia

Objective
Deficient immunity
Impaired healing; altered clotting
Maladaptive stress response
Perspiring [inappropriately]
Dyspnea; cough
Restlessness; immobility
Disorientation
Pressure sores

SAMPLE CLINICAL APPLICATIONS: cancer, AIDS, systemic lupus, substance abuse, tuburculosis, dementia/Alzheimer's disease, anorexia/bulimia nervosa, diabetes mellitus, thrombophlebitis, conditions requiring long-term steroid use (e.g., COPD, asthma, renal failure), major surgery

Authors' note: The purpose of this diagnosis seems to combine multiple NDs under a single heading for ease of planning care when a number of variables may be present. Outcomes/evaluation criteria and interventions are specifically tied to individual related factors that are present, such as:

Extremes of age: Concerns may include body temperature/thermoregulation or thought process/sensory-perceptual alterations, as well as risk for trauma, suffocation, or poisoning; and fluid volume imbalances.

Inadequate nutrition: Brings up issues of nutrition, less than body requirements; infection, altered thought processes, trauma, ineffective coping, and atteration of family processes.

Alcohol abuse: May be situational or chronic with problems ranging from ineffective breathing patterns, decreased cardiac output, and fluid volume deficit to nutritional problems, infection, trauma, altered thought processes, and coping/family process difficulties.

Abnormal blood profile: Suggests possibility of fluid volume deficit, decreased tissue perfusion, impaired gas exchange, activity intolerance, or risk for infection.

Drug therapies, treatments, and disease concerns: Would include risk for infection, fluid volume imbalances, altered skin/tissue integrity, pain, nutritional problems, fatigue, and emotional responses.

- It is suggested that the user refer to specific NDs based on identified related factors and individual concerns for this client to find appropriate outcomes and interventions.

Sample **NOC** linkages:
Cognitive Orientation: Ability to identify person, place, and time
Immune Status: Adequacy of natural and acquired appropriately targeted resistance to internal and external antigens
Abuse Protection: Protection of self or dependent others from abuse

Sample **NIC** linkages:
Postanesthesia Care: Monitoring and management of the patient who has recently undergone general or regional anesthesia
Infection Protection: Minimizing the acquisition and transmission of infectious agents
Environmental Management: Violence Prevention: Monitoring and manipulation of the physical environment to decrease the potential for violent behavior directed toward self, others, or environment

 Cultural Collaborative Community/ Home Care 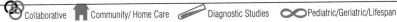 Diagnostic Studies Pediatric/Geriatric/Lifespan Medications

Rape-Trauma Syndrome [specify]

Definition: Sustained maladaptive response to a forced, violent sexual penetration against the victim's will and consent. Note: This syndrome includes the following three subcomponents: [A] Rape-Trauma; [B] Compound Reaction; and [C] Silent Reaction. [All three are presented here.]

[**Note:** Although attacks are most often directed toward women, men also may be victims.]

RELATED FACTORS

Rape [actual/attempted forced sexual penetration]

DEFINING CHARACTERISTICS

[a] Rape-Trauma

Subjective

Embarrassment; humiliation; shame; guilt; self-blame
Loss of self-esteem; helplessness; powerlessness
Shock; fear; anxiety; anger; revenge
Nightmare and sleep disturbances
Change in relationships; sexual dysfunction

Objective

Physical trauma (e.g., bruising, tissue irritation); muscle tension, and/or spasms
Confusion; disorganization; inability to make decisions
Agitation; hyperalertness; aggression
Mood swings; vulnerability; dependence; depression
Substance abuse; suicide attempts
Denial; phobias; paranoia; dissociative disorders

[b] Compound Reaction

Definition: Forced violent sexual penetration against the victim's will and consent. The trauma syndrome that develops from this attack or attempted attack includes an acute phase of disorganization of the victim's lifestyle and a long-term process of reorganization of lifestyle.

RELATED FACTORS

To be developed by nurse researchers and submitted to NANDA

DEFINING CHARACTERISTICS

Acute pase: Emotional reactions (e.g., anger, embarrassment, fear of physical violence and death, humiliation, self-blame, revenge)
Multiple physical symptoms (e.g., gastrointestinal irritability, genitourinary discomfort, muscle tension, sleep pattern disturbance)
Reactivated symptoms of such previous conditions (i.e., physical/psychiatric illness); reliance on alcohol and/or drugs
Long-term phase: Changes in lifestyle (e.g., changes in residence, dealing with repetitive nightmares and phobias, seeking family/social network support)

[C] Silent Reaction

Definition: Forced violent sexual penetration against the victim's will and consent. The trauma syndrome that develops from this attack or attempted attack includes an acute phase of disorganization of the victim's lifestyle and a long-term process of reorganization of lifestyle.

RELATED FACTORS

To be developed by nurse researchers and submitted to NANDA

DEFINING CHARACTERISTICS

Abrupt changes in relationships with men

Increase in nightmares

Increasing anxiety during interview (i.e., blocking of associations, long periods of silence; minor stuttering, physical distress)

Pronounced changes in sexual behavior

No verbalization of the occurrence of rape

Sudden onset of phobic reactions

SAMPLE CLINICAL APPLICATIONS: sexual assualt, abuse

DESIRED OUTCOMES/EVALUATION CRITERIA

Sample **NOC** linkages:

Abuse Recovery: Emotional: Healing of psychologic injuries due to abuse

Coping: Actions to manage stressors that tax an individual's resources

Abuse Recovery: Sexual: Healing following sexual abuse or exploitation

Client Will (Include Specific Time Frame)

- Deal appropriately with emotional reactions as evidenced by behavior and expression of feelings.
- Report absence of physical complications, pain, and discomfort.
- Verbalize a positive self-image.
- Verbalize recognition that incident was not of own doing.
- Identify behaviors/situations within own control that may reduce risk of recurrence.
- Deal with practical aspects (e.g., court appearances).
- Demonstrate appropriate changes in lifestyle (e.g., change in job/residence) that contribute to recovery and seek/obtain support from SO(s) as needed.
- Interact with individuals/groups in desired and acceptable manner.

ACTIONS/INTERVENTIONS

Sample **NIC** linkages:

Rape-Trauma Treatment: Provision of emotional and physical support immediately following a reported rape

Crisis Intervention: Use of short-term counseling to help the patient cope with a crisis and resume a state of functioning comparable to or better than the pre-crisis state

Counseling: Use of an interactive helping process focusing on the needs, problems, or feelings of the patient and significant others to enhance or support coping, problem-solving, and interpersonal relationships

 Cultural   Collaborative   Community/ Home Care   Diagnostic Studies   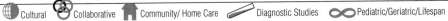 Pediatric/Geriatric/Lifespan   Medications

NURSING PRIORITY NO. 1. To assess trauma and individual reaction, noting length of time since occurrence of event:

- Observe for and elicit information about physical injury and assess stress-related symptoms such as numbness, headache, tightness in chest, nausea, pounding heart, and so forth. *Indicators of degree of/reaction to trauma experienced by the client, which may occur immediately and in the days or weeks following the attack.*[3,4]

- Identify psychological responses: anger, shock, acute anxiety, confusion, denial. Note laughter, crying, calm or agitated, excited (hysterical) behavior, expressions of disbelief and/or self-blame. *Victim may exhibit Expressed response pattern (Compound reaction), displaying these feelings openly and freely as manifestations of experiencing the trauma of rape, and the accompanying feelings of fear of death, violation, powerlessness and helplessness. Or may exhibit controlled (Silent) response pattern with little or no emotion expressed. Any emotion is appropriate, as each person responds in own individual way; however, inappropriate behaviors/acting out may require intervention.*[1,4] Refer to NDs risk for self/other-directed Violence.

- Note silence, stuttering, inability to sit still. May be *signs of increasing anxiety indicating need for further evaluation and intervention. Anxiety is suppressed and client does not talk about the trauma, resulting in an overwhelming emotional burden.*[1]

- Determine degree of disorganization. *Initially the individual may be in shock and disbelief, which is a normal response to the incident. The person may respond by withdrawing, and be unable to manage activities of daily living, especially when the incident was particularly brutal, requiring assistance and treatment to enable her or him to recover and move on.*[4]

- Identify whether incident has reactivated preexisting or coexisting situations (physical/psychological). *The presence of these factors can affect how the client views the current trauma. Previous traumatic incidents which have not been effectively resolved may compound the current incident.*[1]

- Determine disruptions in relationships with men and with others, e.g., family, friends, coworkers, SO(s). *Many women find that they react to men in general in a different way, seeing them as reminders of the rape.*[1]

- Identify development of phobic reactions to ordinary articles (e.g., knives) and situations (e.g., walking in groups of people, strangers ringing doorbell). *These are manifestations of extreme anxiety and client will need to continue treatment to learn how to manage these feelings.*[4]

- Note degree of intrusive repetitive thoughts, sleep disturbances. *Survivor may notice disruptions in activities of daily living, reliving the attack, thoughts of recrimination, self-blame "Why didn't I...?", nightmares. Although these factors are distressing and upsetting, they are part of the normal healing process.*[4]

- Assess degree of dysfunctional coping. *Client may turn to use of alcohol, other drugs, suicidal/homicidal ideation, marked change in sexual behavior in an attempt to cope with traumatic event.*[4]

NURSING PRIORITY NO. 2. To assist client to deal with situation that exists:

- Explore own feeling (nurse/caregiver) regarding rape/incest issue prior to interacting with the client. *Since the feelings related to these incidents are so pervasive, the individual involved in caregiving needs to recognize own biases to prevent imposing them on the client.*[1]

Acute phase/immediate care

- Stay with the client/do not leave child unattended. Listen but do not probe. Tell client you are sorry this has happened and that she or he is safe now. *During this phase the client expe-*

riences a complete disruption of life as she or he has known it and presence of caregiver provides reassurance/sense of safety.[4]

 • Involve rape or sexual assault response team (SART), or sexual assault nurse examiner (SANE) when available. Provide same-sex examiner when appropriate. *Presence of the response team who has been trained to collect evidence appropriately and sensitively provides assurance to the survivor that she or he is being taken care of. Client may react to someone who is the sex of the attacker and use of a same-sex examiner communicates sensitivity to her or his feelings at this difficult time.*[4]

 • Be sensitive to cultural factors that may affect individual client/situation. *May believe incident will bring shame on the family, blame self, some cultures do not allow women to be examined without a male family member being present. These issues need to be considered when treating the survivor.*[6]

 • Evaluate infant/child/adolescent as dictated by age, gender, and developmental level. *Age of the survivor is an important consideration in deciding plan of care and appropriate interventions.*[4]

• Assist with documentation of incident for police/child-protective services reports, explaining each step of the procedure. Maintain sequencing and collection of evidence (chain of evidence), label each specimen, and store/package properly. Be careful to use nonjudgmental language. *It is crucial to maintain chain of evidence to provide accurate information to law enforcement for potential legal proceedings when perpetrator is charged. Words can carry legal implications which may affect subsequent proceedings.*[1]

• Provide environment in which client can talk freely about feelings and fears. *Client needs to talk about the incident and concerns such as issues of relationship with/response of SO(s), pregnancy, sexually transmitted diseases so they may be dealt with in a positive manner.*[4]

• Provide information about emergency birth control and prophylactic treatment for STDs and assist with finding resources for follow-through. *Promotes client's peace of mind and opportunity to prevent these conditions.*[4]

• Provide psychological support by listening and remaining with client. If client does not want to talk, accept silence. *May indicate Silent Reaction to the occurrence in which the individual contains their emotions, using all their energy to maintain composure.*[4]

 • Listen to/investigate physical complaints. Assist with medical treatments as indicated. *Emotional reactions may limit client's ability to recognize physical injury.*[4]

 • Assist with practical realities. *Client may be so emotionally distraught she or he may not be able to attend to needs for such things as safe temporary housing, money, or other issues that may need to be done. Assistance helps individual maintain contact with reality.*[4]

 • Be aware of client's ego strengths and assist client to use them in a positive way by acknowledging client's ability to handle what is happening. *Validation of belief that person can deal with what has happened and move forward with life promotes self-acceptance and helps client begin this process.*[4]

 • Identify supportive persons for this individual. *Client needs to know she or he can go to a strong system of friends and family who will respond with empathy.*[4]

Postacute phase

 • Allow the client to work through own kind of adjustment. May be withdrawn or unwilling to talk (Silent reaction); do not force the issue. *Individuals react in many ways to the traumatic event of rape and no response is abnormal. Factors that influence how the survivor deals with the situation are personality, support system, existing life problems and prior sexual victimization, relationship with the offender, degree of violence used, social and cultural influences, and ability to cope with stress.*[4]

 • Listen for expressions of fear of crowds, men, and so forth. *May reveal developing phobias needing evaluation and appropriate interventions, ongoing therapy.*[4]

 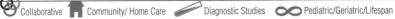

- Discuss specific concerns/fears. Identify appropriate actions and provide information as indicated. *May need diagnostic testing for pregnancy, sexually transmitted diseases or other resources. Meeting these needs and providing information will help client begin the process of recovery.*[4]
- Include written instructions that are concise and clear regarding medical treatments, crisis support services, and so on. Encourage return for follow-up. *Reinforces teaching, provides opportunity to deal with information at own pace. Follow-up appointment provides opportunity for determining how client is managing feelings and what needs may not have been met.*[4]

Long-term phase

- Continue listening to expressions of concern. Note persistence of somatic complaints, (e.g., nausea, anorexia, insomnia, muscle tension, headache). *May need to continue to talk about the assault. Repeating the story helps client to move on, but continued somatic concerns may indicate developing PTSD.*[4]
- Permit free expression of feelings (may continue from the crisis phase). Do not rush client through expressions of feelings too quickly and do not reassure inappropriately. *Client may believe pain and/or anguish is misunderstood and depression may limit responses.*[1]
- Acknowledge reality of loss of self that existed before the incident. Assist client to move toward an acceptance of the potential for growth that exists within individual. *Following this traumatic event, the individual will not be able to go back to the person they were before. Life will always have the memory of what happened and client needs to accept that reality and move on in the best way possible.*[2]
- Continue to allow client to progress at own pace. *The process of grieving is a very individual one and each person needs to know that she or he can take whatever time needed to resolve her or his feelings and move on with life.*[4]
- Give "permission" to express/deal with anger at the perpetrator/situation in acceptable ways. Set limits on destructive behaviors. *Facilitates resolution of feelings without diminishing self-concept.*[5]
- Keep discussion on practical and emotional level rather than intellectualizing the experience. *When the person talks about the incident intellectually, instead of identifying and talking about feelings, client avoids dealing with feelings and can inhibit recovery.*[1]
- Assist in dealing with ongoing concerns about and effects of the incident, such as court appearance, sexually transmitted disease, relationship with SO(s), and so forth. *Depending on degree of disorganization, client will need help to deal with these practical and emotional issues.*[4]
- Provide for sensitive, trained counselors, considering individual needs. *Male/female counselors may be best determined on an individual basis as counselor's gender may be an issue for some clients, affecting ability to disclose and deal with feelings.*[1]

NURSING PRIORITY NO. 3. To promote wellness (Teaching/Discharge Considerations):

- Provide information about what reactions client may expect during each phase. Let client know these are common reactions. Be sure to phrase in neutral terms of "You may or may not...." *Be aware that, although male rape perpetrators are usually heterosexual, the male victim may be concerned about his own sexuality and may exhibit a homophobic response. Such information helps client anticipate and deal with reactions if they are experienced.*[1]
- Assist client to identify factors that may have created a vulnerable situation and that she or he may have power to change to protect self in the future. *While client needs to be assured that she or he is not to blame for incident, the circumstances of the incident need to be assessed*

to identify factors that are within the individual's control to avoid a similar incident occurring.[4]

- Avoid making value judgments. *The survivor is usually blaming self about the incident and agonizing over the circumstances and nonjudgmental language is very important to help the person accept that the fault is not hers or his.*[1]

- Discuss lifestyle changes client is contemplating and how they will contribute to recovery. *Helps client evaluate appropriateness of plans. In the anxiety of the moment, the individual may believe that changing residence, job, or other aspects of her or his environment will be healing. In reality, these changes may not help and may make matters worse.*[4]

- Encourage psychiatric consultation if client is violent, inconsolable, or does not seem to be making an adjustment. Participation in a group may be helpful. *May need intensive professional help to come to terms with the rape.*[1]

- Refer to family/marital counseling as indicated. *When relationships with family members are affected by the incident, counseling may be needed to resolve the issues.*[1]

- Refer to NDs Powerlessness; ineffective Coping, anticipatory/dysfunctional Grieving, Anxiety, Fear.

DOCUMENTATION FOCUS

Assessment/Reassessment
- Individual findings, including nature of incident, individual reactions/fears, degree of trauma (physical/emotional), effects on lifestyle.
- Reactions of family/SO(s).
- Samples gathered for evidence and disposition/storage (chain of evidence).

Planning
- Plan of action and who is involved in planning.
- Teaching plan.

Implementation/Evaluation
- Responses to interventions/teaching and actions performed.
- Attainment/progress toward desired outcome(s).
- Modifications to plan of care.

Discharge Planning
- Long-term needs and who is responsible for actions to be taken.
- Specific referrals made.

References

1. Townsend, M. C. (2003). Psychiatric Mental Health Nursing Concepts of Care, ed 4. Philadelphia: F. A. Davis.
2. Dealing with Rape – Rape Trauma Syndrome. Available at: http://www.rapecrisis.org.za/dealing/trauma.htm. Accessed January 2004.
3. Cox, H. C., et al. (2002). Clinical Applications of Nursing Diagnosis: Adult, Child, Women's, Psychiatric, Gerontic, and Home Health Considerations, ed 4. Philadelphia: F. A. Davis.
4. Rape Trauma Syndrome. Available at: http://www.rapevictimadvocates.org/trauma.html. Accessed January 2004.
5. Doenges, M. E., Moorhouse, M. F., & Geissler-Murr, A. C. (2004). Nurses' Pocket Guide, Diagnoses, Interventions, and Rationales, ed 9. Philadelphia: F. A. Davis.
6. Lipson, J., Dibble, S., & Minarik, P. (1996). Culture & Nursing Care: A Pocket Guide. San Francisco: UCSF Nursing Press.

 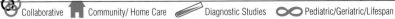

Relocation Stress Syndrome

Definition: Physiologic and/or psychosocial disturbance following transfer from one environment to another

RELATED FACTORS

Past, concurrent, and recent losses
Feeling of powerlessness
Lack of adequate support system; lack of predeparture counseling; unpredictability of experience
Isolation from family/friends; language barrier
Impaired psychosocial health; passive coping
Decreased health status

DEFINING CHARACTERISTICS

Subjective
Anxiety (e.g., separation); anger
Insecurity; worry; fear
Loneliness; depression
Unwillingness to move, or concern over relocation
Sleep disturbance

Objective
Temporary or permanent move; voluntary/involuntary move
Increased [frequency of] verbalization of needs
Pessimism; frustration
Increased physical symptoms/illness (e.g., gastrointestinal disturbances; weight change)
Withdrawal; aloneness; alienation; [hostile behavior/outbursts]
Loss of identity, self-worth, or self-esteem; dependency
[Increased confusion/cognitive impairment]

SAMPLE CLINICAL APPLICATIONS: chronic conditions (e.g., MS, asthma, cystic fibrosis), brain injury/stroke, dementia, schizophrenia, developmental delay, end-of-life/hospice care

DESIRED OUTCOMES/EVALUATION CRITERIA

Sample **NOC** linkages:

Psychosocial Adjustment: Life Change: Psychosocial adaptation of an individual to a life change

Quality of Life: An individual's expressed satisfaction with current life circumstances

Coping: Actions to manage stressors that tax an individual's resources

Client Will (Include Specific Time Frame)
- Verbalize understanding of reason(s) for change.
- Demonstrate appropriate range of feelings and lessened fear.
- Participate in routine and special/social events as able.
- Verbalize acceptance of situation.
- Experience no catastrophic event.

ACTIONS/INTERVENTIONS

Sample **NIC** linkages:

Coping Enhancement: Assisting a patient to adapt to perceived stressors, changes, or threats that interfere with meeting life demands and roles

Hope Instillation: Facilitation of the development of a positive outlook in a given situation

Family Involvement Promotion: Facilitating family participation in the emotional and physical care of the patient

NURSING PRIORITY NO. 1. To assess degree of stress as perceived/experienced by client and determine issues of safety:

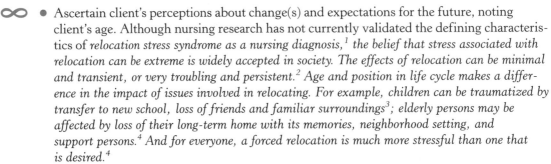

- Ascertain client's perceptions about change(s) and expectations for the future, noting client's age. *Although nursing research has not currently validated the defining characteristics of relocation stress syndrome as a nursing diagnosis,[1] the belief that stress associated with relocation can be extreme is widely accepted in society. The effects of relocation can be minimal and transient, or very troubling and persistent.[2] Age and position in life cycle makes a difference in the impact of issues involved in relocating. For example, children can be traumatized by transfer to new school, loss of friends and familiar surroundings[3]; elderly persons may be affected by loss of their long-term home with its memories, neighborhood setting, and support persons.[4] And for everyone, a forced relocation is much more stressful than one that is desired.[4]*

- Note signs of increased stress in client preparing for relocation or recently relocated: *Client may report/demonstrate anxiety or uncertainty, "new" physical discomfort/pains, increased reliance on medications or drugs/alcohol, start biting nails or grinding teeth, or complain of extreme fatigue.[2,5]*

- Determine involvement of family/SO(s). Note availability/use of support systems and resources. Ascertain presence/absence of comprehensive information and planning (e.g., when/how move will take place, if the environment for the client will be similar or greatly changed, etc.). *These factors can greatly affect client's ability to cope with change.[4]*

- Identify cultural and/or religious concerns *that may affect client's coping, and/or impact social interactions, expectations, and business dealings.[2] This issue also affects the healthcare provider who must try to reduce the client's confusion and feelings of alienation while communicating with client of another primary language, or client who is displaced from cultural, familial or religious attachments.[6]*

NURSING PRIORITY NO. 2. To assist client to deal with situation/changes:

- *Provide information to client/SO as early in process as possible* to eliminate misconceptions and facilitate decision-making process. This can include obtaining audiovisual materials about the city/region/country or new home.[7]

- Encourage contact with someone (friend, family, business associate) who has been to/lived in new area/resides in facility where move is being planned *to absorb some of their experience and knowledge.[7]*

- Obtain interpreter where indicated *to improve communication with client regarding relocation and to obtain information from the client/SO regarding residence/relocation wishes.[6]*

- Involve client in placement choices when possible (e.g., move to nursing home or adult foster care) *to provide client with some control over the situation.[8]*

- Plan ahead *to reduce anxiety and confusion of last-minute rushing.*

- Encourage visit *to new surroundings before transfer when possible. Provides opportunity to "get acquainted" with new situation, reducing fear of unknown.*

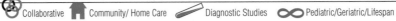 Cultural Collaborative Community/ Home Care Diagnostic Studies Pediatric/Geriatric/Lifespan Medications

- Place in private room, if appropriate, and include SO(s)/family into care activities, meal-time, etc. *Keeping client secluded may be needed under some circumstances (e.g., advanced Alzheimer's disease with fear or aggressive reactions) to decrease the client's stress reactions to new environment.*
- Determine client's usual schedule of activities and incorporate into facility routine as possible. *Reinforces sense of importance of individual.*
- Orient to surroundings/schedules and repeat directions as needed.
- Introduce to new staff members, roommate/residents.
- Provide clear, honest information about actions/events.
- Provide consistency in daily routine; maintain same staff with client in new facility as possible during adjustment phase.
- Anticipate variety of emotions and reactions. *May vary from insomnia and loss of appetite to becoming involved with alcohol/other drugs, or exacerbation of health problems/onset of serious illness or behavioral problems.*[9]
- Anticipate and address feelings of distress in family/caregivers when placing loved one in a different environment (e.g., nursing home, foster care).
- Encourage free expression of feelings, both positive and negative. *Bringing feelings out into the open helps clarify emotion and make feelings easier to deal with.*[10]
- Encourage client to listen to "self-talk" and give self encouraging messages for accomplishments.
- Acknowledge reality of situation and maintain hopeful attitude regarding move/change.
- Identify strengths/successful coping behaviors the individual has used previously. *Incorporating these into problem solving builds on past successes.*
- Address ways to preserve lifestyle *(e.g., usual bath/bed times in new facility, involvement in church activities). Helps reduce the sense of loss associated with move.*
- Encourage individual/family to personalize area with pictures, own belongings, and the like as soon as possible. *Enhances sense of belonging, self-expression and creating of personal space (health impact).*
- Introduce socialization and diversional activities, such as art therapy, music, movies, etc. *Involvement increases opportunity to interact with others/form new friendships, thus decreasing isolation and stress reactions.*
- Encourage client to maintain contact with friends (e.g., telephone, letters, e-mail, video/audio tapes, arranged visits) *to reduce sense of isolation.*[10]
- Encourage hugging and use of touch unless client is paranoid or agitated at the moment. *Human connection reaffirms acceptance of individual.*
- Deal with aggressive behavior by imposing calm, firm limits. Control environment and protect others from client's disruptive behavior. *Promotes safety for client/others.*
- Remain calm, place in a quiet environment, providing time-out, *to prevent escalation into panic state and violent behavior.*
- Assist child/encourage parent to:
  Discuss relocation/move with child. *Information for child must be aimed at level of understanding and interest.*[3] *Child lacks ability to put problem into perspective, so minor mishap may seem catastrophic. Also, child is more vulnerable to stress because he/she has less control over environment than most adults.*[2]
  If child is adolescent, avoid moving in middle of school year, when possible. *Adolescent is vulnerable to emotional, social, and cognitive dysfunction because of the great importance of peer group and loss of friends and social standing caused by relocation.*[11]
  Take practical steps to alleviate stress. *Walking together to school, visiting new classroom, rehearsing boarding the school bus, contacting friends child left behind, driving past places of interest to child, finding a safe play place, unpacking child's favorite toys, inviting neighbor-*

hood children to a get-acquainted party, etc, helps child to maintain ties and develop new ones, reducing sense of loss and shifting focus to the future.[3]

 • Provide client with information/list of organizations/community services (Welcome Wagon, senior citizens or teen clubs, churches, singles' groups, sports leagues, etc.) *to provide contacts for client to develop new relationships and learn more about the new setting.*[10]

• Suggest/refer for professional counseling if more serious difficulties develop (e.g., depression, alcohol/drug abuse, deteriorating behavior of children) *to prevent long-lasting problems from developing.*[7]

NURSING PRIORITY NO. 3. To promote wellness (Teaching/Discharge Considerations):

• Involve client in formulating goals and plan of care when possible. *Supports independence and commitment to achieving outcomes.*

• Encourage communication between client/family/SO *to provide mutual support and problem-solving opportunities.*[7]

• Discuss benefits of adequate nutrition, rest, and exercise *to maintain physical well-being and reduce adverse effects of stressful situation.*

• Instruct in anxiety-and stress-reduction activities (e.g., meditation, relaxation techniques, exercise) as able *to enhance psychological well-being and coping abilities.*

• Encourage participation in activities/hobbies/personal interactions as appropriate. *Promotes creative endeavors, stimulating the mind.*

• Support self-responsibility and coping strategies *to foster sense of control and self-worth.*

DOCUMENTATION FOCUS

Assessment/Reassessment
• Assessment findings, individual's perception of the situation/changes, specific behaviors.
• Safety issues.

Planning
• Note plan of care, who is involved in planning, and who is responsible for proposed actions.
• Teaching plan.

Implementation/Evaluation
• Response to interventions (especially time-out/seclusion)/teaching and actions performed.
• Sentinel events.
• Attainment/progress toward desired outcome(s).
• Modifications to plan of care.

Discharge Planning
• Long-term needs and who is responsible for actions to be taken.
• Specific referrals made.

References

1. Mallick, M. J., & Whipple, T. W. (2000). Validity of the nursing diagnosis of relocation stress syndrome. Nurs Res, 49(2), 97–100.

 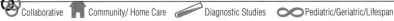

2. Conquering relocation stress. (2001). Public information article by the U.S. Army for military families. Available at: http://www.usarec.army. Accessed September 2003.
3. Chiaro, C. (2003). Preventing relocation stress, easing children's transition. Special report for The Colorado Springs Business Journal.
4. Health impacts of relocation. (2002). Summary Evidence Review Series: No. 11. Health Impact Assessment. Available at: http://online.northumbria.ac.uk/faculties/hswe/hia/evidence/eleven.htm. Accessed September 2003.
5. Solomon, A. (2000). Relocation stress: The warning signs. Article for Psych Bytes. Available at: http://www.therapyinla.com. Accessed January 2004.
6. Purnell's Model for Cultural Competence. In Purnell, L. D., & Paulanka, B. J. (1998). Transcultural Health Care: A Culturally Competent Approach. Philadelphia: F. A. Davis, pp 11, 14.
7. Solomon, A. (2000). Coping with the stress of relocation. Article for Psych Bytes. Available at: http://www.therapyinla.com. Accessed January 2004.
8. Npaver, J. M., Titus, M., & Brugler, C. J. (1996). Patient transfer to rehabilitation: Just another move? Relocation stress syndrome. Rehabil Nurs, 21(2), 94–97.
9. Stress. Article for Youth Center, Army Community Services. Available at: http://www.armycommunityservices.org. Accessed January 2004.
10. ND. (2002). Relocation Stress Syndrome, risk for. In Cox, H. C., et al. Clinical Applications of Nursing Diagnosis: Adult, Child, Women's, Psychiatric, Gerontic, and Home Health Considerations, ed 4. Philadelphia: F. A. Davis.
11. Puskar, K. R., & Dvorsak, K. G. (1991). Relocation stress in adolescents: Helping teenagers cope with a moving dilemma. Pediatr Nurs, 17(3), 298–297.

risk for Relocation Stress Syndrome

Definition: At risk for physiologic and/or psychosocial disturbance following transfer from one environment to another

RISK FACTORS

Moderate to high degree of environmental change (e.g., physical, ethnic, cultural)

Temporary and/or permanent moves; voluntary/involuntary move

Lack of adequate support system/group; lack of predeparture counseling

Passive coping; feelings of powerlessness

Moderate mental competence (e.g., alert enough to experience changes)

Unpredictability of experiences

Decreased psychosocial or physical health status

Past, current, recent losses

NOTE: A risk diagnosis is not evidenced by signs and symptoms, as the problem has not occurred and nursing interventions are directed at prevention.

SAMPLE CLINICAL APPLICATIONS: chronic conditions (e.g., MS, asthma, cystic fibrosis), brain injury/stroke, dementia, schizophrenia, developmental delay

DESIRED OUTCOMES/EVALUATION CRITERIA

Sample **NOC** linkages:

Psychosocial Adjustment: Life Change: Psychosocial adaptation of an individual to a life change

Quality of Life: An individual's expressed satisfaction with current life circumstances

Grief Resolution: Adjustment to actual or impending loss

Client Will (Include Specific Time Frame)
- Verbalize understanding of reason(s) for change.
- Express feelings and concerns openly and appropriately.
- Experience no catastrophic event.

ACTIONS/INTERVENTIONS

Sample **NIC** linkages:

Discharge Planning: Preparation for moving a patient from one level of care to another within or outside the current healthcare agency

Emotional Support: Provision of reassurance, acceptance, and encouragement during times of stress

Socialization Enhancement: Facilitation of another persons's ability to interact with others

NURSING PRIORITY NO. 1. To assess causative/contributing factors:

 • Evaluate client for current and potential losses related to relocation, noting age, developmental level, role in family, and physical/emotional health status. *Although nursing research has not currently validated the defining characteristics of relocation stress syndrome as a nursing diagnosis,[1] the belief that stress associated with relocation can be extreme is widely accepted in society. The effects of relocation can be minimal and transient, or very troubling and persistent.[2]*

• Ascertain client's perception about change(s) and expectations for the future, noting client's age. *Age and position in life cycle makes a difference in the impact of issues involved in relocating. For example, children can be traumatized by transfer to new school, loss of friends and familiar surroundings[3]; elderly persons may be affected by loss of their long-term home with its memories, neighborhood setting and support persons. And for everyone, a forced relocation is much more stressful than one that is desired.[4]*

• Note whether relocation will be temporary (e.g., extended care for rehabilitation therapies) or long-term/permanent (e.g., move from home of many years, placement in nursing home). *To some degree, a temporary relocation is usually easier to cope with than a permanent relocation. However, any anticipated disruption of the client's usual way of living is upsetting, and emotional responses aren't always congruent with the magnitude of the event.*

• Identify cultural and/or religious concerns *that may affect client's coping, and/or impact social interactions, expectations, and business dealings.[2] These issues also affect the healthcare provider who must try to reduce the client's confusion and feelings of alienation while communicating, with client of another primary language, or client who is displaced from cultural, familial or religious attachments.*

• Determine involvement of family/SO(s). Note availability/use of support systems and resources. Ascertain presence/absence of comprehensive information and planning (e.g., when/how move will take place, if the environment for the client will be similar or greatly changed, etc.) *These factors can greatly affect client's ability to cope with change.[4]*

• Evaluate client/caregiver's resources and coping abilities. Determine family/SO degree of involvement and willingness to be involved.

• Determine issues of safety that need to be addressed.

NURSING PRIORITY NO. 2. To prevent/minimize adverse response to change:

• **Refer to Relocation Stress Syndrome for additional Action/Interventions and Documentation Focus.**

References

1. Mallick, M. J., & Whipple, T. W. (2000). Validity of the nursing diagnosis of relocation stress syndrome. Nurs Res, 49(2), 97–100.

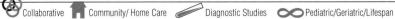 Cultural   Collaborative   Community/ Home Care   Diagnostic Studies   Pediatric/Geriatric/Lifespan   Medications

2. Conquering relocation stress. (2001). Public information article by the U.S. Army for military families. Available at: http://www.usarec.army. Accessed September 2003.
3. Chiaro, C. (2003). Preventing relocation stress, easing children's transition. Special report for The Colorado Springs Business Journal.
4. Health impacts of relocation. (2002). Summary Evidence Review Series: No. 11. Health Impact Assessment. Available at: http://online.northumbria.ac.uk/faculties/hswe/hia/evidence/eleven.htm. Accessed September 2003.

Ineffective Role Performance

Definition: Patterns of behavior and self-expression that do not match the environmental context, norms, and expectations. Note: There is a typology of roles: sociopersonal (friendship, family, marital, parenting, community), home management, intimacy (sexuality, relationship building), leisure/exercise/recreation, self-management, socialization (developmental transitions), community contributor, and religious.

RELATED FACTORS

Social
Inadequate role socialization (e.g., role model, expectations, responsibilities)
Young age, developmental level
Lack of resources; low socioeconomic status; poverty
Stress and conflict; job schedule demands
Family conflict; domestic violence
Inadequate support system; lack of rewards
Inadequate or inappropriate linkage with the healthcare system

Knowledge
Lack of knowledge about role/role skills; lack of or inadequate role model
Inadequate role preparation (e.g., role transition, skill, rehearsal, validation); lack of opportunity for role rehearsal
Education attainment level; developmental transitions
Role transition
Unrealistic role expectations

Physiologic
Health alterations (e.g., physical health, body image, self-esteem, mental health, psychosocial health, cognition, learning style, neurological health); fatigue; pain; low self-esteem; depression
Substance abuse
Inadequate/inappropriate linkage with healthcare system

DEFINING CHARACTERISTICS

Subjective
Altered role perceptions/change in self-perception of role/usual patterns of responsibility/capacity to resume role/other's perception of role
Inadequate opportunities for role enactment
Role dissatisfaction; overload; denial
Discrimination [by others]; powerlessness

Objective

Inadequate knowledge; role competency and skills; adaptation to change or transition; inappropriate developmental expectations

Inadequate confidence; motivation; self-management; coping

Inadequate opportunities/external support for role enactment

Role strain; conflict; confusion; ambivalence; [failure to assume role]

Uncertainty; anxiety or depression; pessimistic

Domestic violence; harassment; system conflict

SAMPLE CLINICAL APPLICATIONS: chronic conditions (e.g., MS, pain, fatigue syndrome), cancer, substance abuse, brain/spinal cord injury, major surgery, major depression, bipolar disorder, borderline personality disorder, schizophrenia

DESIRED OUTCOMES/EVALUATION CRITERIA

Sample **NOC** linkages:

Role Performance: Congruence of an individual's role behavior with role expectations

Coping: Actions to manage stressors that tax an individual's resources

Psychosocial Adjustment: Life Change: Psychosocial adaptation of an individual to a life change

Client Will (Include Specific Time Frame)

- Verbalize realistic perception and acceptance of self in changed role.
- Verbalize understanding of role expectations/obligations.
- Talk with family/SO(s) about situation and changes that have occurred and limitations imposed.
- Develop realistic plans for adapting to new role/role changes.

ACTIONS/INTERVENTIONS

Sample **NIC** linkages:

Role Enhancement: Assisting a patient, significant other, and/or family to improve relationships by clarifying and supplementing specific role behaviors

Normalization Promotion: Assisting parents and other family members of children with chronic diseases or disabilities in providing normal life experiences for their children and families

Values Clarification: Assisting another to clarify her/his own values in order to facilitate effective decision making

NURSING PRIORITY NO. 1. To assess causative/contributing factors:

• Identify type of role dysfunction. *Life changes such as developmental (adolescent to adult); situational (husband to father, gender identity); health-illness transitions can affect how client functions in usual role. This information is important to developing a plan of care and appropriate interventions and goals.*[1]

• Determine client role in family constellation. *How client has functioned in the past (i. e., husband/father, wife/mother), provides a beginning point of reference for understanding changes that have occurred due to health alterations (mental or physical), lack of knowledge about role/role skills, lack of role model or what other situation has occurred to bring about a role change.*[1]

• Identify how client sees self as a man/woman in usual lifestyle/role functioning. *Each*

Cultural Collaborative Community/ Home Care Diagnostic Studies Pediatric/Geriatric/Lifespan Medications

person has a perception of self that is important to know to understand changes that may be occurring.[1]

- Ascertain client's view of sexual functioning. *Changes such as the loss of childbearing ability following hysterectomy, erectile dysfunction following prostate surgery can affect how client views self in role as male or female and may need specific interventions to resolve feelings of loss.*[1]
- Identify cultural factors relating to individual's sexual roles. *Varies with the culture, for instance, for American Indians who are in matrilineal clans or band, women may make important decisions, male roles include ritual to protect family and community well-being. In Arab-American families, men are expected to be responsible for financial affairs and women typically assume caregiving roles.*[4]
- Determine client's perceptions/concerns about current situation. *May believe current role is more appropriate for the opposite sex (e.g., passive role of the client may be somewhat less threatening for women).*[2]
- Interview SO(s) regarding their perceptions and expectations. *The beliefs of the individuals who will be directly involved with the client and the situation (such as parent's bringing a new baby home from the hospital) are important to understanding the new roles the parents are undertaking. Conflicts can arise when expectations vary from individual to individual.*[5]

NURSING PRIORITY NO. 2. To assist client to deal with existing situation:

- Discuss perceptions and significance of the situation as seen by client. *Provides opportunity to clarify any misperceptions and discuss changes client may have to make in regard to what has happened (e.g., loss of a limb, disfiguring surgery).*[3]
- Maintain positive attitude toward the client. *Promotes safe relationship in which client can discuss changes that are occurring and plan for a positive future.*[1]
- Provide opportunities for client to exercise control over as much of situation as possible. *Enhances self-concept and promotes commitment to goals.*[1]
- Offer realistic assessment of situation and communicate hope. *Client may or may not accept reality but opportunity to discuss issues and have a sense of hope can help client begin to accept reality.*[6]
- Discuss and assist the client/SO(s) to develop strategies for dealing with changes in role related to past transitions, cultural expectations, and value/belief challenges. *Helps those involved deal with differences between individuals (e.g., adolescent task of separation in which parents clash with child's choices).*[2]
- Acknowledge reality of situation related to role change and help client to express feelings of anger, sadness, and grief. Encourage celebration of positive aspects of change and expressions of feelings. *Changes in role necessitated by illness/accident, or by changes in family structure (new baby, child leaving home for college, elderly parent needing care), or any other circumstance, results in a sense of loss and need to deal with the feelings that accompany the change.*[1,5]
- Provide open environment for client to discuss concerns about sexuality. *Embarrassment can block discussion of sensitive subject and potentially impede progress. (Refer to NDs Sexual Dysfunction, ineffective Sexuality Patterns.)*[7]
- Educate about role expectations using written and audiovisual materials. *Using different modalities enables client to review material at leisure and begin to incorporate information into own thinking.*[2]
- Identify role model for the client. *Promotes opportunity for client to observe how someone else functions in a role that is new to him or her.*[2]

● Use the techniques of role rehearsal to practice new role. *Provides opportunity for the client to try on and develop new skills to cope with anticipated changes.*[7]

NURSING PRIORITY NO. 3. To promote wellness (Teaching/Discharge Considerations):

 ● Make information available (including bibliotherapy, appropriate Web sites) for client to learn about role expectations/demands that may occur. *Provides opportunity to be proactive in dealing with changes, such as classes to help new parents learn about new roles, credible Web sites for additional information regarding individuals' specific concerns.*[5]

 ● Accept client in changed role. Encourage and give positive feedback for changes and goals achieved. *Provides reinforcement and facilitates continuation of efforts.*[7]

● Refer to support groups, employment counselors, Parent Effectiveness classes, counseling/psychotherapy as indicated by individual need(s). *Provides ongoing support to sustain progress.*[6]

● Refer to NDs Self-Esteem [specify] and the Parenting diagnoses.

DOCUMENTATION FOCUS

Assessment/Reassessment
● Individual findings, including specifics of predisposing crises/situation, perception of role change.
● Expectations of SO(s).

Planning
● Plan of care and who is involved in planning.
● Teaching plan.

Implementation/Evaluation
● Responses to interventions/teaching and actions performed.
● Attainment/progress toward desired outcome(s).
● Modifications of plan of care.

Discharge Planning
● Long-term needs and who is responsible for actions to be taken.
● Specific referrals made.

References

1. Townsend, M. C. (2003). Psychiatric Mental Health Nursing Concepts of Care, ed 4. Philadelphia: F. A. Davis.
2. Cox, H. C., et al. (2002). Clinical Applications of Nursing Diagnosis: Adult, Child, Women's, Psychiatric, Gerontic, and Home Health Considerations, ed 4. Philadelphia: F. A. Davis.
3. Doenges, M. E., Moorhouse, M. F., & Geissler-Murr, A. C. (2002). Nurses' Pocket Guide, Diagnoses, Interventions, and Rationales, ed 8. Philadelphia: F. A.Davis.
4. Lipson, J. G., Dibble, S. L., & Minarik, P. A. (1996). Culture & Nursing Care: A Pocket Guide. San Francisco: UCSF Nursing Press.
5. Gjerdingen, D. (2000). Expectant parents' anticipated changes in workload after the birth of their first child. J Fam Pract, 49(11), 993–997.
6. Rice, J., Hicks, P. B., & Wiche, V. (2000). Life care planning: a role for social workers. Soc Work Health Care, 31(1), 85–94.
7. Doenges, M. E., Townsend, M. C., & Moorhouse, M. F. (1998). Psychiatric Care Plans Guidelines for Individualizing Care, ed 3. Philadelphia: F. A. Davis.

 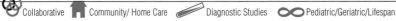

Self-Care Deficit: bathing/hygiene, dressing/grooming, feeding, toileting

Definition: Impaired ability to perform feeding, bathing/ hygiene, dressing and grooming, or toileting activities for oneself [on a temporary, permanent, or progressing basis]

[Note: Self-Care also may be expanded to include the practices used by the client to promote health, the individual responsibility for self, a way of thinking. Refer to NDs impaired Home Maintenance, ineffective Health Maintenance.]

RELATED FACTORS

Weakness or tiredness; decreased or lack of motivation
Neuromuscular/musculoskeletal impairment
Environmental barriers
Severe anxiety
Pain, discomfort
Perceptual or cognitive impairment
Inability to perceive body part or spatial relationship [bathing/hygiene]
Impaired transfer ability (self-toileting)
Impaired mobility status (self-toileting)
[Mechanical restrictions such as cast, splint, traction, ventilator]

DEFINING CHARACTERISTICS

Self-feeding deficit
Inability to:
Prepare food for ingestion; open containers
Handle utensils; get food onto utensil safely; bring food from a receptacle to the mouth
Ingest food safely; manipulate food in mouth; chew/swallow food
Pick up cup or glass
Use assistive device
Ingest sufficient food; complete a meal
Ingest food in a socially acceptable manner

Self-bathing/hygiene deficit
Inability to:
Get bath supplies
Wash body or body parts
Obtain or get to water source; regulate temperature or flow of bath water
Get in and out of bathroom [tub]
Dry body

Self-dressing/grooming deficit
Inability to choose clothing, pick up clothing, use assistive devices
Impaired ability to obtain or replace articles of clothing; put on or take off necessary items of clothing on upper/lower body; fasten clothing/use zippers; put on socks/shoes
Inability to maintain appearance at a satisfactory level

Self-toileting deficit
Inability to:
Get to toilet or commode

Manipulate clothing

Sit on or rise from toilet or commode

Carry out proper toilet hygiene

Flush toilet or [empty] commode

SAMPLE CLINICAL APPLICATIONS: arthritis, neuromuscular impairment (e.g., MS, brain injury/stroke, Parkinson's disease, spinal cord injury), chronic pain, chronic fatigue syndrome, depression, dementia, autism, developmental delay, end-of-life/hospice care

DESIRED OUTCOMES/EVALUATION CRITERIA

Sample **NOC** linkages:

Self-Care: Activities of Daily Living (ADL): Ability to perform the most basic physical tasks and personal care activities

Self-Care: Bathing/Hygiene: Ability to cleanse own body/maintain own hygiene

Self-Care: Dressing/Grooming: Ability to dress self/maintain appearance

Self-Care: Eating: Ability to prepare and ingest food

Self-Care: Toileting: Ability to toilet self

Client Will (Include Specific Time Frame)

- Identify individual areas of weakness/needs.
- Verbalize knowledge of healthcare practices.
- Demonstrate techniques/lifestyle changes to meet self-care needs.
- Perform self-care activities within level of own ability.
- Identify personal/community resources that can provide assistance.

ACTIONS/INTERVENTIONS

Sample **NIC** linkages:

Self-Care Assistance: [specify]: Assisting another to perform activities of daily living

Bathing: Cleaning of the body for the purpose of relaxation, cleanliness, and healing

Hair/Nail Care: Promotion of neat, clean, attractive hair/nails and prevention of skin lesions related to improper care of nails

Feeding: Providing nutritional intake for patient who is unable to feed self

Bowel/Urinary Elimination Management: Establishment and maintenance of a regular pattern of bowel elimination/Maintenance of an optimum urinary elimination pattern

NURSING PRIORITY NO. **1.** To identify causative/contributing factors:

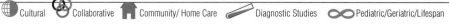

- Determine existing conditions/health problems, age/developmental level, and cognitive/psychological factors affecting ability of individual to care for own needs. *Self-care deficits range from a total deficit to very specific areas of deficit. There are a wide variety of factors that can impact self-care, some of which may be 1) invariable or permanent (e.g., quadriplegia or advanced dementia); 2) temporary (e.g., fractures requiring immobilization, or mild stroke with potential for good recovery) and 3) variable (e.g., person having episode of severe depression or episodes of remitting/exacerbating type MS).*[1]
- Note concomitant medical factors *that impact self-care, or level of needed assistance (e.g., stroke, heart or kidney failure, malnutrition, pain, trauma, surgery, mental illness, and/or medications client is taking).*[1]
- Identify other etiologic factors present, including language barriers, speech impairment, visual acuity, loss of visual/spatial orientation, hearing problem, emotional instability/lability *that can both affect and be affected by self-care needs and deficits.*
- Assess barriers to participation in regimen *that can limit use of resources/choice of options*

(e.g., lack of information, insufficient time for discussion; psychological and/or intimate family problems that may be difficult to share, fear of appearing stupid or ignorant, social/economic limitations, work/home environment problems).[1]

NURSING PRIORITY NO. 2. To assess degree of disability:

- Identify degree of individual impairment/functional level according to a functional level scale as below[1]:
  0—Completely independent
  1—Requires use of equipment or device
  2—Requires help from another person for assistance, supervision, or teaching
  3—Requires help from another person and equipment device
  4—Dependent, does not participate in activity
- Assess cognitive functioning (memory, intelligence, concentration, ability to attend to task, etc.) *to determine client's potential ability to return to normal functioning, or to learn/relearn tasks.[1]*
- Note developmental level to which client has regressed/progressed. *Assists in setting realistic goals and creates baseline for evaluating effectiveness of interventions.[3]*
- Determine individual strengths and skills of the client *to incorporate into plan of care enhancing likelihood of achieving outcomes.*

NURSING PRIORITY NO. 3. To assist in correcting/dealing with situation:

General interventions for any deficit:
- Establish "contractual" partnership with client/SO(s), encouraging their input in planning schedules *to ease frustration of loss of independence, and to enhance client's quality of life when desires are considered and incorporated into care.[2]*
- Promote client/SO participation in problem identification and decision-making. *Enhances independence and commitment to plan, optimizing outcomes.*
- Consult with physician and PT/OT/rehabilitation specialists *to develop plan appropriate to individual situation to enhance client's capabilities, maximize rehabilitation potential, and to obtain adaptive devices and support.[1]*
- Teach/review appropriate skills necessary for self-care, using terms understandable to client (e.g., child, adult, cognitively impaired person) and with sensitivity to developmental needs for practice, repetition or reluctance. *Individualized teaching best affords reinforcement of learning. Sensitivity to special needs attaches value to the client's needs.[3]*
- Plan time for listening to the client/SO(s) *to discover barriers to participation in regimen, and to provide encouragement/support.[1]*
- Provide for periodic communication among those who are involved in caring for/assisting the client. *Enhances coordination and continuity of care.*
- Establish remotivation/resocialization programs when indicated *to reduce sense of isolation/boredom.*
- Provide privacy during personal care activities *to preserve client's dignity.[3]*
- Schedule activities *to conform to client's normal schedule as much as possible (e.g., bathing at a relaxing time for client, rather than on a set routine).[1]*
- Note presence of/accommodate for fatigue. *Fatigue can be very debilitating and greatly impact ability to perform ADLs.[2]*
- Plan activities to prevent fatigue and/or exacerbation of pain *to conserve energy and promote maximum participation in self-care.*
- Avoid doing things for client that client can do for self but provide assistance as needed.

Client may be fearful and/or dependent, and although assistance is helpful in preventing frustration (and sometimes easier for the caregiver in terms of their time), it is important for client to do as much as possible for self to regain/maintain self-esteem, reduce helplessness, and promote optimal recovery.[2]

- Maintain a supportive attitude and allow sufficient time for client *to accomplish tasks to fullest extent of ability.*
- Avoid unnecessary conversation/interruptions *that divert focus from the task at hand and can contribute to client's level of frustration.*
- Assist with necessary adaptations *to accomplish ADLs.* Ensure that client has any needed aids (e.g., glasses, dentures, hearing aids, prosthetics) and arrange for assistive devices as necessary (e.g., raised toilet seat/grab bars, buttonhook, and modified eating utensils) *to optimize self-care efforts.*[1,3]
- Anticipate needs and begin with familiar, easily accomplished tasks *to encourage client and build on successes.*
- Cue client, as indicated. *Cognitively impaired or forgetful client can often successfully participate in many activities with cueing, which can enhance their self-esteem and potentiate learning/relearning of self-care tasks.*[1,3]
- Identify energy-saving behaviors *(e.g., sitting instead of standing when possible, organizing needs before beginning tasks).*

- Assist with medication regimen as necessary, noting potential for/presence of side effects. *Client may need assistance with obtaining prescription medications, preparing daily doses, or ingesting correct doses, etc. In addition, client may need medications that are specifically for improving self-care (e.g., vitamins, nutritional supplements, antidepressants, etc.). All prescribed and OTC medications have the potential for side effects, adverse effects and interactions that may be harmful to the client or affect client's ability to provide self-care.*[1]
- Refer/arrange for home visit, as indicated, *to assess environmental concerns that can impact client's abilities to care for self in home. Modifications may be needed there, or client may require temporary/long-term relocation or assistance with care.*[2]
- Arrange for consult with other agencies (e.g., Meals on Wheels, home care/visiting nurse service, nutritionist) *to obtain additional forms of assistance that may improve client's independence and self-care.*[2]

For self-feeding deficit:
- Assess client's need/ability to prepare food as indicated (including shopping, cooking, cutting food, opening containers, etc). *Identifies specific assistance required.*
- Encourage food/fluid choices reflecting individual likes and abilities, and that meet nutritional needs *to maximize food intake.*[4]
- Ascertain that client can swallow safely, checking gag and swallow reflexes, when indicated (Refer to ND impaired Swallowing).
- Assist client to handle utensils, or in guiding utensils to mouth. *May require specialized equipment (e.g., rocker knife, plate guard, built-up handles) to increase independence, or assistance with movement of arms/hands.*[3]
- Assist client with cup/glass/bottle for liquids, using straw or adaptive lids as indicated *to enhance fluid intake while reducing spills.*
- Allow client time for intake of sufficient food *for feeling satisfied or completing a meal.*[1]
- Assist client with social graces when eating with others; provide privacy *when manners might be offensive to others, or client could be embarrassed.*
- Collaborate with nutritionist/physician *for special diets or feeding methods necessary to provide adequate nutrition.*[2]
- Feed client allowing adequate time for chewing and swallowing, *when client is not able to*

 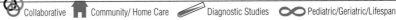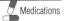

obtain nutrition by self-feeding. Avoid providing fluids until client has swallowed food/mouth is clear. *Prevents "washing down" foods, reducing risk of choking.*[1]

For self-bathing/hygiene deficit:

- Ask client/SO for input on bathing habits/cultural bathing preferences. *Creates opportunities for client to 1) keep long-standing routines (e.g., bathing at bedtime to improve sleep), and 2) exercise control over situation. This enhances self-esteem, while respecting personal and cultural preferences.*[5]
- Bathe or assist client in bathing, providing for any/all hygiene needs, as indicated. *Type (e.g., bed bath, towel bath, tub bath, shower) and purpose (e.g., cleansing, removing odor, or simply soothing agitation) of bath is determined by individual need.*[1]
- Obtain hygiene supplies (soap, toothpaste, toothbrush, mouthwash, lotion, shampoo, razor, towels, etc.) for specific activity to be performed and place in client's easy reach *to provide visual cues and facilitate completion of activity.*
- Ascertain that all safety equipment is in place/properly installed (e.g., grab bars, anti-slip strips, shower chair, hydraulic lift) and that client/caregiver(s) can safely operate equipment *to prevent injury to client and caregivers.*[6]
- Instruct client to request assistance when needed/place call device within easy reach, *so client can summon help if bathing alone;* or stay with client *as dictated by safety needs.*
- Provide for adequate warmth (e.g., covering client during bed bath, or warming bathroom). *Certain individuals (especially infants, the elderly and very thin or debilitated persons) are prone to hypothermia and can experience evaporative cooling during and after bathing.*[7]
- Determine that client can perceive water temperature, adjust water temperature safely, or that water is correct temperature for client's bath or shower *to prevent chilling or burns. This step requires that client is cognitively and physically able to perceive hot and cold and to adjust faucets safely; otherwise, adequate supervision must be available at all times.*[7]
- Assist client in/out of shower/tub as indicated. *Needs are variable (e.g., client may need to get into tub before running water; may require a shower chair, may be independent with one fixture and not another), requiring assessment of individual situations.*[1]
- Assist with/encourage client to complete hygiene steps (oral care, lotion application, cleaning and clipping nails, applying deodorant, washing/styling hair, etc.). *These steps may be completed at same or different time as bathing, but are usually part of a daily routine that is necessary for client's physical well-being and emotional/social comfort.*[1]

For self-dressing/grooming deficit:

- Ascertain that appropriate clothing is available. *Client may not have sufficient clothing, clothing may be inadequate for situation or weather conditions, or clothing may need to be modified for client's particular medical condition or physical limitations.*[2]
- Assist client in choosing clothing, or lay out clothing as indicated. *May be needed when client has cognitive, physical or psychiatric conditions affecting ability to choose appropriate pieces of clothing, or to maintain a satisfactory appearance.*[3]
- Dress client/assist with dressing, as indicated. *Client may need assistance in putting on or taking off items of clothing (e.g., shoes and socks, or over-the-head shirt), or may require partial or complete assistance with fasteners (e.g., buttons, snaps, zippers, shoelaces).*[1,2]
- Allow sufficient time for dressing/undressing *because tasks may be tiring, painful, and difficult to complete.*
- Use adaptive clothing as indicated (e.g., clothing with front closure, wide sleeves and pant legs, Velcro or zipper closures).
- Teach client to dress affected side first, then unaffected side (when client has paralysis or injury to one side of body) *to allow for easier manipulation of clothing.*[2]
- Provide for/assist with grooming activities (e.g., shaving, hair care, makeup) on a routine,

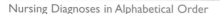

consistent basis. Encourage participation, guiding client's hand through tasks, as indicated. *Experiencing the normal process of a task through established routine and guided practice facilitates optimal relearning.*[8]

 For self-toileting deficit:

- Provide mobility assistance to bathroom or commode; or place on bedpan or offer urinal, as indicated. *Client might be impaired because of age, cognitive problems, weakness, acute injury or illness, requiring a range of interventions from complete care to help with walking.*[1,2]
- Direct cognitively impaired client to bathroom, if needed. *May need directions to the facilities, or reminders to use the bathroom, etc.*[8]
- Observe for behaviors such as pacing, fidgeting, holding crotch *that may be indicative of need for prompt toileting.*[8]
- Provide privacy *to enhance self-esteem, and improve ability to urinate/defecate.*[3]
- Assist with manipulation of clothing if needed, *to decrease incidence of functional incontinence caused by difficulty removing clothing/underwear.*[9]
- Observe need for/assist in obtaining modified clothing or fasteners *to assist client in manipulation of clothing, fostering independence in self-toileting.*
- Provide/assist with use of assistive equipment (e.g., raised toilet seat, support rails, spill-proof urinals, fracture pans, bedside commode) *to promote independence and safety in sitting down or arising from toilet, and/or for aiding elimination when client unable to go to bathroom.*[1,2]
- Keep toilet paper/wipes and hand-washing items within client's easy reach *to enhance self-cleansing efforts.*
- Implement bowel or bladder training/retraining programs as indicated. *This may include developing a schedule for toileting and other interventions as seen in NDs Bowel Incontinence, Constipation, impaired Urinary Elimination, Urinary Incontinence, [specify].*[1,2]

NURSING PRIORITY NO. 4. To promote wellness (Teaching/Discharge Considerations):

 • Assist the client to become aware of rights and responsibilities in health/healthcare and to assess own health strengths—physical, emotional, and intellectual.

 • Support client *in making health-related decisions and assist in developing self-care practices and goals that promote health.*

 • Instruct in relaxation techniques (e.g., deep breathing, meditation, music, yoga) *to reduce frustration/enhance coping.*

 • Provide for ongoing evaluation of self-care program *to note progress and identify needed changes.*

 • Modify program periodically *to accommodate changes in client's abilities. Assists client to adhere to plan of care to fullest extent.*

 • Encourage keeping a journal *to note progress/identify factors affecting ability to perform self-care activities.*[1,3]

 • Review safety concerns. Modify activities/environment *to reduce risk of injury.*

 • Refer to home care provider, social services, physical/occupational therapy, rehabilitation and counseling resources as indicated.

 • Identify additional community resources (e.g., senior services, Meals on Wheels) *to provide long-term support.*[3]

 • Review instructions from other members of the healthcare team and provide written copy. *Provides clarification, reinforcement, and periodic review by client/caregivers.*[1]

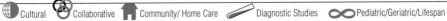

Cultural   Collaborative   Community/ Home Care   Diagnostic Studies   Pediatric/Geriatric/Lifespan   Medications

- Discuss respite/other care options with family. *Allows them free time away from the care situation to renew themselves, enhances coping abilities.*
- Assist/support family with alternative placements as necessary. *Enhances likelihood of finding individually appropriate situation to meet client's needs.*
- Be available for discussion of feelings (e.g., grieving, anger, frustration). *Provides opportunity for client/family to get feelings out in the open, realize the feelings are normal, and begin to problem-solve solutions as indicated.*
- Refer to NDs risk for Injury/Trauma, ineffective Coping, compromised family Coping, situational low Self-Esteem, Constipation, Bowel Incontinence, impaired Urinary Elimination, impaired physical Mobility, Activity Intolerance, Powerlessness.

DOCUMENTATION FOCUS

Assessment/Reassessment
- Individual findings, functional level, and specifics of limitation(s).
- Needed resources/adaptive devices.

Planning
- Plan of care and who is involved in planning.
- Teaching plan.

Implementation/Evaluation
- Response to interventions/teaching and actions performed.
- Attainment/progress toward desired outcome(s).
- Modifications of plan of care.

Discharge Planning
- Long-term needs and who is responsible for actions to be taken.
- Type of and source for assistive devices.
- Specific referrals made.

References

1. ND: Self-Care Deficit: bathing/hygiene, dressing/grooming, feeding, toileting. In Doenges, M. E., Moorhouse, M. F., & Geissler-Murr, A. C. (2004). Nurse's Pocket Guide: Diagnoses, Interventions, and Rationales, ed 9. Philadelphia: F. A. Davis.
2. ND: Self-Care Deficit (specify). In Doenges, M. E., Moorhouse, M. F., & Geissler, Murr, A. C. (2002). Nursing Care Plans: Guidelines for Individualizing Patient Care, ed 6. Philadelphia: F. A. Davis, pp 238, 291, 545, 729.
3. ND: Self Care Deficit (Feeding, Bathing-Hygiene, Dressing-Grooming, Toileting). In Cox, H. C., et al. (2002). Clinical Applications of Nursing Diagnosis: Adult, Child, Women's Psychiatric, Gerontic, and Home Health Considerations, ed 4. Philadelphia: F. A. Davis, pp 331–335.
4. Kayser-Jones, J., & Schell, E. (1997). The mealtime experience of a cognitively impaired elder: ineffective and effective strategies. J Gerontol Nurs, 23(7), 33.
5. Freeman, E. (1997). International perspectives on bathing. J Gerontol Nurs, 22(1), 40–44.
6. Schemm, R. L., & Gitlin, L. N. (1998). How occupational therapists teach older patients to use bathing and dressing devices in rehabilitation. Am J Occup Ther, 52(4), 276–282.
7. Miller, M. (1997). Physically aggressive resident behavior during hygienic care. J Gerontol Nurs, 23(5), 24–39.
8. Sloane, P., et al. (1995). Bathing the Alzheimer's patient in long term care: Results and recommendation from three studies. Am J Alzheimer's Dis, 10(4), 3–11.
9. Penn, C., et al. (1996). Assessment of urinary incontinence. J Gerontol Nurs, 22:8.

Definition: A pattern of perceptions or ideas about the self that is sufficient for well-being and can be strengthened

RELATED FACTORS

To be developed by nurse researchers and submitted to NANDA

DEFINING CHARACTERISTICS

Subjective

Expresses willingness to enhance self-concept
Expresses satisfaction with thoughts about self, sense of worthiness, role performance, body image, and personal identity
Expresses confidence in abilities
Accepts strengths and limitations

Objective

Actions are congruent with expressed feelings and thoughts
SAMPLE CLINICAL APPLICATIONS: as a health seeking behavior the client may be healthy or this diagnosis can occur in any clinical condition

DESIRED OUTCOMES/EVALUATION CRITERIA

Sample **NOC** Linkages:
Self-Esteem: Personal judgment of self-worth
Hope: Presence of internal state of optimism that is personally satisfying and life-supporting
Health Promoting Behavior: Actions to sustain or increase wellness

Client Will (Include Specific Time Frame)

- Verbalize understanding of own sense of self-concept.
- Participate in programs and activities to enhance self-worth.
- Demonstrate behaviors/lifestyle changes to promote positive self-esteem.
- Participate in family/group/community activities to enhance self-concept.

ACTIONS/INTERVENTIONS

Sample **NIC** Linkages:
Self-Modification Assistance: Reinforcement of self-directed change initiated by the patient to achieve personally important goals
Self-Esteem Enhancement: Assisting a patient to increase his/her personal judgment of self-worth
Hope Instillation: Facilitation of the development of a positive outlook in a given situation

NURSING PRIORITY NO. 1. To assess current situation and desire to enhance self-concept:

- Determine current status of individual's belief about self. *Self-concept consists of the physical self (body image), personal self (identity) and self-esteem and information about*

  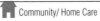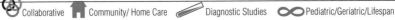

client's current thinking about self provides a beginning for making changes to improve self.[1,2]

- Determine availability/quality of family/SO(s) support. *Presence of supportive people who reflect positive attitudes regarding the individual promotes a positive sense of self.*[1]
- Identify family dynamics, present and past. *Self-esteem begins in early childhood and is influenced by the perceptions of how the individual is viewed by significant others. Provides information about family functioning that will help to develop plan of care for enhancing client's self-concept.*[1,2]
- Note willingness to seek assistance, motivation for change. *An individual who has a sense of their own self-image and is willing to look at themselves realistically, will be able to progress in the desire to improve.*[1]
- Determine client's concept of self in relation to cultural/religious ideals/beliefs. *Culture and religion play a major role in view individual has of self in relation to self worth.*[3]
- Observe nonverbal behaviors and note congruence with verbal expressions. Discuss cultural meanings of nonverbal communication. *Incongruence between verbal and nonverbal communication requires clarification. Interpretation of nonverbal expressions is culturally determined and needs to be identified to avoid misinterpretation.*[1,3]

NURSING PRIORITY NO. 2. To promote client sense of self-esteem:

- Develop therapeutic relationship. Be attentive, validate client's communication, provide encouragement for efforts, maintain open communication, use skills of Active-listening and I-messages. *Promotes trusting situation in which client is free to be open and honest with self and others.*[2,3]
- Accept client's perceptions/view of current status. *Avoids threatening existing self-esteem and provides opportunity for client to develop realistic plan for improving self-concept.*[3]
- Be aware that people are not programmed to be rational. *They must seek information, choosing to learn, to think rather than merely accepting/reacting in order to have respect for self, facts, honesty, and to develop positive self-regard.*[3]
- Discuss client perception of self, confronting misconceptions and identifying negative self-talk. Address distortions in thinking, such as self-referencing (beliefs that others are focusing on individuals' weaknesses/limitations); filtering (focusing on negative and ignoring positive); catastrophizing (expecting the worst outcomes). *Addressing these issues openly allows client to identify things that may negatively affect self-concept and provides an opportunity for change.*[3]
- Have client list current/past successes and strengths. *Emphasizes fact that client is and has been successful in many actions taken.*[1]
- Use positive I-messages rather than praise. *Praise is a form of external control, coming from outside sources, whereas I-messages allow the client to develop internal sense of self-worth.*[4]
- Discuss what behavior does for client (positive intention). Ask what options are available to the client/SO(s). *Encourages thinking about what inner motivations are and what actions can be taken to enhance self-esteem.*[3]
- Give reinforcement for progress noted. *Positive words of encouragement support development of effective coping behaviors.*[3]
- Allow client to progress at own rate. *Adaptation to a change in self-concept depends on its significance to the individual, and disruption to lifestyle.*[3]
- Involve in activities/exercise program of choice, promote socialization. *Enhances sense of well-being/can help to energize client.*[3]

NURSING PRIORITY NO. 3. To promote enhanced sense of personal worth and happiness:

• Assist client to identify goals that are personally achievable. Provide positive feedback for verbal and behavioral indications of improved self-view. *Increases likelihood of success and commitment to change.*[3]

• Refer to vocational/employment counselor, educational resources as appropriate. *Assists with improving development of social/vocational skills.*[3]

• Encourage participation in classes/activities/hobbies that client enjoys or would like to experience. *Provides opportunity for learning new information/skills that can enhance feelings of success, improving self-esteem.*[3,5]

• Reinforce that current decision to improve self-concept is ongoing. *Continued work and support are necessary to sustain behavior changes/personal growth.*[3,5]

• Suggest assertiveness training classes. *Promotes learning to assist with developing new skills to promote self-esteem.*[3]

• Emphasize importance of grooming and personal hygiene and assist in developing skills to improve appearance and dress for success. *Looking your best improves sense of self-worth and presenting a positive appearance enhances how others see you.*[1]

DOCUMENTATION FOCUS

Assessment/Reassessment
- Individual findings, including evaluations of self and others, current and past successes.
- Interactions with others/lifestyle.
- Motivation for/willingness to change.

Planning
- Plan of care and who is involved in planning.
- Educational plan.

Implementation/Evaluation
- Responses to interventions/teaching and actions performed.
- Attainment/progress toward desired outcome(s).
- Modifications to plan of care.

Discharge Planning
- Long-term needs and who is responsible for actions to be taken.
- Specific referrals made.

References

1. Townsend, M. C. (2003). Psychiatric Mental Health Nursing Concepts of Care, ed 4. Philadelphia: F. A. Davis.
2. Doenges, M. E., Townsend, M. C., & Moorhouse, M. F. (1998). Psychiatric Care Plans Guidelines for Individualizing Patient Care, ed 3. Philadelphia: F. A. Davis.
3. Doenges, M. E., Moorhouse, M. F., & Geissler-Murr, A. C. (2004). Nurse's Pocket Guide Diagnoses, Interventions, and Rationales, ed 9. Philadelphia: F. A. Davis.
4. Gordon, T. (2000). Parent Effectiveness Training, (updated ed). New York: Three River Press.
5. National Association of Self-Esteem. Available at: www.self-esteem-nase.org.

chronic low Self-Esteem

Definition: Long-standing negative self-evaluation/feelings about self or self-capabilities

RELATED FACTORS

To be developed by nurse researchers and submitted to NANDA
[Fixation in earlier level of development]
[Continual negative evaluation of self/capabilities from childhood]
[Personal vulnerability]
[Life choices perpetuating failure; ineffective social/occupational functioning]
[Feelings of abandonment by SO; willingness to tolerate possibly life-threatening domestic violence]
[Chronic physical/psychiatric conditions; antisocial behaviors]

DEFINING CHARACTERISTICS

Subjective
(Long-standing or chronic):
Self-negating verbalization
Expressions of shame/guilt
Evaluates self as unable to deal with events
Rationalizes away/rejects positive feedback and exaggerates negative feedback about self

Objective
Hesitant to try new things/situations (long-standing or chronic)
Frequent lack of success in work or other life events
Overly conforming, dependent on others' opinions
Lack of eye contact
Nonassertive/passive; indecisive
Excessively seeks reassurance

SAMPLE CLINICAL APPLICATIONS: chronic health conditions, degenerative diseases, eating disorders, substance abuse, depressive disorders, personality disorders, pervasive developmental disorders

DESIRED OUTCOMES/EVALUATION CRITERIA

Sample **NOC** linkages:
Self-Esteem: Personal judgment of self-worth
Body Image: Positive perception of own appearance and body functions
Hope: Presence of internal state of optimism that is personally satisfying and life-supporting

Client Will (Include Specific Time Frame)
- Verbalize understanding of negative evaluation of self and reasons for this problem.
- Participate in treatment program to promote change in self-evaluation.
- Demonstrate behaviors/lifestyle changes to promote positive self-esteem.
- Verbalize increased sense of self-esteem in relation to current situation.
- Participate in family/group/community activities to enhance change.

ACTIONS/INTERVENTIONS

Sample **NIC** linkages:

Self-Esteem Enhancement: Assisting a patient to increase his/her personal judgment of self-worth

Emotional Support: Provision of reassurance, acceptance, and encouragement during times of stress

Body Image Enhancement: Improving a patient's conscious and unconscious perceptions and attitudes toward his/her body

NURSING PRIORITY NO. 1. To assess causative/contributing factors:

 • Determine factors of low self-esteem that may have been exacerbated by current situation, noting age and developmental level of individual. *Occurrences such as family crises, physical disfigurement from an accident or illness, feelings of abandonment by SO resulting in social isolation are important to identify to develop plan of care and appropriate interventions to help client develop a sense of self-worth.*[1]

 • Assess content of negative self-talk. Note client's perceptions of how others view him or her. *Constant repetition of negative words and thoughts reinforce idea that individual is worthless and belief that others view him or her in a negative manner. Identifying these negative ruminations and bringing them to the client's awareness enables person to begin to replace them with positive thoughts.*[1]

• Determine availability/quality of family/SO(s) support. *Family is an important component of how an individual views self. The development of a positive sense of self depends on how the person relates to members of the family, as they are growing up and in the current situation.*[1,3]

 • Identify family dynamics, present and past. *How family members interact affects an individual's development and sense of self-esteem. If family members are negative and non-supportive, or positive and supportive, affects the needs of the client at this time.*[4]

 • Note nonverbal behavior (e.g., nervous movements, lack of eye contact). *Incongruencies between verbal/nonverbal communication require clarification to assure accuracy of interpretation.*[1]

 • Determine degree of participation and cooperation with therapeutic regimen. *Maintaining scheduled medications, such as antidepressants/antipsychotics, and other aspects of the plan of care indicates need for additional evaluation and possibility of change in regimen.*[1]

 • Note willingness to seek assistance, motivation for change. *Determines client's degree of participation in adhering to therapeutic regimen.*[1]

 • Be alert to client concept of self in relation to cultural/religious ideal(s). *Composition and structure of nuclear family influences individual's sense of who they are in relation to others in the family and in society. Mexican-American culture dictates that family comes first, the father is the authority in the family, and the behavior of the individual reflects on the entire family.*[5]

NURSING PRIORITY NO. 2. To promote client's sense of self-esteem in dealing with situation:

• Develop therapeutic relationship. Be attentive, validate client's communication, provide encouragement for efforts, maintain open communication, use skills of Active-listening and I-messages. *Promotes trusting situation in which client is free to be open and honest with self and therapist so current situation can be dealt with most effectively.*[1]

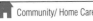 • Address presenting medical/safety issues. *Client's self-esteem may be affected by physical changes of current medical situation. Changes in body, such as weight loss or chronic illness,*

 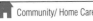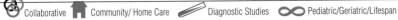

amputation will affect how client sees self as a person. Attitude may contribute to feelings of depression and lack of attention to personal safety needing evaluation and assistance.[1]

- Accept client's perceptions/view of situation. Avoid threatening existing self-esteem. *Promotes trust and allows client to begin to look at options for improving self-esteem.*[2]
- Be aware that people are not programmed to be rational. *They must seek information—choosing to learn; to think rather than merely accepting/reacting—in order to have respect for self, facts, honesty, and to develop positive self-esteem.*[1]
- Discuss client perceptions of self related to what is happening; confront misconceptions and negative self-talk. Address distortions in thinking, such as self-referencing (belief that others are focusing on individual's weaknesses/limitations), filtering (focusing on negative and ignoring positive), catastrophizing (expecting the worst outcomes). *Addressing these issues openly provides opportunity for change.*[7]
- Emphasize need to avoid comparing self with others. Encourage client to focus on aspects of self that can be valued. *Changing negative thinking can be effective in developing positive self-talk to enhance self-esteem.*[2]
- Have client list current/past successes and strengths. *Often in the depths of despair and sense of failure in current situation, individual forgets these aspects of his or her life and bringing them to mind can remind client of these successes, enhancing sense of self-esteem.*[4]
- Use positive I-messages rather than praise. *Praise may be heard as manipulative and insincere and be rejected. Use of positive I-messages communicates a feeling that is genuine and real and allows client to feel good about himself or herself developing internal sense of self-esteem.*[6]
- Discuss what behavior does for client (positive intention). What options are available to the client/SO(s)? *Helping client begin to look at what rewards are gained from current actions and what actions might be taken to achieve the same rewards in a more positive way can provide a realistic and accurate self-appraisal, enhancing sense of competence and self-worth.*[4]
- Assist client to deal with sense of powerlessness. Refer to ND Powerlessness.
- Set limits on aggressive or problem behaviors such as acting out, suicide preoccupation, or rumination. Put self in client's place using empathy not sympathy. *Preventing undesirable behavior prevents feelings of worthlessness. Suicidal thoughts need further evaluation and intervention. Use of empathy helps caregiver to understand client's feelings better.*[1]
- Give reinforcement for progress noted. *Positive words of encouragement support development of coping behaviors.*[2]
- Allow client to progress at own rate. *Adaptation to a change in self-concept depends on its significance to individual, disruption to lifestyle, and length of illness/debilitation.*[4]
- Assist client to recognize and cope with events, alterations, and sense of loss of control. *Incorporating changes accurately into self-concept enhances sense of self-worth.*[1]
- Involve in activities/exercise program, promote socialization. *Enhances sense of well-being/can help energize client.*[1]

NURSING PRIORITY NO. 3. To promote wellness (Teaching/Discharge Considerations):

- Discuss inaccuracies in self-perception with client/SO(s). *Enables client and significant others to begin to look at misperceptions and accept reality and look at options for change to improve sense of self-worth.*[7]
- Prepare client for events/changes that are expected, when possible. *Providing time to adapt to changes allows client to prepare self and feel more confident in ability to manage the changes, enhancing sense of self-worth.*[1]
- Provide structure in daily routine/care activities. *Knowing what to expect promotes a sense of control and ability to deal with activities as they occur.*[1]

- Emphasize importance of grooming and personal hygiene. Assist in developing skills as indicated (e.g., makeup classes, dress for success). *People feel better about themselves when they present a positive outer appearance.*[1,3]
- Assist client to identify goals that are personally achievable. Provide positive feedback for verbal and behavioral indications of improved self-view. *Increases likelihood of success and commitment to change.*[4]
- Refer to vocational/employment counselor, educational resources as appropriate. *Assists with development of social/vocational skills, promoting sense of competence and self-responsibility.*[4]
- Encourage participation in classes/activities/hobbies that client enjoys or would like to experience. *Meaningful accomplishment, assuming self responsibility, and participating in new activities engenders one's sense of competence and self-worth.*[4]
- Reinforce that this therapy is a brief encounter in overall life of the client/SO(s), with continued work and ongoing support being necessary to sustain behavior changes/personal growth. *Provides individual with information and encouragement to build on for the future.*[1]
- Refer to classes to assist with learning new skills, e.g., assertiveness training, positive self-image, communication skills. *These skills can help client develop a sense of competence through realistic and accurate self-appraisal promoting self-esteem.*[4]
- Refer to counseling/therapy, mental health, and special needs support groups as indicated. *May need additional intervention to develop needed changes.*[1]

DOCUMENTATION FOCUS

Assessment/Reassessment
- Individual findings, including early memories of negative evaluations (self and others), subsequent/precipitating failure events.
- Effects on interactions with others/lifestyle.
- Specific medical/safety issues.
- Motivation for/willingness to change.

Planning
- Plan of care and who is involved in planning.
- Teaching plan.

Implementation/Evaluation
- Responses to interventions/teaching and actions performed.
- Attainment/progress toward desired outcome(s).
- Modifications to plan of care.

Discharge Planning
- Long-term needs and who is responsible for actions to be taken.
- Specific referrals made.

References

1. Townsend, M. C. (2003). Psychiatric Mental Health Nursing Concepts of Care, ed 4. Philadelphia: F. A. Davis.
2. Vasconcellos, J., Reasoner, R., Borba, M., Duhl, L., & Canfield, J. In Defense of Self-Esteem. Available at: National Association for Self-Esteem, http://www.self-esteem-nase.org. Accessed January 2004.

 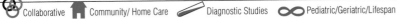

3. Battle, J. (1990). Self-Esteem: The New Revolution. Edmonton, Alberta, Canada: James Battle & Associates.
4. Reasoner, R. (2000). The True Meaning of Self Esteem. Palo Alto, CA: Consulting Psychologists Press.
5. Lipson, J. G., Dibble, S. L, & Minarik, P. A. (1996). Culture & Nursing Care: A Pocket Guide. San Francisco: UCSF Nursing Press.
6. Gordon, T. (2000). Parent Effectiveness Training. New York: Three Rivers Press.
7. Peden, A., et al. (2000). Reducing negative thinking and depressive symptoms in college women. J Nurs Scholarsh, 32:2.

situational low Self-Esteem

Definition: Development of a negative perception of self-worth in response to a current situation (specify)

RELATED FACTORS

Developmental changes (specify); [maturational transitions, adolescence, aging]

Functional impairments; disturbed body image

Loss (specify)[e.g., loss of health status, body part, independent functioning; memory deficit/cognitive impairment]

Social role changes (specify)

Failures/rejections; lack of recognition/rewards; [feelings of abandonment by SO]

Behavior inconsistent with values

DEFINING CHARACTERISTICS

Subjective

Reports current situational challenge to self-worth

Expressions of helplessness and uselessness

Evaluation of self as unable to deal with situations or events

Objective

Self-negating verbalizations

Indecisive, nonassertive behavior

SAMPLE CLINICAL APPLICATIONS: traumatic injuries, surgery, pregnancy, newly diagnosed conditions (e.g., diabetes mellitus), adjustment disorders, substance use, stroke, dementia

DESIRED OUTCOMES/EVALUATION CRITERIA

Sample **NOC** linkages:

Self-Esteem: Personal judgment of self-worth

Psychosocial Adjustment: Life Change: Psychosocial adaptation of an individual to a life change

Abuse Recovery: Emotional: Healing of psychologic injuries due to abuse

Client Will (Include Specific Time Frame)

- Verbalize understanding of individual factors that precipitated current situation.
- Identify feelings and underlying dynamics for negative perception of self.
- Express positive self-appraisal.
- Demonstrate behaviors to restore positive self-esteem.
- Participate in treatment regimen/activities to correct factors that precipitated crisis.

ACTIONS/INTERVENTIONS

Sample **NIC** linkages:

Self-Esteem Enhancement: Assisting a patient to increase his/her personal judgment of self-worth

Coping Enhancement: Assisting a patient to adapt to perceived stressors, changes, or threats that interfere with meeting life demands and roles

Support System Enhancement: Facilitation of support to patient by family, friends, and community

NURSING PRIORITY NO. 1. To assess causative/contributing factors:

 • Determine individual situation (e.g., family crisis, physical disfigurement) related to low self-esteem in the present circumstances. *Essential information needed for planning accurate care.*[1]

 • Identify basic sense of self-esteem of client, image client has of self—existential, physical, psychological. *The components of self-concept consist of the physical self or body image, the personal self or personal identity, and the self-esteem, and each aspect plays a role in the client's ability to deal with current situation/crisis.*[1]

 • Assess degree of threat/perception of client in regard to crisis. *How individuals perceive themselves is based on the self-judgments they make. How the client sees the current situation in relation to ability to cope will affect his or her sense of self-worth and needs to be acknowledged and planned for to help client deal with feelings of low self-esteem that may occur.*[1]

 • Be aware of sense of control client has (or perceives to have) over self and situation. *Degree of control client believes or perceives he or she has may be a critical factor in ability to deal with current situation/crisis.*[1,2]

 • Determine client's awareness of own responsibility for dealing with situation, personal growth, and so forth. *These factors enhance the ability of the client to effectively manage situation in a positive manner.*[4]

 • Assess family/SO(s) dynamics and support of client. *Effective interactions among family members usually lead to positive support for the client in current situation. Dysfunctional interactions may be detrimental to client's ability to deal with what is happening.*[2,3]

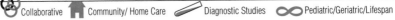 • Be alert to client's concept of self in relation to cultural/religious ideals. *Self-esteem is developed by many factors including genetics and environment. Cultural and religious influences during the individual's life affect beliefs about self, measure of worth and ability to deal with current situation/crisis.*[1,5]

 • Note client's locus of control (internal/external). *Individual's with internal locus of control tend to be more optimistic about their ability to deal with adversity even in the face of current difficulties. Individuals with external locus of control will look to others to solve problems and take care of them.*[1,3]

 • Determine past coping skills in relation to current episode. *Trust is built over time and past experiences with failure or success will affect client's expectations regarding the eventual outcome of dealing with current illness/crisis.*[8,9]

 • Assess negative attitudes and/or self-talk. *An individual who is feeling unimportant, incompetent, and not in control often is unconsciously saying negative things to him or herself contributing to a loss of self-esteem and an attitude of despair affecting current situation.*[1,7]

 • Note nonverbal body language. *Incongruencies between verbal/nonverbal communication require clarification.*[1]

    Cultural    Collaborative   Community/ Home Care   Diagnostic Studies   Pediatric/Geriatric/Lifespan   Medications

- Assess for self-destructive/suicidal behavior. *Client who believes situation is hopeless often begins to consider suicide as an option. Refer to ND risk for Suicide as appropriate.*[1]
- Identify previous adaptations to illness/disruptive events in life. *May be predictive of current outcome.*[1]

NURSING PRIORITY NO. 2. To assist client to deal with loss/change and recapture sense of positive self-esteem:

- Assist with treatment of underlying condition when possible. *For example, cognitive restructuring and improved concentration in mild brain injury often result in restoration of positive self-esteem.*[1]
- Encourage expression of feelings, anxieties. Facilitate grieving the loss. *As client expresses feelings and anxieties he or she begins to deal with the realities of the current situation and the loss that occurs with the changes of illness.*[1]
- Active-listen client's concerns/negative verbalizations without comment or judgment. *Conveys a message of acceptance and confidence in client's ability to deal with whatever occurs.*[6]
- Identify individual strengths/assets and aspects of self that remain intact, can be valued. Reinforce positive traits, abilities, self-view. *Client may not see these in the anxiety and hopelessness of the immediate situation, and reminding client of own positive attributes can help him or her recover hope and develop a positive attitude about situation.*[1,7]
- Help client identify own responsibility and control or lack of control in situation. *Accepting responsibility enables client to realistically look at what is under own control and what is not. When client stops expending energy on issues that cannot be controlled, energy is freed up to concentrate on more productive avenues.*[1]
- Assist client to problem-solve situation, developing plan of action and setting goals to achieve desired outcome. *Personal involvement enhances commitment to plan, optimizing outcomes.*[6]
- Convey confidence in client's ability to cope with current situation. *Validation helps client accept own ability to deal with what is happening.*[1]
- Mobilize support systems. *Feeling hopeless and alone lowers client's ability to manage care and concentrate on healing. Support systems can provide role modeling and the help needed to engender hope and enhance self-esteem.*[1]
- Provide opportunity for client to practice alternative coping strategies, including progressive socialization opportunities. *Involvement with others provides client with situation in which new actions can be tried out, and validated or discarded to enhance feelings of self-worth.*[1,3]
- Encourage use of visualization, guided imagery, and relaxation. *These strategies promote a positive sense of self and enhance client's coping ability.*[1]
- Provide feedback of client's self-negating remarks/behavior, using I-messages. *Allows the client to experience a different view. I-messages are a nonjudgmental way to let individual understand how behavior is perceived/affecting others and self.*[6]
- Encourage involvement in decisions about care when possible. *Promotes sense of control over what is happening, enhancing feelings of self-worth.*[1]

NURSING PRIORITY NO. 3. To promote wellness (Teaching/Discharge Considerations):

- Encourage client to set long-range goals for achieving necessary lifestyle changes. *Supports view that this is an ongoing process, providing client with hope for the future.*[1,3]

• Support independence in ADLs/mastery of therapeutic regimen. *Individuals who are confident are more secure and positive in self-appraisal.*[1]

• Promote attendance in therapy/support group as indicated. *Provides opportunity to discuss own situation and hear how others are dealing with similar problems, promoting new ideas about own ability to deal with issues.*[1]

 • Involve extended family/SO(s) in treatment plan as indicated. *Increases likelihood they will provide appropriate support to client.*[1]

 • Provide information to assist client in making desired changes. *Promotes opportunity for making informed decisions and improving ability to deal with situation.*[1,7]

 • Suggest participation in group/community activities (e.g., assertiveness classes, volunteer work, support groups). *Provides opportunities for learning new information and being appreciated for contributions, enhancing sense of self-worth.*[1]

DOCUMENTATION FOCUS

Assessment/Reassessment
• Individual findings, noting precipitating crisis, client's perceptions, effects on desired lifestyle/interaction with others.

Planning
• Plan of care and who is involved in planning.
• Teaching plan.

Implementation/Evaluation
• Responses to interventions/teaching, actions performed, and changes that may be indicated.
• Attainment/progress toward desired outcome(s).
• Modifications to plan of care.

Discharge Planning
• Long-term needs/goals and who is responsible for actions to be taken.
• Specific referrals made.

References

1. Townsend, M. C. (2003). Psychiatric Mental Health Nursing Cocepts of Care, ed 4. Philadelphia: F. A. Davis.
2. National Association for Self-Esteem. Available at: http://www.self-esteem-nase.org.
3. Battle, J. (1990). Self-Esteem: The New Revolution. Edmonton, Alberta, Canada: James Battle & Associates.
4. Reasoner, R. (2000). The True Meaning of Self Esteem. Palo Alto, CA: Consulting Psychologists Press.
5. Lipson, J. G., Dibble S. L., & Minarik, P. A. (1996). Cullture & Nursing Care: A Pocket Guide. San Francisco: UCSF Nursing Press.
6. Gordon, T. (2000). Parent Effectiveness Training. New York: Three Rivers Press.
7. Peden, A., et al. (2000). Reducing negative thinking and depressive symptoms in college women. J Nurs Scholarsh, 32:2.
8. Munson, P. J. (1991). Life's Decisions – by Chance or by Choice? Adapted from Winning Teachers, Teaching Winners. Santa Cruz, CA: ETR Associates.
9. Vasconcellos, J., Reasoner, R., Borba, M., Duhl, L., & Canfield, J. In Defense of Self-Esteem. Available at: National Association for Self-Esteem, http://www.self-esteem-nase.org. Accessed January 2004.

risk for situational low Self-Esteem

Definition: At risk for developing negative perception of self-worth in response to a current situation (specify)

 Cultural Collaborative Community/ Home Care 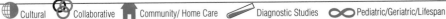 Diagnostic Studies Pediatric/Geriatric/Lifespan Medications

Developmental changes (specify)

Disturbed body image; functional impairment (specify); loss (specify)

Social role changes (specify)

History of learned helplessness; neglect, or abandonment

Unrealistic self-expectations

Behavior inconsistent with values

Lack of recognition/rewards; failures/rejections

Decreased power/control over environment

Physical illness (specify)

NOTE: A risk diagnosis is not evidenced by signs and symptoms, as the problem has not occurred and nursing interventions are directed at prevention.

SAMPLE CLINICAL APPLICATIONS: traumatic injuries, surgery, pregnancy, newly diagnosed conditions (e.g., diabetes mellitus, hypertension), adjustment disorders, substance use, stroke, dementia

DESIRED OUTCOMES/EVALUATION CRITERIA

Sample **NOC** linkages:

Self-Esteem: Personal judgment of self-worth

Psychosocial Adjustment: Life Change: Psychosocial adaptation of an individual to a life change

Abuse Recovery: Emotional: Healing of psychological injuries due to abuse

---

Client Will (Include Specific Time Frame)
- Acknowledge factors that lead to possibility of feelings of low self-esteem.
- Verbalize view of self as a worthwhile, important person who functions well both interpersonally and occupationally.
- Demonstrate self-confidence by setting realistic goals and actively participating in life situation.

ACTIONS/INTERVENTIONS

Self-Esteem Enhancement: Assisting a patient to increase his/her personal judgment of self-worth

Coping Enhancement: Assisting a patient to adapt to perceived stressors, changes, or threats that interfere with meeting life demands and roles

Support System Enhancement: Facilitation of support to patient by family, friends, and community

NURSING PRIORITY NO. 1. To assess causative/contributing factors:

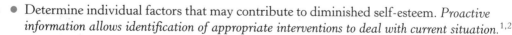
- Determine individual factors that may contribute to diminished self-esteem. *Proactive information allows identification of appropriate interventions to deal with current situation.*[1,2]

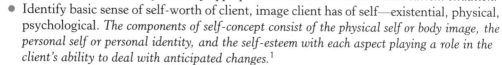
- Identify basic sense of self-worth of client, image client has of self—existential, physical, psychological. *The components of self-concept consist of the physical self or body image, the personal self or personal identity, and the self-esteem with each aspect playing a role in the client's ability to deal with anticipated changes.*[1]
- Note client's perception of threat to self in current situation. *Perception is more important than reality of what is happening. Some individual view a potentially severe situation as something easily handled while another may view a minor problem with anxiety and catastrophizing.*[2,3]

• Be aware of sense of control client has (or perceives to have) over self and situation. *Individual who perceives self in control of what is happening will participate more actively in care and feel more sense of self-worth.*[7,8]

• Determine client awareness of own responsibility for dealing with situation, personal growth, and so forth. *Acceptance of responsibility for self enables client to feel more comfortable with treatment regime and participate more fully, promoting self-esteem.*[1]

• Assess family/SO(s) dynamics and support of client. *How family interacts with one another affects not only the development of self-esteem but also the maintenance of a sense of self-worth when client is facing an illness or crisis.*[1,5]

• Note client concept of self in relation to cultural/religious ideals. *Culture and religion play a major role in view individual has of self in relation to self-worth. Illness may interfere with this view, for instance, males in Mexican-American culture are seen as the head of the household and giving up this role because of illness can diminish self-esteem.*[4]

• Assess negative attitudes and/or self-talk. *Contributes to view of situation as hopeless, difficult.*[3,6]

• Listen for self-destructive/suicidal verbalizations, noting behaviors that indicate these thoughts. *Indicates need for further evaluation and referral for mental health services.*[1,6]

• Note nonverbal body language. *Incongruencies between verbal/nonverbal communication require clarification.*[1]

• Identify previous adaptations to illness/disruptive events in life. *May be predictive of current outcome.*[1]

• Determine availability/use of support systems. *Feeling hopeless and alone lowers client ability to manage care and concentrate on healing. Support systems can provide role modeling and the help needed to engender hope and enhance self-esteem.*[1]

• Refer to NDs situational low Self-Esteem, and chronic low Self-Esteem as appropriate for additional nursing priorities/interventions.

DOCUMENTATION FOCUS

Assessment/Reassessment
• Individual findings, including individual expressions of lack of self-esteem, effects on interactions with others/lifestyle.
• Underlying dynamics and duration (situational or situational exacerbating chronic).

Planning
• Plan of care and who is involved in planning.
• Teaching plan.

Implementation/Evaluation
• Responses to interventions/teaching, actions performed, and changes that may be indicated.
• Attainment/progress toward desired outcome(s).
• Modifications to plan of care.

Discharge Planning
• Long-term needs/goals and who is responsible for actions to be taken.
• Specific referrals made.

 Cultural   Collaborative   Community/ Home Care   Diagnostic Studies   Pediatric/Geriatric/Lifespan   Medications

References

1. Townsend, M. C. (2003). Psychiatric Mental Health Nursing Concepts of Care, ed 4. Philadelphia: F. A. Davis.
2. Battle, J. (1990). Self-Esteem: The New Revolution. Edmonton, Alberta, Canada: James Battle & Associates.
3. Reasoner, R. (2000). The True Meaning of Self Esteem. Palo Alto, CA: Consulting Psychologists Press.
4. Lipson, J. G., Dibble, S. L., & Minarik, P. A. (1996). Culture & Nursing Care: A Pocket Guide. San Francisco: UCSF Nursing Press.
5. Gordon, T. (2000). Parent Effectiveness Training. New York: Three Rivers Press.
6. Peden, A., et al. (2000). Reducing negative thinking and depressive symptoms in college women. J Nurs Scholarsh, 32:2.
7. Munson, P. J. (1991). Life's Decisions – by Chance or by Choice? Adapted from Winning Teachers, Teaching Winners. Santa Cruz, CA: ETR Associates.
8. Vasconcellos, J., Reasoner, R., Borba, M., Duhl, L., & Canfield, J. In Defense of Self-Esteem. Available at: National Association for Self-Esteem, http://www.self-esteem-nase.org. Accessed January 2004.

Self-Mutilation

Definition: Deliberate self-injurious behavior causing tissue damage with the intent of causing nonfatal injury to attain relief of tension

RELATED FACTORS

History of self-injurious behavior; family history of self-destructive behaviors

Feelings of depression, rejection, self-hatred, separation anxiety, guilt, depersonalization

Low or unstable self-esteem/body image; labile behavior (mood swings); feels threatened with actual or potential loss of significant relationship (e.g., loss of parent/parental relationship)

Perfectionism; emotionally disturbed; battered child; substance abuse; eating disorders; sexual identity crisis; childhood illness or surgery; childhood sexual abuse

Adolescence; peers who self-mutilate; isolation from peers

Family divorce; family alcoholism; violence between parental figures

History of inability to plan solutions or see long-term consequences; inadequate coping

Mounting tension that is intolerable; needs quick reduction of stress; impulsivity; irresistible urge to cut/damage self

Use of manipulation to obtain nurturing relationship with others; chaotic/disturbed interpersonal relationships; poor parent-adolescent communication; lack of family confidant

Experiences dissociation or depersonalization; psychotic state (command hallucinations); character disorders; borderline personality disorders; developmentally delayed or autistic individuals

Foster, group, or institutional care; incarceration

DEFINING CHARACTERISTICS

Subjective
Self-inflicted burns (e.g., eraser, cigarette)
Ingestion/inhalation of harmful substances/objects

Objective
Cuts/scratches on body
Picking at wounds
Biting; abrading; severing
Insertion of object(s) into body orifice(s)

Hitting

Constricting a body part

SAMPLE CLINICAL APPLICATIONS: borderline personality, dissociative disorders, developmental delay, autism, eating disorders, substance abuse, physical/psychological abuse, gender identity crisis

DESIRED OUTCOMES/EVALUATION CRITERIA

Sample **NOC** linkages:

Self-Mutilation Restraint: Ability to refrain from intentional self-inflected injury (nonlethal)

Impulse Control: Self-restraint of compulsive or impulsive behaviors

Distorted Thought Control: Self-restraint of disruption in perception, thought processes, and thought content

---

Client Will (Include Specific Time Frame)

- Verbalize understanding of reasons for occurrence of behavior.
- Identify precipitating factors/awareness of arousal state that occurs prior to incident.
- Express increased self-concept/self-esteem.
- Seeks help when feeling anxious and having thoughts of harming self.

ACTIONS/INTERVENTIONS

Sample **NIC** linkages:

Behavior Management: Self-Harm: Assisting the patient to decrease or eliminate self-mutilating or self-abusive behavior

Environmental Management: Safety: Manipulation of the patient's surroundings for therapeutic benefit

Limit Setting: Establishing the parameters of desirable and acceptable patient behavior

NURSING PRIORITY NO. 1. To assess causative/contributing factors:

- Determine underlying dynamics of individual situation as listed in Related Factors. Note previous episodes of self-mutilation behavior. *Although some body piercing (e.g., ears) is generally accepted as decorative, piercing of multiple sites often is an attempt to establish individuality, addressing issues of separation and belonging.*[1]
- Identify previous history of self-mutilative behavior and relationship to stressful events. *Information about previous behavior and precipitating factors is important to understanding and planning care in current situation.*[1]
- Determine presence of inflexible, maladaptive personality traits that reflect personality/character disorder. *Identification of impulsive, unpredictable, or inappropriate behaviors, intense anger or lack of control of anger is important for planning appropriate interventions and plan of care. Clients who have been diagnosed as borderline personality disorder are often unstable and prone to self-injury and need a specific treatment plan to diminish these behaviors.*[1]
- Evaluate history of mental illness (e.g., borderline personality, identity disorder). *These illnesses may be the underlying cause of the self-injurious behavior.*[1]
- Note use/abuse of addicting substances. *May be indicative of attempt to treat self and needs further evaluation and plan of care.*[2]
- Review laboratory findings (e.g., blood alcohol, polydrug screen, glucose, and electrolyte levels). *For identification of drug use that may be affecting behavior negatively.*[1]

 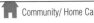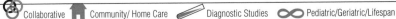

NURSING PRIORITY NO. 2. To structure environment to maintain client safety:

- Assist client to identify feelings leading up to desire for self-mutilation. *Early recognition of recurring feelings provides opportunity to seek other ways of coping.*[5]
- Provide external controls/limit setting. *Decreasing the opportunity to self-mutilate helps the client learn to stop the behavior.*[4]
- Include client in development of plan of care. *Enhances commitment to goals, optimizing outcomes and promoting adherence to the plan.*[2]
- Encourage appropriate expression of feelings. *Helps client to identify feelings and promote understanding of what leads to development of tension and subsequent injurious behavior.*[2]
- Keep client in continuous staff view and do special observation checks during inpatient stay. *Promotes safety by recognizing escalating behaviors and providing timely intervention.*[2]
- Structure inpatient milieu to maintain positive, clear, open communication among staff and clients, with an understanding that "secrets are not tolerated" and will be confronted. *Prevents manipulative behavior, so client does not pit one staff member against another to fulfill own desires.*[1,4]
- Note feelings of healthcare providers/family, such as frustration, anger, defensiveness, need to rescue. *Client may be manipulative, evoking defensiveness and conflict. These feelings need to be identified, recognized, and dealt with openly with staff/family and client.*[4]
- Provide care for client's wounds, when self-mutilation occurs, in a matter-of-fact manner. Do not offer sympathy or additional attention. *A matter-of-fact approach can convey empathy/concern but not undue concern that could provide reinforcement for maladaptive behavior and encourage its repetition.*[2]
- Discuss use of medication, such as clozapine. *This medication has been shown to reduce acts of self-injurious behavior and help client maintain a more stable mood.*[3]
- Develop schedule of/refer to alternative healthy, success-oriented activities. *Groups such as Overeaters Anonymous (OA) or similar 12-step program based on individual needs, self-esteem activities including positive affirmations, visiting with friends, and exercise helps client to practice new behaviors in a supportive environment.*[7]

NURSING PRIORITY NO. 3. To promote movement toward positive changes:

- Develop a contract between client and counselor to enable the client to stay physically safe, such as "I will not cut or harm myself for the next 24 hours." Renew contract on a regular basis and have both parties sign and date each contract. *Making a commitment in writing helps client to think before acting and can prevent new incidents of self-injury.*[4]
- Provide avenues of communication for times when client needs to talk. *Having an opportunity to discuss anxieties helps client to avoid cutting or damaging self.*[4]
- Assist client to learn assertive behavior. Include the use of effective communication skills, focusing on developing self-esteem by replacing negative self-talk with positive comments. *Low self-esteem is a factor in this behavior and by learning new ways of expressing self client can begin to feel better and deal with anxieties in a more positive* manner.[2]
- Use interventions that help the client to reclaim power in own life (e.g., experiential and cognitive). *Beginning to think in a positive manner and then translating that into action provides reinforcement for using power to stop injurious behaviors and develop a more productive lifestyle.*[2]

NURSING PRIORITY NO. **4.** To promote wellness (Teaching/Discharge Considerations):

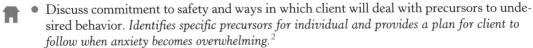

- 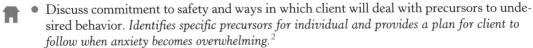 Discuss commitment to safety and ways in which client will deal with precursors to undesired behavior. *Identifies specific precursors for individual and provides a plan for client to follow when anxiety becomes overwhelming.*[2]
- Promote the use of healthy behaviors, identifying the consequences and outcomes of current actions. *As client develops a more positive attitude and accepts the idea that current actions are being destructive to desired lifestyle, new behaviors can help make needed changes.*[2]
- Identify support systems. *Knowing who client can turn to when anxiety becomes a problem helps to avoid injurious behavior.*[1]
- Discuss living arrangements when client is discharged. *May need assistance with transition to changes required to avoid recurrence of self-mutilating behaviors.*[2]
- Involve family/SO(s) in planning for discharge and involve in group therapies as appropriate. *Promotes coordination and continuation of plan, commitment to goals.*[2,6]
- Provide information and discuss the use of medication as appropriate. *Antidepressant medications may be useful, but they need to be weighed against the potential for overdosing.*[1]
- Refer to NDs Anxiety; impaired Social Interaction, Self-Esteem, (specify).

DOCUMENTATION FOCUS

Assessment/Reassessment
- Individual findings, including risk factors present, underlying dynamics, prior episodes.

Planning
- Plan of care and who is involved in planning.
- Teaching plan.

Implementation/Evaluation
- Response to interventions/teaching and actions performed.
- Attainment/progress toward desired outcome(s).
- Modifications to plan of care.

Discharge Planning
- Long-range needs and who is responsible for actions to be taken.
- Community resources, referrals made.

References

1. Townsend, M. C. (2003). Psychiatric Mental Health Nursing Cocepts of Care, ed 4. Philadelphia: F. A. Davis.
2. Doenges, M. E., Townsend, M. C., & Moorhouse, M. F. (1998). Psychiatric Care Plans Guidelines for Individualizing Care, ed 3. Philadelphia: F. A. Davis.
3. Chengappa, K. N., et al. (1999). Clozapine reduces severe self-mutilation and aggression in psychotic patients with borderline personality disorder. J Clin Psychiatry, 60(7):477–484.
4. Clarke, L., & Whittaker, M. (1998). Self-mutilation: culture, contexts, and nursing responses. J Clin Nurs, 7(2)129–137.
5. Dallam, S. J. (1997). The identification and management of self-mutilating patients in primary care. Nurs Pract, 22(5):151–153, 159–165.
6. Selekman, MD. (2004). Adolescent self-harm: A growing epidemic. Family Therapy Magazine, 1(2):34–40.
7. Cox, et al. (2002). Clincal Applications of Nursing Diagnosis: Adult, Child, Women's Psychiatric, Gerontic and Home Health Considerations, ed 4. Philadelphia: F. A. Davis.

 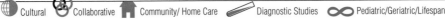

risk for Self-Mutilation

Definition: At risk for deliberate self-injurious behavior causing tissue damage with the intent of causing nonfatal injury to attain relief of tension

RISK FACTORS

Feelings of depression, rejection, self-hatred, separation anxiety, guilt, and depersonalization

Low or unstable self-esteem/body image

Adolescence; isolation from peers; peers who self-mutilate

Perfectionism; childhood illness or surgery; eating disorders; substance abuse; sexual identity crisis

Emotionally disturbed and/or battered children; childhood sexual abuse; developmentally delayed or autistic individual

Inadequate coping; loss of control over problem-solving situations; history of inability to plan solutions or see long-term consequences

Experiences mounting tension that is intolerable; inability to express tension verbally; needs quick reduction of stress

Experiences irresistible urge to cut/damage self; history of self-injurious behavior

Chaotic/disturbed interpersonal relationships; use of manipulation to obtain nurturing relationship with others

Family alcoholism; divorce; history of self-destructive behaviors; violence between parental figures

Loss of parent/parental relationships; feels threatened with actual or potential loss of significant relationship

Character disorders; borderline personality disorders; experiences dissociation or depersonalization; psychotic state (command hallucinations)

Foster, group, or institutional care; incarceration

NOTE: A risk diagnosis is not evidenced by signs and symptoms, as the problem has not occurred and nursing interventions are directed at prevention.

SAMPLE CLINICAL APPLICATIONS: borderline personality, dissociative disorders, developmental delay, autism, eating disorders, substance abuse, physical/psychological abuse, gender identity crisis

DESIRED OUTCOMES/EVALUATION CRITERIA

Sample **NOC** linkages:

Self-Mutilation Restraint: Ability to refrain from intentional self-inflicted injury (nonlethal)

Impulse Control: Self-restraint of compulsive or impulsive behaviors

Distorted Thought Control: Self-restraint of disruption in perception, thought processes, and thought content

Client Will (Include Specific Time Frame)
- Verbalize understanding of reasons for occurrence of behavior.
- Identify precipitating factors/awareness of arousal state that occurs prior to incident.
- Express increased self-concept/self-esteem.
- Demonstrate self-control as evidenced by lessened (or absence of) episodes of self-mutilation.
- Engage in use of alternative methods for managing feelings/individuality.

ACTIONS/INTERVENTIONS

Sample **NIC** linkages:

Behavior Modification: Promotion of a behavior change

Calming Technique: Reducing anxiety in patient experiencing acute distress

Behavior Management: Self-Harm: Assisting the patient to decrease or eliminate self-mutilating or self-abusive behavior

NURSING PRIORITY NO. 1. To assess causative/contributing factors:

 • Determine underlying dynamics of individual situation as listed in Risk Factors. Note previous episodes of self-mutilating behavior (e.g., cutting, scratching, bruising, unconventional body piercings). *Although some body piercing (e.g., ears) is generally accepted as decorative, piercing of multiple sites often is an attempt to establish individuality, addressing issues of separation and belonging and may reflect feelings of anxiety.*[2]

 • Identify conditions that may interfere with ability to control own behavior. *Illnesses such as psychotic states (borderline personality, dissociative disorders), developmental delay, autism may lead to incidents of self-injury.*[1]

• Note beliefs, cultural/religious practices that may be involved in choice of behavior. *Individuals may believe mental illness is the result of unacceptable actions and feelings of guilt may lead to anxiety and subsequent self-injurious behaviors.*[4]

• Determine use/abuse of addictive substances, including alcohol. *Individuals often use these substances to self-medicate feelings of anxiety and may increase the risk of suicide by sixfold.*[2]

• Assess presence of inflexible, maladaptive personality traits. *May reflect personality/character disorder (e.g., impulsive, unpredictable, inappropriate behaviors, intense anger or lack of control of anger) that may lead to self-mutilative behaviors.*[2]

• Note degree of impairment in social and occupational functioning. *May dictate treatment setting (e.g., specific outpatient program, or short-stay inpatient when client is experiencing extreme anxiety).*[1]

• Review laboratory findings (e.g., blood alcohol, polydrug screen, glucose, electrolyte levels). *Identifies conditions that may need further assessment/treatment.*[1]

NURSING PRIORITY NO. 2. To structure environment to maintain client safety:

• Assist client to identify feelings and behaviors that precede desire for self-mutilation. *Early recognition of recurring feelings provides client opportunity to seek other ways of coping.*[2]

• Provide external controls/limit setting as indicated. *Decreases the opportunity to injure self and helps client think about reasons for actions and learn different ways to deal with them.*[1]

• Include client in development of plan of care. *Provides opportunity to reestablish ego boundaries, strengthen commitment to goals and participate in therapy.*[5]

• Encourage client to recognize and appropriately express feelings verbally. *Learning to express feelings enables client not only to recognize them, but to begin to find acceptable/appropriate ways to deal with them.*[6]

• Keep client in continuous staff view and do special observation checks during inpatient stay. *Promotes safety by recognizing escalating behaviors and providing timely intervention.*[2]

• Structure inpatient milieu to maintain positive, clear, open communication among staff and clients, with an understanding that "secrets are not tolerated" and will be confronted.

 Cultural    Collaborative   Community/ Home Care   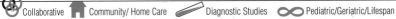 Diagnostic Studies   Pediatric/Geriatric/Lifespan   Medications

Prevents manipulative behavior, so client does not pit one staff member against another to fulfill own desires.[1,4]

- Note feelings of healthcare providers/family, such as frustration, anger, defensiveness, distraction, despair and powerlessness, need to rescue. *Client may be manipulating/splitting providers/family members, which evokes defensiveness and resultant conflict. These feelings need to be identified, recognized, and dealt with openly with staff/family and client.*[1]
- Develop schedule of/refer to alternative healthy, success-oriented activities. *Groups such as Overeaters Anonymous (OA) or similar 12-step program based on individual needs, self-esteem activities including positive affirmations, visiting with friends, and exercise helps client to practice new behaviors in a supportive environment.*[6]

NURSING PRIORITY NO. 3. To promote movement toward positive actions:

- Encourage client involvement in developing plan of care. *Enhances commitment to goals, optimizing outcomes and enhancing self-esteem.*[2]
- Assist client to learn assertive behavior rather than nonassertive/aggressive behavior. Include use of effective communication skills, focusing on developing self-esteem by replacing negative self-talk with positive comments. *By learning these new skills, client can get needs met in positive, acceptable ways and begin to handle anxieties in different ways.*[1]
- Develop a contract between client and counselor to enable the client to stay physically safe, such as "I will not cut or harm myself for the next 24 hours." Contract is renewed on a regular basis and signed and dated by both parties. Contingency arrangements need to be made so client can talk to counselor as needed. *Discussing the contract gets issues out in the open and conveys a sense of acceptance of the client, while placing some of the reponsibility for safety on the client.*[1]
- Discuss with client/family normalcy of adolescent task of separation and ways of achieving. *Helps individual members understand these actions and begin to recognize the normal from the ones that are of concern and need intervention.*[1]
- Promote the use of healthy behaviors, identifying the consequences and outcomes of current actions: "Does this get you what you want?" "How does this behavior help you achieve your goals?" *Provides client with opportunity to look at own behaviors in a different way and begin to understand how they are harmful rather than helpful. Contrasting healthy behaviors versus current actions can help client decide to change them.*[1]
- Use interventions that help the client to reclaim power in own life (e.g., experiential and cognitive). *As client experiences by doing new ways of interacting with others, he or she can begin to think more positively about self-worth and changing behaviors.*[2]
- Involve client/family in group therapies as appropriate. *Group setting aids in promoting diffusion of anger; provides insight as to how negative, aggressive behavior affects others, making feedback easier to digest.*[2]

NURSING PRIORITY NO. 4. To promote wellness (Teaching/Discharge Considerations):

- Discuss commitment to safety and ways in which client will deal with precursors to undesired behavior. *Helps client verbalize anger and anxiety and understand how these feelings lead to desire to injure self and actions that can be taken to prevent this behavior.*[4]
- Mobilize support systems. *These individuals often come from abusive families and unresolved feelings of abandonment remain into adulthood. Positive support by many people in their lives can begin to overcome these feelings.*[1]

- Identify living circumstances client will be going to once discharged. *Will need assistance with transition to changes required to avoid recurrence of anxieties and self-mutilating behaviors.*[4]
- Arrange for continued involvement in group therapy(ies). *Remaining in this supportive environment can help client maintain new behaviors as he or she returns to society.*[2]
- Involve family/SO(s) in planning for discharge. *Promotes coordination and continuation of plan, commitment to goals.*[5,7]
- Discuss and provide information about the use of medication as appropriate. *Antidepressant medications may be useful, but use needs to be weighed against potential for overdosing.*[3]
- Refer to NDs Anxiety; impaired Social Interaction, Self-Esteem (specify).

DOCUMENTATION FOCUS

Assessment/Reassessment
- Individual findings, including risk factors present, underlying dynamics, prior episodes.

Planning
- Plan of care and who is involved in planning.
- Teaching plan.

Implementation/Evaluation
- Response to interventions/teaching and actions performed.
- Attainment/progress toward desired outcome(s).
- Modifications to plan of care.

Discharge Planning
- Long-range needs and who is responsible for actions to be taken.
- Community resources, referrals made.

References

1. Townsend, M. C. (2003). Psychiatric Mental Health Nursing Concepts of Care, ed 4. Philadelphia: F. A. Davis.
2. Doenges, M. E., Townsend, M. C., & Moorhouse, M. F. (1998). Psychiatric Care Plans Guidelines for Individualizing Care, ed 3. Philadelphia: F. A. Davis.
3. Chengappa, K. N., et al. (1999). Clozapine reduces severe self-mutilation and aggression in psychotic patients with borderline personality disorder. J Clin Psychiatry, 60(7):477–484.
4. Clarke, L., & Whittaker, M. (1998). Self-mutilation: culture, contexts, and nursing responses. J Clin Nurs, 7(2):129–137.
5. Dallam, S. J. (1997). The identification and management of self-mutilating patients in primary care. Nurs Pract, 22(5):151–153, 159–165.
6. Cox, et al. (2002). Clincal Applications of Nursing Diagnosis: Adult, Child, Women's Psychiatric, Gerontic and Home Health Considerations, ed 4. Philadelphia: F. A. Davis.
7. Selekman, M. D. (2004). Adolescent self-harm A growing epidemic. Family Therapy Magazine, 1(2): 34–40.

disturbed Sensory Perception (specify: visual, auditory, kinesthetic, gustatory, tactile, olfactory)

Definition: Change in the amount or patterning of incoming stimuli accompanied by a diminished, exaggerated, distorted, or impaired response to such stimuli

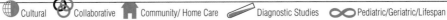 Cultural Collaborative Community/ Home Care Diagnostic Studies Pediatric/Geriatric/Lifespan Medications

Excessive/insufficient environmental stimuli:

[Therapeutically restricted environments (e.g., isolation, intensive care, bedrest, traction, confining illnesses, incubator)]

[Socially restricted environment (e.g., institutionalization, homebound, aging, chronic/ terminal illness, infant deprivation); stigmatized (e.g., mentally ill/developmentally delayed/handicapped); bereaved]

[Excessive noise level such as work environment, client's immediate environment (ICU with support machinery and the like)]

Altered sensory reception, transmission, and/or integration:

[Neurologic disease, trauma, or deficit]

[Altered status of sense organs]

[Inability to communicate, understand, speak, or respond]

[Sleep deprivation]

[Pain, (phantom limb)]

Altered sensory perception

Biochemical imbalances; electrolyte imbalance; biochemical imbalances for sensory distortion (e.g., illusions, hallucinations), [elevated BUN, elevated ammonia, hypoxia], [drugs, (e.g., stimulants or depressants, mind-altering drugs)]

Psychological stress [narrowed perceptual fields caused by anxiety]

DEFINING CHARACTERISTICS

Subjective

Reported change in sensory acuity [e.g., photosensitivity, hypoesthesias/hyperesthesias, diminished/altered sense of taste, inability to tell position of body parts (proprioception)]

Visual/auditory distortions

[Distortion of pain (e.g., exaggerated, lack of)]

Objective

Measured change in sensory acuity

Change in usual response to stimuli, [rapid mood swings, exaggerated emotional responses, anxiety/panic state, motor incoordination, altered sense of balance/falls (e.g., Menière's syndrome)]

Change in problem-solving abilities; poor concentration

Disoriented in time, in place, or with people

Altered communication patterns

Change in behavior pattern

Restlessness, irritability

Hallucinations; [illusions]; [bizarre thinking]

SAMPLE CLINICAL APPLICATIONS: glaucoma, cataract, brain tumor/stroke, traumatic injury, amputation, surgery, immobility, peripheral neuropathy (e.g., diabetes), substance abuse, schizophrenia, developmental delay

DESIRED OUTCOMES/EVALUATION CRITERIA

Sample **NOC** linkages:

Hearing/Vision Compensation: Actions to identify, monitor and compensate for hearing loss/visual impairment

Balance: Ability to maintain body equilibrium

Sensory Function: Taste & Smell: Extent to which chemicals inhaled or dissolved in saliva are sensed

Sensory Function: Cutaneous: Extent to which stimulation of the skin is sensed in an impaired area

---

Client Will (Include Specific Time Frame)
- Regain/maintain usual level of cognition.
- Recognize and correct/compensate for sensory impairments.
- Verbalize awareness of sensory needs and presence of overload and/or deprivation.
- Identify/modify external factors that contribute to alterations in sensory/perceptual abilities.
- Use resources effectively and appropriately.
- Be free of injury.

ACTIONS/INTERVENTIONS
Sample **NIC** linkages:

Communication Enhancement: Hearing/Vision Deficit: Assistance in accepting and learning alternative methods for living with diminished hearing/vision

Nutrition Management: Assisting with or providing a balanced dietary intake of foods and fluids

Environmental Management: Manipulation of the patient's surroundings for therapeutic benefit

Peripheral Sensation Management: Prevention or minimization of injury or discomfort in the patient with altered sensation

NURSING PRIORITY NO. 1. To assess causative/contributing factors and degree of impairment:

- Identify underlying reason for alterations in sensory perception, as noted in Related Factors. Refer to additional NDs Anxiety, disturbed Thought Processes, Unilateral Neglect, acute/chronic Confusion, as appropriate based on findings. *Specific clinical concerns (e.g., neurologic disease or trauma, intensive care unit confinement, surgery, pain, biochemical imbalances, psychosis, substance abuse, toxemia) have the potential for altering one or more of the senses, with resultant change in the reception, sensitivity or interpretation of sensory input.*[1]
- Be aware of clients at risk for loss/alterations in sensory/perceptual senses *because of current diagnosis or treatments (e.g., glaucoma, surgery, immobility, recent stroke, diabetes, mental illness; drug toxicity or side effects (e.g., halos around lights, ringing in ears), middle-ear disturbances (altered sense of balance).*
- 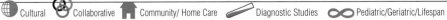 Note age and developmental stage. *Problems with sensory perception may be known to client/caregiver (e.g., child wearing hearing aid, elderly adult with known macular degeneration), where compensatory interventions are in place. Screening/evaluation may be required if sensory impairments are suspected, but not obvious, as might occur when an infant is not progressing developmentally or an older individual has a gradual loss of sensory discrimination associated with aging; or sensory changes associated with a sudden neurologic event.*[2,3]
- Assess ability to speak and response to simple commands *to ascertain client's awareness, developmental level and cognitive functioning.*
- Evaluate sensory awareness. *Screening evaluations can detect changes (e.g., discrimination of*

Cultural   Collaborative   Community/ Home Care   Diagnostic Studies   Pediatric/Geriatric/Lifespan   Medications

hot/cold, dull/sharp; awareness of motion, and location of body parts; visual/hearing acuity, and speech).

- Determine response to touch and painful stimuli, *to note whether response is appropriate to stimulus, and whether it is immediate or delayed. The sense of touch is usually maintained throughout life and may become more needed as other senses diminish. Different types of touch are associated with different meanings, and involves client's sensitivity to touch, and is a means of communication.*[3]

- Observe for behavioral responses (e.g., illusions/hallucinations, delusions, withdrawal, hostility, crying, inappropriate affect, confusion/disorientation) *that may indicate mental/emotional problems, or chemical toxicity (as might occur with digitalis or other drug overdose/reaction), or be associated with brain/neurologic trauma or infection.*

- Ascertain client's perception of problem/changes. Interview SO(s) regarding observations of changes that have occurred and responses of client to changes. *Client may or may not be aware of changes (e.g., diabetic with neuropathy may not realize he or she has lost discrimination for pain in feet; or parents may notice child's problem with coordination or difficulty with words).*

- Refer for/review results of screening tests and laboratory values (e.g., cognitive testing, or laboratory values such as electrolytes, chemical profile, ABGs, serum drug levels).

NURSING PRIORITY NO. 2. To promote normalization of response to stimuli:

- Note degree of alteration/involvement (single/multiple senses) *to determine scope/complexity of condition and needed interventions.*

- Ascertain/validate client's perceptions. Listen to and respect client's expressions of deprivation *to assist in planning of appropriate care, to identify inconsistencies in reception and integration of stimuli, and to provide compassionate regard for client's feelings.*[4]

- Provide feedback *to assist client to separate reality from fantasy/altered perception.*

- Position client to see surroundings and participate in activities as much as possible *to prevent sensory deprivation.*

- Provide sensory stimulation, including familiar smells/sounds, tactile stimulation with a variety of objects, changing of light intensity and other cues (e.g., clocks, calendars).

- Provide diversional activities as able (e.g., TV/radio, conversation, large print or talking books). Refer to ND deficient Diversional Activity.

- Provide means of communication as indicated.

- Note inattention to body parts, segments of environment; lack of recognition of familiar objects/persons. *Loss of comprehension of auditory, visual or other sensations may be indicative of unilateral neglect/inability to recognize and respond to environmental cues.* Refer to ND Unilateral Neglect.

- Protect from bodily harm (e.g., falls, burns, positioning problems), *as client may not perceive pain, or impaired sense of position increases the risk for falls.*

- Identify and encourage use of resources/prosthetic devices (e.g., hearing aids, computerized visual aid/glasses with a level-plumb line for balance). *Useful for augmenting sensory input/interpretation.*

- Provide a stable environment with continuity of care by same personnel as much as possible.

- Provide undisturbed rest/sleep periods *to reduce anxiety, agitation and/or psychosis that can accompany sleep deprivation, particularly when client is confined to bed (e.g., intensive care unit).*

- Address client by name and have personnel wear name tags/reintroduce self as needed *to preserve client's sense of identity and orientation.*

- Document perceptual deficit on chart, and coded on wall in client's room if needed, *so caregivers are aware of specific needs/limitations.*
- Avoid isolation of client, physically or emotionally, *to prevent sensory deprivation/limit confusion.*
- Explain procedures/activities, expected sensations, and outcomes.
- Minimize discussion of negatives (e.g., client and personnel problems) within client's hearing. *Client may misinterpret and believe references are to himself/herself.*
- Eliminate extraneous noise/stimuli, including nonessential equipment, alarms/audible monitor signals when possible. *Reduces anxiety and exaggerated emotional responses/confusion associates with sensory overload.*[4]
- Encourage SO(s) to bring in familiar objects, talk to, and touch the client frequently.
- Involve other health-team members in providing stimulating modalities such as music therapy, sensory training, and remotivation therapy.
- Limit/carefully monitor use of sedation, especially in older population.

Visual deficits:

- Note particular vision problem (e.g., loss of visual field, change in depth perception, double vision, blindness) *that affects client's ability to perceive environment and learn/relearn motor skills.*[3]
- Speak to visually impaired or unresponsive client frequently, especially when entering room/client's presence *to provide auditory stimulation and prevent startle reflex.*
- Approach from visually intact side, position objects to take advantage of intact visual field, use eye patch when needed *to decrease sensory confusion when client has loss of vision or field of vision in one eye.*[3]
- Reorient to time, place, and situation/events as necessary *to reduce confusion and provide sense of normalcy to client's daily life.*
- Encourage family/SO to read client's favorite books, periodicals, or newspapers, and discuss family happenings.
- Provide/encourage listening to music, radio, TV, talking books, and use of talking timepieces.
- Supply adequate lighting for reading and activities.
- Place glasses/contacts where they can be easily found and encourage client to wear corrective lenses during waking hours.
- Arrange bed, personal articles, and food trays to take advantage of functional vision. *Enhances independence and safety.*
- Describe food and placement, feeding or assisting client as necessary (e.g., cooking, cutting food, offering finger food, placing food in clock-position on plate, etc.), *when vision impairments could hinder nutritional intake or cause social discomfort.*
- Assist client with picking out clothing *if problems with color discrimination causes mismatching.*[3]
- Color-code doors and drawers to assist client with low vision *in locating belongings or dwelling, or a particular site (e.g., bathroom).*

Auditory deficits:

- Determine if client reads lips and face client, enunciating words clearly.
- Encourage client's use of hearing aid when one is available.
- Refer for periodic evaluation by audiologist *to note changes in acuity, determine if client might benefit from a hearing aid.*[3]
- Lower the pitch of the voice and speak in tone that does not include shouting *(which increases the pitch of the voice).*[3]

 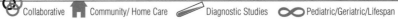

- Speak slowly and distinctly; use simple sentences. Avoid asking multiple questions at one time *to enhance client's comprehension and ability to respond.*
- Use touch to get the client's attention, if needed.
- Be aware/careful of facial expressions.
- Pay attention to background noise and reduce it to a minimum when attempting conversation. *Background noise is often amplified, causing misinterpretation of conversation/inability to hear words, and often resulting in overstimulation of senses.*[3]

Kinesthetic deficits:
- Provide tactile stimulation as care is given, and when communicating with client (respecting cultural and personal preferences). *Communicates presence/connection with other human being, because touching is an important part of caring, and the need for touch is a deep psychological need.*
- Be aware that older clients may be more interested in touching *because they have lost loved ones, their appearance may not be attractive as it once was, and the attitude of the public toward older adults does not encourage physical contact with them.*[3]
- Stimulate sense of touch (e.g., give client objects to touch, grasp; have client practice touching walls/other boundaries). *Aids in retraining sensory pathways to integrate reception and interpretation of stimuli.*[4]
- Provide touch, using level of appropriate intensity (e.g., light, moderate, deep, strong), *depending on the need (e.g., light touch to get client's attention, stroking to convey love to infant).*[3,5]
- Teach client/SO to frequently inspect skin and extremities for pressure points/skin trauma *when client is unable to sense pain and prone to tissue injury.*[4,6]

Taste and smell:
- Be aware that taste and smell dysfunction (loss or distortion of function) is associated with many chronic conditions (e.g., cystic fibrosis, chronic sinusitis, hypothyroidism, MS, Alzheimer's disease, head trauma) or may suggest a new/developing problem (e.g., zinc deficiency, dental conditions, allergies).[7]
- Evaluate client's medications *if reporting changes in tastes of foods (foods taste or smell odd), ability to salivate, or loss of appetite.*[3,8]
- Encourage variety of food colors and textures, flavor enhancers (in addition to good chewing) *to maximize taste sensation.*[3,8]
- Assist client in observing for offensive or dangerous odors (e.g., body odor, spoiled foods, or propane gas or smoke) *if sense of smell is diminished.*[3]
- Remove offensive odors from client's presence, especially *when client is immobile, debilitated, and/or suffering from oversensitivity to odors, nausea or vomiting.*[4]

NURSING PRIORITY NO. 3. To prevent injury/complications:

- Place call bell within reach and be sure client knows where it is/how to use it.
- Provide safety measures (e.g., side rails, bed in low position, furniture always in same place, door left closed or open consistently, ambulate with assistance).
- Protect from thermal injury (e.g., monitor bath water temperature, use of heating pads/lights, ice packs).
- Position doors, rugs, and furniture so they are out of travel path, or strategically place items/grab bars.
- Ambulate with assistance/devices *to enhance balance.*
- Describe where affected body parts are when moving the client.

- Monitor drug regimen postsurgically (e.g., antiemetics, miotics, sympathomimetics, β-blockers) *to prevent increase in or to reduce intraocular pressure.*
- Refer to NDs risk for Injury, risk for Trauma.

NURSING PRIORITY NO. 4. To promote wellness (Teaching/Discharge Considerations):

- Assist client/SO(s) *to learn effective ways of coping with and managing sensory disturbances, anticipating safety needs according to client's sensory deficits and developmental level.*
- Identify alternative ways of dealing with perceptual deficits (e.g., compensation techniques).
- Provide explanations of and plan care with client/SO(s). *Enhances commitment to and continuation of plan, optimizing outcomes.*
- Review home safety measures pertinent to deficits.
- Discuss drug regimen, noting possible toxic side effects of both prescription and OTC drugs. *Prompt recognition of side effects allows for timely intervention/change in drug regimen.*
- Demonstrate use/care of sensory prosthetic devices. Identify resources/community programs for acquiring and maintaining devices.
- Promote meaningful socialization. Refer to ND Social Isolation.
- Encourage out-of-bed/out-of-room/home activities as appropriate.
- Refer to helping resources such as Society for the Blind, Self-Help for the Hard of Hearing (SHHH), or local support groups, screening programs, etc., as indicated.
- Refer to additional NDs Anxiety, disturbed Thought Processes, Unilateral Neglect, acute/chronic Confusion, as appropriate.

DOCUMENTATION FOCUS

Assessment/Reassessment
- Individual findings, noting specific deficit/associated symptoms, perceptions of client/SO(s).
- Assistive device needs.

Planning
- Plan of care including who is involved in planning.
- Teaching plan.

Implementation/Evaluation
- Responses to interventions/teaching and actions performed.
- Attainment/progress toward desired outcome(s).
- Modifications to plan of care.

Discharge Planning
- Long-term needs and who is responsible for actions to be taken.
- Available resources; specific referrals made.

References

1. ND: Sensory Perception, disturbed. In Cox, H.C, et al. (2002). *Clinical Applications of Nursing Diagnosis: Adult, Child, Women's, Psychiatric, Gerontic, and Home Health Considerations,* ed 4. Philadelphia: F. A. Davis, pp 431–438.

 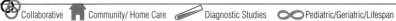

2. Engel, J. (2002). Pocket Guide To Pediatric Assessment, ed 4. St. Louis: Mosby.
3. Gallman, L., & Elfervig, L. S. The aging sensory system. In Stanley, M., & Beare, P. G. (1995). Gerontological Nursing: A Health Promotion/Protection Approach, ed 2. Philadelphia: F. A. Davis, pp 93–101.
4. NDs: Sensory Perception, disturbed (specify). In Doenges, M. E., Moorhouse, M. F., & Geissler-Murr, A. C. (2002). Nursing Care Plans: Guidelines for Individualizing Patient Care, ed 6. Philadelphia: F. A. Davis, pp 236, 272, 395, 773, 789.
5. Infant and family-centered developmental care. (2000). National Association of Neonatal Nurses. Available at: http://www.guideline.gov. Accessed January 2004.
6. Mayfield, J. A., et al. (1998). Preventative foot care in people with diabetes (Technical Review). Diabetes Care, 21:2161–2177.
7. Henkin, R. I. Taste and Smell Clinic Research and Clinical Overview. Available at: http://tasteandsmell.com. Accessed January 2004.
8. Glezos, S. P. Taste and smell loss: Risk for disease? Seminar presentation for the NIH Office of Behavioral and Social Sciences Research (OBSSR). Available at: http://obssr.od.nih.gob. Accessed January 2004.

Sexual Dysfunction

Definition: Change in sexual function that is viewed as unsatisfying, unrewarding, inadequate

RELATED FACTORS

Biopsychosocial alteration of sexuality:
Ineffectual or absent role models; lack of SO
Vulnerability
Misinformation or lack of knowledge
Physical abuse; psychosocial abuse (e.g., harmful relationships)
Values conflict
Lack of privacy
Altered body structure or function (pregnancy, recent childbirth, drugs, surgery, anomalies, disease process, trauma, [paraplegia/quadriplegia], radiation, [effects of aging])

DEFINING CHARACTERISTICS

Subjective

Verbalization of problem [e.g., loss of sexual desire, disruption of sexual response patterns such as premature ejaculation, dyspareunia, vaginismus]
Actual or perceived limitation imposed by disease and/or therapy
Inability to achieve desired satisfaction
Alterations in achieving perceived sex role
Conflicts involving values
Alterations in achieving sexual satisfaction
Seeking confirmation of desirability

Objective

Alteration in relationship with SO
Change of interest in self and others

SAMPLE CLINICAL APPLICATIONS: arthritis, cancer, major surgery, heart disease, hypertension, diabetes mellitus, spinal cord injury, traumatic injury, pregnancy/childbirth, abuse, depression

Sample **NOC** linkages:

Sexual Functioning: Integration of physical, socioemotional and intellectual aspects of sexual expression

Physical Aging Status: Physical changes that commonly occur with adult aging

Abuse Recovery: Sexual: Healing following sexual abuse or exploitation

Client Will (Include Specific Time Frame)

- Verbalize understanding of sexual anatomy/function and alterations that may affect function.
- Verbalize understanding of individual reasons for sexual problems.
- Identify stressors in lifestyle that may contribute to the dysfunction.
- Identify satisfying/acceptable sexual practices and some alternative ways of dealing with sexual expression.
- Discuss concerns about body image, sex role, desirability as a sexual partner with partner/SO.

ACTIONS/INTERVENTIONS

Sample **NIC** linkages:

Sexual Counseling: Use of an interactive helping process focusing on the need to make adjustments to sexual practice or to coping with a sexual event/disorder

Teaching: Sexuality: Assisting individuals to understand physical and psychosocial dimensions of sexual growth and development

Values Clarification: Assisting another to clarify her/his own values in order to facilitate effective decision making

NURSING PRIORITY NO. **1.** To assess causative/contributing factors:

 • Obtain sexual history including usual pattern of functioning and level of desire. *Establishes a database from which a plan of care can be formulated.*[1]

 • Note vocabulary and style of communication used by the individual/SO. Maximizes communication/understanding *of words and meaning in an area that individual may find difficult to discuss. Knowing that male and female brains are organized differently may help with recognizing different styles of communication.*[4]

 • Have client describe problem in own words. *Client's perception of the problem may differ from the care-giver's and plan of care needs to be based on client's perceptions for maximum effectiveness.*[1]

 • Determine importance of sex to individual/partner and client's motivation for change. *Both individuals may have differing levels of desire and expectations that may create conflict in relationship.*[3]

 • Be alert to comments of client as sexual concerns are often disguised as humor, sarcasm, and/or offhand remarks. *Many people are uncomfortable talking about sexual issues but want to discuss them with a caregiver, so they use this method to bring up the subject. It is important for the caregiver to recognize and acknowledge client's concern.*[2]

 • Assess knowledge of client/SO regarding sexual anatomy/function and effects of current situation/condition. *Basic knowledge is essential for understanding the problem and how it is affecting the individual. Lack of knowledge may be contributing to the problem(s).*[3]

 • Determine preexisting problems/conditions that may be factors in current situation.

 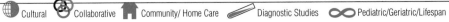 Cultural   Collaborative   Community/ Home Care   Diagnostic Studies   Pediatric/Geriatric/Lifespan   Medications

Physical conditions such as recent myocardial infarction, chronic conditions (e.g., arthritis, MS, hypertension, diabetes mellitus), fatigue may be contributing to sexual problems.[3]

- Identify current stress factors in individual situation (e.g., *marital/job stress, role conflicts*). *These factors may be producing enough anxiety to cause depression or other psychological reaction(s) that would cause physiologic symptoms.*[5]

- Discuss cultural/religious value factors or conflicts present. *Client may feel guilt or shame and feel depressed about sexual difficulties because of belief that they conflict with what they learned in family of origin or in religious studies.*[2]

- Determine pathophysiology, illness/surgery/trauma involved, and impact on (perception of) individual/SO. *These conditions can directly affect sexual functioning, such as presence of a colostomy, or individual can believe that illness precludes sexual activity, such as heart surgery.*[7]

- Review medication regimen/drug use (prescription, OTC, illegal, alcohol) and cigarette use. *Antihypertensives may cause erectile dysfunction; MAO inhibitors and tricyclics can cause erection/ejaculation problems and anorgasmia in women; narcotics/alcohol produce impotence and inhibit orgasm; smoking creates vasoconstriction and may be a factor in erectile dysfunction. Evaluation of drug and individual response is important to determine accurate intervention.*[1]

- Observe behavior/stage of grieving when related to body changes or loss of a body part, (e.g., pregnancy, obesity, amputation, mastectomy). *A change in body image can affect how individual views body in many aspects, but particularly in the sensitive area of sexual functioning and indicates need for information and additional support.*[7]

- Assist with diagnostic studies to determine cause of erectile dysfunction. *More than half of the cases have a physical cause such as diabetes, vascular problems, and so on.* Monitor penile tumescence during REM sleep *to determine physical ability.*[8]

- Explore with client the meaning of client's behavior. *Masturbation, for instance, may have many meanings/purposes, such as for relief of anxiety, sexual deprivation, pleasure, a nonverbal expression of need to talk, a way of alienating.*[3] *Or client's inhibitions may be decreased by changes in cognition.*[12]

- Avoid making value judgments. *They do not help the client to cope with the situation. Nurse needs to be aware of and be in control of own feelings and response to client expressions and/or concerns. Client needs to be free to express concerns in whatever way is comfortable to individual.*[3] *And even clients with limited cognition have a right to engage in intimate behaviors.*[12]

NURSING PRIORITY NO. 2. To assist client/SO(s) to deal with individual situation:

- Establish therapeutic nurse-client relationship. *Promotes treatment and facilitates sharing of sensitive information/feelings in a safe environment.*[1]

- Assist with treatment of underlying medical conditions, including changes in medication regimen, weight management, cessation of smoking, and so forth. *Many conditions (e.g., cardiovascular, diabetes, arthritis) can affect sexual functioning, as well as medication side-effects which may affect sexual ability.*[7]

- Provide factual information about individual condition involved. *Accurate information helps client make informed decisions about own situation.*[2]

- Determine what client wants to know to tailor information to client needs. *Providing too much information may be overwhelming and result in client not remembering something that is essential. Information affecting client safety/consequences of actions may need to be reviewed/reinforced.*[9]

Encourage and accept expressions of concern, anger, grief, fear. *Individuals need to be free to express these feelings and be accepted so they can begin to deal with situation and move on in a positive way.*[6]

 Assist client to be aware/deal with stages of grieving for loss/change. *Sexual dysfunction is often a result of losses such as breast cancer treatment, prostate surgery, and need to be addressed in the context of the whole. Healthcare providers need to be willing to help client understand grieving issues.*[2]

 Encourage client to share thoughts/concerns with partner and to clarify values/impact of condition on relationship. *Helps to identify issues in the relationship that may be related to the sexual dysfunction.*[11]

 Provide for/identify ways to obtain privacy to allow for sexual expression for individual and/or between partners without embarrassment and/or objections of others. *Often caregivers do not think about the importance of providing this basic need for couples, but in any setting privacy may be difficult to provide unless it is thought about and planned for.*[6]

 Discuss client's rights regarding intimacy in residential/extended care settings with SO/family. Review appropriateness of home visists or provision for privacy for intimate contact. *Family members may not realize that the need for sexual expression is not limited by advancing age, declining cognition, or marital status. And, they may be unaware that client has a right to engage in intimate behaviors.*[12]

 Assist client/SO(s) to problem-solve alternative ways of sexual expression. *When illness/condition, such as arthritis, paraplegia interfere with a couple's usual sexual activities, couple needs to learn new ways to achieve satisfaction.*[3]

Provide information about availability of corrective measures including medication, such as papaverine or sildenafil (Viagra), or Levitra for erectile dysfunction, reconstructive surgery (e.g., penile/breast implants), or sensate focus exercises, when indicated. *Sexual problems, such as erectile dysfunction, female orgasmic disorders, female sexual arousal disorders may respond to these interventions providing more satisfactory sexual life.*[8,10]

Refer to appropriate resources as need indicates (e.g., healthcare coworker with greater comfort level and/or knowledge clinical nurse specialist or professional sex therapist, family counseling). *Not all professionals are knowledgeable or comfortable dealing with sexual issues, and referrals to more appropriate resources can provide client/couple with accurate and appropriate help.*[2]

NURSING PRIORITY NO. 3. To promote wellness (Teaching/Discharge Considerations):

 Provide sex education, explanation of normal sexual functioning when necessary. *Many individuals are not knowledgeable about these areas and often providing accurate information can help assuage anxiety about unknowns, such as normal changes of aging, or provide an accurate basis for understanding problems being experienced.*[6]

 Provide written material appropriate to individual needs. Include bibliotherapy or Internet resources related to client's needs. *Provides reinforcement for client to read/access at his or her leisure, when ready to deal with sensitive materials.*[6]

 Encourage ongoing dialogue and take advantage of teachable moments that occur. *Within a therapeutic relationship, comfort is achieved and individual is encouraged to ask questions and be receptive to continuing conversation about sexual issues.*[1]

 Demonstrate and assist client to learn relaxation and/or visualization techniques. *Stress is often a component of sexual dysfunction and using these skills can help with resolution of problems.*[2]

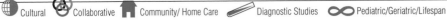 Cultural Collaborative Community/ Home Care Diagnostic Studies Pediatric/Geriatric/Lifespan Medications

- Identify resources for assistive devices/sexual "aids." *These aids can enhance sex life of couple and prevent/help with problems of dysfunction.*[3]
- Assist client to learn regular self-examination as indicated (e.g., breast/testicular examinations). *Encourages client to participate in own health prevention activities, become more aware of potential problems, and become more comfortable with sexual self.*[3,5]
- Identify community resources for further assistance, such as Reach for Recovery, CanSurmount, Ostomy Association.
- Refer for further professional assistance concerning relationship difficulties, low sexual desire/other sexual concerns, such as premature ejaculation, vaginismus, painful intercourse. *May need additional/continuing help to deal with individual situation.*[3]

DOCUMENTATION FOCUS

Assessment/Reassessment
- Individual findings including nature of dysfunction, predisposing factors, perceived effect on sexuality/relationships.
- Response of SO(s).
- Motivation for change.

Planning
- Plan of care and who is involved in planning.
- Teaching plan.

Implementation/Evaluation
- Response to interventions/teaching and actions performed.
- Attainment/progress toward desired outcome(s).
- Modifications to plan of care.

Discharge Planning
- Long-term needs/referrals and who is responsible for actions to be taken.
- Community resources, specific referrals made.

References

1. Townsend, M. C. (2003). Psychiatric Mental Health Nursing Concepts of Care, ed 4. Philadelphia: F. A. Davis.
2. Doenges, M. E., Townsend, M. C., & Moorhouse, M. F. (1998). Psychiatric Care Plans Guidelines for Individualizing Care, ed 3. Philadelphia: F. A. Davis.
3. Hyde, J., & DeLamater, J. (2002). Understanding Human Sexuality, ed 7. New York: McGraw-Hill.
4. Moir, A., & Jessel, D. (1991). Brain Sex, the Real Difference Between Men & Women. New York: Dell.
5. New Our Bodies, Ourselves: Boston Women's Health Staff. (1998). Boston: Smith, Peta.
6. Sexuality in Midlife and Beyond: A Special Health Report (2003). Harvard Medical School.
7. Stanley, M., & Beare, P. G. (1999). Gerontological Nursing, ed 2. Philadelphia: F. A. Davis.
8. Carver, C. (1998). Premature ejaculation: a common and treatable concern. J Am Psy Nurs Assoc, 4(6), 199–204.
9. McEnany, G. (1998). Sexual dysfunction in the pharmacologic treatment of depression: When "don't ask, don't tell" is an unsuitable approach to care. J Am Psy Nurs Assoc, 4(1), 24–29.
10. Phillips, N. A. (2000). Female sexual dysfunction: Evaluation and treatment. Am Family Phys, 62(1), 127–136, 141–142.
11. Cox, H. C., et al. (2002). Clinical Applications of Nursing Diagnosis: Adult, Child, Women's, Psychiatric, Gerontic and Home Health Considerations, ed 4. Philadelphia: F. A. Davis.
12. Sexuality in the nursing home (1997). The Legal Center for People with Disabilities and Older People.

ineffective Sexuality Patterns

Definition: Expressions of concern regarding own sexuality

RELATED FACTORS

Knowledge/skill deficit about alternative responses to health-related transitions, altered body function or structure, illness or medical treatment

Lack of privacy

Impaired relationship with a SO; lack of SO

Ineffective or absent role models

Conflicts with sexual orientation or variant preferences

Fear of pregnancy or of acquiring a sexually transmitted disease

DEFINING CHARACTERISTICS

Subjective

Reported difficulties, limitations, or changes in sexual behaviors or activities

[Expressions of feeling alienated, lonely, loss, powerless, angry]

SAMPLE CLINICAL APPLICATIONS: spinal cord injury, brain injury/stroke, sexually transmitted disease, cancer, mastectomy, hysterectomy, menopause, prostatectomy, gender reassignment

DESIRED OUTCOMES/EVALUATION CRITERIA

Sample **NOC** linkages:

Sexual Identity: Acceptance: Acknowledgment and acceptance of own sexual identity

Child Development: Adolescent: Milestones of physical, cognitive, and psychosocial progression between 12 and 17 years of age

Role Performance: Congruence of an individual's role behavior with role expectations

Client Will (Include Specific Time Frame)

- Verbalize understanding of sexual anatomy and function.
- Verbalize knowledge and understanding of sexual limitations, difficulties, or changes that have occurred.
- Verbalize acceptance of self in current (altered) condition.
- Demonstrate improved communication and relationship skills.
- Identify individually appropriate method of contraception.

ACTIONS/INTERVENTIONS

Sample **NIC** linkages:

Sexual Counseling: Use of an interactive helping process focusing on the need to make adjustments to sexual practice or to coping with a sexual event/disorder

Teaching: Sexuality: Assisting individuals to understand physical and psychosocial dimensions of sexual growth and development

Teaching: Safe Sex: Providing instruction concerning sexual protection during sexual activity

Support System Enhancement: Facilitation of support to patient by family, friends, and community

 Cultural   Collaborative   Community/ Home Care Diagnostic Studies   Pediatric/Geriatric/Lifespan   Medications

NURSING PRIORITY NO. 1. To assess causative/contributing factors:

- Obtain sexual history, as indicated, including perception of normal function, use of vocabulary (*assessing basic knowledge*). Note comments/concerns about sexual identity, dissatisfaction with sexual pattern. *Information about client's perception of the problem is essential to planning appropriate care to meet client's needs.*[1]
- Determine importance of sex and a description of the problem in the client's own words. Be alert to comments of client/SO (e.g., discount of overt or covert sexual expressions such as "He's just a dirty old man"). *Sexual concerns are often disguised as sarcasm, humor, or in offhand remarks.*[1]
- Note cultural/religious value factors and conflicts that may exist. *These factors may create conflicts regarding variant sexual practices with resultant feelings of shame and guilt.*[3]
- Assess stress factors in client's environment that might cause anxiety or psychological reactions. *Sexual variant behaviors, power issues involving SO, adult children, aging, employment, loss of prowess related to illlness/condition are often associated with stress in the client's life.*[1]
- Explore knowledge of effects of altered body function/limitations precipitated by illness and/or medical treatment of alternative sexual responses and expressions (e.g., reassignment procedure). *Client needs to understand when conditions such as undescended testicle in young male, gender change, mutilating cancer surgery have an effect on sexuality.*[10]
- Review substance use history (prescription medication, OTC drugs, alcohol, and illicit drugs). *Substance/prescription drug use may affect sexual functioning, or be used to relieve anxiety of sexually deviant behavior.*[2]
- Explore issues and fears associated with sex. *Possibility of pregnancy, acquiring sexually transmitted diseases; trust/control issues, inflexible beliefs, preference confusion, altered performance need to be addressed so they may be solved.*[3]
- Determine client's interpretation of the altered sexual activity or behavior. *May be a way of controlling, provide relief of anxiety, pleasure, lack of partner. These behaviors, when related to body changes, including pregnancy or weight loss/gain, or loss of body part, may reflect a stage of grieving.*[3]
- Assess life-cycle issues, such as adolescence, young adulthood, menopause, aging. *Stages of maturation bring changes that affect sexual self, and understanding of the normalcy can help individual grow with them.*[3,7]
- Avoid value judgments. *They do not help the client to cope with the situation. Nurse needs to be aware of and in control of own feelings and responses to the client's expressions and/or concerns.*[9]

NURSING PRIORITY NO. 2. To assist client/SO to deal with individual situation:

- Provide atmosphere in which discussion of sexual problems is encouraged/permitted. *Sense of trust/comfort enhances ability to discuss sensitive matters and begin to resolve problems perceived by client.*[5]
- Provide information about individual situation, determining client needs and desires. *Lack of knowledge may contribute to current situation, and providing desired information conveys message of importance and self-responsibility.*[3]
- Encourage discussion of individual situation with opportunity for expression of feelings without judgment. *Provides opportunity for client to talk about variant sexual practices, concern about sexual identity and sexual issues related to illness/condition and possibilities for resolution.*[2]

- Provide specific suggestions about interventions directed toward the identified problems. *Being specific about actions client can take, such as alternate sexual positions when arthritis prevents movement, masturbation when no partner is available, use of condoms when infection is a concern, positive discussion of normalcy of sexual behavior when identity is being questioned, can lead discussion in appropriate direction to provide solutions.*[3]
- Identify alternative forms of sexual expression that might be acceptable to both partners. *Being able to satisfactorily communicate with partner and identifying ways to achieve sexual satisfaction for both is important to the relationship.*[1]
- Discuss ways to manage individual devices/appliances. *Change in body image/medical condition may require the use of devices such as an ostomy bag, breast prostheses, a urinary collection device which may affect how client views sexual activity. Providing information about ways to deal with these issues helps client to refocus attention on achieving satisfactory sexual experience.*[6]
- Discuss use of performance enhancing medications, such as sidenafil citrate (Viagra), Levitra, cialis. *Erectile dysfunction is a common occurrence as men age, and while frequently caused by an underlying physical illness/prescribed medication, psychological issues often accompany this problem. While an accurate diagnosis is necessary, there are many treatments available. Prescription drugs are popular, but the individual needs to feel desire and be sexually stimulated for them to work.*[6]
- Determine concerns of older client regarding sexuality. *Myths abound regarding sexual activity as people grow older, and individual may believe he or she is no longer attractive or a satisfying sex life is no longer possible and accurate information can correct misperceptions.*[6]
- Provide anticipatory guidance about losses that are to be expected. *Surgical procedures resulting in a major change in body image, whether planned as in transsexual surgery, or unplanned as in emergency bowel resection with resultant colostomy, or traumatic amputation, result in a loss of known self, which needs specific intervention to deal with change.*[9]
- Introduce client to individuals who have successfully managed a similar problem, when possible. *Provides a positive role model and support for problem solving.*[9]

NURSING PRIORITY NO. 3. To promote wellness (Teaching/Discharge Considerations):

- Provide factual information about problem(s) as identified by the client. *Specific facts about individual situation will provide client with knowledge needed to deal with what is happening, such as conflict with sexual orientation or variant preferences or impaired relationship with SO.*[9]
- Engage in ongoing dialogue with the client and SO(s) as situation permits. *As communication continues, new insights arise and understanding is enhanced.*[2,4]
- Discuss methods/effectiveness/side effects of contraceptives if indicated. *It is important to provide specific information for the individual to meet needs and desires to plan for and/or prevent pregnancy.*[1]
- Refer to community resources as indicated. *May need additional information and support that can be obtained at resources such as planned parenthood, gender identity clinic, social services, others.*[8,9]
- Refer for intensive individual/group psychotherapy, which may be combined with couple/family and/or sex therapy, as appropriate.
- Refer to NDs Sexual Dysfunction, disturbed Body Image, Self-Esteem (specify).

 Cultural Collaborative Community/ Home Care Diagnostic Studies 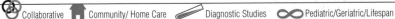 Pediatric/Geriatric/Lifespan Medications

Assessment/Reassessment

- Individual findings, including nature of concern, perceived difficulties/limitations or changes, specific needs/desires.
- Response of SO(s).

Planning

- Plan of care and who is involved in the planning.
- Teaching plan.

Implementation/Evaluation

- Response to interventions/teaching and actions performed.
- Attainment/progress toward desired outcome(s).
- Modifications to plan of care.

Discharge Planning

- Long-term needs/teaching and referrals and who is responsible for actions to be taken.
- Community resources, specific referrals made.

References

1. Townsend, M. C. (2003). Psychiatric Mental Health Nursing Concepts of Care, ed 4. Philadelphia: F. A. Davis.
2. Doenges, M. E., Townsend, M. C., & Moorhouse, M. F. (1998). Psychiatric Care Plans Guidelines for Individualizing Care, ed 3. Philadelphia: F. A. Davis.
3. Hyde, J., & DeLamater, J. (2002). Understanding Human Sexuality, ed 7. New York: McGraw-Hill.
4. Moir, A., & Jessel, D. (1991). Brain Sex: the Real Difference Between Men & Women. New York: Dell.
5. New Our Bodies, Ourselves: Boston Women's Health Staff. (1998). Boston: Smith, Peta.
6. Sexuality in Midlife and Beyond: A Special Health Report. (2003). Harvard Medical School.
7. Stanley, M., & Beare, P. G. Gerontological Nursing, ed 2. Philadelphia: F. A. Davis.
8. Saunders, P., & Pickering, R. (1997). The causes of homosexuality. Available at: http://www.cmf.org.uk/index.htm?pubs/pubs.htm. Accessed March 2002.
9. Becker, J. V., Johnson, B. R., & Kavoussi, R. J. (1999). Sexual and gender identity disorders. In Hales, R. E., & Yudofsky, S. C. (Eds). (1999). Essentials of Clinical Psychiatry. Washington, DC: American Psychiatric Press.
10. Bell, R. (1998). Changing Bodies, Changing Lives, ed 3. New York: Random House.

impaired Skin Integrity

Definition: Altered epidermis and/or dermis [The integumentary system is the largest multifunctional organ of the body.]

RELATED FACTORS

External

Hyperthermia or hypothermia

Chemical substance; radiation; medications

Physical immobilization

Humidity; moisture; [excretions/secretions]

Altered fluid status

Mechanical factors (e.g., shearing forces, pressure, restraint), [trauma: injury/surgery]

Extremes in age

Internal

Altered nutritional state (e.g., obesity, emaciation); metabolic state; fluid status
Skeletal prominence; alterations in turgor (change in elasticity); [presence of edema]
Altered circulation; sensation; pigmentation
Developmental factors
Immunologic deficit
[Psychogenic]

DEFINING CHARACTERISTICS

Subjective

[Reports of itching, pain, numbness of affected/surrounding area]

Objective

Disruption of skin surface (epidermis)
Destruction of skin layers (dermis)
Invasion of body structures

SAMPLE CLINICAL APPLICATIONS: arteriosclerosis, venous insufficiency, hypertension, obesity, diabetes mellitus, malignant neoplasms, traumatic injury, surgery, chronic steroid use (e.g., COPD, asthma), renal failure, burns, radiation therapy, malnutrition

DESIRED OUTCOMES/EVALUATION CRITERIA

Sample **NOC** linkages:

Tissue Integrity: Skin & Mucous Membranes: Structural intactness and normal physiologic function of skin and mucous membranes

Wound Healing: Primary Intention: The extent to which cells and tissues have regenerated following intentional closure

Wound Healing: Secondary Intention: The extent to which cells and tissues in an open wound have regenerated

Client Will (Include Specific Time Frame)

- Display timely healing of skin lesions/wounds/pressure sores without complication.
- Maintain optimal nutrition/physical well-being.
- Participate in prevention measures and treatment program.
- Verbalize feelings of increased self-esteem and ability to manage situation.

ACTIONS/INTERVENTIONS

Sample **NIC** linkages:

Wound Care: Prevention of wound complications and promotion of wound healing

Incision Site Care: Cleansing, monitoring, and promotion of healing in a wound that is closed with sutures, clips, or staples

Pressure Ulcer Care: Facilitation of healing in pressure ulcers

NURSING PRIORITY NO. 1. To assess causative/contributing factors:

 • Identify underlying condition/pathology involved. *Skin integrity problems can be the result of 1) **disease processes** that affect circulation and perfusion of vital organs/tissues (e.g., arteriosclerosis, venous insufficiency, hypertension, obesity, diabetes, malignant neoplasms); 2) **medications** (e.g., anticoagulants, corticosteroids, immunosuppressives, antineoplastics) that adversely affect/impair healing; 3) **burns/radiation** (can break down internal tissues as well*

 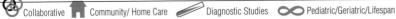

as skin); and 4) **nutrition and hydration** (e.g., malnutrition deprives the body of protein and calories required for cell growth and repair, and dehydration impairs transport of oxygen and nutrients). Disruption in skin integrity can be **intentional** (e.g., surgical incision) or **unintentional** (accidental), and **closed** (e.g., contusion, abrasion, rash) or **open** (e.g., laceration, penetrating wound, ulcerations).[1,2]

- Note general health. *Many factors (e.g., debilitation, immobility, restraints, extremes of age, mental status, dehydration or malnutrition, presence of chronic disease; occupational, treatment, and environmental hazards) can all affect the ability of the skin to perform its functions (e.g., protection, sensation, movement and growth, chemical synthesis, immunity, thermoregulation and excretion).*[3,4]

- Determine client's age and developmental factors/ability to care for self. *Newborn/infant's skin is thin, provides ineffective thermal regulation and nails are thin.*[5] *Babies and children are prone to skin rashes associated with viral, bacterial and fungal infections and allergic reactions. In adolescence, hormones stimulate hair growth and sebaceous gland activity. In adults, it takes longer to replenish epidermis cells, resulting in increased risk of skin cancers and infection. In older adults there is decreased epidermal regeneration, fewer sweat glands, less subcutaneous fat, elastin and collagen, causing skin to become thinner, drier and less responsive to pain sensations.*[1,3,4,6,7]

- Evaluate client's skin care practices and hygiene issues. *Individual's skin may be oily, dry or sensitive, and is affected by bathing frequency (or lack of bathing), temperature of water, types of soap and other cleansing agents. Incontinence (urinary or bowel) and ineffective hygiene can result in serious skin impairment and discomfort.*

- Ascertain allergy history. *Individual may be sensitive or allergic to substances (e.g., insects, grasses, medications, lotions, soaps, foods) that can adversely affect the skin.*

- Inspect skin frequently and palpate during inspection, observing for color, temperature, surface changes, texture and contours. *Systematic inspection can identify impending problems early.*[8]

- Note distribution and scarcity of hair (e.g., loss of hair on lower legs may indicate peripheral vascular disease). (Refer to ND risk for Peripheral Vascular Dysfunction for additional interventions.)

- Assess blood supply (e.g., capillary return time, color and warmth) and sensation of skin surfaces/affected area on a regular basis *to provide comparative baseline and opportunity for timely intervention when problems are noted.*[3,9]

- Evaluate skin color changes in sclera, conjunctiva, nail beds, buccal mucosa, tongue, palms, and soles of feet (areas of least pigmentation).

- Determine areas at risk for injury *because of immobility and/or malnutrition (e.g., pressure points on emaciated and/or elderly client).*

- Note character and color of drainage, when present (e.g., blood, bile, pus, stoma effluent) *which can cause skin irritation/excoriation.*

- Review laboratory results *to evaluate causative factors and/or ability to heal.*

NURSING PRIORITY NO. 2. To assess extent of involvement/injury:

- Obtain a complete history of condition (especially in children where recurrent rash/lesions are common) including age at onset, date of first episode, how long it lasted, original site, characteristics of lesions, and any changes that have occurred. *Common skin manifestations of sensitivity/allergies are hives, eczema, and contact dermatitis. Contagious rashes include measles, rubella, roseola, chickenpox and scarlet fever. Bacterial, viral and fungal infections can also cause skin problems (e.g., impetigo, cellulitis, cold sores, shingles, athlete's foot and candidiasis diaper rashes).*[6]

- Determine anatomic location and depth of injury/damage when wounds are present (e.g., epidermis, dermis, and/or underlying issues) and describe as partial or full-thickness injuries *to provide baseline/document changes.*[3,10]
- Inspect skin surrounding IV/invasive line insertion site *for infiltration (swelling, erythema, coolness and pain, failure of infusion) or evidence of extravasation (e.g., blistering, blanching, skin sloughing).*[4]
- Evaluate skin surrounding restraints (when used), noting any abrasions, contusions, skin breaks, or skin color/temperature changes distal to restraints *suggesting impaired circulation.*
- Monitor periodic laboratory studies (e.g., CBC, serum albumen, transferrin and proteins, wound culture/sensitivities) *reflecting general well-being and status of specific problem.*[1]

NURSING PRIORITY NO. 3. To determine impact of condition:

- Determine if wound is **acute** (e.g., injury from surgery or trauma) or **chronic** (e.g., venous/arterial insufficiency, *which affects healing time and the client's emotional and physical responses. For example an acute and noninfected wound can heal in about 4 weeks, while a chronic wound often does not progress through phases of healing in an orderly or timely fashion.*[10]
- Determine client's level of discomfort (e.g., can vary widely from minor itching or aching, to deep pain with burns, or excoriation associated with drainage) *to clarify intervention needs and priorities.*
- Ascertain attitudes of individual/SO(s) about condition (e.g., cultural values, stigma). Obtain psychological assessment of client's emotional status, noting potential or sexual problems arising from presence of condition. *The healthy wholeness and beauty of skin impacts the client's body image and self-esteem. Lesions and/or wounds that disfigure can be especially devastating.*
- Note presence of compromised vision, hearing, or speech *that may impact client's self-care as relates to skin care (e.g., diabetic with impaired vision probably cannot satisfactorily examine own feet).*[11]

NURSING PRIORITY NO. 4. To assist client with correcting/minimizing condition[3,4,7,9,12,13]:

- Inspect skin on a daily basis (especially over bony prominences) describing changes observed *to allow for early intervention.*
- Practice and instruct client/caregiver(s) in scrupulous hand washing and clean or sterile technique *to reduce incidence of contamination and/or infection.*
- Maintain/instruct in good skin hygiene (e.g., wash thoroughly, pat dry, gently massage with lotion or appropriate cream) *to provide barrier to infection, reduce risk of dermal trauma, improve circulation, and enhance comfort.*
- Encourage/maintain mobility, activity and range-of-motion *to enhance circulation and promote health of skin and other organs.*
- Cleanse skin after incontinent or diaphoretic episodes *to restore normal skin pH and flora and limit potential for infection.*
- Avoid products containing perfumes, dyes, preservatives *(may cause dermatitis reactions)* or alcohol, povidone-iodine, hydrogen peroxide *(may hinder wound healing).*
- Avoid use of latex products *when client has known or suspected sensitivity.* (Refer to ND latex Allergy Response.)
- Limit lengthy/unnecessary sun exposure, use high SPF sun block, avoid use of tanning beds.

 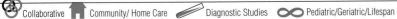

- Use proper turning/transfer techniques. Avoid movements *that cause friction/shearing (e.g., pulling client with parallel force, dragging movements, etc.).*
- Provide foam/flotation/alternating pressure/air mattress *to reduce pressure on skin/tissues and lesions, decreasing tissue ischemia.*
- Use appropriate padding devices (e.g., air/water mattress, egg crate, heel boots, sheepskin) when indicated *to reduce pressure on/enhance circulation to compromised tissues.*
- Encourage early ambulation/mobilization. *Promotes circulation and reduces risks associated with immobility.*
- Limit/avoid use of plastic material (e.g., rubber sheet, plastic-backed linen savers), and remove wet/wrinkled linens promptly. *Moisture potentiates skin breakdown and increases risk for infection.*
- Develop regularly timed repositioning schedule for client with mobility and sensation impairments, using turn sheet as needed; encourage/assist with periodic weight shifts for client in chair *to reduce stress on pressure points and encourage circulation to tissues.*
- Encourage optimum nutrition (including adequate protein, lipids, calories, trace minerals and multivitamins) *to promote skin health/healing and to maintain general good health.*
- Provide/encourage adequate hydration (oral, tube feeding, IV, ambient room humidity, etc.) *to reduce/replenish transepidermal water loss.*
- Instruct client with sensation impairments *in care of skin/extremities during cold or hot weather (e.g., wearing gloves, boots, clean/dry socks, properly fitting shoes/boots, face protection, etc.).*
- Apply hot and cold applications judiciously *to reduce risk of dermal injury in persons with circulatory and neurosensory impairments.*

NURSING PRIORITY NO. 5. To promote optimal healing[1,9,12,13]:

- Assess wound(s) and document for 1) dimensions and depth in centimeters; 2) exudates—color, odor, and amount; 3) margins—fixed or unfixed; 4) tunneling/tracts; 5) evidence of necrosis (e.g., color gray to black) or healing (e.g., pink/red granulation tissue) *to establish comparative baseline/evaluate effectiveness of interventions.*
- Classify pressure ulcer(s) using tool such as Waterlow, Braden, Norton (or similar) Ulcer Classification System. *Provides consistent terminology for assessment and documentation of pressure sores.*
- Photograph lesion(s) as appropriate *to document status/provide visual baseline for future comparisons.*
- Remeasure wound(s) regularly and periodically photograph, and observe incisions/wounds for complications *to monitor progress/failure of healing.*
- Keep surgical area(s) clean/dry; carefully dress wounds; support incision (e.g., use of Steri-Strips, splinting when coughing) and stimulate circulation to surrounding areas *to assist body's natural process of repair.*
- Use appropriate barrier dressings or wound coverings (e.g., semipermeable, occlusive, wet-to-damp, hydrocolloid, hydrogel), drainage appliances, and skin-protective agents for open/draining wounds and stomas *to protect the wound and/or surrounding tissues from excoriating secretions/drainage, and to promote wound healing.*
- Expose moist lesions to air and light (if indicated) *to assist with drying.*
- Assist with débridement/enzymatic therapy as indicated (e.g., burns, severe pressure ulcer).
- Use body-temperature physiologic solutions (e.g., isotonic saline) *to clean or irrigate wounds and prevent washout of electrolytes.*

- Cleanse wound with irrigation syringe or gauze squares, avoiding cotton balls or other products *that shed fibers.*
- Obtain specimen from purulent wounds when appropriate *for culture/sensitivities or Gram's stain to determine appropriate therapy.*
- Consult with wound specialist as indicated *to assist with developing plan of care for problematic or potentially serious wounds.*
- Apply/administer topical/systemic drugs as indicated *to treat skin lesions.*
- Cover open pressure ulcers with appropriate protective dressings (e.g., DuoDerm, Tegaderm, etc.) *to assist with wound débridement and promote healing.*
- Remove adhesive products with care, removing on horizontal plane, and using mineral oil or Vaseline for softening, if needed, *to prevent abrasions or tearing of skin.*
- Secure dressings with tape (e.g., elastic, paper, nonallergic) or Montgomery straps when frequent dressing changes are needed *to limit dermal injury.* Apply tape at center of surgical incision to outer margin of dressings.

NURSING PRIORITY NO. 6. To promote wellness (Teaching/Discharge Considerations):

- Review importance of skin and routine measures *to maintain proper skin functioning.*
- Discuss client's particular conditions (e.g., arteriosclerosis, obesity, diabetes), treatments (e.g., radiation) and medications (e.g., anticoagulants, corticosteroids, immunosuppressives) *that could affect skin health and wound healing.*
- Discuss importance of early detection and reporting to healthcare providers any skin changes and/or failure to heal *for timely evaluation and intervention.*
- Assist the client/SO(s) in understanding and following medical regimen and developing program of preventive care and daily maintenance. *Enhances commitment to plan, optimizing outcomes.*
- Review measures *to avoid spread/reinfection of communicable conditions.*
- Emphasize importance of proper fit of clothing/shoes, use of specially lined shock-absorbing socks or pressure-reducing insoles for shoes *to prevent injury to feet in presence of reduced sensation/circulation.*
- Identify safety factors for use of equipment/appliances (e.g., heating pad, ostomy appliances, padding straps of braces).
- Encourage client to verbalize feelings and discuss how/if condition affects self-concept/self-esteem. (Refer to NDs disturbed Body Image, situational low Self-Esteem.)
- Assist client to work through stages of grief and feelings associated with individual condition.
- Lend psychological support and acceptance of client, using touch, facial expressions, and tone of voice.
- Assist client to learn stress reduction and alternate therapy techniques *to control feelings of helplessness and enhance coping.*
- Refer to dietitian or certified diabetes educator as appropriate *to manage general well-being, enhance healing, reduce risk of recurrence of diabetic ulcers.*

DOCUMENTATION FOCUS

Assessment/Reassessment
- Characteristics of lesion(s)/condition, ulcer classification.
- Causative/contributing factors.
- Impact of condition.

 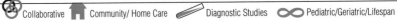

Planning
- Plan of care and who is involved in planning.
- Teaching plan.

Implementation/Evaluation
- Responses to interventions/teaching and actions performed.
- Attainment/progress toward desired outcome(s).
- Modifications to plan of care.

Discharge Planning
- Long-term needs/referrals and who is responsible for actions to be taken.
- Specific referrals made.

References

1. Llewellyn, S. (2002). Skin integrity and wound care, (Lecture materials) Chapel Hills, NC: Cape Fear Community College Nursing Program.
2. Colburn, L. (2001). Prevention for chronic wounds. In Krasner, D, Rodeheaver, G, & Sibbald, RG. Chronic Wound Care: A Clinical Source Book for Healthcare Professionals, ed 2. Wayne, PA: HMP Communications.
3. Calianno, C. (2002). Patient hygiene, part 2-Skin care: Keeping the outside healthy. Nursing, 32(6): June Clinical Supp.
4. Neonatal skin care. Evidence-based clinical practice guideline. (2001). Washington DC: Association of Women's Health, Obstetric and Neonatal Nurses (AWHONN). Available at: http://www.guideline.gov. Accessed September 2003.
5. McGovern, C. (2003). Skin, hair and nail assessment. Unit 2, (Lecture materials). Villanova, PA: Villanova University College of Nursing. Available at: http://www10homepage.villanova.edu/marycarol.mcgovern. Accessed February 2004.
6. Engel, J. (2002). Pocket Guide to Pediatric Assessment, ed 4. St. Louis: Mosby, pp 99–112.
7. Wiersema, L. A., & Stanley, M. The aging integumentary system. In Stanley, M., & Beare, P. G. (1999). Gerontological Nursing: A Health Promotion/Protection Approach, ed 2. Philadelphia: F. A. Davis, pp 102–111.
8. Krasner, D., Rodeheaver, G., & Sibbald, R. G. Advanced wound caring for a new millennium. In Krasner, D., Rodeheaver, G., & Sibbald, R. G. (2001). Chronic Wound Care: A Clinical Source Book for Healthcare Professionals, ed 2. Wayne, PA: HMP Communications.
9. ND: Skin Integrity, impaired. In Doenges, M. E., Moorhouse, M. F., & Geissler-Murr, A. C. (2002). Nursing Care Plans: Guidelines for Individualizing Patient Care, ed 6. Philadelphia: F. A. Davis.
10. Hahn, JF, et al. Wounds: Nursing care and product selection-Part 1, (CE offering). Nursing Spectrum. Available at: http://nsweb.nursingspectrum.com/ce/ce80.htm. Accessed September 2003.
11. Lawrance, D. P. DIABETES FYI-Foot Care, (Monograph 5 in series). Champaign, IL: University of Illinois, McKinley Diabetes Team.
12. McGovern, C. (2003). Skin integrity: Pressure ulcers, wounds and wound healing. Unit 3, (Lecture materials). Villanova, PA: Villanova University College of Nursing. Available at: http://www10homepage.villanova.edu/marycarol.mcgovern. Accessed February 2004.
13. No author listed. Risk factors and prevention. Geriatric Syndromes: Pressure Ulcers. Novartis Foundation for gerontology. Available at: http://geriatricsyllabus.com. Accessed February 2004.

risk for impaired Skin Integrity

Definition: At risk for skin being adversely altered; Note: Risk should be determined by the use of a risk assessment tool (e.g., Braden, Norton [or similar] Scale)

RISK FACTORS

External
Chemical substance; radiation
Hypothermia or hyperthermia

Physical immobilization
Excretions and/or secretions; humidity; moisture
Mechanical factors (e.g., shearing forces, pressure, restraint)
Extremes of age

Internal
Medication
Alterations in nutritional state (e.g., obesity, emaciation), metabolic state, [fluid status]
Skeletal prominence; alterations in skin turgor (change in elasticity); [presence of edema]
Altered circulation, sensation, pigmentation
Developmental factors
Psychogenic
Immunologic
NOTE: A risk diagnosis is not evidenced by signs and symptoms, as the problem has not occurred and nursing interventions are directed at prevention.
SAMPLE CLINICAL APPLICATIONS: arteriosclerosis, venous insufficiency, hypertension, obesity, diabetes mellitus, systemic lupus, malignant neoplasms, chronic steroid use (e.g., COPD, asthma), renal failure, malnutrition

DESIRED OUTCOMES/EVALUATION CRITERIA
Sample **NOC** linkages:
Risk Control: Actions to eliminate or reduce actual, personal, and modifiable health threats
Immobility Consequences: Physiologic: Extent of compromise to physiologic functioning due to impaired physical mobility
Tissue Integrity: Skin & Mucous Membranes: Structural intactness and normal physiologic function of skin and mucous membranes

---

Client Will (Include Specific Time Frame)
- Identify individual risk factors.
- Verbalize understanding of treatment/therapy regimen.
- Demonstrate behaviors/techniques to prevent skin breakdown.

ACTIONS/INTERVENTIONS
Sample **NIC** linkages:
Skin Surveillance: Collection and analysis of patient data to maintain skin and mucous membrane integrity
Pressure Management: Minimizing pressure to body parts
Pressure Ulcer Prevention: Prevention of pressure ulcers for a patient at high risk for developing them

NURSING PRIORITY NO. **1.** To assess causative/contributing factors:

- Note general health. *Many factors (e.g.,* debilitation, reduced mobility, changes in skin and muscle mass associated with aging, poor nutritional status, chronic diseases, incontinence and/or problems of self-care and/or medication/therapy *can all affect the ability of the skin to perform its functions (e.g., protection, sensation, movement and growth, chemical synthesis, immunity, thermoregulation and excretion).*[2,3]
- Note laboratory results pertinent to causative factors (e.g., Hg/Hct, blood glucose, albumin/total protein).
- Calculate ankle-brachial index as appropriate (diabetic clients or clients with impaired

circulation to lower extremities). *Result less than 0.9 is associated with peripheral arterial disease (among other conditions) and need for more aggressive preventive interventions to prevent skin/tissue ulcerations.*[1] Refer to ND risk for Peripheral Neurovascular Dysfunction for additional interventions, if indicated.

NURSING PRIORITY NO. 2. To maintain optimal skin integrity:[2–7]

- Inspect skin on a daily basis (especially over bony prominences), describing changes observed *to allow for early intervention.*
- Observe for reddened/blanched areas and institute treatment immediately. *Reduces likelihood of progression to skin breakdown.*
- Handle infant (especially premature infants) gently. *Epidermis of infants and very young children is thin and lacks subcutaneous depth that will develop with age.*
- Practice and instruct client/caregiver(s) in scrupulous hand washing and clean or sterile technique as appropriate *to reduce incidence of contamination and/or infection.*
- Maintain/instruct in good skin hygiene (e.g., wash thoroughly, pat dry, gently massage with lotion or appropriate cream) *to provide barrier to infection, reduce risk of dermal trauma, improve circulation, and promote comfort.*
- Cleanse skin after incontinent or diaphoretic episodes *to maintain normal skin pH and flora, and limit potential for infection.*
- Develop regularly timed repositioning schedule for client with mobility and sensation impairments, using turn sheet as needed; encourage/assist with periodic weight shifts for client in chair *to reduce stress on pressure points and encourage circulation to tissues.*
- Use proper turning/transfer techniques. *Avoids movements that cause friction/shearing (e.g., pulling client with parallel force, dragging movements, etc.).*
- Encourage/maintain mobility, activity and range-of-motion *to enhance circulation and promote health of skin and other organs.*
- Encourage early ambulation/mobilization. *Promotes circulation and reduces risks associated with immobility.*
- Provide for safety measures during ambulation and other therapies *to reduce risk of dermal injury (e.g., assistive devices and/or sufficient personnel; grab bars, clear pathways, safe chairs; properly fitting hose/footwear, use of heating pads/lamps, restraints).*
- Provide foam/flotation/alternating pressure/air mattress *to reduce pressure on skin/tissues and lesions, decreasing tissue ischemia.*
- Use appropriate padding devices (e.g., air/water mattress, egg crate, heel boots, sheepskin) when indicated *to reduce pressure on/enhance circulation to compromised tissues.*
- Limit/avoid use of plastic material (e.g., rubber sheet, plastic-backed linen savers), and remove wet/wrinkled linens promptly. *Moisture potentiates skin breakdown and increases risk for infection.*
- Avoid products containing perfumes, dyes, preservatives *(may cause dermatitis reactions)* or alcohol, povidone-iodine, hydrogen peroxide *(may hinder wound healing).*
- Avoid use of latex products *when client has known or suspected sensitivity.* Refer to ND latex Allergy Response.
- Limit lengthy/unnecessary sun exposure, use high SPF sun block, avoid use of tanning beds.
- Provide optimum nutrition (including adequate protein, lipids, calories, trace minerals and multivitamins) *to promote skin health/healing and to maintain general good health.*
- Provide/encourage adequate hydration (oral, tube feeding, IV, ambient room humidity, etc.) *to reduce/replenish transepidermal water loss.*
- Instruct in care of skin/extremities during cold or hot weather (e.g., wearing gloves, boots,

clean/dry socks, properly fitting shoes/boots, face protection) *to reduce risk of tissue damage especially in clients with impaired sensation.*

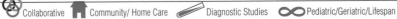

- Apply hot and cold applications judiciously *to reduce risk of dermal injury in persons with circulatory and neurosensory impairments.*
- Provide adequate clothing/covers; protect from drafts *to prevent vasoconstriction and reduction of circulation to skin.*
- Keep bedclothes dry, use nonirritating materials, and keep bed free of wrinkles, crumbs, etc. *to prevent skin irritation.*
- Keep nails cut short, encouraging client *to refrain from scratching.*
- Obtain order for mittens (considered a restraint) if necessary *to prevent dermal injury from scratching.*
- Refer to ND impaired Skin Integrity for additional interventions, as indicated.

NURSING PRIORITY NO. 3. To promote wellness (Teaching/Discharge Considerations):

- Provide information to client/SO(s) about the importance of regular observation and effective skin care *to prevent skin problems.*
- Emphasize importance of adequate nutritional/fluid intake *to maintain general good health and skin turgor.*
- Encourage continuation of regular exercise program (active/assistive) *to enhance circulation.*
- Recommend elevation of lower extremities when sitting *to enhance venous return and reduce edema formation.*
- Encourage restriction/abstinence from tobacco, *which can cause vasoconstriction.*
- Suggest use of ice, colloidal bath, and lotions *to decrease irritable itching.*
- Recommend keeping nails short or wearing gloves *to reduce risk of dermal injury when severe itching is present.*
- Discuss importance of avoiding exposure to sunlight in specific conditions (e.g., systemic lupus, tetracycline/psychotropic drug use, radiation therapy) as well as potential for development of skin cancer.
- Counsel diabetic and neurologically impaired client about importance of skin care, especially of lower extremities.
- Perform periodic assessment using a tool such as Braden Scale *to determine changes in risk status and need for alterations in the plan of care.*

DOCUMENTATION FOCUS

Assessment/Reassessment
- Individual findings, including individual risk factors.

Planning
- Plan of care and who is involved in planning.
- Teaching plan.

Implementation/Evaluation
- Responses to interventions/teaching and actions performed.
- Attainment/progress toward desired outcome(s).
- Modifications to plan of care.

 Cultural Collaborative Community/ Home Care Diagnostic Studies Pediatric/Geriatric/Lifespan Medications

Discharge Planning

- Long-term needs and who is responsible for actions to be taken.

References

1. Murabito, J. M., et al. (2003) The ankle-brachial index can predict the risk of stroke in the elder. Archives of Internal Medicine, September. Available at: http://www.colordohealthsite.org/CHNReports/ABIandstroke-elderly.html. Accessed February 2004.
2. Calianno, C. (2002). Patient hygiene, part 2-Skin care: Keeping the outside healthy. Nursing, 32(6), June Clinical Supp.
3. Neonatal skin care. Evidence-based clinical practice guideline. (2001). Washington DC: Association of Women's Health, Obstetric and Neonatal Nurses (AWHONN). Available at: http://www.guideline.gov. Accessed September 2003.
4. Wiersema, L. A., & Stanley, M. The aging integumentary system. In Stanley, M., & Beare, P.G. (1999). Gerontological Nursing: A Health Promotion/Protection Approach, ed 2. Philadelphia: F. A. Davis, pp 102–111.
5. ND: Skin Integrity, impaired. In Doenges, M. E., Moorhouse, M. F., & Geissler-Murr, A. C. (2002). Nursing Care Plans: Guidelines for Individualizing Patient Care, ed 6. Philadelphia: F. A. Davis.
6. McGovern, C. (2003). Skin integrity: Pressure ulcers, wounds and wound healing. Unit 3. (Lecture materials). Villanova, PA: Villanova University College of Nursing. Available at: http://www10homepage.villanova.edu/marycarol.mcgovern. Accessed February 2004.
7. No author listed. Risk factors and prevention. Geriatric Syndromes: Pressure Ulcers. Novartis Foundation for gerontology. Available at: http://geriatricsyllabus.com. Accessed February 2004.

readiness for enhanced Sleep

Definition: A pattern of natural, periodic suspension of consciousness that provides adequate rest, sustains a desired lifestyle, and can be strengthened

RELATED FACTORS

To be developed by nurse researchers and submitted to NANDA

DEFINING CHARACTERISTICS

Subjective
Expresses willingness to enhance sleep
Expresses a feeling of being rested after sleep
Follows sleep routines that promote sleep habits

Objective
Amount of sleep and REM sleep is congruent with developmental needs
Occasional or infrequent use of medications to induce sleep

SAMPLE CLINICAL APPLICATIONS: postoperative recovery, chronic pain, pregnancy—prenatal/post-partal period, sleep apnea

DESIRED OUTCOMES/EVALUATION CRITERIA
Sample **NOC** Linkages:

Sleep: Extent and pattern of natural periodic suspension of consciousness during which the body is restored

Rest: Extent and pattern of diminished activity for mental and physical rejuvenation

Comfort Level: Extent of physical and psychological ease

Client Will (Include Specific Time Frame)
- Identify individually appropriate interventions to promote sleep.
- Verbalize feeling rested after sleep.
- Adjust lifestyle to accommodate routines that promote sleep.

ACTIONS/INTERVENTIONS

Sample **NIC** Linkages:

Sleep Enhancement: Facilitation of regular sleep/wake cycles

Simple Relaxation Therapy: Use of techniques to encourage and elicit relaxation for the purpose of decreasing undesirable signs and symptoms such as pain, muscle tension, or anxiety

Environmental Management: Manipulation of the patient's surroundings for therapeutic benefit

NURSING PRIORITY NO. 1. To evaluate sleep pattern:

- Listen to client's reports of sleep quantity and quality. *Determines client's experience and expectations regarding sleep. Provides opportunity to address misconceptions/unrealistic expectations and plan for interventions.*
- Observe and/or obtain feedback from client/SO(s) regarding usual bedtime, desired rituals and routines, number of hours of sleep, time of arising, and environmental needs *to determine usual sleep pattern and provide comparative baseline for improvements.*
- Note client report of potential for alteration of habitual sleep time (e.g., change of work pattern/rotating shifts) or change in normal bedtime (e.g., hospitalization). *Helps identify circumstances that are known to interrupt sleep patterns and which could disrupt the person's circadian rhythm. This results in mental and physical fatigue, affecting concentration, interest, energy and appetite.*[1,2,8]

NURSING PRIORITY NO. 2. To promote sleep/rest:

- Discuss client's usual bedtime rituals, expectations for obtaining good sleep time. *Provides information on client's management of the situation and identifies areas that may require modifications.*
- Discuss/implement effective age-appropriate bedtime rituals for infant/child (e.g., rocking, story reading, cuddling, favorite blanket/toy). *Rituals can enhance ability to fall asleep, reinforce that bed is a place to sleep and promote sense of security for child.*[3]
- Investigate use of sleep mask, darkening shades/curtains, earplugs, low-level background(white) noise. *Aids in blocking out light and disturbing noise.*
- Discuss strategies with shift workers: Keep a sleep diary to find best time for sleep, take time to unwind from work before going to bed, defend your sleep time from telephones, doorbells, family and friend interruptions, hire a babysitter during your sleep time. *Planning for optimum sleep can improve sleep habits and quality of rest.*[8]
- Arrange care *to provide for uninterrupted periods for rest.* Explain necessity of disturbances for monitoring vital signs and/or other care when client is hospitalized. Do as much care as possible without waking client during night. *Allows for longer periods of uninterrupted sleep, especially during night.*
- Provide quiet environment and comfort measures (e.g., back rub, washing hands/face, cleaning and straightening sheets). *Promotes relaxation and readiness for sleep.*

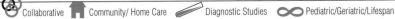 Cultural Collaborative Community/ Home Care Diagnostic Studies Pediatric/Geriatric/Lifespan Medications

- Explore/implement use of warm bath, intake of light protein meal before bedtime, comfortable room termperature, soothing music, favorite calming television show. *Non-pharmacautical aids may enhance falling asleep without the undesired side effects associated with medications.*
- Recommend limiting intake of chocolate and caffeine/alcoholic beverages, especially prior to bedtime. *Subtances known to impair falling or staying asleep. Use of alcohol at bedtime may help individual fall asleep, but ensuing sleep is then fragmented.*[4]
- Suggest limiting fluid intake in evening if nocturia or bedwetting is a problem *to reduce need for nighttime elimination.*
- Assist client in use of necessary equipment, instucting as necessary *Client may use oxygen or CPAP sysem to improve sleep/rest in presence of hypoxia or sleep apnea.*

NURSING PRIORITY NO. 3. To promote optimum wellness:

- Assure client that occasional sleeplessness should not threaten health. *Knowledge that occasional insomnia is universal and usually not harmful, may promote relaxation and relief from worry.*[5]
- Assist client to develop individual program of relaxation (e.g., biofeedback, self-hypnosis, visualization, progressive muscle relaxation). *Methods that reduce sympathetic response and decrease stress can help in inducing sleep, particularly in persons suffering from chronic and long-term sleep disturbances.*[6]
- Encourage participation in regular exercise program during day *to aid in stress control/release of energy. Note: Exercise at bedtime may stimulate rather than relax client and actually interfere with sleep.*[7]
- Recommend inclusion of bedtime snack (e.g., milk or mild juice, crackers, protein source such as cheese/peanut butter) in dietary program *to reduce sleep interference from hunger/hypoglycemia.*
- Advise using barbiturates and/or other sleeping medications sparingly.

DOCUMENTATION FOCUS

Assessment/Reassessment
- Assessment findings, including specifics of sleep pattern (current and past) and effects on lifestyle/level of functioning.
- Medications/interventions, previous therapies.

Planning
Plan of care and who is involved in planning.
Teaching plan.

Implementation/Evaluation
- Client's response to interventions/teaching and actions performed.
- Attainment/progress toward desired outcome(s).
- Modifications to plan of care.

Discharge Planning
- Long-term needs and who is responsible for actions to be taken.
- Specific referrals made.

References

1. Cochran, H. (2003). Diagnose and treat primary insomnia. The Nurse Practitioner, 28(9), 13–27.
2. Spenceley, S. M. (1993). Sleep inquiry: A look with fresh eyes. Image, 25(3), 249–255.
3. Mindell, J. (1997). Sleeping through the night: How infants, toddlers, and their parents can get a good night's sleep. Harper-Collins.
4. Bahr, Sr. R. T. Sleep Disturbances. In Stanley, M., & Beare, P. G. (1999). Gerontological Nursing: A Health Promotion/Protection Approach, ed 2. Philadelphia: F. A. Davis, pp 335–341.
5. Brain basics: Understanding sleep. Available at: National Institute of Neurological Disorders and Stroke (NINDS), http://www.ninds.nih.gov. Accessed February 2004.
6. ND: Sleep Pattern, disturbed. In Cox, H. C., et al. (2002). Clinical Applications of Nursing Diagnosis: Adult, Child, Women's, Psychiatric, Gerontic, and Home Health Considerations, ed 4. Philadelphia: F. A. Davis, pp 375–380.
7. Grandjean, C. K., & Gibbons, S. W. (2000). Assessing ambulatory geriatic sleep complaints. The Nurse Practitioner: Am J Prim Health Care 25(9), 25.
8. Pronitis-Ruotolo, D. (2001). Surviving the night shift: Making Zeitgeber work for you. AJN, 101(7), 63.

Sleep Deprivation

Definition: Prolonged periods without sleep (sustained natural, periodic suspension of relative consciousness)

RELATED FACTORS

Sustained environmental stimulation; unfamiliar or uncomfortable sleep environment

Inadequate daytime activity; sustained circadian asynchrony; aging-related sleep stage shifts; non–sleep-inducing parenting practices

Sustained inadequate sleep hygiene; prolonged use of pharmacologic or dietary antisoporifics

Prolonged physical/psychological discomfort; periodic limb movement (e.g., restless leg syndrome, nocturnal myoclonus); sleep-related: enuresis; painful erections

Nightmares; sleepwalking; sleep terror

Sleep apnea

Sundowner's syndrome; dementia

Idiopathic CNS hypersomnolence; narcolepsy; familial sleep paralysis

DEFINING CHARACTERISTICS

Subjective

Daytime drowsiness; decreased ability to function

Malaise; tiredness; lethargy

Anxious

Perceptual disorders (e.g., disturbed body sensation, delusions, feeling afloat); heightened sensitivity to pain

Objective

Restlessness; irritability

Inability to concentrate; slowed reaction

Listlessness; apathy

Mild, fleeting nystagmus; hand tremors

Acute confusion; transient paranoia; agitated or combative; hallucinations

SAMPLE CLINICAL APPLICATIONS: COPD, heart failure (nocturia), chronic pain, sleep

 Cultural   Collaborative   Community/ Home Care   Diagnostic Studies   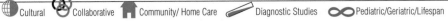 Pediatric/Geriatric/Lifespan   Medications apnea, pregnancy/postpartum, colic, dementia/Alzheimer's disease, anxiety disorders, post-traumatic stress disorder

DESIRED OUTCOMES/EVALUATION CRITERIA

Sample **NOC** linkages:

Sleep: Extent and pattern of natural periodic suspension of consciousness during which the body is rested

Rest: Extent and pattern of diminished activity for mental and physical rejuvenation

Pain Control: Personal actions to control pain

Client Will (Include Specific Time Frame)

- Identify individually appropriate interventions to promote sleep.
- Verbalize understanding of sleep disorders.
- Adjust lifestyle to accommodate chronobiological rhythms.
- Report improvement in sleep/rest pattern.

Sample **NOC** linkage:

Coping: Actions to manage stressors that tax an individual's resources

Family Will (Include Specific Time Frame)

- Deal appropriately with parasomnias.

ACTIONS/INTERVENTIONS

Sample **NIC** linkages:

Sleep Enhancement: Facilitation of regular sleep/wake cycles

Anxiety Reduction: Minimizing apprehension, dread, foreboding, or uneasiness related to an unidentified source or anticipated danger

Environmental Management: Comfort: Manipulation of the patient's surroundings for promotion of optimal comfort

NURSING PRIORITY NO. 1. To assess causative/contributing factors:

- Note client's age and developmental stage. *Newborns normally sleep 14–18 hours a day, developing a more regular sleep pattern at about 4–6 weeks of approximately 10–12 hours. By age 10, a child sleeps around 10 hours; adolescent sleep is irregular but averages 8–10 hours; at age 20, the individual sleeps around 8 hours; pregnant women and new mothers, while needing more sleep, usually are sleep-deprived; menopausal women can experience interrupted sleep because of hot flashes; elderly persons sleep fewer hours, report less restful sleep and need for more sleep.*[1–5]
- Determine presence of physical or psychological stressors: *These include multiple, varying factors, such as night-shift work, pain (acute and chronic), current/recent illness, hospitalization, especially in intensive care unit; death of a spouse, loss of a job; new baby in the home, inadequate sleep-promoting behaviors; etc.*
- Investigate anxious feelings *to help determine basis and appropriate anxiety-reduction techniques.*
- Note presence of current medical diagnoses *that are known to affect sleep (e.g., mental confusion/dementias, certain brain infections (e.g., encephalitis), brain injury, narcolepsy, obsessive/compulsive disorder, anxiety, depression and other major psychological disorders; drug or alcohol abuse; sleep-induced respiratory disorders/obstructive sleep apnea, childhood snoring with sleep apnea).*[6,7]

- Evaluate for use of medications and/or other drugs affecting sleep. *Diet pills/other stimulants, alcohol, sedatives, antidepressants, antihypertensives, diuretics, narcotics, and need for medications requiring nighttime dosing can inhibit getting to sleep or remaining asleep.*[8,9]
- Note environmental factors affecting sleep *(e.g., unfamiliar or uncomfortable sleep environment, excessive noise and light, frequent checking of vital signs, uncomfortable temperature, roommate irritations/actions—snoring, watching television late at night, etc.). Note: Clients in critical care units are known to experience lack of sleep or frequent disruptions, often compounding their illness.*[9]
- Determine presence of parasomnias: nightmares/terrors or somnambulism (e.g., falling asleep while sitting, sleepwalking, sleep paralysis, or other complex behaviors during sleep). *May require more extensive evaluation for serious sleep disorders.*[10]

NURSING PRIORITY NO. 2. To assess degree of impairment:

- Assess client's usual sleep patterns and current sleep disturbance, relying upon client/SO report of problem. Incorporate screening information into in-depth sleep diary or testing if needed. *Usual sleep patterns are individual, but insomnia has been shown to be the most common complaint reported in primary care settings*[4,11]*; therefore, screening for the problem should be routine. Data collected from a comprehensive assessment is needed to determine etiology of challenging sleep disturbances, including the stage of sleep that is impaired.*[9,12]
- Determine client's sleep expectations. *Individual may have faulty beliefs/attitudes about sleep and unrealistic sleep expectations (e.g., "I must get 8 hours of sleep every night, or I can't accomplish anything").*[11]
- Ascertain duration of current problem and effect on life/functional ability. *Client may not get enough sleep and not realize that life functioning is being impaired (e.g., can't concentrate in school, falls asleep when stopped at a light while driving).*[11]
- Listen to subjective reports of sleep quality (e.g., "short, interrupted") and response from lack of good sleep (feeling foggy, sleepy, and woozy, fighting sleep, fatigue, etc.). *Helps clarify client's perception of sleep quantity/quality and response to inadequate sleep.*[11]
- Observe for physical signs of fatigue. *Client may display restlessness, irritability, disorientation, frequent yawning, and/or other changes in mood/behavior or performance. Fatigue, daytime sleepiness and functional impairment have been reported as significant problem in teens.*[3,4,11]
- Determine interventions client has tried to date. *Helps identify appropriate options and may reveal additional interventions that can be attempted.*
- Distinguish client's beneficial bedtime habits from detrimental ones *(e.g., drinking late evening milk versus coffee).*
- Instruct client and/or bed partner to keep a sleep-wake log *to document symptoms and identify factors that are interfering with sleep.*
- Obtain a chronological chart *to determine client's peak performance rhythms.*

NURSING PRIORITY NO. 3. To assist client to establish optimal sleep pattern:[2,4,5,8,9,11,13,14]

- Review medications being taken and their effect on sleep, suggesting modifications in regimen, *if medications are found to be interfering.*
- Restrict caffeine and other stimulating substances from late afternoon/evening intake.

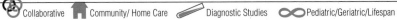 Cultural   Collaborative   Community/ Home Care   Diagnostic Studies   Pediatric/Geriatric/Lifespan   Medications

Recommend avoidance of bedtime alcohol. *Both alcohol and some medications can produce immediate sleep followed by early awakening/difficulty remaining asleep.*

- Avoid eating large evening/late-night meals.
- Recommend light bedtime snack (protein, simple carbohydrate, and low fat) and/or glass of warm milk, for individuals who feel hungry, eaten 15 to 30 minutes before retiring. *Sense of fullness and satiety can encourage sleep.*
- Limit evening fluid intake if nocturia is present *to reduce need for nighttime elimination.*
- Promote adequate physical exercise activity during day, finishing workout at least 3 hours before bedtime. *Enhances expenditure of energy/release of tension so that client feels ready for sleep/rest. Note: Rigorous exercise close to bedtime can delay onset of sleep.*
- Suggest abstaining from daytime naps, or napping in the morning *to improve ability to fall asleep at night.*
- Recommend quiet relaxing activities prior to bedtime such as reading, listening to soothing music, meditation *to reduce stimulation and promote relaxation.*
- Discuss/implement effective age-appropriate bedtime rituals (e.g., going to bed at same time each night, brushing teeth, reading, drinking warm milk, rocking, story reading, cuddling, favorite blanket/toy) *to enhance client's ability to fall asleep, reinforce that bed is a place to sleep, and promote sense of security for child.*
- Provide back massage/other therapeutic touch, as appropriate. *Touch can be relaxing and emotionally pleasing, caregiver's given that the client has undivided attention for a few moments.*
- Provide calm, quiet environment for hospitalized client, *to manage controllable sleep-disrupting factors (e.g., reduce noise and talking, dim lights, shut room door, adjust room temperature as needed, silence/reduce volume on phones, beepers, alarms, television, radios).*
- Administer pain medication first *to make sure client is pain-free,* and then sedatives/other sleep medications *(so that hypnotic will be more effective)* when indicated, noting client's response. Time pain medications for peak effect/duration *to reduce need for redosing during prime sleep hours.*
- Instruct client to get out of bed, leave bedroom, engage in relaxing activities *if unable to fall asleep,* and not return to bed until feeling sleepy.
- Recommend/instruct client in relaxation techniques (e.g., visualization, breathing, yoga).
- Refer for biofeedback, cognitive therapy, etc, *when measures that are more intensive are needed/desired to cope with stressors and promote relaxation.*
- Refer client/collaborate with healthcare team for evaluation/treatment of more serious sleep problems (e.g., obstructive sleep apnea, narcolepsy, sleep paralysis, night terrors).
- Review with the client the physician's recommendations for weight management, medications or surgery (e.g., alteration of facial structures/tracheotomy), and/or oxygenation therapy—continuous positive airway pressure (CPAP) such as Respironics—*when sleep apnea is severe as documented by sleep disorder studies.*

NURSING PRIORITY NO. 4. To promote wellness (Teaching/Discharge Considerations):

- Review possibility of next-day drowsiness/"rebound" insomnia and temporary memory loss *that may be associated with prescription sleep medications.*
- Discuss use/appropriateness of OTC sleep medications/herbal supplements. Note possible side effects and drug interactions.

• Refer to support group/counselor *to help deal with psychological stressors (e.g., grief, sorrow)*. Refer to NDs dysfunctional Grieving, chronic Sorrow.

• Encourage family counseling *to help deal with concerns arising from parasomnias.*

• Refer to sleep specialist/laboratory *when problem is unresponsive to interventions.*

DOCUMENTATION FOCUS

Assessment/Reassessment

• Assessment findings, including specifics of sleep pattern (current and past) and effects on lifestyle/level of functioning.
• Medications/interventions, previous therapies.
• Family history of similar problem.

Planning

• Plan of care and who is involved in planning.
• Teaching plan.

Implementation/Evaluation

• Client's response to interventions/teaching and actions performed.
• Attainment/progress toward desired outcome(s).
• Modifications to plan of care.

Discharge Planning

• Long-term needs and who is responsible for actions to be taken.
• Specific referrals made.

References

1. ND: Sleep Deprivation (developmental considerations). In Cox, H. C., et al. (2002). Clinical Applications of Nursing Diagnosis: Adult, Child, Women's, Psychiatric, Gerontic, and Home Health Considerations, ed 4. Philadelphia: F. A. Davis, pp 368–369.
2. Mindell, J. (1997). Sleeping Through the Night: How Infants, Toddlers, and Their Parents Can Get a Good Night's Sleep. New York: Harper Collins.
3. No author listed. Adolescent sleep needs and patterns: Research report and resource guide. Available at: National Sleep Foundation, http://www.sleepfoundation.org. Accessed February 2004.
4. No author listed. Women and sleep. Available at: National Sleep Foundation, http://www.sleepfoundation.org. Accessed February 2004.
5. Bahr, Sr. R. T. Sleep disturbances. In Stanley, M., & Beare, P. G. (1999). Gerontological Nursing: A Health Promotion/Protection Approach, ed 2. Philadelphia: F. A. Davis, pp 337–341.
6. Sateia, M. J., et al., (2000). Evaluation of chronic insomnia: An American Academy of Sleep Medicine review. Sleep 23(2), 243–308. Available at: http://www.guideline.gov. Accessed February 2004.
7. Clinical practice guideline: Diagnosis and management of childhood obstructive sleep apnea syndrome. (2002). Pediatrics, 109(4), 704–712. Available at: http://www.guideline.gov. Accessed February 2004.
8. Barroso, J. (2003). Living with illness: HIV-related fatigue. AJN, 102(5), 83.
9. Honkus, V. L. (2003). Sleep deprivation in critical care units. Crit Care Nurs Quart, 26(3), 179–191.
10. Cardinal, F. (2004). Sleep disorders-the basics. (Monographs). Available at: What you need to know about Sleep Disorders, http://sleepdisorders.about.com. Accessed February 2004.
11. Cochran, H. (2003). Diagnose and treat primary insomnia. The Nurse Practitioner, 28(9), 13–27.
12. Spenceley, S. M. (1993). Sleep inquiry: A look with fresh eyes. Image, 25(3), 249–255.
13. Pronitis-Ruotolo, D. (2001). Surviving the night shift: Making Zeitgeber work for you. AJN, 101(7), 63.
14. Cmiel, C. A., et al. (2004). Noise control: A nursing team's approach to sleep promotion. AJN, 104(2), 40–48.

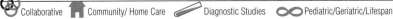   Cultural   Collaborative   Community/ Home Care   Diagnostic Studies   Pediatric/Geriatric/Lifespan   Medications

disturbed Sleep Pattern

Definition: Time-limited disruption of sleep (natural, periodic suspension of consciousness) amount and quality

RELATED FACTORS

Psychological
Daytime activity pattern; fatigue; dietary; body temperature
Social schedule inconsistent with chronotype; shift work; daylight/darkness exposure
Frequently changing sleep-wake schedule/travel across time zones; circadian asynchrony
Childhood onset; aging-related sleep shifts; periodic gender-related hormonal shifts
Inadequate sleep hygiene; maladaptive conditioned wakefulness
Ruminative presleep thoughts; anticipation; thinking about home
Preoccupation with trying to sleep; fear of insomnia
Biochemical agents; medications; sustained use of antisleep agents
Temperament; loneliness; grief; anxiety; fear; boredom; depression
Separation from SOs; loss of sleep partner, life change
Delayed or advanced sleep phase syndrome

Environmental
Excessive stimulation; noise; lighting; ambient temperature, humidity; noxious odors; sleep partner
Unfamiliar sleep furnishings
Interruptions for therapeutics, monitoring, laboratory tests; other-generated awakening
Physical restraint
Lack of sleep privacy/control

Parental
Mother's sleep-wake pattern/emotional support
Parent-infant interaction

Physiologic
Position
Gastroesophageal reflux; nausea
Shortness of breath; stasis of secretions
Fever
Urinary urgency, incontinence
[Upper airway incompetence]
[Pain syndromes]

DEFINING CHARACTERISTICS

Subjective
Verbal complaints [reports] of difficulty falling asleep/not feeling well rested; dissatisfaction with sleep
Sleep onset greater than 30 minutes
Three or more nighttime awakenings; prolonged awakenings

Awakening earlier or later than desired; early morning insomnia
Decreased ability to function; [falling asleep during activities]

Objective
Less than age-normed total sleep time
Increased proportion of stage 1 sleep
Decreased proportion of stages 3 and 4 sleep (e.g., hyporesponsiveness, excess sleepiness, decreased motivation)
Decreased proportion of REM sleep (e.g., REM rebound, hyperactivity, emotional lability, agitation and impulsivity, atypical polysomnographic features)
Sleep maintenance insomnia
Self-induced impairment of normal pattern
[Changes in behavior and performance (increasing irritability, disorientation, listlessness, restlessness, lethargy)]
[Physical signs (mild fleeting nystagmus, ptosis of eyelid, slight hand tremor, expressionless face, dark circles under eyes, changes in posture, frequent yawning)]

SAMPLE CLINICAL APPLICATIONS: Alzheimers/senile dementias, anxiety disorders, bipolar disorders, depression; HIV/AIDs, hyperthyroidism, postoperative recovery, chronic pain, pregnancy—prenatal/post-partal period, pulmonary diseases (e.g., COPD, asthma)

DESIRED OUTCOMES/EVALUATION CRITERIA
Sample **NOC** linkages:
Sleep: Extent and pattern of natural periodic suspension of consciousness during which the body is restored
Rest: Extent and pattern of diminished activity for mental and physical rejuvenation
Comfort Level: Extent of physical and psychological ease

Client Will (Include Specific Time Frame)
- Verbalize understanding of sleep disturbance
- Identify individually appropriate interventions to promote sleep.
- Adjust lifestyle to accommodate chronobiological rhythms.
- Report improvement in sleep/rest pattern.
- Report increased sense of well-being and feeling rested.

ACTIONS/INTERVENTIONS
Sample **NIC** linkages—
Sleep Enhancement: Facilitation of regular sleep/wake cycles
Simple Relaxation Therapy: Use of techniques to encourage and elicit relaxation for the purpose of decreasing undesirable signs and symptoms such as pain, muscle tension, or anxiety
Environmental Management: Manipulation of the patient's surroundings for therapeutic benefit

NURSING PRIORITY NO. 1. To identify causative/contributing factors:

 • Identify presence of factors as listed in Related Factors (e.g., depression, chronic pain, grieving, new baby in household, cardiac surgery); metabolic diseases (e.g., hyperthyroidism and diabetes mellitus); prescribed/OTC drug use (including those that require

 Cultural   Collaborative   Community/ Home Care Diagnostic Studies Pediatric/Geriatric/Lifespan Medications

nighttime dosing); aging (*increased sleep latency and awakenings*); shift work, working long hours, working more than one job (*alters biological rhythms*). *Many factors are involved in causing or contributing to sleep problems. Stress is considered by most to be the number-1 cause of short-term sleeping difficulties.*[1-6]

- Assess sleep pattern disturbances associated with specific underlying health conditions (*e.g., benign prostatic hypertrophy, mental disorders, brain injury, restless leg syndrome, chronic fatigue often impair an individual's ability to fall asleep or result in early arousal*).[2]

- Note whether female is pregnant or has new baby. *Hormonal shifts and tasks involved in parenting newborn can alter sleep.*[1]

- Observe parent-infant-child interactions and sleep-wake patterns. *Knowledge of normal infant cues/problems can identify behaviors that need modifying, can reduce tension interfering with sleep and improve rest during sleep times.*[7]

- Determine whether woman has premenstrual syndrome or is menopausal. *Hormonal shifts, depression, or hot flashes can alter sleep.*[1]

- Review individual sleeping environment especially for elderly client. *More than 50% of adults over age 65 living at home and approximately two thirds of elderly living in care facilities report sleep disturbances.*[2]

- Determine recent traumatic events in client's life (e.g., a death in family, loss of job). *Individual may be coping poorly and need assistance or direction in improving coping skills or dealing with stressors.*[2,3]

- Evaluate use of decongestants, steroids, antihypertensives, some asthma drugs, and sedatives (as well as caffeine and alcoholic beverages). *Use and/or timing of use may be interfering with falling asleep, level of sleep achieved, or staying asleep.*[8]

- Investigate whether client snores and in what position(s) this occurs. Also determine if obese individual experiences loud periodic snoring, along with unusual nighttime activities (e.g. sitting upright, sleepwalking); morning headaches, sleepiness, depression. *Sleep studies (polysomnography) may need to be done to determine if cause is sleep apnea.*[2,4]

NURSING PRIORITY NO. 2. To evaluate sleep pattern and dysfunction(s):

- Listen to subjective reports of sleep quality. Determine client's/SO's expectations of adequate sleep. *Provides opportunity to address misconceptions/unrealistic expectations and plan for interventions.*[9]

- Determine type of insomnia (e.g., transient, short-term, chronic). *Transient episodes are occasional restless nights caused by such factors as jet lag, first night in a new bed, etc. Short term lasts a few weeks and arises from a temporary stressful experience, such as pressures at work, loss of job, death in family and usually resolves over time as client adapts to stressor. Chronic insomnia lasts for more than three weeks and can be caused by many physical and psychological factors as well as use/misuse of medications and drugs.*[5]

- Observe for restlessness, irritability, hand tremors, frequent yawning, thick speech. *Physical signs of fatigue.*[9]

- Observe and/or obtain feedback from client/SO(s) regarding usual bedtime, rituals and routines, number of hours of sleep, time of arising, and environmental needs *to determine usual sleep pattern and provide comparative baseline.*[9]

- Note alteration of habitual sleep time (e.g., change of work pattern/rotating shifts) or change in normal bedtime (e.g., hospitalization). *Helps identify circumstances that are known to interrupt sleep patterns and which cause disruption in the person's circadian rhythm. This results in mental and physical fatigue, affecting concentration, interest, energy and appetite.*[6]

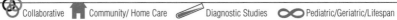

- Assist with diagnostic testing (e.g., electroencephalogram [EEG], electro-oculogram [EOG] and electromyogram [EMG]; psychological assessment/testing, chronological chart). *Polysomnography (the three electrical tests noted previously) are performed in a sleep laboratory to measure several parameters of sleep, including brain wave activity, eye movement and leg muscle tone. These tests may be performed after initial clinical evaluation and/or symptom management fails to discover or resolve a particular sleep disturbance and/or point to appropriate interventions and treatments.*[1,2,4]

NURSING PRIORITY NO. 3. To assist client to establish optimal sleep/rest patterns:

- Arrange care *to provide for uninterrupted periods for rest.* Explain necessity of disturbances for monitoring vital signs and/or other care when client is hospitalized. Do as much care as possible without waking client during night. *Allows for longer periods of sleep, especially during night.*[9]
- Provide quiet environment and comfort measures (e.g., back rub, washing hands/face, cleaning and straightening sheets). *Promotes relaxation and readiness for sleep.*[9]
- Provide warm bath for infant 30–60 minutes before usual bedtime *to enhance relaxation and provide quiet time.*[7]
- Discuss/implement effective age-appropriate bedtime rituals for infant/child (e.g., rocking, story reading, cuddling, favorite blanket/toy) *Rituals can enhance ability to fall asleep, reinforce that bed is a place to sleep and promote sense of security for child.*[7]
- Explore use of warm bath/milk, intake of light protein snack before bedtime, comfortable room termperature, soothing music, favorite television show. *Nonpharmaceutical aids may enhance falling asleep free of concern of side-effects, such as morning hangover or drug dependence.*[5]
- Recommend limiting intake of chocolate and caffeine/alcoholic beverages, especially before bedtime. *Subtances known to impair falling or staying asleep. Use of alcohol at bedtime may help individual fall asleep, but ensuing sleep is then fragmented.*[5]
- Limit fluid intake in evening if bedwetting or nocturia is a problem. *Reduces need for night-time elimination and resultant interruption of sleep.*[10]
- Administer pain and sedative medications (if required) 1 hour before sleep and after therapeutic and daily activities are completed *to relieve discomfort and take maximum advantage of sedative effect.*[3,8]
- Monitor effects of therapeutic use of amphetamines or stimulants (such as may be given for attention deficit disorder or narcolepsy). *Use of these medications can induce or potentiate sleep disturbances.*[8]
- Develop behavioral program for insomnia:[1–6]
  Establish routine bedtime and arising.
  Think relaxing thoughts when in bed.
  Do not nap in the daytime.
  Do not read in bed; get out of bed if not asleep in 15 minutes.
  Limit sleep to 7 hours a night.
  Get up the same time each day—even on weekends/days off.
- Recommend/assist with implementing/facilitating program to "reset" sleep clock (chronotherapy) when client has delayed sleep-onset insomnia. *These sleep-wake schedule problems are common among shift workers and airplane travelers. Shift workers can benefit by adhering to a set routine and ensuring that noises and interruptions are kept to a minimun. Those who travel across country and other long flights that take them across time zones can*

benefit by adjusting their sleep time to match the time zone of their arrival and avoiding caffeine and alcohol.[11]

 ● Refer to sleep specialist/laboratory for treatment as indicated. *Additional evaluation or therapy may be required when routine interventions are unsuccessful.*[2]

NURSING PRIORITY NO. 4. To promote wellness (Teaching/Discharge Considerations):

● Assure client that occasional sleeplessness should not threaten health. *Knowledge that occasional insomnia is universal and usually not harmful may promote relaxation and relief from worry.*[4]

● Discuss effects of dysfunctional sleep pattern on SO/family and identify any potential conflicts with therapeutic interventions. *Lack of restful sleep can result in stressful interactions with other individuals and changes in schedules/routines or habits may impact sleep partner as well.*[10]

● Review effects of aging on sleep pattern. *Understanding that increased sleep latency (time required to fall asleep), decreased sleep efficiency, and increased awakenings are common in the elderly may aid client/family in accepting and coping with change.*[2]

● Encourage individual to develop schedule identified in chronobiological chart. *Takes advantage of peak performance times, enhancing ability to do one's best.*[10]

● Assist client to develop individual program of relaxation. Demonstrate or advise training in relaxation techniques (e.g., biofeedback, self-hypnosis, visualization, progressive muscle relaxation). *Methods that reduce sympathetic response and decrease stress can help induce sleep, particularly in persons suffering from chronic and long-term sleep disturbances.*[3]

● Discuss strategies with shift workers: Keep a sleep diary to find best time for sleep, take time to unwind from work prior to going to bed, defend your sleep time from telephones, doorbells, family and friend interruptions; hire a babysitter during your sleep time. *Planning for optimum sleep can improve sleep habits and quality of rest.*[6]

● Encourage participation in regular exercise program during day *to aid in stress control/release of energy. Note: Exercise at bedtime may stimulate rather than relax client and actually interfere with sleep.*[2]

● Recommend inclusion of bedtime snack (e.g., milk or mild juice, crackers, protein source such as cheese/peanut butter) in dietary program *to reduce sleep interference from hunger/hypoglycemia. Carbohydrates promote release of serotonin, enhancing induction of sleep, and proteins aid in maintaining blood glucose level.*[12]

● Advise using barbiturates and/or other sleeping medications sparingly *to avoid dependence.*[8]

● Recommend diuretic medications be taken in the early morning *to reduce therapeutic effects interfering with sleep.*[8]

● Suggest that bed/bedroom be used only for sleep, not for working, watching television. *Promotes idea of sleep instead of work or other activities.*[10]

● Provide for child's (or impaired individual's) sleep time safety (e.g., infant placed on back or side padded crib; use of bedrails/bed in low position, nonplastic sheets).[7,11]

● Investigate use of sleep mask, darkening shades/curtains, earplugs, low-level background(white) noise. *Aids in blocking out light and disturbing noises.*[11]

● Recommend midmorning nap if one is required. *Napping, especially in the afternoon, can disrupt normal sleep patterns.*[2]

● Assist client to deal with grieving process when loss has occurred. (Refer to ND dysfunctional Grieving.) *Sleep can be used as an avoidance mechanism if individual is not dealing appropriately with loss.*[3]

Assessment/Reassessment

- Assessment findings, including specifics of sleep pattern (current and past) and effects on lifestyle/level of functioning.
- Medications/interventions, previous therapies.

Planning

- Plan of care and who is involved in planning.
- Teaching plan.

Implementation/Evaluation

- Client's response to interventions/teaching and actions performed.
- Attainment/progress toward desired outcome(s).
- Modifications to plan of care.

Discharge Planning

- Long-term needs and who is responsible for actions to be taken.
- Specific referrals made.

References

1. National Sleep Foundation. When you can't sleep: ABCs of ZZZs. Available at: http://www.sleepfoundation.org. Accessed August 2003.
2. Grandjean, C. K., & Gibbons, S. W. (2000). Assessing ambulatory geriatic sleep complaints. Nurse Practitioner: Am J Prim Health Care, 25(9), 25.
3. Sleep pattern, disturbed. In Cox, H. C., Hinz, M. D., Lubano, M. A., et al. (2002). Clinical Applications of Nursing Diagnosis: Adult, Child, Women's, Psychiatric, Gerontic, and Home Health considerations, ed 4. Philadelphia: F. A. Davis, pp 375–380.
4. Brain basics: Understanding sleep. Available at:National Institute of Neurological Disorders and Stroke (NINDS), http://www.ninds.nih.gov. Accessed August 2003.
5. Bahr, Sr R. T. (1999). Sleep disturbances. In Stanley, M., & Beare, P. G. Gerontological Nursing: A Health Promotion/Protection Approach, ed 2. Philadelphia: F. A. Davis, pp 335–341.
6. Pronitis-Ruotolo, D. (2001). Surviving the night shift: Making Zeitgeber work for you. AJN, 101(7):63.
7. Olds, S., London, M., & Ladwig, P. (1999). Maternal-Newborn Nursing: A Family and Community-based Approach, ed 6. Upper Saddle River, NJ: Prentice Hall.
8. Deglin, J. H., & Vallerand, A. H. (2003). Davis's Drug Guide for Nurses, ed 8. Philadelphia: F. A. Davis.
9. Doenges, M. E., Moorhouse, M. F., & Geissler-Murr, A. C. (2004). Nurse's Pocket Guide: Diagnoses, Interventions and Rationales, ed 9. Philadelphia: F. A. Davis.
10. Townsend, M. C. (2000). Psychiatric mental health nursing concepts of care, ed 4. Philadelphia: F. A. Davis.
11. Doenges, M. E., Moorhouse, M. F., & Geissler-Murr, A. C. (2002). Nursing care plans: Guidelines for individualizing patient care, ed 6. Philadelphia: F. A. Davis.
12. Somer, E., & Snyderman, N. L. (1999). Food & Mood: The Complete Guide to Eating Well and Feeling Your Best, ed 2. New York: Owl Books.

impaired Social Interaction

Definition: Insufficient or excessive quantity or ineffective quality of social exchange

RELATED FACTORS

Knowledge/skill deficit about ways to enhance mutuality

Communication barriers [including head injury, stroke, other neurologic conditions affecting ability to communicate]

Self-concept disturbance
Absence of available SO(s) or peers
Limited physical mobility [e.g., neuromuscular disease]
Therapeutic isolation
Sociocultural dissonance
Environmental barriers
Altered thought processes

DEFINING CHARACTERISTICS

Subjective
Verbalized discomfort in social situations
Verbalized inability to receive or communicate a satisfying sense of belonging, caring, interest, or shared history
Family report of change of style or pattern of interaction

Objective
Observed discomfort in social situations
Observed inability to receive or communicate a satisfying sense of belonging, caring, interest, or shared history
Observed use of unsuccessful social interaction behaviors
Dysfunctional interaction with peers, family, and/or others
SAMPLE CLINICAL APPLICATIONS: brain injury/stroke, cancer, neuromuscular disease (e.g., MS), cerebral palsy, substance abuse, Alzheimer's disease, schizophrenia

DESIRED OUTCOMES/EVALUATION CRITERIA
Sample **NOC** linkages:
Social Interaction Skills: An individual's use of effective interaction behaviors
Child Development: (specify age): Milestones of physical, cognitive, and psychosocial progression by [specify] months/years of age
Role Performance: Congruence of an individual's role behavior with role expectations

Client Will (Include Specific Time Frame)
- Verbalize awareness of factors causing or promoting impaired social interactions.
- Identify feelings that lead to poor social interactions.
- Express desire/be involved in achieving positive changes in social behaviors and interpersonal relationships.
- Give self positive reinforcement for changes that are achieved.
- Develop effective social support system; use available resources appropriately.

ACTIONS/INTERVENTIONS
Sample **NIC** linkages:
Socialization Enhancement: Facilitation of another person's ability to interact with others
Behavior Modification: Social Skills: Assisting the patient to develop or improve interpersonal social skills
Complex Relationship Building: Establishing a therapeutic relationship with a patient who has difficulty interacting with others

NURSING PRIORITY NO. 1. To assess causative/contributing factors:

 • Review social history with client/SO(s) and go back far enough in time to note when changes in social behavior or patterns of relating occurred/began. *For example, loss or long-term illness of loved one; failed relationships; loss of occupation, financial, or political (power) position; change in status in family hierarchy (job loss, aging, illness); poor coping/adjustment to developmental stage of life, as with marriage, birth/adoption of child, or children leaving home are situations that may affect quality of social exchange.*[1]

• Ascertain ethnic/cultural or religious implications for the client. *Client may perceive behaviors as normal because of belief system, or may have conflict regarding behaviors that are not accepted by society, such as homosexuality or gender identity disorder.*[1]

• Review medical history noting stressors of physical/long-term illness (e.g., stroke, cancer, MS, head injury, Alzheimer's disease), mental illness (e.g., schizophrenia), medications/substance use, debilitating accidents. *Conditions such as these can isolate individual who feels disconnected from others resulting in difficulty relating in social situations.*[3]

• Note presence of visual or hearing impairments. *Individuals with these conditions may find communication barriers are increased, social interaction is affected and interventions need to be designed to promote involvement with others in positive ways.*[1]

• Review family patterns of relating and social behaviors. Explore possible family scripting of behavioral expectations in the children and how the client was affected. *Family may not have effective patterns of relating to others, and the child learns these skills in this setting. Often child reflects family expectaions rather than own desires and may result in conforming or rebellious behaviors.*[2]

• Observe client while relating to family/SO(s) and note observations of prevalent patterns. *Identification of patterns will help with plan for change.*[2]

• Encourage client to verbalize feeling of discomfort about social situations. Note any causative factors, recurring precipitating patterns, and barriers to using support systems. *Identifies areas of concern and suggests possible ways to learn new skills.*[2]

• Note socioeconomic level, ethnic/religious practices. *Beliefs regarding social interaction are strongly influenced by these factors and identifying what may create feelings of anxiety for the individual can help in developing plan of care.*[5,6]

NURSING PRIORITY NO. 2. To assess degree of impairment:

• Encourage client to verbalize perceptions of reasons for problems. Active-listen to note indications of hopelessness, powerlessness, fear, anxiety, grief, anger, feeling unloved/unlovable; problems with sexual identity; hate (directed or not). *These feelings arise from the anxiety that comes with the need to participate with others in social situations and begin to interfere with work, friendships, and life in general.*[5]

• Observe and describe social/interpersonal behaviors in objective terms, noting speech patterns, body language (a) in the therapeutic setting and (b) in normal areas of daily functioning (if possible): family, job, social/entertainment settings. *Provides information about extent of anxiety client experiences in different settings and identifies appropriate interventions.*[5]

• Determine client's use of coping skills and defense mechanisms. *Symptoms associated with social anxiety affect ability to be involved in social situations, making client's life miserable and seriously interfering with work, friendships, and family life.*[5]

• Evaluate possibility of client being the victim of or using destructive behaviors against self or others. (Refer to ND [actual/]risk for other-directed/self-directed Violence.)

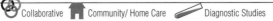

- Interview family, SO(s), friends, spiritual leaders, coworkers, as appropriate. *Obtaining observations of client's behavioral changes from others associated with the individual provides a broader view of actual problems and how behavior affects client's life.*[5]

NURSING PRIORITY NO. 3. To assist client/SO(s) to recognize/make positive changes in impaired social and interpersonal interactions:

- Establish therapeutic relationship using positive regard for the person, Active-listening, and providing safe environment for self-disclosure. *Client who is having difficulty interacting in social situations needs to feel comfortable and accepted before he or she is willing to talk about self and concerns.*[1]
- Have client list behaviors that cause discomfort. *Anxiety usually has physical symptoms such as a racing heart, dry mouth, shaky voice, blushing, sweating, and nausea and once recognized, client can choose to begin treatment to change.*[5,7]
- Have family/SO(s) list client's behaviors that are causing discomfort for them. *Anxiety is contagious and by identifying specific behaviors, all members of the family can begin to deal appropriately with them so they are diminished.*[5,7]
- Review/list negative behaviors observed previously by caregivers, coworkers, and so forth. *Others may see behaviors and the problems assoiacted with them, such as unwillingness to participate in necessary activities (eating in a public place, interviewing for a job) and may provide additional information needed to develop an appropriate plan of care.*[1]
- Compare lists and validate reality of perceptions. Help client prioritize those behaviors needing change. *Each individual may have a different view of what constitutes a problem, and by comparing lists each person hears how others view the problems, enabling the client/family to identify behaviors/concerns to be dealt with.*[1]
- Explore with client and role-play means of making changes in social interactions/behaviors (as determined earlier). *Client needs to learn social skills because they have never learned the elements of interacting with others in social settings. Role-playing one-on-one is less threatening and can help individual identify with another and practice new social skills.*[5]
- Role-play random social situations in therapeutically controlled environment with "safe" therapy group. Have group note behaviors, both positive and negative, and discuss these and any changes needed. *Having client participate in a controlled group environment provides opportunities to try out different behaviors in a built-in social setting where members can make friends and provide mutual advice and comfort.*[5]
- Role-play changes and discuss impact. Include family/SO(s) as indicated. *Provides opportunity for person to recognize changes in feelings and behavior and enhances comfort with new behaviors.*[4]
- Provide positive reinforcement for improvement in social behaviors and interactions. *Encourages continuation of desired behaviors/efforts for change.*[5]
- Participate in multidisciplinary client-centered conferences *to evaluate progress.* Involve everyone associated with client's care, family members, SO(s), and therapy group. *These conferences have the advantage of providing information from and to each participant in an atmosphere of trust where questions can be asked, decisions can be made and goals for the future can be agreed on.*[1]
- Work with the client to alleviate underlying negative self-concepts *because they often impede positive social interactions. By replacing negative thoughts with positive messages, client can reduce anxiety and develop a positive sense of self-esteem. While this is not an easy process, the rewards are great when client is willing to practice consistently.*[2]
- Involve neurologically impaired client in individual and/or group interactions as situation

allows. *Individual may not be able to interact appropriately because of disabilities but involvement in the group provides an opportunity to practice and relearn skills to enable reintegration into social situations.*[1]

 • Refer for family therapy as indicated. *Social behaviors and interpersonal relationships involve more than the individual and family may need additional help to resolve ongoing family problems.*[1]

NURSING PRIORITY NO. 4. To promote wellness (Teaching/Discharge Considerations):

 • Encourage client to keep a daily journal in which social interactions of each day can be reviewed and the comfort/discomfort experienced noted with possible causes/precipitating factors. *Helps client to identify specific problem areas and begin to choose to take responsibility for own behavior(s).*

 • Assist the client to develop positive social skills through practice of skills in real social situations accompanied by a support person. Provide positive feedback with the use of I-messages during interactions with client. *Cognitive and behavioral methods can help individuals overcome fears with the help of a trusted person. I-messages convey a positive message, individual does not feel criticized, and is encouraged to continue new thinking and behaviors.*[1,5]

 • Discuss the use of medications when indicated and monitor for effectiveness and side effects. *Several kinds of drugs have been found to be effective in the treatment of social anxiety problems, selective serotonin reuptake inhibitors (SSRIs), such as paroxetine (Paxil) and sertraline (Zoloft), are the usually the first choice. Anti-anxiety drugs, such as clonazepam (Klonopin) and alprazolam (Xanax), can reduce anxiety and may be used alone or in conjunction with SSRIs. Propranolol (Inderal) has been found to be useful for performance anxiety and when taken an hour before the scheduled event, may suppress the physical symptoms of anxiety.*[5]

 • Seek community programs for client involvement that promote positive behaviors the client is striving to achieve. *Encouraging reading materials, attending classes, community support groups, and lectures for self-help can help to alleviate negative self-concepts that lead to impaired social interactions.*[5]

 • Encourage ongoing family or individual therapy as long as it is promoting growth and positive change. *Be alert to possibility of therapy being used as a crutch. While therapy groups can be useful, individuals can become dependent on the process and not move on to managing on their own.*[1]

 • Provide for occasional follow-up for reinforcement of positive behaviors after professional relationship has ended. *Change is difficult and identifying problems that may arise during these contacts can enhance maintenance and enable client/family to continue to progress.*[2]

 • Refer to/involve psychiatric clinical nurse specialist when indicated. *May need additional assistance to promote long-term change.*[1]

DOCUMENTATION FOCUS

Assessment/Reassessment
- Individual findings, including factors affecting interactions, nature of social exchanges, specifics of individual behaviors.
- Perceptions/response of others.

 Cultural Collaborative 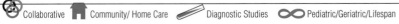 Community/ Home Care Diagnostic Studies Pediatric/Geriatric/Lifespan Medications

Planning
- Plan of care and who is involved in the planning.
- Teaching plan.

Implementation/Evaluation
- Responses to interventions/teaching and actions performed.
- Attainment/progress toward desired outcome(s).
- Modifications to plan of care.

Discharge Planning
- Long-term needs and who is responsible for actions to be taken.
- Community resources, specific referrals made.

References
1. Townsend, M. C. (2003). Psychiatric Mental Health Nursing Concepts of Care, ed 4. Philadelphia: F. A. Davis.
2. Doenges, M. E., Townsend, M. C., & Moorhouse, M. F. (1998). Psychiatric Care Plans Guidelines for Individualizing Care, ed 3. Philadelphia: F. A. Davis.
3. Cox, H., Hinz, M., Lubno, M. A., Newfield, S., Scott-Tilley, D., Slater, M., & Sridaromont, K. (2002). Clinical Applications of Nursing Diagnosis Adult, Child, Women's Psychiatric, Gerontic and Home Health Considerations, ed 4. Philadelphia: F. A. Davis.
4. Drew, N. (1991). Combating the social isolation of chronic mental illness. J Psychosocial Nurs, 29(6), 14–17.
5. Beyond shyness and stage fright: Social anxiety disorder. (October, 2003). Harvard Mental Health Letter.
6. Lipson, J. G., Dibble, S. L, & Minarik, P, A. (1996). Culture & Nursing Care: A Pocket Guide. San Francisco: School of Nursing, UCSF Nursing Press.
7. National Institute of Mental Health (2000). Anxiety Disorders, NIH Publication No. 00–3879. Rockville, Md: author. Available at: www.nimh.nih.gov.anxiety/anxiety.cfm. Accessed December 2003.

Social Isolation

Definition: Aloneness experienced by the individual and perceived as imposed by others and as a negative or threatened state

RELATED FACTORS
Factors contributing to the absence of satisfying personal relationships (e.g., delay in accomplishing developmental tasks); immature interests

Alterations in physical appearance/mental status

Altered state of wellness

Unaccepted social behavior/values

Inadequate personal resources

Inability to engage in satisfying personal relationships

[Traumatic incidents or events causing physical and/or emotional pain]

DEFINING CHARACTERISTICS

Subjective
Expresses feelings of aloneness imposed by others

Expresses feelings of rejection

Expresses values acceptable to the subculture but unacceptable to the dominant cultural group

Inability to meet expectations of others
Experiences feelings of difference from others
Inadequacy in or absence of significant purpose in life
Expresses interests inappropriate to developmental age/stage
Insecurity in public

Objective
Absence of supportive SO(s)—family, friends, group
Sad, dull affect
Inappropriate or immature interests/activities for developmental age/stage
Hostility projected in voice, behavior
Evidence of physical/mental handicap or altered state of wellness
Uncommunicative; withdrawn; no eye contact
Preoccupation with own thoughts; repetitive meaningless actions
Seeking to be alone or existing in a subculture
Showing behavior unaccepted by dominant cultural group

SAMPLE CLINICAL APPLICATIONS: traumatic injuries, facial scarring/acne, chemotherapy, AIDS, dementia, major depression, conduct disorder, developmental delay, paranoid disorders, schizophrenia

DESIRED OUTCOMES/EVALUATION CRITERIA
Sample **NOC** linkages:
Social Involvement: Frequency of an individual's social interactions with persons, groups, or organizations
Loneliness: The extent of emotional, social, or existential isolation response
Social Support: Perceived availability and actual provision of reliable assistance from other persons

Client Will (Include Specific Time Frame)
- Identify causes and actions to correct isolation.
- Verbalize willingness to be involved with others.
- Participate in activities/programs at level of ability/desire.
- Express increased sense of self-worth.

ACTIONS/INTERVENTIONS
Sample **NIC** linkages:
Socialization Enhancement: Facilitation of another person's ability to interact with others
Visitation Facilitation: Promoting beneficial visits by family and friends
Normalization Promotion: Assisting parents and other family members of children with chronic diseases or disabilities in providing normal life experiences for their children and families

NURSING PRIORITY NO. 1. To assess causative/contributing factors:

 • Determine presence of factors as listed in Related Factors and other concerns (e.g., elderly; female; adolescent; ethnic/racial minority; economically/educationally disadvantaged, hearing or visual impairment). *Identifying individual factors allows for developing an accurate plan of care for the client.*[5]

 • Identify blocks to social contacts. *Reluctance to enagage in social activities may be the result*

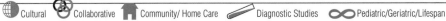 Cultural   Collaborative   Community/ Home Care   Diagnostic Studies   Pediatric/Geriatric/Lifespan   Medications

of problems such as physical immobility, sensory deficits, housebound for any reason, incontinence, financial constraints, transportation difficulties. Individual may be afraid of what others might think of her or him, be concerned of embarrassing self, or of not having money or means of transportation for desired activities.[1]

- Assess factors in client's life that may contribute to sense of helplessness. *Losses, such as a spouse, parent or other, presence of chronic pain/other disabling conditions may cause individual to withdraw, desire to be alone, and refuse to participate in therapeutic activities.*[1]
- Listen to comments of client regarding sense of isolation. Differentiate isolation from solitude and loneliness *that may be acceptable or by choice. Provides clues to what client is thinking and feeling about current situation and what interventions might be appropriate. Client who chooses to be alone and is satisfied may not need further intervention.*[2]
- Assess client's feelings about self, sense of ability to control situation, sense of hope, and coping skills. *Provide basic information for developing an appropriate plan of care. If client is isolating self because of negative feelings, lack of hope, etc., measures to promote self-esteem will need to be taken.*[5]
- Identify support systems available to the client including presence of/relationship with extended family. *People with social anxiety often do not have support systems because of their withdrawal from contact with others. Often the family of origin may be anxious and does not provide the encouragement and support needed by a temperamentally inhibited child. It is difficult for these individuals to ask for help because they are afraid to meet new people and often find support only when they seek help for other conditions, such as depression.*[4]
- Determine drug use (legal/illicit). *Individuals may begin to use drugs such as alcohol or cocaine to control anxiety in social situations. Prescribed medications, such as SSRIs, can be very effective in treating social disorders.*[3]
- Identify behavior response of isolation. *Individual may display behaviors such as excessive sleeping/daydreaming or substance use, which also may potentiate isolation.*[7]
- Review history and elicit information about traumatic events that may have occurred. (Refer to ND Post-Trauma Syndrome.) *While little is known about the origins of social anxiety disorders, clients who have experienced a traumatic event may withdraw from contact and suffer from anxiety when faced with having to deal with social situations.*[1]

NURSING PRIORITY NO. 2. To alleviate conditions that contribute to client's sense of isolation:

- Establish therapeutic nurse-client relationship. *Promotes trust and acceptance, allowing client to feel safe and free to discuss sensitive matters without being judged.*[2]
- Note onset of physical/mental illness and whether recovery is anticipated or condition is chronic/progressive. *Individual may withdraw from activities because of concern about how others view changes that occur due to illness, concern with own thoughts, alterations in physical appearance/mental status. Anticipated length of illness may dictate interventions that are appropriate.*[1]
- Spend time interacting with client, and identify other resources available. *Getting to know client and identifying concerns about being involved in activities with others can lead to appropriate interventions. Other people such as a volunteer, social worker, chaplain may be able to spend time with client, enhancing circle of trusted people.*[4]
- Develop plan of action with client: Look at available resources; support risk-taking behaviors, financial planning, appropriate medical care/self-care, and so forth. *Helping client to learn how to manage these issues of daily living can increase self-confidence and help individual to feel more comfortable in social settings.*[5]

• Introduce client to those with similar/shared interests and other supportive people. *Provides role models and encourages getting to know others who share feelings of anxiety, providing an opportunity to develop social skills and learn some ways of problem solving to deal with anxiety.*[5]

 • Provide positive reinforcement when client makes move(s) toward other(s). *Acknowledges and encourages continuation of efforts, helping client toward independence.*[1]

• Provide for placement in sheltered community when necessary. *The individual who is mentally impaired may be unable to learn to participate in society and display socially acceptable behaviors and will benefit from an environment which offers structure and assistance.*[3]

 • Assist client to problem-solve solutions to short-term/imposed isolation. *Conditions such as communicable disease measures, including compromised host, may require individual to be isolated from others for his or her protection as well as individual's, and working together to decide how to manage loneliness can promote successful outcome.*[3]

• Encourage open visitation when possible and/or telephone contacts. *Maintains involvement with others promoting social involvement, especially when client is unable to go out to activities.*[3]

• Provide environmental stimuli when client is confined. *Open curtains in room, display pictures of family or views of nature, promote television and radio listening to help client feel less isolated.*[3]

 • Promote participation in recreational/special interest activities in setting that client views as safe. *These activities have the advantage of providing physical and mental stimulation for client who feels isolated and anxious in social settings.*[2]

• Identify foreign language resources for client who speaks another language. *A professional interpreter is important to ensure accuracy of interpretation; newspaper, radio programming in appropriate foreign language helps client feel connected with own community.*[6,8]

NURSING PRIORITY NO. 3. To promote wellness (Teaching/Discharge Considerations):

 • Assist client to learn skills as needed. *Enhancing problem solving, communication, social skills, and learning skills to manage ADLs will improve sense of self-esteem.*[4]

 • Encourage and assist client to enroll in classes as appropriate. *Assertiveness, vocational, sex education classes may provide skills to improve ability to engage more effectively in social situations.*[5]

• Involve children and adolescents in programs/activities, as indicated. *Promotes socialization skills and peer contact to enable young person to learn by interacting with others.*[5]

• Help client differentiate between isolation and loneliness or aloneness and discuss how to avoid slipping into an undesired state. *Time for the individual to be alone is important to the maintenance of mental health, but the sadness created by isolation and loneliness needs different interventions.*[2]

  • Involve client in programs directed to correction and prevention of identified causes of problem. *Activities such as senior citizen services, daily telephone contact, house sharing, pets, day-care centers, church resources can help individual move out of isolation and become involved in life.*[5]

• Refer to counselor/therapist as appropriate. *Facilitates grief work, promotes relationship building, and provides opportunity to work toward improvement of individual issues affecting social interactions.*[1]

 Cultural   Collaborative   Community/ Home Care   Diagnostic Studies   Pediatric/Geriatric/Lifespan   Medications

Assessment/Reassessment
- Individual findings, including precipitating factors, effect on lifestyle/relationships, and functioning.
- Client's perception of situation.

Planning
- Plan of care and who is involved in planning.
- Teaching plan.

Implementation/Evaluation
- Responses to interventions/teaching and actions performed.
- Attainment/progress toward desired outcome(s).
- Modifications to plan of care.

Discharge Planning
- Long-term needs/referrals and who is responsible for actions to be taken.
- Available resources, specific referrals made.

References

1. Townsend, M. C. (2003). Psychiatric Mental Health Nursing Concepts of Care, ed 4. Philadelphia: F. A. Davis.
2. Doenges, M. E., Townsend, M. C., & Moorhouse, M. F. (1998). Psychiatric Care Plans Guidelines for Individualizing Care, ed 3. Philadelphia: F. A. Davis.
3. Cox, H., Hinz, M., Lubno, M. A., Newfield, S., Scott-Tilley, D., Slater, M., & Sridaromont, K. (2002). Clinical Applications of Nursing Diagnosis Adult, Child, Women's Psychiatric, Gerontic and Home Health Considerations, ed 4. Philadelphia: F. A. Davis.
4. Drew, N. (1991). Combating the social isolation of chronic mental illness. J Psychosoc Nurs 29(6), 14–17.
5. Harvard Mental Health Letter. Beyond shyness and stage fright: Social anxiety disorder. Oct. 2003.
6. Lipson, J. G., Dibble, S. L., & Minarik, P. A. (1996). Culture & Nursing Care: A Pocket Guide. San Francisco: School of Nursing, UCSF Nursing Press.
7. National Institute of Mental Health. (2000). Anxiety Disorders, NIH Publication No. 00–3879. Rockville, MD: author. Available at: www.nimh.nih.gov.anxiety/anxiety.cfm. Accessed December 2003.
8. Andrulis, D. P. (2002). What a Difference an Interpreter Can Make, Health Care Experiences of Uninsured with Limited English Proficiency, The Access Project. Boston, MA: Brandeis University.

chronic Sorrow

Definition: Cyclical, recurring, and potentially progressive pattern of pervasive sadness experienced (by a parent or caregiver, individual with chronic illness or disability) in response to continual loss, throughout the trajectory of an illness or disability

RELATED FACTORS

Death of a loved one

Experiences chronic physical or mental illness or disability (e.g., mental retardation, MS, prematurity, spina bifida or other birth defects, chronic mental illness, infertility, cancer, Parkinson's disease); one or more trigger events (e.g., crises in management of the illness, crises related to developmental stages, missed opportunities or milestones that bring comparisons with developmental, social, or personal norms)

Unending caregiving as a constant reminder of loss

Subjective

Expresses one or more of the following feelings: anger, being misunderstood, confusion, depression, disappointment, emptiness, fear, frustration, guilt/self-blame, helplessness, hopelessness, loneliness, low self-esteem, recurring loss, overwhelmed
Client expresses periodic, recurrent feelings of sadness

Objective

Feelings that vary in intensity, are periodic, may progress and intensify over time, and may interfere with the client's ability to reach his or her highest level of personal and social well-being
SAMPLE CLINICAL APPLICATIONS: cancer, MS, Parkinson's disease, AIDS, ALS, prematurity, genetic/congenital defects, infertility, dementia/Alzheimer's disease, bipolar disorder, schizophrenia, developmental delay

DESIRED OUTCOMES/EVALUATION CRITERIA

Sample **NOC** linkages:
Depression Level: Severity of level of melancholic mood and loss of interest in life events
Grief Resolution: Adjustment to actual or impending loss
Hope: Presence of internal state of optimism that is personally satisfying and life-supporting

Client Will (Include Specific Time Frame)

- Acknowledge presence/impact of sorrow.
- Demonstrate progress in dealing with grief.
- Participate in work and/or self-care ADLs as able.
- Verbalize a sense of progress toward resolution of sorrow and hope for the future.

ACTIONS/INTERVENTIONS

Sample **NIC** linkages:
Hope Instillation: Facilitation of the development of a positive outlook in a given situation
Grief Work Facilitation: Assistance with the resolution of a significant loss
Coping Enhancement: Assisting a patient to adapt to perceived stressors, changes, or threats that interfere with meeting life demands and roles

NURSING PRIORITY NO. **1.** To assess causative/contributing factors:

 - Determine current/recent events or conditions contributing to client's state of mind, as listed in Related Factors (e.g., death of loved one, chronic physical or mental illness or disability, etc. *Individual information is necessary to formulating a plan of care to address appropriate issues.*[1]

 - Note cues of sadness. *Expressions of feelings of loss, behaviors of sighing, faraway look, unkempt appearance, inattention to conversation, refusing food, etc., can be indicators of sorrow that is not being dealt with.*[5]

 - Determine level of functioning, ability to care for self. *Individual who is coping with chronic illnesses such as Parkinson's, MS, HIV/AIDS may exhibit chronic sorrow related to the illness, fear of death, poverty, and isolation associated with these conditions which may lead to difficulty managing ADLs and need for assistance.*[2,3]

 - Be aware of avoidance behaviors. *Anger, withdrawal, denial are part of the grieving process*

 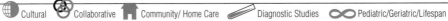

and may be used to avoid dealing with the reality of what has happened. However, in a situation which is unchangeable, such as developmentally disabled child, or the child with diabetes, sorrow is seen as a normal response and will continue to be a factor even as the family copes with the condition.[5]

- Identify cultural factors/religious conflicts. *Expressions of sorrow are influenced by these beliefs and may result in conflicts, for instance, Mexican-American culture believes genetic defects are the will of God, but individual may be angry at God because of occurrence.*[6]

- Ascertain response of family/SOs to client's situation. Assess needs of family/SO. *Parents who have chronically ill children or premature babies; adults who have multiple sclerosis; elderly caregivers of spouses with dementia may continue to have feelings of sorrow even though they may be managing well. Identifying needs of the individuals involved allows for specific interventions to meet them.*[4]

- Refer to NDs dysfunctional Grieving, Caregiver Role Strain, ineffective Coping as appropriate.

NURSING PRIORITY NO. 2. To assist client to move through sorrow:

- Encourage verbalization about situation. *Helpful in beginning resolution and acceptance.* Active-listen feelings and be available *for support/assistance. Individuals involved, client and caregivers, benefit from being able to talk freely about the situation. Active-listening conveys a message of acceptance and helps individual come to own resolution.*[5]

- Encourage expression of anger/fear/anxiety. (Refer to appropriate NDs.) *May need to determine specific interventions for these feelings.*[1]

- Acknowledge reality of feelings of guilt/blame, including hostility toward spiritual power. (Refer to ND Spiritual Distress.) *It had been believed that grief has an end stage but research has shown that individuals in chronic conditions, such as diabetes mellitus, multiple sclerosis, disabling conditions, continue to experience chronic sorrow and lifelong, recurring sadness. Understanding this can help individual accept that feelings of guilt and blame are real and can be dealt with.*[5]

- Provide comfort and availability as well as caring for physical needs. *The way healthcare professionals respond to families is important to helping them cope with the situation as physical care is given.*[5]

- Discuss ways individual has dealt with past losses and reinforce use of previously effective coping skills. *As client begins to look at how they have handled previous situations, effective coping skills can be recalled and applied to current situation.*[2]

- Instruct/encourage use of visualization and relaxation skills. *Learning these stress management skills can help the individual relax promoting ability to deal with feelings of sorrow regarding the long-term situation.*[5]

- Assist SO to cope with client response. *Family/SO may not be dysfunctional, but may be intolerant and lack understanding of individual responses to long-term illness. Grief is unique to each individual and may not always follow a particular course to resolution which may not be understood by all.*[5]

- Include family/SO in setting realistic goals for meeting individual needs. *Inclusion of all family members ensures they all have the same information and are all working toward effective coping strategies.*[5]

NURSING PRIORITY NO. 3. To promote wellness (Teaching/Discharge Considerations):

- Discuss healthy ways of dealing with difficult situations. Providing information about effective communication skills, understanding condition they are dealing with and expectations of the course of the illness/condition can promote personal growth and lead to a positive outcome for the family.[7]

 • Have client identify familial, religious, and cultural factors that have meaning for him or her. *May help bring loss or distressing situation into perspective and promote grief/sorrow understanding.*[6]

 • Encourage involvement in usual activities, exercise, and socialization within limits of physical and psychological state. *Energy is restored and individuals can go on with their lives when they are willing and able to continue activities.*[5,7]

 • Introduce concept of mindfulness (living in the moment). *Promotes feelings of capability and belief that this moment can be dealt with.*[8]

 • Refer to other resources (e.g., pastoral care, counseling, psychotherapy, respite care providers, support groups). *Provides additional help when needed to resolve situation, continue grief work and move on with life.*[3]

DOCUMENTATION FOCUS

Assessment/Reassessment
- Individual findings, including nature of sorrow, effects on participation in treatment regimen.
- Physical/emotional response to conflict.
- Reactions of family/SO.

Planning
- Plan of care and who is involved in planning.
- Teaching plan.

Implementation/Evaluation
- Response to interventions/teaching, and actions performed.
- Attainment/progress toward desired outcome(s).
- Modifications to plan of care.

Discharge Planning
- Long-term needs and who is responsible for actions to be taken.
- Available resources, specific referrals made.

References

1. Doenges, M. E., Moorhouse, M. F., & Geissler-Murr, A. C. (2004). Nurse's Pocket Guide Diagnoses, Interventions and Rationales, ed 9. Philadelphia: F. A. Davis.
2. Lindgren, C. L. (1996). Chronic sorrow in persons with Parkinson's and their spouse caregivers. Scholarly Inquiry for Nursing Practice: An International Journal, 10(4), 351–366.
3. Lichtensten, B., Laska, M. K., & Clair, J. M. (2002). Chronic sorrow in the HIV-positive patient: Issues of race, gender, and social support. Birmingham, Alabama: Department of Sociology, University of Alabama at Birmingham.
4. Kearney, P. (2003). Chronic Grief (Or Is It Periodic Grief?). Available at: http://www.indiana.edu/~famlygrf/units/chronic.html. Accessed February 2004.
5. Lowes, L., & Lyne, P. (2000). Chronic sorrow in parents of children with newly diagnosed diabetes: a review of the literature and discussion of the implications for nursing practice. J Advanced Nurs 32(1), 41–48.
6. Lipson, J. G., Dibble, S. L., & Minarik, P. A. (1996). Culture & Nursing Care: A Pocket Guide. San Francisco: School of Nursing, UCSF Nursing Press.
7. Mallow, G. E., & Bechtel, G. A. (1999). Chronic sorrow: the experience of parents with children who are developmentally disabled. J Psychosoc Nurs 17(7), 31–43.
8. Kabat-Zinn, J. (1994). Wherever You Go There You Are. New York: Hyperion.

 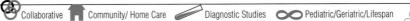

Spiritual Distress

Definition: Impaired ability to experience and integrate meaning and purpose in life through a person's connectedness with self, others, art, music, literature, nature, or a power greater than oneself.

RELATED FACTORS

Loneliness/social alienation; self-alienation; sociocultural deprivation
Anxiety; pain
Life change
Chronic illness of self or others; death and dying of self or others
[Challenged belief/value system (e.g., moral/ethical implications of therapy)]

DEFINING CHARACTERISTICS

Subjective
Connections to Self
Expresses lack of: Hope; meaning and purpose in life; peace/serenity; love; acceptance; forgiveness of self; courage
[Expresses] anger; guilt

Connections to Others
Refuses interactions with friends, family/ spiritual leaders
Verbalizes being separated from their support system
Expresses alienation

Connections with Art, Music, Literature, Nature
Inability to express previous state of creativity (singing/listening to music/writing)
No interest in nature
No interest in reading spiritual literature

Connections with Power Greater Than Self
Inability to pray/participate in religious activities; sudden changes in spiritual practices
Expresses being abandoned by or having anger toward God; without hope, suffering
Requests to see a religious leader

Objective
Connections to Self
Poor coping

Connections with Power Greater Than Self
Inability to be introspective/inward turning; to experience the transcendent

SAMPLE CLINICAL APPLICATIONS: chronic conditions (e.g., rheumatoid arthritis, MS, systemic lupus erythematosus, ALS), cancer, traumatic brain injury/vegetative state, fetal demise, infertility, SIDS

DESIRED OUTCOMES/EVALUATION CRITERIA

Sample **NOC** Linkages:
Spiritual Well-Being: Personal expression of connectedness with self, others, higher power, all life, nature, and the universe that transcend and empower the self

Hope: Presence of internal state of optimism that is personally satisfying and life-supporting

Psychosocial Adjustment: Life Change: Psychosocial adaptation of an individual to a life change

Client Will (Include Specific Time Frame)
- Verbalize increased sense of connectedness and hope for future.
- Demonstrate ability to help self/participate in care.
- Participate in activities with others, actively seek relationships.
- Discuss beliefs/values about spiritual issues.
- Verbalize acceptance of self as not deserving illness/situation, "no one is to blame."

ACTIONS/INTERVENTIONS
Sample **NIC** Linkages:

Spiritual Support: Assisting the patient to feel balance and connection with a greater power

Hope Instillation: Facilitation of the development of a positive outlook in a given situation

Grief Work Facilitation: Assistance with the resolution of a significant loss

NURSING PRIORITY NO. **1.** To assess causative/contributing factors:

- 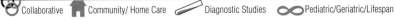 Determine client's religious/spiritual orientation, current involvement, presence of conflicts. *Identification of individual spiritual practices/restrictions that may affect client care or create conflict between spiritual beliefs and treatment provide for more accurate interventions.*[1]

- Listen to client's/SO(s') reports/expressions of anger or concern, alienation from God, belief that illness/situation is a punishment for wrongdoing, and so forth. *Indicates depth of grieving process and possible need for spiritual advisor or other resource to address client's belief system if desired.*[2]

- Determine sense of futility, feelings of hopelessness and helplessness, lack of motivation to help self. *Indicators that client may see no, or only limited, options/alternatives or personal choices available, lacks energy to deal with situation and need for further evaluation.*[1]

- Note expressions of inability to find meaning in life, reason for living. Evaluate suicidal ideation. *Crisis of the spirit/loss of will-to-live places client at increased risk for inattention to personal well-being/harm to self. Indicates need for referral to mental health professional for evaluation/intervention.*[1]

- Note recent changes in behavior (e.g., withdrawal from others/creative or religious activities, dependence on alcohol/medications). *Helpful in determining severity/duration of situation and possible need for additional referrals such as substance withdrawal.*[1]

- Assess sense of self-concept, worth, ability to enter into loving relationships. *Lack of connectedness with self/others impairs client's ability to trust others or feel worthy of trust from others leading to difficulties in relationships with others.*[1]

- Observe behavior indicative of poor relationships with others (e.g., manipulative, nontrusting, demanding). *Manipulation is used for management of client's sense of powerlessness because of distrust of others, interfering with relationships with others.*[3]

- Determine support systems available to client/SO(s) and how they are used. *Provides insight to client's willingness to pursue outside resources.*[1]

- Be aware of influence of caregiver's belief system. *It is still possible to be helpful to client while remaining neutral/not espousing own beliefs because client's beliefs and needs are what is important.*[6]

 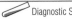

- Assess for influence of cultural beliefs and spiritual values that affect individual in this situation. *Circumstances of illness/situation may conflict with client's view of self, cultural background, and distress over values. For instance, many Mexican Americans are Catholic with strong beliefs in the relationship of illness and religious practices.*[5]

NURSING PRIORITY NO. 2. To assist client/SO(s) to deal with feelings/situation:

- Develop therapeutic nurse-client relationship. Ask how you can be most helpful. Convey acceptance of client's spiritual beliefs/concerns. *Promotes trust and comfort, encouraging client to be open about sensitive matters.*[6]
- Identify inappropriate coping behaviors and associated consequences and discuss with client. *Recognizing consequences of actions may enhance desire to change.*[2]
- Ascertain past coping behaviors. *Helps to determine approaches used previously that may be effective in dealing with current situation, providing encouragement.*[6]
- Problem-solve solutions/identify areas for compromise. *May be useful in resolving conflicts that arise from feelings of anxiety regarding questioning of beliefs and current illness/situation.*[3]
- Establish environment that promotes free expression of feelings and concerns. *Provides opportunity for client to explore own thoughts and make appropriate decisions regarding spiritual issues.*[4]
- Provide calm, peaceful setting when possible. *Promotes relaxation and enhances opportunity for reflection on situation/discussions with others, meditation.*[3]
- Set limits on acting-out behavior that is inappropriate/destructive. *Promotes safety for client/others and helps prevent loss of self-esteem.*[2]
- Make time for nonjudgmental discussion of philosophic issues/questions about spiritual impact of illness/situation and/or treatment regimen. *Open communication can assist client in reality checks of perceptions and help to identify personal options.*[6]
- Involve client in refining healthcare goals and therapeutic regimen as appropriate. *Promotes feelings of control over what is happening, enhancing commitment to plan and optimizing outcomes.*[3]
- Discuss difference between grief and guilt and help client to identify and deal with each. Point out consequences of actions based on guilt. *Aids client in assuming responsibility for own actions and avoids acting out of false guilt.*[6]
- Use therapeutic communication skills of reflection and Active-listening. *Conveys message of competence and helps client find own solutions to concerns.*[7]
- Identify role models (e.g., individual experiencing similar situation). *Provides opportunities for sharing of experiences/hope and identifying new options to deal with situation.*[7]
- Suggest use of journaling. *Provides opportunity to write feelings and happenings; reviewing them over time can assist in clarifying values/ideas, recognizing and resolving feelings/situation.*[6]
- Assist client to learn use of meditation/prayer. *Provides avenue for learning forgiveness to heal past hurts and developing a sense of peace.*[3]
- Provide information that anger with God is a normal part of the grieving process. *Realizing these feelings are not unusual can reduce sense of guilt, encourage open expression, and facilitate resolution of grief.*[3]
- Provide time and privacy to engage in spiritual growth/religious activities as desired (e.g., prayer, meditation, scripture reading, listening to music). *Allows client to focus on self and seek connectedness with spiritual beliefs and values.*[6]

• Encourage/facilitate outings to neighborhood park/nature walks. *Sunshine, fresh air and activity can stimulate release of endorphins, promoting sense of well-being encouraging connection with nature.*[6]

 • Provide play therapy for child that encompasses spiritual data. *Interactive pleasurable activity promotes open discussion and enhances retention of information. Child will act out feelings in play therapy easier than talking. Provides opportunity for child to practice what has been learned and for therapist to evaluate child's progress.*[3]

• Abide by parents' wishes in discussing and implementing child's spiritual support. *Limits confusion for child and prevents conflict of values/beliefs.*[3]

• Refer to appropriate resources (e.g., pastoral/parish nurse or religious counselor, crisis counselor, hospice; psychotherapy; Alcoholics/Narcotics Anonymous). *Useful in dealing with immediate situation and identifying long-term resources for support to help foster sense of connectedness.*[7]

• Refer to NDs ineffective Coping, Powerlessness, Self-Esteem (specify), Social Isolation, risk for Suicide for additional interventions as indicated.

NURSING PRIORITY NO. 3. To promote wellness (Teaching/Discharge Considerations):

• Assist client to develop goals for dealing with life/illness situation. *Involvement in planning for desired outcomes enhances commitment to goal, optimizing outcomes.*[7]

• Encourage life-review by client. Support client in finding a reason for living. *Promotes sense of hope and willingness to continue efforts to improve situation.*[3]

• Assist in developing coping skills *to deal with stressors of illness/necessary changes in lifestyle.*[7]

• Assist client to identify SO(s) and people who could provide support as needed. *Ongoing support is important to enhance sense of connectedness and continue progress toward goals.*[6]

• Assist client to identify spiritual resources that could be helpful (e.g., contact spiritual advisor who has qualifications/experience in dealing with specific problems such as death/dying, relationship problems, substance abuse, suicide). *Provides answers to spiritual questions, assists in the journey of self-discovery, and can help client learn to accept and forgive self.*[6]

DOCUMENTATION FOCUS

Assessment/Reassessment
• Individual findings, including nature of spiritual conflict, effects of participation in treatment regimen.
• Physical/emotional responses to conflict.

Planning
• Plan of care and who is involved in planning.
• Teaching plan.

Implementation/Evaluation
• Responses to interventions/teaching and actions performed.
• Attainment/progress toward desired outcome(s).
• Modifications to plan of care.

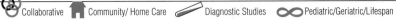

Discharge Planning

- Long-term needs and who is responsible for actions to be taken.
- Available resources, specific referrals made.

References

1. Fallot, R. D. (1998a). Assessment of spirituality and implications for service planning. New Directions in Mental Health Services, 80, 13–23.
2. Moller, M. D. (1999). Meeting spiritual needs on an inpatient unit. J Psychosoc Nurs, 37(11), 5–10.
3. Baldacchino, D., & Draper, P. (2001). Spiritual coping strategies: A review of the nursing research literature. J Adv Nurs, 34(6), 833–841.
4. Cox, H. C., et al. (2002). Clinical Applications of Nursing Diagnosis, ed 4. Philadelphia: F. A. Davis.
5. Lipson, J. G., Dibble, S. L., & Minarik, P. A. (1996). Culture & Nursing Care: A Pocket Guide. San Francisco: UCSF Nursing Press.
6. Ross, L. A. (1994). Spiritual aspects of nursing, J Adv Nurs, 19, 439–447.
7. Townsend, M. C. (2003). Psychiatric Mental Health Nursing Concepts of Care, ed 4. Philadelphia: F. A. Davis.

risk for Spiritual Distress

Definition: At risk for an altered sense of harmonious connectedness with all of life and the universe in which dimensions that transcend and empower the self may be disrupted

RISK FACTORS

Physical or psychological stress; energy-consuming anxiety; physical/mental illness

Situation/maturational losses; loss of loved one

Blocks to self-love; low self-esteem; poor relationships; inability to forgive

Substance abuse

Natural disasters

NOTE: A risk diagnosis is not evidenced by signs and symptoms, as the problem has not occurred and nursing interventions are directed at prevention.

SAMPLE CLINICAL APPLICATIONS: chronic conditions (e.g., rheumatoid arthritis, MS, systemic lupus erythematosus, ALS), cancer, traumatic brain injury/vegetative state, fetal demise, infertility, SIDS

DESIRED OUTCOMES/EVALUATION CRITERIA

Sample **NOC** linkages:

Spiritual Well-Being: Personal expression of connectedness with self, others, higher power, and all life, nature, and the universe that transcend and empower the self

Coping: Actions to manage stressors that tax an individual's resources

Hope: Presence of internal state of optimism that is personally satisfying and life-supporting

Client Will (Include Specific Time Frame)

- Identify meaning and purpose in one's life that reinforces hope, peace, and contentment.
- Verbalize acceptance of self as being worthy, not deserving of illness/situation, and so forth.
- Identify and use resources appropriately.

ACTIONS/INTERVENTIONS

Sample **NIC** linkages:

Spiritual Support: Assisting the patient to feel balance and connection with a greater power

Coping Enhancement: Promotion of deep inhalation by the patient with subsequent generation of high intrathoracic pressures and compression of underlying lung parenchyma for the forceful expulsion of air

Forgiveness Facilitation: Assisting an individual to forgive and/or experience forgiveness in relationship with self, others, and higher power

NURSING PRIORITY NO. 1. To assess causative/contributing factors:

 • Ascertain current situation (e.g., natural disaster, death of a spouse, personal injustice). *Identification of circumstances that put the individual at risk for loss of connectedness with spiritual beliefs are essential to plan for appropriate interventions.*[8]

 • Listen to client's/SO(s') reports/expressions of anger/concern, belief that illness/situation is a punishment for wrongdoing, and so forth. *Identifies need for client to talk about and be listened to in regard to concerns about potential loss of control over his/her life.*[3]

 • Note reason for living and whether it is directly related to situation. *Tragic occurrences such as home and business washed away in a flood/lost in a fire, parent whose only child is terminally ill, loss of a spouse can cause individual to question previous beliefs and how he or she has coped in the past/will cope in future.*[3]

 • Determine client's religious/spiritual orientation, current involvement, presence of conflicts, especially in current circumstances. *Client may be a member of a religious organization and whether he or she is active or whether conflicts have risen in relation to current illness/situation will indicate need for assistance from spiritual advisor, pastor or other resource client would accept.*[1]

 • Assess sense of self-concept, worth, ability to enter into loving relationships. *Lack of connectedness with self and others impairs client's ability to trust others or feel worthy of trust from others.*[1]

 • Observe behavior indicative of poor relationships with others. *Client may be manipulative, nontrusting, and demanding because of distrust of self and others, interfering with relationships with others, indicating need for learning positive ways to interact with others.*[2]

 • Determine support systems available to and used by client/SO(s). *Provides insight into individual's willingness to pursue outside resources.*[6]

 • Ascertain substance use/abuse. *Affects ability to deal with problems in a positive manner and determines severity/duration of problem and need for referral to appropriate treatment programs.*[4]

• Assess for influence of cultural beliefs and spiritual values that affect individual in this situation. *Circumstances of illness/situation may conflict with client's view of self, cultural background, and distress over values. For instance, many Mexican Americans are Catholic with strong beliefs in the relationship of illness and religious practices.*[5]

NURSING PRIORITY NO. 2. To assist client/SO(s) to deal with feelings/situation:

 • Establish environment that promotes free expression of feelings and concerns. *Provides opportunity for client to explore own thoughts and make appropriate decisions regarding spiritual issues and conflicts.*[7]

 • Have client identify and prioritize current/immediate needs. *Helps client focus on what needs to be done and identify manageable steps to take to achieve goals.*[6]

 • Make time for nonjudgmental discussion of philosophical issues/questions about spiritual impact of illness/situation and/or treatment regimen. *Open communication can assist client to make reality checks of perceptions and begin to identify personal options.*[6]

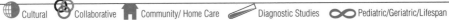

- Discuss difference between grief and guilt and help client to identify and deal with each. *Helps client to assume responsibility for own actions, become aware of the consequences of acting out of false guilt.*[6]
- Use therapeutic communication skills of reflection and Active-listening. *Communicates confidence in client's ability to find own solutions to concerns.*[7]
- Review coping skills used and their effectiveness in current situation. *Identifies strengths to incorporate into plan and techniques needing revision.*[6]
- Identify role model, (e.g., individual experiencing similar situation/disease). *Sharing of experiences/hope provides opportunity for client to look at options as modeled by other and to begin to deal with reality.*[7]
- Suggest use of journaling. *Provides opportunity to write feelings and happenings; reviewing them over time can assist in clarifying values/ideas, recognizing and resolving feelings/ situation.*[6]
- Provide play therapy for child that encompasses spiritual data. *Interactive pleasurable activity promotes open discussion and enhances retention of information. Child will act out feelings in play therapy easier than talking. Provides opportunity for child to practice what has been learned and for therapist to evaluate child's progress.*[3]
- Abide by parents' wishes in discussing and implementing child's spiritual support. *Limits confusion for child and prevents conflict of values/beliefs.*[3]
- Refer to appropriate resources (e.g., crisis counselor, governmental agencies; pastoral/parish nurse or spiritual advisor who has qualifications/experience dealing with specific problems such as death/dying, relationship problems, substance abuse, suicide; hospice, psychotherapy, Alcoholics/ Narcotics Anonymous). *Useful in dealing with immediate situation and identifying long-term resources for support to help foster sense of connectedness.*[7]

NURSING PRIORITY NO. 3. To promote wellness (Teaching/Discharge Considerations):

- Role-play new coping techniques. *Provides opportunity to practice and enhances integration of new skills/necessary lifestyle changes.*[4]
- Assist client to identify SO(s) and individuals/support groups who could provide ongoing support. *This is a daily need requiring lifelong commitment and having sufficient support can help client maintain spiritual resolve.*[6]
- Discuss benefit of family counseling as appropriate. *Issues of this nature (e.g., situational losses, natural disasters, difficult relationships) affect family dynamics and family may find it useful to discuss problems they are experiencing.*[7]

DOCUMENTATION FOCUS

Assessment/Reassessment
- Individual findings, including risk factors, nature of current distress.
- Physical/emotional responses to distress.
- Access to/use of resources.

Planning
- Plan of care and who is involved in planning.
- Teaching plan.

Implementation/Evaluation
- Responses to interventions/teaching and actions performed.
- Attainment/progress toward desired outcome(s).
- Modifications to plan of care.

Discharge Planning
- Long-term needs and who is responsible for actions to be taken.
- Available resources, specific referrals made.

References
1. Fallot, R. D. (1998a). Assessment of spirituality and implications for service planning. New Directions in Mental Health Services, 80, 13–23.
2. Moller, M. D. (1999). Meeting spiritual needs on an inpatient unit. J Psychosoc Nurs, 37(11), 5–10.
3. Baldacchino, D., & Draper, P. (2001). Spiritual coping strategies: A review of the nursing research literature. J Adv Nurs, 34(6), 833–841.
4. Cox, H. C, et al. (2002). Clinical Applications of Nursing Diagnosis: Adult, Child, Women's, Psychiatric, Gerontic, and Home Health Considerations, ed 4. Philadelphia: F. A. Davis.
5. Lipson, J. G., Dibble, S. L., & Minarik, P. A. (1996). Culture & Nursing Care: A Pocket Guide. San Francisco: UCSF Nursing Press.
6. Ross, L. A. (1994). Spiritual aspects of nursing. J Adv Nurs, 19, 439–447.
7. Townsend, M. C. (2003). Psychiatric Mental Health Nursing Concepts of Care, ed 4. Philadelphia: F. A. Davis.
8. Doenges, M. E., Moorhouse, M. F., & Murr, A. C. (2004). Nurse's Pocket Guide Diagnoses, Interventions, and Rationales, ed 9. Philadelphia: F. A. Davis.

readiness for enhanced Spiritual Well-Being

Definition: Ability to experience and integrate meaning and purpose in life through a person's connectedness with self, others, art, music, literature, nature, or a power greater than oneself

RELATED FACTORS
To be developed by nurse researchers and submitted to NANDA

DEFINING CHARACTERISTICS

Subjective
Connections to Self
Desire for enhanced: Hope; meaning and purpose in life; peace/serenity; acceptance; surrender; love; forgiveness of self; satisfying philosophy of life; joy; courage
Meditation

Connections with Others
Requests interactions with friends, family/spiritual leaders
Provides service to others
Requests forgiveness of others

Connections with Powers Greater Than Self
Participates in religious activities; prays
Expresses reverence, [awe]; reports mystical experiences

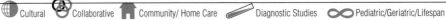

Objective

Connections to Self
Heightened coping

Connections with Others
Provides service to others

Connections with Art, Music, Literature, Nature
Displays creative energy (e.g., writing, poetry); sings/listens to music; reads spiritual literature; spends time outdoors

SAMPLE CLINICAL APPLICATIONS: as a health-seeking behavior the client may be healthy or this diagnosis can occur in any clinical condition

DESIRED OUTCOMES/EVALUATION CRITERIA
Sample **NOC** linkages:

Spiritual Well-Being: Personal expression of connectedness with self, others, higher power, and all life, nature, and the universe that transcend and empower the self

Hope: Presence of internal state of optimism that is personally satisfying and life-supporting

Quality of Life: An individual's expressed satisfaction with current life circumstances

Client Will (Include Specific Time Frame)
- Acknowledge the stabilizing and strengthening forces in one's life needed for balance and well-being of the whole person.
- Identify meaning and purpose in one's life that reinforces hope, peace, and contentment.
- Verbalize a sense of peace/contentment and comfort of spirit.
- Demonstrate behavior congruent with verbalizations that lend support and strength for daily living.

ACTIONS/INTERVENTIONS

Sample **NIC** linkages:

Spiritual Growth Facilitation: Facilitation of growth in patient's capacity to identify, connect with, and call upon the source of meaning, purpose, comfort, strength, and hope in his/her life

Religious Ritual Enhancement: Facilitating participation in religious practices

Meditation Facilitation: Facilitating a person to alter his/her level of awareness by focusing specifically on an image or thought

NURSING PRIORITY NO. 1. To determine spiritual state/motivation for growth:

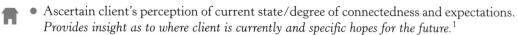

- Ascertain client's perception of current state/degree of connectedness and expectations. *Provides insight as to where client is currently and specific hopes for the future.*[1]
- Review spiritual/religious history, activities/rituals and frequency of participation. *Determines basis to build on for growth/change.*[1]
- Determine relational values of support systems to one's spiritual centeredness. *The client's family of origin may have differing beliefs from those espoused by the individual that may be a source of conflict for the client. Comfort can be gained when family and friends share client's beliefs and support search for spiritual knowledge.*[2]

- Explore meaning/interpretation and relationship of spirituality, life/death, and illness to life's journey. *This information helps client strengthen personal belief system, enabling him or her to move forward and live life to the fullest.*[2,3]
- Clarify the meaning of one's spiritual beliefs/religious practice and rituals to daily living. *Discussing these issues allows client to explore spiritual needs and decide what fits own view of the world to enhance life.*[6]
- Explore ways that spirituality/religious practices have affected one's life and given meaning and value to daily living. Note consequences as well as benefits. *Promotes understanding and appreciation of the difference between spirituality and religion and how each can be used to enhance client's journey of self-discovery.*[3]
- Discuss life's/God's plan (when this is the person's belief) for the individual. *Helpful in determining individual goals/choosing specific options.*[2]

NURSING PRIORITY NO. 2. To assist client to integrate values and beliefs to achieve a sense of wholeness and optimum balance in daily living:

- Explore ways beliefs give meaning and value to daily living. *As client develops understanding of these issues they will provide support for dealing with current/future concerns.*[4]
- Clarify reality/appropriateness of client's self-perceptions and expectations. *Necessary to provide firm foundation for growth. Unrealistic ideas can impede desired improvement.*[2]
- Determine influence of cultural beliefs/values. *Most individuals are strongly influenced by the spiritual/religious orientation of their family of origin which can be a very major determinate for client's choice of activities/receptiveness to various options.*[5]
- Discuss the importance and value of connections to one's daily life. *The contacts that one has with others maintains a feeling of belonging and connection and promotes feelings of wholeness and well-being.*[4,6]
- Identify ways to achieve connectedness or harmony with self, others, nature, higher power (e.g., meditation, prayer, talking/sharing one's self with others; being out in nature/gardening/walking; attending religious activities). *This is a highly individual and personal decision, and no action is too trivial to be considered.*[4]

NURSING PRIORITY NO. 3. To enhance wellness:

- Encourage client to take time to be introspective in the search for peace and harmony. *Finding peace within oneself will carry over to relationships with others and one's outlook on life.*[1]
- Discuss use of relaxation/meditative activities (e.g., yoga, tai chi, prayer). *Helpful in promoting general well-being and sense of connectedness with self/nature/spiritual power.*[4]
- Suggest attendance/involvement in dream-sharing group *to develop/enhance learning of the characteristics of spiritual awareness and facilitate the individual's growth.*[1]
- Identify ways for spiritual/religious expression. *There are multiple options for enhancing spirituality through connectedness with self/others (e.g., volunteering time to community projects, mentoring, singing in the choir, painting, or spiritual writings).*[4]
- Encourage participation in desired religious activities, contact with minister/spiritual advisor. *Validating one's beliefs in an external way can provide support and strengthen the inner self.*[1]
- Discuss and role-play, as necessary, ways to deal with alternative view/conflict that may occur with family/SO(s)/society or cultural group. *Provides opportunity to try out different behaviors in a safe environment and be prepared for potential ities.*[3]

 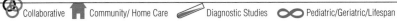

🏠 • Provide bibliotherapy, list of relevant resources (e.g., study groups, parish nurse, poetry society), and possible Web sites *for later reference/self-paced learning and ongoing support.*[3]

DOCUMENTATION FOCUS

Assessment/Reassessment
- Assessment findings, including client perception of needs and desire/expectations for growth/enhancement.

Planning
- Plan for growth and who is involved in planning.

Implementation/Evaluation
- Response to activities/learning and actions performed.
- Attainment/progress toward desired outcome(s).
- Modifications to plan.

Discharge Planning
- Long-range needs/expectations and plan of action.
- Specific referrals made.

References

1. Fallot, R. D. (1998a). Assessment of spirituality and implications for service planning. New Directions in Mental Health Services, 80, 13–23.
2. Moller, M. D. (1999). Meeting spiritual needs on an inpatient unit. J of Psychosoc Nurs, 37(11), 5–10.
3. Baldacchino, D, & Draper, P. (2001). Spiritual coping strategies: A review of the nursing research literature. J Adv Nurs, 34(6), 833–841.
4. Cox, H. C., et al. (2002). Clinical Applications of Nursing Diagnosis, ed 4. Philadelphia: F. A. Davis.
5. Lipson, J. G., Dibble, S. L., & Minarik, P. A. (1996). Culture & Nursing Care: A Pocket Guide. San Francisco: UCSF Nursing Press.
6. Ross, L. A. (1994). Spiritual aspects of nursing. J Adv Nurs, 19, 439–447.

risk for Suffocation

Definition: Accentuated risk of accidental suffocation (inadequate air available for inhalation)

RISK FACTORS

Internal (individual)
Reduced olfactory sensation
Reduced motor abilities
Lack of safety education, precautions
Cognitive or emotional difficulties [e.g., altered consciousness/mentation]
Disease or injury process

External (environmental)
Pillow/propped bottle placed in an infant's crib
Pacifier hung around infant's head

Children playing with plastic bag or inserting small objects into their mouths or noses
Children left unattended in bathtubs or pools
Discarded or unused refrigerators or freezers without removed doors
Vehicle warming in closed garage [faulty exhaust system]; use of fuel-burning heaters not vented to outside
Household gas leaks; smoking in bed
Low-strung clothesline
Person who eats large mouthfuls [or pieces] of food
NOTE: A risk diagnosis is not evidenced by signs and symptoms, as the problem has not occurred and nursing interventions are directed at prevention.
SAMPLE CLINICAL APPLICATIONS: substance use/abuse, spinal cord injury, crushing chest injury, obesity, near-drowning, burn/inhalation injury, sleep apnea, seizure disorder

DESIRED OUTCOMES/EVALUATION CRITERIA
Sample **NOC** linkages:
Risk Control: Actions to eliminate or reduce actual, personal, and modifiable health threats
Aspiration Control: Personal actions to prevent the passage of fluid and solid particles into the lung
Safety Behavior: Personal: Individual or caregiver efforts to control behaviors that might cause physical injury

Client/SO Will (Include Specific Time Frame)
- Verbalize knowledge of hazards in the environment.
- Identify interventions appropriate to situation.
- Correct hazardous situations to prevent/reduce risk of suffocation.
- Demonstrate CPR skills and how to access emergency assistance.

ACTIONS/INTERVENTIONS
Sample **NIC** linkages:
Airway Management: Facilitation of patency of air passages
Aspiration Precautions: Prevention or minimization of risk factors in the patient at risk for aspiration
Teaching Infant Safety: Instruction on safety during first year of life

NURSING PRIORITY NO. 1. To assess causative/contributing factors:

 - Note presence of internal/external factors in individual situation (e.g., seizure activity, inadequate supervision of small child or cognitively impaired individual; comatose client; person with motor or sensory impairments) *with inability to manage own environment or safety issues.*
- Identify client at potential risk (e.g., person with altered level of consciousness, infant/young child, person with trauma, developmental delay, cognitive, or neurologic impairments. *Suffocation can be caused by 1) spasm of airway (e.g., food or water going down wrong way, irritant gases, asthma, 2) airway obstruction (e.g., foreign body, tongue falling back in unconscious person, or swelling of tissues from burn injury), 3) airway compression (e.g., tying rope tightly around neck, hanging, throttling, or smothering), 4) conditions affecting the respiratory mechanism (e.g., epilepsy, tetanus, rabies, nerve diseases causing paralysis of chest wall or diaphragm), 5) conditions affecting respiratory center in brain (e.g., electric shock, stroke/other brain trauma; medications such as morphine, barbiturates), and 6)*

 Cultural   Collaborative   Community/ Home Care Diagnostic Studies Pediatric/Geriatric/Lifespan Medications

compression of the chest (e.g., crushing as might occur with cave-in, auto crash, pressure in a massive crowd). [1]

- Determine client's/SO's knowledge of safety factors/hazards present in the environment *to identify misconceptions and educational needs.*
- Identify level of concern/awareness and motivation of client/SO(s) to correct safety hazards and improve individual situation. *Lack of commitment may limit growth/willingness to make changes, placing dependent individuals at risk.*
- Assess neurologic status. *Factors such as stroke, cerebral palsy, MS, ALS, etc. have potential to compromise airway or affect ability to swallow.*
- Review medication regimen (e.g., analgesics, sedatives, antidepressants), *to note potential for oversedation and respiratory or swallowing impairments.*
- Be alert to/carefully monitor those individuals who are severely depressed, mentally ill, or aggressive and in restraints. *These individuals could be at risk for suicide by suffocation (e.g., inhaled carbon monoxide, or death by strangling or hanging).* [2] (Refer to ND risk for Suicide.)
- Monitor for respiratory distress (e.g., cough, stridor, wheezing, increased work of breathing) *that could indicate swelling/obstruction of airways.* [3] (Refer to NDs: ineffective Airway Clearance, risk for Aspiration, ineffective Breathing Pattern, impaired spontaneous Ventilation as appropriate for additional interventions.)
- Determine use of antiepileptics and how well epilepsy is controlled. *Seizure activity (and especially status epilepticus) is a major risk factor for respiratory inhibition/arrest.* [4]
- Note reports of sleep disturbance and daytime fatigue. *May be indicative of sleep apnea (airway obstruction).* (Refer to ND: disturbed Sleep Pattern.)

NURSING PRIORITY NO. 2. To reverse/correct contributing factors: [2,4–9]

- Discuss with client/SO(s) identified environmental safety hazards and problem-solve methods for resolution (e.g., need for smoke/carbon monoxide alarms, vents for household heater, clean chimney, properly strung clothesline).
- Protect airway at all times, especially if client unable to protect self:
  Use proper positioning, suctioning, use of adjuncts as indicated for infant, comatose or cognitively impaired client.
  Provide seizure precautions and antiseizure medications as indicated.
  Avoid physical and mechanical restraints including vest/waist restraint, side rails, choke hold. *Increases agitation and risk of partial escape, resulting in entrapment of head/hanging.*
  When using oral chemical restraint, administer medication when client is sitting or standing upright and can swallow without difficulty.
  Review importance of chewing carefully, taking small amounts of food, using caution *to prevent aspiration when talking or drinking while eating.*
  Provide diet modifications as indicated by extent of swallowing dysfunction *to reduce risk of aspiration.*
  Emphasize with client/SO the importance of getting help when beginning to choke or feel respiratory distress (e.g., staying with people instead of leaving table, make gestures across throat; making sure someone recognizes the emergency) *in order to provide timely intervention (abdominal thrusts).*
- Refrain from smoking in bed; supervise smoking materials (use, disposal, and storage) in impaired individuals. Keep smoking materials out of reach of children.
- Avoid idling automobile (or using fuel-burning heaters) in closed or unvented spaces.
- Emphasize importance of periodic evaluation and repair of gas appliances/furnace, automobile exhaust system *to prevent exposure to carbon monoxide.*

• Review child protective measures:

Place infant in nonprone position for sleep. (Refer to ND: sudden infant Death Syndrome.)

Do not prop baby bottles in infant crib.

Remove bib before putting baby in bed.

Store/dispose of plastic bag (e.g. shopping, garbage, dry cleaning, and shipping) out of reach of infants/young children.

Avoid use of plastic mattress or crib covers.

Avoid placing infant to sleep on soft surfaces (e.g., beanbag chair, basket with soft sides, soft pillow, water bed) *that baby can sink into or be unable to free face.*

Use a crib with slats that are no more than 2 3/8 inches apart *so that baby cannot get head trapped or slip body through slats.*

Avoid bedsharing with infant/young child *to prevent accidental smothering.*

Provide constant supervision of young children in bathtub or swimming pool.

Make certain that blind and curtain cords, drawstrings on clothing, etc., are out of reach of small children *to prevent accidental hanging.*

Observe young child and impaired individual for objects put in mouth (e.g., food such as raw carrots, nuts, seeds, popcorn, hot dogs; toy parts, buttons, balloons, batteries, coins, etc.) *that can get lodged in airway/cause choking.*

Lock/remove lid or door of chests, trunks, old refrigerators/freezers *to prevent child from being trapped in airless environment.*

NURSING PRIORITY NO. 3. To promote wellness (Teaching/Discharge Considerations):

• Review safety factors identified in individual situation and methods for remediation.
• Develop plan with client/caregiver for long-range management of situation to avoid injuries. *Enhances commitment to plan, optimizing outcomes.*
• Discuss possibility of choking *because of throat muscle relaxation and impaired judgment when drinking alcohol and eating.*
• Involve family members in learning and practicing rescue techniques (e.g., treating of choking or breathing problems, and/or CPR) *to deal with emergency situations (especially when at-home client is at risk on a regular basis).*
• Encourage individuals to read package labels and identify and remove safety hazards such as toys with small parts.
• Promote pool safety, vigilance, and use of approved flotation equipment, fencing/locked gates, etc.
• Discuss safety measures regarding use of heaters, household gas appliances, old/discarded appliances.
• Promote public education in techniques for clearing blocked airways (e.g., abdominal thrusts maneuver, back blows, CPR).

DOCUMENTATION FOCUS

Assessment/Reassessment
• Individual risk factors including individual's cognitive status and level of knowledge.
• Level of concern/motivation for change.
• Equipment/airway adjunct needs.

Planning
• Plan of care and who is involved in planning.
• Teaching plan.

 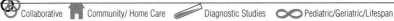

Implementation/Evaluation
- Responses to interventions/teaching and actions performed.
- Attainment/progress toward desired outcome(s).
- Modifications to plan of care.

Discharge Planning
- Long-term needs/referrals, appropriate preventive measures, and who is responsible for actions to be taken.
- Specific referrals made.

References
1. No author listed. Suffocation and artificial respiration. (2000). Fact sheet for WebHealthCentre. Available at: http://webhealthcentre.com. Accessed September 2003.
2. Summary of the practice parameter for the prevention and management of aggressive behavior in child and adolescent psychiatric institutions with special reference to seclusion and restraint. (2002). J Am Acad Child Adoles Psychiatry, Feb; 41(2Suppl), 4S-25S. Available at: http://www.guideline.gov. Accessed February 2004.
3. Kline, A. (2003). Pinpointing the cause of pediatric respiratory distress. Nursing, 33(9), 58–63.
4. ND: Suffocation, risk for in Seizure Disorders. In Doenges, M. E., Moorhouse, M. F., & Geissler-Murr, A. C. (2002). Nursing Care Plans: Guidelines for Individualizing Patient Care, ed 6. Philadelphia: F. A. Davis, pp 201–203.
5. Changing concepts of sudden infant death syndrome: Implications for infant sleeping environment and sleep position. (2001). American Academy of Pediatrics. Task Force on Infant Sleep Position and Sudden Infant Death Syndrome. Available at: http://www.guideline.gov. Accessed February 2004.
6. No author listed. Suffocation. Doctors Book of Home Remedies for Children. Available at: http://www.motherature.com. Accessed September 2003.
7. Green, P. M. (1993). High risk for suffocation. In McFarland, G. K., & McFarlane, E. A. (Eds). Nursing Diagnosis and interventions. St. Louis: Mosby.
8. No author listed. Suffocation. Health Sciences Centre, Winnipeg, Manitoba. Available at: http://www.hsc.mb.ca/impact.suffocation.htm.
9. No author listed. Preventing strangulation and suffocation among infants and children. SAFEUSA. Available at: http://safeusa.org. Accessed September 2003.

risk for Suicide

Definition: At risk for self-inflicted, life-threatening injury

RISK FACTORS

Behavioral
History of suicide attempt
Buying a gun; stockpiling medicines
Making or changing a will; giving away possessions
Sudden euphoric recovery from major depression
Impulsiveness; marked changes in behavior, attitude, school performance

Verbal
Threats of killing oneself; states desire to die/end it all

Situational
Living alone; retired; relocation, institutionalization; economic instability
Presence of gun in home

Adolescents living in nontraditional settings (e.g., juvenile detention center, prison, half-way house, group home)

Psychological
Family history of suicide; abuse in childhood
Alcohol and substance use/abuse
Psychiatric illness/disorder (e.g., depression, schizophrenia, bipolar disorder)
Guilt
Gay or lesbian youth

Demographic
Age: elderly, young adult males, adolescents
Race: white, Native American
Gender: male
Divorced, widowed

Physical
Physical/terminal illness; chronic pain

Social
Loss of important relationship; disrupted family life; poor support systems; social isolation
Grief, bereavement; loneliness
Hopelessness; helplessness
Legal or disciplinary problem
Cluster suicides
NOTE: A risk diagnosis is not evidenced by signs and symptoms, as the problem has not occurred and nursing interventions are directed at prevention.

SAMPLE CLINICAL APPLICATIONS: acute/chronic brain syndrome, hormonal imbalances (e.g., PMS, postpartum psychosis), substance use/abuse, chronic/terminal illness (e.g., ALS, cancer), major depression, schizophrenia, bipolar disorder, panic state

DESIRED OUTCOMES/EVALUATION CRITERIA
Sample **NOC** linkages:
Suicide Self-Restraint: Ability to refrain from gestures and attempts at killing self
Coping: Actions to manage stressors that tax an individual's resources
Hope: Presence of internal state of optimism that is personally satisfying and life-supporting

Client Will (Include Specific Time Frame)
- Acknowledge difficulties perceived in current situation.
- Identify current factors that can be dealt with.
- Be involved in planning course of action to correct existing problems.

ACTIONS/INTERVENTIONS
Sample **NIC** linkages:
Suicide Prevention: Reducing the risk for self-inflicted harm with intent to end life
Behavior Management: Self-Harm: Assisting the patient to decrease or eliminate self-mutilating or self-abusive behavior
Patient Contracting: Negotiating an agreement with a patient that reinforces a specific behavior change

 Cultural Collaborative Community/ Home Care Diagnostic Studies 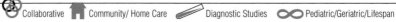 Pediatric/Geriatric/Lifespan Medications

NURSING PRIORITY NO. 1. To assess causative/contributing factors and degree of risk:

- Identify degree of risk/potential for suicide and seriousness of threat. Use a scale of 1–10 and prioritize according to severity of threat, availability of means. *Most people who are contemplating suicide send a variety of signals indicating their intent, and recognizing these warning signs allows for immediate intervention. While women talk about suicide more frequently, men usually succeed more often. Risk of suicide is greater in teens and the elderly, but there is a rising awareness of risk in early childhood.*[4]

- Note behaviors indicative of intent. *Individual may not make statements of intent but gestures, presence of means such as guns, threats, giving away possessions, previous attempts, and presence of hallucinations or delusions may provide clues to intent.*[3]

- Ask directly if person is thinking of acting on thoughts/feelings to determine intent. *Most individuals want someone to see what desperate straits they are in and by bringing the issue into the open, discussion can begin and plans made to keep the person safe.*[3]

- Note withdrawal from usual activities, lack of social interactions. *These are classic behaviors of the individual who is feeling depressed and sad and may be having negative thoughts of worthlessness.*[6]

- Identify conditions such as acute/chronic brain syndrome; panic state; hormonal imbalance (e.g., PMS, postpartum psychosis, drug-induced). *These conditions may interfere with ability to control own behavior leading to impulsive behaviors that may put client at risk.*[1]

- Review laboratory findings (e.g., blood alcohol, blood glucose, ABGs, electrolytes, renal function tests). *Identifies factors that may affect reasoning ability interfering with ability to think clearly about issues that are leading to thoughts of suicide.*[1]

- Assess physical complaints. *Sleeping difficulties, lack of appetite can be indicators of depression and suicidal ideation and need for further evaluation.*[3]

- Note family history of suicidal behavior. *Individual risk is increased when other family members have committed suicide or exhibited symptoms of depression. Studies have shown a possible genetic link toward suicidal behavior.*[3]

- Assess coping behaviors presently used. *Client's current negtive thinking may preclude looking at positive behaviors that have been used in the past that would help in the current situation. Client may believe there is no alternative except suicide.*[6]

- Determine presence of SO(s)/friends who are available for support. *Individuals who have positive support systems whom they can rely on during a crisis situation are less likely to commit suicide and are more apt to return to a successful life.*[3]

- Determine drug use, involvement with judicial system. *The use of alcohol, especially the combination of alcohol and barbiturates, increase the risk of suicide. Feelings of despair over problems with the legal system and lack of hope about outcome can lead to belief that the only solution is suicide.*[3]

- Reevaluate potential for suicide periodically at key times (e.g., mood changes, increasing withdrawal), as well as when client is feeling better and planning for discharge becomes active. *The highest risk is when the client has both suicidal ideation and sufficient energy with which to act.*[6]

NURSING PRIORITY NO. 2. To assist clients to accept responsibility for own behavior and prevent suicide:

- Develop therapeutic nurse-client relationship, providing consistent caregiver. *Promotes sense of trust, allowing individual to discuss feelings openly. Collaborating with the client to better understand the problem affirms the client's ability to solve the current situation.*[3,6]

- Maintain straightforward communication. *By being direct and honest and acknowledging need for attention caregiver can avoid reinforcing manipulative behavior.*[6]
- Explain concern for safety and willingness to help client stay safe. *Clients often believe their concerns will not be taken seriously and stating clearly that they will be listened to sends a clear message of support and caring.*[6]
- Encourage expression of feelings and make time to listen to concerns. *Acknowledges reality of feelings and that they are okay. Helps individual sort out thinking and begin to develop understanding of situation.*[3,6]
- Give permission to express angry feelings in acceptable ways and let client know someone will be available to assist in maintaining control. *Promotes acceptance and sense of safety while client is regaining own control.*[3]
- Acknowledge reality of suicide as an option. Discuss consequences of actions if they follow through on intent. Ask how it will help individual to resolve problems. *Can help client to focus on consequences of actions and begin to discuss the possibility of other options.*[5]
- Maintain observation of client and check environment for hazards that could be used to commit suicide. *Increases client safety/reduces risk of impulsive behavior when client is hospitalized.*[3]
- Help client identify more appropriate solutions/behaviors. *Alternative activities, such as exercise, can lessen sense of anxiety and associated physical manifestations.*[3]
- Provide directions for actions client can take, avoiding negative statements, such as "do nots." *Providing opportunity for client to have control over circumstances can promote a positive attitude and give client some hope for the future.*[3]

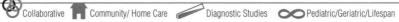

- Determine cultural/religious beliefs that may be affecting client's thinking about life and death. *Family of origin and culture in which individual grew up influence attitudes toward taking one's own life, for instance Protestants commit suicide more frequently than Catholics or Jews, and whites are at highest risk, followed by Native Americans, African Americans, Hispanic Americans, and Asian Americans.*[2,3]

NURSING PRIORITY NO. 3. To assist client to plan course of action to correct/ deal with existing situation:

- Gear interventions to individual involved. *Age, relationships, and current situation determine what is needed to help client deal with feelings of despair and hopelessness.*[6]
- Negotiate contract with client regarding willingness not to do anything lethal for a stated period of time. Specify what caregiver will be responsible for and what client responsibilities are. *Making a contract in which the individual agrees to stay alive for a specified period of time, from day one through the entire course of treatment and written and signed by each party, may help the client to follow through with therapy to find reason for living. Although there is little research on the effectiveness of these contracts, they are frequently used.*[6]
- Specify alternative actions necessary if client is unwilling to negotiate contract. *Client may be willing to agree to other actions (i.e., calling therapist if feelings are overwhelming), even though he or she is not willing to commit to a contract.*[6]
- Discuss losses client has experienced and meaning of those losses. *Unresolved issues may be contributing to thoughts of hopelessness, feelings of despair, and suicidal ideation.*[3,6]
- Consider the use of medications, especially when there may be a significant organic component to the suicidal ideation. *While the use of medications may be helpful in the short term there are some drawbacks, namely, the length of time it takes for most medications to take effect, and the potential for giving a client a means of suicide because of the possibility of a lethal overdose.*[6]

NURSING PRIORITY NO. 4. To promote wellness (Teaching/Discharge Considerations):

- Promote development of internal control. *Helping the client look at new ways to deal with problems can provide a sense of own ability to solve problems, improve situation, and hope for the future.*[3]
- Assist with learning problem solving, assertiveness training, and social skills. *By learning these new skills, client can begin to feel more confidence in own ability to handle problems that arise and deal with the current situation.*[3]
- Engage in physical activity programs. *Promotes release of endorphins and feelings of self-worth, improving sense of well-being and giving client hope.*[3]
- Determine nutritional needs and help client to plan for meeting them. *Enhances general well-being and energy level.*
- Involve family/SO in planning. *Improves understanding and support when family knows the facts and has a part in planning for rehabilitation efforts for the client.*[1]
- Refer to formal resources as indicated. *May need assistance with referrals to individual/group/marital psychotherapy, substance abuse treatment program, or social services when situation involves mental illness, family disorganization.*[3]

DOCUMENTATION FOCUS

Assessment/Reassessment
- Individual findings, including nature of concern (e.g., suicidal/behavioral risk factors and level of impulse control, plan of action/means to carry out plan).
- Client's percesption of situation, motivation for change.

Planning
- Plan of care and who is involved in the planning.
- Details of contract regarding suicidal ideation/plans.
- Teaching plan.

Implementation/Evaluation
- Actions taken to promote safety.
- Response to interventions/teaching and actions performed.
- Attainment/progress toward desired outcome(s).
- Modifications to plan of care.

Discharge Planning
- Long-range needs and who is responsible for actions to be taken.
- Available resources, specific referrals made.

Reference

1. Cox, H. C., et al. (2002). Clinical Applications of Nursing Diagnosis: Adult, Child, Women's, Psychiatric, Gerontic, and Home Health Considerations, ed 4. Philadelphia: F. A. Davis.
2. Lipson, J. G., Dibble, S. L., & Minarik, P. A. (1996). Culture & Nursing Care: A Pocket Guide. San Francisco: UCSF Nursing Press.
3. Townsend, M. C. (2003). Psychiatric Mental Health Nursing Concepts of Care, ed 4. Philadelphia: F. A. Davis.
4. Doenges, M. E., Moorhouse, M. F., & Murr, A. G. (2004). Nurse's Pocket Guide Diagnoses, Interventions, and Rationales, ed 9. Philadelphia: F. A. Davis.

5. Doenges, M., Townsend, M., & Moorhouse, M. (1998). Psychiatric Care Plans: Guidelines for Individualizing Care, ed 3. Philadelphia: F. A. Davis.
6. Jurich, A. P. (2003). The Nature of Suicide. Clinical Update (insert in Family Therapy Magazine), 3(6), 1–8.

delayed Surgical Recovery

Definition: Extension of the number of postoperative days required to initiate and perform activities that maintain life, health, and well-being

RELATED FACTORS

To be developed by nurse researchers and submitted to NANDA

DEFINING CHARACTERISTICS

Subjective
Perception more time needed to recover
Report of pain/discomfort; fatigue
Loss of appetite with or without nausea
Postpones resumption of work/employment activities

Objective
Evidence of interrupted healing of surgical area (e.g., red, indurated, draining, immobile)
Difficulty in moving about; requires help to complete self-care

SAMPLE CLINICAL APPLICATIONS: major surgical procedures, traumatic injuries with surgical intervention, chronic conditions (e.g., diabetes mellitus, cancer, HIV/AIDS, COPD)

DESIRED OUTCOMES/EVALUATION CRITERIA

Sample **NOC** linkages:

Wound Healing: Primary/Secondary Intention: The extent to which cells and tissues have regenerated following intentional closure/cells and tissues in an open wound have regenerated

Self-Care: Activities of Daily Living (ADL): Ability to perform the most basic physical tasks and personal care activities

Endurance: Extent that energy enables a person to sustain activity

Client Will (Include Specific Time Frame)
- Display complete healing of surgical area.
- Be able to perform desired self-care activities.
- Report increased energy, able to participate in usual (work/employment) activities.

ACTIONS/INTERVENTIONS

Sample **NIC** linkages:

Self-Care Assistance: Assisting another to perform activities of daily living

Energy Management: Regulating energy use to treat or prevent fatigue and optimize function

Wound Care: Prevention of wound complications and promotion of wound healing

NURSING PRIORITY NO. 1. To assess causative/contributing factors:

(Note: This diagnosis may occur in the acute care setting or be recognized after discharge. Therefore the interventions identified may be carried out in either setting.)

 Cultural Collaborative Community/ Home Care Diagnostic Studies Pediatric/Geriatric/Lifespan Medications

- Determine general state of health and extent of injury/damage to tissues *to help determine time that may usually be required for client to resume ADLs and other activities, or expectation of time needed for healing. Note: The older adult undergoing surgical treatment is at great risk for problems with delayed recovery because of age-related changes in numerous systems and protective mechanisms that increase the potential for complications.*[1]
- Identify underlying condition/pathology involved (e.g., skin/other cancers, burns, diabetes, hypothyroidism; steroid therapy, multiple trauma, infections, radiation therapy *that can adversely affect healing and prolong recuperation time.*
- Assess circulation and sensation in surgical area *to evaluate for 1) internal bleeding that compromises wound integrity; or 2) loss of blood flow to area, resulting in decreased oxygen supply to tissues, or nerve damage delaying healing.*[2,3]
- Evaluate client's preoperative medications *to ascertain that none could impede healing processes (e.g., aspirin and NSAIDs increase bleeding time; alcohol—a potent vasodilator— and some herbals such as garlic and Ginkgo biloba can also be associated with bleeding complilations.*[3]
- Determine nutritional status and current intake. *Client can be fasting for several days peri-operatively and/or can experience nausea, vomiting and loss of appetite postoperatively, depending on the client's preoperative status, the surgical procedure performed and client's postoperative reactions to medications (e.g., pain medications, antibiotics, etc.).*[2,3]
- Ascertain attitudes/cultural values of individual about condition. *Family and cultural values, stress and fear related to surgery (and the reason for it); possible stigma relative condition/disease or change in body image; or motivation to return to usual role/activities all impact rate and expectations for sick role and recovery.*[6]

NURSING PRIORITY NO. 2. To determine impact of delayed recovery:

- Determine the type and length of procedure, as well as type of surgical wound (e.g., clean, clean-contaminated, or grossly contaminated and acutely infected) *that can affect the pace of healing and/or risk of complications (such as infection, suture reactions, dehiscence).*[3]
- Note length of illness/hospitalization to date/time of discharge and compare with expected length of stay for procedure and situation.
- Determine energy level and current participation in ADLs *to compare with usual level of function.*
- Ascertain whether client usually requires assistance in home setting and who provides it/current availability and capability.
- Obtain psychological assessment of client's emotional status, noting potential problems arising from current situation.

NURSING PRIORITY NO. 3. To promote optimal recovery:

- Assist with care activities as needed. Plan/implement gradual increase in activities to allow client *to increase strength and tolerance for activities.*[1]
- Withhold oral fluids in the immediate postoperative period *to decrease incidence of discomfort associated with vomiting.*[4]
- Provide optimal nutrition and adequate protein intake including nutritional supplement drinks as appropriate *to provide a positive nitrogen balance aiding in healing and to achieve general good health.*
- Ensure/encourage adequate fluid and electrolyte intake *to avoid dehydration of tissues and to promote optimal cellular/organ function.*[2]

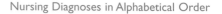

- Encourage ambulation, regular exercise *to promote circulation, improve muscle strength and overall endurance, and reduce risks associated with immobility.*[2]
- Recommend pacing (alternating activity with adequate rest periods) *to prevent fatigue and allow weakened muscles/tissues to recuperate.*[2]
- Administer medications to manage postoperative discomforts (e.g., pain, nausea/vomiting), and other concurrent or underlying conditions such as diabetes, osteoporosis, heart failure, COPD. *Client may be experiencing stubborn infection requiring IV antibiotics, or need insulin or other hormones to support tissue repair, or require management of chronic pain to improve mobility and tissue recovery.*[2]
- Employ nonpharmacologic healing measures as indicated (e.g., breathing exercises, listening to music, relaxation tapes, biofeedback, hot or cold applications) *to promote relaxation of muscles and tissue healing as well as improve coping and outlook for positive healing experience.*[2]
- Monitor activity/provide assistance as indicated when out of bed. *Client may be weak/unsteady, increasing the risk of falls and new injury.*
- Encourage client to adhere to medical regimen and follow-up care *to monitor healing process and provide for timely intervention as needed.*

NURSING PRIORITY NO. 4. To enhance wound healing:

- Practice and instruct client/caregiver(s) in proper handwashing and aseptic technique for incisional care *to reduce incidence of contamination and infection.*[5]
- Inspect incisions/wounds routinely, describing changes. Document healing (e.g., pink/red granulation tissue) or changes in wound indicative of failure to heal (e.g., deepening wound, local or systemic fever; exudates [noting color, amount and odor]; loss of approximation of wound edges) *to establish comparative baseline and allow for early intervention (e.g., antimicrobial therapy, wound irrigation/packing, etc.).*
- Assist with wound care as indicated. *May require chemical or surgical débridement, barrier dressings, wound coverings, skin-protective agents for open/draining wounds.*
- Include wound care specialist/stomal therapist as appropriate *to problem solve healing difficulties.*
- Limit/avoid use of plastics or latex materials as indicated. *Plastics retain heat and may enhance growth of pathogens in wound. Some client may develop sensitivity to repeated exposure to latex products.* (Refer to ND risk for latex Allergy Response.)

NURSING PRIORITY NO. 5. To promote wellness (Teaching/Discharge Considerations):

- Discuss reality of recovery process and client's/SO's expectations. *Individuals are often unrealistic regarding energy and time required for healing and own abilities/responsibilities to facilitate process.*
- Provide postoperative/wound care expectations and instructions in verbal and written forms *to facilitate self-care and reduce likelihood of misinterpretation of information when client/SO is providing care at home.*[3]
- Involve client/SO(s) in setting incremental goals. *Enhances commitment to plan and reduces likelihood of frustration blocking progress.*
- Refer to physical/occupational therapists as indicated *to identify assistive devices to facilitate independence in ADLs.*

• Identify suppliers for dressings/wound care items and assistive devices as needed.

 • Consult dietitian for individual dietary plan *to meet increased nutritional needs that reflect personal situation/resources.*

 • Determine home situation (e.g., lives alone, bedroom/bathroom on second floor, availability of assistance). *Identifies necessary adjustments, such as moving bedroom to first floor, arranging for commode during recovery, obtaining an in-home emergency call system.*

 • Discuss alternative placement (e.g., convalescent/rehabilitation center as appropriate). *Brief stay with concentrated support/therapy may speed recovery/return to home.*

 • Identify community resources (e.g., visiting nurse, home healthcare agency, Meals on Wheels, respite care). *Facilitates adjustment to home setting.*

 • Refer for counseling/support. *May need additional help to overcome feelings of discouragement, deal with changes in life.*

DOCUMENTATION FOCUS

Assessment/Reassessment

• Assessment findings, including individual concerns, family involvement, and support factors/availability of resources.

Planning

• Plan of care and who is involved in planning.
• Teaching plan.

Implementation/Evaluation

• Responses of client/SO(s) to plan/interventions/teaching and actions performed.
• Attainment/progress toward desired outcome(s).
• Modifications to plan of care.

Discharge Planning

• Long-range needs and who is responsible for actions to be taken.
• Specific referrals made.

References

1. ND: Surgical Recovery, delayed. In Cox, H. C., et al. (2002). Clinical Applications of Nursing Diagnosis: Adult, Child, Women's, Psychiatric, Gerontic, and Home Health Considerations, ed 4. Philadelphia: F. A. Davis.
2. No author listed. Post-surgical rehabilitation and healing: benefits of RECOVERY. (Monograph) Surgery, Treatments and Wound Healing with Biostructural Medicine. Available at: http://www.biostructural.com. Accessed September 2003.
3. Semchyshyn, N. & Sengelmann, R. D. (2002). Surgical complications. Available at: http://www.emedicine.com. Accessed February 2004.
4. Haynes, G. R., & Bailey, M. K. (1996). Postoperative nausea and vomiting-review and clinical approaches. South Med J, 89(10), 940–949.
5. Stadelmann, W. K., Degenis, A. G., & Tobin, G. R. (1998). Impediments to wound healing. Am J Surg, 176 (2A suppl), 39S.
6. Purnell, L., & Paulanka, B. (1998). Transcultural Health Care: A Culturally Diverse Approach, ed 2. Philadelphia: F. A. Davis.

impaired Swallowing

Definition: Abnormal functioning of the swallowing mechanism associated with deficits in oral, pharyngeal, or esophageal structure or function

Congenital deficits

Upper airway anomalies; mechanical obstruction (e.g., edema, tracheostomy tube, tumor); history of tube feeding

Neuromuscular impairment (e.g., decreased or absent gag reflex, decreased strength or excursion of muscles involved in mastication, perceptual impairment, facial paralysis); conditions with significant hypotonia; cranial nerve involvement

Respiratory disorders; congenital heart disease

Behavioral feeding problems; self-injurious behavior

Failure to thrive or protein energy malnutrition

Neurologic problems

External/internal traumas; acquired anatomic defects

Nasal or nasopharyngeal cavity defects

Oral cavity or oropharynx abnormalities

Upper airway/laryngeal anomalies; tracheal, laryngeal, esophageal defects

Gastroesophageal reflux disease; achalasia

Premature infants; traumatic head injury; developmental delay; cerebral palsy

DEFINING CHARACTERISTICS

Subjective

Esophageal Phase Impairment

Complaints [reports] of "something stuck"; odynophagia

Food refusal or volume limiting

Heartburn or epigastric pain

Nighttime coughing or awakening

Objective

Oral Phase Impairment

Weak suck resulting in inefficient nippling

Slow bolus formation; lack of tongue action to form bolus; premature entry of bolus

Incomplete lip closure; food pushed out of/falls from mouth

Lack of chewing

Coughing, choking, gagging before a swallow

Piecemeal deglutition; abnormality in oral phase of swallow study

Inability to clear oral cavity; pooling in lateral sulci; nasal reflux; sialorrhea or drooling

Long meals with little consumption

Pharyngeal Phase Impairment

Food refusal

Altered head positions; delayed/multiple swallows; inadequate laryngeal elevation; abnormality in pharyngeal phase by swallow study

Choking, coughing, or gagging; nasal reflux; gurgly voice quality

Unexplained fevers; recurrent pulmonary infections

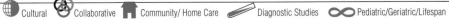 Cultural   Collaborative   Community/ Home Care   Diagnostic Studies   Pediatric/Geriatric/Lifespan   Medications

Esophageal Phase Impairment
Observed evidence of difficulty in swallowing (e.g., stasis of food in oral cavity, coughing/choking); abnormality in esophageal phase by swallow study
Hyperextension of head, arching during or after meals
Repetitive swallowing or ruminating; bruxism
Unexplained irritability surrounding mealtime
Acidic smelling breath; regurgitation of gastric contents or wet burps; vomitus on pillow; vomiting; hematemesis
SAMPLE CLINICAL APPLICATIONS: brain injury/stroke, neuromuscular conditions (e.g., muscular dystrophy, cerebral palsy, Parkinson's disease, ALS, Guillain-Barré syndrome), facial trauma, head/neck cancer, radical neck surgery/laryngectomy, cleft lip/palate, tracheoesophageal fistula, gastroesophageal reflux disease, dementia

DESIRED OUTCOMES/EVALUATION CRITERIA
Sample **NOC** linkages:
Swallowing Status: Extent of safe passage of fluids and/or solids from the mouth to the stomach
Self-Care: Eating: Ability to prepare and ingest food

Client Will (Include Specific Time Frame)
- Verbalize understanding of causative/contributing factors.
- Identify individually appropriate interventions/actions to promote intake and prevent aspiration.
- Demonstrate feeding methods appropriate to the individual situation.
- Pass food and fluid from mouth to stomach safely.
- Maintain adequate hydration as evidenced by good skin turgor, moist mucous membranes, and individually appropriate urine output.
- Achieve and/or maintain desired body weight.

Sample **NOC** linkage:
Risk Control: Actions to eliminate or reduce actual, personal, and modifiable health threats.

Caregiver/SO(s) Will (Include Specific Time Frame)
- Demonstrate emergency measures in the event of choking.

ACTIONS/INTERVENTIONS
Sample **NIC** linkages:
Swallowing Therapy: Facilitating swallowing and preventing complications of impaired swallowing
Aspiration Precautions: Prevention or minimization of risk factors in the patient at risk for aspiration
Airway Suctioning: Removal of airway secretions by inserting a suction catheter into the patient's oral airway and/or trachea

NURSING PRIORITY NO. 1. To assess causative/contributing factors and degree of impairment:

 - Evaluate client's potential for swallowing problems, noting age and medical conditions. *Swallowing disorders are especially common in elderly, possibly due to coexistence of variety of neurologic, neuromuscular, or other conditions. Infants at risk include those*

born with tracheoesophageal fistula, or lip and palate malformation. *Persons with traumatic brain injuries often exhibit swallowing impairments, regardless of gender or age.*[1–4]

- Identify client's usual medications (e.g., anticholinergics, phenothiazides, aminoglycosides, various anticonvulsants, lipid-lowering drugs, calcium channel blockers, certain antidepressants) *that can contribute to swallowing dysfunction.*[1,5]
- Assess for problems related to upper areas of the **mouth and pharynx**:[1,6]

  Obstruction to the passage of food or liquid (e.g., emotional or anxiety disorder; lesions, ulcers or tumors of the mouth/oral cavity and throat; cervical spine injury or disease; congenital esophageal web)

  Nerve and muscle problems (e.g., cerebral hemorrhage and infarction, dementias, Parkinson's or Huntington's disease, multiple sclerosis, amyotrophic lateral sclerosis, myasthenia gravis, muscular dystrophy, poliomyelitis)

  Miscellaneous causes (e.g., poor teeth, ill-fitting dentures, common cold; presence of dry mouth; intubation, surgery of head/neck/jaw; vocal cord paralysis).
- Assess for problems related to the **esophagus**:[1,6]

  Obstruction to the passage of food or liquid (e.g., tumors, strictures that may be caused by radiation, chemical ingestions, medications, ulcers; foreign bodies and gastroesophageal reflux disease (GERD), *which is one of the most common causes of dysphagia.*[6]

  Nerve and muscle problems (e.g., achalasia, esophageal spasm, hypertensive lower esophageal sphincter; scleroderma).
- Assess client's cognitive and sensory-perceptual status. *Sensory awareness, orientation, concentration, motor coordination and ability to move tongue in mouth affect desire and ability to swallow safely and effectively.*[7]
- Inspect oropharyngeal cavity. *Edema, inflammation, altered integrity of oral mucosa or structures, state of detention, and adequacy of oral hygiene can limit swallowing.*
- Evaluate swallow effort:

  Note voice quality and speech. *Abnormal voice (dysphonia) and abnormal speech patterns (dysarthria) are signs of motor dysfunction of structures involved in oral and pharyngeal swallowing.*[1] *Client may have "gurgling or gargly" voice.*[8]

  Ascertain presence and strength of cough and gag reflex. *While absence of gag reflex is not necessarily predictive of client's eventual ability to swallow safely, it certainly increases client's potential for aspiration (overt or silent).*[1,4] *Coughing, drooling, double swallowing, decreased ability to move food in mouth, and throat clearing with/after swallowing is indicative of swallowing dysfunction, and high risk for aspiration.*[1,8,9]

  Assess strength and excursion of muscles involved in chewing and swallowing.

  Place client in upright, seated position. Use small sips of water for initial testing, before using any food.

  Auscultate breath sounds *to evaluate the presence of aspiration, especially if client is coughing with intake.*
- Review laboratory test results for underlying problems (e.g., *Candida*/other infections; Cushing's disease/other metabolic conditions; multiple sclerosis, myasthenia gravis/other neuromuscular conditions) *that can affect swallowing.*[5]
- Prepare for/assist with diagnostic testing of swallowing activity (e.g., transnasal or esophageal endoscopy, fiberoptic endoscopic examination of swallowing techniques (FEEST); barium swallow radiography or videofluoroscopy *to identify the pathophysiology of swallowing disorder.*[1,6]
- Consult with speech pathologist/dysphagia specialist/rehabilitation team as indicated *to identify needs, and/or implement swallow therapy. Client/SO may learn specific retraining or compensatory techniques (e.g., modifying head and neck posture, or strengthening of swallowing muscles, or techniques of food placement in mouth).*[1,6]

 Cultural   Collaborative Community/ Home Care   Diagnostic Studies Pediatric/Geriatric/Lifespan   Medications

NURSING PRIORITY NO. 2. To prevent aspiration and maintain airway patency:

- Withhold oral feedings until appropriate diagnostic workup is completed to determine client's individual factors causing impaired swallowing and identify specific needs.
- Consult with physician/dietitian regarding meeting current nutritional needs. *May need enteral (preferably by gastrostomy [PEG] tube) or parenteral feedings in order to obtain nutrition, while reducing risk of aspiration that could accompany nasogastric feedings.*[10]
- Encourage client to sit in chair for meals/raise head to a 90-degree angle with head in anatomic alignment and slightly flexed forward *during feeding or for secretion management.* Maintain elevation for 30 to 45 minutes after feeding, if possible, *to reduce risk of regurgitation/aspiration.*
- Instruct client to cough and expectorate *when secretion management is of concern.* Suction oral cavity if client cannot clear secretions *to prevent aspiration.*
- Teach client self-suction when appropriate (e.g., drooling, frequent choking, structural changes in mouth/throat). *Promotes independence/sense of control.*

NURSING PRIORITY NO. 3. To enhance swallowing ability to meet fluid and caloric body requirements:

- Collaborate with physician and other providers (e.g., dietitian, gastroenterologist) as indicated for treatment of particular condition. *Therapy may consist of dietary modification, compensatory movements, medical or surgical procedures, etc. For example, medications may help with underlying condition (e.g., swallowing problem associated with Parkinson's disease), surgery (e.g., to correct structural defect in infant) or esophageal dilatation when impaired sphincter function or esophageal strictures impede swallowing.*[1]
- Implement dietary modifications as indicated:
  Provide proper consistency of food/fluid. *Foods that can be formed into a bolus before swallowing such as gelatin desserts prepared with less water than usual, pudding, and custard; thickened liquids (addition of thickening agent, or yogurt, cream soups prepared with less water), thinned purees (hot cereal with water added) or thick drinks such as nectars or fruit juices that have been frozen into "slush" consistency, medium-soft boiled or scrambled eggs, canned fruit, soft-cooked vegetables are most easily swallowed.*
  Feed one consistency and/or texture of food at a time. *Single textured foods (e.g., pudding, hot cereal, pureed food) should be tolerated well before advancing to soft table foods.*[10]
  Avoid milk products and chocolate, *which may thicken oral secretions and impair swallowing.*
  Avoid sticky foods (e.g., peanut butter, white bread) *that are difficult to swallow or need fluids to completely swallow.*[10]
  Ensure temperature (hot or cold versus tepid) of foods/fluid, *which will stimulate sensory receptors.*
  Use a glass with a nose cutout *to avoid posterior head tilting while drinking.*
  Avoid pouring liquid into the mouth or "washing food down" with liquid. *May cause client to lose control of food bolus, increasing risk of aspiration.*
  Feed smaller, more frequent meals *to limit fatigue associated with eating efforts and to promote adequate nutritional intake.*
  Determine food preferences of client and present foods in an appealing, attractive manner. *Client may make effort to overcome swallowing problems when food is appealing and desired.*
  Avoid food within 3 hours of bedtime, eliminate alcohol and caffeine intake, reduce weight if needed, practice stress reduction, and elevate head of bed during sleep *to limit potential for gastric reflux and aspiration.*
- Provide/encourage proper food placement, chewing and swallowing techniques:

Provide cognitive cues and specific directions (e.g., remind client to "open mouth, chew, or swallow now" as indicated) *to enhance concentration and performance of swallowing sequence.*

Focus attention on feeding/swallowing activity and decreasing environmental stimuli, *which may be distracting during feeding. Also, if client is talking and/or laughing while eating, risk of aspiration is increased.*[11]

Position client on the unaffected side when appropriate, placing food in this side of mouth and having client use the tongue *to assist with managing the food when one side of the mouth is affected (e.g., hemiplegia).*

Place food midway in oral cavity; provide medium-sized bites (approximately 15 mL) *to adequately trigger the swallowing reflex.*

Massage the laryngopharyngeal musculature (sides of trachea and neck) gently *to stimulate swallowing.*

Allow ample time for eating (feeding). Incorporate client's eating style and pace when feeding *to avoid fatigue and frustration with process.*

Remain with client during meal *to reduce anxiety and provide assistance if needed.*

Provide positive feedback for client's efforts. *Encourages continuation of efforts/attainment of goals.*

Encourage a rest period before meals *if fatigue is interfering with efforts.*

Provide analgesics, with caution, before feeding as indicated *to enhance comfort, but avoiding decreasing awareness/sensory perception.*

Observe oral cavity after each bite and have client check around cheeks with tongue for remaining/unswallowed food to prevent overloading mouth with food/reduce risk of aspiration.

Discontinue feeding and remove any food from mouth if client choking/unable to swallow *to reduce potential for aspiration.*

- Have suction equipment available during initial feeding attempts and as indicated.
- Monitor intake, output, and body weight *to evaluate adequacy of fluid and caloric intake and need for changes to therapeutic regimen.*
- Discuss use of tube feedings/parenteral solutions as indicated *for the client unable to achieve adequate nutritional intake.*

NURSING PRIORITY NO. 4. To promote wellness (Teaching/Discharge Considerations):

- Consult with dietitian *to establish optimum dietary plan considering specific pathology, nutritional needs, available resources.*
- Consult with pharmacist *to determine if pills may be crushed or if liquids/capsules are available.*
- Administer medication in gelatin, jelly, or puddings as appropriate.
- Instruct client and/or SO in specific feeding techniques and swallowing exercises. *Enhances client safety and independence.*
- Demonstrate emergency measures in event of choking *to prevent aspiration/more serious complications.*
- Encourage continuation of facial exercise program *to maintain/improve muscle strength.*
- Establish routine schedule for obtaining weight (same time of day/clothes). Instruct in specific weight loss/gain to be reported to primary care provider. *Facilitates timely intervention to change regimen as needed.*
- Refer to ND imbalanced Nutrition: risk for less than body requirements.

 Cultural   Collaborative   Community/ Home Care   Diagnostic Studies   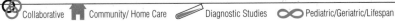 Pediatric/Geriatric/Lifespan   Medications

Assessment/Reassessment

- Individual findings, including degree/characteristics of impairment, current weight/recent changes.
- Effects on lifestyle/socialization and nutritional status.

Planning

- Plan of care and who is involved in planning.
- Teaching plan.

Implementation/Evaluation

- Response to interventions/teaching and actions performed.
- Attainment/progress toward desired outcome(s).
- Modifications to plan of care.

Discharge Planning

- Long-term needs and who is responsible for actions to be taken.
- Available resources and specific referrals made.

References

1. Palmer, J. B., Drennan, J. C., & Baba, M. (2000). Evaluation and treatment of swallowing impairments. Available at: http://www.aafp.org. Accessed September 2003.
2. Engel, J. (2002). Pocket Guide to Pediatric Assessment, ed 4. St. Louis: Mosby, p 158.
3. Kosta, J. C., & Mitchell, C. A. (1998). Current procedures for diagnosing dysphagia in elderly clients. Geriatr Nurs, 19(4), 195.
4. Leder, S. B. (1999) Fiberoptic endoscopic evaluation of swallowing in patients with acute traumatic brain injury. J Head Trauma Rehabil, 14(5), 448–453.
5. No author listed. American Gastroenterological Association medical position statement on management of oropharyngeal dysphagia. (1999). Gastroenterology 116(2), 452–454. Available at: http://www.guideline.gov. Accessed February 2004.
6. No author listed. Swallowing problems (dysphagia). College of Physicians and Surgeons, Department of Otolaryngology/Head and Neck Surgery. Available at: http://www.entcolumbia.org/dysphag.htm. Accessed September 2003.
7. Poertner, L. C., & Coleman, R. F. (1998). Swallowing therapy in adults. Otolaryngol Clin North Am, 31(3), 56.
8. Lugger, K. E. (1994). Dysphagia in the elderly stroke patient. J Neurosci Nurs, 26, 78.
9. Baker, D. M. (1993). Assessment and management of impairments in swallowing. Nurs Clin North Am, 28, 793.
10. Fine, R., & Ackley, B. J. (2002). ND: Impaired Swallowing. In Ackley, BJ, & Ladwig, GB. Nursing Diagnosis Handbook: A Guide to Planning Care, ed 5. St. Louis: Mosby, pp 735, 736.
11. Galvan, T. J. (2001). Dysphagia: Going down and staying down. Am J Nurs, 101(1), 37–42.

effective Therapeutic Regimen Management

Definition: Pattern of regulating and integrating into daily living a program for treatment of illness and its sequelae that is satisfactory for meeting specific health goals

RELATED FACTORS

To be developed by nurse researchers and submitted to NANDA

[Complexity of healthcare management; therapeutic regimen]

[Added demands made on individual or family]

[Adequate social supports]

Subjective

Verbalized desire to manage the treatment of illness and prevention of sequelae

Verbalized intent to reduce risk factors for progression of illness and sequelae

Objective

Appropriate choices of daily activities for meeting the goals of a treatment or prevention program

Illness symptoms are within a normal range of expectation

SAMPLE CLINICAL APPLICATIONS: chronic conditions (e.g., asthma, arthritis, systemic lupus), genetic/congenital conditions (e.g., sickle cell anemia, spina bifida)

DESIRED OUTCOMES/EVALUATION CRITERIA

Sample **NOC** linkages:

Symptom Control: Personal actions to minimize perceived adverse changes in physical and emotional functioning

Knowledge: Treatment Regimen: Extent of understanding conveyed about a specific treatment regimen

Participation: Health Care Decisions: Personal involvement in selecting and evaluating healthcare options

Client Will (Include Specific Time Frame)

- Verbalize understanding of therapeutic regimen for illness/ condition.
- Demonstrate effective problem solving in integration of therapeutic regimen into lifestyle.
- Identify/use available resources.
- Remain free of preventable complications/progression of illness and sequelae.

ACTIONS/INTERVENTIONS

Sample **NIC** linkages:

Health System Guidance: Facilitating a patient's location and use of appropriate health services

Health Education: Developing and providing instruction and learning experiences to facilitate voluntary adaptation of behavior conducive to health in individuals, families, groups, or communities

Anticipatory Guidance: Preparation of patient for an anticipated developmental and/or situational crisis

NURSING PRIORITY NO. 1. To assess situation and individual needs:

- Ascertain client's knowledge/understanding of condition and treatment needs. Note specific health goals. *Provides a basis for determining direction client wants to go and planning individualized care.*[1]
- Identify individual's perceptions of adaptation to treatment/anticipated changes. *How client sees the situation is important to discussing what is happening in regard to the treatment regimen and planning for the future.*[1]
- Note treatments added to present regimen and client's/SO('s) associated learning needs. *As changes are made, client needs to understand what the new medication/treatment is for and what to expect, as well as how it fits into the current regimen. Understanding these issues helps client feel confident in incorporating new treatments.*[3]

 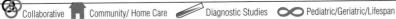

- Determine client's/family's health goals and patterns of healthcare. *Provides information about current behaviors, possible misperceptions, and areas of potential conflict such as values, cultural mores, religious beliefs, or financial concerns.*[1]
- Discuss present resources used by client, and possible need for change. *Continuing to monitor needs, such as hours of home care assistance; access to case manager, and making changes as indicated, supports complex/long-term program.* (3)

NURSING PRIORITY NO. 2. To assist client/SO(s) in developing strategies to meet increased demands of therapeutic regimen:

- Identify steps necessary to reach desired health goal(s). *Promotes understanding that goal(s) can only be reached by knowing what needs to be done as treatment regimen progresses.*[5]
- Accept client's evaluation of own strengths/limitations while working together to improve abilities. *Promotes sense of self-esteem and confidence to continue efforts.*[3]
- Provide information/bibliotherapy and help client/SO(s) identify and evaluate resources they can access on their own. *When referencing the Internet or nontraditional/unproven resources, the individual must exercise some restraint and determine the reliability of the source/information provided before acting on it. Promotes sense of control and confidence in own ability to be able to learn about illness/condition and be in charge of own treatment regimen.*[5]
- Acknowledge individual's efforts/capabilities. *Reinforces movement toward attainment of desired outcomes.*[5]

NURSING PRIORITY NO. 3. To promote wellness (Teaching/Discharge Considerations):

- Promote client/care giver choices and involvement in planning and implementing added tasks/responsibilities. *Individuals gain self-esteem by being involved in the daily planning of care when they have sufficient support and are given options about what they can do.*[3]
- Provide for follow-up contact/home visit as appropriate. *Encourages continuation of therapeutic regimen and opportunity to help family identify needs and solutions as they arise preventing untoward complications.*[3]
- Assist in implementing strategies for monitoring progress/responses to therapeutic regimen. *Promotes proactive problem solving to maintain effectiveness of regimen.*[5]
- Mobilize support systems, including family/SO(s), social, financial, and so on. *When these issues are managed well, family can attend to the process of recovery or in the case of chronic illness, learning to live well with situation.*[1,4]
- Refer to community resources as needed/desired. *Enhances management of effective therapeutic regimen.*[2]

DOCUMENTATION FOCUS

Assessment/Reassessment
- Findings, including dynamics of individual situation.
- Individual strengths/additional needs.

Planning
- Plan of care and who is involved in planning.
- Teaching plan.

Implementation/Evaluation
- Response to interventions/teaching and actions performed.
- Attainment/progress toward desired outcome(s).
- Modifications to plan of care.

Discharge Planning
- Short-range and long-range needs and who is responsible for actions.
- Available resources, specific referrals made

References
1. Cox, H. C, et al. (2002). Clinical Applications of Nursing Diagnosis: Adult, Child, Women's, Psychiatric, Gerontic, and Home Health Considerations, ed 4. Philadelphia: F. A. Davis.
2. Healthy People 2010 Toolkit, A Field Guide to Health Planning. (2002). Washington, DC: Public Health Foundation.
3. Stuifbergen, A. (1997). Health promotion: an essential component of rehabilitation for persons with chronic disabling conditions. ADV Nurs Sci, 19(4), 147–148.
4. Larsen, L. S. (1998). Effectiveness of counseling intervention to assist family caregivers of chronically ill relatives. J Psychosoc Nurs, 36(8), 26.
5. Lai, S. C., & Cohen, M. N. (1999). Promoting lifestyle changes. AJN, 99(4), 63.

ineffective community Therapeutic Regimen Management

Definition: Pattern of regulating and integrating into community processes programs for treatment of illness and the sequelae of illness that are unsatisfactory for meeting health-related goals

RELATED FACTORS
To be developed by nurse researchers and submitted to NANDA
[Lack of safety for community members]
[Economic insecurity]
[Healthcare not available]
[Unhealthy environment]
[Education not available for all community members]
[Does not possess means to meet human needs for recognition, fellowship, security, and membership]

DEFINING CHARACTERISTICS

Subjective
[Community members/agencies verbalize inability to meet therapeutic needs of all members]
[Community members/agencies verbalize overburdening of resources for meeting therapeutic needs of all members]

Objective
Deficits in people and programs to be accountable for illness care of aggregates
Deficits in advocates for aggregates

 Cultural Collaborative  Community/ Home Care Diagnostic Studies Pediatric/Geriatric/Lifespan Medications

Deficit in community activities for [primary medical care/prevention]/secondary and tertiary prevention

Illness symptoms above the norm expected for the number and type of population; unexpected acceleration of illness(es)

Number of healthcare resources insufficient[/unavailable] for the incidence or prevalence of illness(es)

[Deficits in community for collaboration and development of coalitions to address programs for treatment of illness and the sequelae of illness]

SAMPLE CLINICAL APPLICATIONS: HIV/AIDS, substance abuse, sexually transmitted diseases, teen pregnancy, prematurity, acute lead poisoning, influenza, SARS

DESIRED OUTCOMES/EVALUATION CRITERIA

Sample **NOC** linkages:

Community Competence: The ability of a community to collectively problem solve to achieve goals

Community Health Status: The general state of well-being of a community or population

Community Risk Control: [specify e.g., Communicable Disease]: Community actions to eliminate or reduce the spread of infectious agents (bacteria, fungi, parasites, and viruses) that threaten public health

---

Community Will (Include Specific Time Frame)

- Identify both negative and positive factors affecting community treatment programs for meeting health-related goals.
- Participate in problem solving of factors interfering with regulating and integrating community programs.
- Report illness symptoms moving toward norm expected for the incidence or prevalence of illness(es).

ACTIONS/INTERVENTIONS

Sample **NIC** linkages:

Community Health Development: Facilitating members of a community to identify a community's health concerns, mobilize resources, and implement solutions

Program Development: Planning, implementating, and evaluating a coordinated set of activities designed to enhance wellness, or to prevent, reduce, or eliminate one or more health problems of a group or community

Health Policy Monitoring: Surveillance and influence of government and organization regulations, rules, and standards that affect nursing systems and practices to ensure quality care of patients

NURSING PRIORITY NO. 1. To identify causative/precipitating factors:

- Evaluate community healthcare resources for illness/sequelae of illness. *Identifying current available resources provides a starting point to determine needs of the community and plan for future needs.*[1]
- Note reports from members of the community regarding ineffective/inadequate community functioning. *Provides feedback from people who live in the community and avail themselves of resources presenting a realistic picture of how they are functioning.*[2]
- Determine areas of conflict among members of community. *Cultural/religious beliefs, values, social mores may limit dialogue or creative problem solving if not addressed.*[4]

- Investigate unexpected acceleration of illness in the community. *Prompt identification of illness, such as West Nile virus, or HIV allows community to develop plan of care and intervene to prevent further spread with possibility of becoming epidemic.*[2]
- Identify strengths/limitations of community resources and community commitment to change. *Knowledge of these factors is important for developing a plan for community improvement. Without this information any plan will have difficulty succeeding.*[2]
- Ascertain effect of related factors on community activities. *Issues of safety, poor air quality, lack of education/information, lack of sufficient healthcare facilities affect citizens and how they view their community—whether it is a healthy, positive environment in which to live or lacks adequate healthcare/safety resources.*[1]
- Determine knowledge/understanding of treatment regimen. *Citizens need to know and understand what is being done to correct the identified deficiencies, before they are willing to be involved and actively support goals of the treatmemt regimen.*[1]

NURSING PRIORITY NO. 2. To assist community to develop strategies to improve community functioning/management:

- Foster cooperative spirit of community without negating individuality of members/groups. *As individuals feel valued and respected, they are more willing to work together with others to develop plan for identifying and improving healthcare for the community.*[2]
- Involve community in determining healthcare goals and prioritize them to facilitate planning process. *The goal is healthy people in a healthy community and as community members become involved and see that by prioritizing the identified goals progress can be seen as individuals become healthier and needed services become readily available.*[2]
- Plan together with community health and social agencies to problem-solve solutions identified and anticipated problems/needs. *Working together promotes a sense of involvement and control, helping people do more effective problem solving.*[3]
- Identify specific populations at risk or underserved to actively involve them in process. *Populations, such as the homeless, Latino, black, and native american, need to be involved in the problem identification and solutions because they are closely involved in the issues they face every day and can provide important facts to be considered. Being part of the solution empowers these groups and promotes participation in the process.*[3]
- Create teaching plan/form speakers' bureau. *Disseminating information to community members regarding value of treatment/preventive programs helps people know and understand the importance of these actions and be willing to support the programs.*[3]

NURSING PRIORITY NO. 3. To promote wellness (Teaching/Discharge Considerations):

- Assist community to develop a plan for continuing assessment of community needs/functioning and effectiveness of plan. *Promotes proactive approach in planning for the future and continuation of efforts to improve healthy behaviors and necessary services.*[1]
- Encourage community to form partnerships within the community and between the community and the larger society. *Aids in long-term planning for anticipated/projected needs/concerns to assure the quality and accessibility of health services.*[1]

DOCUMENTATION FOCUS

Assessment/Reassessment
- Assessment findings, including members' perceptions of community problems.

 Cultural   Collaborative 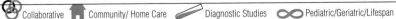 Community/ Home Care   Diagnostic Studies Pediatric/Geriatric/Lifespan   Medications

Planning
- Plan and who is involved in planning process.
- Teaching Plan.

Implementation/Evaluation
- Community's response to plan/interventions and actions performed.
- Attainment/progress toward desired outcome(s).
- Modifications to plan.

Discharge Planning
- Long-range goals and who is responsible for actions to be taken.
- Specific referrals made.

References

1. Environmental Health Competency Project: Draft Recommendations for Non-Technical Competencies at the Local Level. Washington, DC: American Public Health Association. Available at: http://www.apha.org/ppp/phipmain/ehep.htm. Accessed February 2004.
2. Public Health in America. (September, 1994). Washington, DC: American Public Health Association. Available at: http://www.apha.org/ppp/science/ESposter.htm. Accessed February 2004.
3. Healthy People 2010 Toolkit, A Field Guide to Health Planning. (2002). Washington, DC: Public Health Foundation.
4. Cox, H. C., et al. (2002). Clinical Applications of Nursing Diagnosis: Adult, Child, Women's, Psychiatric, Gerontic, and Home Health Considerations, ed 4. Philadelphia: F. A. Davis.

ineffective family Therapeutic Regimen Management

Definition: Pattern of regulating and integrating into family processes a program for treaent of illness and the sequelae of illness that is unsatisfactory for meeting specific health goals

RELATED FACTORS

Complexity of healthcare system
Complexity of therapeutic regimen
Decisional conflicts
Economic difficulties
Excessive demands made on individual or family
Family conflicts

DEFINING CHARACTERISTICS

Subjective
Verbalized difficulty with regulation/integration of one or more effects or prevention of complication; [inability to manage treatment regimen]
Verbalized desire to manage the treatment of illness and prevention of the sequelae
Verbalizes that family did not take action to reduce risk factors for progression of illness and sequelae

Objective
Inappropriate family activities for meeting the goals of a treatment or prevention program
Acceleration (expected or unexpected) of illness symptoms of a family member
Lack of attention to illness and its sequelae

SAMPLE CLINICAL APPLICATIONS: chronic conditions (e.g., COPD, MS, arthritis, chronic pain, substance abuse, end-stage liver/renal failure) or new diagnoses necessitating lifestyle changes

DESIRED OUTCOMES/EVALUATION CRITERIA

Sample **NOC** linkages:

Family Participation in Professional Care: Family involvement in decision making, delivery, and evaluation of care provided by healthcare professionals

Family Health Status: Overall health status and social competence of family unit

Family Functioning: Ability of the family to meet the needs of its members through developmental transitions

Family Will (Include Specific Time Frame)

- Identify individual factors affecting regulation/integration of treatment program.
- Participate in problem solving of factors.
- Verbalize acceptance of need/desire to change actions to achieve agreed-on outcomes or goals of treatment or prevention program.
- Demonstrate behaviors/changes in lifestyle necessary to maintain therapeutic regimen.

ACTIONS/INTERVENTIONS

Sample **NIC** linkages:

Family Involvement Promotion: Facilitating family participation in the emotional and physical care of the patient

Family Mobilization: Utilization of family strengths to influence patient's health in a positive direction

Health System Guidance: Facilitating a patient's location and use of appropriate health services

NURSING PRIORITY NO. 1. To identify causative/precipitating factors:

- Ascertain family's perception of efforts to date. *Perceptions are more important than facts, and by getting family's point of view realistic goals can be set and family can look to the future.*[2]
- Evaluate family activities as related to appropriate family functioning/activities. *Looking at frequency/effectiveness of family communication, promotion of autonomy, adaptation to meet changing needs, health of home environment/lifestyle, problem-solving abilities, ties to community provides information about current problem areas and need for specific interventions.*[1]
- Note family health goals and agreement of individual members. *Presence of conflict interferes with problem solving and needs to be addressed before family can move forward to meet goals.*[2]
- Determine understanding of and value of the treatment regimen to the family. *Individual members may misunderstand either the cause of the illness or the prescribed regimen and may disagree with what is happening, promoting dissension within the family group and causing distress for the identified client.*[1]
- Identify availability and use of resources. *Knowing who is available to help and support the family will help in planning care to maximize positive outcomes.*[2]

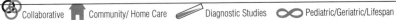

NURSING PRIORITY NO. 2. To assist family to develop strategies to improve management of therapeutic regimen:

- Provide information to aid family in understanding the value of the treatment program. *Accurate information helps individuals make decisions based on that knowledge, see the connection between illness and treatment, and may adhere to therapeutic regimen.*[3]
- Assist family members to recognize inappropriate family activities. Help the members identify both togetherness and individual needs and behavior. *Effective interactions can be enhanced and perpetuated when these factors are identified and used to improve family behaviors.*[2]
- Make a plan jointly with family members to deal with complexity of healthcare regimen/system and other related factors. *Enhances commitment to plan, optimizing outcomes when family and caregivers work together to plan therapeutic regimen.*[2]
- Identify community resources as needed using the three strategies of education, problem solving, and resource-linking to address specific deficits. *Providing information, helping family members learn effective problem-solving techniques and how to access needed resources can help them deal successfully with the chronically ill family member.*[4]

NURSING PRIORITY NO. 3. To promote wellness as related to future health of family members:

- Help family identify criteria to promote ongoing self-evaluation of situation/effectiveness and family progress. *Involvement promotes sense of control and provides the opportunity to be proactive in meeting needs.*[2]
- Make referrals to and/or jointly plan with other health/social and community resources. *Problems often are multifaceted, requiring involvement of numerous providers/agencies to plan appropriate regimen to meet family/individual needs.*[3]
- Provide contact person/case manager for one-to-one assistance as needed. *Having a single contact to coordinate care, provide support, and assist with problem solving maintains continuity and prevents misunderstandings and errors in managing the family's regimen.*[1]
- Refer to NDs Caregiver Role Strain, ineffective Therapeutic Regimen Management, as indicated.

DOCUMENTATION FOCUS

Assessment/Reassessment
- Individual findings, including nature of problem/degree of impairment, family values/health goals, and level of participation and commitment of family members.
- Availability and use of resources.

Planning
- Plan of care and who is involved in planning.
- Teaching Plan.

Implementation/Evaluation
- Response to interventions/teaching and actions performed.
- Attainment/progress toward desired outcome(s).
- Modifications of plan of care.

Discharge Planning
- Long-term needs, plan for meeting and who is responsible for actions.
- Specific referrals made.

References
1. Cox, H. C., et al. (2002). Clinical Applications of Nursing Diagnosis: Adult, Child, Women's, Psychiatric, Gerontic, and Home Health Considerations, ed 4. Philadelphia: F.A. Davis.
2. Healthy People 2010 Toolkit: A Field Guide to Health Planning (2002). Washington, DC: Public Health Foundation.
3. Stuifbergen, A. (1997). Health promotion: An essential component of rehabilitation for persons with chronic disabling conditions. ADV Nurs Sci, 19(4), 147–148.
4. Larsen. L. S. (1998). Effectiveness of counseling intervention to assist family caregivers of chronically ill relatives. J Psychosoc Nurs, 36(8), 26.

ineffective Therapeutic Regimen Management

Definition: Pattern of regulating and integrating into daily living a program for treatment of illness and the sequelae of illness that is unsatisfactory for meeting specific health goals

RELATED FACTORS
Complexity of healthcare system/therapeutic regimen
Decisional conflicts
Economic difficulties
Excessive demands made on individual or family
Family conflict
Family patterns of healthcare
Inadequate number and types of cues to action
Knowledge deficits
Mistrust of regimen and/or healthcare personnel
Perceived seriousness/susceptibility/barriers/benefits
Powerlessness
Social support deficits

DEFINING CHARACTERISTICS

Subjective
Verbalized desire to manage the treatment of illness and prevention of sequelae
Verbalized difficulty with regulation/integration of one or more prescribed regimens for treatment of illness and its effects or prevention of complications
Verbalized that did not take action to include treatment regimens in daily routines/reduce risk factors for progression of illness and sequelae

Objective
Choice of daily living ineffective for meeting the goals of a treatment or prevention program
Acceleration (expected or unexpected) of illness symptoms
SAMPLE CLINICAL APPLICATIONS: chronic conditions (e.g., COPD, MS, arthritis, chronic pain, end-stage liver/renal failure) or new diagnoses necessitating lifestyle changes

 Cultural Collaborative Community/ Home Care Diagnostic Studies 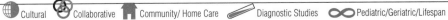 Pediatric/Geriatric/Lifespan Medications

DESIRED OUTCOMES/EVALUATION CRITERIA

Sample **NOC** linkages:

Treatment Behavior: Illness or Injury: Personal actions to palliate or eliminate pathology

Health Beliefs [specify]: Personal convictions that influence health behaviors/that one can influence a health outcome

Adherence Behavior: Self-initiated action taken to promote wellness, recovery, and rehabilitation

Client Will (Include Specific Time Frame)

- Verbalize acceptance of need/desire to change actions to achieve agreed-on outcomes.
- Verbalize understanding of factors/blocks involved in individual situation.
- Participate in problem solving of factors interfering with integration of therapeutic regimen.
- Demonstrate behaviors/changes in lifestyle necessary to maintain therapeutic regimen.
- Identify/use available resources.

ACTIONS/INTERVENTIONS

Sample **NIC** linkages:

Self-Modification Assistance: Reinforcement of self-directed change initiated by the patient to achieve personally important goals

Health System Guidance: Facilitating a patient's location and use of appropriate health services

Patient Contracting: Negotiating an agreement with a patient that reinforces a specific behavior change

NURSING PRIORITY NO. 1. To identify causative/contributing factors:

- Ascertain client's knowledge/understanding of condition and treatment needs. *Provides a baseline so planning care can begin where the client is in relation to condition/illness and current regimen.*[1]
- Determine client's/family's health goals and patterns of healthcare. *Provides information about current behaviors/misperceptions that may be potential areas of conflict, values, cultural mores, religious beliefs, or financial considerations.*[1]
- Identify individual perceptions and expectations of treatment regimen. *May reveal misinformation, unrealistic expectations, other factors that may be interfering with client's willingness to follow therapeutic regimen.*[1]
- Note availability/use of resources for assistance, caregiving/respite care. *Client may not have or be aware of resources or not know how to access resources that may be available.*[6]

NURSING PRIORITY NO. 2. To assist client/SO(s) to develop strategies to improve management of therapeutic regimen:

- Use therapeutic communication skills to assist client to problem-solve solution(s). *Active listening promotes accurate identification of the problem, ensuring that problem solving is directed to the correct solution.*[7]
- Explore client involvement in or lack of mutual goal setting. *Understanding client's willingness to be involved or not provides insight into the reasons for these actions and appropriate interventions.*[7]

- Identify steps necessary to reach desired goal(s). *Specifying steps to take requires discussion and the use of critical thinking skills to determine how to best reach the goals.*[4]
- Contract with the client for participation in care. *By making a contract, client commits self to therapeutic regimen and is more likely to follow through because of commitment.*[6]
- Accept client's evaluation of own strengths/limitations while working together to improve abilities. State belief in client's ability to cope and/or adapt to situation. *Individuals often minimize own strengths and exaggerate limitations when faced with the difficulties of a chronic illness. By helping in concrete ways, client can begin to accept reality of strengths. Stating your belief in positive terms lets client hear someone else's evaluation and begin to accept that he or she can manage the situation.*[3]
- Acknowledge individual efforts/capabilities. *Encourages continuation of desired behaviors and reinforces movement toward attainment of desired outcomes.*[5,7]
- Provide information as well as help client to know where and how to find it on own. Reinforce previous instructions and rationale, using a variety of learning modalities, including role playing, demonstration, written materials, and so forth. *Various modalities promote retention of information. Developing client's skill at finding own information encourages self-sufficiency and sense of self-worth.*[2]

NURSING PRIORITY NO. 3. To promote wellness (Teaching/Discharge Considerations):

- Emphasize importance of client knowledge and understanding of the need for treatment/medication as well as consequences of actions/choices. *Reinforces client's role in success of therapeutic regimen, encouraging continuation of competent behaviors.*[1]
- Promote client/caregiver/SO(s) participation in planning and evaluating process. *Enhances commitment to plan, optimizing outcomes.*[1]
- Assist client to develop strategies for monitoring therapeutic regimen. *Promotes early recognition of changes, allowing proactive response.*[5]
- Mobilize support systems, including family/SO(s), social, financial, and so on. *Success of therapeutic regimen is enhanced by using support systems effectively, avoiding stress and worry of dealing with unresolved problems.*[2]
- Refer to counseling/therapy (group and individual) as indicated. *May need additional help to deal with stress and anxiety of chronic condition/illness.*[1]
- Identify home and community-based nursing services. *Provides services for assessment, follow-up care, and education in client's home to promote continuation of effective management of therapeutic regimen.*[1]

DOCUMENTATION FOCUS

Assessment/Reassessment
- Findings including underlying dynamics of individual situation, client's perception of problem/needs.
- Family involvement/needs.
- Individual strengths/limitations.
- Availability/use of resources.

Planning
- Plan of care and who is involved in planning.
- Teaching plan.

 Cultural   Collaborative   Community/ Home Care   Diagnostic Studies   Pediatric/Geriatric/Lifespan   Medications

Implementation/Evaluation
- Response to interventions/teaching and actions performed.
- Attainment/progress toward desired outcome(s).
- Modifications to plan of care.

Discharge Planning
- Long-range needs and who is responsible for actions to be taken.
- Available resources, specific referrals made.

References

1. Cox, H. C., et al. (2002). Clinical Applications of Nursing Diagnosis: Adult, Child, Women's, Psychiatric, Gerontic, and Home Health Considerations, ed 4. Philadelphia: F. A. Davis.
2. Healthy People 2010 Toolkit: A Field Guide to Health Planning. (2002). Washington, DC: Public Health Foundation.
3. Stuifbergen, A. (1997). Health promotion: an essential component of rehabilitation for persons with chronic disabling conditions. ADV Nurs Sci, 19(4), 147–148.
4. Larsen L. S. (1998). Effectiveness of counseling intervention to assist family caregivers of chronically ill relatives. J Psychosoc Nurs, 36(8), 26.
5. Lai, S. C., & Cohen, M. N. (1999). Promoting lifestyle changes. AJN, 99(4), 63.
6. Miller, J. F. (1999). Coping with Chronic Illness: Overcoming Powerlessness, ed 3. Philadelphia: F. A. Davis.
7. Townsend, M. C. (2003). Psychiatric Mental Health Nursing Concepts of Care, ed 4. Philadelphia: F. A. Davis.

readiness for enhanced Therapeutic Regimen Management

Definition: A pattern of regulating and integrating into daily living a program(s) for treatment of illness and its sequelae that is sufficient for meeting health-related goals and can be strengthened

RELATED FACTORS
To be developed by nurse researchers and submitted to NANDA

DEFINING CHARACTERISTICS

Subjective
Expresses desire to manage the treatment of illness and prevention of sequelae
Expresses little to no difficulty with regulation/integration of one or more prescribed regimens for treatment of illness or prevention of complications
Describes reduction of risk factors for progression of illness and sequelae

Objective
Choices of daily living are appropriate for meeting the goals of treatment or prevention
No unexpected acceleration of illness symptoms

SAMPLE CLINICAL APPLICATIONS: diabetes mellitus, CHF, COPD/asthma, MS, systemic lupus, HIV positive/AIDS, prematurity

DESIRED OUTCOMES/EVALUATION CRITERIA
Sample **NOC** linkages:
Symptom Control: Personal actions to minimize perceived adverse changes in physical and emotional functioning

Knowledge: Treatment Regimen: Extent of understanding conveyed about a specific treatment regimen

Participation: Health Care Decisions: Personal involvement in selecting and evaluating healthcare options

---

Client Will (Include Specific Time Frame)

- Assume responsibility for managing treatment regimen.
- Demonstrate proactive management by anticipating and planning for eventualities of condition/potential complications.
- Identify/use additional resources as appropriate.
- Remain free of preventable complications/progression of illness and sequelae.

ACTIONS/INTERVENTIONS

Sample **NIC** linkages:

Health System Guidance: Facilitating a patient's location and use of appropriate health services

Health Education: Developing and providing instruction and learning experiences to facilitate voluntary adaptation of behavior conducive to health in individuals, families, groups, or communities

Anticipatory Guidance: Preparation of patient for an anticipated developmental and/or situational crisis

NURSING PRIORITY NO. **1.** To determine motivation for continued growth:

- Verify client's level of knowledge/understanding of therapeutic regimen. Note specific health goals. *Provides opportunity to assure accuracy and completeness of knowledge base for future learning.*[1]
- Determine individual's perceptions of adaptation to treatment/anticipated changes. *How client sees the situation is important to discussing what is happening in regard to the treatment regimen and planning for the future.*[1]
- Identify individual's expectations of long-term treatment needs/anticipated changes. *Knowing expectations identifies understanding and acceptance of what is realistic for own situation.*[3]
- Discuss present resources used by client. *Noting whether changes can be arranged (e.g., increased hours of home care assistance; access to case manager to support complex/long-term program) helps with planning for improved therapeutic regimen.*[3]
- Determine influence of cultural beliefs on client/caregiver(s) participation in regimen. *For instance, some Mexican Americans may not believe in usual health maintenance and prevention because of their traditional present-time orientation and belief that the future is in God's hands and may have difficulty adhering to a long-term health care regimen.*[7]

NURSING PRIORITY NO. **2.** To assist client/SO(s) to develop plan to meet individual needs:

- Identify steps necessary to reach desired health goal(s). *Understanding the process enhances commitment and the likelihood of achieving the goals.*[4]
- Accept client's evaluation of own strengths/limitations while working together to improve abilities. *Promotes sense of self-esteem and confidence to continue efforts to manage therapeutic regimen more effectively, such as diabetes, multiple sclerosis.*[6]

 Cultural   Collaborative   Community/ Home Care   Diagnostic Studies   Pediatric/Geriatric/Lifespan   Medications

- Provide information/bibliotherapy and help client/SO(s) identify and evaluate resources they can access on their own. *Promotes sense of confidence in own ability to learn about illness/condition. When referencing the Internet or nontraditional/unproven resources, the individual must exercise some restraint and determine the reliability of the source/information provided before acting on it.*[5]
- Acknowledge individual efforts/capabilities to reinforce movement toward attainment of desired outcomes. *Provides positive reinforcement, encouraging continued progress toward desired goals to enhance therapeutic regimen.*[3]

NURSING PRIORITY NO. 3. To promote optimum functioning:

- Promote client/caregiver choices and involvement in planning for and implementing added tasks/responsibilities. *Being involved in planning and knowing that he or she can make own choices promotes commitment to program and enhances probability that client will follow through with regimen.*[1]
- Assist in implementing strategies for monitoring progress/responses to therapeutic regimen. *Promotes proactive problem solving enabling client/caregiver to identify problems as they arise and deal appropriately with them so regimen is maintained.*[1]
- Identify additional community resources/support groups. *Provides additional opportunities for role-modeling, skill training, anticipatory problem solving, etc.*[2,6]

DOCUMENTATION FOCUS

Assessment/Reassessment
- Findings, including dynamics of individual situation.
- Individual strengths/additional needs.

Planning
- Plan of care and who is involved in planning.
- Teaching Plan.

Implementation/Evaluation
- Response to interventions/teaching and actions performed.
- Attainment/progress toward desired outcome(s).
- Modifications to plan of care.

Discharge Planning
- Short-range and long-range needs and who is responsible for actions.
- Available resources, specific referrals made.

References

1. Cox, H. C., et al. (2002). Clinical Applications of Nursing Diagnosis: Adult, Child, Women's, Psychiatric, Gerontic, and Home Health Considerations, ed 4. Philadelphia: F. A. Davis.
2. Healthy People 2010 Toolkit: A Field Guide to Health Planning. (2002). Washington, DC: Public Health Foundation.
3. Stuifbergen, A. (1997). Health promotion: An essential component of rehabilitation for persons with chronic disabling conditions. ADV Nurs Sci, 19(4), 147–148.
4. Larsen L. S. (1998). Effectiveness of counseling intervention to assist family caregivers of chronically ill relatives. J Psychosoc Nurs, 36(8), 26.

5. Lai, S. C., & Cohen, M. N. (1999). Promoting lifestyle changes. AJN, 99(4), 63.

6. Miller, J.F. (1999). Coping with Chronic Illness: Overcoming Powerlessness, ed 3. Philadelphia: F. A. Davis.

7. Lipson, J. G., Dibble, S. L., & Minarik, P. A. (1996). Culture & Nursing Care: A Pocket Guide. San Francisco: UCSF Nursing Press.

ineffective Thermoregulation

Definition: Temperature fluctuation between hypothermia and hyperthermia

RELATED FACTORS

Trauma or illness [e.g., cerebral edema, CVA, intracranial surgery, or head injury]

Immaturity, aging [e.g., loss/absence of brown adipose tissue]

Fluctuating environmental temperature

[Changes in hypothalamic tissue causing alterations in emission of thermosensitive cells and regulation of heat loss/production]

[Changes in metabolic rate/activity; changes in level/action of thyroxine and catecholamines]

[Chemical reactions in contracting muscles]

DEFINING CHARACTERISTICS

Objective

Fluctuations in body temperature above or below the normal range

Tachycardia

Reduction in body temperature below normal range; cool skin; pallor (moderate); shivering (mild); piloerection; cyanotic nail beds; slow capillary refill; hypertension

Warm to touch; flushed skin; increased respiratory rate; seizures/convulsions

SAMPLE CLINICAL APPLICATIONS: prematurity, brain injury/CVA/intracranial surgery (cerebral edema), infections/sepsis, major surgical procedures

DESIRED OUTCOMES/EVALUATION CRITERIA

Sample **NOC** linkages:

Thermoregulation: Individual or caregiver efforts to control behaviors that might cause physical injury

Thermoregulation: Neonate: Balance among heat production, heat gain, and heat loss during the neonatal period

Client/Caregiver Will (Include Specific Time Frame)

- Verbalize understanding of individual factors and appropriate interventions.
- Demonstrate techniques/behaviors to correct underlying condition/situation.
- Maintain body temperature within normal limits.

ACTIONS/INTERVENTIONS

Sample **NIC** linkages:

Temperature Regulation: Attaining and/or maintaining body temperature within a normal range

Temperature Regulation: Intraoperative: Attaining and/or maintaining desire intraoperative body temperature

 Cultural   Collaborative   Community/ Home Care  Diagnostic Studies 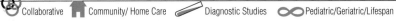 Pediatric/Geriatric/Lifespan   Medications

Fever Treatment: Management of a patient with hyperpyrexia caused by nonenvironmental factors

NURSING PRIORITY NO. 1. To identify causative/contributing factors:

- Assist with measures to identify causative factor(s)/underlying condition (e.g., obtaining history concerning present symptoms, correlation with past history/family history, diagnostic studies). *Thermoregulation is a controlled process that maintains the body's core temperature in the range in which most biochemical processes work best (99 °F to 99.6 °F).*[1] *Thermoregulation is affected in two ways: 1)* **endogenous** *factors (via diseases or conditions of body/organ systems) and 2)* **exogenous factors** *(via medications and nutrition).*[2] *Exercise, behavioral impulses, metabolic and hormonal changes influence changes in body temperature, leading to loss or gain of heat.*
- Determine if present illness/condition results from exposure to environmental factors, surgery, infection, or trauma. *Helps to determine the scope of interventions that may be needed (e.g., simple addition of warm blankets after surgery, or hypothermia therapy following brain trauma).*[4]
- Note client's age (e.g., premature neonate, young child, or aging individual), *as it can directly impact ability to maintain/regulate body temperature and respond to changes in environment.*[3]
- Monitor laboratory values (e.g., tests indicative of infection, thyroid/other endocrine tests, drug screens) *to identify potential internal causes of temperature imbalances.*

NURSING PRIORITY NO. 2. To assist with measures to correct/treat underlying cause:

- Monitor temperature by appropriate route (e.g., tympanic, rectal, oral), noting variation from client's usual/normal temperature. *Rectal and tympanic temperatures most closely approximate core temperature; however, shell temperatures (oral, axillary, touch) are often measured at home and are predictive of fever or subnormal temperatures. Rectal temperature measurement may be the most accurate, but is not always expedient (e.g., client declines, is agitated, has rectal lesions or surgery, etc.). Abdominal temperature monitoring may be done in the premature neonate.*
- Ascertain if client has the potential for/is demonstrating signs of cold stress (e.g., low body temperature, cool, pale, or blue skin, shivering, hypertension, tachycardia), or signs of heat stress (e.g., fever, tachycardia, hyperventilation, dry skin/mucous membranes, decreased sweating and urine output). Refer to NDs: risk for imbalanced Body Temperature, Hypothermia, or Hyperthermia for interventions to restore/maintain body temperature within normal range.
- Administer fluids, nutrition, electrolytes, and medications as indicated *to restore or maintain body/organ function.*
- Maintain ambient temperature in comfortable range *to prevent/compensate for client's heat production or heat loss (e.g., may need to add or remove clothing or blankets, reduce or increase room temperature).*
- Place newborn infant under radiant warmer *to prevent heat loss.*
- Monitor use of heating pads, ice bags, and hypothermia blankets, especially in pediatric/geriatric clients *who are more susceptible to temperature fluctuations.*
- Discuss with client/caregivers dressing appropriately such as:
  Wear layers of clothing that can be removed or added, hat/gloves in cold weather, light

loose protective clothing in hot weather, or water resistant outer gear to protect from wet weather chill.[1]

Cover infant's head with knit cap, use layers of lightweight blankets. *Newborns/infants can have temperature instability. Heat loss is greatest through head and by evaporation and convection.*[5]

- Prepare client for/assist with procedures (e.g., surgical intervention, neoplastic agent, antibiotics) *to treat underlying cause of hypothermia or hyperthermia.*
- Ascertain that cooling and warming equipment and supplies are available during/following procedures and surgery.

NURSING PRIORITY NO. 3. To promote wellness (Teaching/Discharge Considerations):

- Review causative/related factors with client/SO(s). *Provides information about what, if any, measures can be implemented to protect client from harm, and/or limit potential for problems associated with ineffective thermoregulation.*
- Provide oral and written information concerning client's disease processes, current therapies, and postdischarge precautions, as appropriate to situation. *Allows for early intervention and implementation of preventive or corrective measures.*
- Discuss use of/identify resources for heating/cooling measures as needed such as space heater or air conditioner/fans.
- Refer at-risk persons to appropriate community resources (e.g., home care, social services, Foster Adult Care, housing agencies) *to provide assistance to meet individual needs.*
- Refer to teaching in NDs risk for imbalanced Body Temperature, Hypothermia, or Hyperthermia as appropriate.

DOCUMENTATION FOCUS

Assessment/Reassessment
- Individual findings, including nature of problem, degree of impairment/fluctuations in temperature.

Planning
- Plan of care and who is involved in planning.
- Teaching Plan.

Implementation/Evaluation
- Responses to interventions/teaching actions performed.
- Attainment/progress toward desired outcome(s).
- Modifications to plan of care.

Discharge Planning
- Long-term needs and who is responsible for actions to be taken.
- Specific referrals made.

References

1. Worfolk, J. (1997). Keep frail elders warm! Geriatr Nurs 18(1), 7–11.
2. Kneis, R. C. (1996). Geriatric trauma: What you need to know. Int J Traum Nurs, 2(3), 85–91.
3. Cox, H. C., et al. (2002). Clinical Applications of Nursing Diagnosis: Adult, Child, Women's, Psychiatric, Gerontic, and Home Health Considerations, ed 4. Philadelphia: F. A. Davis.

4. ND: Surgical Intervention. In Doenges, M. E., Moorhouse, M. F., & Geissler-Murr, A. C. (2002). Nursing Care Plans: Guidelines for Individualizing Patient Care, ed 6. Philadelphia: F. A. Davis.
5. Early discharge of the term newborn. Guideline from National Association of Neonatal Nurses. Glenview, IL. 1999. Retrieved October 2003, from National Guideline Clearinghouse website, www.guideline.gov.

disturbed Thought Processes

Definition: Disruption in cognitive operations and activities

RELATED FACTORS

To be developed by nurse researchers and submitted to NANDA
[Physiologic changes, aging, hypoxia, head injury, malnutrition, infections]
[Biochemical changes, medications, substance abuse]
[Sleep deprivation]
[Psychological conflicts, emotional changes, mental disorders]

DEFINING CHARACTERISTICS

Subjective
[Ideas of reference, hallucinations, delusions]

Objective
Inaccurate interpretation of environment
Inappropriate/nonreality-based thinking
Memory deficit/problems, [disorientation to person, place, time, circumstances and events, loss of short-term/remote memory]
Hypervigilance or hypovigilance
Cognitive dissonance [decreased ability to grasp ideas, make decisions, problem-solve, use abstract reasoning or conceptualize, calculate; disordered thought sequencing]
Distractibility, [altered attention span]
Egocentricity
[Confabulation]
[Inappropriate social behavior]

SAMPLE CLINICAL APPLICATIONS: brain injury/CVA, CNS infections, anorexia nervosa, substance abuse, septicemia, cirrhosis of liver, delirium, dementia, schizophrenia, dissociative disorders, paranoid disorder, obsessive-compulsive disorder

DESIRED OUTCOMES/EVALUATION CRITERIA

Sample **NOC** linkages:

Distorted Thought Control: Self-restraint of disruption in perception, thought processes, and thought content

Cognitive Orientation: Ability to identify person, place, and time

Memory: Ability to cognitively retrieve and report previously stored information

Client Will (Include Specific Time Frame)
- Recognize changes in thinking/behavior.
- Verbalize understanding of causative factors when known/able.
- Identify interventions to deal effectively with situation.
- Demonstrate behaviors/lifestyle changes to prevent/minimize changes in mentation.
- Maintain usual reality orientation.

ACTIONS/INTERVENTIONS

Sample **NIC** linkages:

Dementia Management: Provision of a modified environment for the patient who is experiencing a chronic confusional state

Delusion Management: Promoting the comfort, safety, and reality orientation of a patient experiencing false, fixed beliefs that have little or no basis in reality

Environmental Management: Safety: Manipulation of the patient's surroundings for therapeutic benefit

NURSING PRIORITY NO. 1. To assess causative/contributing factors:

- Identify factors present: *Disturbances in thinking can be the result of a wide variety of conditions (e.g., acute/chronic brain syndrome—recent CVA, dementias, retardation; traumatic brain injury with increased intracranial pressure, brain/CNS infections, malnutrition, metabolic problems such as acid-base imbalances, diabetes, renal/hepatic failure; sensory deprivation or overstimulation; toxins including drug interactions/reactions, substance use/abuse, overdose, accidental exposures; emotional/psychiatric illness).*[2]
- Interview client and SO(s) *to determine aspects of current problem (e.g., usual thinking ability, changes in behavior, discrepancies in age and mastery of developmental milestones, etc.).* Note length of time problem has existed, and other pertinent information, *to provide baseline for comparison.*[6]
- Assist with/review results of diagnostic testing (e.g., MRI, CT scan, spinal tap) *to identifying etiology of thinking impairment.*
- Assess for presence/severity of pain, as well as use and/or need for analgesics. *Both pain and the treatments for pain can diminish the acuity of client's thinking processes. Untreated pain can increase confusion and agitation.*[1]
- Determine client's medication/drug use (prescription/OTC/illicit/herbal). *May have adverse side and/or cumulative effects that alter thought processes and sensory perception.*[2]
- Note schedule of drug administration. *May be significant when evaluating cumulative effects/interactions.*
- Assess dietary intake/nutritional status. *Good nutrition is essential for optimal brain functioning. Persons with anorexia, major depression, substance use and chronic debilitating conditions may have problems with thinking related to deficits in nutrients, vitamins, electrolytes, and minerals.*[2]
- Evaluate impact of environment. *Excessive noise, multiple people in client's surroundings, chaotic lifestyle, rapid changes in routines, etc., can result in overstimulation/confusion clouding client's thinking and impairing coping abilities.*
- Monitor laboratory values. *Abnormalities such as metabolic alkalosis, hypokalemia, anemia, elevated ammonia levels, and signs of infection may be affecting thought processes.*

NURSING PRIORITY NO. 2. To assess degree of impairment:

- Perform neurologic assessments as indicated and compare with baseline. Note changes in level of consciousness and cognition, such as increased lethargy, confusion, drowsiness, irritability; changes in ability to communicate. *Early recognition of changes promotes proactive modifications to plan of care.*[2]
- Evaluate mental status using appropriate tools *(establishes baseline and comparative functional level according to age, developmental stage and neurologic status),* noting[5]:
  extent of impairment in thinking ability. *Varies widely, with impairments being overt or diffi-*

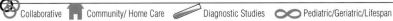 Cultural   Collaborative   Community/ Home Care   Diagnostic Studies   Pediatric/Geriatric/Lifespan   Medications

cult to identify. *Long time periods and sophisticated neuropsychiatric testing may be required to more fully identify nature of this impairment.*

remote/recent memory. *Remote memory is often intact, while recent/short term memory may be lost or impaired.*

orientation to person/place/time. *Confusion may be short-term, long-term or permanent and can be stable or progressive.* Refer to NDs acute/chronic Confusion.

insight and judgment. *Client may/may not be aware of changes in these areas, but family, friends or colleagues may report concerns.*

changes in personality or response to stimuli. *Can range from lethargy and withdrawal to anger, agitation and violent responses.*

attention span/distractibility and ability to make decisions or problem-solve. *Determines ability to participate in planning/executing care.*

ability to receive, send, and appropriately interpret communications. Note absence of speech or changes in speech patterns (e.g., slowing and/or slurring of speech, problems with word finding, presence of aphasia, etc.). *Speech and communication difficulties are both indicators and consequences of impaired thought processes.*

client's anxiety level (from mild to panic level) *that both causes and potentiates alterations in thought processes.*[2]

occurrence of paranoia and delusions, hallucinations. *Can occur with brain injury, mental illness, metabolic and electrolyte disturbances, alcohol/other drug use/overdose, dementias, etc., reflecting escalation of thought disturbances.*[2]

NURSING PRIORITY NO. 3. To prevent further deterioration, maximize level of function:

- Assist with treatment for underlying problems such as anorexia, increased intracranial pressure, sleep disorders, biochemical imbalances. *Cognition often improves with correction of medical problems.*[6]
- Establish alternate means for self-expression. *Provides way of determining thinking ability if unable to communicate verbally.* Refer to ND impaired verbal Communication.
- Reorient to person/place/time as needed *to reinforce/maintain reality of the moment. Note: Inability to maintain orientation is a sign of deterioration.*
- Note behavior that may be indicative of potential for violence and take appropriate actions *to prevent harm to client/others. Clients with brain injuries often have lowered impulse control, problems with anger management, and the potential for violent outbursts, requiring specific interventions designed to help the client learn to control these behaviors.*[7] Refer to ND risk for other-directed Violence.
- Stay with client when agitated, frightened. *Support may provide calming effect, reducing anxiety and risk of injury.*[2]
- Provide safety measures—cautious use of side rails, padding as necessary; bed in low position/on floor, close supervision, seizure precautions—as indicated. *May help to prevent accidents/injury to client.*[2]
- Schedule structured activity and rest periods. *Provides stimulation without undue fatigue, helping to maintain orientation and sense of reality.*[3]
- Encourage/provide opportunities for adequate sleep. *Sleep deprivation can increase confusion. Regular sleep routine reinforces the idea of bedtime, and adequate rest can enhance clarity of thinking.*[6] Refer to ND Sleep Deprivation.

- Monitor medication regimen, limit use of sedatives and drugs affecting the nervous system *that have shown correlation with episodes of confusion.*[1–3]

- Encourage family/SO(s) to participate in reorientation and provide ongoing input (e.g., current news and family happening). *Promotes sense of normalcy, maintains contact with family.*

- Refer to appropriate rehabilitation providers. Cognitive retraining program, speech therapist, psychosocial resources, biofeedback, counselor may help client to enhance degree of functioning.[6]

NURSING PRIORITY NO. 4. To create therapeutic milieu and assist client/SO(s) to develop coping strategies (especially when condition is irreversible):

- Provide opportunities for SO(s) to ask questions and obtain information. *SOs frequently have difficulty accepting and dealing with client's aberrant behavior and may require assistance in understanding and coping with the situation.*[2]
- Maintain a pleasant, quiet environment and approach in a slow, calm manner. *Client may respond with anxious or aggressive behaviors if startled or overstimulated.*
- Maintain reality-oriented relationship and environment. *Using aids such as clocks, calendars, personal items, and seasonal decorations helps individual maintain current reality.*[6]
- Present reality concisely and briefly and do not challenge illogical thinking. *Helps client stay focused on the present. Client may react defensively if thinking is challenged.*[6]
- Give simple directions, using short words and simple sentences. *Provides for processing of basic communication when thinking is impaired.*[3]
- Listen with regard to client's verbalizations in spite of speech pattern/content *to convey interest and worth to individual, enhancing self-esteem and encouraging continued efforts.*[3]
- Reduce provocative stimuli, negative criticism, arguments, and confrontations *to avoid triggering fight/flight responses.*
- Refrain from forcing activities and communications. *Client may feel threatened and may withdraw or rebel.*
- Respect individuality and personal space. *Conveys concern for the person regardless of the circumstances.*[3]

- Use touch judiciously, respecting personal needs, but keeping in mind physical and psychological importance of touch. *Touch is a powerful communication tool and can have positive and negative reactions, and the appropriateness of its use is culturally determined.*[5]
- Provide nutritionally well-balanced diet incorporating client's preferences as able. Encourage client to eat, provide pleasant environment, and allow sufficient time to eat. *Enhances intake promoting nutritional status and general well-being.*[6]
- Allow more time for client to respond to questions/comments and make simple decisions. *Processing information takes more time when thinking is impaired, and allowing more time promotes communication and client's sense of self-esteem.*[6]

- Inform family/caregiver of the meaning of/reasons for common behaviors observed in client with disturbed thought processes, as well as the probable course of disease process and plan of care. *Helps them to understand and cope with situation and assists them in providing a safe environment for the client.*[4]

- Support client/SO(s) with grieving for loss of self/abilities as in Alzheimer's disease. *Progressive loss of mental abilities is difficult for family members to deal with as they grieve the loss of the person they knew. Providing opportunity for individuals to talk about feelings of grief will promote coping abilities.*[4]Refer to ND anticipatory/dysfunctional Grieving.

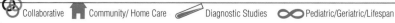

- Encourage participation in resocialization activities/groups as appropriate. *Can help the individual maintain/regain some degree of social skills. Even in conditions of dementia, client can benefit from these activities.*[6]

Cultural   Collaborative   Community/ Home Care   Diagnostic Studies   Pediatric/Geriatric/Lifespan   Medications

NURSING PRIORITY NO. 5. To promote wellness (Teaching/Discharge Considerations):

- Assist in identifying ongoing treatment needs/rehabilitation program for the individual *to maintain gains and continue progress if able.*[6]
- Stress importance of cooperation with therapeutic regimen. *Client and SOs benefit from maintaining regimen as agreed on and working together benefits everyone.*[6]
- Promote socialization within individual limitations. *Client may have difficulty tolerating large or even small groups of people, unfamiliar or noisy surroundings.* Refer to ND disturbed Sensory Perception.
- Identify problems related to aging that are remediable and assist client/SO(s) to seek appropriate assistance/access resources. *Encourages problem solving to improve condition when possible rather than accept the status quo.*
- Help client/SO(s) develop plan of care to meet ADLs *when problem is progressive/long-term.* Refer to ND Self-Care Deficit (specify).
- Refer to community resources (e.g., social services, daycare programs, support groups, drug/alcohol rehabilitation) *to provide assistance and support for client/caregivers.*

DOCUMENTATION FOCUS

Assessment/Reassessment
- Individual findings, including nature of problem, current and previous level of function, effect on independence and lifestyle.

Planning
- Plan of care and who is involved in planning.
- Teaching Plan.

Implementation/Evaluation
- Response to interventions/teaching and actions performed.
- Attainment/progress toward desired outcome(s).
- Modifications to plan of care.

Discharge Planning
- Long-term needs/referrals and who is responsible for actions to be taken.
- Available resources, specific referrals made.

References

1. Foreman, M. (1989). Complexities of acute confusion. Geriatr Nurs, 3, 136.
2. ND:Thought Processes, disturbed. In Doenges, M. E., Moorhouse, M. F., & Geissler-Murr. (2002). Nursing Care Plans: Guidelines for Individualizing Patient Care, ed 6. Philadelphia: F. A. Davis, pp 217, 369, 410, 535, 715, 773.
3. Dellasaga, C., & Stricklin, M. L. (1993). Cognitive impairment in the elderly home health clients. Home Health Care Serve Q, 14:81.
4. Smart, G. , & Sundeen, S. (1991). Pocket Guide to Psychiatric Assessment. St Louis: Mosby.
5. Doenges, M. E., Townsend, M. C., & Moorhouse, M. F. (1998). Psychiatric Care Plans Guidelines for Individualizing Care, ed 3. Philadelphia: F. A. Davis.
6. Cox, H. C., et al. (2002). Clinical Applications of Nursing Diagnosis: Adult, Child, Women's, Psychiatric, Gerontic, and Home Health Considerations, ed 4. Philadelphia: F. A. Davis.
7. Johnson, G. (1998). Traumatic brain injury survival guide. Retrieved February 2004, from Neuro-Recovery Head Injury Program. Available at: http://www.triguide.com.

impaired Tissue Integrity

Definition: Damage to mucous membrane, corneal, integumentary, or subcutaneous tissues

RELATED FACTORS
Altered circulation
Nutritional deficit/excess; [metabolic, endocrine dysfunction]
Fluid deficit/excess
Knowledge deficit
Impaired physical mobility
Irritants, chemical (including body excretions, secretions, medications); radiation (including therapeutic radiation)
Thermal (temperature extremes)
Mechanical (e.g., pressure, shear, friction), [surgery]
[Infection]

DEFINING CHARACTERISTICS

Objective
Damaged or destroyed tissue (e.g., cornea, mucous membrane, integumentary, or subcutaneous)

SAMPLE CLINICAL APPLICATIONS: trauma, burns, diabetes mellitus, peripheral vascular disease, venous insufficiency, AIDS, cancer, radiation therapy, sickle cell crisis, cocaine use, scleroderma, infections, borderline personality or obsessive-compulsive disorders

DESIRED OUTCOMES/EVALUATION CRITERIA
Sample **NOC** linkages:
Tissue Integrity: Skin & Mucous Membranes: Structural intactness and normal physiologic function of skin and mucous membranes
Tissue Perfusion: Peripheral: Extent to which blood flows through the small vessels of the extremities and maintains tissue function

Client/Caregiver Will (Include Specific Time Frame)
- Verbalize understanding of condition and causative factors.
- Identify interventions appropriate for specific condition.
- Demonstrate behaviors/lifestyle changes to promote healing and prevent complications/recurrence.

Sample **NOC** linkage:
Wound Healing: Primary/Secondary Intention: The extent to which cells and tissues have regenerated following intentional closure/cells and tissues in an open wound have regenerated

Client Will (Include Specific Time Frame)
- Display progressive improvement in wound/lesion healing.

ACTIONS/INTERVENTIONS
Sample **NIC** linkages:
Wound Care: Prevention of wound complications and promotion of wound healing

 Cultural Collaborative  Community/ Home Care Diagnostic Studies 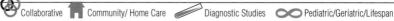 Pediatric/Geriatric/Lifespan Medications

Incision Site Care: Cleansing, monitoring, and promotion of healing in a wound that is closed with sutures, clips, or staples

Pressure Ulcer Care: Facilitation of healing in pressure ulcers

NURSING PRIORITY NO. **1.** To identify causative/contributing factors:

- Obtain history of condition: including characteristics of previous episode(s), if any, other symptoms that have accompanied episodes, characteristics of tissue lesions and changes/differences between past and current lesions/episodes.
- Assess for individual factors *that increase risk of circulatory insufficiency and occlusion, for example: 1) trauma to extremity that causes internal tissue damage such as high-velocity and penetrating trauma, fractures (especially long-bone fractures) with hemorrhage, or external pressures from burn eschar; 2) immobility (e.g., long-term bedrest, tight dressings, splints or casting); 3) presence of conditions affecting peripheral circulation, such as atherosclerosis, Buerger's disease, Raynaud's disease, or diabetes; 4) women older than age 60; 5) smoking; 6) obese and sedentary individuals; 7) high levels of homocysteine and cholesterol; 8) use of anti-coagulants; and 9) vigorous exercise.*[1-3]
- Identify underlying condition/pathology involved. *Tissue impairment can be the result of 1) **disease processes** that affect circulation and perfusion of vital organs/tissues (e.g., arteriosclerosis, venous insufficiency, hypertension, obesity, diabetes, malignant neoplasms); 2) **medications** (e.g., anticoagulants, corticosteroids, immunosuppressives, antineoplastics that adversely affect healing); 3) **burns/radiation** (can break down internal tissues); and 4) **nutrition and hydration** (e.g., malnutrition deprives the body of protein and calories required for cell growth and repair, and dehydration impairs transport of oxygen and nutrients).*[4,5]
- Note race/ethnic background and family history *for genetic conditions such as sickle cell anemia.*
- Assess skin/tissue color, temperature and sensation *for adequacy of blood supply and nerve innervation.*
- Note use of prosthetic, diagnostic or external devices. *Artificial limbs, contacts, dentures, endotracheal airways, indwelling catheters, esophageal dilators, etc., may cause pressure on/injure delicate tissues or provide entry point for infectious agents.*
- Evaluate client for poor health/safety practices. *Lack of cleanliness, frequent use of enemas, poor nutrition, unsafe sexual practices, failure to use safety equipment for occupational or sports related hazards (e.g., need for protective eyewear during contact with toxic chemicals/welding or racketball); lack of/poor dental hygiene, ill-fitting dentures can place client at risk for injury to tissues and/or impaired function.*
- Assess skin turgor, status of mucous membranes; note degree of edema (1+ to 4+), urine characteristics and output. *Determines presence of fluid deficit or overload that can adversely affect cell/tissue strength and organ function. Note: Edematous tissues are prone to breakdown.* (Refer to ND: risk for impaired Fluid Balance.)
- Inspect mucous membranes and skin for signs of ulceration (*suggestive of impaired circulation or presence of infection that can affect underlying tissues*), or evidence of other organ/tissue involvement (*e.g., a draining fistula through the integumentary and subcutaneous tissue may involve a bone infection*).
- Review recent/current drug regimen, noting use of anticoagulants and vasoactive agents *that can affect blood supply to tissues/organs.*
- Assist with diagnostic procedures (e.g., cultures, endoscopy, scans, biopsies). *May be necessary to determine cause for/extent of impairment.*

NURSING PRIORITY NO. 2. To assess degree of impairment:

- Assess wound(s), when present, and document 1) **dimensions and depth** in cm, 2) **exudates**—color, odor, and amount; 3) **margins**-fixed or unfixed; 4) **tunneling/tracts**—*(full extent of lesions of mucous membranes or subcutaneous tissue may not be visually discernible);* 5) evidence of **necrosis** (e.g., color gray to black) or **healing** (e.g., pink/red granulation tissue) *in order to clarify treatment needs and establish a comparative baseline.*[4,5]
- Classify pressure ulcer(s) using tool such as Waterlow, Braden, Norton (or similar) Ulcer Classification System. *Provides consistent terminology for assessment and documentation of pressure ulcers.*[6]
- Measure/photograph wound(s) periodically *to evaluate progress, development of complications/delayed healing.*
- Obtain specimens of wound exudate/lesions for culture/sensitivity and Gram stain when appropriate *to identify effective antimicrobial therapies.*
- Monitor laboratory studies (e.g., CBC, electrolytes, glucose, cultures) *for systemic changes indicative of healing or infection/complications.*
- Determine psychological effects of condition on the client and family. *For example, embarrassment about visual appearance may affect interaction with others, or pain associated with ulceration of vaginal mucosa can impair sexual functioning.*

NURSING PRIORITY NO. 3. To facilitate healing:[10,11,13,14]

- Keep surgical area(s) clean/dry, change dressings/drainage appliances frequently as indicated *to prevent accumulation of secretions/excretions that can cause skin/tissue excoriation.*
- Practice aseptic technique for cleansing/dressing/medicating wounds or lesions. *Reduces risk of cross-contamination.*
- Protect incision/wound approximation (e.g., use of Steri-Strips, splinting when coughing) and stimulate circulation to surrounding areas, *to assist body's natural process of repair.*
- Apply appropriate barrier dressings or wound coverings (e.g., semipermeable, occlusive, wet-to-damp, hydrocolloid, hydrogel), drainage appliances, and skin-protective agents for open/draining wounds and stomas *to protect the wound and/or surrounding tissues from excoriating secretions/drainage and to enhance healing.*
- Assist with débridement/enzymatic therapy as indicated (e.g., burns, severe pressure ulcer).
- Cover open pressure ulcers with appropriate protective dressings (e.g., DuoDerm, Tegaderm, etc.) *to assist with wound débridement necessary for growth of healthy tissues.*
- Remove adhesive products with care, removing on horizontal plane, and using mineral oil or Vaseline for softening, if needed, *to prevent abrasions or tearing of skin/damage to underlying tissues.*
- Inspect lesions/wounds daily for changes (e.g., signs of infection/complications or healing). *Promotes timely intervention/revision of plan of care.*
- Collaborate with other healthcare providers (e.g., physician, wound specialist, and/or ostomy nurse) as indicated *to assist with developing plan of care for problematic or potentially serious wounds.*
- Refer to NDs impaired Skin Integrity, risk for Infection, risk for Injury for additional interventions.

NURSING PRIORITY NO. 4. To correct hazards/minimize impairment:[4–6,8–12]

- Modify/eliminate factors contributing to condition, if possible.
- Assist with treatment of underlying condition(s) as appropriate.

 Cultural Collaborative Community/ Home Care 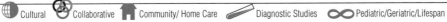 Diagnostic Studies Pediatric/Geriatric/Lifespan Medications

- Assess IV site on regular basis for erythema, edema, tenderness, burning, etc., *which indicate infiltration and/or phlebitis requiring immediate discontinuation of site use and/or interventions to heal the area.*
- Use appropriate catheter (e.g., peripheral or central venous) when infusing anticancer or other toxic drugs and ascertain that IV is infusing well *to prevent infiltration and extravasation with resulting tissue damage.*
- Inspect skin/tissues routinely around incisions *(for progress of healing)*, and cast edges and traction devices *to ensure proper application/function and note possible development of pressure points.*
- Monitor for correct placement of tubes, catheters, other devices, and assess skin tissues around these devices for effects of tape/fasteners or pressure from the devices *to prevent damage to skin and tissues as a result of pressure, friction or shear forces.*
- Observe for tissue bleeding and/or spread of hematoma formation in injured areas, *which can result in compressed blood vessels and impaired circulation, aggravating injury to tissues.*[1,2]
- Encourage early mobility *to stimulate circulation, enhance organ function, and prevent/limit potential complications of immobility.*
- Develop regularly timed repositioning schedule for client with mobility and sensation impairments, using turn sheet as needed; encourage/assist with periodic weight shifts for client in chair *to reduce stress on pressure points and encourage circulation to tissues.*
- Use/demonstrate proper turning and transfer techniques *to avoid movements that cause friction/shearing (e.g., pulling client with parallel force, dragging movements).*
- Provide foam/flotation/alternating pressure/air mattress and appropriate padding devices (e.g., foam boots, heel protectors, sheepskin) when indicated *to reduce tissue pressure and enhance circulation to compromised tissues.*
- Limit use of plastic material (e.g., rubber sheet, plastic-backed linen savers), and remove wet/wrinkled linens promptly. *Moisture potentiates skin/underlying tissues, increasing risk of breakdown/infection.*
- Restrict/avoid use of restraints; use adequate padding and evaluate circulation, movement and sensation of extremity frequently, when restraints are required. *Reduces risk of impaired circulation/tissue ischemia.*
- Elevate linens over affected extremity with bed cradle *to reduce pressure on/irritation of compromised tissues.*
- Provide adequate clothing/covers; protect from drafts *to prevent vasoconstriction that can compromise circulation.*
- Encourage optimum nutrition (including adequate protein, lipids, calories, trace minerals and multivitamins) *to promote tissue health/healing* and adequate hydration (oral, IV, ambient room humidity, etc.) *to reduce/replenish cellular water loss and enhance circulation.*
- Instruct client/caregiver in proper care of extremities during cold or hot weather. *Individuals with impaired sensation or young children/individuals unable to verbalize discomfort require special attention to deal with extremes in weather (e.g., dressing in layers, wearing gloves, boots, clean/dry socks, properly fitting shoes/boots, face mask in winter; or use of sunscreen and light clothing to protect from dermal injury in summer).*

NURSING PRIORITY NO. 5. To promote wellness (Teaching/Discharge Considerations):

- Encourage verbalizations of feelings and expectations regarding present condition.
- Assist client and family to identify/implement effective coping mechanisms.
- Discuss importance of regular monitoring and reporting of changes in condition or any

 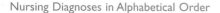

unusual physical discomforts/changes. *Promotes early detection of developing complications and timely intervention.*

• Calculate ankle-brachial index as appropriate (e.g., diabetic clients or clients with impaired circulation to lower extremities). *Result less than 0.9 is associated with peripheral arterial disease (among other conditions) and need for more aggressive interventions to prevent skin/tissue ulcerations.* [7]

• Instruct in aseptic/clean techniques for dressing changes and proper disposal of soiled dressings *to prevent spread of infectious agent.*

• Review medical regimen (e.g., proper use of topical sprays, creams, ointments, soaks, or irrigations).

• Identify required changes in lifestyle, occupation, or environment *necessitated by limitations imposed by condition or to avoid causative factors.*

• Refer to community/governmental resources as indicated (e.g., Public Health Department, OSHA, National Association for the Prevention of Blindness) *for information regarding specific conditions/report hazards.*

DOCUMENTATION FOCUS

Assessment/Reassessment
- Individual findings, including history of condition, characteristics of wound/lesion, evidence of other organ/tissue involvement.
- Impact on functioning/lifestyle.

Planning
- Plan of care and who is involved in planning.
- Teaching Plan.

Implementation/Evaluation
- Responses to interventions/teaching, actions performed.
- Attainment/progress toward desired outcome(s).
- Modifications to plan of care.

Discharge Planning
- Long-term needs/referrals and who is responsible for actions to be taken.
- Specific referrals made.

References

1. Fort, C. W. (2003). How to combat 3 deadly trauma complications. Nursing, 33(5), 58–63.
2. Paula, R. (2002). Compartment syndrome, extremity. Available at: http://www.emedicine.com. Accessed January 2004.
3. Peripheral vascular disease. (Public information sheet). Available at: http://ivillagehealth.com. Accessed January 2004.
4. Llewellyn, S. (2002). Skin integrity and wound care. (Lecture materials). Chapel Hills, NC: Cape Fear Community College Nursing Program.
5. Colburn, L. (2001). Prevention for chronic wounds. In Krasner, D., Rodeheaver, G., & Sibbald, R. G.: Chronic Wound Care: A Clinical Source Book for Healthcare Professionals, ed 2. Wayne, PA: HMP Communications.
6. No author listed. Risk factors and prevention. Geriatric Syndromes: Pressure Ulcers. Available at: http://geri-atricsyllabus.com. Accessed February 2004.
7. Murabito, J. M., et al. (2003). The ankle-brachial index can predict the risk of stroke in the elder. Archives of Internal Medicine, September. Available at: http://www.coloradohealthsite.org/CHNReports/ABIandstroke-elderly.html. Accessed February 2004.

  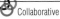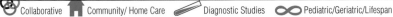

8. Calianno, C. (2002). Patient hygiene, part 2-Skin care: Keeping the outside healthy. Nursing, 32(6), June Clinical Supp.
9. Wiersema, L. A., & Stanley, M. The aging integumentary system. In Stanley, M, and Beare, PG, (1999). Gerontological Nursing: A Health Promotion/Protection Approach, ed 2. Philadelphia: F. A. Davis, pp 102–111.
10. NDs: Skin Integrity, impaired and Tissue Integrity, impaired. In Doenges, M. E., Moorhouse, M. F., & Geissler-Murr, A. C. (2002). Nursing Care Plans: Guidelines for Individualizing Patient Care, ed 6. Philadelphia: F. A. Davis.
11. McGovern, C. (2003). Skin integrity: Pressure ulcers, wounds and wound healing. Unit 3. (Lecture materials) for Villanova, PA: Villanova University College of Nursing. Available at: http://www10homepage.villanova.edu/ marycarol.mcgovern. Accessed February 2004.
12. Faller, N., & Beitz, J. (2001). When a wound isn't a wound: Tubes, drains, fistulas and draining wounds. In Krasner, D., Rodeheaver, G., & Sibbald, R. G.: Chronic Wound Care: a Clinical Source Book for Healthcare Professionals, ed 2. Wayne, PA: HMP Communications.
13. Peripheral Arterial Occlusive Disease. (Fact sheet). Available at: http://www.fpnotebook.com. Accessed January 2004.
14. Guideline for management of wounds in patients with lower-extremity arterial disease. (2002). Wound Ostomy and Continence Nurses Society (WOCN), Clinical practice guideline series; No 1. Available at: http://www.guideline.gov. Accessed September 2003.

ineffective Tissue Perfusion (specify type: renal, cerebral, cardiopulmonary, gastrointestinal, peripheral)

Definition: Decrease in oxygen resulting in the failure to nourish the tissues at the capillary level [Tissue perfusion problems can exist without decreased cardiac output; however, there may be a relationship between cardiac output and tissue perfusion.]

RELATED FACTORS

Interruption of flow—arterial, venous
Exchange problems
Hypervolemia, hypovolemia
Mechanical reduction of venous and/or arterial blood flow
Decreased Hb concentration in blood
Altered affinity of hemoglobin for O_2; enzyme poisoning
Impaired transport of the O_2 across alveolar and/or capillary membrane
Mismatch of ventilation with blood flow
Hypoventilation

DEFINING CHARACTERISTICS

Renal
Objective
Altered blood pressure outside of acceptable parameters
Oliguria or anuria; hematuria
Arterial pulsations, bruits
Elevation in BUN/Cr ratio

Cerebral

Objective
Altered mental status; speech abnormalities
Behavioral changes; [restlessness]; changes in motor response; extremity weakness or paralysis

Changes in pupillary reactions
Difficulty in swallowing

Cardiopulmonary
Subjective
Chest pain
Dyspnea
Sense of "impending doom"

Objective
Dysrhythmias
Capillary refill >3 seconds
Altered respiratory rate outside of acceptable parameters
Use of accessory muscles; chest retraction; nasal flaring
Bronchospasm
Abnormal ABGs
[Hemoptysis]

Gastrointestinal
Subjective
Nausea
Abdominal pain or tenderness

Objective
Hypoactive or absent bowel sounds
Abdominal distention
[Melena]

Peripheral
Subjective
Claudication

Objective
Altered skin characteristics (hair, nails, moisture)
Skin temperature changes
Skin discolorations; color diminished; color pale on elevation, color does not return on lowering the leg
Altered sensations
BP changes in extremities; weak or absent pulses; diminished arterial pulsations; bruits
Edema
Delayed healing
Positive Homans' sign

SAMPLE CLINICAL APPLICATIONS: atherosclerosis, coronary artery disease, CHF, myocardial infarction, pulmonary embolus, anemia, Raynaud's disease, peripheral vascular disease, brain injury/CVA, trauma/compartment syndrome, thrombophlebitis, diabetes mellitus, necrotizing enterocolitis

DESIRED OUTCOMES/EVALUATION CRITERIA
Sample **NOC** linkages:
Urinary Elimination: Ability of the urinary system to filter wastes, conserve solutes, and collect and discharge urine in a healthy pattern

 Cultural Collaborative Community/ Home Care Diagnostic Studies 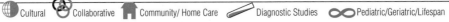 Pediatric/Geriatric/Lifespan Medications

Tissue Perfusion: Cerebral: Extent to which blood flows through the cerebral vasculature and maintains brain function

Tissue Perfusion: Cardiac: Extent to which blood flows through the coronary vasculature and maintains heart function

Tissue Perfusion: Pulmonary: Extent to which blood flows through intact pulmonary vasculature with appropriate pressure and volume, perfusing alveoli/capillaries

Tissue Perfusion: Abdominal Organs: Extent to which blood flows through the small vessels of the abdominal viscera and maintains organ function

Tissue Perfusion: Peripheral: Extent to which blood flows through the small vessels of the extremities and maintains tissue function

---

Client Will (Include Specific Time Frame)

- Verbalize understanding of condition, therapy regimen, side effects of medications, and when to contact healthcare provider.
- Demonstrate behaviors/lifestyle changes to improve circulation (e.g., cessation of smoking, relaxation techniques, exercise/dietary program).
- Demonstrate increased perfusion as individually appropriate (e.g., skin warm/dry, peripheral pulses present/strong, vital signs within client's normal range, alert/oriented, balanced intake/output, absence of edema, free of pain/discomfort).

ACTIONS/INTERVENTIONS

Sample **NIC** linkages:

Fluid/Electrolyte Management: Promotion of fluid/electrolyte balance and prevention of complications resulting from abnormal or undesired fluid/serum electrolyte levels

Cerebral Perfusion Promotion: Promotion of adequate perfusion and limitation of complications for a patient experiencing or at risk for inadequate cerebral perfusion

Cardiac Care: Limitation of complications resulting from an imbalance between myocardial oxygen supply and demand for a patient with symptoms of impaired cardiac function

Gastrointestinal Intubation: Insertion of a tube into the gastrointestinal tract

Circulatory Care: Arterial/Venous Insufficiency: Promotion of arterial/venous circulation

NURSING PRIORITY NO. 1. To assess causative/contributing factors:

- Determine factors related to individual situation. *For example, previous history of/at risk for formation of thrombus or emboli, fractures, diagnosis of Raynaud's or Buerger's disease, or situations that can affect all body systems (e.g., Addison's disease, congestive heart failure, pheochromocytoma/other endocrine imbalances, sepsis) can decrease circulation but require different interventions to enhance perfusion.*
- Evaluate for signs of infection especially when immune system is compromised, *as sepsis/septic shock can occur, resulting in decreased cardiac output/systemic perfusion with multiple organ involvement and critical consequences.*
- Observe for sudden onset of chest pain, cyanosis, respiratory distress, hemoptysis, diaphoresis, hypoxia, anxiety, restlessness. *Signs of pulmonary emboli requiring prompt evaluation/intervention.*

NURSING PRIORITY NO. 2. To note degree of impairment/organ involvement:

- Determine duration of problem, frequency of recurrence, precipitating or aggravating factors.

- Identify changes (e.g., altered mentation, vital signs, postural blood pressure changes; pain, changes in skin/tissue/organ function, signs of metabolic imbalances) *reflecting systemic and/or peripheral alterations in circulation.*
- Note customary baseline data (e.g., usual BP, weight, mentation, cardiac and respiratory status; oxygen saturation/ABGs, and other appropriate laboratory study values). *Provides comparison with current findings (e.g., while confusion may reflect decreased cerebral perfusion, it may be usual in the client with Alzheimer's disease).*
- Ascertain impact on functioning/lifestyle. *For example, claudication may prevent client from shopping for groceries, impaired peripheral sensation or decreased mentation may place client at risk for injury, or reduced cardiac circulation may lead to angina with exertion.*

Renal[1]

- Ascertain usual voiding pattern and compare with current situation *to note changes (e.g., low output such as may occur with renal failure associated with hypovolemia or disease/injury to kidneys; hematuria, or use/need for diuretics, etc.).*
- Note characteristics of urine (e.g., concentrated, dilute) and measure specific gravity *to evaluate kidney's ability to concentrate the urine.*
- Measure urine output on a regular schedule. *Intake may be calculated against output to monitor renal function and to determine replacement needs.*
- Weigh daily or on regular basis *to ascertain if fluid is being retained.*
- Observe for dependent/generalized edema. *Edema (on scale of +1 to +4) occurs primarily in dependent tissues (hands, feet, lumbosacral area) and becomes generalized over body as kidneys fail.*
- Note level of consciousness, mentation, and behavior. *Adverse changes may be the consequence of fluid shifts, accumulation of toxins, acidosis, electrolyte imbalances, and/or increased BUN/Cr.*
- Auscultate BP, ascertain client's usual range. *Hypertension is often associated with chronic renal failure; hypotension (and hypovolemia) can result in decreased glomerular filtration rate (GFR) that initially may increase rennin and raise BP, before shock state causes BP to fall.*

- Review laboratory studies (e.g., BUN/Cr levels, protein, specific gravity, electrolytes) *to assess status of renal function; evaluate progression of renal dysfunction/failure and effects on body/organ function.*

Cerebral[1]

- Determine presence of changes in vision or sensory/motor responses, hemiparesis, headache, dizziness, altered mental status, problems with speech and swallowing; behavioral changes *indicative of ineffective cerebral perfusion (e.g., brain trauma, TIA or CVA from hemorrhage or clot).*
- Note history of brief/intermittent periods of confusion/blackout. *Suggests conditions such as orthostatic hypotension, syncope, TIA.*
- Evaluate blood pressure. *Blood pressure is an inadequate parameter because it is a function of cardiac output and systemic vascular resistance, rather than perfusion.[2] However, blood pressure can be indicative of certain perfusion impairments. For example, chronic or severe acute hypertension can precipitate cerebrovascular spasm and stroke. Fluctuations in blood pressure can accompany traumatic brain injury and stroke. Low blood pressure/severe hypotension causes inadequate perfusion of brain, with adverse changes in consciousness/mentation.*
- Monitor fluid and electrolyte status. *Imbalances in fluid and electrolytes have a direct bearing on brain perfusion and cortical function.*

 Cultural Collaborative Community/ Home Care 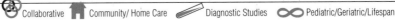 Diagnostic Studies Pediatric/Geriatric/Lifespan Medications

- Review medication regimen. *Failure to take prescribed antihypertensives, adverse side effects/interactions, drug overdose, inappropriate medications can affect brain functioning.*

Cardiopulmonary[1]

- Investigate reports of chest pain/angina; note precipitating factors, changes in vital signs and characteristics of pain episodes *to evaluate for potential myocardial ischemia or inadequate systemic oxygenation/perfusion of organs.*
- Determine cardiac rhythm, presence of dysrhythmias. *Can be caused by inadequate myocardial perfusion, electrolyte imbalances or be associated with brain injury (e.g., bradycardia can accompany traumatic injury; or stroke can be precipitated by dysrhythmias).*
- Investigate reports of difficulty breathing; note respiratory rate outside of acceptable parameters, use of accessory muscles to breath. *Indicative of oxygen exchange problems or ventilation/perfusion mismatch.*[3]
- Inspect for pallor, mottling, cool/clammy skin and diminished pulses. *Systemic vasoconstriction resulting from reduced cardiac output may be evidenced by poor skin/tissue perfusion and diminished pulses.*
- Note presence/degree of dyspnea, cyanosis, hemoptysis, sense of impending doom *that may indicate pulmonary embolus.*
- Review diagnostic studies (e.g., ECG, echocardiogram, angiography, Doppler ultrasound, chest radiography; pulse oximetry/oxygen saturation/capnometry/ABGs, electrolytes, BUN/Cr, cardiac enzymes) *to identify conditions requiring treatment, and/or to evaluate response to therapies.*[1–3]

Gastrointestinal[1]

- Note reports of nausea/vomiting, verify location/type/intensity of pain. *May reflect hypoperfusion of the gastrointestinal tract which is particularly vulnerable to even small decreases in circulating volume.*[2]
- Auscultate bowel sounds. *May be hypoactive or absent as result of surgery, or ileus/other obstruction, or hyperactive as might occur with GI bleeding.*
- Measure abdominal girth and compare with client's customary waist size/belt length *to monitor development/progression of distention possibly reflecting intra-abdominal bleeding, infection, or edema associated with toxins.*
- Note changes in stool characteristics/presence of blood. *May indicate breakdown of mucosa due to ischemia/necrotizing enterocolitis.*
- Observe for symptoms of peritonitis, ischemic colitis, abdominal angina.

Peripheral

- Identify high-risk behaviors/conditions (e.g., smoking, hyperlipidemia, diabetes, hyperviscous blood, sepsis, hypotension, low cardiac output/MI, atrial fibrillation; aneurysms, aortic dissection, and underlying atherosclerotic narrowing of arteries; prolonged periods of immobility). *Places client at greater risk for developing peripheral vascular disease (PVD) and/or complications of PVD.*[4]
- Ascertain history/characteristics of extremity problems such as pain (with/without activity); temperature/color changes, paresthesia. Determine time (day/night) that symptoms are worse and precipitating/aggravating events (e.g., walking) and relieving factors (e.g., rest, sitting down) *to help isolate and differentiate problems (e.g., intermittent claudication vs. loss of function and pain due to ischemia related to loss of perfusion).*[4]
- Palpate for presence and quality of pulses. Note pulselessness, paralysis, paresthesia, pain, and pallor *suggestive of peripheral vascular disease.*[4]

- Measure capillary refill *to determine adequacy of distal circulation.*
- Inspect lower extremities for skin texture (e.g., atrophic, shiny appearance, lack of hair, dry/scaly, reddened skin), and skin breaks/ulcerations *that often accompany diminished peripheral circulation.*[4]
- Check for calf tenderness or pain on dorsiflexion of foot (Homans' sign), swelling and redness. *Indicators of deep vein thrombosis (DVT), although DVT can be present without a positive Homans' sign.*[1]
- Measure circumference of extremities as indicated. *Useful in identifying edema in involved extremity.*[1]
- Auscultate for systolic/continuous bruits below obstruction in extremities.
- Review laboratory studies (e.g., clotting times, Hb/Hct, renal/cardiac function tests) and diagnostic studies (e.g., Doppler ultrasound, MRI/other scan, angiography, ankle-brachial index [ABI]) *to evaluate effectiveness of perfusion and determine degree of impairment.*[4,5]

NURSING PRIORITY NO. 3. To maximize tissue perfusion:

Renal[1]

- Administer medication (e.g., antihypertensive agents, diuretics, anticoagulants in presence of thrombosis, steroids in membranous nephropathy) as indicated *to treat underlying condition.*
- Provide for fluid and diet restrictions, as indicated, while providing adequate calories and hydration *to meet the body's needs without overtaxing kidney function.*
- Provide psychological support for client/SO(s), especially when progression of disease and resultant treatment (dialysis) may be long term. *Enhances coping skills and promotes adjustment to changes in lifestyle.*
- Refer to NDs decreased Cardiac Output, deficient/excess Fluid Volume, impaired Urinary Elimination for additional interventions.

Cerebral[1]

- Elevate HOB (e.g., 10 degrees) and maintain head/neck in midline or neutral position *to promote circulation/venous drainage.*
- Administer medications as indicated to treat underlying condition. *For example, steroids/diuretics may be used to decrease edema, anticoagulants may be required for cerebral embolus.*
- Assist with/monitor hypothermia therapy *that may be used to decrease metabolic and oxygen needs associated with hypermetabolic state/hyperthermia.*
- Prepare client for surgery as indicated (e.g., carotid endarterectomy, evacuation of hematoma/space-occupying lesion).
- Refer to NDs decreased Cardiac Output, decreased Intracranial Adaptive Capacity for additional interventions.

Cardiopulmonary[1]

- Monitor vital signs, hemodynamic pressures, heart sounds, and cardiac rhythm.
- Encourage quiet, restful atmosphere. *Conserves energy/lowers tissue O_2 demands.*
- Caution client to avoid strenuous activities *that increase cardiopulmonary workload (e.g., straining at stool, heavy lifting).*
- Provide perfusion support as indicated (e.g., oxygen by appropriate delivery method; IV fluids, blood) *to increase circulating volume and oxygenation.*

 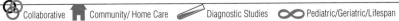

- Administer medications (e.g., antidysrhythmics, vasopressors, cardiotonics, fibrinolytic agents, anticoagulants, respiratory drugs) *to treat underlying condition.*

- Prepare for/assist with emergency procedures (e.g., arteriography, placement of cardiac stents, CABG surgery, thrombectomy, placement of vena cava filter) as indicated *to treat underlying/life-threatening conditions.*[3]
- Refer to NDs: decreased Cardiac Output, ineffective Breathing Pattern, impaired Gas Exchange for additional interventions.

Gastrointestinal[1]

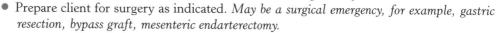

- Withhold oral food/fluids *when nausea or vomiting or intestinal pain is present.*
- Maintain gastric/intestinal decompression; when indicated, measure output periodically, and note characteristics of drainage.
- Provide small/easily digested food and fluids when oral intake tolerated.
- Encourage rest after meals *to maximize blood flow to digestive system.*
- Prepare client for surgery as indicated. *May be a surgical emergency, for example, gastric resection, bypass graft, mesenteric endarterectomy.*
- Refer to NDs Nausea, imbalanced Nutrition: Less than body requirements for additional interventions.

Peripheral[1]

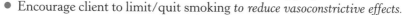

- Perform assistive/active range of motion exercises (e. g., Buerger and Buerger-Allen).
- Encourage early ambulation when possible. *Enhances venous return.*
- Discourage sitting/standing for long periods, wearing constrictive clothing, crossing legs *that can restrict circulation and lead to edema.*
- Elevate the legs when sitting, but avoid sharp angulation of the hips or knees *to enhance venous return/minimize edema formation.*
- Avoid use of knee gatch on bed; elevate entire foot as indicated *to reduce risk of thrombosis.*
- Provide air mattress, sheepskin padding, bed/foot cradle *to reduce excessive tissue pressure that could lead to skin breakdown.*
- Elevate HOB at night *to increase gravitational blood flow.*
- Apply/instruct client/SO in application/periodic removal of antithromboembolic devices/hose to lower extremities *to limit venous stasis, improve venous return and reduce risk of DVT in client who is limited in activity.*
- Avoid massaging the leg *in presence of thrombosis to reduce risk for embolus.*
- Exercise caution in use of hot water bottles or heating pads. *Tissues may have decreased sensitivity due to ischemia, increasing risk of dermal injury. Heat also increases the metabolic demands of already compromised tissues.*
- Apply ice cautiously and elevate injured limb as appropriate *to reduce edema.*
- Encourage client to limit/quit smoking *to reduce vasoconstrictive effects.*

- Assist with/prepare for medical procedures (e.g., sympathectomy, vein graft) *to improve peripheral circulation.*
- Monitor closely for signs of shock following sympathectomy *(result of unmediated vasodilation).*
- Administer medications with caution (e.g., vasodilators, papaverine, antilipemics, anticoagulants). *Drug response, half-life, toxic levels may be altered by decreased tissue perfusion.*
- Monitor for signs of bleeding during use of fibrinolytic agents *to provide timely intervention and reversal of bleeding diathesis.*
- Refer to ND risk for Peripheral Neurovascular Dysfunction for additional interventions.

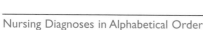

NURSING PRIORITY NO. 4. To promote wellness (Teaching/Discharge Considerations):

 • Discuss the risk factors and potential outcomes of atherosclerosis. *Information necessary for client to make informed choices and commit to lifestyle changes as appropriate.*

 • Encourage discussion of feelings regarding prognosis/long-term effects of condition. *Major/unplanned life changes can strain coping abilities, impairing functioning and jeopardizing relationships, and may even result in depression.*

 • Identify necessary changes in lifestyle and assist client to incorporate disease management into ADLs. *Promotes independence, enhances self-concept regarding ability to deal with change and manage own needs.*

 • Encourage client to quit smoking, join Smoke-out, other stop-smoking programs. *Smoking causes vasoconstriction compromising perfusion.*

 • Demonstrate/encourage use of relaxation techniques, exercises/techniques *to decrease tension level.* Establish regular exercise program *to enhance circulation and promote general well-being.*

• Review specific dietary changes/restrictions with client (e.g., reduction of cholesterol and triglycerides, high or low in protein, avoidance of rye in Buerger's disease).

 • Discuss care of dependent limbs, body hygiene, foot care as appropriate. *When circulation is impaired, changes in sensation place client at risk for development of lesions/ulcerations that are often slow to heal.*

• Recommend avoidance of vasoconstricting herbals/drugs.

 • Discourage massaging of calf in presence of varicose veins/thrombophlebitis *to prevent embolization.*

• Emphasize importance of avoiding use of aspirin, some OTC drugs, vitamins containing potassium, mineral oil, or alcohol *when taking anticoagulants.*

 • Review medical regimen and appropriate safety measures. *For example, use of electric razor for shaving, wearing gloves for gardening, or avoiding forceful blowing of nose when taking anticoagulants to decrease risk of trauma resulting in prolonged bleeding.*

 • Discuss preventing exposure to cold, dressing warmly and use of natural fibers *to retain heat more efficiently and reduce risk of hypothermia/dermal injury.*

• Provide preoperative teaching appropriate for the situation.

• Refer to specific support groups, counseling as appropriate *to assist with problem solving, provide role model, enhance coping ability.*

DOCUMENTATION FOCUS

Assessment/Reassessment
• Individual findings, noting nature/extent and duration of problem, effect on independence/lifestyle.
• Characteristics of pain, precipitators, and what relieves pain.
• Vital signs, cardiac rhythm/dysrhythmias.
• Pulses/BP, including above/below suspected lesion as appropriate.
• I/O and weight as indicated.

Planning
• Plan of care and who is involved in planning.
• Teaching plan.

 Cultural   Collaborative   Community/ Home Care  Diagnostic Studies 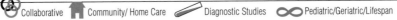 Pediatric/Geriatric/Lifespan   Medications

Implementation/Evaluation
- Response to interventions/teaching, actions performed.
- Attainment/progress toward desired outcome(s).
- Modifications to plan of care.

Discharge Planning
- Long-term needs and who is responsible for actions to be taken.
- Available resources, specific referrals made.

References

1. ND: Tissue Perfusion, ineffective (specify). In Doenges, M. E., Moorhouse, M. F., & Geissler-Murr, A. C. (2002). Nursing Care Plans: Guidelines for Individualizing Patient Care, ed 6. Philadelphia: F. A. Davis.
2. Schulman, C. (2002). End points of resuscitation: Choosing the right parameters to monitor. Dimens Crit Care Nurs, 21(1), 2–10.
3. No author listed (2000). Guidelines on diagnosis and management of acute pulmonary embolism. Task Force on Pulmonary Embolism, European Society of Cardiology. Available at: http://www.guideline.gov. Accessed February 2004.
4. Stephens, E. (2003). Peripheral vascular disease. Available at: http://www.emedicine.com. Accessed February 2004.
5. No author listed. (1999). Antithrombotic therapy: A national clinical guideline. Scottish Intercollegiate Guidelines Network (SIGN). Available at: http://www.guideline.gov. Accessed February 2004.

impaired Transfer Ability

Definition: Limitation of independent movement between two nearby surfaces

RELATED FACTORS
To be developed by nurse researchers and submitted to NANDA
[Conditions that result in poor muscle tone]
[Cognitive impairment]
[Fractures, trauma, spinal cord injury]

DEFINING CHARACTERISTICS

Subjective or Objective
Impaired ability to transfer: from bed to chair and chair to bed, chair to car or car to chair, chair to floor or floor to chair, standing to floor or floor to standing; on or off a toilet or commode; in and out of tub or shower, between uneven levels

Specify level of independence—[refer to ND impaired physical Mobility for suggested functional level classification]

SAMPLE CLINICAL APPLICATIONS: arthritis, fractures, amputation, neuromuscular diseases (e.g., MS, ALS, Guillian-Barré syndrome), paralysis, glaucoma, macular degeneration, dementias

DESIRED OUTCOMES/EVALUATION CRITERIA
Sample **NOC** linkages:
Transfer Performance: Ability to change body locations
Balance: Ability to maintain body equilibrium
Body Positioning: Self-Initiated: Ability to change own body position

Client/Caregiver Will (Include Specific Time Frame)
- Verbalize understanding of situation and appropriate safety measures.
- Master techniques of transfer successfully.
- Make desired transfer safely.

ACTIONS/INTERVENTIONS

Sample **NIC** linkages:

Transport: Moving a patient from one location to another

Body Mechanics Promotion: Facilitating the use of posture and movement in daily activities to prevent fatigue and musculoskeletal strain or injury

Exercise Promotion: Strength Training: Facilitation of regular physical exercise to maintain or advance to a higher level of fitness and health

[Refer also to NDs impaired bed/physical/wheelchair Mobility, unilateral Neglect, or impaired Walking for additional interventions.]

NURSING PRIORITY NO. 1. To assess causative/contributing factors:

- Determine diagnoses for conditions that contribute to transfer problems. *Neuromuscular and musculoskeletal problems such as MS, fractures, back injuries, quadriplegia/paraplegia, agedness (arthritis, decreased muscle mass/tone/strength), and effects of dementias, brain injury, etc., can seriously impact balance, physical, and psychological well-being.*[1,5]
- Note factors complicating current situation. *Recent surgery, fractures, amputation, contractures, traction apparatus, mechanical ventilation, multiple IV/indwelling tubings can restrict movement.*
 Review medication regimen/schedule *to determine possible side effects or drug interactions impairing balance and/or muscle tone.*

NURSING PRIORITY NO. 2. To assess functional ability:

- Perform "Get-up and Go" test, as indicated, *to assess client's ability to transfer and ambulate safely. In this test, the client is asked to get up from a seated position in a chair, stand still momentarily, walk forward 10 feet, turn around, walk back to the chair, turn, and sit down. Factors assessed include sitting balance, ability to transfer from sitting to standing and back to sitting, the pace and stability of ambulation, and the ability to turn without staggering. If the client is not safe with ambulation, assistance may also be required with transfers.*[2]
- Determine degree of impairment in relation to 0–4 scale, noting muscle strength and tone, joint mobility, cardiovascular status, balance and endurance. *Identifies strengths and deficits (e.g., ability to ambulate with assistive devices, or problems with balance, failure to attend to one side, inability to transfer safely from bed to wheelchair) and may provide information regarding potential for recovery.*[5]
- Evaluate perceptual/cognitive impairments and ability to follow directions. *Problems in this area that may require interventions related to age, chronic or acute nature of condition (e.g., client with severe brain injury may have permanent limitations because of impaired cognition affecting memory, judgment, problem solving and motor coordination, requiring more intensive inpatient and long-term care).*
- Observe movement when client is unaware of observation *to note any incongruence with reported abilities.*
- Note emotional/behavioral responses of client/SO to problems of immobility. *Restrictions and/or limitations imposed by immobility can cause physical, social, emotional, and financial difficulties for everyone.*

 Cultural   Collaborative Community/ Home Care   Diagnostic Studies   Pediatric/Geriatric/Lifespan   Medications

NURSING PRIORITY NO. 3. To promote optimal level of movement:

- Assist with treatment of underlying condition causing dysfunction. *Treatment of condition (e.g., surgery for hip replacement, therapy for unilateral neglect following stroke) can alleviate or improve difficulties with transfer activity.*

- Consult with PT/OT/rehabilitation team *to develop general and specific muscle strengthening and range-of-motion (ROM) exercises, transfer training and techniques, as well as recommendations/provision of assistive devices.*[2]
- Provide/instruct in use of siderails, overhead trapeze, safety grab bars, hydraulic lift, transfer board, devices on the bed/chair (e.g., call light, bed-positioning switch in easy reach), and extra personnel as necessary *to protect client and/or care providers from injury during transfers/movements.*
- Provide instruction/reinforcing verbal cues for client and caregivers regarding body and equipment positioning *to improve/maintain balance during transfers.*
- Monitor body alignment and balance and encourage wide base of support *when standing to transfer.*
- Use full-length mirror as needed *to facilitate client's view of own postural alignment.*

NURSING PRIORITY NO. 4. To promote wellness (Teaching/Discharge Considerations):

- Demonstrate/reinforce safety measures as individually indicated. *Proper use of transfer board, locking wheels on bed/chair; correct placement of equipment for optimal body mechanics of client and/or careprovider(s); use of gait belt, supportive/nonslip footwear, good lighting, clearing floor of clutter, and so forth is important to facilitating transfers, and reducing the possibility of fall and subsequent injury to client and caregiver.*[3]
- Discuss need for and sources of care/supervision. *Homecare agency, before and after school programs, elderly day care, personal companions, etc., may be required to assist with/monitor activity.*[4]
- Refer to appropriate community resources *for evaluation and modification of environment (e.g., roll-in-shower/tub, correction of uneven floor surfaces/steps, installation of ramps, use of standing tables/lifts, etc.).*

DOCUMENTATION FOCUS

Assessment/Reassessment
- Individual findings, including level of function/ability to participate in desired transfers.

Planning
- Plan of care and who is involved in the planning.
- Teaching Plan.

Implementation/Evaluation
- Responses to interventions/teaching and actions performed.
- Attainment/progress toward desired outcome(s).
- Modifications to plan of care.

Discharge Planning
- Discharge/long-range needs, noting who is responsible for each action to be taken.
- Specific referrals made.
- Sources of/maintenance for assistive devices.

References

1. Mass, M. L. (1989). Impaired physical mobility. (Unpublished manuscript). Cited in research article for National Institutes for Health.
2. Cruise, C. M., & Koval, K. J. (1998). Rehabilitation of the elderly. Arch Am Acad Orthop Surg, 2(1), 103–107.
3. No author listed. (2000). Patient safety during transfers. Policy/Operations Manual. UTMB Department of Rehabilitation Services.
4. Hogue, C. C. (1984). Falls and mobility late in life. An ecological model. J Am Geriatr Soc, 32, 858–861.
5. Tinetti, M. E. Williams, T. F., and Mayewski, R. (1986). Fall risk index for elderly patients based on number of chronic disabilities. Am J Med, 80, 429–434.

risk for Trauma

Definition: Accentuated risk of accidental tissue injury (e.g., wound, burn, fracture)

RISK FACTORS

Internal (individual)
Weakness; balancing difficulties; reduced large or small muscle coordination, hand/eye coordination

Poor vision

Reduced temperature and/or tactile sensation

Lack of safety education/precautions

Insufficient finances to purchase safety equipment or to effect repairs

Cognitive or emotional difficulties

History of previous trauma

External (environmental) [includes but is not limited to]:
Slippery floors (e.g., wet or highly waxed; unanchored rug; litter or liquid spills on floors or stairways; snow or ice collected on stairs, walkways)

Bathtub without handgrip or antislip equipment

Use of unsteady ladder or chairs

Obstructed passageways; entering unlighted rooms

Unsturdy or absent stair rails; children playing without gates at top of stairs

Unanchored electric wires

High beds; inappropriate call-for-aid mechanisms for bed-resting client

Unsafe window protection in homes with young children

Pot handles facing toward front of stove; bathing in very hot water (e.g., unsupervised bathing of young children)

Potential igniting gas leaks; delayed lighting of gas burner or oven

Unscreened fires or heaters; wearing plastic apron or flowing clothing around open flames; highly flammable children's toys or clothing

Smoking in bed or near oxygen; grease waste collected on stoves

Children playing with matches, candles, cigarettes

Playing with fireworks or gunpowder; guns or ammunition stored unlocked

Experimenting with chemical or gasoline; inadequately stored combustibles or corrosives (e.g., matches, oily rags, lye; contact with acids or alkalis)

Overloaded fuse boxes; faulty electrical plugs, frayed wires, or defective appliances; overloaded electrical outlets

Exposure to dangerous machinery; contact with rapidly moving machinery, industrial belts, or pulleys

 Cultural Collaborative Community/ Home Care Diagnostic Studies 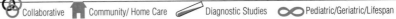 Pediatric/Geriatric/Lifespan Medications

Sliding on coarse bed linen or struggling within bed [/chair] restraints

Contact with intense cold; overexposure to sun, sunlamps, radiotherapy

Use of thin or worn-out pot holders [or mitts]

Use of cracked dishware or glasses

Knives stored uncovered; children playing with sharp-edged toys

Large icicles hanging from roof

High-crime neighborhood and vulnerable clients

Driving a mechanically unsafe vehicle; driving at excessive speeds; driving without necessary visual aids

Driving after partaking of alcoholic beverages or [other] drugs

Children riding in the front seat of car, nonuse or misuse of seat restraints/ [unrestrained infant/child riding in car]

Misuse [or nonuse] of necessary headgear for motorized cyclists or young children carried on adult bicycles

Unsafe road or road-crossing conditions; playing or working near vehicle pathways (e.g., driveways, lanes, railroad tracks)

NOTE: A risk diagnosis is not evidenced by signs and symptoms, as the problem has not occurred and nursing interventions are directed at prevention.

SAMPLE CLINICAL APPLICATIONS: substance intoxication/abuse, peripheral neuropathy, cataracts/glaucoma/macular degeneration, Parkinson's disease, seizure disorder, dementia, major depression, developmental delay

DESIRED OUTCOMES/EVALUATION CRITERIA

Sample **NOC** linkages:

Safety Status: Physical Injury: Severity of injuries from accidents and trauma

Abuse Protection: Protection of self or dependent others from abuse

Knowledge: Personal Safety: Extent of understanding conveyed about preventing unintentional injuries

Client/Caregiver Will (Include Specific Time Frame)

- Identify and correct potential risk factors in the environment.
- Demonstrate appropriate lifestyle changes to reduce risk of injury.
- Identify resources to assist in promoting a safe environment.
- Recognize need for/seek assistance to prevent accidents/injuries.

ACTIONS/INTERVENTIONS

In reviewing this ND, it is apparent there is much overlap with other diagnoses. We have chosen to present generalized interventions. Although there are commonalities to trauma situations, we suggest that the reader refer to other primary diagnoses as indicated, such as Activity Intolerance, risk for imbalanced Body Temperature, acute/chronic Confusion, risk for Falls, ineffective Health Maintenance, impaired Home Maintenance, Hypothermia; Hyperthermia; impaired Mobility (specify type), risk for Injury/Poisoning/Suffocation, impaired Skin Integrity, disturbed Sensory Perception, disturbed Thought Processes.

Sample **NIC** linkages:

Environmental Management: Safety: Manipulation of the patient's surroundings for therapeutic benefit

Environmental Management: Worker Safety: Monitoring and manipulation of the work-site environment to promote safety and health of workers

Teaching: Infant/Toddler Safety: Instruction on safety during first/second and third years of life

Surveillance: Safety: Purposeful and ongoing collection and analysis of information about the patient and the environment for use in promoting and maintaining patient safety

NURSING PRIORITY NO. 1. To assess causative/contributing factors:

- Determine factors related to individual situation and extent of risk for trauma. *Safety is dynamic and is a constant in every life and situation. Clients interfacing with the healthcare system are at higher risk for trauma for any number of reasons (e.g., age/developmental stage, illness, cognitive function, family structure, information and training, etc.), and require protection in numerous ways.*[1]
- Note age of individual, mentation, agility, impairment of mobility *to determine individual's ability to recognize danger and/or to protect self.*
- Evaluate environment (home/work/transportation) *for obvious safety hazards, as well as situations that can exacerbate injury or adversely affect the client's health. Unsafe factors include a vast array of things (e.g., unsafe heating appliances, smoking materials, toxic substances and chemicals, open flames, knives, improperly stored guns, overloaded electrical outlets, tools and machinery, dangerous neighborhoods, unsupervised children).*[1]
- Assess client/caregiver interest in and understanding of safety concerns, and ways of looking at and improving the client's environment. *Lack of appreciation of significance of individual hazards increases risk of traumatic injury.*[1]
- Note history of accidents during given period, noting circumstances of the accident (e.g., time of day that falls occur, activities going on, who was present). *Investigation of such events can provide clues for client's risk for subsequent events, which have the potential for being prevented by a change in the people or environment involved (e.g., client may need assistance when getting up at night, or child/frail elder may require placement if being injured in family setting).*
- Assess influence of stressors (e.g., physical, mental, work-related, financial, etc.) *that can impair judgment/greatly increase client's potential for injury.*
- Review potential environmental/occupational risk factors (e.g., noise level/use of headphones, working with chemicals/various inhalants and length of exposure time, etc.).
- Review laboratory studies and observe for electrolyte imbalances *that may result in/exacerbate conditions, such as confusion, tetany, pathologic fractures, etc.*

NURSING PRIORITY NO. 2. To promote safety measures required by individual situation:

- Provide safe environment for client while in acute care[2–11]:
  Provide adequate supervision and frequent observation.
  Orient client to environment.
  Place confused client, children, person with dementia near nurses' station
  Demonstrate use and place call bell/light within client's reach.
  Provide for appropriate communication tools (e.g., call bell, writing implements and paper; alphabet picture board, etc.).
  Encourage client's use of corrective vision and hearing aids.
  Keep bed in low position or place mattress on floor as appropriate.
  Maintain correct body alignment and mechanics.
  Provide positioning as required by situation (e.g., immobilization of fractures).
  Implement appropriate measures to maintain skin and tissue health.
  Make certain that client with sensory impairments is protected from injury due to heat and cold.

 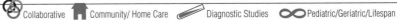

Use side rails with caution, pad rails as indicated.

Provide seizure precautions when indicated.

Lock wheels on bed/movable furniture.

Assist with activities and transfers as needed.

Provide well-fitting, nonskid footwear.

Demonstrate/monitor use of assistive devices, such as cane, walker, crutches, wheelchair, safety bars.

Clear travel paths, remove scatter rugs, pick up small items from floor; keep furniture in one place and door in one position (completely open or closed).

Provide adequate area lighting.

Apply/monitor use of restraints when required (e.g., vest, limb, belt, mitten).

Administer treatments, medications and therapies in a therapeutic manner.

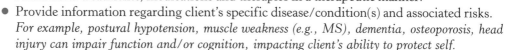

- Provide information regarding client's specific disease/condition(s) and associated risks. *For example, postural hypotension, muscle weakness (e.g., MS), dementia, osteoporosis, head injury can impair function and/or cognition, impacting client's ability to protect self.*

- Identify interventions/safety devices to promote safe physical environment and individual safety. *This can include a wide variety of interventions, including (but not limited to) stand assist/repositioning/lifting devices, back safety classes and injury-prevention devices/exercises; seat raisers for chairs; ergonomic beds, chairs, workstations; locked institutional wards or home areas when client can wander away; adequate lighting; electrical and fire safety devices, extinguishers, and alarms; proper storage/disposal of volatile liquids; appropriate use of car restraints, bicycle/skating/skiing helmets; installation of proper ventilation for use when mixing/using toxic substances; use of safety glasses/goggles; electrical outlet covers/lockouts; first aid/CPR classes, door and window locks, obtaining visual aids, communication devices (telephone, computer, hearing aid, medical alert devices, etc.); mobility devices (e.g., canes, wheelchair, crutches, walkers); installed handrails, ramps, bathroom safety tapes; oxygen safety rules; swimming pool fencing and supervision; childproof cabinets and medication/toxic substance containers; use of trigger locks/gun safes.*

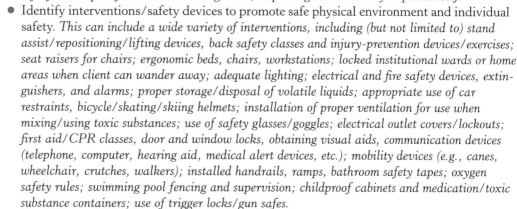

NURSING PRIORITY NO. 3. To treat underlying medical/psychiatric condition:

- Review client's usual level of physical activity. Encourage use of warm-up/stretching exercises before engaging in strenuous exercise/athletic activities *to prevent muscle injuries.*

- Assist with treatments for endocrine/electrolyte imbalance conditions. *May improve cognition/muscle tone and general well-being.*

- Provide quiet environment and reduced stimulation as indicated. *Helps limit confusion or overstimulation for clients at risk for such conditions as seizures, tetany, autonomic hyperreflexia.*

- Refer to physical or occupational therapist as appropriate *to identify high-risk tasks, conduct site visits, select/create/modify equipment and provide education about body mechanics and musculoskeletal injuries, as wells as provide needed therapies.*[3]

- Initiate appropriate teaching and wellness counseling/referrals *if reckless behavior is occurring/likely to occur (e.g., smoking in bed, driving without safety belts, high-risk sex practices, working with chemicals without safety goggles, etc.).*

- Discuss importance of self-monitoring of conditions/emotions that can contribute to occurrence of injury to self/others (e.g., fatigue, anger, irritability). *Client/SO may be able to modify risk through monitoring of actions, or postponement of certain actions, especially during times when client is likely to be highly stressed.*

- Demonstrate/encourage use of techniques to reduce/manage stress and vent emotions such as anger, hostility.

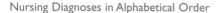

• Encourage participation in self-help programs *to address individual risks (e.g., assertiveness training, positive self-image to enhance self-esteem; smoking cessation; weight management)*.

• Refer to counseling/psychotherapy, as need indicates, *especially when individual is "accident-prone" or self-destructive behavior is noted*. Refer to NDs [actual/] risk for self-directed Violence.

NURSING PRIORITY NO. 4. To promote wellness (Teaching/Discharge Considerations):

• Review expectations caregivers have of children, cognitively impaired, and/or elderly family members *to identify needed information, required assistance with care, follow-up that may be needed to provide safe environment for client.*

• Discuss need for/sources of adult supervision (e.g., elderly day care, home health aide or companion, etc.).

• Problem-solve with client/parent *to provide adequate child supervision after school, during working hours, and on school holidays.*

• Explore behaviors related to use of alcohol, tobacco, and recreational drugs and other substances. *Provides opportunity to review consequences of previously determined risk factors (e.g., increase in oral cancer among teenagers using smokeless tobacco, potential consequences of illegal activities, person needing surgery who is smoking and has heart disease; occurrence of spontaneous abortion, fetal alcohol syndrome/neonatal addiction in prenatal women using tobacco, alcohol, and other drugs).*

• Discuss necessary environmental changes in the home (e.g., decals on glass doors *to show when they are closed*, lowering temperature on hot water heater *to prevent scalding*, adequate lighting of stairways *to reduce risk of falls*).

• Encourage development of fire safety program. *Participation in family fire drills, use of smoke detectors, yearly chimney cleaning, purchase of fire-retardant clothing (especially children's nightwear), fireworks safety, etc., enhances home safety.*

• Review/recommend transportation safety needs (e.g., use of seat belts, fitted helmets for cyclists, approved infant seat; avoidance of hitchhiking) as indicated.

• Recommend accident prevention programs (e.g., driver training, parenting classes, firearms safety, and so forth).

• Refer to other resources as indicated (e.g., counseling/psychotherapy, budget counseling, and parenting classes).

• Provide client/caregiver with emergency contact numbers as individually indicated (e.g., doctor, 911, poison control, police).

• Provide client/caregiver with bibliotherapy/written resources *for later review and self-paced learning.*

NURSING PRIORITY NO. 5. To enhance community awareness and correction of identified needs:

• Promote community education programs *geared to increasing awareness of safety measures and resources available to the individual.*

• Promote community awareness about the problems of design of buildings, equipment, transportation, and workplace practices *that contribute to accidents.*

• Develop community resources/identify neighbors or friends *to assist elderly/handicapped individuals in providing such things as structural maintenance, snow and ice removal from walks and steps, etc.*

 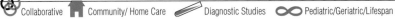

🏠 • Encourage involvement in community self-help programs such as Neighborhood Watch, Helping Hand.

Assessment/Reassessment
- Individual risk factors, past/recent history of injuries, awareness of safety needs.

Planning
- Plan of care and who is involved in the planning.
- Teaching Plan.

Implementation/Evaluation
- Responses to interventions/teaching, actions performed.
- Attainment/progress toward desired outcome(s).
- Modifications to plan of care.

Discharge Planning
- Long-term needs and who is responsible for actions to be taken.
- Available resources, specific referrals made.

References

1. Ebright, P. R., Patterson, E. S., & Render, M. L. (2002). The "New Look" approach to patient safety: A guide for clinical specialist leadership. Clin Nurs Spec, 16(5), 247–253.
2. ND: Trauma, risk for. In Doenges, M. E., Moorhouse, M. F., & Geissler-Murr, A. C. (2002). Nurse's Pocket Guide: Diagnoses, Interventions, and Rationales, ed 8. Philadelphia: F. A. Davis.
3. Nelson, A., et al. (2003). Safe patient handling & movement. AJN, 103(3), 32–43.
4. Walton, J. (2001). Helping high-risk surgical patients beat the odds. Nursing, 31(3), 54.
5. Mion, L. C., & Mercurio, A. T. (1992). Methods to reduce restraints: Process, outcomes and future directions. J Gerontol Nurs, 20(10), 5.
6. Wright, A. (1998). Nursing interventions with advanced osteoporosis. Home Health Nurs, 16(3), 145.
7. Kuang, T., & Kedlaya, D. (2002). Assistive devices to improve independence. Available at: http://www.emedicine.com. Accessed March 2004.
8. Safety for older consumers' home safety checklist. (Document #701). Available at: Consumer Product Safety Commission (CPSC), http://www.cpsc.gov. Accessed September 2003.
9. Nursing Care Plan: Extended Care, Falls, risk for. In Doenges, M. E., Moorhouse, M. F., & Geissler-Murr, A. C. (2002). Nursing Care Plans: Guidelines for Individualizing Patient Care, ed 6. (CD-ROM). Philadelphia: F. A. Davis.
10. Daus, C. (1999). Maintaining mobility: Assistive equipment helps the geriatric population stay active and independent. Rehab Management, 12(5), 58–61.
11. Horn, L. B. (2000). Reducing the risk of falls in the elderly. Rehab Management, 13(3), 36–38.

impaired Urinary Elimination

Definition: Disturbance in urine elimination

RELATED FACTORS

Multiple causality; sensory motor impairment; anatomical obstruction; UTI; [mechanical trauma; fluid/volume states; psychogenic factors; surgical diversion]

Subjective
Frequency; urgency
Hesitancy
Dysuria
Nocturia, [enuresis]

Objective
Incontinence
Retention

SAMPLE CLINICAL APPLICATIONS: urinary tract infection, prostate disease (BPH), bladder cancer, spinal cord injury, MS, pregnancy/childbirth, pelvic trauma, abdominal surgery, dementia/Alzheimer's disease

DESIRED OUTCOMES/EVALUATION CRITERIA
Sample **NOC** linkages:
Urinary Elimination: Ability of the urinary system to filter wastes, conserve solutes, and collect and discharge urine in a healthy pattern
Urinary Continence: Control of the elimination of urine
Self-Care: Toileting: Ability to toilet self

Client Will (Include Specific Time Frame)
- Verbalize understanding of condition.
- Identify causative factors. (Refer to specific NDs for incontinence/retention as appropriate.)
- Achieve normal elimination pattern or participate in measures to correct/compensate for defects.
- Demonstrate behaviors/techniques to prevent urinary infection.
- Manage care of urinary catheter, or stoma and appliance following urinary diversion.

ACTIONS/INTERVENTIONS

Sample **NIC** linkages:
Urinary Elimination Management: Maintenance of an optimum urinary elimination pattern
Urinary Catheterization: Insertion of a catheter into the bladder for temporary or permanent drainage of urine
Perineal Care: Maintenance of perineal skin integrity and relief of perineal discomfort

NURSING PRIORITY NO. **1.** To assess causative/contributing factors:

- Review medical history *for conditions that may impact elimination such as surgery (including urinary diversion); neurologic deficits such as MS, paraplegia/tetraplegia; mental/emotional dysfunction; prostate disease; recent/multiple pregnancies; cardiovascular disease; pelvic trauma; use of penile clamps (may result in urethral trauma). Information essential to developing plan of care.*[1]
- Determine whether problem is due to loss of neurologic functioning or disorientation (e.g., Alzheimer's disease). *Identifies direction for further evaluation/treatment options to discover specifics of individual situation.*[2]

 Cultural   Collaborative   Community/ Home Care   Diagnostic Studies ∞ Pediatric/Geriatric/Lifespan   Medications
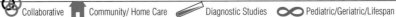

- Determine pathology of bladder dysfunction relative to identified medical diagnosis. *In neurologic/demyelinating diseases such as MS, problem may be failure to store urine, empty bladder, or both. Therapeutic measures can be taken which are directed at underlying pathology.*[3]
- Inspect stoma of urinary diversion. *Factors such as edema, scarring, presence of congealed mucus can interfere with urinary flow and indicate need for intervention directed at specific cause.*[4]
- Review drug regimen *to note use of drugs that may be nephrotoxic (e.g., aminoglycosides, tetracyclines), especially in clients who are immunosuppressed or medications that may result in retention (e.g., atropine, belladonna).*
- Note age and sex of client. *Urinary tract infections (UTIs) are more prevalent in women and older men.*[5]
- Rule out gonorrhea in men. *This infection needs to be considered when urethritis with a penile discharge is present and there are no bacteria in the urine.*[3]
- Assist with antibody-coated bacteria assay. *Diagnosis of bacterial infection of the kidney or prostate is important for immediate treatment to prevent damage to these organs.*[3]
- Review laboratory tests for hyperparathyroidism, changes in renal function, presence of infection. *Identification of these conditions is crucial for correct treatment regimen.*[3]
- Strain all urine for calculi and describe stones expelled and/or send to laboratory for analysis. *Retrieval of calculi allows identification of type of stone and influences choice of therapy.*[3]

NURSING PRIORITY NO. 2. To assess degree of interference/disability:

- Determine client's previous pattern of elimination and compare with current situation. Note reports of frequency, urgency, burning, incontinence, nocturia/enuresis, size and force of urinary stream. *Provides information about degree of interference with elimination or may indicate bladder infection.*[3]
- Palpate bladder to assess retention. *Fullness over bladder following voiding is indicative of inadequate emptying/retention and requires intervention.*[3]
- Investigate pain, noting location, duration, intensity; presence of bladder spasms, back or flank pain, etc., *which may be indicative of infection.*
- Determine client's usual daily fluid intake (both amount and beverage choices/use of caffeine). Note condition of skin and mucous membranes, color of urine *to determine level of hydration.*[5]

NURSING PRIORITY NO. 3. To assist in treating/preventing urinary alteration:

- Encourage fluid intake up to 3000–4000 mL/day (within cardiac tolerance), including cranberry juice. *Maintains renal function, prevents infection and formation of urinary stones, avoids encrustation around indwelling catheter, or may be used to flush urinary diversion appliance.*[5]
- Assist with developing toileting routines as appropriate. *For adults who are cognitively intact and physically capable of self-toileting, bladder training, timed voiding, and habit retraining may be beneficial.*[5]
- Encourage client to void in sitz bath after surgical procedures of the perineal area. *Warm water helps relax muscles and soothe sore tissues, facilitating voiding.*[3]
- Observe for signs of infection—cloudy, foul odor; bloody urine. Send urine (midstream clean-voided specimen) for culture and sensitivity as indicated. *Prompt treatment is important to prevent serious complications; colony count over 100,000 indicates need for treatment.*[3]

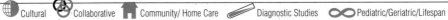

- Encourage client to verbalize fear/concerns (e.g., disruption in sexual activity, inability to work, concern about involvement in social activities). *Open expression allows client to talk about, deal with feelings, and begin to solve the identified problems.*[6]
- Note influence of culture/ethnicity or gender on client's view of problems of incontinence. *Limited evidence exists to understand and help people cope with the physical and psychosocial consequences of this chronic, socially isolating and potentially devastating disorder.*[6]
- Monitor medication regimen, antimicrobials (single-dose is frequently used for UTI), sulfonamides, antispasmodics, etc. *Evaluates client's response to medication, need to modify treatment if results are unsatisfactory.*[3]
- Discuss surgical procedures and review medical regimen needed for specific situation. *Although preventive and restorative measures may suffice, client with benign prostatic hypertrophy, bladder/prostatic cancer, and large cystoceles in women benefit from appropriate surgical intervention.*[6]
- Refer to specific NDs Urinary Incontinence (specify); [acute/chronic] Urinary Retention for additional interventions/treatment regimens.

NURSING PRIORITY NO. **4.** To assist in management of long-term urinary alterations:

- Keep bladder deflated by use of an indwelling catheter connected to closed drainage. Investigate alternatives when possible. *Measures such as intermittent catheterization, surgical interventions, urinary drugs, voiding maneuvers, condom catheter may be preferable to the indwelling catheter to provide more effective control and prevent possibility of recurrent infections.*[3,7]
- Provide latex-free catheter and care supplies. *Reduces risk of developing sensitivity to latex, which often develops in individuals requiring frequent catheterization or who have long-term indwelling catheters.*[8]
- Check frequently for bladder distention and observe for overflow. *Requires immediate intervention to reduce risk of infection and/or autonomic hyperreflexia.*[3]
- Maintain acidic environment of the bladder by the use of agents such as vitamin C, Mandelamine when appropriate. *There is some evidence that the acidic environment discourages bacterial growth by preventing bacteria from adhering to the bladder wall.*[3]
- Adhere to a regular bladder/diversion appliance emptying schedule. *Avoids accidents and prevents embarrassment to the individual.*[4]
- Provide for routine diversion appliance care, and assist client to recognize and deal with problems such as alkaline salt encrustation, ill-fitting appliance, malodorous urine, infection, etc. *Provides information and promotes competence in care increasing self-confidence in dealing with appliance on a regular basis.*[4]

NURSING PRIORITY NO. **5.** To promote wellness (Teaching/Discharge Considerations):

- Emphasize importance of keeping area clean and dry. *Reduces risk of infection and/or skin breakdown.*[3]
- Instruct female clients with urinary tract infection to drink large amounts of fluid, void immediately after intercourse, wipe from front to back, promptly treat vaginal infections, and take showers rather than tub baths. *These measures can limit risk of/avoid reinfection.*[5]
- Encourage SO(s) who participate in routine care to recognize complications (including

 Cultural   Collaborative   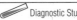 Community/ Home Care   Diagnostic Studies   Pediatric/Geriatric/Lifespan   Medications

latex allergy) necessitating medical interventions. *Client may be too embarrassed to discuss symptoms, and caregivers need to be alert to changes that necessitate evaluation and treatment.*[6]

● Instruct in proper application and care of appliance for urinary diversion. Encourage liberal fluid intake, avoidance of foods/medications that produce strong odor, use of white vinegar or deodorizer in pouch to promote odor control. *These measures help to ensure patency of device and prevent embarrassing situations for client.*[4]

● Identify sources for supplies, programs/agencies providing financial assistance. *Lack of access to necessities can be a barrier to management of incontinence and having help to obtain needed equipment can assist with daily care.*[6]

● Recommend avoidance of gas-forming foods in presence of ureterosigmoidostomy. *Flatus can cause urinary incontinence.*[2]

● Recommend use of silicone catheter. *These catheters are more comfortable and have fewer problems with infection when permanent/long-term catheterization is required.*[3]

● Demonstrate proper positioning of catheter drainage tubing and bag. *Facilitates drainage/prevents reflux and complications of infection.*[2]

● Refer client/SO(s) to appropriate community resources such as ostomy specialist, support group, sex therapist, psychiatric clinical nurse specialist, and so on. *May be necessary to deal with changes in body image/function.*[6]

DOCUMENTATION FOCUS

Assessment/Reassessment

● Individual findings, including previous and current pattern of voiding, nature of problem, effect on desired lifestyle.

Planning

● Plan of care and who is involved in planning.
● Teaching Plan.

Implementation/Evaluation

● Response to interventions/teaching, actions performed.
● Attainment/progress toward desired outcome(s).
● Modifications to plan of care.

Discharge Planning

● Long-term needs and who is responsible for actions to be taken.
● Available resources/specific referrals made.
● Individual equipment needs and sources.

References

1. ND: Urinary Elimination, impaired. In Doenges, M. E., Moorhouse, M. F., & Murr, A. C. (2004). Nurse's Pocket Guide: Diagnoses, Interventions, and Rationales, ed 9. Philadelphia: F. A. Davis.
2. Cox, H. C., et al. (2002). Clinical Applications of Nursing Diagnosis: Adult, Child, Women's, Psychiatric, Gerontic, and Home Health Considerations, ed 4. Philadelphia: F. A. Davis.
3. ND: Urinary Elimination, impaired. In Doenges, M. E., Moorhouse, M. F., & Geissler-Murr, A. C. (2002). Nursing Care Plans, Guidelines for Individualizing Patient Care, ed 6. Philadelphia: F. A. Davis.
4. Colwell, J. C., et al. (2001). The state of the standard diversion. J Wound Ostomy Continence Nurs, 28(1), 6–17.
5. Wyman, J. F. (2003). Treatment of urinary incontinence in men and older women. In Newman, D. K., & Palmer, M. H. (Eds). The State of the Science on Urinary Incontinence. Am J Nurs, 293 3(suppl), 20.
6. Newman, D. K., & Palmer, M. H. (Eds). (2003). The state of the science on urinary incontinence. Am J Nurs, 293 3(suppl), 20

7. Beers, M. H., & Berkow, R. (Eds). (1999). The Merck Manual of Diagnosis and Therapy, ed 17. Whitehouse Station, NJ: Merck Research Laboratories.
8. Statement on natural latex allergies and SB latex. Available at: http://www.occupationalhazards.com. Accessed February 2003.

readiness for enhanced Urinary Elimination

Definition: A pattern of urinary functions that is sufficient for meeting eliminatory needs and can be strengthened

RELATED FACTORS

To be developed by nurse researchers and submitted to NANDA

DEFINING CHARACTERISTICS

Subjective
Expresses willingness to enhance urinary elimination
Positions self for emptying of bladder

Objective
Urine is straw colored with no odor
Specific gravity is within normal limits
Amount of output is within normal limits for age and other factors
Fluid intake is adequate for daily needs

SAMPLE CLINICAL APPLICATIONS: spinal cord injury, MS, pregnancy/childbirth, pelvic trauma, abdominal surgery, prostate disease

DESIRED OUTCOMES/EVALUATION CRITERIA

Sample **NOC** Linkages:

Urinary Continence: Control of the elimination of urine

Knowledge: Disease Process: Extent of understanding conveyed about a specific disease process

Symptom Control: Personal actions to minimize perceived adverse changes in physical and emotional functioning

Client Will (Include Specific Time Frame)
- Verbalize understanding of condition that has potential for altering elimination.
- Achieve normal elimination pattern, voiding in appropriate amounts.
- Alter environment to accommodate individual needs.

ACTIONS/INTERVENTIONS

Sample NIC Linkages:

Urinary Elimination Management: Maintenance of an optimum urinary elimination pattern

Prompted Voiding: Promotion of urinary continence through the use of timed verbal toileting reminders and positive social feedback for successful toileting

Urinary Habit Training: Establishing a predictable pattern of bladder emptying to prevent incontinence for persons with limited cognitive ability who have urge, stress, or functional incontinence

 Cultural Collaborative Community/ Home Care 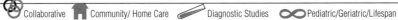 Diagnostic Studies Pediatric/Geriatric/Lifespan Medications

NURSING PRIORITY NO. 1. To assess situation and adaptive skills being used by client:

- Review medical history *for conditions that may have impacted client's elimination patterns (e.g., surgery, childbirth, recent/multiple pregnancies, pelvic trauma, stroke, mental/emotional dysfunction, prostate disease).*[1]
- Determine client's previous pattern of elimination and compare with current situation *to determine how pattern can be improved.*[1]
- Observe current voiding patterns, time, color and amount voided as indicated (e.g., post-surgical client) *to document normalization of elimination.*[1]
- Ascertain methods of self-management (e.g., limiting or increasing liquid intake, regular voiding times) *to determine degree of success of current interventions.*[2]
- Determine client's usual daily fluid intake. *Both amount and beverage choices are important in managing elimination.*[2–4]
- Note condition of skin and mucous membranes, color of urine *to help determine level of hydration.*[1]

NURSING PRIORITY NO. 2. To assist client to strengthen management of urinary elimination:

- Encourage fluid intake, including water and cranberry juice, *to help maintain renal function, prevent infection.*[1]
- Regulate liquid intake at prescheduled times *to promote predictable voiding pattern.*[2,3]
- Suggest restricting fluid intake 2–3 hours before bedtime *to reduce voiding during the night.*[2,4,5]
- Assist with modifying current routines, as appropriate. *Client may benefit from additional information in enhancing success, such as regarding cues/urge to void, adjusting schedule of voiding (shorter or longer), relaxation and/or distraction techniques, standing or sitting upright during voiding, to ensure that bladder is completely empty, and/or practicing pelvic muscle strengthening exercises (Kegels).*[2,4–6]
- Provide assistance/devices as indicated. *Having means of summoning assistance; placement of bedside commode, urinal, or bedpan within client's reach (especially when client is frail or mobility impaired), elevated toilet seats, or mobility devices enhances client's ability to maintain urinary function.*[5]
- Modify/recommend diet changes if indicated. *Client may benefit from reduction of caffeine because of its bladder irritant effect, or weight reduction may help reduce overactive bladder symptoms and incontinence by decreasing pressure on the bladder.*[2,4–6]
- Modify medication regimens as appropriate. For example, administer prescribed diuretics in the morning *to lessen nighttime voiding, reduce or eliminate use of hypnotics if possible as client may be too sedated to recognize/respond to urge to void.*[5]

NURSING PRIORITY NO. 3. To enhance wellness:

- Encourage continuation of successful toileting program.
- Instruct client/SO/caregivers in cues that client needs (e.g., voiding on routine schedule; showing client location of the bathroom, providing adequate room lighting, signs, color coding of door, *to assist client in continued continence, especially when in unfamiliar surroundings.*[3–5]
- Review signs/symptoms of urinary complications and need for medical follow-up *to monitor condition/provide timely intervention.*

Assessment/Reassessment
- Findings/adaptive skills being used.

Planning
- Plan of care and who is involved in planning.
- Teaching plan.

Implementation/Evaluation
- Responses to treatment plan/interventions and actions performed.
- Attainment/progress toward desired outcome(s).
- Modifications to plan of care.

Discharge Planning
- Available resources, equipment needs/sources.

References

1. ND: Urinary Elimination, readiness for enhanced. In Doenges, M. E., Moorhouse, M. F., & Murr, A. C. (2004). Nurse's Pocket Guide: Diagnoses, Interventions and Rationales, ed 9. Philadelphia: F. A. Davis.
2. Sampselle, C. M. (2003). Behavioral interventions in young and middle-age women. In Newman, D. K., & Palmer, M. H. (eds). The state of the science on urinary incontinence. AJN, 293(suppl), 9–19.
3. Lyons, S. S., & Specht, J. K. P. (1999). Prompted voiding for persons with urinary incontinence. University of Iowa Gerontological Nursing Interventions Research Center. Available at: http://www.guideline.gov. Accessed June 2003.
4. Wyman, J. F., et al. (1998). Comparative efficacy of behavioral interventions in the management of female urinary incontinence. Am J Obstet Gynecol, 179(4), 999–1007.
5. Wyman, J. F. Treatment of urinary incontinence in men and older women. In Newman, D. K., & Palmer, M. H. (eds). The state of the science on urinary incontinence. AJN, 293(suppl), 26–35.
6. Burgio, K. L., et al. (1989). Behavioral training for post-prostatectomy urinary incontinence. J Urol, 141(2), 303–306.

functional Urinary Incontinence

Definition: Inability of usually continent person to reach toilet in time to avoid unintentional loss of urine

RELATED FACTORS
Altered environmental factors [e.g., poor lighting or inability to locate bathroom]
Neuromuscular limitations
Weakened supporting pelvic structures
Impaired vision/cognition
Psychological factors; [reluctance to use call light or bedpan]
[Increased urine production]

DEFINING CHARACTERISTICS

Subjective
Senses need to void
[Voiding in large amounts]

 Cultural   Collaborative   Community/ Home Care   Diagnostic Studies 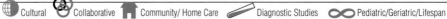 Pediatric/Geriatric/Lifespan   Medications

Objective

Loss of urine before reaching toilet; amount of time required to reach toilet exceeds length of time between sensing urge and uncontrolled voiding

Able to completely empty bladder

May only be incontinent in early morning

SAMPLE CLINICAL APPLICATIONS: diabetes mellitus, congestive heart failure (diuretic use), arthritis, bladder prolapse/cystocele, stroke

DESIRED OUTCOMES/EVALUATION CRITERIA

Sample **NOC** linkages:

Urinary Continence: Control of the elimination of urine

Urinary Elimination: Ability of the urinary system to filter wastes, conserve solutes, and collect and discharge urine in a healthy pattern

Self-Care Toileting: Ability to toilet self

Client Will (Include Specific Time Frame)

- Verbalize understanding of condition and identify interventions to prevent incontinence.
- Alter environment to accommodate individual needs.
- Report voiding in individually appropriate amounts.
- Urinate at acceptable times and places.

ACTIONS/INTERVENTIONS

Sample **NIC** linkages:

Prompted Voiding: Promotion of urinary continence through the use of timed verbal toileting reminders and positive social feedback for successful toileting

Urinary Habit Training: Establishing a predictable pattern of bladder emptying to prevent incontinence for persons with limited cognitive ability who have urge, stress, or functional incontinence

Self-Care Assistance: Toileting: Assisting another with elimination

NURSING PRIORITY NO. 1. To assess causative/contributing factors:

- Determine if client is voluntarily postponing urination. *Often the demands of the work setting, either because of restrictions on bathroom breaks, working alone (e.g., pharmacist, nurse, teacher), demands of the job (heavy workload and unable to find time for a bathroom break) make it difficult for individuals to go to the bathroom when the need arises, resulting in frequent urinary tract infections and incontinence.*[1]
- Review medical history *for conditions or use of medication/substances known to increase urine output and/or alter bladder tone. Diabetes mellitus, prolapsed bladder, diuretics, alcohol, caffeine are a few of the factors that can affect frequency of urination and ability to hold urine until individual can reach the bathroom.*[1]
- Test urine with Chemstix to note presence of glucose. *Hyperglycemia can cause polyuria and overdistention of the bladder, resulting in problem with incontinence.*[2]
- Determine the difference between the time it takes to get to the bathroom/remove clothing and the time between urge and involuntary loss of urine. *Information helpful for planning interventions necessary to avoid incontinent episodes.*[1]
- Evaluate cognition. *Disease processes/medications can affect mental status/orientation to place, recognition of urge to void, and/or its significance, leading to problems with incontinence.*[1]

- Identify environmental conditions that interfere with timely access to bathroom/successful toileting process. *Factors such as unfamiliar surroundings, dexterity problems, poor lighting, improperly fitted chair walker, low toilet seat, absence of safety bars, and travel distance to toilet may affect self-care ability.*[1]

NURSING PRIORITY NO. 2. To assess degree of interference/disability:

- Assist client to keep voiding diary. Determine the frequency and timing of continent/incontinent voids. *Information will be used to plan program to manage incontinence.*[3]
- Measure/estimate amount of urine voided or lost with incontinence. *Provides information that can be useful to planning care and managing incontinence.*[1]
- Examine urine for signs of infection. *Cloudy/hazy, foul-smelling urine is a sign of infection and need for treatment.*[2]
- Ascertain effect on lifestyle (including socialization and sexuality) and self-esteem. *There is a general belief that incontinence is an inevitable result of aging and that nothing can be done about it. However, those with incontinence problems are often embarrassed, withdraw from social activities and relationships, and hesitate to discuss the problem—even with their health-care provider.*[1]

NURSING PRIORITY NO. 3. To assist in treating/preventing incontinence:

- Administer prescribed diuretics in the morning. *The effect of these medications is diminished by bedtime and nighttime voidings are lessened.*[2]
- Reduce or eliminate use of hypnotics if possible. *Client may be too sedated to recognize/respond to urge to void.*[4]
- Provide means of summoning assistance. *The ready placement of a call light when hospitalized or a bell in the home setting enables the client to obtain toileting help as needed.*[4]
- Adapt clothes for quick removal. *Velcro fasteners, full skirts, crotchless panties or no panties, suspenders or elastic waists instead of belts on pants facilitate toileting once urge to void is noted.*[4]
- Use night-lights to mark bathroom location. *Elderly person may become confused upon arising and be unable to locate bathroom in the dark and lighting will facilitate access, reducing the possibility of accidents.*[4]
- Provide cues such as adequate room lighting, signs, color coding of door. *Assists client who is disoriented to find the bathroom.*[4]
- Remove throw rugs, excess furniture in travel path to bathroom. *Reduces risk of falls, facilitates access to bathroom, and avoids loss of urine.*[4]
- Raise chair and/or toilet seat or provide bedside commode, urinal, or bedpan as indicated. *Facilitates toileting when individual has difficulty with movement.*[1]
- Schedule voiding on regular time schedule (e.g., every 3 hours). *Emptying bladder on a regular schedule minimizes pressure, reducing overflow voiding.*[1]
- Restrict fluid intake 2–3 hours before bedtime. *Reduces need to waken to void during the night.*[1]
- Instruct in pelvic floor strengthening exercises as appropriate. *Kegel exercises strengthen the pelvic floor muscles, promoting increased ability to contract them and prevent incontinence.*[1]
- Implement bladder training program as indicated. *May be helpful to gradually increase the interval between voidings with a goal of overall decreasing voiding frequency between waking and sleeping hours.*[1]
- Include physical/occupational therapist in determining ways to alter environment, appropriate assistive devices. *Useful in meeting individual needs of client.*[1]

 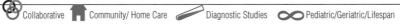

NURSING PRIORITY NO. 4. To promote wellness (Teaching/Discharge Considerations):

- Discuss need to respond immediately to urge to void and to take advantage of any opportunity to void. *Emptying bladder frequently prevents buildup of pressure and inevitable loss of urine.*[1]
- Suggest limiting intake of coffee, tea, and alcohol. *Diuretic effect of these substances impacts voiding pattern and can contribute to incontinence.*[1]
- Review use/intake of foods, fluids, and supplements containing potassium. *Potassium deficiency can negatively affect bladder tone.*[4]
- Emphasize importance of perineal care following voiding. *Promotes cleanliness and reduces possibility of infection.*[1]
- Maintain positive regard when incontinence occurs. *Reduces embarrassment associated with incontinence, need for assistance, use of bedpan.*[1]
- Promote participation in developing long-term plan of care. *Encourages involvement in follow-through of plan, increasing possibility of success and confidence in own ability to manage program.*[1]
- Refer to NDs reflex/stress/total/or urge Urinary Incontinence for additional interventions as appropriate.

DOCUMENTATION FOCUS

Assessment/Reassessment
- Current elimination pattern/assessment findings and effect on lifestyle and self-esteem.

Planning
- Plan of care and who is involved in planning.
- Teaching plan.

Implementation/Evaluation
- Response to interventions/teaching and actions performed.
- Attainment/progress toward desired outcome(s).
- Modifications to plan of care.

Discharge Planning
- Long-term needs and who is responsible for actions to be taken.
- Specific referrals made.

References

1. Newman, D. K., & Palmer, M. H. (Eds). (2003). The state of the science on urinary incontinence. Am J Nurs, 293, 3(suppl), 20
2. Doenges, M. E., Moorhouse, M. F., & Geissler-Murr, A. C. (2002). Nursing Care Plans: Guidelines for Individualizing Patient Care, ed 6. Philadelphia: F. A. Davis.
3. Wyman, J. F. (2003). Treatment of urinary incontinence in men and older women. In Newman, D. K., & Palmer, M. H. (Eds). The state of the science on urinary incontinence. Am J Nurs, 293, 3(suppl), 20.
4. Cox, H. C., et al. (2002). Clinical Applications of Nursing Diagnosis: Adult, Child, Women's, Psychiatric, Gerontic, and Home Health Considerations, ed 4. Philadelphia: F. A. Davis.

reflex Urinary Incontinence

Definition: Involuntary loss of urine at somewhat predictable intervals when a specific bladder volume is reached

Tissue damage from radiation cystitis, inflammatory bladder conditions, or radical pelvic surgery

Neurologic impairment above level of sacral or pontine micturition center

DEFINING CHARACTERISTICS

Subjective
No sensation of bladder fullness/urge to void/voiding

Sensation of urgency without voluntary inhibition of bladder contraction

Sensations associated with full bladder such as sweating, restlessness, and abdominal discomfort

Objective
Predictable pattern of voiding

Inability to voluntarily inhibit or initiate voiding

Complete emptying with [brain] lesion above pontine micturition center

Incomplete emptying with [spinal cord] lesion above sacral micturition center

SAMPLE CLINICAL APPLICATIONS: spinal cord injury, MS, bladder/pelvis cancer, dementia

DESIRED OUTCOMES/EVALUATION CRITERIA

Sample **NOC** linkages:

Urinary Continence: Control of the elimination of urine

Neurologic Status: Autonomic: Extent to which the autonomic nervous system coordinates visceral function

Urinary Elimination: Ability of the urinary system to filter wastes, conserve solutes, and collect and discharge urine in a healthy pattern

Client Will (Include Specific Time Frame)
- Verbalize understanding of condition/contributing factors.
- Establish bladder regimen appropriate for individual situation.
- Demonstrate behaviors/techniques to control condition and prevent complications.
- Urinate at acceptable times and places.

ACTIONS/INTERVENTIONS
Sample **NIC** linkages:

Urinary Bladder Training: Improving bladder function for those with urge incontinence by increasing the bladder's ability to hold urine and the patient's ability to suppress urination

Urinary Catheterization: Intermittent: Regular periodic use of a catheter to empty the bladder

Urinary Incontinence Care: Assistance in promoting continence and maintaining perineal skin integrity

NURSING PRIORITY NO. 1. To assess degree of interference/disability:

- Note causative/disease process as listed in Related Factors. *Identification of individual situation and concerns is critical to developing appropriate plan of care.*[1]

 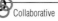

- Evaluate for concomitant urinary retention. *Often the bladder is not completely emptied because there is no voluntary control of the bladder.*[2]
- Assess ability to sense bladder fullness, awareness of incontinence. *Individuals with neurologic impairments often lose control of their bladder without warning and may have little to no awareness of need to void.*[3]
- Review voiding diary, if available, or record frequency and time of urination. Compare timing of voidings, particularly in relation to liquid intake and medications. *Aids in targeting interventions to meet individual situation.*[4]
- Measure amount of each voiding. *Incontinence often occurs once a specific bladder volume is reached and may indicate need for insertion of a permanent/intermittent catheter.*[5]
- Evaluate ability to manipulate/use urinary collection device or catheter. *Type and degree of neurologic impairment (i.e., spinal cord injury, multiple sclerosis, dementia) may interfere with client's ability to be self sufficient.*[3]
- Refer to urologist/appropriate specialist for testing of sphincter control and volumes. *A thorough physical examination and diagnostic tests, including urinalysis, ultrasound, radiographs, and urine flowmetry to measure urine flow is standard. A urodynamic evaluation measuring bladder capacity, pressure, and rate of urinary flow may also be indicated based on results of other testing.*[6]

NURSING PRIORITY NO. 2. To assist in managing incontinence:

- Encourage minimum of 1500–2000 mL of fluid intake daily. Regulate liquid intake at prescheduled times (with and between meals). *Promotes a predictable voiding pattern to help with treatment regimen.*[6]
- Restrict fluids 2–3 hours before bedtime. *Can reduce need to void during the night, preventing incontinence/interruption of sleep.*[6]
- Direct client to, or take to, toilet before the expected time of incontinence. *May stimulate the reflex for voiding.*[4]
- Instruct in measures such as pouring warm water over perineum, running water in sink, stimulating/massaging skin of lower abdomen, thighs, and so on. *May stimulate voiding reflexes and voiding, preventing loss of urine at unpredictable times.*[7]
- Set alarm to awaken during night to maintain schedule, or use external catheter as appropriate. *Developing a regular time for voiding will empty the bladder, preventing incontinence during the night.*[6]
- Demonstrate application of external collection device or intermittent self-catheterization using small-lumen straight catheter. *If neurologic condition indicates, can drain urine from bladder, preventing loss of urine at inconvenient times.*[3]
- Establish intermittent catheterization schedule. *Basing catherization on client's activity schedule as indicated enables client to maintain a normal lifestyle when incontinence is a permanent problem.*[4]
- Measure postvoid residuals/catheterization volumes. *Determines frequency for emptying bladder.*[4]

NURSING PRIORITY NO. 3. To promote wellness (Teaching/Discharge Considerations):

- Encourage continuation of regular toileting program. *May be able to establish a schedule that takes advantage of whatever ability remains, even though the neurologic impairment is affecting bladder sensation.*[6]

● Suggest use of incontinence pads/pants during day and social contact, if appropriate. *Depending on client's activity level, amount of urine loss, manual dexterity, and cognitive ability these devices provide security and comfort and protect the skin and clothing from urine leakage, reduce odor and are generally unnoticeable under clothing.*[6]

 ● Stress importance of perineal care following voiding and frequent changing of incontinence pads if used. *Maintains cleanliness and prevents skin irritation/breakdown and odor.*[6]

 ● Encourage limited intake of coffee, tea, and alcohol. *Diuretic effect of these substances may affect predictability of voiding pattern.*[2]

 ● Instruct in proper care of catheter and clean techniques. *Reduces risk of infection.*[3]

● Review signs/symptoms of urinary complications and need for medical follow-up. *Provides immediate attention preventing exacerbation of problem or extension of infection into kidneys.*

DOCUMENTATION FOCUS

Assessment/Reassessment
● Findings/degree of disability and effect on lifestyle.

Planning
● Plan of care and who is involved in planning.
● Teaching plan.

Implementation/Evaluation
● Responses to treatment plan/interventions and actions performed.
● Attainment/progress toward desired outcome(s).
● Modifications to plan of care.

Discharge Planning
● Long-term needs and who is responsible for actions to be taken.
● Available resources, equipment needs/sources.

References

1. ND: Urinary Incontinence, reflex. In Doenges, M. E., Moorhouse, M. F., & Murr, A. C. (2004). Nurse's Pocket Guide: Diagnoses, Interventions, and Rationales, ed 9. Philadelphia: F. A. Davis.
2. What is urinary incontinence? Available at: http://ourworld.compuserve.com/homepages/nacs/INCONT.HTM. Accessed February 2004.
3. Doenges, M. E., Moorhouse, M. F., & Geissler-Murr, A. C. (2002). Nursing Care Plans, Guidelines for Individualizing Patient Care, ed 6. Philadelphia: F. A. Davis.
4. Newman, D. K., & Palmer, M. H. (Eds). (2003). The state of the science on urinary incontinence. Am J Nurs, 293, 3(suppl), 20.
5. Cox, H. C., et al. (2002). Clinical Applications of Nursing Diagnosis: Adult, Child, Women's, Psychiatric, Gerontic, and Home Health Considerations, ed 4. Philadelphia: F. A. Davis.
6. Urinary Incontinence. Available at: http://www.hmc.psu.edu/healthinfo/uz/urinaryincontinence.htm. Accessed February 2004.
7. Beers, M. H., & Berkow, R. (eds). (1999). The Merck Manual of Diagnosis and Therapy, ed 17. Whitehouse Station, NJ: Merck Research Laboratories.

stress Urinary Incontinence

Definition: Loss of less than 50 mL of urine occurring with increased abdominal pressure

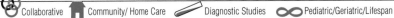 Cultural   Collaborative   Community/ Home Care Diagnostic Studies Pediatric/Geriatric/Lifespan   Medications

Degenerative changes in pelvic muscles and structural supports associated with increased age [e.g., poor closure of urethral sphincter, estrogen deficiency]

High intra-abdominal pressure (e.g., obesity, gravid uterus)

Incompetent bladder outlet; overdistention between voidings

Weak pelvic muscles and structural supports [e.g., straining with chronic constipation]

[Neural degeneration, vascular deficits, surgery, radiation therapy]

DEFINING CHARACTERISTICS

Subjective

Reported dribbling with increased abdominal pressure [e.g., coughing, sneezing, lifting, impact aerobics, changing position]

Urinary urgency; frequency (more often than every 2 hours)

Objective

Observed dribbling with increased abdominal pressure

SAMPLE CLINICAL APPLICATIONS: obesity, pregnancy, cystocele, menopause, prostate surgery, abdominal/pelvic trauma, cancer/radiation therapy

DESIRED OUTCOMES/EVALUATION CRITERIA

Sample **NOC** linkages:

Urinary Continence: Control of the elimination of urine

Symptom Control: Personal actions to minimize perceived adverse changes in physical and emotional functioning

Self-Care: Hygiene: Ability to maintain own hygiene

Client Will (Include Specific Time Frame)

- Verbalize understanding of condition and interventions for bladder conditioning.
- Demonstrate behaviors/techniques to strengthen pelvic floor musculature.
- Remain continent even with increased intra-abdominal pressure.

ACTIONS/INTERVENTIONS

Sample **NIC** linkages:

Pelvic Muscle Exercise: Strengthening and training the levator ani and urogenital muscles through voluntary repetitive contraction to decrease stress, urge, or mixed types of urinary incontinence

Urinary Incontinence Care: Assistance in promoting continence and maintaining perineal skin integrity

Urinary Habit Training: Establishing a predictable pattern of bladder emptying to prevent incontinence for persons with limited cognitive ability who have urge, stress, or functional incontinence

NURSING PRIORITY NO. 1. To assess causative/contributing factors:

- Identify physiologic causes of increased intra-abdominal pressure (e.g., obesity, gravid uterus). Note contributing history such as multiple births, bladder or pelvic trauma/repairs, weak pelvic muscles. *Identification of specifics of individual situation provides for developing an accurate plan of care.*[1]

• Assess for urine loss with coughing or sneezing, relaxed pelvic musculature and support, noting inability to start/stop stream while voiding, bulging of perineum when bearing down. *Severity of symptoms may indicate need for more specialized evaluation.*

 • Refer to urologic specialists. *Diagnosing urinary incontinence requires a comprehensive history and physical examination, as well as specific laboratory and diagnostic tests (e.g., urinalysis, urine culture/sensitivity and cytology, postvoid residuals, pelvic ultrasound, radiographs, and cystogram). A urodynamic evaluation (measuring bladder filling and capacity, cough stress test, and rate of urinary flow) may also be ordered to differentiate stress incontinence from other types.*[2–4]

• Catheterize as indicated. *May be needed to rule out the possibility of postvoid residuals that would require further evaluation.*[5]

NURSING PRIORITY NO. 2. To assess degree of interference/disability:

 • Observe voiding patterns, time and amount voided, and note the stimulus provoking incontinence. Review voiding diary if available. *Provides information that can help determine type of incontinence and type of treatment indicated.*[6]

• Prepare for/assist with appropriate testing, (e.g., cystoscopy, cystometrogram). *Providing information about what is to be expected; ensuring privacy reduces anxiety client may have about testing.*[3,4,7]

 • Determine effect on lifestyle (including socialization and sexuality) and self-esteem. *Untreated incontinence can have emotional and physical consequences. Urinary tract infections, skin rashes, and sores can occur. Self-esteem is affected and the client may suffer from depression and withdraw from social activities.*[6]

 • Ascertain methods of self-management. *Client may already be limiting liquid intake, voiding before any activity, and/or using undergarment protection.*[6]

 • Assess for concomitant urge or functional incontinence, noting whether bladder irritability, reduced bladder capacity, or voluntary overdistention is present. (Refer to NDs: impaired Urinary Elimination, Urinary Incontinence (specify functional, reflex, or total). *Mixed incontinence, consisting of two or more kinds of incontinence, may occur and impacts treatment choices.*[6]

NURSING PRIORITY NO. 3. To assist in treating/preventing incontinence:

• Assist with medical treatment of underlying urologic condition as indicated. *Stress incontinence may be treated with surgical intervention (e.g., bladder neck suspension, pubovaginal sling, gynecologic or prostate surgery) and nonsurgical therapies (e.g., pelvic floor exercise, biofeedback, electric stimulation, medications).*[8,9]

 • Suggest client urinate at least every 3 hours during the day to reduce bladder pressure. Recommend consciously delaying voiding as appropriate to slowly achieve desired 3- to 4-hour intervals between voids. *Training the bladder by gradually increasing the time between voidings can promote larger bladder capacity and more acceptable time between bathroom breaks.*[6]

 • Suggest starting and stopping stream two or three times during voiding, when client is doing bladder retraining. *Isolates muscles involved in voiding process so client can begin exercise training (Kegel exercises).*[10]

 • Encourage regular pelvic floor strengthening exercises (Kegel exercises or use of vaginal cones). Combine activity with biofeedback as appropriate *to enhance training for controlling pelvic muscles. Muscle toning exercises can help alleviate stress incontinence in both men and women. These exercises involve tightening the muscles of the pelvic floor and need to be done numerous times throughout the day.*[6]

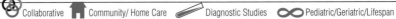 Cultural　Collaborative　Community/ Home Care　Diagnostic Studies　Pediatric/Geriatric/Lifespan　Medications

- Incorporate "bent-knee sit-ups" into exercise program. *Increasing abdominal muscle tone can help relieve stress incontinence.*[11]
- Restrict intake 2–3 hours before bedtime. *Decreasing the amount of evening fluid intake reduces the need for awakening to void, resulting in more restful sleep.*[5]
- Administer medications as indicated (e.g., alpha-adrenergic drugs *to increase bladder outlet contractions;* estrogens *to increase urethral muscle tone,* tricyclic antidepressants *to treat mixed bladder dysfunction, etc.)*[9]

NURSING PRIORITY NO. 4. To promote wellness (Teaching/Discharge Considerations):

- Encourage limiting use of coffee/tea and alcohol. *Diuretic effect of these substances may lead to bladder distention, increasing likelihood of incontinence.*[12]
- Suggest use of incontinence pads/pants as needed. *Considering client's activity level, amount of urine loss, physical size, manual dexterity, and cognitive ability to determine specific product choices best suited to individual situation and needs may be necessary when leakage continues to occur in spite of other measures.*[9,13]
- Stress importance of perineal care following voiding and frequent changing of incontinence pads. Recommend application of oil-based emollient. *Prevents infection and protects skin from irritation.*[13]
- Avoid/limit participation in activities such as heavy lifting, impact aerobics. Substitute swimming, bicycling, or low-impact exercise. *These activities increase intra-abdominal pressure, increasing possibility of the occurrence of incontinence.*[12]
- Refer to weight-loss program/support group. *When obesity is a contributing factor, losing weight may reduce intra-abdominal pressure and improve problems of incontinence.*[7]
- Review use of drugs, if prescribed, such as estrogen hormone replacement, anticholinergics, (i.e., propantheline or Pro-Banthine), antispasmodics (i.e., oxybutynin or Ditropan). *May improve resting tone of the bladder neck and proximal urethra and relax the bladder muscles.*[6,14]

DOCUMENTATION FOCUS

Assessment/Reassessment
- Findings/pattern of incontinence and physical factors present.
- Effect on lifestyle and self-esteem.
- Client understanding of condition.

Planning
- Plan of care and who is involved in the planning.
- Teaching plan.

Implementation/Evaluation
- Responses to interventions/teaching, actions performed, and changes that are identified.
- Attainment/progress toward desired outcome(s).
- Modifications to plan of care.

Discharge Planning
- Long-term needs, referrals, and who is responsible for specific actions.
- Specific referrals made.

References

1. Doenges, M. E., Moorhouse, M. F., & Geissler-Murr, A. C. (2004). Nurse's Pocket Guide: Diagnoses, Interventions, and Rationales, ed 9. Philadelphia: F. A. Davis.
2. Urinary Incontinence. Available at: http://www.hmc.psu.edu/healthinfo/uz/urinaryincontinence.htm. Accessed February 2004.
3. No author listed. (1996). Urinary incontinence. American Medical Directors Association (AMDA). Available at: http://www.guidleine.gov. Accessed September 2003.
4. Guerrero, P., & Sinert, R. (2002). Urinary incontinence. Available at: http://www.emedicine.com. Accessed September 2003.
5. Doenges, M. E., Moorhouse, M. F., & Geissler-Murr, A. C. (2002): Nursing Care Plans: Guidelines for Individualizing Patient Care, ed 6. Philadelphia: F. A. Davis.
6. Ford-Martin, P. A. (1999). Urinary Incontinence. Gale Encyclopedia of Medicine. Gale Research. Available at: http://www.findarticles.com/cf_0/g2601001430/p3/article.jhtml?term. Accessed September 2003.
7. Beers, M. H., & Berkow, R. (Eds). (1999). The Merck Manual of Diagnosis and Therapy, ed 17. Whitehouse Station, NJ: Merck Research Laboratories.
8. Choe, J. M. (2003). Incontinence, urinary: Surgical therapies. Available at: http://www.emedicine.com. Accessed September 2003.
9. Choe, J. M. (2002). Incontinence, urinary: Nonsurgical therapies. Available at: http://www.emedicine.com. Accessed September 2003.
10. Wyman, J. F. (2003). Treatment of urinary incontinence in men and older women. In Newman, D. K., & Palmer, M. H. (eds). The state of the science on urinary incontinence. Am J Nurs, 293, 3(suppl), 20.
11. ND: Urinary Incontinence, stress. In Cox, H. C., et al. (2002). Clinical Applications of Nursing Diagnosis: Adult, Child, Women's, Psychiatric, Gerontic, and Home Health Considerations, ed 4. Philadelphia: F. A. Davis.
12. Newman, D. K., & Palmer, M. H. (eds). (2003). The state of the science on urinary incontinence. Am J Nurs, 293, 3(suppl), 20.
13. What is urinary incontinence? Available at: http://ourworld.compuserve.com/homepages/nacs/INCONT.HTM. Accessed September 2003.
14. Booth, C. (2002). Introduction to Urinary Incontinence. Hosp Pharmacist, 9(3), 65–68.

total Urinary Incontinence

Definition: Continuous and unpredictable loss of urine

RELATED FACTORS

Neuropathy preventing transmission of reflex [signals to the reflex arc] indicating bladder fullness

Neurologic dysfunction [e.g., cerebral lesions] causing triggering of micturition at unpredictable times

Independent contraction of detrusor reflex due to surgery

Trauma or disease affecting spinal cord nerves [destruction of sensory or motor neurons below the injury level]

Anatomic (fistula)

DEFINING CHARACTERISTICS

Subjective

Constant flow of urine at unpredictable times without uninhibited bladder contractions/ spasm or distention

Nocturia

Lack of perineal or bladder filling awareness

Unawareness of incontinence

Objective

Unsuccessful incontinence refractory treatments

 Cultural Collaborative  Community/ Home Care Diagnostic Studies 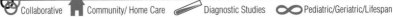 Pediatric/Geriatric/Lifespan 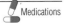 Medications

SAMPLE CLINICAL APPLICATIONS: spinal cord injury/nerve compression, spina bifida, myelomeningocele, Guillain-Barré, brain injury/stroke, hydrocephalus, MS, cerebral palsy, Parkinson's disease, diabetes mellitus, abdominal trauma, dementia

DESIRED OUTCOMES/EVALUATION CRITERIA

Sample **NOC** linkages:

Urinary Continence: Control of the elimination of urine

Self-Care: Hygiene: Ability to maintain own hygiene

Tissue Integrity: Skin & Mucous Membranes: Structural intactness and normal physiologic function of skin and mucous membranes

Client/Caregiver Will (Include Specific Time Frame)

- Verbalize awareness of causative/contributing factors.
- Establish bladder regimen for individual situation.
- Demonstrate behaviors, techniques to manage condition and to prevent complications.
- Manage incontinence so that social functioning is regained/maintained.

ACTIONS/INTERVENTIONS

Sample **NIC** linkages:

Urinary Incontinence Care: Assistance in promoting continence and maintaining perineal skin integrity

Urinary Catheterization: Insertion of a catheter into the bladder for temporary or permanent drainage of urine

Perineal Care: Maintenance of perineal skin integrity and relief of perineal discomfort

NURSING PRIORITY NO. **1.** To assess causative/contributing factors:

- Identify client with condition(s) causing actual/potential for total incontinence as listed in Related Factors: *High-risk persons include frail elderly, women, presence of brain lesions/disease (e.g., stroke, cancer, Parkinson's disease, cerebral palsy, hydrocephalus, dementia); spinal cord injury (e.g., quadriplegia, paraplegia, herniated disk, pelvic crush injury); chronic neurologic diseases (e.g., multiple sclerosis, child with myelomeningocele), pregnancy, prolonged labor, early postpartum period; genitourinary surgery/trauma(e.g., radical hysterectomy, abdominoperineal resection); peripheral neuropathy (e.g., diabetes mellitus, AIDS, poliomyelitis, Guillain-Barré); and lifestyle issues (e.g., certain medications, irritating foods, fluid intake, mobility limitations).* [1,2]
- Determine if client is aware of incontinence. *In the presence of neurologic or cognitive impairment, client may not be able to sense loss of urine.* [3]
- Be aware of/note effect of medical history of global neurologic impairment, neuromuscular trauma after surgery/radiation therapy or childbirth, or presence of fistula. *Injury to the nerves supplying the bladder can result in constant loss of urine because of loss of integrity of lower urinary tract function. Presence of vesicovaginal fistula may also cause incontinence.* [3]
- Check for perineal sensation and fecal impaction *to determine whether sensation and reflexes are impaired when neurologic condition is present.* [1,4]
- Determine concomitant chronic retention through palpation of bladder, ultrasound scan/catheterize for residual. *Rather than relaxing when the bladder contracts, the outlet contracts leading to severe outlet obstruction.* [3]
- Observe for overflow incontinence *due to chronic urinary retention or secondary to flaccid bladder associated with obstructive or neuropathic lesion.* [1,2]
- Assess for continuous incontinence (i.e., involuntary loss of urine at all times and in all positions), *usually associated with urinary tract fistula or genital malformation.* [1,2]

- Carry out/assist with procedures/tests (e.g., postvoid residual, urine flow rate, pressure flow studies, cystoscopy, filling and voiding cystogram). *Establishes diagnosis/identifies appropriateness of surgical repair/other treatments.*[1,5]

NURSING PRIORITY NO. 2. To assess degree of interference/disability:

- Have client/care provider(s) keep an incontinence chart. Note times of voiding and incontinence. *Determines pattern of urination and whether there is any control.*[1,4]
- Ascertain effect of condition on lifestyle and self-esteem. *Incontinence is embarrassing and distressing and may severely affect the quality of life for the individual and even family members.*[6]
- Inspect skin for areas of erythema/excoriation. *Constant loss of urine can abraid the skin causing breakdown if not cared for frequently.*[5]
- Review history for past episodes of impaired urinary elimination. *Provides information about interventions that were successful previously and could help manage current situation.*[5]

NURSING PRIORITY NO. 3. To assist in preventing/managing incontinence:

- Collaborate with physician/urologist/rehabilitation team to implement bladder training program and/or incontinence management, as indicated:

  Provide ready access to bathroom, commode, bedpan, or urinal

  Encourage at least 1500–2000 mL liquid intake per day. Regulate liquid intake at prescheduled times (with and between meals). *Ensures an adequate fluid intake and promotes a predictable voiding pattern where possible.*[4]

  Restrict intake 2–3 hours before bedtime. *Reduces need for wakening during the night for voiding and/or limits nighttime incontinence.*[4]

  Establish voiding schedule by toileting at same time as recorded voidings and 30 minutes earlier than recorded time of incontinence. *Bladder training may be an effective strategy when neurologic impairment is not extensive.*[6]

  Encourage measures such as pouring warm water over perineum, running water in sink, massaging lower abdomen. *These measures can stimulate voiding; however they may not be successful if reflex is not intact.*[6]

  Adjust schedule, once continent, by increasing voiding time in 30-minute increments to achieve desired 3- to 4-hour intervals between voids. *Depending on degree of neurologic impairment, bladder training may be helpful to individual client.*[7]

  Use condom catheter or female cone during the day and pad the bed during the night if external device is not tolerated. *Maintains dry clothing and bedding, preventing skin irritation, odor with resultant embarrassment.*[4]

  Implement catheterization appropriate to client's conditions (e.g., indwelling urethral or suprapubic catheter *as might be needed to 1) promote comfort for terminally ill; 2) to avoid contamination or to promote healing of severe pressure ulcers; 3) severely impaired indiviual in whom other interventions (e.g., bladder training, self-catheterization) are not an option; 4) person lives alone and cannot provide own supportive care.*[2]

  Demonstrate techniques of clean intermittent self-catheterization (CISC) using small-lumen straight catheter (or Mitrofanoff continent urinary channel for clients not able to catheterize themselves) as indicated. *In the presence of neurologic damage and when client is cognitively competent, these measures can assure a successful management program.*[8,9]

  Implement dietary changes where indicated. *Client may need to eliminate foods that are highly spicy or acidic and foods or fluids containing caffeine.*[9]

 Cultural   Collaborative   Community/ Home Care   Diagnostic Studies 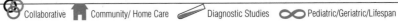 Pediatric/Geriatric/Lifespan   Medications

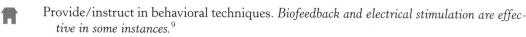

Provide/instruct in behavioral techniques. *Biofeedback and electrical stimulation are effective in some instances.*[9]

Administer medications as indicated. *Various categories and combinations of drugs may be used to treat symptoms, depending on the type(s) of incontinence diagnosed.*[9]

Discuss/prepare for surgical intervention when indicated. *Many forms of surgical repair have been developed depending on underlying cause (e.g., to treat urethral hypermobility, to suspend the bladder, to repair vaginal walls, remove obstructions; provide artificial sphincter or bladder reservoir).*[7,10]

Refer to ND: functional/stress/reflex Urinary Incontinence for additional interventions specfic to diagnosis.

NURSING PRIORITY NO. 4. To promote wellness (Teaching/Discharge Considerations):

- Assist client to identify regular period of time for voiding. *Can be helpful to establish elimination program that meets individual needs.*[6]
- Suggest use of incontinence pads/adult briefs as indicated. *Provides protection during social contacts and enhances confidence when other measures have not been successful.*[7]
- Stress importance of pericare after voiding (using alcohol-free products) and application of oil-based emollient. *Protects the skin from irritation from the constant flow of urine.*[5]
- Instruct in proper care of catheter and clean technique. *Reduces risk of infection when client is using catheterization on a regular basis.*[6]
- Recommend use of silicone catheter. *When long-term/continuous placement is indicated after other measures/bladder training have failed, silicone catheter has less problems with deterioration and infection than latex products.*[5]
- Encourage self-monitoring of catheter patency and avoidance of reflux of urine. *Reduces risk of infection.*[5]
- Suggest intake of acidifying juices, such as cranberry. *Discourages bacterial growth/adherence to bladder wall preventing recurrent infections.*[5]

DOCUMENTATION FOCUS

Assessment/Reassessment
- Current elimination pattern.
- Assessment findings including effect on lifestyle and self-esteem.

Planning
- Plan of care/interventions, including who is involved in planning.
- Teaching plan.

Implementation/Evaluation
- Response to interventions/teaching and actions performed.
- Attainment/progress toward desired outcome(s).
- Modifications to plan of care.

Discharge Planning
- Discharge plan/long-term needs and who is responsible for actions to be taken.
- Specific referrals made.

References

1. Guerrero, P., & Sinert, R. (2002). Urinary incontinence. Available at: http://www.emedicine.com. Accessed September 2003.
2. Choe, J. M., & Mardovin, W. Neurogenic bladder. Available at: http://www.emedicine.com. Accessed September 2003.
3. Beers, M. H., & Berkow, R. (eds). (1999). The Merck Manual of Diagnosis and Therapy, ed 17. Whitehouse Station, NJ: Merck Research Laboratories.
4. ND: Urinary Incontinence. In Cox, H. C., et al. (2002). Clinical Applications of Nursing Diagnosis: Adult, Child, Women's Psychiatric, Gerontic, and Home Health Considerations, ed 4. Philadelphia: F. A. Davis.
5. Doenges, M. E., Moorhouse, M. F., & Geissler-Murr, A. C. (2002). Nursing Care Plans: Guidelines for Individualizing Patient Care, ed 6. Philadelphia: F. A. Davis.
6. Newman, D. K., & Palmer, M. H. (eds). (2003). The state of the science on urinary incontinence. Am J Nurs, 293, 3(suppl), 20.
7. Booth, C. (2002). Introduction to urinary incontinence. Hospital Pharmacist, 9(3), 65–68.
8. Understanding Female Urinary Incontinence. Family Doctor Series. Available at: http://www.familydoctor.co.uk. Accessed September 2003.
9. Choe, J. M. (2002). Incontinence, urinary: Nonsurgical therapies. Available at: http://www.emedicine.com. Accessed September 2003.
10. Choe, J. M. (2003). Incontinence, urinary: Surgical therapies. Available at: http://www.emedicine.com. Accessed September 2003.

urge Urinary Incontinence

Definition: Involuntary passage of urine occurring soon after a strong sense of urgency to void

RELATED FACTORS

Decreased bladder capacity (e.g., history of pelvic inflammatory disease—PID, abdominal surgeries, indwelling urinary catheter)

Irritation of bladder stretch receptors causing spasm (e.g., bladder infection, [atrophic urethritis, vaginitis]; alcohol, caffeine, increased fluids; increased urine concentration; overdistention of bladder

[Medication use, such as diuretics, sedatives, anticholinergic agents]

[Constipation/stool impaction]

[Restricted mobility; psychological disorder such as depression, change in mentation/confusional state, e.g., stroke, dementia, Parkinson's disease]

DEFINING CHARACTERISTICS

Subjective
Urinary urgency
Frequency (voiding more often than every 2 hours)
Bladder contracture/spasm
Nocturia (more than 2 times per night)

Objective
Inability to reach toilet in time
Voiding in small amounts (<100 cc) or in large amounts (>550 cc)

SAMPLE CLINICAL APPLICATIONS: abdominal trauma/surgery, PID, recurrent UTIs, brain injury/stroke, MS, Parkinson's disease, diabetes mellitus, dementia

DESIRED OUTCOMES/EVALUATION CRITERIA
Sample **NOC** linkages:
Urinary Continence: Control of the elimination of urine

 Cultural Collaborative Community/ Home Care Diagnostic Studies 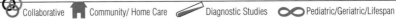 Pediatric/Geriatric/Lifespan Medications

Cognitive Ability: Ability to execute complex mental processes
Self-Care: Toileting: Ability to toilet self

Client Will (Include Specific Time Frame)
- Verbalize understanding of condition.
- Demonstrate behaviors/techniques to control/correct situation.
- Report increase in interval between urge and involuntary loss of urine.
- Void every 3–4 hours in individually appropriate amounts.

ACTIONS/INTERVENTIONS
Sample **NIC** linkages:

Urinary Habit Training: Establishing a predictable pattern of bladder emptying to prevent incontinence for persons with limited cognitive ability who have urge, stress, or functional incontinence

Urinary Incontinence Care: Assistance in promoting continence and maintaining perineal skin integrity

Perineal Care: Maintenance of perineal skin integrity and relief of perineal discomfort

NURSING PRIORITY NO. **1.** To assess causative/contributing factors:

- Assess for signs and symptoms of cloudy, odorous urine; bacteriuria. *Indicative of bladder infection and need for treatment. Incontinence often leads to/or reflects urinary tract infections.*[1]
- Determine use/presence of bladder irritants. *Significant intake of alcohol or caffeine can result in increased output or concentrated urine that may make the bladder more irritable.*[2]
- Determine whether there is a history of long-standing habits or medical conditions such as severe PID, abdominal surgeries, recent/lengthy use of indwelling urinary catheter, or frequent voluntary voiding. *May reduce bladder capacity resulting in loss of urine at unexpected times.*[1]
- Note factors that may affect ability to respond to urge to void. *Impaired mobility, use of sedation, cognitive impairments may result in client not recognizing need to void or moving too slowly to make it to the bathroom, with subsequent loss of urine.*[3]
- Clinitest urine for glucose. *Presence of glucose in urine causes polyuria, resulting in overdistention of the bladder and inability to hold urine until reaching the bathroom.*[4]
- Assess for concomitant functional incontinence. Refer to ND functional Urinary Incontinence.
- Palpate bladder for overdistention. Rule out high postvoid residuals via palpation/catheterization/ultrasound. *An overdistended bladder, detrusor underactivity may result in urinary retention that must be ruled out before starting treatment.*[5]
- Prepare for/assist with appropriate testing. *Urinalysis, ultrasound and cystometry are a few of the tests that can be used to identify the type of incontinence and appropriate treatment.*[3,4]

NURSING PRIORITY NO. **2.** To assess degree of interference/disability:

- Measure amount of urine voided, especially noting amounts less than 100 cc or greater than 550 cc. *Provides information about amount of urine required to initiate desire to void and loss of urine and interventions indicated.*[6]
- Record frequency and degree of urgency. *Maintaining a voiding diary identifies degree of difficulty being experienced by client.*[7]
- Note length of warning time between initial urge and loss of urine. *Overactivity or irritabil-*

ity decreases the length of time between urge and loss and helps clarify the type of incontinence.[2]

- Ascertain effect on lifestyle. *There is a considerable reduction in the quality of life of individuals with an incontinence problem, affecting socialization and view of themselves as sexual beings and sense of self-esteem.*[4]

NURSING PRIORITY NO. 3. To assist in treating/preventing incontinence:

- Increase fluid intake to 1500–2000 mL/day. *Sufficient fluid intake is important for kidney and bladder functioning and promotes successful bladder training program.*[7]
- Regulate liquid intake at prescheduled times, with and between meals. *Promotes a predictable voiding pattern to enhance bladder training.*[8]
- Provide assistance/devices as indicated for clients who are mobility impaired. *Providing means of summoning assistance, placing bedside commode, urinal, or bedpan within reach helps to avoid unintended loss of urine and promotes sense of control over situation.*[7]
- Establish schedule for voiding based on client's usual voiding pattern. *Bladder training program is highly successful in the control of urge incontinence.*[7]
- Instruct client to tighten pelvic floor muscles before arising from bed. *Helps prevent loss of urine as abdominal pressure changes.*[7]
- Suggest starting and stopping stream two or more times during voiding. *Isolates muscles involved in voiding process for exercise training (Kegel's) that is highly successful for controlling incontinence.*[7]
- Encourage regular pelvic floor strengthening exercise (Kegel exercises or use of vaginal cones). Combine activity with biofeedback as appropriate. *Enhances effectiveness of training and success at controlling incontinence.*[7]
- Set alarm to awaken during night if indicated. *May be necessary to continue voiding schedule.*[7]
- Recommend consciously delaying voiding to gradually increase intervals between voiding to every 2–4 hours. *Expands the capacity of the bladder and allows individual to successfully wait for longer periods between voidings.*[4]
- Suggest client take advantage of every opportunity to use the bathroom. *Emptying the bladder frequently can prevent overdistention and unexpected loss of urine.*[9]

NURSING PRIORITY NO. 4. To promote wellness (Teaching/Discharge Considerations):

- Suggest limiting intake of coffee/tea and alcohol. *These substances have an irritating effect on the bladder and may be worth a trial to see if there is any benefit.*[2]
- Recommend use of incontinence pads/pants if necessary. *Considering client's level of activity, amount of urine loss, physical size, manual dexterity, and cognitive ability will identify correct type and size of pads/pants to use for maximum protection.*[8]
- Suggest wearing loose fitting or especially adapted clothing. *Facilitates response to voiding urge especially in older individuals who may have difficulty managing restrictive clothing fasteners.*[8]
- Emphasize importance of perineal care after each voiding. *Prevents skin irritation and reduces potential for bladder infection.*[9]
- Identify signs/symptoms indicating urinary complications and need for medical follow-up. *Helps client be aware and seek intervention in a timely manner to prevent more serious problems from developing.*[7]
- Review use of anticholinergics, if prescribed. *These drugs are used to increase warning time*

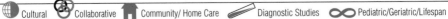

by blocking impulses within the sacral reflex arc and when used along with bladder training can provide a substantial reduction in symptoms.[4]

 • Discuss possible surgical intervention or use of electronic stimulation therapy. *May be appropriate when conservative measures have failed, to induce bladder contraction/inhibit detrusor overactivity as appropriate. Different surgical interventions have been developed to cure various forms of incontinence and minimize surgical trauma, decreasing the length of hospitalization.*[4]

DOCUMENTATION FOCUS

Assessment/Reassessment
- Individual findings, including pattern of incontinence, effect on lifestyle and self-esteem.

Planning
- Plan of care/interventions and who is involved in planning.
- Teaching plan.

Implementation/Evaluation
- Response to interventions/teaching and actions performed.
- Attainment/progress toward desired outcome(s).
- Modifications to plan of care.

Discharge Planning
- Discharge needs/referrals and who is responsible for actions to be taken.
- Specific referrals made.

References

1. Wyman, J. F. (2003). Treatment of urinary incontinence in men and older women. In Newman, D. K, & Palmer, M. H. (eds). The state of the science on urinary incontinence. Am J Nurs, 293, 3(suppl), 20.
2. What is urinary incontinence? Available at: http://ourworld.compuserve.com/homepages/nacs/INCONT.HTM. Accessed September 2003.
3. Urinary incontinence. Available at: http://www.hmc.psu.edu/healthinfo/uz/urinaryincontinence.htm. Accessed February 2004.
4. Booth, C. (2002). Introduction to urinary incontinence. Hosp Pharmacist, 9(3), 65–68.
5. Beers, M. H., & Berkow, R. (eds). (1999). The Merck Manual of Diagnosis and Therapy, ed 17. Whitehouse Station, NJ: Merck Research Laboratories.
6. Doenges, M. E., Moorhouse, M. F., & Geissler-Murr, A. C. (2004). Nurse's Pocket Guide: Diagnoses, Interventions, and Rationales, ed 9. Philadelphia: F. A. Davis.
7. Newman, D. K., & Palmer, M. H. (eds). (2003). The state of the science on urinary incontinence. Am J Nurs, 293, 3(suppl), 20.
8. Ford-Martin, P. A. (1999). Urinary incontinence. Gale Encyclopedia of Medicine. Gale Research. Available at: http://www.findarticles.com/cf_0/g2601001430/p3/article.jhtml?term. Accessed September 2003.
9. ND: Urinary Incontinence. In Cox, H. C., et al. (2002). Clinical Applications of Nursing Diagnosis: Adult, Child, Women's, Psychiatric, Gerontic, and Home Health Considerations, ed 4. Philadelphia: F. A. Davis.

risk for urge Urinary Incontinence

Definition: At risk for an involuntary loss of urine associated with a sudden, strong sensation or urinary urgency

RISK FACTORS

Effects of medications; caffeine; alcohol

Detrusor hyperreflexia from cystitis, urethritis, tumors, renal calculi, CNS disorders above pontine micturition center

---

Detrusor muscle instability with impaired contractility; involuntary sphincter relaxation

Ineffective toileting habits

Small bladder capacity

NOTE: A risk diagnosis is not evidenced by signs and symptoms, as the problem has not occurred and nursing interventions are directed at prevention.

SAMPLE CLINICAL APPLICATIONS: MS, BPH, recurrent UTIs, renal calculi, pelvic surgery/ radiation, Guillain-Barré, dementia, major depression

DESIRED OUTCOMES/EVALUATION CRITERIA

Sample **NOC** linkages:

Urinary Continence: Control of the elimination of urine

Risk Control: Actions to eliminate or reduce actual, personal, and modifiable health threats

Neurologic Status: Autonomic: Extent to which the autonomic nervous system coordinates visceral function

---

Client Will (Include Specific Time Frame)

- Identify individual risk factors and appropriate interventions.
- Demonstrate behaviors or lifestyle changes to prevent development of problem.

ACTIONS/INTERVENTIONS

Sample **NIC** linkages:

Urinary Habit Training: Establishing a predictable pattern of bladder emptying to prevent incontinence for persons with limited cognitive ability who have urge, stress, or functional incontinence

Self-Care Assistance: Toileting: Assisting another with elimination

Prompted Voiding: Promotion of urinary continence through the use of timed verbal toileting reminders and positive social feedback for successful toileting

NURSING PRIORITY NO. 1. To assess potential for developing incontinence:

- Assess client for potential problem with urge incontinence when taking health history, as appropriate. *The elderly, frail adult in long-term care institutions, women, individuals with cognitive, neurologic and mobility impairments; persons with history of frequent bladder infections; women in prolonged labor or undergoing pelvic surgery; men with prostatic hyperplasia or prostate surgery, are at highest risk of developing incontinence (either temporary or permanent).*[1]

- Review history for long-standing habits or current conditions that may affect bladder capacity or function. *Impaired mobility, use of certain drugs (e.g., diuretics, sedatives, alcohol); neurologic conditions (stroke, multiple sclerosis, spinal cord injury); delirium or dementias; abdominal surgery or distention, fecal impaction, etc. may impair bladder function leading to possibility of incontinence.*[2,3]

- Note factors that may affect ability to respond to urge to void: *1) Impaired mobility such as in stroke, spinal cord injury, 2) lack of access to toilet, 3) impaired awareness (either cognition or sensation), 4) restraints, 5) drugs that affect the bladder (i.e., beta-blockers and cholinergic drugs can cause increased detrusor tone; neuroleptics, antidepressants, sedatives, hypnotics, opiates, calcium antagonists can cause detrusor relaxation; antiepileptics, muscle relaxants and psychoactive drugs can cause sphincter relaxation) can all affect the bladder and the client's ability to respond in a timely manner.*[2,4]

- Determine use/presence of bladder irritants. *A significant intake of alcohol or caffeine can*

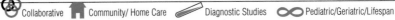

result in increased output or concentrated urine and contribute to the possibility of incontinence.[5]

• Prepare for/assist with appropriate testing. *Accurate assessment and diagnosis (e.g., urinalysis, urine culture, urine/serum glucose, voiding cystometrogram) can evaluate voiding pattern and identify pathology, which may lead to the development of incontinence.*[2,4]

NURSING PRIORITY NO. 2. To prevent occurrence of problem:

• Measure amount of urine voided, especially noting amounts less than 100 mL or greater than 550 mL. *Provides information about amount of urine required to initiate desire to void, as well as potential for dehydration or excessive fluid loss if large voidings are frequent.*[6]

• Record intake and frequency/degree of urgency of voiding. *May reveal developing incontinence problem when need to void is more frequent and urgent in relation to normal fluid intake.*[7]

• Ascertain client's awareness/concerns about developing problem and whether lifestyle is affected (e.g., socialization, sexual patterns). *Provides information regarding the degree of concern client is experiencing and need for preventive measures to be instituted.*[8]

• Regulate liquid intake at prescheduled times (with and between meals). *Promotes a predictable voiding pattern to establish a bladder-training program to prevent incontinence.*[5]

• Establish schedule for voiding. *Bladder training program based on client's usual voiding pattern and strengthening perineal area muscles can successfully reduce risk for incontinence.*[8]

• Provide assistance/devices as indicated for clients who are mobility impaired. *Providing means of summoning assistance; placing bedside commode, urinal, or bedpan within client's reach can promote sense of control by managing voiding by self.*[9]

• Instruct client to tighten pelvic floor muscles before arising from bed. *Helps prevent loss of urine as abdominal pressure changes.*[9]

• Suggest starting and stopping stream two or more times during voiding. *Isolates and identifies muscles involved in voiding process for training, so client can exercise control and avoid unwanted loss of urine.*[10]

• Encourage regular pelvic floor strengthening exercise (Kegel exercises or use of vaginal cones). Combine activity with biofeedback, as appropriate. *Enhances effectiveness of training, preventing progression of incontinence problem.*[5]

NURSING PRIORITY NO. 3. To promote wellness (Teaching/Discharge Considerations):

• Recommend limiting intake of coffee/tea and alcohol. *These substances have an irritating effect on the bladder and may contribute to incontinence.*[7]

• Suggest wearing loose fitting or especially adapted clothing. *Facilitates response to voiding urge, especially in elderly or infirm individuals, enabling them to reach the bathroom without unwanted loss of urine.*[11]

• Emphasize importance of perineal care after each voiding. *Reduces risk of ascending infection.*[12]

• Discuss use of hormone (conjugated estrogens—Premarin) cream vaginally. *Strengthens urethral tissues, enabling women to control passage of urine more effectively.*[13]

Assessment/Reassessment
Individual findings, including specific risk factors and pattern of voiding.

Planning
Plan of care/interventions and who is involved in planning.
Teaching plan.

Implementation/Evaluation
Response to interventions/teaching and actions performed.
Attainment/progress toward desired outcome(s).
Modifications to plan of care.

Discharge Planning
Discharge needs/referrals and who is responsible for actions to be taken.
Specific referrals made.

References

1. Guerrero, P., & Sinert, R. (2002). Urinary incontinence. Available at: http://www.emedicine.com. Accessed September 2003.
2. Booth, C. (2002). Introduction to urinary incontinence. Hosp Pharmacist, 9(3), 65–68.
3. No author listed. (2000). Evidence-based clinical practice guideline—Continence for women. Washington: DC: Association of Women's Health, Obstetric and Neonatal Nurses (AWHONN). Available at: http://guideline.gov. Accessed January 2004.
4. No author listed. (1996). Urinary incontinence. American Medical Directors Association (AMDA). Available at: http://www.guidleine.gov. Accessed September 2003.
5. Newman, D. K., & Palmer, M. H. (eds). (2003). The state of the science on urinary incontinence. Am J Nurs, 293, 3(suppl), 20.
6. Doenges, M. E, Moorhouse, M. F., and Geissler-Murr, A. C. (2004). Nurse's Pocket Guide: Diagnoses, Interventions, and Rationales, ed 9. Philadelphia: F. A. Davis.
7. What is urinary incontinence? Available at: http://ourworld.compuserve.com/homepages/nacs/INCONT.HTM. Accessed September 2003.
8. Ford-Martin, P. A. Urinary Incontinence. (1999). Gale Encyclopedia of Medicine. Gale Research. Available at: http://www.findarticles.com/cf_0/g2601001430/p3/article.jhtml?term. Accessed September 2003.
9. ND: Urinary Incontinence. In Cox, H. C., et al. (2002). Clinical Applications of Nursing Diagnosis: Adult, Child, Women's, Psychiatric, Gerontic, and Home Health Considerations, ed 4. Philadelphia: F. A. Davis.
10. Urinary Incontinence. Available at: http://www.hmc.psu.edu/healthinfo/uz/urinaryincontinece.htm. Accessed February 2004.
11. Wyman, J. F. (2003). Treatment of urinary incontinence in men and older women. In Newman, D. K., & Palmer, M. H. (eds). The state of the science on urinary incontinence. Am J Nurs, 293, 3(suppl), 20.
12. Doenges, M. E., Moorhouse, M. F., & Geissler-Murr, A. C. (2002). Nursing Care Plans: Guidelines for Individualizing Patient Care, ed 6. Philadelphia: F. A. Davis.
13. Beers, M. H., & Berkow, R. (eds). (1999). The Merck Manual of Diagnosis and Therapy, ed 17. Whitehouse Station, NJ: Merck Research Laboratories.

[acute/chronic] Urinary Retention

Definition: Incomplete emptying of the bladder

RELATED FACTORS
High urethral pressure caused by weak[/absent] detrusor
Inhibition of reflex arc

 Cultural Collaborative Community/ Home Care Diagnostic Studies Pediatric/Geriatric/Lifespan Medications

Strong sphincter; blockage [e.g., benign prostatic hypertrophy-BPH, perineal swelling]
[Habituation of reflex arc]
[Infections]
[Neurologic diseases/trauma]
[Use of medications with side effect of retention (e.g., atropine, belladonna, psychotropics, antihistamines, opiates)]

DEFINING CHARACTERISTICS

Subjective
Sensation of bladder fullness
Dribbling
Dysuria

Objective
Bladder distention
Small, frequent voiding or absence of urine output
Residual urine [150 mL or more]
Overflow incontinence
[Reduced stream]

SAMPLE CLINICAL APPLICATIONS: BPH, prostatitis, cancer, perineal surgery/birth trauma, urethral calculi, MS, spinal cord compression, UTI, genital herpes

DESIRED OUTCOMES/EVALUATION CRITERIA

Sample **NOC** linkages:

Urinary Elimination: Ability of the urinary system to filter wastes, conserve solutes, and collect and discharge urine in a healthy pattern

Symptom Control: Personal actions to minimize perceived adverse changes in physical and emotional functioning

Knowledge: Disease Process: Extent of understanding conveyed about a specific disease process

Client Will (Include Specific Time Frame)
- Verbalize understanding of causative factors and appropriate interventions for individual situation.
- Demonstrate techniques/behaviors to alleviate/prevent retention.
- Void in sufficient amounts with no palpable bladder distention; experience no postvoid residuals greater than 50 mL; have no dribbling/overflow.

ACTIONS/INTERVENTIONS

Acute
Sample **NIC** linkages:

Urinary Catheterization: Insertion of a catheter into the bladder for temporary or permanent drainage of urine

Fluid Monitoring: Collection and analysis of patient data to regulate fluid balance

NURSING PRIORITY NO. 1. To assess causative/contributing factors:

- Note presence of pathological conditions such as neurologic disease (e.g., MS, stroke), bladder/kidney infection, bladder stone formation; and reaction to medications, diagnostic dye, or anesthesia *that can cause mechanical obstruction, nerve dysfunction, ineffective contraction or decompensation of detrusor musculature, resulting in ineffective emptying of the bladder and urine retention.*[1]

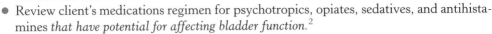

- Review client's medications regimen for psychotropics, opiates, sedatives, and antihistamines *that have potential for affecting bladder function.*[2]
- Determine anxiety level. *Client may be too embarrassed to void in presence of others, or to talk about problem with care providers.*[2]
- Examine for fecal impaction, surgical site swelling, postpartal edema, vaginal or rectal packing, enlarged prostate or other "mechanical" factors *that may produce a blockage of the urethra.*[2]
- Evaluate general hydration status.

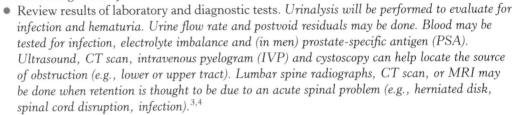

- Review results of laboratory and diagnostic tests. *Urinalysis will be performed to evaluate for infection and hematuria. Urine flow rate and postvoid residuals may be done. Blood may be tested for infection, electrolyte imbalance and (in men) prostate-specific antigen (PSA). Ultrasound, CT scan, intravenous pyelogram (IVP) and cystoscopy can help locate the source of obstruction (e.g., lower or upper tract). Lumbar spine radiographs, CT scan, or MRI may be done when retention is thought to be due to an acute spinal problem (e.g., herniated disk, spinal cord disruption, infection).*[3,4]

NURSING PRIORITY NO. 2. To determine degree of interference/disability:

- Ascertain if client can empty bladder completely, partially, or not at all, in spite of urge to urinate. *Signs of urinary retention, caused by either 1) blockage of the urethra, or 2) disruption of complex system of nerves that connects the urinary tract with the brain. In men, blockage is most commonly caused by enlargement of the prostate, cancer, stones, and urethral stricture. Causes that can occur in both sexes include scar tissue, injury (as in car accident or fall), blood clots, infection, tumors, and stones (rare). Disruption of nerves, or nerve transmission, or interpretation of signals can be caused by injury (e.g., spinal cord injury or tumor, herniated disc, stroke), pelvic infections, surgery, and certain medications.*[3]
- Catheterize/perform ultrasound for bladder residual after voiding *to determine presence/degree of urine retention.*[1]
- Determine if there has been any significant urine output in the previous 6–8 hours. *Small amount of urine may leak out of bladder, but generally not enough to relieve symptoms.*[3]
- Note recent amount/type of fluid intake. *Fluids may initially need to be restricted to prevent bladder distention until adequate urine flow is established.*[1]
- Palpate height of the bladder. Ascertain whether client has sensation of bladder fullness, level of discomfort. *Most people with acute retention also feel pain in lower abdomen (pelvis). Back pain, fever, and painful urination may be present with retention if the cause is urinary tract infection.*[3]

NURSING PRIORITY NO. 3. To assist in treating/preventing retention:

- Catheterize with intermittent or indwelling catheter *to resolve acute retention.*[2]
- Drain bladder slowly with straight catheter in increments of 200 mL at a time *to prevent possibility of occurrence of hematuria, syncope.*[2]
- Relieve pain by administering appropriate medications and measures *to reduce swelling/treat underlying cause.*[2]
- Sit client upright on bedpan/commode or stand *to provide functional position of voiding.*[2]

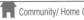 Cultural Collaborative Community/ Home Care Diagnostic Studies 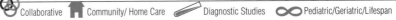 Pediatric/Geriatric/Lifespan Medications

- Encourage good urination habits (e.g., 4–6 times/day). *Frequent holding of urination for prolonged periods can, over time, weaken bladder muscles because of overstretching.*[3]
- Teach client with mild or moderate obstructive symptoms to "double void" by urinating, resting on toilet for 3–5 minutes, and then making a second attempt to urinate. *Promotes more efficient bladder evacuation by allowing the detrusor to contract initially, then rest and contract again.*[5]
- Use ice techniques, spirits of wintergreen, stroking inner thigh, running water in sink or warm water over perineum *to stimulate reflex arc.*[2]
- Remove blockage if possible (e.g., vaginal packing, bowel impaction), *when mechanical obstruction is restricting urine output.*[2]
- Provide adequate fluid intake, including use of acidifying fruit juices or ingestion of vitamin C/Mandelamine *to discourage bacterial growth and stone formation.*[2]
- Prepare for more aggressive intervention (e.g., reconstructive surgery, lithotripsy, prostatectomy, etc.) as indicated *to remove source of obstruction, reconstruct sphincter, or provide for urinary diversion.*[2]
- Reduce recurrences *by controlling causative/contributing factors when possible (e.g., ice to perineum to limit welling timed voiding, use of electrical stimulation, use of stool softeners/laxatives, change of medication/dosage, etc.).*[2]

NURSING PRIORITY NO. 4. To promote wellness (Teaching/Discharge Considerations):

- Encourage client to report problems immediately *so treatment can be instituted promptly.*[2]
- Emphasize need for adequate fluid intake.

Chronic

Sample **NIC** linkages:

Urinary Retention Care: Assistance in relieving bladder distention

Exercise Therapy: Muscle Control: Use of specific activity or exercise protocols to enhance or restore controlled body movement

NURSING PRIORITY NO. 1. To assess causative/contributing factors:

- Review medical history for diagnoses such as prostatic hypertrophy, scarring, recurrent stone formation *that may suggest detrusor muscle atrophy and/or chronic overdistention because of outlet obstruction.*[2]
- Determine presence of weak or absent sensory and/or motor impulses (as with CVAs, spinal injury, or diabetes) *that predispose client to compromised enervation or interpretation of sensory signals resulting in impaired urination.*[2]
- Evaluate customary fluid intake.
- Assess client's medication regimen (e.g., psychotropic, antihistamines, atropine, belladonna,) and consult with physician *regarding client's continued use of those that are known to potentiate urinary retention.*[2]
- Strain urine for presence of stones/calculi *to ascertain if stones are causing outlet obstruction, and/or to note when treatments are being effective in stone breakup/removal.*[1]

NURSING PRIORITY NO. 2. To determine degree of interference/disability:

- Ascertain effect of condition on functioning/lifestyle. *Chronic urinary retention is usually painless, is often caused by a weak bladder muscle which develops slowly, or chronic obstruc-*

---

tion, or nerve diseases that contribute to chronic voiding problems and/or urinary retention. Chronic retention can lead to incontinence and life-threatening complications (e.g., intractable urinary tract infections and kidney failure).[3]

- Measure amount voided and postvoid residuals (via ultrasound or catheterizing after voiding).
- Instruct client/SO to maintain voiding log *to determine severity of condition:*[5]
  Determine frequency and timing of dribbling and/or voiding.
  Note size and force of urinary stream.
  Determine presence/severity (0–10 scale) of bladder spasms, pelvic pain, and other discomforts.

NURSING PRIORITY NO. 3. To assist in treating/preventing retention:

- Teach client/SO to manage voiding problems:
  Attempt voiding in complete privacy *to reduce embarrassment and distractions.*[2]
  Void on timed schedule *to prevent overdistention of bladder.*[2]
  Exercise good urination habits (e.g., four to six times/day). *Frequent holding of urine for prolonged periods can, over time, weaken bladder muscles because of overstretching.*[3]
  Sit client upright on bedpan/commode or stand *to provide functional position of voiding.*[2]
  Take warm sitz bath or shower, voiding in tub/shower, if need be. *Warm water stimulates bladder to relax and may facilitate voiding.*[2]
  Teach client with mild or moderate obstructive symptoms to "double void" by urinating, resting on toilet for 3–5 minutes, and then making a second attempt to urinate. *Promotes more efficient bladder evacuation by allowing the detrusor to contract initially, then rest and contract again.*[5]
  Demonstrate and instruct client/SO(s) in use of Credé's maneuver *to facilitate emptying of the bladder.*[2]
  Encourage client to use Valsalva's maneuver if appropriate *to increase intra-abdominal pressure.*[2]
  Establish regular self-catheterization program, as indicated, *to prevent reflux and increased renal pressures. Note: Clean intermittent cauterization (CIC) is a treatment option for individuals who can urinate, but cannot completely empty the bladder.*[3]
- Consult with urologist/prepare for more aggressive intervention (e.g., reconstructive surgery, lithotripsy, prostatectomy, etc.) as indicated *to remove source of obstruction, reconstruct sphincter, or provide for urinary diversion.*[2]

NURSING PRIORITY NO. 4. To promote wellness (Teaching/Discharge Considerations):

- Establish regular schedule for bladder emptying whether voiding or using catheter.
- Instruct client/SO(s) in clean intermittent catheterization (CIC) techniques *so that more than one individual is able to assist the client in care of elimination needs.*[2]
- Instruct client/SO in care when client has indwelling (urethral or suprapubic catheter) or urinary diversion device (e.g., clean technique, emptying and cleaning of leg bag/drainage bag; irrigation and replacement, etc.) *to enhance safe self-care and prevent complications.*[2]
- Stress need for adequate fluid intake, including use of acidifying fruit juices or ingestion of vitamin C/Mandelamine *to discourage bacterial growth and stone formation.*[2]
- Review signs/symptoms of complications *to promote timely contact with healthcare provider for evaluation/intervention.*

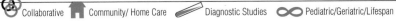 Cultural   Collaborative   Community/ Home Care   Diagnostic Studies   Pediatric/Geriatric/Lifespan   Medications

Assessment/Reassessment
- Individual findings, including nature of problem, degree of impairment, and whether client is incontinent.

Planning
- Plan of care and who is involved in planning.
- Teaching Plan.

Implementation/Evaluation
- Response to interventions.
- Attainment/progress toward desired outcome(s).
- Modifications to plan of care.

Discharge Planning
- Long-term needs/referrals and who is responsible for actions to be taken.
- Specific referrals made.

References

1. ND: Urinary Retention. In Doenges, M. E., Moorhouse, M. F., & Geissler-Murr, A. C. (2002). Nursing Care Plans: Guidelines for Individualizing Patient Care, ed 6. Philadelphia: F. A. Davis.
2. ND: Urinary Retention. In Doenges, M. E., Moorhouse, M. F., & Murr, A. C. (2004). Nurse's Pocket Guide: Diagnoses, Interventions, and Rationales, ed 9. Philadelphia: F. A. Davis.
3. Gaynes, S. M., & Hale, K. L. (2003). Inability to urinate. Available at: http://emedicinehealth.com. Accessed March 2004.
4. No author listed. (2003). The management of benign prostatic hyperplasia. Baltimore, MD: American Urological Association, Inc. Available at: http://www.guideline.com. Accessed March 2004.
5. Gray, M. (2000b). Urinary retention: Management in the acute care setting, (part 2). Am J Nurs, 100(8), 36–44.

impaired spontaneous Ventilation

Definition: Decreased energy reserves results in an individual's inability to maintain breathing adequate to support life

RELATED FACTORS
Metabolic factors; [hypermetabolic state (e.g., infection), nutritional deficits/depletion of energy stores]
Respiratory muscle fatigue
[Airway size/resistance; problems with secretion management]

DEFINING CHARACTERISTICS

Subjective
Dyspnea
Apprehension

Objective
Increased metabolic rate
Increased heart rate

Increased restlessness

Decreased cooperation

Increased use of accessory muscles

Decreased tidal volume

Decreased PO_2; SaO_2

Increased PCO_2

SAMPLE CLINICAL APPLICATIONS: COPD, asthma, pulmonary embolus, acute respiratory distress syndrome, brain injury, chest trauma/surgery, Guillian-Barré syndrome, ALS

DESIRED OUTCOMES/EVALUATION CRITERIA

Sample **NOC** linkages:

Respiratory Status: Ventilation: Movement of air in and out of the lungs

Neurologic Status: Central Motor Control: Extent to which skeletal muscle activity (body movement) is coordinated by the central nervous system

Endurance: Extent that energy enables a person to sustain activity

Client Will (Include Specific Time Frame)

- Reestablish/maintain effective respiratory pattern via ventilator with absence of retractions/use of accessory muscles, cyanosis, or other signs of hypoxia; and with ABGs/SaO_2 within acceptable range.
- Participate in efforts to wean (as appropriate) within individual ability.

Sample **NOC** linkage:

Energy Conservation: Extent of active management of energy to initiate and sustain activity

Caregiver Will (Include Specific Time Frame)

- Demonstrate behaviors necessary to maintain respiratory function

ACTIONS/INTERVENTIONS

Sample **NIC** linkages:

Ventilation Assistance: Promotion of an optimal spontaneous breathing pattern that maximizes oxygen and carbon dioxide exchange in the lungs

Mechanical Ventilation: Use of an artificial device to assist a patient to breath

Respiratory Monitoring: Collection and analysis of patient data to ensure airway patency and adequate gas exchange

NURSING PRIORITY NO. **1.** To determine degree of impairment:

- Investigate client's current status and etiology of respiratory failure (e.g., exacerbation of chronic obstructive lung disease (COPD), pneumonia, pulmonary embolus (PE), heart failure, trauma) *to determine client's care needs, future capabilities, ventilation needs/most appropriate type of ventilatory support.*[1]
- Ascertain desires of client/SOs regarding plan for treatment of respiratory failure, as indicated. *Client may have advance directives, prior stated decisions about the level of therapy aggressiveness that he or she desires if situation is chronic/long-term. Family members may help in decision-making processes if client is minor or incapacitated.*[2]
- Assess spontaneous respiratory pattern, noting rate, depth, rhythm, symmetry of chest movement, and use of accessory muscles. *Tachypnea, shallow breathing,*

 Cultural Collaborative Community/ Home Care Diagnostic Studies 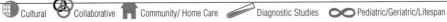 Pediatric/Geriatric/Lifespan Medications demonstrated/reports of dyspnea (using 0–10 scale); increased heart rate/dysrhythmias; pallor or cyanosis, and intercostal retractions/use of accessory muscles indicate increased work of breathing and/or gas exchange impairment.[3]

- Auscultate breath sounds, noting presence/absence and equality of breath sounds, adventitious breath sounds (e.g., wheezing) *to evaluate presence/degree of ventilatory impairment.*[1]

- Obtain ABGs, bedside O_2 saturation readings, pulmonary function studies, as appropriate *to ascertain presence/degree of respiratory distress for comparative baseline.*

- Review results of chest radiography and MRI/CT, if done. *Provides information about source and significance of condition.*

- Note response to current measures/respiratory therapy (e.g., bronchodilators, supplemental oxygen, IPPB treatments). *Client with ventilatory impairments (e.g., exacerbation of COPD) may already be receiving treatments to maintain airway patency and enhance gas exchange or may have respiratory failure associated with sudden event (e.g., severe trauma, sudden onset respiratory illness, surgery with complications).*[1]

NURSING PRIORITY NO. 2. To provide/maintain ventilatory support:[1]

- Collaborate with physician, respiratory care practitioners regarding effective mode of ventilation (e.g., noninvasive oxygenation) or intubation and mechanical ventilation (e.g., continuous mandatory [CMV], assist control [ACV], intermittent mandatory [IMV], pressure support [PSV]). *Specific mode is determined by client's respiratory requirements, presence of underlying disease process, and the extent to which client can participate in ventilatory efforts.*

- Observe overall breathing pattern, distinguishing between spontaneous respirations and ventilator breaths. *Client may be completely dependent on the ventilator, or able to take breaths but have poor oxygen saturation without the ventilator, or may be improving to the point of showing readiness for weaning. The client on noncontrolled ventilation mode can still experience hyper/hypoventilation or "air hunger" and attempt to correct deficiency by overbreathing.*

- Verify that client's respirations are in phase with the ventilator. *Decreases work of breathing, maximizes O_2 delivery when client is not fighting the ventilator.*

- Inflate tracheal/endotracheal tube cuff properly using minimal leak/occlusive technique *to ensure adequate ventilation/delivery of desired tidal volume.*

- Check cuff inflation periodically per facility protocol, and whenever cuff is deflated/reinflated *to prevent risks associated with under/overinflation.*

- Check tubings for obstruction (e.g., kinking or accumulation of water) *that can impede flow of oxygen.* Drain tubing as indicated; avoid draining toward the client, or back into the reservoir, *which can result in contamination/provide medium for growth of bacteria.*

- Check ventilator alarms for proper functioning. Do not turn off alarms, even for suctioning. Remove from ventilator and ventilate manually if source of ventilator alarm cannot be quickly identified and rectified. Verify that alarms can be heard in the nurses' station by care providers *to prevent failure of careprovider being alerted to emergent situation/ventilator disconnect.*

- Verify that oxygen line is in proper outlet/tank; monitor inline oxygen analyzer or perform periodic oxygen analysis *to deliver an acceptable oxygen percentage and saturation for client's specific needs.*

- Note tidal volume (usually 10–15 mL/kg). Verify proper function of spirometer, bellows, or computer readout of delivered volume. Note alterations from desired volume delivery to accommodate alteration in lung compliance or leakage through machine/around tube cuff (if used).

- Monitor airway pressure *for developing complications/equipment problems (e.g., increased airway resistance, retained secretions, decreased lung compliance, client out of phase/off ventilator).*
- Note inspired humidity and temperature; maintain hydration *to prevent excessive drying of mucosa and to liquefy secretions facilitating removal.*
- Auscultate breath sounds periodically. Note frequent crackles or rhonchi that do not clear with coughing/suctioning. *May indicate developing complications (e.g., atelectasis, pneumonia, acute bronchospasm, pulmonary edema).*
- Suction as needed *to clear secretions if client is unable to clear airways, is coughing excessively, has visible secretions, or is tripping high-pressure alarm on ventilator.*
- Note changes in chest symmetry. *May indicate improper placement of ET tube, development of barotrauma.*
- Keep resuscitation bag at bedside *to allow for manual ventilation whenever indicated (e.g., if client is removed from ventilator or troubleshooting equipment problems).*
- Administer and monitor response to medications *that promote airway patency and gas exchange to determine efficacy/need for change.*
- Refer to NDs: ineffective Airway Clearance, ineffective Breathing Pattern, and impaired Gas Exchange for additional interventions.

NURSING PRIORITY NO. 3. To prepare for/assist with weaning process if appropriate:

- Determine client's physical/psychological readiness to wean. *Weaning readiness testing should begin soon after intubation, whenever possible, to limit complications associated with long-term mechanical ventilation. Weaning parameters include 1) evidence for some reversal of the underlying cause of respiratory failure; 2) adequate oxygenation and normal pH; 3) hemodynamic stability; 4) capability and willingness to initiate inspiratory effort; 5) absence of excessive secretions; and 6) nutritionally stable.*[1,4–7]
- Determine mode for weaning. *Recent studies indicate that pressure support mode or multiple daily T-piece trials may be superior to IMV, low level pressure support may be beneficial for unassisted breathing trials, and early extubation and institution of noninvasive positive pressure ventilation may have substantial benefits in alert cooperative client.*[5,7]
- Explain to client/SO weaning activities/techniques, individual plan and expectations. *Reduces fear of unknown, provides opportunities to deal with concerns, clarifies reality of fears, and helps reduce anxiety to a more manageable level).*[1,6]
- Elevate head of bed/place in orthopedic chair if possible, or position *to alleviate dyspnea and to facilitate oxygenation.*
- Assist client in "taking control" of breathing *when weaning is attempted or ventilatory support is interrupted during procedure/activity.*[1]
- Coach client to take slower, deeper breaths, practice abdominal/pursed-lip breathing, assume position of comfort, and use relaxation techniques *to maximize respiratory function and reduce anxiety.*
- Instruct in/assist client to perform effective coughing techniques. *Necessary for secretion management after extubation.*
- Provide quiet environment, calm approach, and undivided attention of nurse. *Promotes relaxation, decreasing energy/oxygen requirements.*

 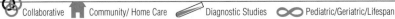

- Involve family/SO(s) as appropriate. Provide diversional activity. *Helps client focus on something other than breathing.*
- Instruct client in use of energy-saving techniques during care activities *to limit oxygen consumption and fatigue associated with work of breathing.*
- Acknowledge and provide ongoing encouragement for client's efforts. Communicate hope for successful weaning response (even partial). *Emotional support can enhance client's commitment to continue weaning activity, maximizing outcomes.*[1]

NURSING PRIORITY NO. 4. To prepare for discharge on ventilator when indicated:

- Collaborate with physician, social worker to plan for discharge placement (e.g., return home, short-term admission to sub-acute/rehabilitation center or permanent placement in extended care facility). *Helps to determine care needs and fiscal impact of home care versus extended care facility.*[8]
- Determine specific equipment needs. Identify resources for equipment needs/maintenance and arrange for delivery before client discharge.
- Review layout of home, noting size of rooms, doorways; placement of furniture, number/type of electrical outlets *to identify necessary modifications.*
- Obtain no-smoking signs to be posted in home. Remind family members to refrain from smoking.
- Have family/SO(s) notify utilities company and fire department of presence of ventilator in home. *Client will be placed in high-risk list for follow-up in case of power outage or fire.*[9]
- Train family members/caregivers in necessary care tasks, and technical aspects of ventilator. Allow sufficient opportunity for SO(s)/family to practice new skills *to become proficient in care tasks.*
- Review and provide written materials regarding proper ventilator management, maintenance, and safety for reference in home setting. *Provides information to enhance client's/SO's level of comfort with challenging tasks.*
- Role-play potential crisis situations *to enhance confidence in ability to handle client's needs.*
- Provide positive feedback and encouragement for efforts of SO(s)/family. *Promotes continuation of desired behaviors.*
- Identify signs/symptoms requiring prompt medical evaluation/intervention. *Timely treatment may prevent progression of problem.*
- List names and phone numbers for identified contact persons/resources. Refer to individual(s) who have managed home ventilation. *Round-the-clock availability reduces sense of isolation and enhances likelihood of obtaining appropriate information when needed.*

NURSING PRIORITY NO. 5. To promote wellness (Teaching/Discharge Considerations):

- Discuss impact of specific activities on respiratory status and problem-solve solutions *to maximize weaning effort, and/or to reduce incidence of respiratory distress/failure.*
- Engage client in specialized exercise program *to enhance respiratory muscle strength and general endurance.*
- Monitor health of visitors, persons involved in care *to protect client from sources of infection.*

● Recommend involvement in support group, introduce to individuals dealing with similar problems *to provide role models, assistance for problem solving.*

 ● Encourage time-out/respite for careproviders *so they may attend to personal needs, wellness, and growth.*

 ● Provide opportunities for client/SO(s) to discuss advance directives. *Clarifies parameters for termination of therapy and/or other end-of-life decisions as desired.*

 ● Identify for client/SO other ventilator-dependent individuals who are successfully managing condition if desired/needed *to answer questions, assist with problem solving, and encouragement/hope for the future.*

 ● Refer to additional resources (e.g., spiritual advisor, counselor).

DOCUMENTATION FOCUS

Assessment/Reassessment
● Baseline findings, subsequent alterations in respiratory function.
● Results of diagnostic testing.
● Individual risk factors/concerns.

Planning
● Plan of care and who is involved in planning.
● Teaching Plan.

Implementation/Evaluation
● Client's/other's responses to interventions, teaching, and actions performed.
● Skill level/assistance needs of SO(s)/family.
● Attainment, progress toward desired outcome(s).
● Modifications to plan of care.

Discharge Planning
● Discharge plan, including appropriate referrals, action taken, and who is responsible for each action.
● Equipment needs and source.
● Resources for support persons/home care providers.

References

1. CP: Ventilatory assistance (mechanical). In Doenges, M. E., Moorhouse, M. F., & Geissler-Murr, A. C. (2002). Nursing Care Plans: Guidelines for Individualizing Patient Care, ed 6. Philadelphia: F. A. Davis, pp 167–179.
2. Campbell, M., & Thill-Baharozian, M. (1994). Impact of the DNR therapeutic plan on patient care requirements. Am J Crit Care, 3, 202.
3. Gift, A., & Narsavage, G. (1998). Validity of the numeric rating scale as a measure of dyspnea. Am J Crit Care, 7(3), 200.
4. Epstein, S. K. (2002). Weaning from mechanical ventilation. Respir Care, 47(4), 454–466.
5. MacIntyre, N. R., et al. (2001). Evidence-based guidelines for weaning and discontinuation of ventilatory support. (Collective task force facilitated by the American College of Chest Physicians; the American Association for Respiratory Care; and the American College of Critical Care Medicine) Chest, 120(6suppl), 385S–484S.
6. Tasota, F. J., & Dobbin, D. (2000). Weaning your patient from mechanical ventilation. Nursing, 30(10), 41.
7. Cook, D. J., et.al. (2000). Weaning from mechanical ventilation. For the McMaster Evidence-Based Practice Center. Agency for Healthcare Research and Quality. Available at: http://www.chestnet.org. Accessed September 2003.
8. Lysaght, L. Ventilation, impaired spontaneous. In Ackley, B. J., & Ladwig, G. B. (2002). Nursing Diagnosis Handbook: A Guide to Planning Care, ed 5. St. Louis: Mosby.
9. Humphrey, C. (1994). Home Care Nursing Handbook, ed 2. Gaithersburg, MD: Aspen.

 Cultural    Collaborative   Community/ Home Care    Diagnostic Studies   Pediatric/Geriatric/Lifespan   Medications

dysfunctional Ventilatory Weaning Response

Definition: Inability to adjust to lowered levels of mechanical ventilator support that interrupts and prolongs the weaning process

RELATED FACTORS

Physical
Ineffective airway clearance
Sleep pattern disturbance
Inadequate nutrition
Uncontrolled pain or discomfort
[Muscle weakness/fatigue, inability to control respiratory muscles; immobility]

Psychological
Knowledge deficit of the weaning process, client's role
Client's perceived inefficacy about the ability to wean
Decreased motivation
Decreased self-esteem
Anxiety (moderate, severe); fear; insufficient trust in the nurse [careproviders]
Hopelessness; powerlessness
[Unprepared for weaning attempt]

Situational
Uncontrolled episodic energy demands or problems
Inappropriate pacing of diminished ventilator support
Inadequate social support
Adverse environment (noisy, active environment, negative events in the room, low nurse-client ratio; extended nurse absence from bedside, unfamiliar nursing staff)
History of ventilator dependence >1 week
History of multiple unsuccessful weaning attempts

DEFINING CHARACTERISTICS
Responds to lowered levels of mechanical ventilator support with:

Mild DVWR
Subjective
Expressed feelings of increased need for O_2; breathing discomfort; fatigue, warmth
Queries about possible machine malfunction

Objective
Restlessness
Slight increased respiratory rate from baseline
Increased concentration on breathing

Moderate DVWR
Subjective
Apprehension

Objective
Slight increase from baseline blood pressure (<20 mm Hg)
Slight increase from baseline heart rate (<20 beats/min)
Baseline increase in respiratory rate (<5 breaths/min)
Hypervigilance to activities
Inability to respond to coaching/cooperate
Diaphoresis
Eye widening, "wide-eyed look"
Decreased air entry on auscultation
Color changes; pale, slight cyanosis
Slight respiratory accessory muscle use

Severe DVWR
Objective
Agitation
Deterioration in ABGs from current baseline
Increase from baseline BP (>20 mm Hg)
Increase from baseline heart rate (>20 beats/min)
Respiratory rate increases significantly from baseline
Profuse diaphoresis
Full respiratory accessory muscle use; shallow, gasping breaths; paradoxical abdominal breathing
Discoordinated breathing with the ventilator
Decreased level of consciousness
Adventitious breath sounds, audible airway secretions
Cyanosis

SAMPLE CLINICAL APPLICATIONS: traumatic brain injury/stroke, substance overdose, COPD, crushing chest trauma, respiratory/cardiac arrest

DESIRED OUTCOMES/EVALUATION CRITERIA
Sample **NOC** linkages:
Respiratory Status: Ventilation: Movement of air in and out of the lungs
Muscle Function: Adequacy of muscle contraction needed for movement
Respiratory Status: Gas Exchange: Alveolar exchange of CO_2 or O_2 to maintain blood gas concentration

Client Will (Include Specific Time Frame)
- Actively participate in the weaning process.
- Reestablish independent respiration with ABGs within client's normal range and be free of signs of respiratory failure.
- Demonstrate increased tolerance for activity/participate in self-care within level of ability.

ACTIONS/INTERVENTIONS
Sample **NIC** linkages:
Mechanical Ventilation: Use of an artificial device to assist a patient to breathe
Mechanical Ventilatory Weaning: Assisting the patient to breathe without the aid of a mechanical ventilator
Energy Management: Regulating energy use to treat or prevent fatigue and optimize function

 Cultural Collaborative Community/ Home Care Diagnostic Studies 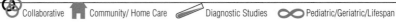 Pediatric/Geriatric/Lifespan Medications

NURSING PRIORITY NO. 1. To identify contributing factors/degree of dysfunction:

- Note length of time on mechanical ventilation (MV) and/or ventilator dependence. Review previous episodes of dependence/weaning. *Although most individuals requiring MV remain on the ventilator for 7 days or less, some require support for several weeks or more. Weaning is more difficult in those clients and may require multiple attempts.*[1]
- Assess physical factors involved in weaning, including vital signs, secretion management, nutritional status, etc. *Major factors adversely affecting client's ability to initiate/maintain spontaneous respirations include: 1) the primary respiratory problem persists; 2) hemodynamic instability; 3) inadequate gas exchange, 4) excessive secretions; 5) poor nutritional status; 6) abnormal electrolytes; and 7) subjective discomfort.*[1–3]
- Ascertain client's/SO's understanding of weaning process, expectations, and concerns. *Unrealistic expectations or unvoiced concerns may impair weaning process or willingness to participate.*
- Determine psychological readiness, presence/degree of anxiety. *Weaning provokes anxiety regarding ability to breathe on own, and likelihood of ventilator dependence. The client must be highly motivated, be able to actively participate in the weaning process, and be physically comfortable enough to work at weaning.*[4]
- Review laboratory studies (e.g., CBC) *to determine number/integrity of red blood cells for O_2 transport;* electrolytes and nutritional markers (e.g., serum protein and albumen) *to determine if client has optimal organ function and/or sufficient energy to meet demands of weaning.*[1]
- Review chest radiograph/pulse oximetry, capnometry, and ABGs. *Before weaning attempts, chest radiograph should show clear lungs or marked improvement in pulmonary congestion. ABGs should document satisfactory oxygenation on an FIO_2 of 40% or less.*[4] *Capnometry is used to measure end-tidal carbon dioxide values and can be used to confirm correct placement of ET, monitor integrity of ventilation equipment, etc.*[5]

NURSING PRIORITY NO. 2. To support weaning process:

- Determine type of tube present (e.g., ET or tracheostomy). *Although an ET is commonly used for short-term MV, it is uncomfortable and often necessitates use of sedation and analgesia. Tracheostomy is commonly used in clients who require prolonged MV, to provide a more comfortable long-term airway, to facilitate earlier weaning, and to improve client's mobility and communication efforts.*[6]
- Explain weaning techniques such as T-piece, pressure support, SIMV, CPAP. Discuss individual plan and expectations. *Prepares client for process, reduces fear of unknown, enhances sense of trust.*[1,2] *An increasing body of research suggests that the key to successful weaning lies not in the use of a particular method but rather in the use of a coordinated approach by a skilled multidisciplinary team.*[7]
- Consult with dietitian, nutritional support team *for adjustments of composition of diet to prevent excessive production of CO_2, which could alter respiratory drive. Individuals on long-term ventilation may require tube-feeding per enteral feedings with high intake of carbohydrates, protein and calories to improve respiratory muscle function.*[4]
- Provide undisturbed rest/sleep periods. Avoid stressful procedures/situations or nonessential activities *to maximize energy for weaning process, promote relaxation, and limit fatigue and oxygen consumption.*[4]
- Time medications during weaning efforts *to minimize sedative effects.*

- Provide quiet room; calm approach, undivided attention of nurse. *Enhances relaxation, conserving energy.*
- Involve SO(s)/family as appropriate (e.g., sit at bedside, provide encouragement, and help monitor client status). *Increases sense of security.*
- Note response to activity/client care during weaning and limit as indicated *to prevent excessive O_2 consumption/demand with increased possibility of failure.*
- Acknowledge and provide ongoing encouragement for client's efforts. *Focusing client's attention on gains and progress to date may help reduce frustration and promote weaning progress.*
- Suspend weaning (take a "holiday") periodically as individually appropriate (e.g., initially may "rest" 45 or 50 minutes each hour, progressing to a 20-minute rest every 4 hours, then weaning during daytime and resting during night).
- Collaborate with physician, respiratory care/other team members *to determine when 1) client cannot be weaned (needs placement on long-term ventilator care, or was already on a ventilator at time of admission), 2) can be partially weaned (e.g., needs some period of time on the ventilator), or 3) must be discontinued from MV even though death may occur (end of life decision).*[8]

NURSING PRIORITY NO. 3. To promote wellness (Teaching/Discharge Considerations):

- Discuss impact of specific activities on respiratory status and problem-solve solutions *to maximize weaning effort.*
- Engage in rehabilitation program *to enhance respiratory muscle strength and general endurance needed for weaning, or being able to sustain respiratory function off the ventilator.*
- Encourage client/SOs to evaluate impact of ventilatory dependence on their lifestyle and what changes they are willing or unwilling to make, if client is to be discharged on ventilator. *Quality of life must be resolved by the ventilator-dependent client and SOs, who need to understand that ventilatory support is a 24-hour job that affects everyone.*[4] *Findings may dictate alternate placement such as foster care or extended care facility.*
- Ascertain that all needed equipment is in place, careproviders are trained, and that safety concerns have been addressed (e.g., alternative power source, backup equipment, client call/alarm system) *to ease the transfer when client is going home on ventilator.*[4]
- Teach client/SO(s) to monitor health of visitors, persons involved in care; avoid crowds during flu season; and obtain immunizations, etc., *to protect client from sources of infection.*
- Identify conditions requiring immediate medical intervention *to treat developing complications/prevent respiratory failure.*
- Evaluate caregiver capabilities and burden when client is on long-term ventilator in the home *to determine potential or presence of skill-related problems or emotional issues (e.g., careprovider overload, burnout, or depression).*[9]
- Discuss importance of time for self and identify appropriate sources for respite care. *Initially, careproviders have limited understanding of the magnitude of the demands on their time and energy. Knowing support is available enhances coping abilities.* Refer to ND risk for Caregiver Role Strain.
- Introduce client/SO(s) to individual who has shared similar experiences with successful management of situation. Refer to support group. *Promotes hope for future, reinforces that situation is not impossible, enhances problem solving and coping.*
- Contact community/facility-based services (e.g., suppliers of home equipment, physical and respiratory therapy providers, emergency power provider, social and financial services, home care agencies) *to facilitate transition to home, and/or to maintain client safely in home setting.*[4]

 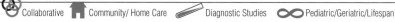

Assessment/Reassessment
- Baseline findings and subsequent alterations.
- Results of diagnostic testing/procedures.
- Individual risk factors.

Planning
- Plan of care/interventions and who is involved in the planning.
- Teaching Plan.

Implementation/Evaluation
- Client response to interventions.
- Attainment of/progress toward desired outcome(s).
- Modifications to plan of care.

Discharge Planning
- Status at discharge, long-term needs and referrals, indicating who is to be responsible for each action.
- Equipment needs/supplier.

References

1. Tasota, F. J., & Dobbin, K. (2000). Weaning your patient from mechanical ventilation. Nursing, 30(10), 41.
2. No author listed. Weaning from mechanical ventilation: Protocols and beyond. Available at: http://www.ed4nurse.com/weaning.htm. Accessed September 2003.
3. MacIntyre, N. R., et al. (2001). Evidence-based guidelines for weaning and discontinuation of ventilatory support. A collective task force facilitated by the American College of Chest Physicians; the American Association for Respiratory Care; and the American College of Critical Care Medicine. Chest, 120(6suppl), 385S–484S.
4. CP: Ventilatory assistance (mechanical). In Doenges, M. E., Moorhouse, M. F., & Geissler-Murr, A. C. (2002). Nursing Care Plans: Guidelines for Individualizing Patient Care, ed 6. Philadelphia: F. A. Davis, pp 167–179.
5. Frakes, M. A. (2001). Measuring end-tidal carbon dioxide: Clinical applications and usefulness. Crit Care Nurse, 21(5), 23–35.
6. Brook, A. D. (2000). Early versus late tracheostomy in patients who require prolonged mechanical ventilation. Am J Crit Care, 9(5), 352–359.
7. Henneman, E. A. (2001). Liberating patients from mechanical ventilation: A team approach. Crit Care Nurse, 21(3), 25–33.
8. Iregui, M., et al. (2002). Determinants of outcome for patients admitted to a long-term ventilator unit. South Med J, 95(3), 310–317.
9. Douglas, S. L., & Daly, B. J. (2003). Caregivers of long-term ventilator patients: Physical and psychological outcomes. Chest, 123:1073–1081.

risk for [/actual] other-directed Violence

Definition: At risk for behaviors in which an individual demonstrates that he/she can be physically, emotionally, and/or sexually harmful to others

NOTE: NANDA has separated the diagnosis of Violence into its two elements: "directed at others" and "self-directed." However, the interventions in general address both situations and have been left in one block following the definition and supporting data of the two diagnoses.

History of violence:

Against others (e.g., hitting, kicking, scratching, biting or spitting, or throwing objects at someone; attempted rape, rape, sexual molestation; urinating/defecating on a person)

Threats (e.g., verbal threats against property/person, social threats, cursing, threatening notes/letters or gestures, sexual threats)

Antisocial behavior (e.g., stealing, insistent borrowing, insistent demands for privileges, insistent interruption of meetings; refusal to eat or to take medication, ignoring instructions)

Indirect (e.g., tearing off clothes, urinating/defecating on floor, stamping feet, temper tantrum; running in corridors, yelling, writing on walls, ripping objects off walls, throwing objects, breaking a window, slamming doors; sexual advances)

Other factors:

Neurologic impairment (e.g., positive EEG, CT, or MRI; head trauma; positive neurologic findings; seizure disorders, [temporal lobe epilepsy])

Cognitive impairment (e.g., learning disabilities, attention deficit disorder, decreased intellectual functioning); [organic brain syndrome]

History of childhood abuse/witnessing family violence, [negative role modeling]; cruelty to animals; firesetting

Prenatal and perinatal complications/abnormalities

History of drug/alcohol abuse; pathological intoxication, [toxic reaction to medication]

Psychotic symptomatology (e.g., auditory, visual, command hallucinations; paranoid delusions; loose, rambling, or illogical thought processes); [panic states; rage reactions; catatonic/manic excitement]

Motor vehicle offenses (e.g., frequent traffic violations, use of motor vehicle to release anger)

Suicidal behavior; impulsivity; availability and/or possession of weapon(s)

Body language: rigid posture, clenching of fists and jaw, hyperactivity, pacing, breathlessness, threatening stances)

[Hormonal imbalance (e.g., premenstrual syndrome—PMS, postpartum depression/psychosis)]

[Expressed intent/desire to harm others directly or indirectly]

[Almost continuous thoughts of violence]

NOTE: A risk diagnosis is not evidenced by signs and symptoms, as the problem has not occurred and nursing interventions are directed at prevention.

SAMPLE CLINICAL APPLICATIONS: psychotic conditions (e.g., schizophrenia, paranoia), antisocial personality disorder, dementia, substance abuse (e.g., PCP, delerium tremens), postpartum psychosis, PMS, brain injured

Risk factors [indicators]* for self-directed violence

Employment (unemployed, recent job loss/failure); occupation (executive, administrator/owner of business, professional, semi-skilled worker)

Conflictual interpersonal relationships

Family background (chaotic or conflictual, history of suicide)

Sexual orientation: bisexual (active), homosexual (inactive)

Physical health (hypochondriac, chronic or terminal illness)

Mental health (severe depression, psychosis, severe personality disorder, alcoholism, or drug abuse), [bipolar disorder]

Emotional status (hopelessness, [lifting of depressed mood], despair, increased anxiety,

 Cultural Collaborative 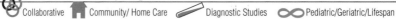 Community/ Home Care   Diagnostic Studies 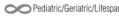 Pediatric/Geriatric/Lifespan Medications panic, anger, hostility); history of multiple suicide attempts; suicidal ideation (frequent, intense prolonged); suicide plan (clear and specific; lethality, method and availability of destructive means)

Personal resources (poor achievement, poor insight, affect unavailable and poorly controlled)

Social resources (poor rapport, socially isolated, unresponsive family)

Verbal clues (e.g., talking about death, "better off without me," asking questions about lethal dosages of drugs)

Behavioral clues (e.g., writing forlorn love notes, directing angry messages at an SO who has rejected the person, giving away personal items, taking out a large life insurance policy), people who engage in autoerotic sexual acts [e.g., asphyxiation]

NOTE: A risk diagnosis is not evidenced by signs and symptoms, as the problem has not occurred and nursing interventions are directed at prevention.

SAMPLE CLINICAL APPLICATIONS: major depression, postpartum depression/psychosis, Munchausen syndrome, psychosis, substance abuse (e.g., PCP), abuse/neglect

DESIRED OUTCOMES/EVALUATION CRITERIA [FOR DIRECTED AT OTHERS/SELF-DIRECTED VIOLENCE]
Sample **NOC** linkages:

Aggression Control: Self-restraint of assualtive, combative, or destructive behavior toward others

Abusive Behavior Self-Control: Self-restrain of own behaviors to avoid abuse and neglect of dependents or significant others

Impulse Control: Self-restraint of compulsive or impulsive behaviors

Client Will (Include Specific Time Frame)
- Acknowledge realities of the situation.
- Verbalize understanding of why behavior occurs.
- Identify precipitating factors.
- Express realistic self-evaluation and increased sense of self-esteem.
- Participate in care and meet own needs in an assertive manner.
- Demonstrate self-control as evidenced by relaxed posture, nonviolent behavior.
- Use resources and support systems in an effective manner.

ACTIONS/INTERVENTIONS
(Address both "directed at others" and "self-directed")
Sample **NIC** linkages:

Anger Control Assistance: Facilitation of the expression of anger in an adaptive, nonviolent manner

Environmental Management: Violence Prevention: Monitoring and manipulation of the physical environment to decrease the potential for violent behavior directed toward self, others, or environment

Behavior Modification: Self-Harm: Assisting the patient to decrease or eliminate self-mutilating or self-abusive behavior

NURSING PRIORITY NO. 1. To assess causative/contributing factors:

- Determine underlying dynamics as listed in the Risk Factors.
- Ascertain client's perception of self/situation. Note use of defense mechanisms. *Individuals who are prone to violent behavior may see themselves as victims (denial), blaming others (projection), not following social norms, and impulsive.*[1]

- Observe/listen for early cues of distress/increasing anxiety. *Behaviors such as irritability,*

lack of cooperation, demanding behavior, body posture/expression may signal escalating potential for violent behavior and need for immediate intervention.[1]

- Identify conditions such as acute/chronic brain syndrome; panic state; hormonal imbalance. *PMS, postpartum psychosis, drug-induced psychotic states, postsurgical/postseizure confusion; psychomotor seizure activity may interfere with ability to control own behavior and lead to violent episodes.*[1]

- Review laboratory findings (e.g., blood alcohol, blood glucose, ABGs, electrolytes, renal function tests). *Provides information about possible treatable sources of behavior.*[6]

- Observe for signs of suicidal/homicidal intent. *Perceived morbid or anxious feelings while with the client; warning from the client, "It doesn't matter," "I'd/They'd be better off dead"; mood swings; "accident-prone"/self-destructive behavior; possession of alcohol and/or other drug(s) in known substance abuser need to be noted, taken seriously and treated appropriately.*[6] (Refer to ND risk for Suicide)

- Note family history of suicidal/homicidal behavior. *Family dynamics in family of origin/ current family, parental deprivation and/or abuse in the early years of an individual's life seem to be contributing factors to violent behavior in current situation.*[1]

- Ask directly if the person is thinking of acting on thoughts/feelings. *Can determine reality and urgency of violent intent and importance of immediate intervention.*[6]

- Determine availability of suicidal/homicidal means. *Identifies urgency of situation and need to intervene by removing lethal means, possibly hospitalizing client or other measures to ensure safety of client and others.*[6]

- Assess client coping behaviors. (Note: Client believes there are no alternatives other than violence.) *Client has been dealing with frustration and anger in unacceptable ways, yelling, hitting and other violent behaviors and needs to learn alternative coping skills.*[1]

- Identify risk factors and assess for indicators of child abuse/neglect: unexplained/frequent injuries, failure to thrive, and so forth. *Visible evidence of physical abuse/neglect makes it more easily recognized; however, behaviors of withdrawal, acting out may also signal the presence of abuse.*[6]

- Determine presence, extent, and acceptance of violence in the client's culture. *Youth violence has become a national concern with widely publicized school shootings and an increase in arrests of both boys and girls for violent crimes and weapons violations. Young people who are at risk for violence need to be identified, and positive programs aimed at promoting emotional wellness need to be instituted in schools, parent education meetings, churches, and community centers.*[3,7]

NURSING PRIORITY NO. 2. To assist client to accept responsibility for impulsive behavior and potential for violence:

- Develop therapeutic nurse-client relationship. Provide consistent caregiver when possible. *Promotes sense of trust, allowing client to discuss feelings openly and begin to identify sources of anger and more acceptable ways of dealing with it.*[1]

- Maintain straightforward communication. *Avoids reinforcing manipulative behavior. Manipulation is used for management of powerlessness because of distrust of others, fear of loss of power/control, fear of intimacy, and search for approval.*[6]

- Note motivation for change (e.g., failing relationships, job loss, involvement with judicial system). *Crisis situation can provide impetus for change, but requires timely therapeutic intervention to sustain efforts.*[7]

- Help client recognize that own actions may be in response to own fear (may be afraid of

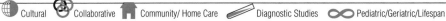 Cultural Collaborative Community/ Home Care Diagnostic Studies ∞ Pediatric/Geriatric/Lifespan Medications

own behavior, loss of control), dependency, and feeling of powerlessness. *Promotes understanding of self and ability to deal with feelings in acceptable ways.*[6]

- Make time to listen to expressions of feelings. Acknowledge reality of client's feelings and that feelings are okay. (Refer to ND Self-Esteem, specify.) *Understanding how feelings lead to actions and how individual is responsible for controlling behavior in acceptable ways.*[6]

- Confront client's tendency to minimize situation/behavior. *Individuals often want to say that things "are not as bad" as portrayed or "it was just a small argument" and "I didn't think I hit him (or her) that hard." By confronting this minimalization, the reality of the situation can be brought out and discussed, leading to better understanding of the situation and changes in behavior.*[6]

- Identify factors (feelings/events) involved in precipitating violent behavior. *By identifying the factors, individual/family, peer conflict, aggressive behavior, individual's view of self, hallucinations, involved in current situation an appropriate plan can be made to change actions to prevent future violent behavior.*[7]

- Discuss impact of behavior on others/consequences of actions. *Discussing these issues openly can help client to develop empathy and understand other person's reactions and begin to change behaviors that can lead to violence.*[8]

- Acknowledge reality of suicide/homicide as an option. Discuss consequences of actions if they were to follow through on intent. Ask how it will help client to resolve problems. *Acknowledging the reality of individual's thoughts provides opportunity to look at how actions would affect others, ability to control own behavior and make choices to make a better life for self.*[6]

- Accept client's anger without reacting on emotional basis. Give permission to express angry feelings in acceptable ways and let client know that staff will be available to assist in maintaining control. *Promotes acceptance and sense of safety. Client's anger is usually directed at the situation and not at the caregiver and by remaining separate the therapist can be more helpful for resolution of the anger.*[6]

- Help client identify more appropriate solutions/behaviors. *Motor activities/exercise can lessen sense of anxiety and associated physical manifestations, diminishing feelings of anger.*[8]

- Provide directions for actions client can take, avoiding negatives, such as "do nots." *Discussing positive ideas to help client begin to look toward a better future can provide hope that violent behaviors can be changed, promoting feelings of self-worth and belief in control of own self.*[5]

NURSING PRIORITY NO. 3. To assist client in controlling behavior:

- Contract with client regarding safety of self/others. *Making a contract in which the individual agrees to refrain from any violent behavior for a specified period of time, from day one through the entire course of treatment, and written and signed by each party, may help the client to follow through with therapy to find more effective ways of resolving conflict. Although there is little research on the effectiveness of these contracts, they are frequently used.*[7]

- Give client as much control as possible within constraints of individual situation. *Since control issues are a factor in violent behavior, giving client control in appropriate ways can enhance self-esteem, promote confidence in ability to change behavior.*[7]

- Be truthful when giving information and dealing with individual. *Builds trust, enhancing therapeutic relationship.*[5]

- Identify current/past successes and strengths. Discuss effectiveness of coping techniques used and possible changes. (Refer to ND ineffective Coping.) *Client is often not aware of positive aspects of life, and once recognized, they can be used as a basis for change.*[8]

- Assist client to distinguish between reality and hallucinations/delusions. *Violent behavior in clients with major mental disorders (schizophrenia, mania) may be responding to command hallucinations and may need more aggressive treatment/hospitalization until behavior is under control.*[1]
- Approach in positive manner, acting as if the client has control and is responsible for own behavior. Be aware, though, that the client may not have control, especially if under the influence of drugs (including alcohol). *Individuals will often respond to a positive expectation reducing threatening actions. Staff needs to be trained in management of this behavior and be prepared to take control of the situation if client is out of control.*[1]
- Maintain distance and do not touch client when situation indicates client does not tolerate such closeness. *Individuals who have experienced traumatic events such as rape or suffer from post-trauma response may fear close contact even with trusted persons.*[1]
- Remain calm and state limits on inappropriate behavior (including consequences) in a firm manner. *Calm manner enables client to de-escalate anger, and knowing what the consequences will be gives an opportunity to choose to change behavior and deal appropriately with situation. Consequences need to be decided beforehand and agreed to by client, or they may sound like punishment and be counterproductive.*[1]
- Direct client to stay in view of staff. *Intervention may be needed to maintain safety of client and others.*[1] (Refer to risk for Suicide.)
- Administer prescribed medications (e.g., antianxiety/antipsychotic), taking care not to oversedate client. *May be least restrictive way to help client control violent behaviors while learning new coping skills to handle anger and impulsive behavior.*[1]
- Monitor for possible drug interactions, cumulative effects of drug regimen (e.g., anticonvulsants/antidepressants). *May be contributory factor in violent behavior.*[1]
- Give positive reinforcement for client's efforts. *Encourages continuation of desired behaviors.*[1]
- Develop violence prevention and emotional literacy programs in the schools and community. *These programs are based on the premise that intelligent management of emotions is critical to successful living. Aggressive youth lack skills in arousal management and nonviolent problem solving which can be learned in programs and reinforced by the adults in their lives.*[7]

NURSING PRIORITY NO. 4. To assist client/SO(s) to correct/deal with existing situation:

- Gear interventions to individual(s) involved, based on age, relationship, and so forth. *Conflict resolution skills can be learned by all age groups when age-appropriate materials are used.*[5,8]
- Maintain calm, matter-of-fact, nonjudgmental attitude. *Decreases defensive response allowing individual to think about own responsibility in the conflict and choose positive behaviors instead of usual angry reaction.*[4,5,8]
- Notify potential victims in the presence of serious homicidal threat in accordance with legal/ethical guidelines. *Therapists are legally required to provide this notice when client expresses homicidal intent overtly or covertly in addition to helping the client realize that the proposed action is not wise or in his or her own best interest.*[1]
- Discuss situation with abused/battered person, providing accurate information about choices and effective actions that can be taken. *Promotes understanding of options, giving hope and support for planning for a violence-free future.*[2]
- Assist individual to understand that angry, vengeful feelings are appropriate in the situation, need to be expressed and not acted on. (Refer to ND Post-Trauma Syndrome, as

 Cultural   Collaborative   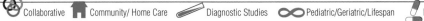 Community/ Home Care   Diagnostic Studies   Pediatric/Geriatric/Lifespan   Medications psychological responses may be very similar.) *Helps client accept feelings as natural, begin to learn effective coping skills and promotes sense of control over situation.*[2]

 • Identify resources available for assistance (e.g., battered women's shelter, social services, financial). *Helps client to manage immediate needs such as food, shelter and safety with a long-range goal of attaining/maintaining independence and violence-free life.*[2]

NURSING PRIORITY NO. 5. To promote safety in event of violent behavior:

- Provide a safe, quiet environment and remove items from the client's environment that could be used to inflict harm to self/others. *Reducing stimuli can help client to calm down and removing articles provides for safety of client and staff.*[1]
- Maintain distance from client who is striking out/hitting and take evasive/controlling actions as indicated. *Staff safety is of prime importance and avoiding physical confrontation until client regains control or Take-down team is assembled can prevent injury.*[6]
- Call for additional staff/security personnel. *Having sufficient people available to handle the situation may defuse client's anger, allowing situation to calm down without further action. All personnel need to be trained in Take-down techniques.*[6]
- Approach aggressive/attacking client from the front, just out of reach, in a commanding posture with palms down. *Safety is a prime concern and these actions may defuse the situation.*[6]
- Tell client to Stop in a firm voice. *This may be sufficient to help client control own actions.*[6]
- Maintain direct/constant eye contact when appropriate. *Assists in identifying client's intentions and conveys sense of caring. Eye contact may be perceived as threatening so it needs to be used cautiously.*[2]
- Speak in a low, commanding voice. *Tone of voice conveys message of control, concern and can help to calm the client's anger.*[6]
- Provide client with a sense that care giver is in control of the situation. *Client is feeling out of control and seeing that staff are in control provides a feeling of safety.*[6]
- Maintain clear route for staff and client and be prepared to move quickly. *Safety for all is of prime importance and staff may need to leave the room to regroup, while continuing to protect the client. Take-down needs to be done quickly to gain control of the individual.*[6]

 • Hold client, using restraints or seclusion when necessary until client regains self-control. *Brief period of physical restraint may be required until client regains control/other therapeutic interventions take effect.*

 • Administer medication as indicated. *Client may require chemical restraint until control is regained.*

- Discuss situation with client after situation is calmed down and control is regained. *Helping client to understand how feelings of anger had gotten out of control and what can be done to prevent a recurrence can provide a learning opportunity for the individual.*[2,6]

NURSING PRIORITY NO. 6. To promote wellness (Teaching/Discharge Considerations):

 • Promote client involvement in planning care within limits of situation, allowing for meeting own needs for enjoyment. *Individuals often believe they are not entitled to pleasure and good things in their lives and need to learn how to meet these needs in acceptable ways.*[6]

 • Assist client to learn assertive behaviors. *Manipulative, nonassertive/aggressive behaviors lead to anger, which can result in violence. Learning assertiveness skills can facilitate change, increase self-esteem, and promote interpersonal relationships.*[1]

- Provide information about conflict-resolution skills and help client learn how to use them effectively. *Conflict is always present in human relationships and learing how to manage conflict is one of the most important tools we can use to solve disagreements and improve relationships.*[4,5,8]
- Discuss reasons for client's behavior with SO(s). Determine desire/commitment of involved parties to sustain current relationships. *Family members may believe individual is purposefully behaving in angry ways, and understanding underlying reasons for behavior can defuse feelings of anger on their part, leading to willingness to resolve problems.*[1,4]
- Develop strategies to help parents learn more effective parenting skills. *Participating in parenting classes and learning appropriate ways of dealing with frustrations can improve family relationships and prevent angry interactions and the possibility of violent behavior.*[4,5]
- Identify support systems. *Presence of family/friends, clergy who can serve as mentors, listen to individual nonjudgmentally, can help client defuse angry feelings and learn appropriate ways of dealing with them.*[1]
- Refer to formal resources as indicated. *May need individual/group psychotherapy, substance abuse treatment program, social services, safe house facility to facilitate change.*[1]
- Refer to NDs impaired Parenting, family Coping, [specify]; Post-Trauma Syndrome.

DOCUMENTATION FOCUS

Assessment/Reassessment
- Individual findings, including nature of concern (e.g., suicidal/homicidal), behavioral risk factors and level of impulse control, plan of action/means to carry out plan.
- Client's perception of situation, motivation for change.

Planning
- Plan of care and who is involved in the planning.
- Details of contract regarding violence to self/others.
- Teaching Plan.

Implementation/Evaluation
- Actions taken to promote safety, including notification of parties at risk.
- Response to interventions/teaching and actions performed.
- Attainment/progress toward desired outcome(s).
- Modifications to plan of care.

Discharge Planning
- Long-range needs and who is responsible for actions to be taken.
- Available resources, specific referrals made.

References

1. Townsend, M. C. (2003). Psychiatric Mental Health Nursing Concepts of Care, ed 4. Philadelphia: F. A. Davis.
2. Cox, H. C., et al. (2002). Clinical Applications of Nursing Diagnosis, ed 4. Philadelphia: F. A. Davis.
3. Lipson, J. G., Dibble, S. L., & Minarik, P. A. (1996). Culture & Nursing Care: A Pocket Guide. San Francisco: UCSF Nursing Press.
4. Gordon, T. (1989). Teaching Children Self-discipline: At Home and At School. New York: Random House.
5. Gordon, T. (2000). Family Effectiveness Training Video. Solana Beach, CA: Gordon Training Intn'l.
6. Doenges, M. E., Townsend, M. C., & Moorhouse, M. F. (1998). Psychiatric Care Plans Guidelines for Individualizing Care, ed 3. Philadelphia: F. A. Davis.

 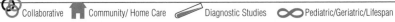

7. Thomas, S. P. (2003). Identifying and intervening with girls at risk for violence. J School Nurs, 19(3), 130–139.
8. Porter-O'Grady, T. (2003). Managing conflict in the workplace. NSNA/Imprint, 48(4), 66–68.

impaired Walking

Definition: Limitation of independent movement within the environment on foot

RELATED FACTORS

To be developed by nurse researchers and submitted to NANDA
[Condition affecting muscles/joints impairing ability to walk]

DEFINING CHARACTERISTICS

Subjective or Objective

Impaired ability to walk required distances, walk on an incline/decline, or on uneven surfaces, to navigate curbs, climb stairs
[Specify level of independence—refer to ND impaired physical Mobility for suggested functional level classification]

SAMPLE CLINICAL APPLICATIONS: arthritis, obesity, amputation, brain injury/stroke, traumatic injury/fractures, chronic pain, peripheral vascular disease, spinal nerve compression, MS, cerebral palsy, Parkinson's disease, macular degeneration, dementia

DESIRED OUTCOMES/EVALUATION CRITERIA

Sample **NOC** linkages:

Ambulation: Walking: Ability to walk from place to place
Mobility Level: Ability to move purposefully
Balance: Ability to maintain body equilibrium

Client Will (Include Specific Time Frame)

- Be able to move about within environment as needed/desired within limits of ability or with appropriate adjuncts.
- Verbalize understanding of situation/risk factors and safety measures.

ACTIONS/INTERVENTIONS

Sample **NIC** linkages:

Exercise Therapy: Ambulation: Promotion and assistance with walking to maintain or restore autonomic and voluntary body functions during treatment and recovery from illness or injury
Body Mechanics Promotion: Facilitating the use of posture and movement in daily activities to prevent fatigue and musculoskeletal strain or injury
Exercise Therapy: Balance: Use of specific activities, postures, and movements to maintain, enhance, or restore balance

Refer also to NDs impaired Mobility [specify] for additional assessments and interventions.

NURSING PRIORITY NO. 1. To assess causative/contributing factors:

- Identify conditions/diagnoses (e.g., advanced age, acute illness, weakness/chronic illness, recent surgery, trauma, arthritis, brain injury, vision impairments, pain, fatigue, cognitive dysfunction) *that contribute to walking impairment and identify specific needs and appropriate interventions.*

- Determine ability to follow directions, and note emotional/behavioral responses *that may be affecting client's ability to engage in activity.*

NURSING PRIORITY NO. 2. To assess functional ability:

- Determine degree of immobility in relation to 0–4 scale, noting muscle strength and tone, joint mobility, cardiovascular status, balance and endurance. *Identifies strengths and deficits (e.g., ability to ambulate with/without assistive devices) and may provide information regarding potential for recovery (e.g., client with severe brain injury may have permanent limitations because of impaired cognition affecting memory, judgment, problem solving and motor planning, requiring more intensive inpatient and long-term care).*
- Note whether impairment is temporary or permanent. *Condition may be caused by reversible condition (e.g., weakness associated with acute illness, or fractures/surgery with weight-bearing restrictions); or walking impairment can be permanent (e.g., congenital anomalies, amputation, severe rheumatoid arthritis).*[1]
- Note emotional/behavioral responses of client/SO to problems of mobility. *Can negatively affect self-concept and self-esteem, autonomy and independence. Feelings of frustration and powerlessness may impede attainment of goals. Social, occupational and relationship roles can change, leading to isolation, depression and economic consequences.*[8,9]

NURSING PRIORITY NO. 3. To promote safe, optimal level of independence in walking:

- Assist with treatment of underlying condition (e.g., heart failure, fatigue associated with cancer therapies, brain trauma, amputation) as needed/indicated by individual situation. *Treatment can, many times, reverse or limit dysfunction.*
- Monitor client's tolerance for walking, as indicated by cardiopulmonary condition. *Increased pulse rate (e.g., >50 bpm above baseline), chest pain, breathlessness, irregular heartbeat) is indicative of cardiac/respiratory intolerance.* Refer to ND: Activity Intolerance.
- Consult with PT/OT/rehabilitation team *to develop individual mobility/walking program (e.g., to improve general conditioning, coordination and balance, perform range of motion exercises, specific muscle strengthening, and to instruct in specific tasks, such as stair climbing or gait-training, etc.), and identify/develop appropriate adjunctive devices (e.g., customized cane, crutches, or walker).*[2]
- Implement fall precautions for high-risk clients (e.g., frail or ill elderly, visually or cognitively impaired, person on multiple medications, presence of dizziness, syncope, etc.) *to reduce risk of accidental injury.* Refer to ND risk for Falls.
- Use adequate personnel and assistive devices (e.g., gait belt, nonslip shoes) when ambulating *to prevent injury to client or caregivers.*
- Limit distractions, provide safe environment *to prevent falls and allow the client to concentrate on walking activities or learning use of assistive devices.*[2]
- 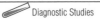 Instruct in proper application/encourage use of prostheses, immobilizers, splints, or braces before walking *to maintain joint stability or immobilization, and/or to maintain alignment during movement.*[3,4]
- Demonstrate/remind client to properly use adjunctive devices (e.g., walker, cane, crutches) *that may be prescribed to improve balance, reduce limb pain/dysfunction, and provide support during ambulation.*[2]

🌐 Cultural   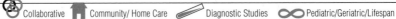 Collaborative   🏠 Community/ Home Care   Diagnostic Studies   ∞ Pediatric/Geriatric/Lifespan   Medications

- Provide cueing as indicated. *Client may need reminders (e.g., lift foot higher, look where going, walk tall, etc.) to concentrate on/perform tasks of walking, especially when balance or cognition is impaired.*[5]
- Provide positive, constructive feedback *to encourage continuation of efforts and enhance client's self-sufficiency.*[6]
- Schedule walking/exercise activities interspersed with adequate rest periods *to reduce problems associated with fatigue, or leg pain associated with claudication, etc.*[7]
- Provide ample time to perform mobility-related tasks and advance levels of exercise as able.
- Assist client to obtain needed information such as handicapped sticker for close-in parking, sources for mobility scooter, special public transportation options, etc., when indicated *to deal with temporary or permanent disability access.*

NURSING PRIORITY NO. 4. To promote wellness (Teaching/Discharge Considerations):

- Evaluate client's home (or work) environment for barriers to walking (e.g., uneven surfaces, many steps, no ramps, long distances between places client needs to walk, etc.) *to determine needed changes, make recommendations for client safety.*
- Provide information/facilitate progressive walking program and self-monitoring methods *to clients contemplating or beginning walking for exercise.*[6]
- Foster emotional and social support (spouse, family members, friends, coworkers) *to offer encouragement and overcome barriers to exercise.*
- Involve client/SO in care, assisting them to learn ways of managing deficits *to enhance safety for client with long-term/permanent impairments.*
- Identify appropriate resources for obtaining and maintaining appliances, equipment, and environmental modifications *to promote safe mobility.*
- Instruct client/SO in safety measures in home, as individually indicated (e.g., maintaining safe travel pathway, proper lighting, wearing glasses, handrails on stairs, grab bars in bathroom, using walker instead of cane when sleepy or walking on uneven surface, etc.) *to reduce risk of falls.*
- Discuss need for emergency call/support system (e.g., Lifeline, HealthWatch) *to provide immediate assistance for falls, other home emergencies when client lives alone.*

DOCUMENTATION FOCUS

Assessment/Reassessment
- Individual findings, including level of function/ability to participate in specific/desired activities.

Planning
- Plan of care and who is involved in the planning.
- Teaching Plan.

Implementation/Evaluation
- Responses to interventions/teaching and actions performed.
- Attainment/progress toward desired outcome(s).
- Modifications to plan of care.

Discharge Planning
- Discharge/long-range needs, noting who is responsible for each action to be taken.

- Specific referrals made.
- Sources of/maintenance for assistive devices.

References

1. ND: Walking impaired. In Doenges, M. E., Moorhouse, M. F., & Geissler-Murr, A. C. (2002). Nursing Care Plans: Guidelines for Individualizing Patient Care, ed 6. Philadelphia: F. A. Davis.
2. Kuang, T., & Kedlaya, D. (2002). Assistive devices to improve independence. Available at: http://www.emedicine.com. Accessed August 2004.
3. Teplicky, R., Law, M., & Russell, D. (2002). The effectiveness of casts, orthotics, and splints for children with neurological disorders. Infants & Young Children, 15(1), 42–50.
4. Wilson, G. B. (1988). Progressive mobilization. In Sine, R. D., et al. (eds). Basic Rehabilitation Techniques: A Self-Instructional Guide, ed 3. Gaithersburg, MD: Aspen.
5. Gee, Z. I., & Passarella, P. M. (1985). Nursing Care of the Stroke Patient: A Therapeutic Approach. Pittsburgh, PA: AREN.
6. Jitramontree, N. (2001). Evidence-based protocol. Exercise promotion: Walking in elders. Iowa City (IA): University of Iowa Gerontological Nursing Interventions Research Center, Research Dissemination Core; Feb; 53.
7. Eberhardt, R. T. (2002). Editorial-Exercise for intermittent claudication: Walking for life? J Cardiopulm Rehab, 22(3), 199–200.
8. Mass, M. L. (1989). Impaired physical mobility. Unpublished manuscript. Cited in research article for National Institutes for Health.
9. Hogue, C. C. (1984). Falls and mobility late in life: An ecological model. J Am Geriatr Soc, 32,858–861.

Wandering [specify sporadic or continual]

Definition: Meandering, aimless, or repetitive locomotion that exposes the individual to harm; frequently incongruent with boundaries, limits, or obstacles

RELATED FACTORS

Cognitive impairment, specifically memory and recall deficits, disorientation, poor visuo-constructive (or visuospatial) ability, language (primarily expressive) defects
Cortical atrophy
Premorbid behavior (e.g., outgoing, sociable personality; premorbid dementia)
Separation from familiar people and places
Emotional state, especially frustration, anxiety, boredom, or depression (agitation)
Physiologic state or need (e.g., hunger/thirst, pain, urination, constipation)
Over/understimulating social or physical environment; sedation
Time of day

DEFINING CHARACTERISTICS

Objective

Frequent or continuous movement from place to place, often revisiting the same destinations
Persistent locomotion in search of "missing" or unattainable people or places; scanning, seeking, or searching behaviors
Haphazard locomotion; fretful locomotion or pacing; long periods of locomotion without an apparent destination
Locomotion into unauthorized or private spaces; trespassing
Locomotion resulting in unintended leaving of a premise
Inability to locate significant landmarks in a familiar setting; getting lost
Locomotion that cannot be easily dissuaded or redirected; following behind or shadowing a caregiver's locomotion
Hyperactivity

 Cultural Collaborative Community/ Home Care Diagnostic Studies 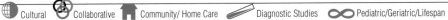 Pediatric/Geriatric/Lifespan Medications

Periods of locomotion interspersed with periods of non-locomotion (e.g., sitting, standing, sleeping)

SAMPLE CLINICAL APPLICATIONS: brain injury, dementias, developmental delays, major depression, substance abuse, amnesia, fugue

DESIRED OUTCOMES/EVALUATION CRITERIA
Sample **NOC** linkage:
Safety Status: Physical Injury: Severity of injuries from accidents and trauma

Client Will (Include Specific Time Frame)
- Be free of injury, or unplanned exits.

Sample NOC linkages:
Risk Control: Actions to eliminate or reduce actual, personal, and modifiable health threats
Safety Behavior: Home Physical Environment: Individual or caregiver actions to minimize environmental factors that might cause physical harm or injury in the home

Caregiver(s) Will (Include Specific Time Frame)
- Modify environment as indicated to enhance safety.
- Provide for maximal independence of client.

ACTIONS/INTERVENTIONS

Sample **NIC** linkages:
Elopement Precautions: Minimizing the risk of a patient leaving a treatment setting without authorization when departure presents a threat to the safety of patient or others
Area Restriction: Limitation of patient mobility to a specified area for purposes of safety or behavior management
Environmental Management: Safety: Manipulation of the patient's surroundings for therapeutic benefit

NURSING PRIORITY NO. 1. To assess degree of impairment/stage of disease process:

- Ascertain history of client's memory loss and cognitive changes.
- Review/evaluate responses of collaborative diagnostic examinations (e.g., cognition, functional capacity, behavior, memory impairments, reality orientation, general physical health and quality of life). *A combination of tests is often needed to complete an evaluation of client's overall condition relating to chronic/irreversible condition. These tests include (but are not limited to) Mini-Mental State Examination (MMSE), Alzheimer's Disease Assessment Scale, cognitive subsection (ADAS-cog), Functional Assessment Questionnaire (FAQ), Clinical Global Impression of Change (CGIC), Neuropsychiatric Inventory (NPI).*[1]
- Evaluate client's past history (e.g., individual was very active physically and socially, or reacted to stress with physical activity rather than emotional reactions) *to help identify likelihood of wandering.*[2]
- Determine from client/SO or testing if client is depressed. *Research supports the idea that wandering develops more often in depressed client with Alzheimer's disease.*[2]
- Evaluate client's mental status during both daytime and nighttime, noting when client's confusion is most pronounced, and when/how long client sleeps. *Information about cognition and behavioral habits can reveal circumstances under which client is likely to wander.*[3]

- Assess frequency and pattern of wandering behavior (using Algase Wandering Scale [AWS]), as indicated. *Knowledge of patterns can prompt caregivers to anticipate need for personal attention.[3] Note: AWS is a useful adjunct tool for clinical assessment, as it quantifies wandering in several domains (as reported by caregivers) to determine individual risks/safety needs.[2]*
- Identify client's reason for wandering if possible. *Client may demonstrate searching behavior (e.g., looking for lost item, or pursuing certain unattainable activity), or demonstrate inexhaustible drive to do things/remain busy, or be experiencing sensations (e.g., hunger, thirst, or discomfort) without ability to express the actual need.[2]*
- Identify client's travel patterns. *Activity may be 1) direct (from one location to another without diversion, 2) random (random direction with no obvious stopping point), 3) pacing (back and forth within limited area) or 4) lapping (circling large areas).[2]*
- Monitor client's use/need for assistive devices such as glasses, hearing aids, cane, safe walking shoes, comfortable clothing, etc. *Wandering client is at high risk of falls due to cognitive impairments and the fatigue related to functional decline, or forgetting necessary assistive devices or how to properly use them.[4]*

NURSING PRIORITY NO. 2. To assist client/caregiver to deal with situations:

- Provide a structured daily routine:
  Encourage participation in family activities and familiar routines such as folding laundry, listening to music, walking outdoors. *Activities and exercises may reduce anxiety, depression, and restlessness. Note: Repetitive activity (e.g., rocking, folding laundry or paperwork may help client with "lapping" wandering to reduce energy expenditure and fatigue.)[3]*
  Offer food, fluids, toileting on a regular schedule when client is unable to verbalize, *as agitation, pacing or wandering may be associated with these basic needs.[3]*
  Sit with client and talk *when client is socially gregarious, enjoys conversation, and/or reminiscence is calming.*
  Provide television/radio/music. *Note: Music may be more effective than talking or reading to decrease wandering.[1]*
  Monitor activities, loud conversations, number of visitors at one time, or new care providers/roommate *to prevent overstimulation/increased agitation.*
  Remove items from immediate environment (e.g., coat, hat, keys, etc.) *to reduce stimulus for leaving the site.[3]*
- Provide safe place for client to wander:
  Remove environmental safety hazards such as hot water faucets, knobs on kitchen stove; gate or block open stairways, etc.[1–3]
  Keep area free of clutter; place comfortable furniture and other items against the wall/out of travel path *to accommodate safe walking and promote rest periods.[1]*
  Install safety locks/latches on doors and windows; door latches are complex and less accessible; equip exits with alarms (that are always turned on).[1–3]
- Enroll client in SafeReturn Program administered by the Alzheimer's Association. *Program registers persons with dementia and mans a 24-hour help line to facilitate the return of lost persons. [800–272–3900].[5]*
- Monitor activity when hospitalized/admitted to facility:
  Place in room near monitoring station; check client location on frequent basis.
  Assign consistent staff as much as possible.
  Create "Wanderer's lounge," or large safe walking area with inaccessible exits or outside gated area.[1–3]

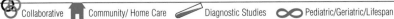

Provide 24-hour supervision and reality orientation. *Client can be awake at any time and fail to recognize day/night routines.*

- Use technology to promote safety:

  Use pressure-sensitive bed/chair alarms *to alert caregivers of movement, especially when client frequently gets up at night, or when no one is present.*

  Provide client ID bracelet or necklace with updated photograph, client name and emergency contact *to assist with identification efforts, particularly when progressive dementia produces marked changes in client's appearance.*[3,5]

  Obtain electronic locator devices *to find client when there is the potential for client to get lost/go missing.*[4,5]

  Install verbal door alarm system. *Voice command is more effective at redirecting client and less likely to increase agitation than loud sound.*[1]

- Use universal symbols, large-print signs, portrait-like photographs, pictures and signs *to assist in finding way, especially when client has diminished ability or has lost ability to read.*[3]

- Avoid using physical or chemical restraints (sedatives) to control wandering behavior. *May increase agitation, sensory deprivation, and falls, and can aggravate wandering behavior.*

NURSING PRIORITY NO. 3. To Promote Wellness (Teaching/Discharge Considerations):

- Identify problems that are remediable and assist client/SO to seek appropriate assistance and access resources. *Encourages problem solving to improve condition rather than accept the status quo.*

- Notify neighbors about client's condition and request that they contact client's family or local police if they see client outside alone. *Community awareness can prevent/reduce risk of client being lost or hurt.*

- Help client/SO and family members develop plan of care when problem is progressive. *Client may initially need part-time assistance at home, progressing to enrollment in day care program, then full-time home care or placement in care facility.*

- Refer to community resources such as day care programs, support groups, respite care, etc. *Careprovider(s) will require access to multiple kinds of assistance and opportunities to promote problem solving, enhance coping, and obtain necessary respite.*

- Refer to NDs: acute/chronic Confusion, disturbed Sensory Perception (specify), impaired Thought Processes, risk for Injury/Falls.

DOCUMENTATION FOCUS

Assessment/Reassessment
- Assessment findings, including individual concerns, family involvement, and support factors/availability of resources.

Planning
- Plan of care and who is involved in planning.
- Teaching plan.

Implementation/Evaluation
- Responses of client/SO(s) to plan interventions and actions performed.
- Attainment/progress toward desired outcome(s).
- Modifications to plan of care.

Discharge Planning
- Long-range needs and who is responsible for actions to be taken.
- Specific referrals made.

References

1. About Alzheimer's. (2003). Physicians and Care Professionals. Various Educational Materials. Available at: http://www.alz.org. Accessed 2003.
2. Futrell, M., & Melillo, K. D. (2002). Evidence-based protocol. Wandering. Iowa City, IA: University of Iowa Gerontological Nursing Interventions Research Center, Research Dissemination Core. Available at: http://www.guideline.gov. Accessed September 2003.
3. ND: Wandering. In Cox, H. C., et al. (2002). Clinical Applications of Nursing Diagnosis: Adult, Child, Women's Psychiatric, Gerontic, and Home Health Considerations, ed 4. Philadelphia: F. A. Davis.
4. Brody, E., et al. (1984). Predictors of falls among institutionalized females with Alzheimer's disease. J Am Geriatr, 32, 877–882.
5. Rowe, M. A. (2003). People with dementia who become lost. AJN, 103(7), 32–39.

 Cultural Collaborative Community/ Home Care 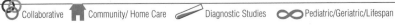 Diagnostic Studies Pediatric/Geriatric/Lifespan Medications

Chapter 6

Health Conditions & Client Concerns with Associated Nursing Diagnoses

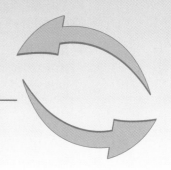

This chapter presents approximately 800 disorders/health conditions reflecting all specialty areas, with associated nursing diagnoses written as client problem/need statements that include "related to" and "evidenced by" statements.

This section will facilitate and help validate the assessment and diagnosis steps of the nursing process. Because the nursing process is perpetual and ongoing, other nursing diagnoses may be appropriate based on changing individual situations. Therefore, the nurse must continually assess, identify, and validate new client needs and evaluate subsequent care.

To facilitate access to the health conditions/concerns and nursing diagnoses, the client needs have been listed alphabetically and coded to identify nursing specialty areas.

MS: Medical-Surgical
PED: Pediatric
OB: Obstetric
CH: Community/Home
PSY: Psychiatric/Behavioral

A separate category for geriatrics was not made because geriatric concerns/conditions actually are subsumed under the other specialty areas, because elderly persons are susceptible to the majority of these problems.

Abdominal hysterectomy   **MS**
(Refer to Hysterectomy)

Abdominal perineal resection   **MS**
(Also refer to Surgery, general)

disturbed Body Image may be related to presence of surgical wounds possibly evidenced by
   verbalizations of feelings/perceptions, fear of reaction by others, preoccupation with
   change.
risk for Constipation: risk factors may include decreased physical activity/gastric motility,
   abdominal muscle weakness, insufficient fluid intake, change in usual foods/eating
   pattern.
risk for Sexual Dysfunction: risk factors may include altered body structure/function, radical
   resection/treatment procedures, vulnerability/psychological concern about response of
   significant other(s), and disruption of sexual response pattern (e.g., erection difficulty).

Abortion, elective termination   **OB**

risk for Decisional Conflict: risk factors may include unclear personal values/beliefs, lack of
   experience or interference with decision making, information from divergent sources, deficient support system.
deficient Knowledge [Learning Need] regarding reproduction, contraception, self-care, Rh factor
   may be related to lack of exposure/recall or misinterpretation of information possibly
   evidenced by request for information, statement of misconception, inaccurate follow-
   through of instructions, development of preventable events/complications.
risk for Spiritual Distress: risk factors may include perception of moral/ethical implications of
   therapeutic procedure.
Anxiety [specify level] may be related to situational/maturational crises, unmet needs, unconscious conflict about essential values/beliefs possibly evidenced by increased tension,
   apprehension, fear of unspecific consequences, sympathetic stimulation, focus on self.
acute Pain/[Discomfort] may be related to after effects of procedure/drug effect possibly
   evidenced by verbal report, distraction behaviors, changes in muscle tone, autonomic
   responses/changes in vital signs.
risk for maternal Injury: risk factors may include surgical procedure, effects of
   anesthesia/medications.

Abortion, spontaneous termination   **OB**

deficient Fluid Volume [isotonic] may be related to excessive blood loss, possibly evidenced by
   decreased pulse volume and pressure, delayed capillary refill, or changes in sensorium.
risk for Spiritual Distress: risk factors may include need to adhere to personal religious
   beliefs/practices, blame for loss directed at self or God.
*deficient Knowledge [Learning Need] regarding cause of abortion, self-care, contraception/future
   pregnancy* may be related to lack of familiarity with new self/healthcare needs, sources for
   support, possibly evidenced by requests for information and statement of concern/
   misconceptions, development of preventable complications.
[effective] Grieving related to perinatal loss, possibly evidenced by crying, expressions of
   sorrow, or changes in eating habits/sleep patterns.
risk for ineffective Sexuality Patterns: risk factors may include increasing fear of pregnancy
   and/or repeat loss, impaired relationship with significant other(s), self-doubt regarding
   own femininity.

Abruptio placentae   **OB**
(Also refer to Hemorrhage, prenatal)

deficient Fluid Volume [isotonic] may be related to excessive blood loss, possibly evidenced by hypotension, increased heart rate, decreased pulse volume and pressure, delayed capillary refill, or changes in sensorium.

Fear related to threat of death (perceived or actual) to fetus/self, possibly evidenced by verbalization of specific concerns, increased tension, sympathetic stimulation.

acute Pain may be related to collection of blood between uterine wall and placenta, possibly evidenced by verbal reports, abdominal guarding, muscle tension, or alterations in vital signs.

impaired fetal Gas Exchange may be related to altered uteroplacental O_2 transfer, possibly evidenced by alterations in fetal heart rate and movement.

Abscess, brain (acute)   MS

acute Pain may be related to inflammation, edema of tissues, possibly evidenced by reports of headache, restlessness, irritability, and moaning.

risk for Hyperthermia: risk factors may include inflammatory process/hypermetabolic state and dehydration.

acute Confusion may be related to physiologic changes (e.g., cerebral edema/altered perfusion, fever), possibly evidenced by fluctuation in cognition/level of consciousness, increased agitation/restlessness, hallucinations.

risk for Suffocation/Trauma: risk factors may include development of clonic/tonic muscle activity and changes in consciousness (seizure activity).

Abscess, gingival   CH

impaired Dentition may be related to ineffective oral hygiene, access/economic barriers to professional care possibly evidenced by toothache, root caries, purulent drainage.

risk for imbalanced Nutrition: less than body requirements: risk factors may include decreased intake.

Abscess, skin/tissue   CH/MS

impaired Skin/Tissue Integrity may be related to immunological deficit/infection possibly evidenced by disruption of skin, destruction of skin layers/tissues, invasion of body structures.

risk for Infection [spread]: risk factors may include broken skin/traumatized tissues, chronic disease, malnutrition, insufficient knowledge.

Abuse, physical   CH/PSY

(Also refer to Battered child syndrome)

risk for Trauma: risk factors may include vulnerable client, recipient of verbal threats, history of physical abuse.

Powerlessness may be related to abusive relationship, lifestyle of helplessness as evidenced by verbal expressions of having no control, reluctance to express true feelings, apathy, passivity.

chronic low Self-Esteem may be related to continual negative evaluation of self/capabilities, personal vulnerability, willingness to tolerate possible life-threatening domestic violence as evidenced by self-negative verbalization, evaluates self as unable to deal with events, rationalizes away/rejects positive feedback.

ineffective Coping may be related to situational or maturational crisis, overwhelming threat to self, personal vulnerability, inadequate support systems, possibly evidenced by verbalized concern about ability to deal with current situation, chronic worry, anxiety, depression, poor self-esteem, inability to problem-solve, high illness rate, destructive behavior toward self/others.

Sexual Dysfunction may be related to ineffectual/absent role model, vulnerability, physical abuse possibly evidenced by verbalizations, change in sexual behaviors/activities, inability to achieve desired satisfaction.

Abuse, psychological   CH/PSY

ineffective Coping may be related to situational or maturational crisis, overwhelming threat to self, personal vulnerability, inadequate support systems, possibly evidenced by verbalized concern about ability to deal with current situation, chronic worry, anxiety, depression, poor self-esteem, inability to problem-solve, high illness rate, destructive behavior toward self/others.

Powerlessness may be related to abusive relationship, lifestyle of helplessness as evidenced by verbal expressions of having no control, reluctance to express true feelings, apathy, passivity.

Sexual Dysfunction may be related to ineffectual/absent role model, vulnerability, psychological abuse (harmful relationship) possibly evidenced by reported difficulties, inability to achieve desired satisfaction, conflicts involving values, seeking confirmation of desirability.

Achalasia (cardiospasm)   MS

impaired Swallowing may be related to neuromuscular impairment, possibly evidenced by observed difficulty in swallowing or regurgitation.

imbalanced Nutrition: less than body requirements may be related to inability and/or reluctance to ingest adequate nutrients to meet metabolic demands/nutritional needs, possibly evidenced by reported/observed inadequate intake, weight loss, and pale conjunctiva and mucous membranes.

acute Pain may be related to spasm of the lower esophageal sphincter, possibly evidenced by reports of substernal pressure, recurrent heartburn, or gastric fullness (gas pains).

Anxiety [specify level]/Fear may be related to recurrent pain, choking sensation, altered health status, possibly evidenced by verbalizations of distress, apprehension, restlessness, or insomnia.

risk for Aspiration: risk factors may include regurgitation/spillover of esophageal contents.

deficient Knowledge [Learning Need] regarding condition, prognosis, self-care and treatment needs may be related to lack of familiarity with pathology and treatment of condition, possibly evidenced by requests for information, statement of concern, or development of preventable complications.

Acidosis, metabolic   MS

(Refer to underlying cause/condition, e.g., Diabetic ketoacidosis; Renal dialysis)

Acidosis, respiratory   MS

(Also refer to underlying cause/condition)

impaired Gas Exchange may be related to ventilation perfusion imbalance (decreased oxygen-carrying capacity of blood, altered oxygen-supply, alveolar-capillary membrane changes) possibly evidenced by dyspnea with exertion, tachypnea, changes in mentation, irritability, tachycardia, hypoxia, hypercapnia.

Acne   CH/PED

impaired Skin Integrity may be related to secretion, infectious process as evidenced by disruptions of skin surface.

disturbed Body Image may be related to change in visual appearance as evidenced by fear of rejection of others, focus on past appearance, negative feelings about body, change in social involvement.

situational low Self-Esteem may be related to adolescence, negative perception of appearance as evidenced by self-negating verbalizations, expressions of helplessness.

Acoustic neuroma   MS

(Also refer to Surgery, general)

disturbed auditory Sensory Perception may be related to altered sensory reception (compression of eighth cranial nerve) possibly evidenced by unilateral sensorineural hearing loss/ tinnitis.

risk for Falls: risk factors may include hearing difficulties, dizziness, sense of unsteadiness.

Acquired immune deficiency syndrome   CH
(Refer to AIDS)

Acromegaly   CH
chronic Pain may be related to soft tissue swelling, joint degeneration, peripheral nerve compression possibly evidenced by verbal reports, altered ability to continue previous activities, changes in sleep pattern, fatigue.

disturbed Body Image may be related to biophysical illness/changes possibly evidenced by verbalization of feelings/concerns, fear of rejection or of reaction of others, negative comments about body, actual change in strcture/appearance, change in social involvement.

risk for Sexual Dysfunction: risk factors may include altered body structure, changes in libido.

Adams-Stokes syndrome   CH
(Refer to Dysrhythmia)

ADD   PEDS
(Refer to Attention deficit disorder)

Addiction   CH/PSY
(Refer to specific substances; Substance dependence/abuse rehabilitation)

Adjustment disorder   PSY
moderate to severe Anxiety may be related to situational/maturational crisis, threat to self-concept, unmet needs, fear of failure, dysfunctional family system, fixation in earlier level of development possibly evidenced by overexcitement/restlessness, increased tension, insomnia, feelings of inadequacy, focus on self, difficulty concentrating, continuous attention-seeking behaviors, numerous physical complaints.

risk for self/other-directed Violence: risk factors may include depressed mood, hopelessness, powerlessness, inability to tolerate frustration, rage reactions, unmet needs, negative role modeling, substance use/abuse, history of suicide attempt.

ineffective Coping may be related to situational/maturational crisis, dysfunctional family system, negative role modeling, unmet dependency needs, retarded ego development possibly evidenced by inability to problem-solve, chronic worry, depressed/anxious mood, manipulation of others, destructive behaviors, increased dependency, refusal to follow rules.

dysfunctional Grieving may be related to real or perceived loss of any concept of value to individual, bereavement overload/cumulative grief, thwarted grieving response, feelings of guilt generated by ambivalent relationship with the lost concept/person possibly evidenced by difficulty in expressing/denial of loss, excessive/inappropriately expressed anger, labile affect, developmental regression, changes in concentration/pursuit of tasks.

Hopelessness may be related to lifestyle of helplessness (repeated failures, dependency), incomplete grief work of losses in life, lost belief in transcendent values/God possibly evidenced by verbal cues/despondent content, apathy/passivity, decreased response to stimuli, lack of initiative, nonparticipation in care or decision making.

Addison's disease   MS
deficient Fluid Volume [hypotonic] may be related to vomiting, diarrhea, increased renal losses, possibly evidenced by delayed capillary refill, poor skin turgor, dry mucous membranes, report of thirst.

decreased Cardiac Output may be related to hypovolemia and altered electrical conduction (dysrhythmias) and/or diminished cardiac muscle mass, possibly evidenced by alterations in vital signs, changes in mentation, and irregular pulse or pulse deficit.

CH

Fatigue may be related to decreased metabolic energy production, altered body chemistry (fluid, electrolyte, and glucose imbalance), possibly evidenced by unremitting overwhelming lack of energy, inability to maintain usual routines, decreased performance, impaired ability to concentrate, lethargy, and disinterest in surroundings.

disturbed Body Image may be related to changes in skin pigmentation, mucous membranes, loss of axillary/pubic hair, possibly evidenced by verbalization of negative feelings about body and decreased social involvement.

risk for impaired physical Mobility: risk factors may include neuromuscular impairment (muscle wasting/weakness) and dizziness/syncope.

imbalanced Nutrition: less than body requirements may be related to glucocorticoid deficiency; abnormal fat, protein, and carbohydrate metabolism; nausea, vomiting, anorexia, possibly evidenced by weight loss, muscle wasting, abdominal cramps, diarrhea, and severe hypoglycemia.

risk for impaired Home Maintenance: risk factors may include effects of disease process, impaired cognitive functioning, and inadequate support systems.

Adenoidectomy   PED/MS

Anxiety [specify level]/Fear may be related to separation from supportive others, unfamiliar surroundings, and perceived threat of injury/abandonment, possibly evidenced by crying, apprehension, trembling, and sympathetic stimulation (pupil dilation, increased heart rate).

risk for ineffective Airway Clearance: risk factors may include sedation, collection of secretions/blood in oropharynx, and vomiting.

risk for deficient Fluid Volume: risk factors may include operative trauma to highly vascular site/hemorrhage.

acute Pain may be related to physical trauma to oronasopharynx, presence of packing, possibly evidenced by restlessness, crying, and facial mask of pain.

Adjustment disorder   PED/PSY
(Refer to Anxiety disorders—PED)

Adoption/loss of child custody   PSY

risk for dysfunctional Grieving: risk factors may include actual loss of child, expectations for future of child/self, thwarted grieving response to loss.

risk for Powerlessness: risk factors may include perceived lack of options, no input into decision process, no control over outcome.

Adrenal crisis, acute   MS
(Also refer to Addison's disease; Shock)

deficient Fluid Volume [hypotonic] may be related to failure of regulatory mechanism (damage to/suppression of adrenal gland), inability to concentrate urine possibly evidenced by decreased venous filling/pulse volume and pressure, hypotension, dry mucous membranes, changes in mentation, decreased serum sodium.

acute Pain may be related to effects of disease process/metabolic imbalances, decreased tissue perfusion possibly evidenced by reports of severe pain in abdomen, lower back, or legs.

impaired physical Mobility may be related to neuromuscular impairment, decreased muscle strength/control possibly evidenced by generalized weakness, inability to perform desired activities/movements.

risk for Hyperthermia: risk factors may include presence of illness/infectious process, dehydration.

risk for ineffective Protection: risk factors may include hormone deficiency, drug therapy, nutritional/metabolic deficiencies.

Adrenalectomy   MS
altered Tissue Perfusion, (specify) may be related to hypovolemia and vascular pooling of blood (vasodilation), possibly evidenced by diminished pulse, pallor/cyanosis, hypotension, and changes in mentation.

risk for Infection: risk factors may include inadequate primary defenses (incision, traumatized tissues), suppressed inflammatory response, invasive procedures.

deficient Knowledge [Learning Need] regarding condition, prognosis, self-care and treatment needs may be related to unfamiliarity with long-term therapy requirements, possibly evidenced by request for information and statement of concern/misconceptions.

Adrenal insufficiency   CH
(Refer to Addison's disease)

Affective disorder   PSY
(Refer to Bipolar disorder; Depressive disorders, major)

Affective disorder, seasonal   PSY
(Also refer to Depressive disorders, major)
intermittent ineffective Coping may be related to situational crisis (fall/winter season), disturbance in pattern of tension release, and inadequate resources available possibly evidenced by verbalizations of inability to cope, changes in sleep pattern (too little or too much), reports of lack of energy/fatigue, lack of resolution of problem, behavioral changes (irritability, discouragement).

risk for imbalanced Nutrition: more/less than body requirements: risk factors may include eating in response to internal cues other than hunger, alteration in usual coping patterns, change in usual activity level, decreased appetite, lack of energy/interest to prepare food.

Agoraphobia   PSY
(Also refer to Phobia)
Anxiety [panic] may be related to contact with feared situation (public place/crowds) possibly evidenced by tachycardia, chest pain, dyspnea, gastrointestinal distress, faintness, sense of impending doom.

Agranulocytosis   MS
risk for infection: risk factors may include suppressed inflammatory response.
risk for impaired Oral Mucous Membrane: risk factors may include infection.
risk for imbalanced Nutrition: less than body requirements: risk factors may include inability to ingest food/fluids (lesions of oral cavity).

AIDS (acquired immunodeficiency syndrome)   MS
(Also refer to HIV infection)
risk for Infection, [progression to sepsis/onset of new opportunistic infection]: risk factors ay include depressed immune system, use of antimicrobial agents, inadequate primary defenses; broken skin, traumatized tissue; malnutrition and chronic disease processes.

---

risk for deficient Fluid Volume: risk factors may include excessive losses: copious diarrhea, profuse sweating, vomiting, hypermetabolic state or fever; and restricted intake (nausea, anorexia; lethargy).

acute/chronic Pain may be related to tissue inflammation/destruction: infections, internal/external cutaneous lesions, rectal excoriation, malignancies, necrosis, peripheral neuropathies, myalgias and arthralgias, possibly evidenced by verbal reports, self-focusing/narrowed focus, alteration in muscle tone, paresthesias, paralysis, guarding behaviors, changes in vital signs (acute), autonomic responses, and restlessness.

CH

imbalanced Nutrition: less than body requirements may be related to altered ability to ingest, digest, and/or absorb nutrients (nausea/vomiting, hyperactive gag reflex, intestinal disturbances); increased metabolic activity/nutritional needs (fever, infection), possibly evidenced by weight loss, decreased subcutaneous fat/muscle mass; lack of interest in food/aversion to eating, altered taste sensation; abdominal cramping, hyperactive bowel sounds, diarrhea, sore and inflamed buccal cavity.

Fatigue may be related to decreased metabolic energy production, increased energy requirements (hypermetabolic state), overwhelming psychological/emotional demands; altered body chemistry (side effects of medication, chemotherapy), possibly evidenced by unremitting/ overwhelming lack of energy, inability to maintain usual routines, decreased performance; impaired ability to concentrate, lethargy/restlessness, and disinterest in surroundings.

ineffective Protection may be related to chronic disease affecting immune and neurologic systems, inadequate nutrition, drug therapies, possibly evidenced by deficient immunity, impaired healing, neurosensory alterations, maladaptive stress response, fatigue, anorexia, disorientation.

PSY

Social Isolation may be related to changes in physical appearance/mental status, state of wellness, perceptions of unacceptable social or sexual behavior/values, physical isolation, phobic fear of others (transmission of disease); possibly evidenced by expressed feelings of aloneness/rejection, absence of supportive significant other(s)—(SOs), and withdrawal from usual activities.

disturbed Thought Processes/chronic Confusion may be related to physiologic changes (hypoxemia, central nervous system—CNS—infection by HIV, brain malignancies, and/or disseminated systemic opportunistic infection); altered drug metabolism/excretion, accumulation of toxic elements (renal failure, severe electrolyte imbalance, hepatic insufficiency), possibly evidenced by clinical evidence of organic impairment, altered attention span, distractibility, memory deficit, disorientation, cognitive dissonance, delusional thinking, impaired ability to make decisions/problem-solve, inability to follow complex commands/mental tasks, loss of impulse control and altered personality.

AIDS dementia   CH

(Also refer to Dementia, HIV)

impaired Environmental Interpretation Syndrome may be related to dementia, depression possibly evidenced by consistent disorientation, inability to follow simple directions/instructions, loss of social functioning from memory decline.

ineffective Protection may be related to chronic disease affecting immune and neurologic systems, inadequate nutrition, drug therapies, possibly evidenced by deficient immunity, impaired healing, neurosensory alterations, maladaptive stress response, fatigue, anorexia, disorientation.

Alcohol abuse/withdrawal   **CH/MS/PSY**
(Refer to Alcohol intoxication, acute; Delirium tremens; Substance dependency/abuse reha-
    bilitation)

Alcohol intoxication, acute   **MS**
(Also refer to Delirium tremens)
acute Confusion may be related to substance abuse, hypoxemia possibly evidenced by halluci-
    nations, exaggerated emotional response, fluctuation in cognition/level of consciousness,
    increased agitation.
risk for ineffective Breathing Pattern: risk factors may include neuromuscular
    impairment/CNS depression.
risk for Aspiration: risk factors may include reduced level of consciousness, depressed
    cough/gag reflexes, delayed gastric emptying.

Alcoholism   **CH**
(Refer to Substance dependency/abuse rehabilitation)

Aldosteronism, primary   **MS**
deficient Fluid Volume [isotonic] may be related to increased urinary losses, possibly evidenced
    by dry mucous membranes, poor skin turgor, dilute urine, excessive thirst, weight loss.
impaired physical Mobility may be related to neuromuscular impairment, weakness, and pain,
    possibly evidenced by impaired coordination, decreased muscle strength, paralysis, and
    positive Chvostek's and Trousseau's signs.
risk for decreased Cardiac Output: risk factors may include hypovolemia and altered electrical
    conduction/dysrhythmias.

Alkalosis, metabolic   **MS**
(Refer to underlying cause/condition, e.g., Renal dialysis)

Alkalosis, respiratory   **MS**
(Also refer to underlying cause/condition)
impaired Gas Exchange may be related to ventilation perfusion imbalance (decreased oxygen-
    carrying capacity of blood, altered oxygen supply, alveolar-capillary membrane changes)
    possibly evidenced by dyspnea, tachypnea, changes in mentation, tachycardia, hypoxia,
    hypocapnia.

Allergies, seasonal   **CH**
(Refer to Hay fever)

Alopecia   **CH**
disturbed Body Image may be related to effects of illness/therapy or aging process, change in
    appearance possibly evidenced by verbalization of feelings/concerns, fear of
    rejection/reaction of others, focus on past appearance, preoccupation with change, feelings
    of helplessness.

ALS   **CH**
(Refer to Amyotrophic Lateral Sclerosis)

Alzheimer's disease   **CH**
(Also refer to Dementia, presenile/senile)
risk for Injury/Trauma: risk factors may include inability to recognize/identify danger in
    environment, disorientation, confusion, impaired judgment, weakness, muscular incoordi-
    nation, balancing difficulties, and altered perception.

chronic Confusion, related to physiologic changes (neuronal degeneration); possibly evidenced by inaccurate interpretation of/response to stimuli, progressive/long-standing cognitive impairment, short-term memory deficit, impaired socialization, altered personality, and clinical evidence of organic impairment.

disturbed Sensory Perception (specify) may be related to altered sensory reception, transmission, and/or integration (neurologic disease/deficit), socially restricted environment (homebound/institutionalized), sleep deprivation possibly evidenced by changes in usual response to stimuli, change in problem-solving abilities, exaggerated emotional responses (anxiety, paranoia, hallucinations), inability to tell position of body parts, diminished/altered sense of taste.

disturbed Sleep Pattern may be related to sensory impairment, changes in activity patterns, psychological stress (neurologic impairment), possibly evidenced by wakefulness, disorientation (day/night reversal); increased aimless wandering, inability to identify need/time for sleeping, changes in behavior/performance, lethargy; dark circles under eyes, and frequent yawning.

ineffective Health Maintenance may be related to deterioration affecting ability in all areas including coordination, communication, cognition; ineffective individual/family coping, possibly evidenced by reported or observed inability to take responsibility for meeting basic health practices, lack of equipment/financial or other resources, and impairment of personal support system.

PSY

compromised family Coping/Caregiver Role Strain may be related to family disorganization, role changes, family/caregiver isolation, long-term illness/complexity and amount of homecare needs exhausting supportive/financial capabilities of family member(s), lack of respite; possibly evidenced by verbalizations of frustrations in dealing with day-to-day care, reports of conflict, feelings of depression, expressed anger/guilt directed toward client, and withdrawal from interaction with client/social contacts.

risk for Relocation Stress Syndrome: risk factors may include little or no preparation for transfer to a new setting, changes in daily routine, sensory impairment, physical deterioration, separation from support systems.

Amenorrhea (secondary or pathologic) **GYN**
(Also refer to Anorexia nervosa)

imbalanced Nutrition: less than body requirements may be related to inability to ingest/digest food or absorb nutrients possibly evidenced by verbal reports, aversion to eating, lack of interest in food, weight loss, excessive hair growth/lanugo, pale conjuntiva/mucous membranes, abnormal lab studies.

risk for Sexual Dysfunction: risk factors may include altered body function.

Amphetamine abuse **PSY**
(Refer to Stimulant abuse)

Amputation **MS**

risk for ineffective peripheral Tissue Perfusion: risk factors may include reduced arterial/venous blood flow; tissue edema, hematoma formation; hypovolemia.

acute Pain may be related to tissue and nerve trauma, psychological impact of loss of body part, possibly evidenced by reports of incisional/phantom pain, guarding/protective behavior, narrowed/self-focus, and autonomic responses.

impaired physical Mobility may be related to loss of limb (primarily lower extremity), altered sense of balance, pain/discomfort, possibly evidenced by reluctance to attempt movement, impaired coordination; decreased muscle strength, control, and mass.

disturbed Body Image may be related to loss of a body part, possibly evidenced by verbalization of feelings of powerlessness, grief, preoccupation with loss, and unwillingness to look at/touch stump.

Amyotrophic lateral sclerosis (ALS)   MS

impaired physical Mobility may be related to muscle wasting/weakness, possibly evidenced by impaired coordination, limited range of motion, and impaired purposeful movement.

ineffective Breathing Pattern/impaired spontaneous Ventilation may be related to neuromuscular impairment, decreased energy, fatigue, tracheobronchial obstruction, possibly evidenced by shortness of breath, fremitus, respiratory depth changes, and reduced vital capacity.

impaired Swallowing may be related to muscle wasting and fatigue, possibly evidenced by recurrent coughing/choking and signs of aspiration.

PSY

Powerlessness [specify level] may be related to chronic/debilitating nature of illness, lack of control over outcome, possibly evidenced by expressions of frustration about inability to care for self and depression over physical deterioration.

anticipatory Grieving may be related to perceived potential loss of self/physiopsychosocial well-being, possibly evidenced by sorrow, choked feelings, expression of distress, changes in eating habits/sleeping patterns, and altered communication patterns/libido.

CH

impaired verbal Communication may be related to physical barrier (neuromuscular impairment), possibly evidenced by impaired articulation, inability to speak in sentences, and use of nonverbal cues (changes in facial expression).

risk for Caregiver Role Strain: risk factors may include illness severity of care receiver, complexity and amount of homecare needs, duration of caregiving required, caregiver is spouse, family/caregiver isolation, lack of respite/recreation for caregiver.

Anaphylaxis   CH

(Also refer to Shock)

ineffective Airway Clearance may be related to airway spasm (bronchial), laryngeal edema possibly evidenced by diminished/adventitious breath sounds, cough ineffective or absent, difficulty vocalizing, wide-eyed.

decreased Cardiac Output may be related to decreased preload—increased capillary permeability (third spacing) and vasodilation possibly evidenced by tachycardia/palpitations, changes in BP, anxiety, restlessness.

Anecephaly   OB

(Also refer to Fetal demise)

Anxiety [specify level] may be related to situational crisis, threat of fetal death, interpersonal transmission/contagion possibly evidenced by increased tension, apprehension, feelings of inadequacy, somatic complaints, difficulty sleeping.

risk for decisional Conflict [specify]: risk factors may include threat to value/belief system, multiple or divergent sources of information, support system deficit, feelings of guilt (particularly regarding ethical issues such as termination of pregnancy, organ donation).

Anemia   CH

Activity Intolerance may be related to imbalance between O_2 supply (delivery) and demand, possibly evidenced by reports of fatigue and weakness, abnormal heart rate or blood pressure (BP) response, decreased exercise/activity level, and exertional discomfort or dyspnea.

imbalanced Nutrition: less than body requirements may be related to failure to ingest/inability to digest food or absorb nutrients necessary for formation of normal red blood cells (RBCs); possibly evidenced by weight loss/weight below normal for age, height, body build; decreased triceps skinfold measurement, changes in gums/oral mucous membranes; decreased tolerance for activity, weakness, and loss of muscle tone.

deficient Knowledge [Learning Need] regarding condition, prognosis, self-care and treatment needs may be related to inadequate understanding or misinterpretation of dietary/physiologic needs, possibly evidenced by inadequate dietary intake, request for information, and development of preventable complications.

risk for delayed Surgical Recovery: risk factors may include decreased O_2 delivery to tissues.

Anemia, iron-deficiency   CH

(Also refer to Anemia)

risk for deficient Fluid Volume: risk factors may include active fluid loss/hemorrhage.

risk for impaired Oral Mucous Membrane: risk factors may include dehydration, malnutrition, vitamin deficiency.

Anemia, pernicious   CH

(Also refer to Anemia)

disturbed kinesthetic/visual Sensory Perception may be related to changes in reception/perception possibly evidenced by paresthesia, inability to tell position of extremities (proprioception), loss of vibratory sensation, changes in sensory acuity (yellow-blue color blindness).

risk for Constipation/Diarrhea: risk factors may include muscular weakness, changes in GI motility, neurologic impairment.

risk for Injury/Falls: risk factors may include generalized weakness, paresthesia of extremeties, loss of proprioception, ataxia.

Anemia, sickle cell   MS

impaired Gas Exchange may be related to decreased O_2-carrying capacity of blood, reduced RBC life span, abnormal RBC structure, increased blood viscosity, predisposition to bacterial pneumonia/pulmonary infarcts, possibly evidenced by dyspnea, use of accessory muscles, cyanosis/signs of hypoxia, tachycardia, changes in mentation, and restlessness.

ineffective Tissue Perfusion: (specify) may be related to stasis, vasoocclusive nature of sickling, inflammatory response, atrioventricular (AV) shunts in pulmonary and peripheral circulation, myocardial damage (small infarcts, iron deposits, fibrosis), possibly evidenced by signs and symptoms dependent on system involved, for example: renal: decreased specific gravity and pale urine in face of dehydration; cerebral: paralysis and visual disturbances; peripheral: distal ischemia, tissue infarctions, ulcerations, bone pain; cardiopulmonary: angina, palpitations.

                                                                       CH

acute/chronic Pain may be related to intravascular sickling with localized vascular stasis, occlusion, infarction/necrosis and deprivation of O_2 and nutrients, accumulation of noxious metabolites, possibly evidenced by reports of localized, generalized, or migratory joint and/or abdominal/back pain; guarding and distraction behaviors (moaning, crying, restlessness), facial grimacing, narrowed focus, and autonomic responses.

deficient Knowledge [Learning Need] regarding disease process, genetic factors, prognosis, self-care and treatment needs may be related to lack of exposure/recall, misinterpretation of information, unfamiliarity with resources, possibly evidenced by questions, statement of concern/misconceptions, exacerbation of condition, inadequate follow-through of therapy instructions, and development of preventable complications.

delayed Growth and Development may be related to effects of physical condition, possibly evidenced by altered physical growth and delay/difficulty performing skills typical of age group.

compromised family Coping may be related to chronic nature of disease/disability, family disorganization, presence of other crises/situations impacting significant person/parent, lifestyle restrictions, possibly evidenced by significant person/parent expressing preoccupation with own reaction and displaying protective behavior disproportionate to client's ability or need for autonomy.

Aneurysm, abdominal aortic   MS
(Refer to Aortic aneurysm, abdominal)

Aneurysm, cerebral   MS
(Refer to Cerebrovascular accident)

Aneurysm, ventricular   MS
decreased Cardiac Output may be related to altered stroke volume (decreased contractility, increased systemic vascular resistance), changes in heart rate/rhythm possibly evidenced by dyspnea, adevtitious breath sounds, S_3/S_4 heart sounds, changes in hemodynamic measurements, dysrhythmias.

ineffective Tissue Perfusion (specify) may be related to decreased arterial blood flow possibly evidenced by BP changes, diminished pulses, edema, dyspnea, dysrhythmias, altered mental status, decreased renal function.

Activity Intolerance may be related to imbalance between oxygen supply and demand possibly evidenced by weakness, fatigue, abnormal heart rate/BP response to activity, ECG changes (dysrhythmias, ischemia).

Angina pectoris   MS
acute Pain may be related to decreased myocardial blood flow, increased cardiac workload/O_2 consumption, possibly evidenced by verbal reports, narrowed focus, distraction behaviors (restlessness, moaning), and autonomic responses (diaphoresis, changes in vital signs).

decreased Cardiac Output may be related to inotropic changes (transient/prolonged myocardial ischemia, effects of medications), alterations in rate/rhythm and electrical conduction, possibly evidenced by changes in hemodynamic readings, dyspnea, restlessness, decreased tolerance for activity, fatigue, diminished peripheral pulses, cool/pale skin, changes in mental status, and continued chest pain.

Anxiety [specify level] may be related to situational crises, change in health status and/or threat of death, negative self-talk possibly evidenced by verbalized apprehension, facial tension, extraneous movements, and focus on self.

CH
Activity Intolerance may be related to imbalance between O_2 supply and demand, possibly evidenced by exertional dyspnea, abnormal pulse/BP response to activity, and electrocardiogram (ECG) changes.

deficient Knowledge [Learning Need] regarding condition, prognosis, self-care and treatment needs may be related to lack of exposure, inaccurate/misinterpretation of information, possibly evidenced by questions, request for information, statement of concern, and inaccurate follow-through of instructions.

risk for impaired Adjustment: risk factors may include condition requiring long-term therapy/change in lifestyle, assault to self-concept, and altered locus of control

Anorexia nervosa   MS

imbalanced Nutrition: less than body requirements may be related to psychological restrictions of food intake and/or excessive activity, self-induced vomiting, laxative abuse, possibly evidenced by weight loss, poor skin turgor/muscle tone, denial of hunger, unusual hoarding or handling of food, amenorrhea, electrolyte imbalance, cardiac irregularities, hypotension.

risk for deficient Fluid Volume: risk factors may include inadequate intake of food and liquids, chronic/excessive laxative or diuretic use, self-induced vomiting.

PSY

disturbed Thought Processes may be related to severe malnutrition/electrolyte imbalance, psychological conflicts; possibly evidenced by impaired ability to make decisions, problem-solve, nonreality-based verbalizations, ideas of reference, altered sleep patterns, altered attention span/distractibility; perceptual disturbances with failure to recognize hunger, fatigue, anxiety, and depression.

disturbed Body Image/chronic low Self-Esteem may be related to altered perception of body, perceived loss of control in some aspect of life, unmet dependency needs, personal vulnerability, dysfunctional family system, possibly evidenced by negative feelings, distorted view of body, use of denial, feeling powerless to prevent/make changes, expressions of shame/guilt, overly conforming, dependent on others' opinions.

interrupted Family Processes may be related to ambivalent family relationships and ways of transacting issues of control, situational/maturational crises possibly evidenced by enmeshed family, dissonance among family members, family developmental tasks not being met, family members acting as enablers.

Anthrax, cutaneous   MS/CH

impaired Skin/Tissue Integrity may be related to infectious agent possibly evidenced by disruption of skin surface, damage to tissues.

[Discomfort] may be related to local edema, effects of circulating toxins possibly evidenced by reports of headache, muscle aches, nausea, malaise.

risk for Infection [spread/sepsis]: risk factors may include broken skin, tissue destruction, lack of immunity, presence of infective agent.

Anthrax, gastrointestinal   MS

Anxiety [moderate to severe]/Fear may be related to situational crisis, change in health status/threat of death, interpersonal transmission/contagion possibly evidenced by expressed concerns, apprehension, uncertainty, fearful, increased tension, restlessness, blocking of thought.

risk for deficient Fluid Volume: risk factors may include decreased intake (nausea), excessive loss (bloody vomiting/diarrhea), hypermetabolic state.

imbalanced Nutrition: less than body requirements may be related to inability to ingest food/absorb nutrients, increased metabolic demands possibly evidenced by reports of loss of appetite/nausea, abdominal pain; vomiting, diarrhea.

impaired Oral Mucous Membranes may be related to effects of infection, dehydration possibly evidenced by oropharyngeal ulcerations, oral pain, difficulty swallowing.

Anthrax, inhalation (pulmonary)   **MS**

(Also refer to Ventilator assist/dependence)

[Discomfort] may be related to effects of inflammatory response possibly evidenced by fever, malaise, weakness, fatigue, mild chest pain.

Anxiety [moderate to severe]/Fear may be related to situational crisis, change in health status/threat of death, interpersonal transmission/contagion possibly evidenced by expressed concerns, apprehension, uncertainty, fearful, increased tension, restlessness, blocking of thought.

impaired Gas Exchange may be related to alveolar-capillary membrane changes (fluid collection/shifts into interstitial space/alveoli) possibly evidenced by dyspnea, restlessness, irritability, abnormal rate/depth of respirations, cyanosis, hypoxia, lethargy, confusion.

risk for impaired spontaneous Ventilation: risk factors may include problems with secretion management, mechanical compression of lungs (widening of mediastinum), depletion of energy stores.

Antisocial personality disorder   **PSY**

risk for other-directed Violence: risk factors may include contempt for authority/rights of others, inability to tolerate frustration, need for immediate gratification, easy agitation, vulnerable self-concept, inability to verbalize feelings, use of maladjusted coping mechanisms including substance use.

ineffective Coping may be related to very low tolerance for external stress, lack of experience of internal anxiety (e.g., guilt/shame), personal vulnerability, unmet expectations, multiple life changes possibly evidenced by choice of aggression and manipulation to handle problems conflicts, inappropriate use of defense mechanisms (e.g., denial, projection), chronic worry, anxiety, destructive behaviors, high rate of accidents.

chronic low Self-Esteem may be related to lack of positive and/or repeated negative feedback, unmet dependency needs, retarded ego development dysfunctional family system possibly evidenced by acting-out behaviors (e.g., substance abuse, sexual promisicuity, feelings of inadequacy, nonparticipation in therapy.

compromised/disabled family Coping may be related to family disorganization/role changes, highly ambivalent family relationships, client providing little support in turn for the primary person(s), history of abuse/neglect in the home possibly evidenced by expressions of concern or complaints, preoccupation of primary person with own reactions to situation, display of protective behaviors disproportionate to client's abilities or need for autonomy.

impaired Social Interaction may be related to inadequate personal resources (shallow feelings), immature interests, underdeveloped conscience, unaccepted social values possibly evidenced by difficulty meeting expectations of others, lack of belief that rules pertain to self, sense of emptiness/inadequacy covered by expressions of self-conceit/arrogance/contempt, behavior unaccepted by dominant cultural group.

Anxiety disorder, generalized   **PSY**

Anxiety [specify level]/Powerlessness may be related to real or perceived threat to physical integrity or self-concept (may or may not be able to identify the threat), unconscious conflict about essential values/beliefs and goals of life, unmet needs, negative self-talk, possibly evidenced by sympathetic stimulation, extraneous movements (foot shuffling, hand/arm fidgeting, rocking movements, restlessness), persistent feelings of apprehension and uneasiness, a general anxious feeling that client has difficulty alleviating, poor eye contact, focus on self, impaired functioning, free-floating anxiety, impaired functioning, and nonparticipation in decision making.

ineffective Coping may be related to level of anxiety being experienced by the client, personal vulnerability; unmet expectations/unrealistic perceptions, inadequate coping methods and/or support systems possibly evidenced by verbalization of inability to cope/problem-solve, excessive compulsive behaviors (e.g., smoking, drinking), and emotional/muscle tension, alteration in societal participation, high rate of accidents.

disturbed Sleep Pattern may be related to psychological stress, repetitive thoughts, possibly evidenced by reports of difficulty in falling asleep/awakening earlier or later than desired, reports of not feeling rested, dark circles under eyes, and frequent yawning.

risk for compromised family Coping: risk factors may include inadequate/incorrect information or understanding by a primary person, temporary family disorganization and role changes, prolonged disability that exhausts the supportive capacity of significant other(s).

impaired Social Interaction/Social Isolation may be related to low self-concept, inadequate personal resources, misinterpretation of internal/external stimuli, hypervigilance possibly evidenced by discomfort in social situations, withdrawal from or reported change in pattern of interactions, dysfunctional interactions; expressed feelings of difference from others; sad, dull affect.

Anxiety disorders   PED/PSY

Anxiety [severe/panic] may be related to situational/maturational crisis, internal transmission/contagion, threat to physical integrity/self-concept, unmet needs, dysfunctional family system, independence conflicts possibly evidenced by somatic complaints, nightmares, excessive psychomotor activity, refusal to attend school, persistent worry/fear of catastrophic doom to family/self.

ineffective Coping may be related to maturational crisis, multiple life changes/losses, personal vulnerability, lack of self confidence possibly evidenced by inability to problem-solve, persistent/overwhelming fears, inability to meet role expectations, social inhibition, panic attacks.

impaired Social Interaction may be related to excessive self-consciousness, inability to interact with unfamiliar people, altered thought processes possibly evidenced by verbalized/observed discomfort in social situations, inability to receive/communicate a satisfying sense of belonging/caring/interest, use of unsuccessful social interaction behaviors.

risk for Self-Mutilation/self-directed Violence: risk factors may include panic states, dysfunctional family, history of self-destructive behaviors, emotional disturbance, increasing motor activity.

compromised/disabled family Coping may be related to situational/developmental crisis (e.g., divorce, addition to family, midlife crisis), unrealistic parental expectations, frequent disruptions in living arrangements, high-risk family situations (neglect/abuse, substance abuse) possibly evidenced by SO reports frustration with clinging behaviors, emotional lability, harsh/punitive response to tyrannical behaviors, disproportionate protective behaviors.

Anxiolytic abuse   PSY
(Refer to Depressant abuse)

Aortic aneurysm, abdominal (AAA)   MS

risk for ineffective peripheral Tissue Perfusion: risk factors may include interruption of arterial blood flow [embolus formation, spontaneous blockage of aorta].

risk for Infection: risk factors may include turbulent blood flow through arteriosclerotic lesion.

acute Pain may be related to vascular enlargement-dissection/rupture possibly evidenced by verbal coded reports, guarding behavior, facial mask, change in abdominal muscle tone.

Aortic aneurysm repair, abdominal   MS
(Also refer to Surgery, general)

Fear related to threat of injury/death, surgical intervention possibly evidenced by verbal
    reports, apprehension, decreased self-assurance, increased tension, changes in vital signs.
risk for deficient Fluid Volume: risk factors may include weakening of vascular wall, failure of
    vascular repair.
risk for ineffective renal/peripheral Tissue Perfusion: risk factors may include interruption of
    arterial blood flow, hypovolemia.

Aortic insufficiency   MS/CH
(Refer to Valvular heart disease)

Aortic stenosis   MS
(Also refer to Valvular heart disease)

decreased Cardiac Output may be related to structural changes of heart valve, left ventricular
    outflow obstruction, alteration of afterload (increased left ventricular end-diastolic pres-
    sure and systemic vascular resistance—SVR), alteration in preload/increased atrial pres-
    sure and venous congestion, alteration in electrical conduction, possibly evidenced by
    fatigue, dyspnea, changes in vital signs/hemodynamic parameters, and syncope.
risk for impaired Gas Exchange: risk factors may include alveolar-capillary membrane
    changes/congestion.

                                        CH

risk for acute Pain: risk factors may include episodic ischemia of myocardial tissues and
    stretching of left atrium.
Activity Intolerance may be related to imbalance between O_2 supply and demand
    (decreased/fixed cardiac output), possibly evidenced by exertional dyspnea, reported
    fatigue/weakness, and abnormal blood pressure or ECG changes/dysrhythmias in
    response to activity.

Aplastic anemia   CH
(Also refer to Anemia)

risk for ineffective Protection: risk factors may include abnormal blood profile (leukopenia,
    thrombocytopenia), drug therapies (antineoplastics, antibiotics, NSAIDs, anticonvul-
    sants).
Fatigue may be related to anemia, disease states, malnutrition possibly evidenced by verbal-
    ization of overwhelming lack of energy, inability to maintain usual routines/level of physi-
    cal activity, tired, decreased libido, lethargy, increase in physical complaints.

Appendectomy   MS
(Also refer to Surgery, general)

risk for Infection: risk factors may include release of pathogenic organisms into peritoneal
    cavity (prior to or at time of surgery).

Appendicitis   MS

acute Pain may be related to distention of intestinal tissues by inflammation, possibly
    evidenced by verbal reports, guarding behavior, narrowed focus, and autonomic responses
    (diaphoresis, changes in vital signs).
risk for deficient Fluid Volume: risk factors may include nausea, vomiting, anorexia, and
    hypermetabolic state.
risk for Infection: risk factors may include release of pathogenic organisms into peritoneal
    cavity.

ARDS   MS
(Refer to Respiratory distress syndrome, acute)

Arrhythmia, cardiac   MS/CH
(Refer to Dysrhythmia, cardiac)

Arterial occlussive disease, peripheral   CH
ineffective peripheral Tissue Perfusion may be related to decreased arterial blood flow possibly
    evidenced by skin discolorations, temperature changes, altered sensation, claudication,
    delayed healing.
risk for impaired Walking: risk factors may include presence of circulatory problems, pain
    with activity.
risk for inpaired Skin/Tissue Integrity: risk factors may include altered circulation/sensation.

Arthritis, gouty   CH
(Refer to Gout)

Arthritis, juvenile rheumatoid   PED/CH
(Also refer to Arthritis, rheumatoid)
risk for delayed Development: risk factors may include effects of physical disability and
    required therapy.
risk for Social Isolation: risk factors may include delay in accomplishing developmental task,
    altered state of wellness, and changes in physical appearance.

Arthritis, rheumatoid   CH
acute/chronic Pain, may be related to accumulation of fluid/inflammatory process, degenera-
    tion of joint, and deformity, possibly evidenced by verbal reports, narrowed focus, guard-
    ing/protective behaviors, and physical and social withdrawal.
impaired physical Mobility may be related to musculoskeletal deformity, pain/discomfort,
    decreased muscle strength, possibly evidenced by limited range of motion, impaired
    coordination, reluctance to attempt movement, and decreased muscle strength/control
    and mass.
Self-Care Deficit [specify] may be related to musculoskeletal impairment, decreased
    strength/endurance and range of motion, pain on movement, possibly evidenced by inabil-
    ity to manage activities of daily living (ADLs).
disturbed Body Image/Role Performance ineffective may be related to change in body struc-
    ture/function, impaired mobility/ability to perform usual tasks, focus on past
    strength/function/appearance, possibly evidenced by negative self-talk, feelings of help-
    lessness, change in lifestyle/physical abilities, dependence on others for assistance,
    decreased social involvement.

Arthritis, septic   CH
acute Pain may be related to joint inflammation possibly evidenced by verbal/coded reports,
    guarding behaviors, restlessness, narrowed focus.
impaired physical Mobility may be related to joint stiffness, pain/discomfort, reluc-
    tance to initiate movement possibly evidenced by limited range of motion, slowed
    movement.
Self-Care Deficit [specify] may be related to musculosketeal impairment, pain/discomfort,
    decreased strength, impaired coordination possibly evidenced by inability to perform
    desired ADLs.
risk for Infection spread: risk factors may include presence of infectious process, chronic
    disease states, invasive procedures.

Arthroplasty   MS

risk for Infection: risk factors may include breach of primary defenses (surgical incision), stasis of body fluids at operative site, and altered inflammatory response.

risk for deficient Fluid Volume [isotonic]: risk factors may include surgical procedure/trauma to vascular area.

impaired physical Mobility may be related to decreased strength, pain, musculoskeletal changes, possibly evidenced by impaired coordination and reluctance to attempt movement.

acute Pain may be related to tissue trauma, local edema, possibly evidenced by verbal reports, narrowed focus, guarded movement, and autonomic responses (diaphoresis, changes in vital signs).

Arthroscopy   MS

deficient Knowledge [Learning Need] regarding procedure/outcomes and self-care needs may be related to unfamiliarity with information/resources, misinterpretations, possibly evidenced by questions and requests for information, misconceptions.

risk for impaired Walking: risk factors may include joint stiffness, discomfort, prescribed movement restrictions, use of assistive devices/crutches for ambulation.

Asbestosis   CH

impaired Gas Exchange may be related to alveolar-capillary membrane changes, ventilation perfusion imbalance possibly evidenced by dyspnea, tachypnea, restlessness, clubbing of fingers, abnormal ABGs.

Activity Intolerance may be related to imbalance between oxygen supply/demand possibly evidenced by exertional dyspnea, decreased exercise tolerance/abnormal cardiopulmonary response to activity.

ineffective Airway Clearance may be related to inflammatory response to inhaled foreign body (asbestos fibers), smoking/second-hand smoke, infection possibly evidenced by dyspnea, adventitious breath sounds, increased sputum.

risk for Infection: risk factors may include decrease in ciliary action, stasis of body fluids, chronic disease, malnutrition, insufficient knowledge to avoid exposure.

acute Pain may be related to inflammation/irritation of the parietal pleura, possibly evidenced by verbal reports, guarding/distraction behaviors, self-focus, and autonomic responses (changes in vital signs).

Asperger's disorder   PED/PSY

impaired Social Interaction may be related to skill deficit about ways to enhance mutuality, communication barriers (poor pragmatic language skills), preoccupations/compulsions/repetitive motor mannerisms possibly evidenced by observed discomfort in social situations, dysfunctional interactions with others, inability to receive/communicate satisfying sense of belonging.

risk for Injury: risk factors may include rituals/repetitive motor mannerisms, clumsiness/poor coordination, vulnerability to manipulation/peer pressure.

Aspiration, foreign body   CH

ineffective Airway Clearance may be related to presence of foreign body possibly evidenced by dyspnea, ineffective cough, diminished or adventitious breath sounds.

Anxiety [specify] may be related to situational crisis, perceived threat of death possibly evidenced by apprehension, anxious, fearful, scared.

risk for Suffocation: risk for lack of safety education/precautions, eating large mouthfuls/pieces of food.

Asthma   MS

(Also refer to Emphysema)

ineffective Airway Clearance may be related to increased production/retained pulmonary
secretions, bronchospasm, decreased energy/fatigue, possibly evidenced by wheezing,
difficulty breathing, changes in depth/rate of respirations, use of accessory muscles, and
persistent ineffective cough with or without sputum production.

impaired Gas Exchange may be related to altered delivery of inspired O_2/air trapping, possibly evidenced by dyspnea, restlessness, reduced tolerance for activity, cyanosis, and
changes in ABGs and vital signs.

Anxiety [specify level] may be related to perceived threat of death, possibly evidenced by
apprehension, fearful expression, and extraneous movements.

CH

Activity Intolerance may be related to imbalance between O_2 supply and demand, possibly
evidenced by fatigue and exertional dyspnea.

Atelectasis   MS

impaired Gas Exchange may be related to inflammatory process, stasis of secretions affecting
O_2 exchange across alveolar membrane, and hypoventilation possibly evidenced by rest-
lessness/changes in mentation, dyspnea, tachycardia, pallor, cyanosis, and ABGs/oxime-
try evidence of hypoxia.

Athlete's foot   CH

impaired Skin Integrity may be related to fungal invasion, humidity, secretions, possibly
evidenced by disruption of skin surface, reports of painful itching.

risk for Infection [spread]: risk factors may include multiple breaks in skin, exposure to
moist/warm environment.

Atherosclerosis   CH/MS

(Refer to Coronary artery disease, Peripheral vascular disease)

Atrial fibrillation   CH

(Also refer to Dysrhythmias)

Activity Intolerance may be related to imbalance between oxygen supply/demand possibly
evidenced by dyspnea, dizziness, presyncope/syncopal episodes.

risk for ineffective cerebral Tissue Perfusion: risk factors may include interruption of arterial
flow (micro emboli).

Atrial flutter   CH

(Also refer to Dysrhythmias)

Anxiety [specify] may be related to threat to/change in health status possibly evidenced by
expressed concerns, apprehension, awareness of physiologic symptoms (palpitations,
dizziness, presyncope/syncopal episodes), focus on self.

Atrial tachycardia   CH

(Refer to Dysrhythmias)

Attention deficit disorder   PED/PSY

ineffective Coping may be related to situational/maturational crisis, retarded ego development,
low self-concept possibly evidenced by easy distraction by extraneous stimuli, shifting
between uncompleted activities.

chronic low Self-Esteem may be related to retarded ego development, lack of positive/repeated negative feedback, negative role models possibly evidenced by lack of eye contact, derogatory self-comments, hesitance to try new tasks, inadequate level of confidence.

deficient Knowledge regarding condition, prognosis, therapy may be related to misinformation/misinterpretations, unfamiliarity with resources possibly evidenced by verbalization of problems/misconceptions, poor school performance, unrealistic expectations of medication regimen.

Autistic disorder   PED/PSY

impaired Social Interaction may be related to abnormal response to sensory input/inadequate sensory stimulation, organic brain dysfunction; delayed development of secure attachment/trust, lack of intuitive skills to comprehend and accurately respond to social cues, disturbance in self-concept, possibly evidenced by lack of responsiveness to others, lack of eye contact or facial responsiveness, treating persons as objects, lack of awareness of feelings in others, indifference/aversion to comfort, affection, or physical contact; failure to develop cooperative social play and peer friendships in childhood.

impaired verbal Communication may be related to inability to trust others, withdrawal into self, organic brain dysfunction, abnormal interpretation/response to and/or inadequate sensory stimulation, possibly evidenced by lack of interactive communication mode, no use of gestures or spoken language, absent or abnormal nonverbal communication; lack of eye contact or facial expression; peculiar patterns of speech (form, content, or speech production), and impaired ability to initiate or sustain conversation despite adequate speech.

risk for Self-Mutilation: risk factors may include organic brain dysfunction, inability to trust others, disturbance in self-concept, inadequate sensory stimulation or abnormal response to sensory input (sensory overload); history of physical, emotional, or sexual abuse; and response to demands of therapy, realization of severity of condition.

disturbed Personal Identity may be related to organic brain dysfunction, lack of development of trust, fixation at presymbiotic phase of development, possibly evidenced by lack of awareness of the feelings or existence of others, increased anxiety resulting from physical contact with others, absent or impaired imitation of others, repeating what others say, persistent preoccupation with parts of objects, obsessive attachment to objects, marked distress over changes in environment; autoerotic/ritualistic behaviors, self-touching, rocking, swaying.

compromised/disabled family Coping may be related to family members unable to express feelings; excessive guilt, anger, or blaming among family members regarding child's condition; ambivalent or dissonant family relationships, prolonged coping with problem exhausting supportive ability of family members, possibly evidenced by denial of existence or severity of disturbed behaviors, preoccupation with personal emotional reaction to situation, rationalization that problem will be outgrown, attempts to intervene with child are achieving increasingly ineffective results, family withdraws from or becomes overly protective of child.

Bacteremia   MS
(Refer to Sepsis)

Barbiturate abuse   CH/PSY
(Refer to Depressant abuse)

Battered child syndrome   PED/CH
(Also refer to Abuse)

risk for Trauma: risk factors may include dependent position in relationship(s), vulnerability (e.g., congenital problems/chronic illness), history of previous abuse/neglect, lack/nonuse of support systems by caregiver(s).

---

delayed Growth and Development may be related to inadequate caretaking/neglect, indifference, inconsistent responsiveness, environmental/stimulation deficiencies possibly evidenced by delay/difficulty in performing age appropriate skills, altered physical growth, loss of previously acquired skills, precocious/accelerated sexual awareness, flat affect, decreased responses.

interrupted Family Processes / impaired Parenting may be related to poor role model/identity, unrealistic expectations, presence of stressors, and lack of support, possibly evidenced by verbalization of negative feelings, inappropriate caretaking behaviors, and evidence of physical/psychological trauma to child.

PSY

chronic low Self-Esteem may be related to deprivation and negative feedback of family members, personal vulnerability, feelings of abandonment, possibly evidenced by lack of eye contact, withdrawal from social contacts, discounting own needs, nonassertive/passive, indecisive, or overly conforming behaviors.

Post-Trauma Syndrome may be related to sustained/recurrent physical or emotional abuse; possibly evidenced by acting-out behavior, development of phobias, poor impulse control, and emotional numbness.

Bed sores   CH/MS
(Refer to Ulcer, pressure)

Bedwetting   PED
(Refer to Enuresis)

Benign prostatic hyperplasia   CH/MS

[acute/chronic] Urinary Retention may be related to mechanical obstruction (enlarged prostate), decompensation of detrusor musculature, inability of bladder to contract adequately, possibly evidenced by frequency, hesitancy, inability to empty bladder completely, incontinence/dribbling, bladder distention, residual urine.

acute Pain may be related to mucosal irritation, bladder distention, colic, urinary infection, and radiation therapy, possibly evidenced by verbal reports (bladder/rectal spasm), narrowed focus, altered muscle tone, grimacing, distraction behaviors, restlessness, and autonomic responses.

risk for deficient Fluid Volume: risk factors may include postobstructive diuresis, endocrine/electrolyte imbalances.

Fear/Anxiety [specify level] may be related to change in health status (possibility of surgical procedure/malignancy); embarrassment/loss of dignity associated with genital exposure before, during, and after treatment, and concern about sexual ability, possibly evidenced by increased tension, apprehension, worry, expressed concerns regarding perceived changes, and fear of unspecific consequences.

Biliary calculus   CH/MS
(Refer to Cholelithiasis)

Biliary cancer   MS
(Also refer to Cancer)

imbalanced Nutrition: less than body requirements may be related to inability to ingest/absorb nutrients (anorexia, nausea, indigestion), abnormal discomfort, possibly evidenced by aversion to eating, observed lack of intake, muscle wasting, weight loss, and imbalances in nutritional studies.

risk for impaired Skin Integrity: risk factors may include accumulation of bile salts in skin, poor skin turgor, skeletal prominence.

death Anxiety may be related to lack of successful treatment options, poor prognosis possibly evidenced by fear of the process of dying, leaving SO/family alone after death, negative death images, concern of overworking caregiver, deep sadness.

Binge-eating disorder PSY
(Refer to Bulimia nervosa)

Bipolar disorders PSY
risk for other-directed Violence: risk factors may include irritability, impulsive behavior; delusional thinking; angry response when ideas are refuted or wishes denied; manic excitement, with possible indicators of threatening body language/verbalizations, increased motor activity, overt and aggressive acts; hostility.

imbalanced Nutrition: less than body requirements may be related to inadequate intake in relation to metabolic expenditures, possibly evidenced by body weight 20% or more below ideal weight, observed inadequate intake, inattention to mealtimes, and distraction from task of eating; laboratory evidence of nutritional deficits/imbalances.

risk for Poisoning [lithium toxicity]: risk factors may include narrow therapeutic range of drug, client's ability (or lack of) to follow through with medication regimen and monitoring, and denial of need for information/therapy.

disturbed Sleep Pattern may be related to psychological stress, lack of recognition of fatigue/need to sleep, hyperactivity, possibly evidenced by denial of need to sleep, interrupted nighttime sleep, one or more nights without sleep, changes in behavior and performance, increasing irritability/restlessness, and dark circles under eyes.

disturbed Sensory Perception (specify) [overload] may be related to decrease in sensory threshold, endogenous chemical alteration, psychological stress, sleep deprivation, possibly evidenced by increased distractibility and agitation, anxiety, disorientation, poor concentration, auditory/visual hallucination, bizarre thinking, and motor incoordination.

interrupted Family Processes may be related to situational crises (illness, economics, change in roles); euphoric mood and grandiose ideas/actions of client, manipulative behavior and limit testing, client's refusal to accept responsibility for own actions, possibly evidenced by statements of difficulty coping with situation, lack of adaptation to change or not dealing constructively with illness; ineffective family decision-making process, failure to send and to receive clear messages, and inappropriate boundary maintenance.

Bladder cancer MS
(Also refer to Cancer; Urinary diversion)
impaired Urinary Elimination may be related to presence of tumor possibly evidenced by frequency, burning, dysuria.

acute/chronic Urinary Retention may be related to blockage of urethra possibly evidenced by sensation of fullness, bladder distension, residual urine, dysuria.

Body dismorphic disorder PSY
(Refer to Hypochondriasis)

Bone cancer MS/CH
(Also refer to Myeloma, multiple; Amputation)
acute Pain may be related to bone destruction, pressure on nerves possibly evidenced by verbal or coded report, protective behavior, autonomic responses.

risk for Trauma: risk factors may include increased bone fragility, general weakness, balancing difficulties.

Bone marrow transplantation   **MS/CH**
(Also refer to Transplantation, recipient)
risk for Injury: risk factors may include immune dysfunction/supression, abnormal blood
    profile, action of donor T cells.

Borderline personality disorder   **PSY**
risk for self/other-directed Violence/Self-Mutilation: risk factors may include use of projection
    as a major defense mechanism, pervasive problems with negative transference, feelings of
    guilt/need to "punish" self, distorted sense of self, inability to cope with increased psycho-
    logical/physiologic tension in a healthy manner.
Anxiety [severe to panic] may be related to unconscious conflicts (experience of extreme
    stress), perceived threat to self-concept, unmet needs, possibly evidenced by easy frustra-
    tion and feelings of hurt, abuse of alcohol/other drugs, transient psychotic symptoms and
    performance of self-mutilating acts.
chronic low Self-Esteem/disturbed Personal Identity may be related to lack of positive feedback,
    unmet dependency needs, retarded ego development/fixation at an earlier level of develop-
    ment, possibly evidenced by difficulty identifying self or defining self-boundaries, feelings
    of depersonalization, extreme mood changes, lack of tolerance of rejection or of being
    alone, unhappiness with self, striking out at others, performance of ritualistic self-
    damaging acts, and belief that punishing self is necessary.
Social Isolation may be related to immature interests, unaccepted social behavior, inade-
    quate personal resources, and inability to engage in satisfying personal relationships,
    possibly evidenced by alternating clinging and distancing behaviors, difficulty meeting
    expectations of others, experiencing feelings of difference from others, expressing interests
    inappropriate to developmental age, and exhibiting behavior unaccepted by dominant
    cultural group.

Botulism (food borne)   **MS**
deficient Fluid Volume [isotonic] may be related to active losses—vomiting, diarrhea;
    decreased intake—nausea, dysphagia, possibly evidenced by reports of thirst; dry
    skin/mucous membranes, decreased B/P and urine output, change in mental state,
    increased Hct.
impaired physical Mobility may be related to neuromuscular impairment possibly evidenced
    by limited ability to perform gross/fine motor skills.
Anxiety [specify level]/Fear may be related to threat of death, interpersonal transmission
    possibly evidenced by expressed concerns, apprehension, awareness of physiologic symp-
    toms, focus on self.
risk for impaired spontaneous Ventilation: risk factors may include neuromuscular impairment,
    presence of infectious process.

                                                   CH
risk for Poisoning: risk factors may include lack of proper precautions in food storage/prepara-
    tion.

Bowel obstruction   **MS**
(Refer to Ileus)

Bowel resection   **CH**
(Refer to Intestinal surgery [without diversion])

BPH   **CH/MS**
(Refer to Benign prostatic hypertrophy)

Brachytherapy (radioactive implants)   MS

risk for Injury: risk factors may include radiation emitted by client (depending on type of procedure), accidental dislodgement or removal of radiation source.

risk for impaired physical Mobility: risk factors may include prescribed restrictions (48 hours for low-dose implants), reluctance to move (fear of dislodging implants), decreased strength/endurance, depressed mood.

Bradycardia   CH
(Refer to Dysrhythmia, cardiac)

Brain tumor   MS
(Also refer to Cancer)

acute Pain may be related to pressure on brain tissues, possibly evidenced by reports of headache, facial mask of pain, narrowed focus, and autonomic responses (changes in vital signs).

disturbed Thought Processes may be related to altered circulation to and/or destruction of brain tissue, possibly evidenced by memory loss, personality changes, impaired ability to make decisions/conceptualize, and inaccurate interpretation of environment.

disturbed Sensory Perception (specify) may be related to compression/displacement of brain tissue, disruption of neuronal conduction, possibly evidenced by changes in visual acuity, alterations in sense of balance/gait disturbance, and paresthesia.

risk for deficient Fluid Volume: risk factors may include recurrent vomiting from irritation of vagal center in medulla and decreased intake.

Self-Care Deficit [specify] may be related to sensory/neuromuscular impairment interfering with ability to perform tasks, possibly evidenced by unkempt/disheveled appearance, body odor, and verbalization/observation of inability to perform activities of daily living.

Breast cancer   MS/CH
(Also refer to Cancer)

Anxiety [specify level] may be related to change in health status, threat of death, stress, interpersonal transmission possibly evidenced by expressed concerns, apprehension, uncertainty, focus on self, diminished productivity.

deficient Knowledge regarding diagnosis, prognosis, and treatment options may be related to lack of exposure/unfamiliarity with information resources, information misinterpretation, cognitive limitation/anxiety possibly evidenced by verbalizations, statements of misconceptions, inappropriate behaviors.

risk for disturbed Body Image: risk factors may include significance of body part with regard to sexual perceptions.

risk for ineffective Sexual Patterns: risk factors may include health-related changes, medical treatments, concern about relationship with SO.

Bronchitis   CH

ineffective Airway Clearance may be related to excessive, thickened mucous secretions, possibly evidenced by presence of rhonchi, tachypnea, and ineffective cough.

Activity Intolerance [specify level] may be related to imbalance between O_2 supply and demand, possibly evidenced by reports of fatigue, dyspnea, and abnormal vital sign response to activity.

acute Pain may be related to localized inflammation, persistent cough, aching associated with fever, possibly evidenced by reports of discomfort, distraction behavior, and facial mask of pain.

Bronchogenic carcinoma   MS/CH
(Also refer to Cancer)

impaired Gas Exchange may be related to ventilation perfusion imbalance (bronchial narrowing with air trapping, atelectasis), presence of inflammatory exudate possibly evidenced by dyspnea, diminished/adventitious breath sounds, decreased chest expansion (depth of breathing), abnormal ABGs.

risk for ineffective Airway Clearance: risk factors may include retained secretions, inflammatory exudate, bronchial narrowing, pain, smoking/second-hand smoke, infection.

risk for Infection: risk factors may include stasis of body fluids, tissue destruction, chronic disease, malnutrition.

Bronchopneumonia   MS/CH
(Also refer to Bronchitis)

ineffective Airway Clearance may be related to tracheal bronchial inflammation, edema formation, increased sputum production, pleuritic pain, decreased energy, fatigue, possibly evidenced by changes in rate/depth of respirations, abnormal breath sounds, use of accessory muscles, dyspnea, cyanosis, effective/ineffective cough—with or without sputum production.

impaired Gas Exchange may be related to inflammatory process, collection of secretions affecting O_2 exchange across alveolar membrane, and hypoventilation, possibly evidenced by restlessness/changes in mentation, dyspnea, tachycardia, pallor, cyanosis, and ABGs/oximetry evidence of hypoxia.

risk for Infection [spread]: risk factors may include decreased ciliary action, stasis of secretions, presence of existing infection.

Buck's traction   MS
(Refer to Traction)

Buerger's disease   CH
(Refer to Peripheral vascular disease)

Bulimia nervosa   PSY/MS
(Also refer to Anorexia nervosa)

impaired Dentition may be related to dietary habits, poor oral hygiene, chronic vomiting possibly evidenced by erosion of tooth enamel, multiple caries, abraided teeth.

impaired Oral Mucous Membrane may be related to malnutrition or vitamin deficiency, poor oral hygiene, chronic vomiting possibly evidenced by sore, inflamed buccal mucosa; swollen salivary glands, ulcerations of mucosa, reports of constant sore mouth/throat.

risk for deficient Fluid Volume: risk factors may include consistent self-induced vomiting, chronic/excessive laxative/diuretic use, esophageal erosion or tear (Mallory-Weiss syndrome).

deficient Knowledge [Learning Need] regarding condition, prognosis, complication, treatment may be related to lack of exposure to/unfamiliarity with information about condition, learned maladaptive coping skills possibly evidenced by verbalization of misconception of relationship of current situation and behaviors, distortion of body image, bingeing and purging behaviors, verbalized need for information/desire to change behaviors.

Bunion   CH

impaired Walking may be related to inflammation/degeneration of joint, inappropriate footware possibly evidenced by inability to walk required distances.

Bunionectomy   **MS**

(Also refer to Surgery, general; Postoperative recovery period)

impaired Walking may be related to surgical intervention, restrictive therapy possibly
   evidenced by inability to walk required distances, to navigate curbs, climb stairs.

Burns (dependent on type, degree, and severity of the injury) MS/CH

risk for deficient Fluid Volume: risk factors may include loss of fluids through wounds, capillary damage and evaporation, hypermetabolic state, insufficient intake, hemorrhagic
   losses.

risk for ineffective Airway Clearance: risk factors may include mucosal edema and loss of
   ciliary action (smoke inhalation), direct upper airway injury by flame, steam, chemicals.

risk for Infection: risk factors may include loss of protective dermal barrier,
   traumatized/necrotic tissue, decreased hemoglobin, suppressed inflammatory response,
   environmental exposure/invasive procedures.

acute/chronic Pain may be related to destruction of/trauma to tissue and nerves, edema
   formation, and manipulation of impaired tissues, possibly evidenced by verbal reports,
   narrowed focus, distraction and guarding behaviors, facial mask of pain, and autonomic
   responses (changes in vital signs).

risk for imbalanced Nutrition: less than body requirements: risk factors may include
   hypermetabolic state in response to burn injury/stress, inadequate intake, protein
   catabolism.

Post-Trauma Syndrome may be related to life-threatening event, possibly evidenced by reexperiencing the event, repetitive dreams/nightmares, psychic/emotional numbness, and
   sleep disturbance.

ineffective Protection may be related to extremes of age, inadequate nutrition, anemia,
   impaired immune system, possibly evidenced by impaired healing, deficient immunity,
   fatigue, anorexia.

                                                                    PED

deficient Diversional Activity may be related to long-term hospitalization, frequent lengthy
   treatments, and physical limitations, possibly evidenced by expressions of boredom, restlessness, withdrawal, and requests for something to do.

risk for delayed Development: risk factors may include effects of physical disability, separation
   from SO(s), and environmental deficiencies.

Bursitis   **CH**

acute/chronic Pain may be related to inflammation of affected joint, possibly evidenced by
   verbal reports, guarding behavior, and narrowed focus.

impaired physical Mobility may be related to inflammation and swelling of joint, and pain,
   possibly evidenced by diminished range of motion, reluctance to attempt movement, and
   imposed restriction of movement by medical treatment.

CABG   **MS**

(Refer to Coronary artery bypass surgery)

CAD   **CH/MS**

(Refer to Coronary artery disease)

Calculi, urinary   **CH/MS**

acute Pain may be related to increased frequency/force of ureteral contractions, tissue disten-
   sion/trauma and edema formation, cellular ischemia possibly evidenced by reports of

sudden, severe, colicky pains; guarding and distraction behaviors, self-focus, and autonomic responses.

impaired Urinary Elimination may be related to stimulation of the bladder by calculi, renal or ureteral irritation, mechanical obstruction of urinary flow, edema formation, inflammation possibly evidenced by urgency and frequency; oliguria (retention); hematuria.

risk for deficient Fluid Volume: risk factors may include stimulation of renal-intestinal reflexes causing nausea, vomiting, and diarrhea; changes in urinary output, postoperative diuresis; and decreased intake.

risk for Infection: risk factors may include stasis of urine.

deficient Knowledge [Learning Need] regarding condition, prognosis, self-care and treatment needs may be related to lack of exposure/recall and information misinterpretation, possibly evidenced by requests for information, statements of concern, and recurrence/development of preventable complications.

Cancer   MS
(Also refer to Chemotherapy; Radiation therapy)

Fear/death Anxiety may be related to situational crises, threat to/change in health/socioeconomic status, role functioning, interaction patterns; threat of death, separation from family, interpersonal transmission of feelings, possibly evidenced by expressed concerns, feelings of inadequacy/helplessness, insomnia; increased tension, restlessness, focus on self, sympathetic stimulation.

anticipatory Grieving may be related to potential loss of physiologic well-being (body part/function), perceived separation from SO(s)/lifestyle (death), possibly evidenced by anger, sadness, withdrawal, choked feelings, changes in eating/sleep patterns, activity level, libido, and communication patterns.

acute/chronic Pain may be related to the disease process (compression of nerve tissue, infiltration of nerves or their vascular supply, obstruction of a nerve pathway, inflammation), or side effects of therapeutic agents, possibly evidenced by verbal reports, self-focusing/narrowed focus, alteration in muscle tone, facial mask of pain, distraction/guarding behaviors, autonomic responses, and restlessness.

Fatigue may be related to decreased metabolic energy production, increased energy requirements (hypermetabolic state), overwhelming psychological/emotional demands, and altered body chemistry (side effects of medications, chemotherapy), possibly evidenced by unremitting/overwhelming lack of energy, inability to maintain usual routines, decreased performance, impaired ability to concentrate, lethargy/listlessness, and disinterest in surroundings.

impaired Home Maintenance may be related to debilitation, lack of resources, and/or inadequate support systems, possibly evidenced by verbalization of problem, request for assistance, and lack of necessary equipment or aids.

                                                             PED
compromised/disabled family Coping may be related to chronic nature of disease and disability, ongoing treatment needs, parental supervision, and lifestyle restrictions, possibly evidenced by expression of denial/despair, depression, and protective behavior disproportionate to client's abilities or need for autonomy.

readiness for enhanced family Coping may be related to the fact that the individual's needs are being sufficiently gratified and adaptive tasks effectively addressed, enabling goals of self-actualization to surface, possibly evidenced by verbalizations of impact of crisis on own values, priorities, goals, or relationships.

Candidiasis   **CH**
(Also refer to Thrush)

impaired Skin/Tissue Integrity may be related to infectious lesions possibly evidenced by
    disruption of skin surfaces/mucous membranes.

acute Pain/[Discomfort] may be related to exposure of irritated skin/mucous membranes to
    excretions (urine/feces) possibly evidenced by verbal/coded reports, restlessness, guarding
    behaviors.

risk for Sexual Dysfunction: risk factors include presence of infectious process/vaginal
    discomfort.

Cannabis abuse   **CH**
(Refer to Depressant abuse)

Carbon monoxide poisoning   **MS**

impaired Gas Exchange may be related to altered oxygen-carrying capacity of blood possibly
    evidenced by headache, confusion, somnolence, elevated CO levels.

Activity Intolerance may be related to imbalance between oxygen supply/demand possibly
    evidenced by fatigue, exertional dyspnea.

risk for Injury: risk factors may include therapeutic intervention (hyperbaric oxygen therapy).

risk for Trauma/Suffocation: risk factors may include cognitive limitations/altered conscious-
    ness, loss of large- or small-muscle coordination (seizure).

                                                                             CH

disturbed Thought Processes may be related to period of hypoxia/altered affinity of hemoglobin
    for oxygen possibly evidenced by memory disturbances, difficulty concentrating

Cardiac catheterization   **MS**

Anxiety [specify] may be related to threat to/change in health status, stress, family
    heredity possibly evidenced by expressed concerns, apprehension, uncertainty, focus
    on self.

risk for decreased Cardiac Output: risk factors may include altered heart rate/rhythm
    (vasovagal response, ventricular dysrhythmias), decreased myocardial contractility
    (ischemia).

risk for ineffective Tissue Perfusion: risk factors may include mechanical reduction of arterial
    blood flow, local hematoma formation, thrombosis, emboli, allergic dye response.

Cardiac conditions, prenatal   **OB**

risk for Cardiac Output [decompensation]: risk factors may include increased circulat-
    ing volume, dysrhythmias, altered myocardial contractility, inotropic changes in
    the heart.

risk for excess Fluid Volume: risk factors may include increasing circulating volume, changes
    in renal function, dietary indiscretion.

risk for ineffective uteroplacental Tissue Perfusion: risk factors may include changes in circulat-
    ing volume, right-to-left shunt.

risk for Activity Intolerance: risk factors may include presence of circulatory problems, previ-
    ous episodes of intolerance, deconditioned status.

risk for maternal Infection: risk factors may include inadequate primary/secondary defenses,
    chronic condition, insufficient information to avoid exposure to pathogens.

Cardiac inflammatory disease   **MS**
(Refer to Endocarditis; Myocarditis; Pericarditis)

Cardiac surgery **MS/PED**

Anxiety [specify level]/Fear may be related to change in health status and threat to self-concept/of death, possibly evidenced by sympathetic stimulation, increased tension, and apprehension.

risk for decreased Cardiac Output: risk factors may include decreased preload (hypovolemia), depressed myocardial contractility, changes in SVR (afterload), and alterations in electrical conduction (dysrhythmias).

deficient Fluid Volume [isotonic] may be related to intraoperative bleeding with inadequate blood replacement; bleeding related to insufficient heparin reversal, fibrinolysis, or platelet destruction; or volume depletion effects of intraoperative/postoperative diuretic therapy, possibly evidenced by increased pulse rate, decreased pulse volume/pressure, decreased urine output, hemoconcentration.

risk for impaired Gas Exchange: risk factors may include alveolar-capillary membrane changes (atelectasis), intestinal edema, inadequate function or premature discontinuation of chest tubes, and diminished oxygen-carrying capacity of the blood.

acute Pain/[Discomfort] may be related to tissue inflammation/ trauma, edema formation, intraoperative nerve trauma, and myocardial ischemia, possibly evidenced by reports of incisional discomfort/pain in chest and donor site; paresthesia/pain in hand, arm, shoulder, anxiety, restlessness, irritability; distraction behaviors, and autonomic responses.

impaired Skin/Tissue Integrity related to mechanical trauma (surgical incisions, puncture wounds) and edema evidenced by disruption of skin surface/tissues.

Cardiogenic shock **MS**
(Refer to Shock, cardiogenic)

Cardiomyopathy **CH/MS**

decreased Cardiac Output may be related to altered contractility possibility evidenced by dyspnea, fatigue, chest pain, dizziness, syncope.

Activity Intolerance may be related to imbalance between oxygen supply and demand possibly evidenced by weakness/fatigue, dyspnea, abnormal heart rate/BP response to activity, ECG changes.

ineffective Role Performance may be related to changes in physical health, stress, demands of job/life possibly evidenced by change in usual patterns of responsibility, role strain, change in capacity to resume role.

Carotid endarterectomy **MS**
(Also refer to Surgery, general)

risk for ineffective cerebral Tissue Perfusion: risk factors may include interruption of arterial flow (wound hematoma, emboli), pressure changes with edema formation (hyperperfusion syndrome).

Carpal tunnel syndrome **CH/MS**

acute/chronic Pain may be related to pressure on median nerve, possibly evidenced by verbal reports, reluctance to use affected extremity, guarding behaviors, expressed fear of reinjury, altered ability to continue previous activities.

impaired physical Mobility may be related to neuromuscular impairment and pain, possibly evidenced by decreased hand strength, weakness, limited range of motion, and reluctance to attempt movement.

risk for Peripheral Neurovascular Dysfunction: risk factors may include mechanical compression (e.g., brace, repetitive tasks/motions), immobilization.

deficient Knowledge [Learning Need] regarding condition, prognosis and treatment/safety needs may be related to lack of exposure/recall, information misinterpretation, possibly evidenced by questions, statements of concern, request for information, inaccurate follow-through of instructions/development of preventable complications.

Casts   CH/MS
(Also refer to Fractures)

risk for Peripheral Neurovascular Dysfunction: risk factors may include presence of fracture(s), mechanical compression (cast), tissue trauma, immobilization, vascular obstruction.

risk for impaired Skin Integrity: risk factors may include pressure of cast, moisture/debris under cast, objects inserted under cast to relieve itching, and/or altered sensation/circulation.

Self-Care Deficit [specify] may be related to impaired ability to perform self-care tasks, possibly evidenced by statements of need for assistance and observed difficulty in performing activities of daily living.

Cataract   CH

disturbed visual Sensory Perception may be related to altered sensory reception/status of sense organs possibly evidenced by diminished acuity, visual distortions, and change in usual response to stimuli.

risk for Trauma: risk factors may include poor vision, reduced hand/eye coordination.

Anxiety [specify level]/Fear may be related to alteration in visual acuity, threat of permanent loss of vision/independence, possibly evidenced by expressed concerns, apprehension, and feelings of uncertainty.

deficient Knowledge [Learning Need] regarding ways of coping with altered abilities, therapy choices, lifestyle changes may be related to lack of exposure/recall, misinterpretation, or cognitive limitations, possibly evidenced by requests for information, statement of concern, inaccurate follow-through of instructions/development of preventable complications.

Cataract extraction (postoperative care)   MS

risk for Injury: risk factors may include increased intraocular pressure, intraocular hemorrhage, vitreous loss.

risk for Infection: risk factors may include invasive procedure/surgical manipulation, presence of chronic disease.

disturbed visual Sensory Perception may be related to altered sensory reception (use of eye drops/cataract glasses), therapeutically restricted environment (surgical procedure, patching), possibly evidenced by visual distortions/blurring, visual confusion/change in depth perception.

Cat scratch disease   CH

acute Pain may be related to effects of circulating toxins (fever, headache, and lymphadenitis), possibly evidenced by verbal reports, guarding behavior, and autonomic response (changes in vital signs).

Hyperthermia may be related to inflammatory process, possibly evidenced by increased body temperature, flushed warm skin, tachypnea and tachycardia.

Celiac disease   CH

imbalanced Nutrition: less than body requirements may be related to inability to absorb nutrients (mucosal damage, loss of villi, proliferation of crypt cells, shortened transit time through GI tract) possibly evidenced by weight loss, abdominal distention, steatorrhea, evidence of anemia/vitamin deficiencies.

Diarrhea may be related to irritation, malabsorption possibly evidenced by abdominal pain, hyperactive bowel sounds, at least 3 loose stools per day.

risk for deficient Fluid Volume: risk factors may include mild to massive steatorrhea/diarrhea.

Cellulitis   CH/MS

risk for Infection [abscess, bacteremia]: risk factors may inlcude broken skin, chronic disease, presence of pathogens, insufficient knowledge to avoid exposure to pathogens.

acute Pain[/Discomfort] may be related to inflammatory process, circulating toxins possibly evidenced by reports of localized pain/headache, guarding behaviors, restlessness, autonomic responses.

Cerebral embolism   MS/CH

(Refer to Cerebrovascular accident)

Cerebral palsy   PED/CH

(Refer to Palsy, cerebral [spastic hemiplegia])

Cerebrovascular accident   MS

ineffective cerebral Tissue Perfusion may be related to interruption of blood flow (occlusive disorder, hemorrhage, cerebral vasospasm/edema), possibly evidenced by altered level of consciousness, changes in vital signs, changes in motor/sensory responses, restlessness, memory loss; sensory, language, intellectual, and emotional deficits.

impaired physical Mobility may be related to neuromuscular involvement (weakness, paresthesia, flaccid/hypotonic paralysis, spastic paralysis), perceptual/cognitive impairment, possibly evidenced by inability to purposefully move involved body parts/limited range of motion; impaired coordination, and/or decreased muscle strength/control.

impaired verbal [and/or written] Communication may be related to impaired cerebral circulation, neuromuscular impairment, loss of facial/oral muscle tone and control; generalized weakness/fatigue, possibly evidenced by impaired articulation, does not/cannot speak (dysarthria); inability to modulate speech, find and/or name words, identify objects and/or inability to comprehend written/spoken language; inability to produce written communication.

Self-Care Deficit [specify] may be related to neuromuscular impairment, decreased strength/endurance, loss of muscle control/coordination, perceptual/cognitive impairment, pain/discomfort, and depression, possibly evidenced by stated/observed inability to perform ADLs, requests for assistance, disheveled appearance, and incontinence.

risk for impaired Swallowing: risk factors may include muscle paralysis and perceptual impairment.

risk for Unilateral Neglect: risk factors may include sensory loss of part of visual field with perceptual loss of corresponding body segment.

                                                                 CH

impaired Home Maintenance may be related to condition of individual family member, insufficient finances/family organization or planning, unfamiliarity with resources, and inadequate support systems, possibly evidenced by members expressing difficulty in managing home in a comfortable manner/requesting assistance with home maintenance, disorderly surroundings, and overtaxed family members.

situational low Self-Esteem/disturbed Body Image/ineffective Role Performance may be related to biophysical, psychosocial, and cognitive/perceptual changes, possibly evidenced by actual change in structure and/or function, change in usual patterns of responsibility/physical capacity to resume role; and verbal/nonverbal response to actual or perceived change.

Cervix, dysfunctional   OB
(Refer to Dilation of Cervix, premature)

Cesarean birth   OB
(Also refer to Cesarean birth, unplanned/postpartal)

deficient Knowledge [Learning Need] regarding surgical procedure/expectation, postoperative routines/therapy, and self-care needs may be related to lack of information/misinterpretation, possibly evidenced by statements of concern, questions, and misconceptions.

risk for deficient Fluid Volume: risk factors may include restrictions of oral intake, blood loss.

risk for impaired parent/infant Attachment: risk factors may include separation, existing health conditions maternal/infant, lack of privacy.

Cesarean birth, postpartal   OB
(Also refer to Postpartal period)

risk for impaired parent/infant Attachment: risk factors may include developmental transition/gain of a family member, situational crisis (e.g., surgical intervention, physical complications interfering with initial acquaintance/interaction, negative self-appraisal).

acute Pain/[Discomfort] may be related to surgical trauma, effects of anesthesia, hormonal effects, bladder/abdominal distension possibly evidenced by verbal reports (e.g., incisional pain, cramping/afterpains, spinal headache), guarding/distraction behaviors, irritability, facial mask of pain.

risk for situational low Self-Esteem: risk factors may include perceived "failure" at life event, maturational transition, perceived loss of control in unplanned delivery.

risk for Injury: risk factors may include biochemical or regulatory functions (e.g., orthostatic hypotension, development of PIH or eclampsia), effects of anesthesia, thromboembolism, abnormal blood profile (anemia/excessive blood loss, rubella sensitivity, Rh incompatibility), tissue trauma.

risk for Infection: risk factors may include tissue trauma/broken skin, decreased Hb, invasive procedures and/or increased environmental exposure, prolongs rupture of amniotic membranes, malnutrition.

Self-Care Deficit (specify) may be related to effects of anesthesia, decreased strength and endurance, physical discomfort possibly evidenced by verbalization of inability to perform desired ADL(s).

Cesarean birth, unplanned   OB
(Also refer to Cesarean birth, postpartal)

deficient Knowledge [Learning Need] regarding underlying procedure, pathophysiology, and self-care needs may be related to incomplete/inadequate information, possibly evidenced by request for information, verbalization of concerns/misconceptions and inappropriate/exaggerated behavior.

Anxiety [specify level] may be related to actual/perceived threat to mother/fetus, emotional threat to self-esteem, unmet needs/expectations, interpersonal transmission, possibly evidenced by increased tension, apprehension, feelings of inadequacy, sympathetic stimulation, and narrowed focus, restlessness.

Powerlessness may be related to interpersonal interaction, perception of illness-related regimen, lifestyle of helplessness possibly evidenced by verbalization of lack of control, lack of participation in care or decision making, passivity.

risk for impaired fetal Gas Exchange: risk factors may include altered blood flow to placenta and/or through umbilical cord.

risk for acute Pain: risk factors may include increased/prolonged contractions, psychological reaction.

risk for Infection: risk factors may include invasive procedures, rupture of amniotic membranes, break in skin, decreased hemoglobin, exposure to pathogens.

Chemical dependence PSY/CH
(Refer to specific agents; Substance dependency/abuse rehabilitation)

Chemotherapy MS/CH
(Also refer to Cancer)

risk for deficient Fluid Volume: risk factors may include gastrointestinal losses (vomiting), interference with adequate intake (stomatitis/anorexia), losses through abnormal routes (indwelling tubes, wounds, fistulas), hypermetabolic state.

imbalanced Nutrition: less than body requirements may be related to inability to ingest adequate nutrients (nausea, stomatitis, and fatigue), hypermetabolic state, possibly evidenced by weight loss (wasting), aversion to eating, reported altered taste sensation, sore, inflamed buccal cavity; diarrhea and/or constipation.

impaired Oral Mucous Membrane may be related to side effects of therapeutic agents/radiation, dehydration, and malnutrition, possibly evidenced by ulcerations, leukoplakia, decreased salivation, and reports of pain.

disturbed Body Image may be related to anatomical/structural changes; loss of hair and weight, possibly evidenced by negative feelings about body, preoccupation with change, feelings of helplessness/hopelessness, and change in social environment.

ineffective Protection may be related to inadequate nutrition, drug therapy/radiation, abnormal blood profile, disease state (cancer), possibly evidenced by impaired healing, deficient immunity, anorexia, fatigue.

Chickenpox CH/PED
(Refer to Measles)

Chlamydia trachomatis infection CH
(Refer to Sexually transmitted diseases)

Cholecystectomy MS

acute Pain may be related to interruption in skin/tissue layers with mechanical closure (sutures/staples) and invasive procedures (including T-tube/nasogastric—NG—tube), possibly evidenced by verbal reports, guarding/distraction behaviors, and autonomic responses (changes in vital signs).

ineffective Breathing Pattern may be related to decreased lung expansion (pain and muscle weakness), decreased energy/fatigue, ineffective cough, possibly evidenced by fremitus, tachypnea, and decreased respiratory depth/vital capacity.

risk for deficient Fluid Volume: risk factors may include vomiting/NG aspiration, medically restricted intake, altered coagulation.

Cholelithiasis CH

acute Pain may be related to inflammation and distortion of tissues, ductal spasm, possibly evidenced by verbal reports, guarding/distraction behaviors, and autonomic responses (changes in vital signs).

imbalanced Nutrition: less than body requirements may be related to inability to ingest/absorb adequate nutrients (food intolerance/pain, nausea/vomiting, anorexia), possibly evidenced by aversion to food/decreased intake and weight loss.

deficient Knowledge [Learning Need] regarding pathophysiology, therapy choices, and self-care needs may be related to lack of information, misinterpretation, possibly evidenced by verbalization of concerns, questions, and recurrence of condition.

Cholera   CH/MS

deficient Fluid Volume [isotonic] may be related to active volume loss (profuse watery diarrhea, vomiting) possibly evidenced by intense thirst, marked loss of tissue turgor, decreased urine output (oliguria/anuria), change in mental state, hemoconcentration.

risk for impaired Tissue Perfusion: risk factors may include hypovolemia, exchange problems (severe metabolic acidosis).

Chronic obstructive lung disease   CH/MS

impaired Gas Exchange may be related to altered O_2 delivery (obstruction of airways by secretions/bronchospasm, air trapping) and alveoli destruction, possibly evidenced by dyspnea, restlessness, confusion, abnormal ABG values, and reduced tolerance for activity.

ineffective Airway Clearance may be related to bronchospasm, increased production of tenacious secretions, retained secretions, and decreased energy/fatigue, possibly evidenced by presence of wheezes, crackles, tachypnea, dyspnea, changes in depth of respirations, use of accessory muscles, cough (persistent), and chest radiograph findings.

Activity Intolerance may be related to imbalance between O_2 supply and demand, and generalized weakness, possibly evidenced by verbal reports of fatigue, exertional dyspnea, and abnormal vital sign response.

imbalanced Nutrition: less than body requirements may be related to inability to ingest adequate nutrients (dyspnea, fatigue, medication side effects, sputum production, anorexia), possibly evidenced by weight loss, reported altered taste sensation, decreased muscle mass/subcutaneous fat, poor muscle tone, and aversion to eating/lack of interest in food.

risk for Infection: risk factors may include decreased ciliary action, stasis of secretions, and debilitated state/malnutrition.

Circumcision   PEDS

deficient Knowledge [Learning Need] regarding surgical procedure, prognosis, and treatment may be related to lack of exposure, misinterpretation, unfamiliarity with information resources possibly evidenced by request for information, verbalization of concern/misconceptions, inaccurate follow-through of instructions.

acute Pain may be related to trauma to/edema of tender tissues possibly evidenced by crying, changes in sleep pattern, refusal to eat.

impaired urinary Elimination may be related to tissue injury/inflammation, or development of urethral fistula possibly evidenced by edema, difficulty voiding.

risk for Injury [hemorrhage]: risk factors may include decreased clotting factors immediately after birth, previously undiagnosed problems with bleeding/clotting.

risk for Infection: risk factors may include immature immune system, invasive procedure/tissue trauma, environmental exposure.

Cirrhosis   MS

(Also refer to Substance Dependence/Abuse Rehabilitation; Hepatitis, acute viral)

risk for acute Confusion: risk factors may include alcohol abuse, increased serum ammonia level, and inability of liver to detoxify certain enzymes/drugs.

risk for Injury [hemorrhage]: risk factors may include abnormal blood profile (altered clotting factors), portal hypertension/development of esophageal varices.

imbalanced Nutrition: less than body requirements may be related to inability to ingest/absorb nutrients (anorexia, nausea, indigestion, early satiety), abnormal bowel function, impaired storage of vitamins, possibly evidenced by aversion to eating, observed lack of intake, muscle wasting, weight loss, and imbalances in nutritional studies.

excess Fluid Volume may be related to compromised regulatory mechanism (e.g., syndrome of inappropriate antidiuretic hormone—SIADH, decreased plasma proteins/malnutrition) and excess sodium/fluid intake, possibly evidenced by generalized or abdominal edema, weight gain, dyspnea, B/P changes, positive hepatojugular reflex change in mentation, altered electrolytes, changes in urine specific gravity, and pleural effusion.

risk for impaired Skin Integrity: risk factors may include altered circulation/metabolic state, poor skin turgor, skeletal prominence, and presence of edema/ascites, accumulation of bile salts in skin.

situational low Self-Esteem/disturbed Body Image may be related to biophysical changes/altered physical appearance, uncertainty of prognosis, changes in role function, personal vulnerability, self-destructive behavior (alcohol-induced disease), possibly evidenced by verbalization of changes in lifestyle, fear of rejection/reaction of others, negative feelings about body/abilities, and feelings of helplessness/hopelessness/powerlessness.

Cleft lip/palate   PED/MS

(Also refer to Newborn, special needs)

ineffective Infant Feeding Pattern may be related to anatomical abnormality possibly evidenced by inability to sustain an effective suck, inability to coordinate sucking/swallowing/breathing.

risk for Aspiration: risk factors may include impaired swallowing, regurgitation.

risk for impaired verbal Communication: risk factors may include anatomic defect, developmental delay.

risk for disturbed Body Image/Social Isolation: risk factors may include altered appearance/anatomic deficit, significance of body part (face).

Cocaine hydrochloride poisoning, acute   MS

(Also refer to Stimulant abuse; Substance dependence/abuse rehabilitation)

ineffective Breathing Pattern may be related to pharmacological effects on respiratory center of the brain, possibly evidenced by tachypnea, altered depth of respiration, shortness of breath, and abnormal ABGs.

risk for decreased Cardiac Output: risk factors may include drug effect on myocardium (degree dependent on drug purity/quality used), alterations in electrical rate/rhythm/conduction, preexisting myocardiopathy.

Coccidioidomycosis (San Joaquin/Valley Fever)   CH

acute Pain may be related to inflammation, possibly evidenced by verbal reports, distraction behaviors, and narrowed focus.

Fatigue may be related to decreased energy production; states of discomfort, possibly evidenced by reports of overwhelming lack of energy, inability to maintain usual routine, emotional lability/irritability, impaired ability to concentrate, and decreased endurance/libido.

deficient Knowledge [Learning Need] regarding nature/course of disease, therapy and self-care needs may be related to lack of information, possibly evidenced by statements of concern and questions.

Colectomy   MS

(Refer to Intestinal surgery [without diversion])

Colitis, ulcerative   MS

Diarrhea may be related to inflammation or malabsorption of the bowel, presence of toxins and/or segmental narrowing of the lumen, possibly evidenced by increased bowel sounds/peristalsis, urgency, frequency/watery stools (acute phase), changes in stool color, and abdominal pain/cramping.

acute/chronic Pain may be related to inflammation of the intestines/hyperperistalsis and anal/rectal irritation, possibly evidenced by verbal reports, guarding/distraction behaviors.

risk for deficient Fluid Volume: risk factors may include continued GI losses (diarrhea, vomiting, capillary plasma loss), altered intake, hypermetabolic state.

CH

imbalanced Nutrition: less than body requirements may be related to altered intake/absorption of nutrients (medically restricted intake, fear that eating may cause diarrhea) and hypermetabolic state, possibly evidenced by weight loss, decreased subcutaneous fat/muscle mass, poor muscle tone, hyperactive bowel sounds, steatorrhea, pale conjunctiva and mucous membranes, and aversion to eating.

ineffective Coping may be related to chronic nature and indefinite outcome of disease, multiple stressors (repeated over time), personal vulnerability, severe pain, inadequate sleep, lack of/ineffective support systems, possibly evidenced by verbalization of inability to cope, discouragement, anxiety; preoccupation with physical self, chronic worry, emotional tension; depression, and recurrent exacerbation of symptoms.

risk for Powerlessness: risk factors may include unresolved dependency conflicts, feelings of insecurity/resentment, repression of anger and aggressive feelings, lacking a sense of control in stressful situations, sacrificing own wishes for others, and retreat from aggression or frustration.

Collagen disorders   CH

(Refer to Arthritis, rheumatoid/juvenile rheumatoid; Lupus erythematosus, systemic; Polyarteritis nodosa; Temporal arteritis)

Colorectal cancer   MS

(Refer to Cancer; Colostomy)

Colostomy   MS

risk for impaired Skin Integrity: risk factors may include absence of sphincter at stoma and chemical irritation from caustic bowel contents, reaction to product/removal of adhesive, and improperly fitting appliance.

risk for Diarrhea/Constipation: risk factors may include interruption/alteration of normal bowel function (placement of ostomy), changes in dietary/fluid intake, and effects of medication.

CH

deficient Knowledge [Learning Need] regarding changes in physiologic function and self-care/treatment needs may be related to lack of exposure/recall, information misinterpretation, possibly evidenced by questions, statement of concern, and inaccurate follow-through of instruction/development of preventable complications.

disturbed Body Image may be related to biophysical changes (presence of stoma; loss of control of bowel elimination) and psychosocial factors (altered body structure, disease process/associated treatment regimen, e.g., cancer, colitis), possibly evidenced by verbalization of change in perception of self, negative feelings about body, fear of rejection/reaction of others, not touching/looking at stoma, and refusal to participate in care.

impaired Social Interaction may be related to fear of embarrassing situation secondary to altered bowel control with loss of contents, odor, possibly evidenced by reduced participation and verbalized/observed discomfort in social situations.

risk for Sexual dysfunction: risk factors may include altered body structure/function, radical resection/treatment procedures, vulnerability/psychological concern about response of significant other(s), and disruption of sexual response pattern (e.g., erection difficulty).

Coma   MS

risk for Suffocation: risk factors may include cognitive impairment/loss of protective reflexes and purposeful movement.

risk for deficient Fluid Volume/imbalanced Nutrition: less than body requirements: risk factors may include inability to ingest food/fluids, increased needs/hypermetabolic state.

total Self-Care Deficit may be related to cognitive impairment and absence of purposeful activity, evidenced by inability to perform ADLs.

risk for ineffective Tissue Perfusion: cerebral: risk factors may include reduced or interrupted arterial/venous blood flow (direct injury, edema formation, space-occupying lesions), metabolic alterations, effects of drug/alcohol overdose, hypoxia/anoxia.

risk for Infection: risk factors may include stasis of body fluids (oral, pulmonary, urinary), invasive procedures, and nutritional deficits.

Coma, diabetic   MS
(Refer to Diabetic Ketoacidosis)

Compartment syndrome   MS

acute Pain may be related to increasing pressure within muscle possibly evidenced by reports of progressing pain distal to injury unrelieved by routine analgesics.

ineffective peripheral Tissue Perfusion may be related to interruption of arterial blood flow/elevated tissue pressures possibly evidenced by absent/deminished distal pulses, erythema, pain

risk for Peripheral Neurovascular dysfunction: risk factors may include reduction/interruption of blood flow (direct vascular injury, tissue trauma, excessive edema/elevated tissue pressures, hypovolemia).

Complex regional pain syndrome   CH
(Refer to Reflex sympathetic dystrophy)

Concussion of brain   CH
(Also refer to Postconcussion syndrome)

acute Pain may be related to trauma to/edema of cerebral tissue, possibly evidenced by reports of headache, guarding/distraction behaviors, and narrowed focus.

risk for deficient Fluid Volume: risk factors may include vomiting, decreased intake, and hypermetabolic state (fever).

risk for disturbed Thought Processes: risk factors may include trauma to/edema of cerebral tissue.

deficient Knowledge [Learning Need] regarding condition, treatment/safety needs, and potential complications may be related to lack of recall, misinterpretation, cognitive limitation, possibly evidenced by questions/statement of concerns, development of preventable complications.

Conduct disorder (childhood, adolescence)   PSY/PED

risk for self/other-directed Violence: risk factors may include retarded ego development, antisocial character, poor impulse control, dysfunctional family system, loss of significant relationships, history of suicidal/acting-out behaviors.

defensive Coping may be related to inadequate coping strategies, maturational crisis, multiple life changes/losses, lack of control of impulsive actions, and personal vulnerability, possibly evidenced by inappropriate use of defense mechanisms, inability to meet role expectations, poor self-esteem, failure to assume responsibility for own actions, hypersensitivity to slight or criticism, and excessive smoking/drinking/drug use.

disturbed Thought Processes may be related to physiologic changes, lack of appropriate psychological conflict, biochemical changes, as evidenced by tendency to interpret the intentions/actions of others as blaming and hostile; deficits in problem-solving skills, with physical aggression the solution most often chosen.

chronic low Self-Esteem may be related to life choices perpetuating failure, personal vulnerability, possibly evidenced by self-negating verbalizations, anger, rejection of positive feedback, frequent lack of success in life events.

CH

compromised/disabled family Coping may be related to excessive guilt, anger, or blaming among family members regarding child's behavior; parental inconsistencies; disagreements regarding discipline, limit setting, and approaches; and exhaustion of parental resources (prolonged coping with disruptive child), possibly evidenced by unrealistic parental expectations, rejection or overprotection of child; and exaggerated expressions of anger, disappointment, or despair regarding child's behavior or ability to improve or change.

impaired Social Interaction may be related to retarded ego development, developmental state (adolescence), lack of social skills, low self-concept, dysfunctional family system, and neurologic impairment, possibly evidenced by dysfunctional interaction with others (difficulty waiting turn in games or group situations, not seeming to listen to what is being said), difficulty playing quietly and maintaining attention to task or play activity, often shifting from one activity to another and interrupting or intruding on others.

Congestive heart failure   MS
(Refer to Heart Failure, chronic)

Conjunctivitis, bacterial   CH

acute Pain/[Discomfort] may be related to inflammation, ocular irritation, edema possibly evidenced by verbal reports, irritability, guarding behavior.

risk for Infection[spread]: risk factors may include purulent discharge, insufficient knowledge to avoid spread.

risk for ineffective Therapeutic Regimen Management: risk factors may include length of therapy, perceived benefit.

Connective tissue disease   CH
(Refer to Arthritis, rheumatoid/juvenile rheumatoid; Lupus erythematosus, systemic; Polyarteritis nodosa; Temporal arteritis)

Conn's syndrome   MS/CH
(Refer to Aldosteronism, primary)

Constipation   CH
Constipation may be related to weak abdominal musculature, GI obstructive lesions, pain on defecation, diagnostic procedures, pregnancy, possibly evidenced by change in

character/frequency of stools, feeling of abdominal/rectal fullness or pressure, changes in bowel sounds, abdominal distention.

acute Pain may be related to abdominal fullness/pressure, straining to defecate, and trauma to delicate tissues, possibly evidenced by verbal reports, reluctance to defecate, and distraction behaviors.

deficient Knowledge [Learning Need] regarding dietary needs, bowel function, and medication effect may be related to lack of information/misconceptions, possibly evidenced by development of problem and verbalization of concerns/questions.

Conversion disorder   PSY
(Refer to Somatoform disorders)

Convulsions   CH
(Refer to Seizure disorder)

COPD   CH
(Refer to Chronic obstructive lung disease)

Corneal transplantation   MS
risk for Injury: risk factors may include intraocular hemorrhage, edema/swelling, changes in visual acuity, increased intraocular pressure/glaucoma.

risk for Infection: risk factors may include surgical manipulation, use of corticosteroids, presence of chronic disease.

disturbed visual Sensory Perception may be related to altered sensory reception (use of eye drops, edema/swelling), therapeutically restricted environment (patching), possibly evidenced by visual distortions/blurring, change in acuity.

Coronary artery bypass surgery   MS
risk for decreased Cardiac Output: risk factors may include decreased myocardial contractility, diminished circulating volume (preload), alterations in electrical conduction, and increased SVR (afterload).

acute Pain may be related to direct chest tissue/bone trauma, invasive tubes/lines, donor site incision, tissue inflammation/edema formation, intraoperative nerve trauma, possibly evidenced by verbal reports, autonomic responses (changes in vital signs), and distraction behaviors/(restlessness), irritability.

disturbed Sensory Perception (specify) may be related to restricted environment (postoperative/acute), sleep deprivation, effects of medications; continuous environmental sounds/activities, and psychological stress of procedure, possibly evidenced by disorientation, alterations in behavior, exaggerated emotional responses, and visual/auditory distortions.

                                                                   CH
ineffective Role Performance may be related to situational crises (dependent role)/recuperative process, uncertainty about future, possibly evidenced by delay/alteration in physical capacity to resume role, change in usual role or responsibility, change in self/others' perception of role.

Coronary artery disease   CH
Activity Intolerance may be related to imbalance between oxygen supply/demand, sedentary lifestyle possibly evidenced by exertional discomfort/pain, fatigue, abnormal heart rate response, ECG changes (dysrhythmias, ischemia).

risk for decreased Cardiac Output: risk factors may include altered heart rate/rhythm, altered contractility, increased peripheral vascular resistance.

Cor pulmonale   CH/MS

(Also refer to Heart failure, chronic; Chronic obstructive lung disease)

Activity Intolerance may be related to imbalance between O_2 supply/demand, generalized weakness, chest pain possibly evidenced by exertional dyspnea, fatigue, cyanosis.

excess Fluid Volume may be related to compromised regulatory mechanism possibly evidenced by shortness of breath, dependent edema, jugular vein distention, positive hepatojugular reflux, abnormal breath sounds, change in mental status.

impaired Gas Exchange may be related to ventilation perfusion imbalance (heart failure) possibly evidenced by dyspnea, restlessness, lethargy, cyanosis, abnormal ABG values (hypoxemia, hypercapnia, acidosis), polycythemia.

Cradle cap   CH

(Refer to Dermatitis, seborrheic)

Craniotomy   MS

(Also refer to Surgery, general)

risk for decreased Intracranial Adaptive Capacity: risk factors may include brain injuries/surgical procedure, systemic hypotension with intracranial hypertension.

disturbed Sensory Perception (specify) may be related to altered sensory reception, transmission and/or integration (neurologic deficit) possibly evidenced by disorientation to time, place, person; motor incoordination, altered communication patterns, restlessness/irritability, change in behavior pattern.

risk for disturbed Thought Processes: risk factors may include trauma to/manipulation of brain tissue, changes in circulation/perfusion, increased intracranial pressure.

risk for Infection: risk factors may include traumatized tissues, broken skin, invasive procedures, nutritional deficits, altered integrity of closed system (CSF leak).

Creutzfeldt-Jakob disease   CH

impaired Memory may be related to neurologic deficits possibly evidenced by observed experiences of forgetting, inability to perform previously learned skills, inability to recall factual information or recent/past events.

Fear may be related to decreases in functional abilities, progressive deterioration, lack of treatment options possibly evidenced by apprehension, irritability, defensiveness, suspiciousness, aggressive behavior, social isolation.

impaired Walking may be related to changes in muscle coordination/balance, visual changes, impaired judgment, myoclonic seizures possibly evidenced by inability to walk desired distances, climb stairs, navigate uneven surfaces.

disturbed visual Sensory Perception may be related to altered sensory reception/integration (neurologic disease) possibly evidenced by change in sensory acuity (visual field defects, diplopia, dimness/blurring, visual agnosia), change in usual response to stimuli.

total Self-Care Deficit may be related to cognitive decline, physical limitations, frustration over loss of independence, depression possibly evidenced by impaired ability to perform ADLs, unkempt appearance/poor hygiene, apathy.

risk for Caregiver Role Strain: risk factors may include illness severity of care receiver, duration of caregiving required, care receiver exhibiting deviant/bizarre behavior; family/caregiver isolation, lack of respite/recreation, spouse is caregiver.

Crohn's disease   MS/CH

(Also refer to Colitis, ulcerative)

imbalanced Nutrition: less than body requirements may be related to intestinal pain after eating; and decreased transit time through bowel, possibly evidenced by weight loss, aversion to eating, and observed lack of intake.

Diarrhea may be related to inflammation of small intestines, presence of toxins, particular dietary intake, possibly evidenced by hyperactive bowel sounds, cramping, and frequent loose liquid stools.

deficient Knowledge [Learning Need] regarding condition, nutritional needs, and prevention of recurrence may be related to insufficient information/misinterpretation, unfamiliarity with resources, possibly evidenced by statements of concern/questions, inaccurate follow-through of instructions, and development of preventable complications/exacerbation of condition.

Croup   PED/CH

ineffective Airway Clearance may be related to presence of thick, tenacious mucus and swelling/spasms of the epiglottis, possibly evidenced by harsh/brassy cough, tachypnea, use of accessory breathing muscles, and presence of wheezes.

deficient Fluid Volume [isotonic] may be related to decreased ability/aversion to swallowing, presence of fever, and increased respiratory losses, possibly evidenced by dry mucous membranes, poor skin turgor, and scanty/concentrated urine.

Croup membranous   PED/CH
(Also refer to Croup)

risk for Suffocation: risk factors may include inflammation of larynx with formation of false membrane.

Anxiety [specify level]/Fear may be related to change in environment, perceived threat to self (difficulty breathing), and transmission of anxiety of adults, possibly evidenced by restlessness, facial tension, glancing about, and sympathetic stimulation.

C-Section   OB
(Refer to Cesarean birth, unplanned)

Cubital tunnel syndrome   CH

acute/chronic Pain may be related to pressure on ulnar nerve at elbow, possibly evidenced by verbal reports, reluctance to use affected extremity, guarding behaviors, expressed fear of reinjury, altered ability to continue previous activities.

impaired physical Mobility may be related to neuromuscular impairment and pain, possibly evidenced by decreased pinch/grasp strength, hand fatigue, and reluctance to attempt movement.

risk for Peripheral Neurovascular Dysfunction: risk factors may include mechanical compression (e.g., brace, repetitive tasks/motions), immobilization.

Cushing's syndrome   CH/MS

risk for excess Fluid Volume: risk factors may include compromised regulatory mechanism (fluid/sodium retention).

risk for Infection: risk factors may include immunosuppressed inflammatory response, skin and capillary fragility, and negative nitrogen balance.

imbalanced Nutrition: less than body requirements may be related to inability to utilize nutrients (disturbance of carbohydrate metabolism), possibly evidenced by decreased muscle mass and increased resistance to insulin.

Self-Care Deficit [specify] may be related to muscle wasting, generalized weakness, fatigue, and demineralization of bones, possibly evidenced by statements of/observed inability to complete or perform ADLs.

disturbed Body Image may be related to change in structure/appearance (effects of disease process, drug therapy), possibly evidenced by negative feelings about body, feelings of helplessness, and changes in social involvement.

Sexual Dysfunction may be related to loss of libido, impotence, and cessation of menses, possibly evidenced by verbalization of concerns and/or dissatisfaction with and alteration in relationship with significant other.

risk for Trauma [fractures]: risk factors may include increased protein breakdown, negative protein balance, demineralization of bones.

CVA   MS/CH
(Refer to Cerebrovascular accident)

Cyclothymic disorder   PSY
(Refer to Bipolar disorder)

Cystic fibrosis   CH/PED
ineffective Airway Clearance may be related to excessive production of thick mucus and decreased ciliary action, possibly evidenced by abnormal breath sounds, ineffective cough, cyanosis, and altered respiratory rate/depth.

risk for Infection: risk factors may include stasis of respiratory secretions and development of atelectasis.

imbalanced Nutrition: less than body requirements may be related to impaired digestive process and absorption of nutrients, possibly evidenced by failure to gain weight, muscle wasting, and retarded physical growth.

deficient Knowledge [Learning Need] regarding pathophysiology of condition, medical management, and available community resources may be related to insufficient information/misconceptions, possibly evidenced by statements of concern, questions; inaccurate follow-through of instructions, development of preventable complications.

compromised family Coping may be related to chronic nature of disease and disability, inadequate/incorrect information or understanding by a primary person, and possibly evidenced by significant person attempting assistive or supportive behaviors with less than satisfactory results, protective behavior disproportionate to client's abilities or need for autonomy.

Cystitis   CH
acute Pain may be related to inflammation and bladder spasms, possibly evidenced by verbal reports, distraction behaviors, and narrowed focus.

impaired Urinary Elimination may be related to inflammation/irritation of bladder, possibly evidenced by frequency, nocturia, and dysuria.

deficient Knowledge [Learning Need] regarding condition, treatment, and prevention of recurrence may be related to inadequate information/misconceptions, possibly evidenced by statements of concern and questions; recurrent infections.

Cytomegalic inclusion disease   CH
(Refer to Cytomegalovirus infection)

Cytomegalovirus (CMV) infection   CH
risk for disturbed visual Sensory Perception: risk factors may include inflammation of the retina.

risk for fetal Infection: risk factors may include transplacental exposure, contact with blood/body fluids.

Deep Vein Thrombosis   CH/MS
(Refer to Thrombophlebitis)

Degenerative disc disease   **CH/MS**
(Refer to Herniated nucleus pulposus)

Degenerative joint disease   **CH**
(Refer to Arthritis, rheumatoid)
(Although this is a degenerative process versus the inflammatory process of rheumatoid
  arthritis, nursing concerns are the same.)

Dehiscence, abdominal wound   **MS**
impaired Skin Integrity may be related to altered circulation, altered nutritional state
  (obesity/malnutrition), and physical stress on incision, possibly evidenced by
  poor/delayed wound healing and disruption of skin surface/wound closure.
risk for Infection: risk factors may include inadequate primary defenses (separation of incision, traumatized intestines, environmental exposure).
risk for impaired Tissue Integrity: risk factors may include exposure of abdominal contents to
  external environment.
Fear/Anxiety [severe] may be related to crises, perceived threat of death, possibly evidenced
  by fearfulness, restless behaviors, and sympathetic stimulation.
deficient Knowledge [Learning Need] regarding condition/prognosis and treatment needs may be
  related to lack of information/recall and misinterpretation of information, possibly
  evidenced by development of preventable complications, requests for information, and
  statement of concern.

Dehydration   **PED**
deficient Fluid Volume [specify] may be related to etiology as defined by specific situation,
  possibly evidenced by dry mucous membranes, poor skin turgor, decreased pulse
  volume/pressure, and thirst.
risk for impaired Oral Mucous Membrane: risk factors may include dehydration and decreased
  salivation.
deficient Knowledge [Learning Need] regarding fluid needs may be related to lack of informa-
  tion/misinterpretation, possibly evidenced by questions, statement of concern, and inadequate follow-through of instructions/development of preventable complications.

Delirium tremens   **MS/PSY**
(Also refer to Alcohol intoxication, acute)
Anxiety [severe/panic]/Fear may be related to cessation of alcohol intake/physiologic withdrawal, threat to self-concept, perceived threat of death, possibly evidenced by increased
  tension, apprehension, fear of unspecified consequences; identifies object of fear.
disturbed Sensory Perception (specify) may be related to exogenous (alcohol
  consumption/sudden cessation)/endogenous (electrolyte imbalance, elevated ammonia
  and blood urea nitrogen—BUN) chemical alterations, sleep deprivation, and psychological
  stress, possibly evidenced by disorientation, restlessness, irritability, exaggerated emotional
  responses, bizarre thinking, and visual and auditory distortions/hallucinations.
risk for decreased Cardiac Output: risk factors may include direct effect of alcohol on heart
  muscle, altered SVR, presence of dysrhythmias.
risk for Trauma: risk factors may include alterations in balance, reduced muscle coordination,
  cognitive impairment, and involuntary clonic/tonic muscle activity.
imbalanced Nutrition: less than body requirements may be related to poor dietary intake, effects
  of alcohol on organs involved in digestion, interference with absorption/metabolism of
  nutrients and amino acids, possibly evidenced by reports of inadequate food intake, altered
  taste sensation, lack of interest in food, debilitated state, decreased subcutaneous

fat/muscle mass, signs of mineral/electrolyte deficiency including abnormal laboratory findings.

Delivery, precipitous/out of hospital   OB
(Also refer to Labor, precipitous; Labor stages I-IV)

risk for deficient Fluid Volume: risk factors may include presence of nausea/vomiting, lack of intake, excessive vascular loss.

risk for Infection: risk factors may include broken/traumatized tissue, increased environmental exposure, rupture of amniotic membranes.

risk for fetal Injury: risk factors may include rapid descent/pressure changes, compromised circulation, environmental exposure.

Delusional disorder   PSY

risk for self/other-directed Violence: risk factors may include perceived threats of danger, increased feelings of anxiety, acting out in an irrational manner.

[severe] Anxiety may be related to inability to trust possibly evidenced by rigid delusional system, frightened of other people and own hostility.

Powerlessness may be related to lifestyle of helplessness, feelings of inadequacy, interpersonal interaction possibly evidenced by verbal expressions of no control/influence over situation(s), use of paranoid delusions, aggressive behavior to compensate for lack of control.

disturbed Thought Processes may be related to psychological conflicts, increasing anxiety/fear possibly evidenced by interference with ability to think clearly/logically, fragmentation and autistic thinking, delusions, beliefs and behaviors of suspicion/violence.

impaired Social Interaction may be related to mistrust of others/delusional thinking, lack of knowledge/skills to enhance mutuality possibly evidenced by discomfort in social situations, difficulty in establishing relationships with others, expression of feelings of rejection, no sense of belonging.

Dementia, HIV   CH/PSY
(Also refer to Dementia, presenile/senile)

acute/chronic Confusion may be related to direct CNS infection with HIV, disseminated systemic opportunistic infection, hypoxemia, brain malignancies, CVA, vasculitis, altered drug metabolism/excretion, electrolyte imbalance, sleep deprivation possibly evidenced by fluctuation of cognition, progressive cognitive impairment, increased agitation, restlessness, altered interpretation/response to stimuli, clinical evidence of organic impairment.

[mild to severe] Anxiety may be related to threat to self-concept, unmet needs, perceived threat /change in health status, interpersonal transmission/contagion possibly evidenced by reports of feeling scared, shaky, increased tension, loss of control/"going crazy," apprehension, increased warinesss, extraneous movements/tremors, increased somatic complaints.

ineffective family Coping (specify) may be related to prolonged disease progression that exhausts the supportive capacity of SOs, highly ambivalent family relationship, sense of shame/guilt related to diagnosis, other crises SOs may be facing possibly evidenced by intolerance, rejection, abandonment, neglectful relationships with other family members, SO preoccupied with personal reaction, distortion of reality of health problem.

Dementia, presenile/senile   CH/PSY
(Also refer to Alzheimer's disease)

impaired Memory may be related to neurologic disturbances, possibly evidenced by observed experiences of forgetting, inability to determine if a behavior was performed, inability to perform previously learned skills, inability to recall factual information or recent/past events.

Fear may be related to decreases in functional abilities, public disclosure of disabilities, further mental/physical deterioration possibly evidenced by social isolation, apprehension, irritability, defensiveness, suspiciousness, aggressive behavior.

Self-Care Deficit [specify] may be related to cognitive decline, physical limitations, frustration over loss of independence, depression, possibly evidenced by impaired ability to perform ADLs.

risk for Trauma: risk factors may include changes in muscle coordination/balance, impaired judgment, seizure activity.

risk for Caregiver Role Strain: risk factors may include illness severity of care receiver, duration of caregiving required, care receiver exhibiting deviant/bizarre behavior; family/caregiver isolation, lack of respite/ recreation, spouse is caregiver.

Dementia, vascular CH/PSY
(Refer to Alzheimer's disease)

Depersonalization disorder PSY
(Refer to Dissociative disorders)

Depressant abuse CH/PSY
(Also refer to Drug overdose, acute [depressants])

ineffective Denial may be related to weak underdeveloped ego, unmet self-needs possibly evidenced by inability to admit impact of condition on life, minimizes symptoms/problem, refuses healthcare attention.

ineffective Coping may be related to weak ego possibly evidenced by abuse of chemical agents, lack of goal-directed behavior, inadequate problem solving, destructive behavior towards self.

imbalanced Nutrition: less than body requirements may be related to use of substance in place of nutritional food possibly evidenced by loss of weight, pale conjunctiva and mucous membranes, electrolyte imbalances, anemias.

risk for Injury: risk factors may include changes in sleep, decreased concentration, loss of inhibitions.

Depression, major PSY
risk for self-directed Violence: risk factors may include depressed mood and feeling of worthlessness and hopelessness.

[moderate to severe] Anxiety/disturbed Thought Processes may be related to psychological conflicts, unconscious conflict about essential values/goals of life, unmet needs, threat to self-concept, sleep deprivation, interpersonal transmission/contagion, possibly evidenced by reports of nervousness or fearfulness, feelings of inadequacy; agitation, angry/tearful outbursts, rambling/discoordinated speech, restlessness, hand rubbing or wringing, tremulousness; poor memory/concentration, decreased ability to grasp ideas, inability to follow/impaired ability to make decisions, numerous/repetitious physical complaints without organic cause, ideas of reference, hallucinations/delusions.

disturbed Sleep Pattern may be related to biochemical alterations (decreased serotonin), unresolved fears and anxieties, and inactivity, possibly evidenced by difficulty in falling/remaining asleep, early morning awakening/awakening later than desired, reports of not feeling rested, physical signs (e.g., dark circles under eyes, excessive yawning); hypersomnia (using sleep as an escape).

Social Isolation/impaired Social Interaction may be related to alterations in mental status/thought processes (depressed mood), inadequate personal resources, decreased energy/inertia, difficulty engaging in satisfying personal relationships, feelings of worthlessness/low self-concept, inadequacy in or absence of significant purpose in life, and knowledge/skill deficit about social interactions, possibly evidenced by decreased involvement with others, expressed feelings of difference from others, remaining in home/room/bed, refusing invitations/suggestions of social involvement, and dysfunctional interaction with peers, family, and/or others.

interrupted Family Processes may be related to situational crises of illness of family member with change in roles/responsibilities, developmental crises (e.g., loss of family member/relationship), possibly evidenced by statements of difficulty coping with situation, family system not meeting needs of its members, difficulty accepting or receiving help appropriately, ineffective family decision-making process, and failure to send and to receive clear messages.

Depression, postpartum   OB/PSY
(Also refer to Depressive disorders)

risk for impaired parent/infant Attachment: risk factors may include anxiety associated with the parent role, inability to meet personal needs, perceived guilt regarding relationship with infant.

risk for other-directed Violence: risk factors may include hopelessness, increased anxiety, mood swings, despondency, severe depression/psychosis.

Depressive disorders   PSY
(Refer to Depression, major, Bipolar disorder, Premenstrual Dysphoric disorder)

de Quervain's syndrome   CH
acute/chronic Pain may be related to inflammation of tendon sheath base of thumb, swelling possibly evidenced by verbal reports, reluctance to use affected hand, guarding behaviors, expressed fear of reinjury, altered ability to continue previous activities.

impaired physical Mobility may be related to musculoskeletal impairment/swelling and pain, numbness of thumb/index finger possibly evidenced by decreased grasp/pinch strength, weakness, limited range of motion of thumb, and reluctance to attempt movement.

Dermatitis, contact   CH
acute Pain/[Discomfort] may be related to cutaneous inflammation and irritation, possibly evidenced by verbal reports, irritability, and scratching.

impaired Skin Integrity may be related to exposure to chemicals/environmental alllergens, pruritis possibly evidenced by inflammation, epidermal edema, development of vesicles/bullae.

risk for Infection: risk factors may include broken skin and tissue trauma.

Social Isolation may be related to alterations in physical appearance, possibly evidenced by expressed feelings of rejection and decreased interaction with peers.

Dermatitis, seborrheic   CH
impaired Skin Integrity may be related to chronic inflammatory condition of the skin, possibly evidenced by disruption of skin surface with dry or moist scales, yellowish crusts, erythema, and fissures.

Developmental disorders, pervasive   PED/PSY
(Refer to Autistic disorder; Rett's syndrome; Asperger's disorder)

Diabetes, gestational   OB
(Also refer to Diabetes mellitus)

risk for fetal Injury: risk factors may include elevated maternal serum glucose levels, changes in circulation.

risk for maternal Injury: risk factors may include changes in diabetic control, abnormal blood profile/anemia, tissue hypoxia, altered immune response.

deficient Knowledge [Learning Need] regarding diabetic condition, prognosis, self-care treatment needs may be related to lack of resources/exposure to information, misinformation, lack of recall possibly evidenced by questions, statements of misconception, inaccurate follow-through of instructions, development of preventable complications.

Diabetes insipidus   MS/CH

deficient Fluid Volume [hypertonic] may be related to failure of regulatory mechanisms/ hormone imbalance (e.g., brain injury, medication, sickle cell anemia, hypothyroidism) possibly evidenced by urinary frequency, thirst/polydipsia, dilute urine, dry skin/mucous membranes, decreased skin turgor, nocturia, increased serum sodium.

risk for ineffective Therapeutic Regimen Management: risk factors may include complexity of medication regimen, presence of side effects, economic difficulties, inadequate knowledge, perceived seriousness/benefits.

Diabetes, juvenile   PED

(Also refer to Diabetes mellitus)

risk for Injury: risk factors may include ineffective control/swings in serum glucose level, changes in mentation, developmental age, risk-taking behaviors.

ineffective Coping may be related to maturational crisis (desire to be like peers), inadequate level of perception of control, gender differences in coping strategies possibly evidenced by use of forms of coping that impede adaptive behavior, inadequate problem solving, risk taking, destructive behavior toward self (loss of/inadequate diabetic control).

risk for ineffective Therapeutic Regimen Management: risk factors may include complexity/duration of treatmemt, perceived excessive demands made on individual, powerlessness, perceived susceptibility to complications.

Diabetes mellitus   CH/PED

deficient Knowledge [Learning Need] regarding disease process/treatment and individual care needs may be related to unfamiliarity with information/lack of recall, misinterpreta-tion, possibly evidenced by requests for information, statements of concern/misconcep-tions, inadequate follow-through of instructions, and development of preventable complications.

imbalanced Nutrition: less than body requirements may be related to inability to utilize nutrients (imbalance between intake and utilization of glucose) to meet metabolic needs, possibly evidenced by change in weight, muscle weakness, increased thirst/urination, and hyper-glycemia.

risk for impaired Adjustment: risk factors may include all-encompassing change in lifestyle, self-concept requiring lifelong adherence to therapeutic regimen and internal/altered locus of control.

risk for Infection: risk factors may include decreased leukocyte function, circulatory changes, and delayed healing.

risk for disturbed Sensory Perception (specify): risk factors may include endogenous chemical alteration (glucose/insulin and/or electrolyte imbalance).

compromised family Coping may be related to inadequate or incorrect information or under-standing by primary person(s), other situational/developmental crises or situations the significant person(s) may be facing, lifelong condition requiring behavioral changes impacting family, possibly evidenced by family expressions of confusion about what to do, verbalizations that they are having difficulty coping with situation; family does not meet physical/emotional needs of its members; SO(s) preoccupied with personal reaction (e.g., guilt, fear), display protective behavior disproportionate (too little/too much) to client's abilities or need for autonomy.

Diabetes mellitus, intrapartum   OB
(Also refer to Diabetes mellitus)

risk for Trauma/impaired fetal Gas Exchange: risk factors may include inadequate maternal diabetic control, presence of macrosomia or intrauterine growth retardation (IUGR).

risk for maternal Injury: risk factors may include inadequate diabetic control (hypertension, severe edema, ketoacidosis, uterine atony/overdistension, dystocia).

[mild to moderate] Anxiety may be related to situational "crisis"/threat to health status (maternal or fetus) possibly evidenced by increased tension, apprehension, fear of unspecific consequences, sympathetic stimulation.

Diabetes mellitus, postpartum   OB

risk for imbalanced Nutrition: less than body requirements: risk factors may include inability to ingest/utilize nutrients appropriately, increased metabolic demands (recuperation, lactation).

risk for Injury: risk factors may include biochemical or regulatory complications (e.g., uterine hemorrhage, hypertension, hyperglycemia).

risk for impaired parent/infant Attachment: risk factors may include interruption in bonding process, physical illness/changes in physical abilities.

Diabetic ketoacidosis   CH/MS

deficient Fluid Volume [specify] may be related to hyperosmolar urinary losses, gastric losses and inadequate intake, possibly evidenced by increased urinary output/dilute urine; reports of weakness, thirst; sudden weight loss, hypotension, tachycardia, delayed capillary refill, dry mucous membranes, poor skin turgor.

imbalanced Nutrition: less than body requirements that may be related to inadequate utilization of nutrients (insulin deficiency), decreased oral intake, hypermetabolic state, possibly evidenced by recent weight loss, reports of weakness, lack of interest in food, gastric fullness/abdominal pain, and increased ketones, imbalance between glucose/insulin levels.

Fatigue may be related to decreased metabolic energy production, altered body chemistry (insufficient insulin), increased energy demands (hypermetabolic state/infection), possibly evidenced by overwhelming lack of energy, inability to maintain usual routines, decreased performance, impaired ability to concentrate, listlessness.

risk for Infection: risk factors may include high glucose levels, decreased leukocyte function, stasis of body fluids, invasive procedures, alteration in circulation/perfusion.

Dialysis, general   CH
(Also refer to Dialysis, peritoneal; hemodialysis)

imbalanced Nutrition: less than body requirements may be related to inadequate ingestion of nutrients (dietary restrictions, anorexia, nausea/vomiting, stomatitis), loss of peptides and amino acids (building blocks for proteins) during procedure, possibly evidenced by reported inadequate intake, aversion to eating, altered taste sensation, poor muscle tone/weakness, sore/inflamed buccal cavity, pale conjunctiva/mucous membranes.

anticipatory Grieving may be related to actual or perceived loss, chronic and/or fatal illness, and thwarted grieving response to a loss, possibly evidenced by verbal expression of distress/unresolved issues, denial of loss; altered eating habits, sleep and dream patterns, activity levels, libido; crying, labile affect; feelings of sorrow, guilt, and anger.

disturbed Body Image/situational low Self-Esteem may be related to situational crisis and chronic illness with changes in usual roles/body image, possibly evidenced by verbalization of changes in lifestyle, focus on past function, negative feelings about body, feelings of helplessness/powerlessness, extension of body boundary to incorporate environmental objects (e.g., dialysis setup), change in social involvement, overdependence on others for care, not taking responsibility for self-care/lack of follow-through, and self-destructive behavior.

Self-Care Deficit [specify] may be related to perceptual/cognitive impairment (accumulated toxins); intolerance to activity, decreased strength and endurance; pain/discomfort, possibly evidenced by reported inability to perform ADLs, disheveled/unkempt appearance, strong body odor.

Powerlessness may be related to illness-related regimen and healthcare environment, possibly evidenced by verbal expression of having no control, depression over physical deterioration, nonparticipation in care, anger, and passivity.

compromised/disabled family Coping may be related to inadequate or incorrect information or understanding by a primary person, temporary family disorganization and role changes, client providing little support in turn for the primary person, and prolonged disease/disability progression that exhausts the supportive capacity of significant persons, possibly evidenced by expressions of concern or reports about response of SO(s)/family to client's health problem, preoccupation of SO(s) with own personal reactions, display of intolerance/rejection, and protective behavior disproportionate (too little or too much) to client's abilities or need for autonomy.

Dialysis, peritoneal   **MS/CH**
(Also refer to Dialysis, general)

risk for excess Fluid Volume: risk factors may include inadequate osmotic gradient of dialysate, fluid retention (dialysate drainage problems/inappropriate osmotic gradient of solution, bowel distention), excessive PO/IV intake.

risk for Trauma: risk factors may include improper placement during insertion or manipulation of catheter.

acute Pain may be related to procedural factors (catheter irritation, improper catheter placement), presence of edema/abdominal distention, inflammation, or infection, rapid infusion/infusion of cold or acidic dialysate, possibly evidenced by verbal reports, guarding/distraction behaviors, and self-focus.

risk for Infection [peritonitis]: risk factors may include contamination of catheter/infusion system, skin contaminants, sterile peritonitis (response to composition of dialysate).

risk for ineffective Breathing Pattern: risk factors may include increased abdominal pressure with restricted diaphragmatic excursion, rapid infusion of dialysate, pain/discomfort, inflammatory process (e.g., atelectasis/pneumonia).

Diaper rash   **PED**
(Refer to Candidiasis)

Diaphragmatic Hernia   **CH/MS**
(Refer to Hernia, hiatal)

Diarrhea   **PED/CH**
deficient Knowledge [Learning Need] regarding causative/contributing factors and therapeutic needs may be related to lack of information/misconceptions, possibly evidenced by statements of concern, questions, and development of preventable complications.

risk for deficient Fluid Volume: risk factors may include excessive losses through GI tract, altered intake.

acute Pain may be related to abdominal cramping and irritation/excoriation of skin, possibly evidenced by verbal reports, facial grimacing, and autonomic responses.

impaired Skin Integrity may be related to effects of excretions on delicate tissues, possibly evidenced by reports of discomfort and disruption of skin surface/destruction of skin layers.

DIC   MS
(Refer to Disseminated intravascular coagulation)

Diffuse axonal (brain) injury   MS
(Refer to Traumatic brain injury; Cerebrovascular accident)

Digitalis toxicity   MS/CH
decreased Cardiac Output may be related to altered myocardial contractility/electrical conduction, properties of digitalis (long half-life and narrow therapeutic range), concurrent medications, age/general health status and electrolyte/acid-base balance, possibly evidenced by changes in rate/rhythm/conduction (development/worsening of dysrhythmias), changes in mentation, worsening of heart failure, elevated serum drug levels.

risk for imbalanced Fluid Volume: risk factors may include excessive losses from vomiting/diarrhea, decreased intake/nausea, decreased plasma proteins, malnutrition, continued use of diuretics; excess sodium/fluid retention.

deficient Knowledge [Learning Need] regarding condition/therapy and self-care needs may be related to information misinterpretation and lack of recall, possibly evidenced by inaccurate follow-through of instructions and development of preventable complications.

risk for disturbed Thought Processes: risk factors may include physiologic effects of toxicity/reduced cerebral perfusion.

Dilation of Cervix, premature   OB
(Also refer to Preterm labor)

Anxiety [specify level] may be related to situational crisis, threat of death/fetal loss possibly evidenced by increased tension, apprehension, feelings of inadequacy, sympathic stimulation, and repetitive questioning.

risk for maternal Injury: risk factors may include surgical intervention, use of tocolytic drugs.

risk for fetal Injury: risk factors may include premature delivery, surgical procedure.

anticipatory Grieving may be related to perceived potential fetal loss possibly evidenced by expression of distress, guilt, anger, choked feelings.

Dilation and curettage (D and C)   OB/GYN
(Also refer to Abortion, elective or spontaneous termination)

deficient Knowledge [Learning Need] regarding surgical procedure, possible postprocedural complications, and therapeutic needs may be related to lack of exposure/unfamiliarity with information, possibly evidenced by requests for information and statements of concern/misconceptions.

Dislocation/subluxation of joint   CH
acute Pain may be related to lack of continuity of bone/joint, muscle spasms, edema possibly evidenced by verbal or coded reports, guarded/protective behaviors, narrowed focus, autonomic responses.

risk for Injury: risk factors may include nerve impingement, improper fitting of splint device.

impaired physical Mobility may be related to immobilization device/activity restrictions, pain, edema, decreased muscle strength possibly evidenced by limited range of motion, limited ability to perform motor skills, gait changes.

Disruptive behavior disorder   PED/PSY
(Refer to Oppositional defiant disorder)

Disseminated intravascular coagulation   MS
risk for deficient Fluid Volume: risk factors may include failure of regulatory mechanism (coagulation process) and active loss/hemorrhage.

ineffective Tissue Perfusion (specify) may be related to alteration of arterial/venous flow (microemboli throughout circulatory system, and hypovolemia), possibly evidenced by changes in respiratory rate and depth, changes in mentation, decreased urinary output, and development of acral cyanosis/focal gangrene.

Anxiety [specify level]/Fear may be related to sudden change in health status/threat of death, interpersonal transmission/contagion, possibly evidenced by sympathetic stimulation, restlessness, focus on self, and apprehension.

risk for impaired Gas Exchange: risk factors may include reduced oxygen-carrying capacity, development of acidosis, fibrin deposition in microcirculation, and ischemic damage of lung parenchyma.

acute Pain may be related to bleeding into joints/muscles, with hematoma formation, and ischemic tissues with areas of acral cyanosis/focal gangrene, possibly evidenced by verbal reports, narrowed focus, alteration in muscle tone, guarding/distraction behaviors, restlessness, autonomic responses.

Dissociative disorders   PSY
[severe/panic] Anxiety/Fear may be related to a maladaptation or ineffective coping continuing from early life, unconscious conflict(s), threat to self-concept, unmet needs, or phobic stimulus, possibly evidenced by maladaptive response to stress (e.g., dissociating self/fragmentation of the personality), increased tension, feelings of inadequacy, and focus on self, projection of personal perceptions onto the environment.

risk for self/other-directed Violence: risk factors may include dissociative state/conflicting personalities, depressed mood, panic states, and suicidal or homicidal behaviors.

disturbed Personal Identity may be related to psychological conflicts (dissociative state), childhood trauma/abuse, threat to physical integrity/self-concept, and underdeveloped ego, possibly evidenced by alteration in perception or experience of the self, loss of one's own sense of reality/the external world, poorly differentiated ego boundaries, confusion about sense of self, purpose or direction in life; memory loss, presence of more than one personality within the individual.

compromised family Coping may be related to multiple stressors repeated over time, prolonged progression of disorder that exhausts the supportive capacity of significant person(s), family disorganization and role changes, high-risk family situation possibly evidenced by family/SO(s) describing inadequate understanding or knowledge that interferes with assistive or supportive behaviors; relationship and marital conflict.

Diverticulitis   CH
acute Pain may be related to inflammation of intestinal mucosa, abdominal cramping, and presence of fever/chills, possibly evidenced by verbal reports, guarding/distraction behaviors, autonomic responses, and narrowed focus.

Diarrhea/Constipation may be related to altered structure/function and presence of inflammation, possibly evidenced by signs and symptoms dependent on specific problem (e.g., increase/decrease in frequency of stools and change in consistency).

*deficient Knowledge [Learning Need] regarding disease process, potential complications, thera-
peutic and self-care needs* may be related to lack of information/misconceptions, possibly
evidenced by statements of concern, request for information, and development of preventable complications.

risk for Powerlessness: risk factors may include chronic nature of disease process and recurrent
episodes despite cooperation with medical regimen.

Down syndrome   PED/CH
(Also refer to Mental retardation)

delayed Growth and Development may be related to effects of physical/mental disability, possibly evidenced by altered physical growth; delay/inability in performing skills and self-
care/self-control activities appropriate for age.

risk for Trauma: risk factors may include cognitive difficulties and poor muscle tone/coordi-
nation, weakness.

imbalanced Nutrition: less than body requirements may be related to poor muscle tone and
protruding tongue, possibly evidenced by weak and ineffective sucking/swallowing and
observed lack of adequate intake with weight loss/failure to gain.

interrupted Family Processes may be related to situational/maturational crises requiring
incorporation of new skills into family dynamics, possibly evidenced by confusion
about what to do, verbalized difficulty coping with situation, unexamined family
myths.

risk for dysfunctional Grieving: risk factors may include loss of "the perfect child," chronic
condition requiring long-term care, and unresolved feelings.

risk for impaired parent/infant/child Attachment: risk factors may include ill infant/child who
is unable to effectively initiate parental contact due to altered behavioral organization,
inability of parents to meet the personal needs.

risk for Social Isolation: risk factors may include withdrawal from usual social interactions
and activities, assumption of total child care, and becoming overindulgent/overprotective.

Dressler's syndrome   CH

acute Pain may be related to tissue inflammation and presence of effusion, possibly
evidenced by verbal reports of chest pain affected by movement/position and deep breathing, guarding/distraction behaviors, self-focus, and autonomic responses (changes in vital
signs).

Anxiety [specify level] may be related to threat to/change in health status possibly evidenced
by increased tension, apprehension, restlessness, and expressed concerns.

risk for ineffective Breathing Pattern: risk factors may include pain on inspiration.

risk for impaired Gas Exchange: risk factors may include ventilation perfusion imbalance
(pleural effusion, pulmonary infiltrates).

Drug overdose, acute (depressants)   MS/PSY
(Also refer to Substance dependence/abuse rehabilitation)

ineffective Breathing Pattern/impaired Gas Exchange may be related to neuromuscular impair-
ment/CNS depression, decreased lung expansion, possibly evidenced by changes in respirations, cyanosis, and abnormal ABGs.

risk for Trauma/Suffocation/Poisoning: risk factors may include CNS depression/agitation,
hypersensitivity to the drug(s), psychological stress.

risk for self/other-directed Violence: risk factors may include suicidal behaviors, toxic reactions
to drug(s).

risk for Infection: risk factors may include drug injection techniques, impurities in injected
drugs, localized trauma; malnutrition, altered immune state.

Drug withdrawal   **CH/MS**

disturbed Thought Processes may be related to substance abuse/cessation, sleep deprivation, malnutrition possibly evidenced by inaccurate interpretation of environment, inappropriate/nonreality-based thinking, paranoia.

risk for Injury: risk factors may include CNS agitation (depressants).

risk for Suicide: risk factors may include alcohol/substance abuse, legal/disciplinary problems, depressed mood (stimulants).

acute Pain/[Discomfort] may be related to biochemical changes associated with cessation of drug use possibly evidenced by reports of muscle aches, fever, diaphoresis, rhinorrhea/lacrimation, malaise.

Self-Care Deficit (specify) may be related to perceptual/cognitive impairment, therapeutic management (restraints) possibly evidenced by inability to meet own physical needs.

disturbed Sleep Pattern may be related to cessation of substance use, fatigue possibly evidenced by reports of insomnia/hypersomnia, decreased ability to function, increased irritability.

Fatigue may be related to altered body chemistry (drug withdrawal), sleep deprivation, malnutrition, poor physical condition possibly evidenced by verbal reports of overwhelming lack of energy, inability to maintain usual level of physical activity, inability to restore energy after sleep, compromised concentration.

DTs   **MS/PSY**
(Refer to Delirium tremens)

Duchenne's muscular dystrophy   **PED/CH**
(Refer to Muscular dystrophy [Duchenne's])

Duodenal ulcer   **MS/CH**
(Refer to Ulcer, peptic)

DVT   **CH/MS**
(Refer to Thrombophlebitis)

Dysmenorrhea   **GYN**

acute Pain may be related to exaggerated uterine contractibility, possibly evidenced by verbal reports, guarding/distraction behaviors, narrowed focus, and autonomic responses (changes in vital signs).

risk for Activity Intolerance: risk factors may include severity of pain and presence of secondary symptoms (nausea, vomiting, syncope, chills), depression.

ineffective Coping may be related to chronic, recurrent nature of problem; anticipatory anxiety, and inadequate coping methods, possibly evidenced by muscular tension, headaches, general irritability, chronic depression, and verbalization of inability to cope, report of poor self-concept.

Dyspareunia   **GYN/PSY**

Sexual Dysfunction may be related to physical and/or psychological alteration in function (menopausal involution, allergy to contraceptive, abnormalities of genital tract, guilt, control issues), possibly evidenced by verbalization of problem, inability to achieve desired satisfaction, sexual aversion, alteration in relationship with significant other.

Anxiety [specify] may be related to situational crisis, stress, unconscious conflict about essential values, unmet needs possibly evidenced by expressed concerns, distressed, feelings of inadequacy.

Dysrhythmia, cardiac   CH/MS

risk for decreased Cardiac Output: risk factors may include altered electrical conduction and
   reduced myocardial contractility.

Anxiety [specify level] may be related to perceived threat of death, possibly evidenced by
   increased tension, apprehension, and expressed concerns.

deficient Knowledge [Learning Need] regarding medical condition/therapy needs may be related
   to lack of information/misinterpretation and unfamiliarity with information resources,
   possibly evidenced by questions, statement of misconception, failure to improve on previous regimen, and development of preventable complications.

risk for Activity Intolerance: risk factors may include imbalance between myocardial O_2
   supply and demand, and cardiac depressant effects of certain drugs (b-blockers, antidysrhythmics).

risk for Poisoning [digitalis toxicity]: risk factors may include limited range of therapeutic
   effectiveness, lack of education/proper precautions, reduced vision/cognitive limitations.

Dysthymic disorder   PSY/CH

(Refer to Depression, major)

Dystocia   OB

(Also refer to Labor, stage I [latent/active phases])

risk for maternal Injury: risk factors may include alteration of muscle tone/contractile pattern,
   mechanical obstruction to fetal descent, maternal fatigue.

risk for fetal Injury: risk factors may include prolonged labor, fetal malpresentations, tissue
   hypoxia/acidosis, abnormalities of the maternal pelvis, CPD.

risk for deficient Fluid Volume: risk factors may include hypermetabolic state, vomiting,
   profuse diaphoresis, restricted oral intake, mild diuresis associated with oxytocin administration.

ineffective Coping may be related to situational crisis, personal vulnerability, unrealistic
   expectations/perceptions, inadequate/exhausted support systems possibly evidenced
   by verbalizations and behavior indicative of inability to cope (loss of control, inability
   to problem-solve and/or meet role expectations), irritability, reports of fatigue/
   tension.

Eating disorders   CH/PSY

(Refer to Anorexia nervosa; Bulimia nervosa)

Ebola   MS

(Also refer to Disseminated intravascular coagulation; Multiple organ dysfunction
   syndrome)

acute Pain/[Discomfort] may be related to infectious process possibly evidenced by reports of
   headache, myalgia, abdominal or chest pain, sore throat; fever.

Hyperthermia may be related to inflammatory process possibly evidenced by increased body
   temperature, flushes/warm skin, headache.

risk for deficient Fluid Volume: risk factors may include inadequate intake (nausea, painful
   swallowing, abdominal pain), increased losses (vomiting, diarrhea, hemorrhage/DIC),
   hypermetabolic state (fever).

risk for [spread of/secondary] Infection: risk factors may include mode of transmission, invasive monitoring/procedures, debilitated state, malnutrition, insufficient
   knowledge/resources to avoid exposure to pathogens.

acute Confusion may be related to infectious process, hypoxemia possibly evidenced by
   fluctuations in cognition, agitation, change in level of consciousness (stupor/coma).

Eclampsia   **OB**

(Also refer to Pregnancy-Induced hypertension)

Anxiety [specify]/Fear may be related to situational crisis, threat of change in health status/
   death (self/fetus), separation from support system, interpersonal contagion possibly
   evidenced by expressed concerns, apprehension, increased tension, decreased self-
   assurance, difficulty concentrating.

risk for maternal Injury: risk factors may include tissue edema/hypoxia, tonic-clonic convulsions, abnormal blood profile and/or clotting factors.

impaired physical Mobility may be related to prescribed bedrest, discomfort, anxiety possibly
   evidenced by difficulty turning, postural instability.

risk for Self-Care Deficit (specify): risk factors may include weakness, discomfort, physical
   restrictions.

ECT   **PSY**

(Refer to Electroconvulsive therapy)

Ectopic pregnancy (tubal)   **OB**

(Also refer to Abortion, spontaneous termination)

acute Pain may be related to distention/rupture of fallopian tube, possibly evidenced by
   verbal reports, guarding/distraction behaviors, facial mask of pain, and autonomic
   responses (diaphoresis, changes in vital signs).

risk for deficient Fluid Volume [isotonic]: risk factors may include hemorrhagic losses and
   decreased/restricted intake.

Anxiety [specify level]/Fear may be related to threat of death and possible loss of ability to
   conceive, possibly evidenced by increased tension, apprehension, sympathetic stimulation,
   restlessness, and focus on self.

Eczema   **CH**

(Refer to Dermatitis, contact/seborrheic)   CH

Pain/[Discomfort] may be related to cutaneous inflammation and irritation, possibly
   evidenced by verbal reports, irritability, and scratching.

risk for Infection: risk factors may include broken skin and tissue trauma.

Social Isolation may be related to alterations in physical appearance, possibly evidenced by
   expressed feelings of rejection and decreased interaction with peers.

Edema, pulmonary   **MS**

excess Fluid Volume may be related to decreased cardiac functioning, excessive fluid/sodium
   intake, possibly evidenced by dyspnea, presence of crackles (rales), pulmonary congestion
   on radiograph, restlessness, anxiety, and increased central venous pressure
   (CVP)/pulmonary pressures.

impaired Gas Exchange may be related to altered blood flow and decreased alveolar/capillary
   exchange (fluid collection/shifts into interstitial space/alveoli), possibly evidenced by
   hypoxia, restlessness, and confusion.

Anxiety [specify level]/Fear may be related to perceived threat of death (inability to breathe),
   possibly evidenced by responses ranging from apprehension to panic state, restlessness,
   and focus on self.

Elder abuse   **CH/PSY**

(Refer to Abuse, physical/psychological)

Electrical injury   **MS**

(Also refer to Burns)

risk for decreased Cardiac Output: risk factors may include altered heart rate/rhythm (ventricular fibrillation/asystole).

impaired [internal] Tissue Integrity may be related to thermal injury (along path of current), altered circulation (massive edema) possibly evidenced by damaged or destroyed tissue/necrosis.

risk for impaired peripheral Tissue Perfusion: risk factors may include reduction of venous/arterial blood flow (vein coagulation, muscle edema), increased tissue pressure (compartment syndrome).

risk for Trauma/Suffocation: risk factors may include muscle paralysis (CNS damage), loss of large- or small-muscle coordination (seizures).

Electroconvulsive therapy   PSY

decisional Conflict may be related to lack of relevant or multiple/divergent sources of information, mistrust of regimen/healthcare personnel, sense of powerlessness, support system deficit.

risk for Injury [effects of electroconvulsive therapy (ECT)]: risk factors may include effects of therapy on the cardiovascular, respiratory, musculoskeletal, and nervous systems; and pharmacological effects of anesthesia.

acute Confusion may be related to CNS effects of electric shock and medications/anesthesia possibly evidenced by fluctuation in cognition, agitation.

impaired Memory may be related to neurologic disturbance (electrical shock) possibly evidenced by reported/observed experiences of forgetting, difficulty recalling recent events/factual information.

Emphysema   CH/MS

impaired Gas Exchange may be related to alveolar capillary membrane changes/destruction, possibly evidenced by dyspnea, restlessness, changes in mentation, abnormal ABG values.

ineffective Airway Clearance may be related to increased production/retained tenacious secretions, decreased energy level, and muscle wasting, possibly evidenced by abnormal breath sounds (rhonchi), ineffective cough, changes in rate/depth of respirations, and dyspnea.

Activity Intolerance may be related to imbalance between O_2 supply and demand, possibly evidenced by reports of fatigue/weakness, exertional dyspnea, and abnormal vital sign response to activity.

imbalanced Nutrition: less than body requirements may be related to inability to ingest food (shortness of breath, anorexia, generalized weakness, medication side effects), possibly evidenced by lack of interest in food, reported altered taste, loss of muscle mass and tone, fatigue, and weight loss.

risk for Infection: risk factors may include inadequate primary defenses (stasis of body fluids, decreased ciliary action), chronic disease process, and malnutrition.

Powerlessness may be related to illness-related regimen and healthcare environment, possibly evidenced by verbal expression of having no control, depression over physical deterioration, nonparticipation in therapeutic regimen; anger, and passivity.

Encephalitis   MS

risk for ineffective cerebral Tissue Perfusion: risk factors may include cerebral edema altering/interrupting cerebral arterial/venous blood flow, hypovolemia, exchange problems at cellular level (acidosis).

Hyperthermia may be related to increased metabolic rate, illness, and dehydration, possibly evidenced by increased body temperature, flushed/warm skin, and increased pulse and respiratory rates.

acute Pain may be related to inflammation/irritation of the brain and cerebral edema, possibly evidenced by verbal reports of headache, photophobia, distraction behaviors, restlessness, and autonomic response (changes in vital signs).

risk for Trauma/Suffocation: risk factors may include restlessness, clonic/tonic activity, altered sensorium, cognitive impairment; generalized weakness, ataxia, vertigo.

Encopresis   PSY/PED

disturbed Body Image/chronic low Self-Esteem may be related to negative view of self, maturational expectations, social factors, stigma attached to loss of body function in public, family's belief condition is volitional, shame related to body odor possibly evidenced by angry outbursts/oppositional behavior, verbalization of powerlessness, reluctance to engage in social activities.

Bowel Incontinence may be related to situational/maturational crisis, psychogenic factors (predisposing vulnerability, threat to physical integrity—child/sexual abuse) possibly evidenced by involuntary passage of stool at least once monthly, strong odor of feces on client, hiding soiled clothing in inappropriate places.

compromised/disabled family Coping may be related to inadequate/incorrect information or understanding of condition, belief that behavior is volitional, disagreement regarding treatment/coping strategies possibly evidenced by attempts to intervene with child are increasingly ineffective, significant person describes preoccupation with personal reaction (excessive guilt, anger, blame regarding child's condition/behavior), overprotective behavior.

Endocarditis   MS

risk for decreased Cardiac Output: risk factors may include inflammation of lining of heart and structural change in valve leaflets.

Anxiety [specify level] may be related to change in health status and threat of death, possibly evidenced by apprehension, expressed concerns, and focus on self.

acute Pain may be related to generalized inflammatory process and effects of embolic phenomena, possibly evidenced by verbal reports, narrowed focus, distraction behaviors, and autonomic responses (changes in vital signs).

risk for Activity Intolerance: risk factors may include imbalance between O_2 supply and demand, debilitating condition.

risk for ineffective Tissue Perfusion (specify): risk factors may include embolic interruption of arterial flow (embolization of thrombi/ valvular vegetations).

End of life care   CH
(Refer to Hospice care)

Endometriosis   GYN

acute/chronic Pain may be related to pressure of concealed bleeding/formation of adhesions, possibly evidenced by verbal reports (pain between/with menstruation), guarding/distraction behaviors, and narrowed focus.

Sexual Dysfunction may be related to pain secondary to presence of adhesions, possibly evidenced by verbalization of problem, and altered relationship with partner.

deficient Knowledge [Learning Need] regarding pathophysiology of condition and therapy needs may be related to lack of information/misinterpretations, possibly evidenced by statements of concern and misconceptions.

Enteral feeding   MS/CH

risk for Infection: risk factors may include invasive procedure/surgical placement of feeding tube, malnutrition, chronic disease.

risk for Aspiration: risk factors may include presence of feeding tube, bolus tube feedings, increased intragastric pressure, delayed gastric emptying, medication administration.

risk for imbalanced Fluid Volume: risk factors may include active loss/failure of regulatory mechanisms (specific to underlying disease process/trauma), inability to obtain/ingest fluids.

Fatigue may be related to decreased metabolic energy production, increased energy requirements (hypermetabolic state, healing process), altered body chemistry (medications, chemotherapy) possibly evidenced by overwhelming lack of energy, inability to maintain usual routines/accomplish routine tasks, lethargy, impaired ability to concentrate.

Enteritis   MS/CH
(Refer to Colitis, ulcerative; Crohn's disease)

Enuresis   PSY/PED
impaired Urinary Elimination may be related to situational/maturational crisis, psychogenic factors (predisposing vulnerability, threat to physical integrity—child/sexual abuse) possibly evidenced by nocturnal/diurinal enuresis, strong odor of urine on client, hiding soiled clothing in inappropriate places.

disturbed Body Image/chronic low Self-Esteem may be related to negative view of self, maturational expectations, social factors, stigma attached to loss of body function in public, family's belief condition is volitional, shame related to body odor possibly evidenced by angry outbursts/oppositional behavior, verbalization of powerlessness, reluctance to engage in social activities.

ineffective family Coping (specify) may be related to inadequate/incorrect information or understanding of condition, belief that behavior is volitional, disagreement regarding treatment/coping strategies possibly evidenced by attempts to intervene with child are increasingly ineffective, significant person describes preoccupation with personal reaction (excessive guilt, anger, blame regarding child's condition/behavior), overprotective behavior.

Epididymitis   MS
acute Pain may be related to inflammation, edema formation, and tension on the spermatic cord, possibly evidenced by verbal reports, guarding/distraction behaviors (restlessness), and autonomic responses (changes in vital signs).

risk for Infection [spread]: risk factors may include presence of inflammation/infectious process, insufficient knowledge to avoid spread of infection.

deficient Knowledge [Learning Need] regarding pathophysiology, outcome, and self-care needs may be related to lack of information/misinterpretations, possibly evidenced by statements of concern, misconceptions, and questions.

Epilepsy   CH
(Refer to Seizure disorder)

Episiotomy   OB
acute Pain may be related to tissue trauma/edema, surgical incision possibly evidenced by verbalizations, guarding behavior, self-focusing.

risk for Infection: risk factors may include broken skin, traumatized tissue, body excretions, inadequate hygiene.

risk for Sexual Dysfunction: risk factors may include recent childbirth, presence of incision.

Epistaxis CH

[mild to moderate] Anxiety may be related to situational crisis, threat to health status, interpersonal transmission possibly evidenced by expressed concerns, apprehension, anxious.

risk for Aspiration: risk factors may include uncontrolled nasal bleeding.

risk for impaired Tissue Integrity: risk factors may include altered circulation/mechanical compression.

Epstein-Barr virus CH

(Refer to Mononucleosis, infectious)

Erectile dysfunction CH/PSY

Sexual Dysfunction may be related to altered body function, side effects of medication possibly evidenced by reports of disruption of sexual response pattern, inability to achieve desired satisfaction.

situational low Self-Esteem may be related to functional impairment, perceived failure to perform satisfactorily, rejection of other(s) possibly evidenced by self-negating verbalizations, expressions of helplessness/powerlessness.

Esophageal reflux disease CH

(Refer to Gastroesophageal reflux disease)

Esophageal varcies CH/MS

(Refer to Varcies, esophageal)

Esophagitis CH

(Refer to Gastroesophageal reflux disease; Achalasia)

ETOH withdrawal MS/CH

(Refer to Alcohol intoxication, acute; substance dependence/abuse rehabilitation)

Evisceration MS

(Refer to Dehiscence, abdominal)

Facial reconstructive surgery MS/CH

(Also refer to Surgery, general; Intermaxillary fixation)

risk for ineffective Airway Clearance: risk factors may include soft tissue edema, airway trauma , retained secretions.

impaired Skin Integrity may be related to traumatic injury, surgical procedure (incisions/grafts), edema, altered circulation possibly evidenced by disruption/destruction of skin layers.

Fear/Anxiety may be related to situational crisis, memory of traumatic event, threat to self-concept (disfigurement) possibly evidenced by expressed concerns, apprehension, uncertainty, decreased self-assurance, restlessness.

disturbed Body Image may be related to traumatic event, disfigurement possibly evidenced by negative feelings about self, fear of rejection reaction by others, preoccupation with change, change in social involvement.

risk for Social Isolation: risk factors may include change in physical appearance.

Failure to thrive PED

imbalanced Nutrition: less than body requirements may be related to inability to ingest/digest/absorb nutrients (defects in organ function/metabolism, genetic factors), physical deprivation/psychosocial factors, possibly evidenced by lack of appropriate weight gain/weight loss, poor muscle tone, pale conjunctiva, and laboratory tests reflecting nutritional deficiency.

delayed Growth and Development may be related to inadequate caretaking (physical/emotional neglect or abuse); indifference, inconsistent responsiveness, multiple caretakers; environmental and stimulation deficiencies, possibly evidenced by altered physical growth, flat affect, listlessness, decreased response; delay or difficulty in performing skills or self-control activities appropriate for age group.

risk for impaired Parenting: risk factors may include lack of knowledge, inadequate bonding, unrealistic expectations for self/infant, and lack of appropriate response of child to relationship.

deficient Knowledge [Learning Need] regarding pathophysiology of condition, nutritional needs, growth/development expectations, and parenting skills may be related to lack of information/misinformation or misinterpretation, possibly evidenced by verbalization of concerns, questions, misconceptions; or development of preventable complications.

CH/MS

adult Failure to Thrive may be related to depression, apathy, aging process, fatigue, degenerative condition possibly evidenced by expressed lack of appetite, difficulty performing self-care tasks, altered mood state, inadequate intake, weight loss, physical decline.

ineffective Protection may be related to inadequate nutrition, anemia, extremes of age possibly evidenced by fatigue, weakness, deficient immunity, impaired healing, pressure sores.

Fat embolism syndrome   MS
(Refer to Pulmonary embolism; Respiratory distress syndrome, acute)

Fatigue syndrome, chronic   CH
Fatigue may be related to disease state, inadequate sleep, possibly evidenced by verbalization of unremitting/overwhelming lack of energy, inability to maintain usual routines, listless, compromised concentration.

chronic Pain may be related to chronic physical disability possibly evidenced by verbal reports of headache, sore throat, arthralgias, abdominal pain, muscle aches; altered ability to continue previous activities, changes in sleep pattern.

Self-Care Deficit [specify] may be related to tiredness, pain/discomfort possible evidenced by reports of inability to perform desired ADLs.

risk for ineffective Role Performance: risk factors may include health alterations, stress.

Febrile seizure   PED
Hyperthermia may be related to illness, dehydration, decreased ability to perspire possibly evidenced by increase in body temperature, flushed/warm skin, seizures.

Fecal diversion   MS/CH
(Refer to Colostomy)

Fecal impaction   CH
Constipation may be related to irregular defecation habits, decreased activity, dehydration, abdominal muscle weakness, neurologic impairment possibly evidenced by inability to pass stool, abdominal distension/tenderness/pain, nausea/vomiting, anorexia.

Femoral popliteal bypass   MS

(Also refer to Surgery, general)

risk for ineffective peripheral Tissue Perfusion: risk factors may include interruption of arterial blood flow, hypovolemia.

risk for Peripheral Neurovascular Dysfunction: risk factors may include vascular obstruction, immobilization, mechanical compression/dressings.

impaired Walking may be related to surgical incisions, dressings possibly evidenced by inability to walk desired distance, climb stairs, negotiate inclines.

Fetal alcohol syndrome   PED

risk for Injury [CNS damage]: risk factors may include external chemical factors (alcohol intake by mother), placental insufficiency, fetal drug withdrawal in utero/postpartum and prematurity.

disorganized Infant Behavior may be related to prematurity, environmental overstimulation, lack of containment/boundaries, possibly evidenced by change from baseline physiologic measures; tremors, startles, twitches, hyperextension of arms/legs, deficient self-regulatory behaviors, deficient response to visual/auditory stimuli.

risk for impaired Parenting: risk factors may include mental and/or physical illness, inability of mother to assume the overwhelming task of unselfish giving and nurturing, presence of stressors (financial/legal problems), lack of available or ineffective role model, interruption of bonding process, lack of appropriate response of child to relationship.

                                       PSY

ineffective [maternal] Coping may be related to personal vulnerability, low self-esteem, inadequate coping skills, and multiple stressors (repeated over period of time), possibly evidenced by inability to meet basic needs/fulfill role expectations/problem-solve, and excessive use of drug(s).

dysfunctional Family Processes: alcoholism may be related to lack of/insufficient support from others, mother's drug problem and treatment status, together with poor coping skills, lack of family stability/overinvolvement of parents with children and multigenerational addictive behaviors, possibly evidenced by abandonment, rejection, neglectful relationships with family members, and decisions and actions by family that are detrimental.

Fetal demise   OB

effective Grieving may be related to death of fetus/infant (wanted or unwanted), inability to meet personal expectations possibly evidenced by verbal expressions of distress, anger, loss; crying; alteration in eating habits or sleep pattern.

situational low Self-Esteem may be related to perceived "failure" at a life event, possibly evidenced by negative self-appraisal in response to life event in a person with a previous positive self-evaluation, verbalization of negative feelings about the self (helplessness, uselessness), difficulty making decisions.

risk for ineffective Role Performance: risk factors may include stress, family conflict, inadequate support system.

risk for interrupted Family Processes: risk factors may include situational crisis, developmental transition [loss of child], family roles shift.

risk for Spiritual Distress: risk factors may include loss of loved one, blame for loss directed at self/God, alienation from other/support systems, challenged belief and value system (birth is supposed to be the beginning of life, not of death) and intense suffering.

Fibrocytic breast disease   **CH**

[mild to moderate] Anxiety may be related to situational crisis, threat to health status, family
    heredity, interpersonal transmission possibly evidenced by expressed concerns, apprehen-
    sion, uncertainty, fearful, focus on self, increased tension.

acute/chronic Pain may be related to physical agents (edema formation, nerve irritation) possi-
    bly evidenced by verbal reports, guarded/protective behavior, expressive behavior, self-
    focusing.

risk for ineffective Coping: risk factors may include situational crisis, perceived high degree of
    threat, inadequate resources/social supports.

Fibroids, uterine   **GYN**

(Refer to Uterine myomas)

Fibromyalgia syndrome, primary   **CH**

acute/chronic Pain may be related to idiopathic diffuse condition possibly evidenced by
    reports of achy pain in fibrous tissues (muscles, tendons, ligamants), muscle
    stiffness/spasm, disturbed sleep, guarding behaviors, fear of reinjury/exacerbation, rest-
    lessness, irritability, self-focusing, reduced interaction with others.

Fatigue may be related to disease state, stress, anxiety, depression, sleep deprivation possibly
    evidenced by verbalization of overwhelming lack of energy, inability to maintain usual
    routines/level of physical activity, tired, feelings of guilt for not keeping up with responsi-
    bilities, increase in physical complaints, listless.

risk for Hopelessness: risk factors may include chronic debilitating physical condition,
    prolonged activity restriction (possibly self-induced) creating isolation, lack of specific
    therapeutic cure, prolonged stress.

Flail chest   **MS**

(Refer to Hemothroax; Pneumothorax)

Food poisoning   **CH/MS**

(Refer to Gastroenteritis)

Fractures   **MS/CH**

(Also refer to Casts; Traction)

risk for Trauma [additional injury]: risk factors may include loss of skeletal integrity/move-
    ment of skeletal fragments, use of traction apparatus.

acute Pain may be related to muscle spasms, movement of bone fragments, tissue
    trauma/edema, traction/immobility device, stress, and anxiety, possibly evidenced by
    verbal reports, distraction behaviors, self-focusing/narrowed focus, facial mask of pain,
    guarding/protective behavior, alteration in muscle tone, and autonomic responses (changes
    in vital signs).

risk for Peripheral Neurovascular Dysfunction: risk factors may include reduction/interruption
    of blood flow (direct vascular injury, tissue trauma, excessive edema, thrombus formation,
    hypovolemia).

impaired physical Mobility may be related to neuromuscular/skeletal impairment,
    pain/discomfort, restrictive therapies (bedrest, extremity immobilization), and psychologi-
    cal immobility, possibly evidenced by inability to purposefully move within the physical
    environment, imposed restrictions, reluctance to attempt movement, limited range of
    motion, and decreased muscle strength/control.

risk for impaired Gas Exchange: risk factors may include altered blood flow, blood/fat
    emboli, alveolar/capillary membrane changes (interstitial/pulmonary edema,
    congestion).

---

deficient Knowledge [Learning Need] regarding healing process, therapy requirements, potential complications, and self-care needs may be related to lack of exposure, misinterpretation of information, possibly evidenced by statements of concern, questions, and misconceptions.

Frostbite   MS/CH

impaired Tissue Integrity may be related to altered circulation and thermal injury, possibly evidenced by damaged/destroyed tissue.

acute Pain may be related to diminished circulation with tissue ischemia/necrosis and edema formation, possibly evidenced by verbal reports, guarding/distraction behaviors, narrowed focus, and autonomic responses (changes in vital signs).

risk for Infection: risk factors may include traumatized tissue/tissue destruction, altered circulation, and compromised immune response in affected area.

Fusion, cervical   MS
(Refer to Laminectomy, cervical)

Fusion, lumbar   MS
(Refer to Laminectomy, lumbar)

Gallstones   CH
(Refer to Cholelithiasis)

Gangrene, dry   MS

ineffective peripheral Tissue Perfusion may be related to interruption in arterial flow, possibly evidenced by cool skin temperature, change in color (black), atrophy of affected part, and presence of pain.

acute Pain may be related to tissue hypoxia and necrotic process, possibly evidenced by verbal reports, guarding/distraction behaviors, narrowed focus, and autonomic responses (changes in vital signs).

Gangrene, gas   MS

impaired Tissue Integrity may be related to trauma/surgery, infection, altered circulation possibly evidenced by edema, brown/serous exudate, bronze or blackish green skin color, gas bubbles/crepitation, pain.

[severe] Anxiety/Fear may be related to situational crisis, interpersonal transmission, threat of death possibly evidenced by expressed concerns, distress, apprehension, fearful, restlessness, irritability, focus on self.

risk for impaired renal Tissue Perfusion: risk factors may include effects of circulating toxins, altered circulation/shock.

risk for Injury: risk factors may include therapeutic intervention (hyperbaric oxygen therapy).

Gas, lung irritant   MS/CH

ineffective Airway Clearance may be related to irritation/inflammation of airway, possibly evidenced by marked cough, abnormal breath sounds (wheezes), dyspnea, and tachypnea.

risk for impaired Gas Exchange: risk factors may include irritation/inflammation of alveolar membrane (dependent on type of agent and length of exposure).

Anxiety [specify level] may be related to change in health status and threat of death, possibly evidenced by verbalizations, increased tension, apprehension, and sympathetic stimulation.

Gastrectomy, subtotal   **MS**
(Also refer to Surgery, general)

risk for imbalanced Nutrition: less than body requirements: risk factors may include restricted oral intake/early satiety, change in digestive process/malabsorption of nutrients, fear of complications (e.g., dumping syndrome, reactive hypoglycemia).

risk for Fatigue: risk factors may include malnutrition, anemia.

risk for Diarrhea: risk factors may include malabsorption.

Gastric partitioning   **MS**
(Refer to Gastroplasty)

Gastric resection   **MS**
(Refer to Gastrectomy, subtotal)

Gastric ulcer   **MS/CH**
(Refer to Ulcer, peptic)

Gastrinoma   **MS/CH**
(Refer to Zollinger-Ellison syndrome)

Gastritis, acute   **MS**

acute Pain may be related to irritation/inflammation of gastric mucosa, possibly evidenced by verbal reports, guarding/distraction behaviors, and autonomic responses (changes in vital signs).

risk for deficient Fluid Volume [isotonic]: risk factors may include excessive losses through vomiting and diarrhea, continued bleeding, reluctance to ingest/restrictions of oral intake.

Gastritis, chronic   **CH**

risk for imbalanced Nutrition: less than body requirements: risk factors may include inability to ingest adequate nutrients (prolonged nausea/ vomiting, anorexia, epigastric pain).

deficient Knowledge [Learning Need] regarding pathophysiology, psychological factors, therapy needs, and potential complications may be related to lack of information/misinterpretation, possibly evidenced by verbalization of concerns, questions, misconceptions, and continuation of problem.

Gastroenteritis   **CH/MS**

Diarrhea may be related to toxins, contaminants, travel, infectious process, parasites possibly evidenced by at least 3 loose liquid stools/day, hyperactive bowel sounds, abdominal pain.

risk for deficient Fluid Volume: risk factors may include excessive losses (diarrhea, vomiting), hypermetabolic state (infection), decreased intake (nausea, anorexia), extremes of age/weight.

risk for Infection [transmission]: risk factors may include insufficient knowledge to prevent contamination (inappropriate handwashing and food handling).

Gastroesophageal reflux disease (GERD)   **CH**

acute/chronic Pain may be related to acidic irritation of mucosa, muscle spasm, recurrent vomiting possibly evidenced by reports of heartburn, distraction behaviors.

impaired Swallowing may be related to GERD, esophageal defects, achalasia possibly evidenced by reports of heartburn/epigastric pain, "something stuck" when swallowing, food refusal/volume limiting, nighttime coughing or awakening.

risk for imbalanced Nutrition: less than body requirements: risk factors may include limiting intake, recurrent vomiting.

---

risk for disturbed Sleep Pattern: risk factors may include nighttime heartburn, regurgitation of stomach contents.

risk for Aspiration: risk factors may include incompetent lower esophageal sphincter, regurgitation of gastric acid.

Gastrointestinal hemorrhage   MS
(Refer to Gastritis, acute or chronic; Ulcer, peptic; Colitis, ulcerative; Crohn's disease; Varices, esophageal)

Gastroplasty   MS
(Also refer to Surgery, general)

ineffective Breathing Pattern may be related to decreased lung expansion, pain, anxiety, decreased energy/fatigue, tracheobronchial obstruction possibly evidenced by dyspnea, tachypnea, changes in respiratory depth, reduced vital capacity, wheezes, rhonchi, abnormal ABGs.

risk for ineffective peripheral Tissue Perfusion: risk factors may include diminished blood flow, hypovolemia, immobility/bedrest, interruption of venous blood flow (thrombus).

risk for deficient Fluid Volume: risk factors may include excessive gastric losses, nasogastric suction, diarrhea, reduced intake.

risk for imbalanced Nutrition: less than body requirements: risk factors may include decreased intake, dietary restrictions, early satiety, increased metabolic rate/healing, malabsorption of nutrients/impaired absorption of vitamins.

Diarrhea may be related to changes in dietary fiber/bulk, inflammation, irritation, malabsorption of bowel possibly evidenced by loose/liquid stools, increased frequency, hyperactive bowel sounds.

Gender identity disorder   PSY
(For individuals experiencing persistent and marked distress regarding uncertainty about issues relating to personal identity, e.g., sexual orientation and behavior.)

Anxiety [specify level] may be related to unconscious/conscious conflicts about essential values/beliefs (ego-dystonic gender identification), threat to self-concept, unmet needs, possibly evidenced by increased tension, helplessness, hopelessness, feelings of inadequacy, uncertainty, insomnia and focus on self, and impaired daily functioning.

ineffective Role Performance/disturbed Personal Identity may be related to crisis in development in which person has difficulty knowing/accepting to which sex he or she belongs or is attracted, sense of discomfort and inappropriateness about anatomic sex characteristics, possibly evidenced by confusion about sense of self, purpose or direction in life, sexual identification/preference, verbalization of desire to be/insistence that person is the opposite sex, change in self-perception of role, and conflict in roles.

ineffective Sexuality Patterns may be related to ineffective or absent role models and conflict with sexual orientation and/or preferences, lack of/impaired relationship with an SO, possibly evidenced by verbalizations of discomfort with sexual orientation/role, and lack of information about human sexuality.

risk for compromised/disabled family Coping: risk factors may include inadequate/incorrect information or understanding, significant other unable to perceive or to act effectively in regard to client's needs, temporary family disorganization and role changes, and client providing little support in turn for primary person.

readiness for enhanced family Coping may be related to individual's basic needs being sufficiently gratified and adaptive tasks effectively addressed to enable goals of self-actualization to surface, possibly evidenced by family member(s) attempts to describe growth/impact of crisis on own values, priorities, goals, or relationships; family member(s) is moving in direction of health-promoting and enriching lifestyle that supports client's search for self; and choosing experiences that optimize wellness.

Genetic disorder   CH/OB

Anxiety may be related to presence of specific risk factors (e.g., exposure to teratogens), situational crisis, threat to self-concept, conscious or unconscious conflict about essential values and life goals possibly evidenced by increased tension, apprehension, uncertainty, feelings of inadequacy, expressed concerns.

deficient Knowledge [Learning Need] regarding purpose/process of genetic counseling may be related to lack of awareness of ramifications of diagnosis, process necessary for analyzing available options, and information misinterpretation possibly evidenced by verbalization of concerns, statement of misconceptions, request for information.

risk for interrupted Family Processes: risk factors may include situational crisis, individual/family vulnerability, difficulty reaching agreement regarding options.

Spiritual Distress may be related to intense inner conflict about the outcome, normal grieving for the loss of the perfect child, anger that is often directed at God/greater power, religious beliefs/moral convictions possibly evidenced by verbalization of inner conflict about beliefs, questioning of the moral and ethical implications of therapeutic choices, viewing situation as punishment, anger, hostility, and crying.

Genital herpes   CH
(Refer to Herpes simplex; Sexually transmitted disease)

Genital warts (human papillomavirus)   CH
(Refer to Sexually transmitted disease)

GERD   CH
(Refer to Gastroesophageal reflux disease)

GI bleeding   MS
(Refer to Gastritis, acute or chronic; Ulcer, peptic)

Gigantism   CH
(Refer to Acromegaly)

Gingivitis   CH

impaired Oral Mucous Membrane may be related to ineffective oral hygiene, ill-fitting dentures, decreased salivation, hormonal changes possibly evidenced by edema, gingival bleeding, hyperplasia, oral pain.

Glaucoma   CH

disturbed visual Sensory Perception may be related to altered sensory reception and altered status of sense organ (increased intraocular pressure/atrophy of optic nerve head), possibly evidenced by progressive loss of visual field.

Anxiety [specify level] may be related to change in health status, presence of pain, possibility/reality of loss of vision, unmet needs, and negative self-talk, possibly evidenced by apprehension, uncertainty, and expressed concern regarding changes in life event.

Glomerulonephritis   PED

excess Fluid Volume may be related to failure of regulatory mechanism (inflammation of glomerular membrane inhibiting filtration), possibly evidenced by weight gain, edema/anasarca, intake greater than output, and blood pressure changes.

acute Pain may be related to effects of circulating toxins and edema/distention of renal capsule, possibly evidenced by verbal reports, guarding/distraction behaviors, and autonomic responses (changes in vital signs).

imbalanced Nutrition: less than body requirements may be related to anorexia and dietary restrictions, possibly evidenced by aversion to eating, reported altered taste, weight loss, and decreased intake.

deficient Diversional Activity may be related to treatment modality/restrictions, fatigue, and malaise, possibly evidenced by statements of boredom, restlessness, and irritability.

risk for disproportionate Growth: risk factors may include infection, malnutrition, chronic illness.

Goiter CH

disturbed Body Image may be related to visible swelling in neck possibly evidenced by verbalization of feelings, fear of reaction of others, actual change in structure, change in social involvement.

Anxiety may be related to change in health status/progressive growth of mass, perceived threat of death.

risk for imbalanced Nutrition: less than body requirements: risk factors may include decreased ability to ingest/difficulty swallowing.

risk for ineffective Airway Clearance: risk factors may include tracheal compression/obstruction.

Gonorrhea CH

(Also refer to Sexually Transmitted Disease—STD)

risk for Infection [dissemination/bacteremia]: risk factors may include presence of infectious process in highly vascular area and lack of recognition of disease process

acute Pain may be related to irritation/inflammation of mucosa and effects of circulating toxins, possibly evidenced by verbal reports of genital or pharyngeal irritation, perineal/pelvic pain, guarding/distraction behaviors.

deficient Knowledge [Learning Need] regarding disease cause/transmission, therapy, and self-care needs may be related to lack of information/misinterpretation, denial of exposure, possibly evidenced by statements of concern, questions, misconceptions, and inaccurate follow-through of instructions/development of preventable complications.

Gout CH

acute Pain may be related to inflammation of joint(s), possibly evidenced by verbal reports, guarding/distraction behaviors, and autonomic responses (changes in vital signs).

impaired physical Mobility may be related to joint pain/edema, possibly evidenced by reluctance to attempt movement, limited range of motion, and therapeutic restriction of movement.

deficient Knowledge [Learning Need] regarding cause, treatment, and prevention of condition may be related to lack of information/misinterpretation, possibly evidenced by statements of concern, questions, misconceptions, and inaccurate follow-through of instructions.

Grand mal seizures CH/PED

(Refer to Seizure disorder)

Grave's disease CH

(Refer to Hyperthyroidism)

Guillain-Barré syndrome (acute polyneuritis)　　MS

risk for ineffective Breathing Pattern/Airway Clearance: risk factors may include weakness/paralysis of respiratory muscles, impaired gag/swallow reflexes, decreased energy/fatigue.

disturbed Sensory Perceptual: (specify) may be related to altered sensory reception/transmission/integration (altered status of sense organs, sleep deprivation), therapeutically restricted environment, endogenous chemical alterations (electrolyte imbalance, hypoxia), and psychological stress, possibly evidenced by reported or observed change in usual response to stimuli, altered communication patterns, and measured change in sensory acuity and motor coordination.

impaired physical Mobility may be related to neuromuscular impairment, pain/discomfort, possibly evidenced by impaired coordination, partial/complete paralysis, decreased muscle strength/control.

Anxiety [specify level]/Fear may be related to situational crisis, change in health status/threat of death, possibly evidenced by increased tension, restlessness, helplessness, apprehension, uncertainty, fearfulness, focus on self, and sympathetic stimulation.

risk for Disuse Syndrome: risk factors include paralysis and pain.

Gulf War syndrome　　CH/MS

[chronic] Fatigue may be related to unknown environmental exposure, stress, anxiety, disease state possibly evidenced by overwhelming lack of energy, inability to maintain usual routines/level of physical activity, lethargic, compromised concentration.

Anxiety [specify] may be related to exposure to toxins, change in health status, threat of death, change in role function/economic status, unmet needs possibly evidenced by expressed concerns, apprehension, uncertainty, fear of unspecific consequences, sleep disturbance, irritability, preoccupation.

impaired Memory may be related to neurologic disturbances possibly evidenced by reported/observed experiences of forgetting, inability to recall recent events.

chronic Pain may be related to chronic physical condition possibly evidenced by verbal reports of muscle/joint pain, headaches, altered ability to continue previous activities, fatigue, reduced interaction with others.

Diarrhea may be related to environmental exposure to toxins, high stress levels/anxiety possibly evidenced by liquid stools, abdominal pain.

disturbed visual Sensory Perception may be related to altered sensory reception possibly evidenced by blurred vision, photosensitivity.

Hallucinogen abuse　　CH/PSY

(Also refer to Substance dependence/abuse rehabilitation)

disturbed Thought Processes may be related to physiologic changes associated with drug use, impaired judgement, memory loss possibly evidenced by inaccurate interpretation of environment, bizarre thinking, disorientation, inability to make decisions, unpredictible behavior, distractibility, non-reality based thinking.

Anxiety/Fear may be related to situational crisis, threat to/change in health status, perceived threat of death, inexperience/unfamiliarity with effects of drug possibly evidenced by assumptions of "losing my mind/control", apprehension, preoccupation with feelings of impending doom, sympathetic stimulation.

Self-Care Deficit (specify) may be related to perceptual/cognitive impairment, therapeutic management (restraints) possibly evidenced by inability to meet own physical needs.

Hantavirus　　MS

(Refer to Hemorrhagic fever)

Hantavirus pulmonary syndrome   **MS**
(Also refer to Disseminated intravascular coagulation)

acute Pain/[Discomfort] may be related to inflammatory process/circulating toxins possibly evidenced by reports of headache, myalgia, GI distress, fever.

impaired Gas Exchange may be related to alveolar-capillary membrane changes (fluid collection/shifts into interstitial space/alveoli) possibly evidenced by dyspnea, restlessness, irritability, abnormal rate/depth of respirations, lethargy, confusion.

[moderate to severe] Anxiety may be related to change in health status, threat of death, interpersonal transmission possibly evidenced by expressed concerns, distressed, apprehension, extraneous movement.

risk for impaired spontaneous Ventilation: risk factors may include respiratory muscle fatigue, problems with secretion management.

Hashimoto's thyroiditis   **CH**
(Refer to Hypothyroidism; Goiter)

Hay fever   **CH**

acute Pain/[Discomfort] may be related to irritation/inflammation of upper airway mucous membranes and conjunctiva, possibly evidenced by verbal reports, irritability, and restlessness.

deficient Knowledge [Learning Need] regarding underlying cause, appropriate therapy, and required lifestyle changes may be related to lack of information, possibly evidenced by statements of concern, questions, and misconceptions.

Headache   **CH/MS**
(Also refer to Temporal arteritis)

acute/chronic Pain may be related to stress/tension, nerve irritation/pressure, vasospasm, increased intracranial pressure possibly evidenced by verbal/coded reports, pallor, facial mask of pain, guarding/distraction behaviors, restlessness, self-focusing, changes in sleep pattern/appetite, preoccupation with pain.

risk for ineffective Coping: risk factors may include situational crisis, personal vulnerability, inadequate support systems, work overload/no vacations, inadequate relaxation, severe pain, overwhelming threat to self.

deficient Knowledge [Learning Need] regarding condition, prognosis, treatment needs may be related to lack of exposure/recall, unfamiliarity with information/resources, cognitive limitations possibly evidenced by request for information, statement of misconceptions, inaccurate follow-through of instructions, development of preventable complications.

Head injury   **MS/CH**
(Refer to Traumatic brain injury)

Heart attack   **MS**
(Refer to Myocardial infarction)

Heart failure, chronic   **MS**

decreased Cardiac Output, may be related to altered myocardial contractility/inotropic changes; alterations in rate, rhythm, and electrical conduction; and structural changes (valvular defects, ventricular aneurysm), possibly evidenced by tachycardia/dysrhythmias, changes in blood pressure, extra heart sounds, decreased urine output, diminished peripheral pulses, cool/ashen skin, orthopnea, crackles; dependent/generalized edema and chest pain.

excess Fluid Volume may be related to reduced glomerular filtration rate/increased ADH production, and sodium/water retention, possibly evidenced by orthopnea and abnormal breath sounds, S$_3$ heart sound, jugular vein distention, positive hepatojugular reflex, weight gain, hypertension, oliguria, generalized edema.

risk for impaired Gas Exchange: risk factors may include alveolar-capillary membrane changes (fluid collection/shifts into interstitial space/alveoli).

CH

Activity Intolerance may be related to imbalance between O$_2$ supply/demand, generalized weakness, and prolonged bedrest/sedentary lifestyle, possibly evidenced by reported/observed weakness, fatigue; changes in vital signs, presence of dysrhythmias; dyspnea, pallor, and diaphoresis.

deficient Knowledge [Learning Need] regarding cardiac function/disease process, therapy and self-care needs may be related to lack of information/misinterpretation, possibly evidenced by questions, statements of concern/misconceptions; development of preventable complications or exacerbations of condition.

Heart transplantation　　　　　　　　　　**MS/CH**
(Refer to Cardiac surgery; Transplantation, recipient)

Heat exhaustion　　　　　　　　　　　　**CH/MS**
deficient Fluid Volume may be related to excessive losses (profuse sweating), hypermetabolic state (core temperature 101°F to 105°F/38.3°C to 40.6°C), lack of intake, extremes of age possibly evidenced by weakness/fatigue, slow pulse/decreased BP, changes in mentation.

Heatstroke　　　　　　　　　　　　　　**MS**
Hyperthermia may be related to prolonged exposure to hot environment/vigorous activity with failure of regulating mechanism of the body, possibly evidenced by high body temperature (greater than 105°F/40.6°C), flushed/hot skin, tachycardia, and seizure activity.

decreased Cardiac Output may be related to functional stress of hypermetabolic state, altered circulating volume/venous return, and direct myocardial damage secondary to hyperthermia, possibly evidenced by decreased peripheral pulses, dysrhythmias/tachycardia, and changes in mentation.

Hematoma, epidural　　　　　　　　　　**MS**
acute Confusion may be related to head injury possibly evidenced by fluctuation in cognition/level of consciousness.

risk for decreased Intracranial Adaptive Capacity: risk factors may include brain injuries, decreased cerebral perfusion pressure, systemic hypotension with intracranial hypertension.

risk for ineffective Breathing Pattern: risk factors may include neuromuscular dysfunction (injury to respiratory center of brain), perception/cognitive impairment.

risk for deficient Fluid Volume: risk factors may include restricted oral intake, hypermetabolic state, loss of fluid through normal/abnormal routes.

Hematoma, subdural-acute　　　　　　　**MS**
(Refer to Traumatic brain injury)

Hematoma, subdural-chronic　　　　　　**CH**
acute/chronic Pain may be related to physical agent (space-occupying clot) possibly evidenced by reports of increasing daily headache.

acute/chronic Confusion may be related to head injury, alcohol abuse possibly evidenced by fluctuations in cognition, increased agitation/restlessness, misperceptions, inappropriate responses.

impaired physical Mobility may be related to neuromuscular impairment (hemiparesis), decreased muscle strength, cognitive impairment possibly evidenced by limited ability to perform gross/fine motor skills, gait changes, postural instability.

Hemodialysis   MS/CH
(Also refer to Dialysis, general)

risk for Injury [loss of vascular access]: risk factors may include clotting/thrombosis, infection, disconnection/hemorrhage.

risk for deficient Fluid Volume: risk factors may include excessive fluid losses/shifts via ultrafiltration, hemorrhage (altered coagulation/disconnection of shunt), and fluid restrictions.

risk for excess Fluid Volume: risk factors may include excessive fluid intake; rapid IV, blood/ plasma expanders/saline given to support BP during procedure.

ineffective Protection may be related to chronic disease state, drug therapy, abnormal blood profile, inadequate nutrition, possibly evidenced by altered clotting, impaired healing, deficient immunity, fatigue, anorexia.

Hemophilia   PED
risk for deficient Fluid Volume [isotonic]: risk factors may include impaired coagulation/ hemorrhagic losses.

risk for acute/chronic Pain: risk factors may include nerve compression from hematomas, nerve damage or hemorrhage into joint space.

risk for impaired physical Mobility: risk factors may include joint hemorrhage, swelling, degenerative changes, and muscle atrophy.

ineffective Protection may be related to abnormal blood profile, possibly evidenced by altered clotting.

compromised family Coping may be related to prolonged nature of condition that exhausts the supportive capacity of significant person(s), possibly evidenced by protective behaviors disproportionate to client's abilities/need for autonomy.

Hemorrhage, postpartum   OB
deficient Fluid Volume [isotonic] may be related to excessive vascular loss possibly evidenced by hypotension, tachycardia, dry skin/mucous membranes, decreased/concentrated urine, delayed capillary refill, change in mentation.

ineffective Tissue Perfusion may be related to hypovolemia possibly evidenced by diminished arterial pulsations, cold extremities, changes in vital signs, changes in sensorium, decreased milk production.

[moderate] Anxiety may be related to situational crisis, threat of change in health status/death, interpersonal transmission/contagion, physiologic response (catecholamine release) possibly evidenced by increased tension, apprehension, feelings of inadequacy/helplessness, sympathetic stimulation, self-focus.

risk for Infection: risk factors may include traumatized tissue, stasis of body fluids (lochia), decreased Hb, invasive procedures.

risk for impaired parent/infant Attachment: risk factors may include interruption in bonding process, physical condition, perceived threat to own survival.

Hemorrhage, prenatal   OB
deficient Fluid Volume [isotonic] may be related to excessive vascular loss possibly evidenced by hypotension, increased pulse rate, decreased pulse pressure, decreased/concentrated urine, decreased venous filling, change in mentation.

ineffective uteroplacental Tissue Perfusion may be related to hypovolemia possibly evidenced by changes in FHR and/or activity.

Fear may be related to threat of death [perceived or actual] to self/fetus possibly evidenced by verbalizations of specific concerns, increased tension, sympathetic stimulation.

risk for maternal Injury: risk factors may include tissue/organ hypoxia, abnormal blood profile, impaired immune system.

acute Pain may be related to muscle contractions/cervical dilatation, tissue trauma (fallopian tube rupture) possibly evidenced by reports, distraction behaviors, autonomic responses (change in BP/pulse).

Hemorrhagic fever, viral   MS
(Refer to Ebola; Hantavirus pulmonary syndrome)

Hemorrhoidectomy   MS/CH
acute Pain may be related to edema/swelling and tissue trauma, possibly evidenced by verbal reports, guarding/distraction behaviors, focus on self, and autonomic responses (changes in vital signs).

risk for Urinary Retention: risk factors may include perineal trauma, edema/swelling, and pain.

deficient Knowledge [Learning Need] regarding therapeutic treatment and potential complications may be related to lack of information/misconceptions, possibly evidenced by statements of concern and questions.

Hemorrhoids   CH/OB
acute Pain may be related to inflammation and edema of prolapsed varices, possibly evidenced by verbal reports, and guarding/distraction behaviors.

Constipation may be related to pain on defecation and reluctance to defecate, possibly evidenced by frequency, less than usual pattern, and hard, formed stools.

Hemothorax   MS
(Also refer to Pneumothorax)

risk for Trauma/Suffocation: risk factors may include concurrent disease/injury process, dependence on external device (chest drainage system), and lack of safety education/precautions.

Anxiety [specify level] may be related to change in health status and threat of death, possibly evidenced by increased tension, restlessness, expressed concern, sympathetic stimulation, and focus on self.

Hepatitis, acute viral   MS/CH
Fatigue may be related to decreased metabolic energy production and altered body chemistry, possibly evidenced by reports of lack of energy/inability to maintain usual routines, decreased performance, and increased physical complaints.

imbalanced Nutrition: less than body requirements may be related to inability to ingest adequate nutrients (nausea, vomiting, anorexia); hypermetabolic state, altered absorption and metabolism, possibly evidenced by aversion to eating/lack of interest in food, altered taste sensation, observed lack of intake, and weight loss.

acute Pain/[Discomfort] may be related to inflammation and swelling of the liver, arthralgias, urticarial eruptions, and pruritus, possibly evidenced by verbal reports, guarding/distraction behaviors, focus on self, and autonomic responses (changes in vital signs).

risk for Infection: risk factors may include inadequate secondary defenses and immunosuppression, malnutrition, insufficient knowledge to avoid exposure to pathogens/spread to others.

risk for impaired Tissue Integrity: risk factors may include bile salt accumulation in the tissues.

risk for impaired Home Management: risk factors may include debilitating effects of disease process and inadequate support systems (family, financial, role model).

deficient Knowledge [Learning Need] regarding disease process/transmission, treatment needs, and future expectations may be related to lack of information/recall, misinterpretation, unfamiliarity with resources, possibly evidenced by questions, statement of concerns/ misconceptions, inaccurate follow-through of instructions, and development of preventable complications.

Hepatorenal syndrome   MS
(Refer to Cirrhosis; Renal failure, acute)

Hernia, hiatal   CH
chronic Pain may be related to regurgitation of acidic gastric contents, possibly evidenced by verbal reports, facial grimacing, and focus on self.

deficient Knowledge [Learning Need] regarding pathophysiology, prevention of complications and self-care needs may be related to lack of information/misconceptions, possibly evidenced by statements of concern, questions, and recurrence of condition.

Hernia, inguinal   MS
(Refer to Herniorrhaphy)

Herniated nucleus pulposus   CH/MS
acute/chronic Pain may be related to nerve compression/irritation and muscle spasms, possibly evidenced by verbal reports, guarding/distraction behaviors, preoccupation with pain, self/narrowed focus, and autonomic responses (changes in vital signs when pain is acute), altered muscle tone/function, changes in eating/sleeping patterns and libido, physical/social withdrawal.

impaired physical Mobility may be related to pain (muscle spasms), therapeutic restrictions (e.g., bedrest, traction/braces), muscular impairment, and depression, possibly evidenced by reports of pain on movement, reluctance to attempt/difficulty with purposeful movement, decreased muscle strength, impaired coordination, and limited range of motion.

deficient Diversional Activity may be related to length of recuperation period and therapy restrictions, physical limitations, pain and depression, possibly evidenced by statements of boredom, disinterest, "nothing to do," and restlessness, irritability, withdrawal.

Herniorrhaphy   MS/PED
acute Pain may be related to disruption of skin, tissue, and muscle integrity possibly evidenced by verbal/coded reports, alteration in muscle tone, distraction/guarding behaviors, narrowed focus, and autonomic responses.

risk for Injury: risk factors may include surgical repair, insertion of graft, increased intraabdominal pressure (straining at stool, heavy lifting, strenuous activity).

Heroin abuse   CH
risk for Infection: risk factors may include injection /reuse or sharing of needles, malnutrition, environmental exposure, insufficient knowledge/motivation to avoid pathogens.

imbalanced Nutrition: less than body requirements may be related to inadequate intake possibly evidenced by anorexia, lack of food/methods to prepare food, economic difficulties, weight loss, poor muscle tone/decreased muscle mass.

risk for Trauma: risk factors may include personal vulnerability, cigarette smoking, lack of safety precautions, driving impaired/under the influence, high-crime neighborhood.

risk for ineffective Protection: risk factors may include effects of substance use, malnutrition, chronic disease, lifestyle choices, unhealthy environment.

Heroin withdrawal   CH/MS

acute Pain/[Discomfort] may be related to cessation of drug, muscle tremors/twitching, possibly evidenced by reports of muscle aches, hot/cold flashes, diaphoresis, lacrimation, rhinorrhea, drug cravings.

severe Anxiety may be related to CNS hyperactivity possibly evidenced by apprehension, pervasive anxious feelings, jittery, restlessness, weakness, insomnia, anorexia.

risk for ineffective Therapeutic Regimen Management: risk factors may include protracted withdrawal, economic difficulties, family/social support deficits, perceived barriers/benefits.

Herpes simplex   CH

acute Pain may be related to presence of localized inflammation and open lesions, possibly evidenced by verbal reports, distraction behaviors, and restlessness.

risk for [secondary] Infection: risk factors may include broken/traumatized tissue, altered immune response, and untreated infection/treatment failure.

risk for ineffective Sexuality Patterns: risk factors may include lack of knowledge, values conflict, and/or fear of transmitting the disease.

Herpes zoster (shingles)   CH

acute Pain may be related to inflammation/local lesions along sensory nerve(s), possibly evidenced by verbal reports, guarding/distraction behaviors, narrowed focus, and autonomic responses (changes in vital signs).

deficient Knowledge [Learning Need] regarding pathophysiology, therapeutic needs, and potential complications may be related to lack of information/misinterpretation, possibly evidenced by statements of concern, questions, and misconceptions.

High altitude pulmonary edema (HAPE)   MS
(Also refer to Mountain sickness, acute)

impaired Gas Exchange may be related to ventilation perfusion imbalance, alveolar-capillary membrane changes, altered oxygen supply possibly evidenced by dyspnea, confusion, cyanosis, tachycardia, abnormal ABGs.

excess Fluid Volume may be related to compromised regulatory mechanism possibly evidenced by shortness of breath, anxiety, edema, abnormal breath sounds, pulmonary congestion.

High altitude sickness   MS
(Refer to Mountain sickness, acute; High altitude pulmonary edema)

High-risk pregnancy   OB
(Refer to Pregnancy, high-risk)

Hip replacement   MS
(Refer to Total joint replacement)

HIV infection   CH
(Also refer to AIDS)

impaired Adjustment may be related to life-threatening, stigmatizing condition/disease; assault to self-esteem, altered locus of control, inadequate support systems, incomplete grieving, medication side effects (fatigue/depression), possibly evidenced by verbalization of nonacceptance/denial of diagnosis, nonexistent or unsuccessful involvement in problem solving/goal setting; extended period of shock and disbelief or anger; lack of future-oriented thinking.

deficient Knowledge [Learning Need] regarding disease, prognosis, and treatment needs may be related to lack of exposure/recall, information misinterpretation, unfamiliarity with information resources, or cognitive limitation, possibly evidenced by statement of misconception/request for information, inappropriate/exaggerated behaviors (hostile, agitated, hysterical, apathetic), inaccurate follow-through of instructions/development of preventable complications.

Hodgkin's disease   **CH/MS**

(Also refer to Cancer; Chemotherapy)

Anxiety [specify level]/Fear may be related to threat of self-concept and threat of death, possibly evidenced by apprehension, insomnia, focus on self, and increased tension.

deficient Knowledge [Learning Need] regarding diagnosis, pathophysiology, treatment, and prognosis may be related to lack of information/ misinterpretation, possibly evidenced by statements of concern, questions, and misconceptions.

acute Pain/[Discomfort] may be related to manifestations of inflammatory response (fever, chills, night sweats) and pruritus, possibly evidenced by verbal reports, distraction behaviors, and focus on self.

risk for ineffective Breathing Pattern/Airway Clearance: risk factors may include tracheobronchial obstruction (enlarged mediastinal nodes and/or airway edema).

Hospice care   **CH**

acute/chronic Pain may be related to biological, physical, psychological agent possibly evidenced by verbal/coded report, changes in appetite/eating, sleep pattern; protective behavior, restlessness, irritability.

Activity Intolerance/Fatigue may be related to generalized weakness, bedrest/immobility, pain, imbalance between oxygen supply and demand possibly evidenced by inability to maintain usual routine, verbalized lack of desire/interest in activity, decreased performance, lethargy.

anticipatory Grieving/death Anxiety may be related to anticipated loss of physiologic well-being, perceived threat of death.

compromised/disabled family Coping/Caregiver Role Strain may be related to prolonged disease/disability progression, temporary family disorganization and role changes, unrealistic expectations, inadequate or incorrect information or understanding by primary person.

Huntington's disease   **CH**

Hopelessness may be related to chronic progressive debilitating condition possibly evidenced by despondant verbalizations, withdrawal from environs, angry outbursts.

impaired Walking may be related to movement disorder (altered gait, ataxia, dystonia) possibly evidenced by inability to walk required distances, navigate curbs/uneven surfaces, climb stairs.

disturbed Thought Processes may be related to degenerative physiologic changes possibly evidenced by inaccurate interpretation of environment, cognitive dissonance, inappropriate social behavior.

imbalanced Nutrition: less than body requirements may be related to inability to ingest food (difficulty swallowing, cognitive decline) possibly evidenced by aversion to eating, inadequate food intake, weight loss, decreased subcutaneous fat/muscle mass.

total Self-Care Deficit may be related to neuromuscular impairment, cognitive decline possibly evidenced by inability to perform desired ADLs.

risk for Caregiver Role Strain: risk factors may include progressive deterioration (physical and mental) of care receiver, duration of caregiving required, complexity/amount of caregiving tasks, caregiver's competing role commitments, family isolation, lack of respite/recreation for caregiver, bizarre behavior of care receiver.

Hydrocephalus   **PED/MS**

ineffective cerebral Tissue Perfusion may be related to decreased arterial/ venous blood flow (compression of brain tissue), possibly evidenced by changes in mentation, restlessness, irritability, reports of headache, pupillary changes, and changes in vital signs.

disturbed visual Sensory Perception may be related to pressure on sensory/motor nerves, possibly evidenced by reports of double vision, development of strabismus, nystagmus, pupillary changes, and optic atrophy.

risk for impaired physical Mobility: risk factors may include neuromuscular impairment, decreased muscle strength, and impaired coordination.

risk for decreased Intracranial Adaptive Capacity: risk factors may include brain injury, changes in perfusion pressure/intracranial pressure.

CH

risk for Infection: risk factors may include invasive procedure/presence of shunt.

deficient Knowledge [Learning Need] regarding condition, prognosis, and long-term therapy needs/medical follow-up may be related to lack of information/misperceptions, possibly evidenced by questions, statement of concern, request for information, and inaccurate follow-through of instruction/development of preventable complications.

Hydrophobia   **CH/MS**
(Refer to Rabies)

Hyperactivity disorder   **PED/PSY**

defensive Coping may be related to mild neurologic deficits, dysfunctional family system, abuse/neglect possibly evidenced by denial of obvious problems, projection of blame/responsibility, grandiosity, difficulty in reality testing perceptions.

impaired Social Interaction may be related to retarded ego development, negative role models, neurologic impairment possibly evidenced by discomfort in social situations, interrupts/ intrudes on others, difficulty waiting turn in games/group activities, difficulty maintaining attention to task.

disabled family Coping may be related to excessive guilt, anger, or blaming among family members, parental inconsistencies, disagreements regarding discipline/limit-setting/approaches, exhaustion of parental expectations possibly evidenced by unrealistic parental expectations, rejection or overprotection of child, exaggerated expression of feelings, despair regarding child's behavior.

Hyperbilirubinemia   **PED**

risk for Injury [CNS involvement]: risk factors may include prematurity, hemolytic disease, asphyxia, acidosis, hyponatremia, and hypoglycemia.

risk for Injury [effects of treatment]: risk factors may include physical properties of phototherapy and effects on body regulatory mechanisms, invasive procedure (exchange transfusion), abnormal blood profile, chemical imbalances.

deficient Knowledge [Learning Need] regarding condition prognosis, treatment/safety needs may be related to lack of exposure/recall and information misinterpretation, possibly evidenced by questions, statement of concern, and inaccurate follow-through of instructions/development of preventable complications.

Hyperemesis gravidarum   OB

deficient Fluid Volume [isotonic] may be related to excessive gastric losses and reduced intake, possibly evidenced by dry mucous membranes, decreased/concentrated urine, decreased pulse volume and pressure, thirst, and hemoconcentration.

imbalanced Nutrition: less than body requirements may be related to inability to ingest/digest/absorb nutrients (prolonged vomiting), possibly evidenced by reported inadequate food intake, lack of interest in food/aversion to eating, and weight loss.

risk for ineffective Coping: risk factors may include situational/maturational crisis (pregnancy, change in health status, projected role changes, concern about outcome).

Hyperparathyroidism, primary   MS

risk for deficient Fluid Volume: risk factors may include excessive losses through normal routes (vomiting, diarrhea, gastric bleed).

impaired Urinary Elimination may be related to anatomical obstruction (renal calculi) possibly evidenced by decreased renal function.

risk for Trauma: risk factors may include decreased calcium levels/bone fragility.

Hypertension   CH

deficient Knowledge [Learning Need] regarding condition, therapeutic regimen, and potential complications may be related to lack of information/recall, misinterpretation, cognitive limitations, and/or denial of diagnosis, possibly evidenced by statements of concern/ questions, and misconceptions, inaccurate follow-through of instructions, and lack of BP control.

impaired Adjustment may be related to condition requiring change in lifestyle, altered locus of control, and absence of feelings/denial of illness, possibly evidenced by verbalization of nonacceptance of health status change and lack of movement toward independence.

risk for Sexual Dysfunction: risk factors may include side effects of medication.

MS

risk for decreased Cardiac Output: risk factors may include increased afterload (vasoconstriction), fluid shifts/hypovolemia, myocardial ischemia, ventricular hypertrophy/ rigidity.

acute Pain may be related to increased cerebrovascular pressure, possibly evidenced by verbal reports (throbbing pain located in suboccipital region, present on awakening and disappearing spontaneously after being up and about), reluctance to move head, avoidance of bright lights and noise, increased muscle tension.

Hypertension, intrapartum   OB

risk for imbalanced Fluid Volume: risk factors may include compromised regulatory mechanism/fluid shifts, excessive fluid intake, effects of drug therapy (oxytocin infusion).

risk for impaired fetal Gas Exchange: risk factors may include altered blood flow, vasospasms, prolonged uterine contractions.

impaired Urinary Elimination may be related to fluid shifts, hormonal changes, effects of medication possibly evidenced by changes in amount/frequency of voiding, bladder distention, changes in urine specific gravity, presence of albumin.

risk for maternal Injury: risk factors may include tonic-clonic convulsions, altered clotting factors (release of thromboplastin from placenta).

acute Pain may be related to intensification of uterine activity, myometrial hypoxia, anxiety possibly evidenced by verbalizations, altered muscle tone, distraction behaviors, autonomic responses, facial mask.

Hypertension, prenatal OB
(Refer to Pregnancy-induced hypertension)

Hypertension, pulmonary CH/MS
(Refer to Pulmonary hypertension)

Hyperthyroidism CH
(Also refer to Thyrotoxicosis)
Fatigue may be related to hypermetabolic imbalance with increased energy requirements, irritability of CNS, and altered body chemistry, possibly evidenced by verbalization of overwhelming lack of energy to maintain usual routine, decreased performance, emotional lability/irritability, and impaired ability to concentrate.
Anxiety [specify level] may be related to increased stimulation of the CNS (hypermetabolic state, pseudocatecholamine effect of thyroid hormones), possibly evidenced by increased feelings of apprehension, overexcitement/distress, irritability/emotional lability, shakiness, restless movements, tremors.
risk for imbalanced Nutrition: less than body requirements: risk factors may include inability to ingest adequate nutrients for hypermetabolic rate/constant activity, impaired absorption of nutrients (vomiting/diarrhea), hyperglycemia/relative insulin insufficiency.
risk for impaired Tissue Integrity: risk factors may include altered protective mechanisms of eye related to periorbital edema, reduced ability to blink, eye discomfort/dryness, and development of corneal abrasion/ulceration.

Hypervolemia CH/MS
excess Fluid Volume may be related to excess fluid/sodium intake, compromised regulatory mechanisms (renal failure, increased ADH), decreased plasma proteins, rapid/excessive administration of isotonic parenteral fluids possibly evidenced by edema, abnormal breath sounds, S_3 heart sound, shortness of breath, positive hepatojugular reflex/elevated CVP, change in mental status.

Hypochondriasis PSY
(Refer to Somatoform disorders)

Hypoglycemia CH
disturbed Thought Processes may be related to inadequate glucose for cellular brain function and effects of endogenous hormone activity, possibly evidenced by irritability, changes in mentation, memory loss, altered attention span, and emotional lability.
risk for imbalanced Nutrition: less than body requirements: risk factors may include inadequate glucose metabolism and imbalance of glucose/insulin levels.
deficient Knowledge [Learning Need] regarding pathophysiology of condition and therapy/self-care needs may be related to lack of information/recall, misinterpretations, possibly evidenced by development of hypoglycemia and statements of questions/misconceptions.

Hypoparathyroidism (acute) MS
risk for Injury: risk factors may include neuromuscular excitability/tetany and formation of renal stones.
acute Pain may be related to recurrent muscle spasms and alteration in reflexes, possibly evidenced by verbal reports, distraction behaviors, and narrowed focus.
risk for ineffective Airway Clearance: risk factors may include spasm of the laryngeal muscles.
Anxiety [specify level] may be related to threat to, or change in, health status, physiologic responses.

Hypophysectomy   MS

(Also refer to Surgery, general; Cancer)

Fear/Anxiety may be related to situational crisis (nature of diagnosis/procedure), change in health status, perceived threat of death, separation from support system possibly evidenced by expressed concerns, apprehension, being scared, increased tension, extraneous movement, difficulty concentrating.

risk for deficient Fluid Volume: risk factors may include failure of regulatory mechanism (decreased ADH).

risk for Infection: risk factors may include traumatized tissue, invasive procedure, CSF leak.

Sexual Dysfunction may be related to altered body function (loss of anterior pituitary) possibly evidenced by sterility, decreased libido, impotence (male); infertility, atrophy of vaginal mucosa (female).

Hypothermia (systemic)   CH

(Also refer to Frostbite)

Hypothermia may be related to exposure to cold environment, inadequate clothing, age extremes (very young/elderly), damage to hypothalamus, consumption of alcohol/medications causing vasodilation, possibly evidenced by reduction in body temperature below normal range, shivering, cool skin, pallor.

deficient Knowledge [Learning Need] regarding risk factors, treatment needs, and prognosis may be related to lack of information/recall, misinterpretation, possibly evidenced by statement of concerns/misconceptions, occurrence of problem, and development of complications.

Hypothyroidism   CH

(Also refer to Myxedema)

impaired physical Mobility may be related to weakness, fatigue, muscle aches, altered reflexes, and mucin deposits in joints and interstitial spaces, possibly evidenced by decreased muscle strength/control and impaired coordination.

Fatigue may be related to decreased metabolic energy production, possibly evidenced by verbalization of unremitting/overwhelming lack of energy, inability to maintain usual routines, impaired ability to concentrate, decreased libido, irritability, listlessness, decreased performance, increase in physical complaints.

disturbed Sensory Perception (specify) may be related to mucin deposits and nerve compression, possibly evidenced by paresthesias of hands and feet or decreased hearing.

Constipation may be related to decreased peristalsis/physical activity, possibly evidenced by frequency less than usual pattern, decreased bowel sounds, hard dry stools, and development of fecal impaction.

Hypovolemia   CH/MS

deficient Fluid Volume may be related to active fluid loss (hemorrhage, vomiting/gastric intubation, diarrhea, burns, wounds/fistulas), regulatory failure (adrenal disease, recovery phase of ARF, DKA, HHNC, diabetes insipidus, sepsis) possibly evidenced by thirst, weight loss, poor skin turgor, dry mucous membranes, tachycardia, tachypnea, fatigue, decreased CVP.

Hysterectomy   GYN/MS

(Also refer to Surgery, general)

acute Pain may be related to tissue trauma/abdominal incision, edema/hematoma formation, possibly evidenced by verbal reports, guarding/distraction behaviors, and autonomic responses (changes in vital signs).

risk for perioperative-position Injury: risk factors may include immobilization/lithotomy position.

impaired Urinary Elimination/risk for [acute] Urinary Retention: risk factors may include mechanical trauma, surgical manipulation, presence of localized edema/hematoma, or nerve trauma with temporary bladder atony.

ineffective Sexuality Patterns/risk for Sexual Dysfunction: risk factors may include concerns regarding altered body function/structure, perceived changes in femininity, changes in hormone levels, loss of libido, and changes in sexual response pattern.

Ileal conduit   MS/CH
(Refer to Urinary diversion)

Ileocolitis   MS/CH
(Refer to Crohn's disease)

Ileostomy   MS/CH
(Refer to Colostomy)

Ileus   MS

acute Pain may be related to distention/edema and ischemia of intestinal tissue, possibly evidenced by verbal reports, guarding/distraction behaviors, narrowed focus, and autonomic responses (changes in vital signs).

Diarrhea/Constipation may be related to presence of obstruction/changes in peristalsis, possibly evidenced by changes in frequency and consistency or absence of stool, alterations in bowel sounds, presence of pain, and cramping.

risk for deficient Fluid Volume: risk factors may include increased intestinal losses (vomiting and diarrhea), and decreased intake.

Immersion foot   MS

impaired Skin/Tissue Integrity may be related to exposure to cold and wet environment (above freezing), altered circulation, presence of infection possibly evidenced by tissue maceration, pain, soggy edema.

disturbed peripheral Sensory Perception may be related to altered sensory reception possibly evidenced by paresthesia/numbness.

risk for ineffective Health Maintenance: risk factors may include lack of material resources, poor coping skills, inadequate knowledge of safety needs.

Impetigo   PED/CH

impaired Skin Integrity may be related to presence of infectious process and pruritus, possibly evidenced by open/crusted lesions.

acute Pain may be related to inflammation and pruritus, possibly evidenced by verbal reports, distraction behaviors, and self-focusing.

risk for [secondary] Infection: risk factors may include broken skin, traumatized tissue, altered immune response, and virulence/contagious nature of causative organism.

risk for Infection [transmission]: risk factors may include virulent nature of causative organism, insufficient knowledge to prevent infection of others.

Impotence   CH
(Refer to Erectile dysfunction)

Infant (at 4 weeks)   PED

readiness for enhanced Knowledge regarding infant care, developmental expectations, safety and well-being may be related to changing needs of infant possibly evidenced by questions, expressed concerns/desire to learn more, behaviors congruent with expressed knowledge.

risk for acute Pain: risk factors may include accumulation of gas in confined space with cramping of intestinal musculature.

risk for Infection: risk factors may include immature immunologic response, increased environmental exposure.

risk for sudden infant Death Syndrome: risk factors may include sleeping position, second hand smoke exposure, type of bedding used.

risk for disturbed Sensory Perception: risk factors may include immature development of sensory organs, inappropriate/inadequate environmental stimuli, prenatal/intrapartal complications, postpartal course.

risk for imbalanced Nutrition: more than body requirements: risk factors may include obesity in one/both parents, rapid transition across growth percentiles.

Infant of addicted mother   OB/PED

risk for Injury [CNS damage]: risk factors may include prematurity, hypoxia, effects of medications/substance use/withdrawal, possible exposure to infectious agents (prenatal/intrapartal).

ineffective Airway Clearance/impaired Gas Exchange may be related to excess mucus production, depression of cough reflex and respiratory center, intrauterine asphyxia possibly evidenced by tachypnea, tachycardia, cyanosis, nasal flaring, grunting respirations, hypoxia, acidosis.

risk for Infection: risk factors may include presence of maternal infections (GBS, STDs).

risk for imbalanced Nutrition: less than body requirements: risk factors may include inability to ingest/digest/absorb adequate nutrients to meet metabolic needs (e.g., poor/uncoordinated sucking and swallowing, frequent GI irritation with vomiting, diarrhea, repeated regurgitation; frequent hyperactivity).

risk for impaired Skin Integrity: risk factors may include mechanical factors (continual rubbing of face/knees against bedding, scratching face with hands), presence of excretions.

impaired Parenting may be related to lack of available or ineffective role model, unmet emotional maturation needs of parent, lack of support between/from SO, interruption in bonding process, lack of appropriate response of infant possibly evidenced by reports of role inadequacy/inability to care for infant, inattention to infant needs, inappropriate caretaking behaviors, lack of parental attachment behaviors.

disabled family Coping may be related to significant person with chronically unexpressed feelings of guilt, anxiety, hostility, despair; dissonant discrepancy of coping styles, high-risk family situations possibly evidenced by intolerance, rejection, abandonment/desertion, neglectful relationships between family members, neglectful care of infant, distortion of reality of parent's health problem/substance use.

Infant of HIV-positive mother   OB/PED
(Also refer to AIDS)

risk for Infection: risk factors may include immature immune system, inadequate acquired immunity, suppressed inflammatory response, invasive procedures, malnutrition.

imbalanced Nutrition: risk for less than body requirements: risk factors may include inability to ingest, digest, or absorb nutrients (e.g., impaired suck/swallow, GI infection, malabsorption, diarrhea).

risk for delayed Growth and Development: risk factors may include separation from SO, inadequate caretaking, inconsistent responsiveness/multiple caretakers, environmental and stimulation deficiencies, effects of chronic condition/disabilities.

deficient Knowledge [Learning Need] regarding condition, prognosis, treatment needs may be related to lack of exposure, misinterpretation, unfamiliarity with resources, lack of recall/interest in learning possibly evidenced by questions, statements of misconceptions, inaccurate follow-through of instructions, development of preventable complications.

Infection, ear   PED
(Refer to Otitis media)

Infection, wound   MS/CH
risk for Infection [sepsis]: risk factors may include presence of infection, broken skin, and/or traumatized tissues, stasis of body fluids, invasive procedures, and/or increased environmental exposure, chronic disease (e.g., diabetes, anemia, malnutrition), altered immune response, and untoward effect of medications (e.g., opportunistic/secondary infection).
impaired Skin/Tissue Integrity may be related to altered circulation, presence of infection, wound drainage, nutritional deficit possibly evidenced by delayed healing, damaged tissues, invasion of body structures.
risk for delayed Surgical Recovery: risk factors may include presence of infection, activity restrictions/limitations, nutritional deficiency.

Infection, prenatal   OB
(Also refer to AIDS)
risk for maternal/fetal Infection: risk factors may include inadequate primary defenses (e.g., broken skin, stasis of body fluids), inadequate secondary defenses (e.g., decreased hemoglobin, immunosuppression), inadequate acquired immunity, environmental exposure, malnutrition, rupture of amniotic membranes.
deficient Knowledge regarding treatment/prevention, prognosis of condition may be related to lack of exposure to information and/or unfamiliarity with resources, misinterpretation possibly evidenced by verbalization of problem, inaccurate follow-through of instructions, development of preventable complications/continuation of infectious process.
[Discomfort] may be related to body response to infective agent, properties of infection (e.g., skin/tissue irritation, development of lesions) possibly evidenced by verbal reports, restlessness, withdrawal from social contacts.

Infection, puerperal   OB/CH
risk for Infection [spread/sepsis]: risk factors may include presence of infection, broken skin/traumatized tissues, high vascularity of involved area, invasive procedures/increased environmental exposure, anemia, chronic disease.
acute Pain may be related to body response to infective agent/toxins possibly evidenced by verbalizations, restlessness, guarding behavior, self-focusing, autonomic responses.
imbalanced Nutrition: less than body requirements may be related to insufficient intake to meet metabolic demands (anorexia, nausea/vomiting, medical restrictions) possibly evidenced by aversion to eating, decreased/lack of oral intake, unanticipated weight loss.
risk for impaired parent/infant Attachment: risk factors may include interruption in bonding process/separation, physical barriers, maternal fatigue/apathy.

Infertility   CH
situational low Self-Esteem may be related to functional impairment (inability to conceive), unrealistic self-expectations, sense of failure possibly evidenced by self-negating verbalizations, expressions of helplessness, perceived inability to deal with situation.

chronic Sorrow may be related to perceived physical disability (inability to conceive) possibly evidenced by expressions of anger, disappointment, emptiness, self-blame, helplessness, sadness, feelings interfering with client's ability to achieve maximum well-being.

risk for Spiritual Distress: risk factors may include energy-consuming anxiety, low self-esteem, deteriorating relationship with SO, viewing situation as deserved/punishment for past behaviors.

Inflammatory bowel disease   CH
(Refer to Colitis, ulcerative; Crohn's disease)

Influenza   CH
acute Pain/[Discomfort] may be related to inflammation and effects of circulating toxins, possibly evidenced by verbal reports, distraction behaviors, and narrowed focus.

risk for deficient Fluid Volume: risk factors may include excessive gastric losses, hypermetabolic state, and altered intake.

Hyperthermia may be related to effects of circulating toxins and dehydration, possibly evidenced by increased body temperature, warm/flushed skin, and tachycardia.

risk for ineffective Breathing: risk factors may include response to infectious process, decreased energy/fatigue.

Inhalant intoxication/abuse   CH/PSY
(Refer to Stimulant abuse)

Insomnia, acute   CH
disturbed Sleep Pattern may be related to daytime activity pattern, social/work schedule inconsistent with chronotype, travel across time zones, fatigue, life change, physical conditions (dyspnea, gastroesophageal reflux, night sweats) possibly evidenced by verbal reports of difficulties/not feeling well rested, less than age-normed total sleep time, changes in behavior and performance, physical signs (dark circles under eyes, frequent yawning).

Insomnia, chronic   CH
Sleep Deprivation may be related to sustained environmental stimulation, sustained circadian asynchrony, prolonged use of pharmacologic/dietary antisoporifics, prolonged pain, sleep apnea, dementia, narcolepsy possibly evidenced by daytime drowsiness, decreased ability to perform, lethargy, slowed reaction, apathqy.

Insulin shock   MS/CH
(Refer to Hypoglycemia)

Intermaxillary fixation   MS/CH
(Also refer to Surgery, general)

risk for ineffective Airway Clearance: risk factors may include soft tissue trauma, retained secretions.

risk for Aspiration: risk factors may include facial trauma/surgery, wired jaws, difficulty swallowing.

impaired Tissue Integrity may be related to tissue trauma/damage, intraoperative manipulation, mechanical/fixation device, altered circulation, nutritional deficit possibly evidenced by edema, hematoma/ecchymosis, erythema, inflammation, delayed healing.

impaired verbal Communication may be related to wiring of jaws, edema of mouth and surrounding structures, pain possibly evidenced by inability/reluctance to talk.

risk for imbalanced Nutrition: less than body requirements: risk factors may include facial/tissue edema, inability to chew, difficulty swallowing, decreased appetite, increased metabolic needs.

Intervertebral disc excision   **MS**
(Refer to Laminectomy, cervical/lumbar)

Intestinal obstruction   **MS**
(Refer to Ileus)

Intestinal surgery (without diversion)   **MS**
(Also refer to Surgery, general)
risk for deficient Fluid Volume: risk factors may include excessive losses normal routes (vomiting, diarrhea), excessive losses through abnormal routes (indwelling drains, NG/intestinal suctioning, hemorrhage), insufficient replacement, fever.
risk for Infection: risk factors may include chronic disease, malnutrition, opening of abdominal cavity/bowel, stasis of body fluids, altered peristalsis.
Constipation/Diarrhea may be related to effects of anesthesia, surgical manipulation, decreased dietary intake/bulk, physical inactivity, irritation, malabsorption, pain, effects of medication possibly evidenced by change in bowel habits, change in stool characteristics, hyper/hypoactive bowel sounds, abdominal pain.

Intracranial infections   **MS**
(Refer to Abscess, brain (acute); Encephalitis; Meningitis)

Irritable bowel syndrome   **CH**
acute Pain may be related to abnormally strong intestinal contractions, increased sensitivity of intestine to distention, hypersensitivity to hormones gastrin and cholecystokinin, skin/tissue irritation/perirectal excoriation possibly evidenced by verbal reports, guarding behavior, expressive behavior (restlessness, moaning, irritability).
Constipation may be related to motor abnormalities of longitudinal muscles/changes in frequency and amplitude of contractions, dietary restrictions, stress possibly evidenced by change in bowel pattern/decreased frequency, sensation of incomplete evacuation, abdominal pain/distention.
Diarrhea may be related to motor abnormalities of longitudinal muscles/changes in frequency and amplitude of contractions, stress possibly evidenced by precipitous passing of liquid stool on rising or immediately after eating, rectal urgency/incontinence, bloating.

Kanner's syndrome   **PED/PSY**
(Refer to Autistic disorder)

Kaposi's sarcoma, AIDS-related   **CH/MS**
(Also refer to Chemotherapy)
disturbed Body Image may be related to widely disseminated lesions of varied color in skin/mucous membranes possibly evidenced by verbalizations, fear of rejection/ reaction of others, negative feelings about body, hiding body parts, change in social involvement.
risk for deficient Fluid Volume: risk factors may include extensive bleeding of visceral lesions.

Kawasaki disease   **PED**
Hyperthermia may be related to increased metabolic rate and dehydration, possibly evidenced by increased body temperature greater than normal range, flushed skin, increased respiratory rate, and tachycardia.
acute Pain may be related to inflammation and edema/swelling of tissues, possibly evidenced by verbal reports, restlessness, guarding behaviors, and narrowed focus.
impaired Skin Integrity may be related to inflammatory process, altered circulation, and

edema formation, possibly evidenced by disruption of skin surface including macular rash and desquamation.

impaired Oral Mucous Membrane may be related to inflammatory process, dehydration, and mouth breathing, possibly evidenced by pain, hyperemia, and fissures of lips.

risk for decreased Cardiac Output: risk factors may include structural changes/inflammation of coronary arteries and alterations in rate/rhythm or conduction.

Ketoacidosis   CH
(Refer to Diabetic ketoacidosis)

Kidney failure, acute   MS
(Refer to Renal failure, acute)

Kidney failure, chronic   CH/MS
(Refer to Renal failure, chronic)

Kidney stone(s)   CH
(Refer to Calculi, urinary)

Knee replacement   MS
(Refer to Total joint replacement)

Kwashiorkor   PED
imbalanced Nutrition: less than body requirements may be related to financial/resource limitations possibly evidenced by inadequate food intake less than recommended daily allowances, lack of food, weight loss, poor muscle tone, decreased subcutaneous fat/muscle mass, abnormal laboratory studies.

risk for Infection: risk factors may include malnutrition.

risk for disproportionate Growth: risk factors may include malnutrition, caregiver maladaptive feeding behaviors, deprivation/poverty, impaired insulin response, infection.

Labor, breech presentation   OB
Anxiety [specify level] may be related to situational crisis, threat to self/fetus, interpersonal transmission possibly evidenced by increased tension, apprehension, fearful, restlessness, sympathetic stimulation.

risk for fetal Injury: risk factors may include entrapment of head, stretching of brachial plexus or spinal cord (nerve damage), hypoxia (brain damage).

Labor, dysfunctional   OB
(Refer to Dystocia)

Labor, induced/augmented   OB
deficient Knowledge [Learning Need] regarding procedure, treatment needs, and possible outcomes may be related to lack of exposure/recall, information misinterpretation, and unfamiliarity with information resources, possibly evidenced by questions, statement of concern/misconception, and exaggerated behaviors.

risk for maternal Injury: risk factors may include adverse effects/response to therapeutic interventions.

risk for impaired fetal Gas Exchange: risk factors may include altered placental perfusion/cord prolapse.

acute Pain may be related to altered characteristics of chemically stimulated contractions, psychological concerns, possibly evidenced by verbal reports, increased muscle tone, distraction/guarding behaviors, and narrowed focus.

Labor, precipitous   **OB**

Anxiety [specify level] may be related to situational crisis, threat to self/fetus, interpersonal transmission possibly evidenced by increased tension; scared, fearful, restless/jittery; sympathetic stimulation.

risk for impaired Skin/Tissue Integrity: risk factors may include rapid progress of labor, lack of necessary equipment.

acute Pain may be related to occurrence of rapid, strong muscle contractions; psychological issues possibly evidenced by verbalizations of inability to use learned pain-management techniques, sympathetic stimulation, distraction behaviors (e.g., moaning, restlessness).

Labor, preterm   **OB/CH**

Activity Intolerance may be related to muscle/cellular hypersensitivity, possibly evidenced by continued uterine contractions/irritability.

risk for Poisoning: risk factors may include dose-related toxic/side effects of tocolytics.

risk for fetal Injury: risk factors may include delivery of premature/immature infant.

Anxiety [specify level] may be related to situational crisis, perceived or actual threats to self/fetus and inadequate time to prepare for labor, possibly evidenced by increased tension, restlessness, expressions of concern, and autonomic responses (changes in vital signs).

deficient Knowledge [Learning Need] regarding preterm labor treatment needs and prognosis may be related to lack of information and misinterpretation, possibly evidenced by questions, statements of concern, misconceptions, inaccurate follow-through of instruction, and development of preventable complications.

Labor, stage I (latent phase)   **OB**

deficient Knowledge [Learning Need] regarding progression of labor, available options may be related to lack of exposure/recall, information misinterpretation possibly evidenced by questions, statements of misconceptions, inaccurate follow-through of instructions.

risk for mild Anxiety: risk factors may include situational crisis, unmet needs, stress.

risk for ineffective Coping: risk factors may include personal vulnerability, inadequate support systems and/or coping methods.

Labor, stage I (active phase)   **OB**

acute Pain/[Discomfort] may be related to contraction-related hypoxia, dilation of tissues, and pressure on adjacent structures combined with stimulation of both parasympathetic and sympathetic nerve endings, possibly evidenced by verbal reports, guarding/distraction behaviors (restlessness), muscle tension, and narrowed focus.

impaired Urinary Elimination may be related to altered intake/dehydration, fluid shifts, hormonal changes, hemorrhage, severe intrapartal hypertension, mechanical compression of bladder, and effects of regional anesthesia, possibly evidenced by changes in amount/frequency of voiding, urinary retention, slowed progression of labor, and reduced sensation.

risk for ineffective [individual/couple] Coping: risk factors may include situational crises, personal vulnerability, use of ineffective coping mechanisms, inadequate support systems, and pain.

Labor, stage I (transition phase)   **OB**

acute Pain may be related to mechanical pressure of presenting part, tissue dilation/stretching and hypoxia, stimulation of parasympathetic and sympathetic nerves; emotional and muscular tension.

Health Conditions & Client Concerns with Associated Nursing Diagnoses   **777**

Fatigue may be related to discomfort/pain, overwhelming psychological emotional demands, increased energy requirements, decreased caloric intake possibly evidenced by verbalizations, impaired ability to concentrate, emotional lability or irritability, lethargy, altered coping ability.

risk for ineffective [individual/couple] Coping: risk factors may include sense of "work overload," personal vulnerability, inadequate/exhausted support system.

risk for imbalanced Fluid Volume: risk factors may include reduced intake, excess fluid loss/hemorrhage, excess fluid retention, rapid fluid administration.

risk for decreased Cardiac Output: risk factors may include decreased venous return, hypovolemia, changes in systemic vascular resistence.

Labor, stage II (expulsion)   OB

acute Pain may be related to strong uterine contractions, tissue stretching/dilation and compression of nerves by presenting part of the fetus, and bladder distention, possibly evidenced by verbalizations, facial grimacing, guarding/distraction behaviors (restlessness), narrowed focus, and autonomic responses (diaphoresis).

Cardiac Output [fluctuation] may be related to changes in SVR, fluctuations in venous return (repeated/prolonged Valsalva's maneuvers, effects of anesthesia/medications, dorsal recumbent position occluding the inferior vena cava and partially obstructing the aorta), possibly evidenced by decreased venous return, changes in vital signs (BP, pulse), urinary output, fetal bradycardia.

risk for impaired fetal Gas Exchange: risk factors may include mechanical compression of head/cord, maternal position/prolonged labor affecting placental perfusion, and effects of maternal anesthesia, hyperventilation.

risk for impaired Skin/Tissue Integrity: risk factors may include untoward stretching/lacerations of delicate tissues (precipitous labor, hypertonic contractile pattern, adolescence, large fetus) and application of forceps.

risk for Fatigue: risk factors may include pregnancy, stress, anxiety, sleep deprivation, increased physical exertion, anemia, humidity/temperature, lights.

Labor, stage III (placental expulsion)   OB

acute Pain may be related to tissue trauma, psychological response following delivery possibly evidenced by verbalizations, changes in muscle tone, restlessness.

risk for deficient Fluid Volume: risk factors may include lack/restriction of oral intake, vomiting, diaphoresis, increased insensible water loss, uterine atony, lacerations of the birth canal, retained placental fragments.

risk for maternal Injury: risk factors may include positioning during delivery/transfers, difficulty with placental separation, abnormal blood profile.

risk for impaired parent/infant Attachment: risk factors may include physical barriers/separation, anxiety associated with the parent role.

Labor, stage IV (first 4 hr following delivery of placenta)   OB

Fatigue may be related to increased physical exertion, sleep deprivation, stress, environmental stimuli, hormonal changes possibly evidenced by verbalization of overwhelming lack of energy, compromised concentration, listlessness.

acute Pain may be related to effects of hormones/medications, mechanical trauma/tissue edema, physical and psychological exhaustion, anxiety possibly evidenced by reports of cramping (after pains), muscle tremors, guarding/distraction behaviors, facial mask.

risk for deficient Fluid Volume: risk factors may include myometrial fatigue/failure of homeostatic mechanisms (e.g., continued uteroplacental circulation, incomplete vasoconstriction, effects of PIH).

risk for impaired parent/infant Attachment: risk factors may include maternal fatigue, physical barriers/separation, lack of privacy, anxiety associated with the parent role.

Laceration   CH

impaired Skin/Tissue Integrity may be related to trauma possibly evidenced by disruption of skin layers, invasion of body structures.

risk for Infection: risk factors may include trauma, tissue destruction, increased environmental exposure.

Laminectomy, cervical   MS

(Also refer to Laminectomy, lumbar)

risk for perioperative-positioning Injury: risk factors may include immobilization, muscle weakness, obesity, advanced age.

risk for ineffective Airway Clearance: risk factors may include retained secretions, pain, muscular weakness.

risk for impaired Swallowing: risk factors may include operative edema, pain, neuromuscular impairment.

Laminectomy, lumbar   MS

(Also refer to Surgery, general)

ineffective Tissue Perfusion (specify) may be related to diminished/interrupted blood flow (dressing, edema/hematoma formation), hypovolemia, possibly evidenced by paresthesia, numbness; decreased range of motion, muscle strength.

risk for [spinal] Trauma: risk factors may include temporary weakness of spinal column, balancing difficulties, changes in muscle tone/coordination.

acute Pain may be related to traumatized tissues, localized inflammation, and edema, possibly evidenced by altered muscle tone, verbal reports, and distraction/guarding behaviors, autonomic changes.

impaired physical Mobility may be related to imposed therapeutic restrictions, neuromuscular impairment, and pain, possibly evidenced by limited range of motion, decreased muscle strength/control, impaired coordination, and reluctance to attempt movement.

risk for [acute] Urinary Retention: risk factors may include pain and swelling in operative area and reduced mobility/restrictions of position.

Laryngectomy   MS

(Also refer to Cancer; Chemotherapy)

ineffective Airway Clearance may be related to partial/total removal of the glottis, temporary or permanent change to neck breathing, edema formation, and copious/thick secretions, possibly evidenced by dyspnea/difficulty breathing, changes in rate/depth of respiration, use of accessory respiratory muscles, weak/ineffective cough, abnormal breath sounds, and cyanosis.

impaired Skin/Tissue Integrity may be related to surgical removal of tissues/grafting, effects of radiation or chemotherapeutic agents, altered circulation/reduced blood supply, compromised nutritional status, edema formation, and pooling/continuous drainage of secretions, possibly evidenced by disruption of skin/tissue surface and destruction of skin/tissue layers.

impaired Oral Mucous Membrane may be related to dehydration/absence of oral intake, poor/inadequate oral hygiene, pathological condition (oral cancer), mechanical trauma (oral surgery), decreased saliva production, difficulty swallowing and pooling/drooling of secretions, and nutritional deficits, possibly evidenced by xerostomia (dry mouth), oral discomfort, thick/mucoid saliva, decreased saliva production, dry and crusted/coated tongue, inflamed lips, absent teeth/gums, poor dental health and halitosis.

impaired verbal Communication may be related to anatomic deficit (removal of vocal cords), physical barrier (tracheostomy tube), and required voice rest, possibly evidenced by inability to speak, change in vocal characteristics, and impaired articulation.

risk for Aspiration: risk factors may include impaired swallowing, facial/neck surgery, presence of tracheostomy/feeding tube.

Laryngitis   CH/PED
(Refer to Croup)

Latex allergy   CH
latex Allergy Response may be related to no immune mechanism response possibly evidenced by contact dermatitis—erythema, blisters; delayed hypersensitivity—eczema, irritation; hypersensitivity—generalized edema, wheezing/bronchospasm, hypotension, cardiac arrest.

Anxiety [specify level]/Fear may be related to threat of death possibly evidenced by expressed concerns, hypervigilance, restlessness, focus on self.

risk for impaired Adjustment: risk factors may include health status requiring change in occupation.

Laxative abuse   CH
perceived Constipation may be related to health beliefs, faulty apprasial, impaired cognition/thought processes possibly evidenced by expectation of daily bowel movement, expected passage of stool at same time every day.

Lead poisoning, acute   PED/CH
(Also refer to Lead poisoning, chronic)
risk for Trauma: risk factors may include loss of coordination, altered level of consciousness, clonic or tonic muscle activity, neurologic damage.

risk for deficient Fluid Volume: risk factors may include excessive vomiting, diarrhea, or decreased intake.

deficient Knowledge [Learning Need] regarding sources of lead and prevention of poisoning may be related to lack of information/misinterpretation, possibly evidenced by statements of concern, questions, and misconceptions.

Lead poisoning, chronic   CH
(Also refer to Lead Poisoning, acute)
imbalanced Nutrition: less than body requirements may be related to decreased intake (chemically induced changes in the GI tract), possibly evidenced by anorexia, abdominal discomfort, reported metallic taste, and weight loss.

disturbed Thought Processes may be related to deposition of lead in CNS and brain tissue, possibly evidenced by personality changes, learning disabilities, and impaired ability to conceptualize and reason.

chronic Pain may be related to deposition of lead in soft tissues and bone, possibly evidenced by verbal reports, distraction behaviors, and focus on self.

Legionnaires' disease   CH/MS
Hyperthermia may be related to illness/inflammatory process possibly evidenced by increased body temperature, flushed/warm skin, chills.

acute Pain/[Discomfort] may be related to infectious agent/inflammatory response, effects of circulating toxins possibly evidenced by reports of headache, myalgia, high fever, diaphoresis.

ineffective Airway Clearance may be related to tracheal bronchial inflammation, edema formation, increased sputum production, pleuritic pain, decreased energy, fatigue, possibly evidenced by changes in rate/depth of respirations, abnormal breath sounds, use of accessory muscles, dyspnea, cyanosis, effective/ineffective cough—with or without sputum production.

impaired Gas Exchange may be related to inflammatory process, collection of secretions affecting O_2 exchange across alveolar membrane, and hypoventilation, possibly evidenced by restlessness/changes in mentation, dyspnea, tachycardia, pallor, cyanosis, and ABGs/oximetry evidence of hypoxia.

Diarrhea may be related to infectious process possibly evidenced by liquid stools, abdominal cramping.

risk for Infection [spread]: risk factors may include decreased ciliary action, stasis of secretions, presence of existing infection; improper disposal of contaminated materials.

Leukemia, acute   MS
(Also refer to Chemotherapy)

risk for Infection: risk factors may include inadequate secondary defenses (alterations in mature white blood cells, increased number of immature lymphocytes, immunosuppression and bone marrow suppression), invasive procedures, and malnutrition.

Anxiety [specify level]/Fear may be related to change in health status, threat of death, and situational crisis, possibly evidenced by sympathetic stimulation, apprehension, feelings of helplessness, focus on self, and insomnia.

Activity Intolerance [specify level] may be related to reduced energy stores, increased metabolic rate, imbalance between O_2 supply and demand, therapeutic restrictions (bedrest)/effect of drug therapy, possibly evidenced by generalized weakness, reports of fatigue and exertional dyspnea; abnormal heart rate or BP response.

acute Pain may be related to physical agents (infiltration of tissues/organs/CNS, expanding bone marrow) and chemical agents (antileukemic treatments), possibly evidenced by verbal reports (abdominal discomfort, arthralgia, bone pain, headache); distraction behaviors, narrowed focus, and autonomic responses (changes in vital signs).

risk for deficient Fluid Volume: risk factors may include excessive losses (vomiting, hemorrhage, diarrhea), decreased intake (nausea, anorexia), increased fluid need (hypermetabolic state/fever), predisposition for kidney stone formation/tumor lysis syndrome.

Leukemia, chronic   CH

ineffective Protection may be related to abnormal blood profiles, drug therapy (cytotoxic agents, steroids), radiation treatments possibly evidenced by deficient immunity, impaired healing, altered clotting, weakness.

Fatigue may be related to disease state, anemia possibly evidenced by verbalizations, inability to maintain usual routines, listlessness.

imbalanced Nutrition: less than body needs may be related to inability to ingest nutrients possibly evidenced by lack of interest in food, anorexia, weight loss, abdominal fullness/pain.

Lightning injury   MS
(Also refer to Electrical injury)

risk for disturbed visual/auditory Sensory Perception: risk factors may include altered sensory reception (corneal laceration, retinal damage, development of cataracts, rupture of tympanic membrane).

acute Confusion may be related to CNS involvement possibly evidenced by change in level of consciousness.

impaired Memory may be related to acute hypoxia, decreased cardiac output, electrolyte imbalance, neurologic disturbance possibly evidenced by inability to recall recent events, amnesia.

Liver failure   MS/CH
(Refer to Cirrhosis; Hepatitis, acute viral)

Liver transplantation   MS/CH
(Refer to Transplantation, recipient)

Lockjaw   MS
(Refer to Tetanus)

Long-term care   CH
(Also refer to condition requiring/contributing to need for facility placement)

Anxiety [specify level]/Fear may be related to change in health status, role functioning, interaction patterns, socioeconomic status, environment; unmet needs, recent life changes, and loss of friends/SO(s), possibly evidenced by apprehension, restlessness, insomnia, repetitive questioning, pacing, purposeless activity, expressed concern regarding changes in life events, and focus on self.

anticipatory Grieving may be related to perceived/actual or potential loss of physiopsychosocial well-being, personal possessions and significant other(s); as well as cultural beliefs about aging/debilitation, possibly evidenced by denial of feelings, depression, sorrow, guilt; alterations in activity level, sleep patterns, eating habits, and libido.

risk for Poisoning [drug toxicity]: risk factors may include effects of aging (reduced metabolism, impaired circulation, precarious physiologic balance, presence of multiple diseases/organ involvement) and use of multiple prescribed/OTC drugs.

disturbed Thought Processes may be related to physiologic changes of aging (loss of cells and brain atrophy, decreased blood supply); altered sensory input, pain, effects of medications, and psychological conflicts (disrupted life pattern), possibly evidenced by slower reaction times, memory loss, altered attention span, disorientation, inability to follow, altered sleep patterns, and personality changes.

disturbed Sleep Pattern may be related to internal factors (illness, psychological stress, inactivity) and external factors (environmental changes, facility routines), possibly evidenced by reports of difficulty in falling asleep/not feeling rested, interrupted sleep/awakening earlier than desired; change in behavior/performance, increasing irritability, and listlessness.

risk for ineffective Sexuality Patterns: risk factors may include biopsychosocial alteration of sexuality; interference in psychological/physical well-being, self-image, and lack of privacy/SO.

risk for Relocation Stress Syndrome: risk factors may include multiple losses, feeling of powerlessness, lack of/inappropriate use of support system, changes in psychosocial/physical health status.

LSD (lysergic acid diethylamide) intoxication   MS/PSY

(Also refer to Hallucinogen abuse)

risk for Trauma: risk factors may include perceptual distortion, impaired judgement, dangerous decision making, changes in mood.

Anxiety [panic attack] may be related to drug side effects possibly evidenced by severe apprehension, fear of unspecific consequences, CNS excitation, central autonomic hyperactivity.

Lung cancer   MS/CH
(Refer to Bronchogenic carcinoma)

Lung transplantation   **MS/CH**

(Also refer to Transplantation, recipient)

risk for impaired Gas Exchange: risk factors may include ventilation/perfusion mismatch, poor healing/stenosis of bronchial or tracheal anastomosis.

risk for Infection: risk factors may include medically induced immunosuppression, suppressed inflammatory response, antibiotic therapy, invasive procedures, effects of chronic/debilitating disease.

Lupus erythematosus, systemic   **CH**

Fatigue may be related to inadequate energy production/increased energy requirements (chronic inflammation), overwhelming psychological or emotional demands, states of discomfort, and altered body chemistry (including effects of drug therapy), possibly evidenced by reports of unremitting and overwhelming lack of energy/inability to maintain usual routines, decreased performance, lethargy, and decreased libido.

acute Pain may be related to widespread inflammatory process affecting connective tissues, blood vessels, serosal surfaces and mucous membranes, possibly evidenced by verbal reports, guarding/distraction behaviors, self-focusing, and autonomic responses (changes in vital signs).

impaired Skin/Tissue Integrity may be related to chronic inflammation, edema formation, and altered circulation, possibly evidenced by presence of skin rash/lesions, ulcerations of mucous membranes and photosensitivity.

disturbed Body Image may be related to presence of chronic condition with rash, lesions, ulcers, purpura, mottled erythema of hands, alopecia, loss of strength, and altered body function, possibly evidenced by hiding body parts, negative feelings about body, feelings of helplessness, and change in social involvement.

Lyme disease   **CH/MS**

acute/chronic Pain may be related to systemic effects of toxins, presence of rash, urticaria, and joint swelling/inflammation, possibly evidenced by verbal reports, guarding behaviors, autonomic responses, and narrowed focus.

Fatigue may be related to increased energy requirements, altered body chemistry, and states of discomfort evidenced by reports of overwhelming lack of energy/inability to maintain usual routines, decreased performance, lethargy, and malaise.

risk for decreased Cardiac Output: risk factors may include alteration in cardiac rate/rhythm/conduction.

Lymphedema   **CH**

disturbed Body Image may be related to physical changes (chronic swelling of lower extremity) possibly evidenced by verbalizations, fear of reaction of others, negative feelings about body, hiding body part, change in social involvement.

impaired Walking may be related to chronic/progressive swelling of lower extremity possibly evidenced by difficulty walking required distances, climbing stairs, navigating uneven surfaces/declines.

risk for impaired Skin Integrity: risk factors may include altered circulation, significant edema, changes in sensation.

Macular degeneration   **CH**

disturbed visual Sensory Perception may be related to altered sensory reception possibly evidenced by reported/measured change in sensory acuity, change in usual response to stimuli.

Anxiety [specify level]/Fear may be related to situational crisis, threat to or change in health status and role function possibly evidenced by expressed concerns, apprehension, feelings of inadequacy, diminished productivity, impaired attention.

risk for impaired Home Maintenance: risk factors may include impaired cognitive functioning, inadequate support systems.

risk for impaired Social Interaction: risk factors may include limited physical mobility, environmental barriers.

Malaria   MS/CH

Hyperthermia may be related to illness/inflammatory process possibly evidenced by increased body temperature (106° F), flushed/warm skin, tachycardia, headache, altered consciousness.

acute Pain/[Discomfort] may be related to infectious agent/inflammatory response possibly evidenced by reports of headache, backache, myalgia, malaise, high fever, shaking chills, abdominal discomfort.

risk for deficient Fluid Volume: risk factors may include decreased intake (nausea, abdominal pain, prostration), excessive losses (vomiting, diarrhea), hypermetabolic state.

Fatigue may be related to disease state, anemia, lack of restful sleep possibly evidenced by verbalization of unremitting/overwhelming lack of energy, inability to restore energy even after sleep, lethargy.

Mallory-Weiss syndrome   MS
(Also refer to Achalasia)

risk for deficient Fluid Volume [isotonic]: risk factors may include excessive vascular losses, presence of vomiting, and reduced intake.

deficient Knowledge [Learning Need] regarding causes, treatment, and prevention of condition may be related to lack of information/misinterpretation, possibly evidenced by statements of concern, questions, and recurrence of problem.

Malnutrition   CH
(Also refer to Anorexia nervosa)

adult Failure to Thrive may be related to depression, apathy, aging process, fatigue, degenerative condition possibly evidenced by expressed lack of appetite, difficulty performing self-care tasks, altered mood state, inadequate intake, weight loss, physical decline.

ineffective Protection may be related to inadequate nutrition, anemia, extremes of age possibly evidenced by fatigue, weakness, deficient immunity, impaired healing, pressure sores.

Marburg disease   MS
(Refer to Ebola)

Mastectomy   MS

impaired Skin/Tissue Integrity may be related to surgical removal of skin/tissue, altered circulation, drainage, presence of edema, changes in skin elasticity/sensation, and tissue destruction (radiation), possibly evidenced by disruption of skin surface and destruction of skin layers/subcutaneous tissues.

impaired physical Mobility may be related to neuromuscular impairment, pain, and edema formation, possibly evidenced by reluctance to attempt movement, limited range of motion, and decreased muscle mass/strength.

bathing/dressing Self-Care Deficit may be related to temporary loss/altered action of one or both arms, possibly evidenced by statements of inability to perform/complete self-care tasks.

disturbed Body Image may be related to loss of body part denoting femininity, possibly evidenced by not looking at/touching area, negative feelings about body, preoccupation with loss, and change in social involvement/relationship.

Mastitis   OB/GYN

acute Pain may be related to erythema and edema of breast tissues, possibly evidenced by verbal reports, guarding/distraction behaviors, self-focusing, autonomic responses (changes in vital signs).

risk for Infection [spread/abscess formation]: risk factors may include traumatized tissues, stasis of fluids, and insufficient knowledge to prevent complications.

deficient Knowledge [Learning Need] regarding pathophysiology, treatment, and prevention may be related to lack of information/misinterpretation, possibly evidenced by statements of concern, questions, and misconceptions.

risk for ineffective Breastfeeding: risk factors may include inability to feed on affected side/interruption in breastfeeding.

Mastoidectomy   PED/MS

risk for Infection [spread]: risk factors may include preexisting infection, surgical trauma, and stasis of body fluids in close proximity to brain.

acute Pain may be related to inflammation, tissue trauma, and edema formation, possibly evidenced by verbal reports, distraction behaviors, restlessness, self-focusing, and autonomic responses (changes in vital signs).

disturbed auditory Sensory Perception may be related to presence of surgical packing, edema, and surgical disturbance of middle ear structures, possibly evidenced by reported/tested hearing loss in affected ear.

Measles   CH/PED

acute Pain may be related to inflammation of mucous membranes, conjunctiva, and presence of extensive skin rash with pruritus, possibly evidenced by verbal reports, distraction behaviors, self-focusing, and autonomic responses (changes in vital signs).

Hyperthermia may be related to presence of viral toxins and inflammatory response, possibly evidenced by increased body temperature, flushed/warm skin, and tachycardia.

risk for [secondary] Infection: risk factors may include altered immune response and traumatized dermal tissues.

deficient Knowledge [Learning Need] regarding condition, transmission, and possible complications may be related to lack of information/misinterpretation, possibly evidenced by statements of concern, questions, misconceptions, and development of preventable complications.

Measles, German   PED/CH
(Refer to Rubella)

Melanoma, malignant   MS/CH
(Refer to Cancer; Chemotherapy)

Menière's disease   CH
(Also refer to Vertigo)

disturbed auditory Sensory Perception may be related to altered state of sensory organ/sensory reception possibly evidenced by change in sensory acuity, tinnitus, vertigo.

Nausea may be related to inner ear disturbance possibly evidenced by verbal reports, vomiting.

risk for total Self-Care Deficit: risk factors may include perceptual impairment, recurrent nausea, general weakness.

Meningitis, acute meningococcal — MS

risk for Infection [spread]: risk factors may include hematogenous dissemination of pathogen, stasis of body fluids, suppressed inflammatory response (medication-induced), and exposure of others to pathogens.

risk for ineffective cerebral Tissue Perfusion: risk factors may include cerebral edema altering/interrupting cerebral arterial/venous blood flow, hypovolemia, exchange problems at cellular level (acidosis).

Hyperthermia may be related to infectious process (increased metabolic rate) and dehydration, possibly evidenced by increased body temperature, warm/flushed skin, and tachycardia.

acute Pain may be related to inflammation/irritation of the meninges with spasm of extensor muscles (neck, shoulders, and back), possibly evidenced by verbal reports, guarding/distraction behaviors, narrowed focus, photophobia, and autonomic responses (changes in vital signs).

risk for Trauma/Suffocation: risk factors may include alterations in level of consciousness, possible development of clonic/tonic muscle activity (seizures), and generalized weakness/prostration, ataxia, vertigo.

Meniscectomy — MS/CH

impaired Walking may be related to pain, joint instability, and imposed medical restrictions of movement, possibly evidenced by impaired ability to move about environment as needed/desired.

deficient Knowledge [Learning Need] regarding postoperative expectations, prevention of complications, and self-care needs may be related to lack of information, possibly evidenced by statements of concern, questions, and misconceptions.

Menopause — GYN

ineffective Thermoregulation may be related to fluctuation of hormonal levels possibly evidenced by skin flushed/warm to touch, diaphoresis, night sweats; cold hands/feet.

Fatigue may be related to change in body chemistry, lack of sleep, depression possibly evidenced by reports of lack of energy, tired, inability to maintain usual routines, decreased performance.

risk for ineffective Sexuality Patterns: risk factors may include perceived altered body function, changes in physical response, myths/inaccurate information, impaired relationship with SO.

risk for stress urinary Incontinence: risk factors may include degenerative changes in pelvic muscles and structural support.

Health-Seeking Behaviors: management of life-cycle changes may be related to maturational change possibly evidenced by expressed desire for increased control of health practice, demonstrated lack of knowledge in health promotion.

Mental retardation — CH

(Also refer to Down Syndrome)

impaired verbal Communication may be related to developmental delay/impairment of cognitive and motor abilities, possibly evidenced by impaired articulation, difficulty with phonation, and inability to modulate speech/find appropriate words (dependent on degree of retardation).

risk for Self-Care Deficit [specify]: risk factors may include impaired cognitive ability and motor skills.

risk for imbalanced Nutrition: more than body requirements: risk factors may include decreased metabolic rate coupled with impaired cognitive development, dysfunctional eating patterns, and sedentary activity level.

impaired Social Interaction may be related to impaired thought processes, communication barriers, and knowledge/skill deficit about ways to enhance mutuality, possibly evidenced by dysfunctional interactions with peers, family, and/or SO(s), and verbalized/observed discomfort in social situation.

compromised family Coping may be related to chronic nature of condition and degree of disability that exhausts supportive capacity of SO(s), other situational or developmental crises or situations SO(s) may be facing, unrealistic expectations of SO(s), possibly evidenced by preoccupation of SO with personal reaction, SO(s) withdraw(s) or enter(s) into limited interaction with individual, protective behavior disproportionate (too much or too little) to client's abilities or need for autonomy.

impaired Home Maintenance may be related to impaired cognitive functioning, insufficient finances/family organization or planning, lack of knowledge, and inadequate support systems, possibly evidenced by requests for assistance, expression of difficulty in maintaining home, disorderly surroundings, and overtaxed family members.

risk for Sexual Dysfunction: risk factors may include biopsychosocial alteration of sexuality, ineffectual/absent role models, misinformation/lack of knowledge, lack of SO(s), and lack of appropriate behavior control.

Mesothelioma   CH/MS
(Also refer to Asbestosis; Cancer)

acute Pain may be related to tissue distruction possibly evidenced by reports of chest pain (initially nonpleuritic), irritability, self-focusing, autonomic responses.

Activity Intolerance may be related to imbalance between oxygen supply/demand possibly evidenced by dyspnea, fatigue.

Migraine   CH/MS
(Refer to Headache)

Miscarriage   OB
(Refer to Abortion, spontaneous termination)

Mitral insufficiency   MS/CH
(Refer to Valvular heart disease)

Mitral valve prolapse (MVP)   CH
(Refer to Valvular heart disease)

Mitral stenosis   MS/CH

Activity Intolerance may be related to imbalance between O_2 supply and demand, possibly evidenced by reports of fatigue, weakness, exertional dyspnea, and tachycardia.

impaired Gas Exchange may be related to altered blood flow, possibly evidenced by restlessness, hypoxia, and cyanosis (orthopnea/paroxysmal nocturnal dyspnea).

decreased Cardiac Output may be related to impeded blood flow as evidenced by jugular vein distention, peripheral/dependent edema, orthopnea/paroxysmal nocturnal dyspnea.

deficient Knowledge [Learning Need] regarding pathophysiology, therapeutic needs, and potential complications may be related to lack of information/recall, misinterpretation, possibly evidenced by statements of concern, questions, inaccurate follow-through of instructions, and development of preventable complications.

Mononucleosis, infectious   CH

Fatigue may be related to decreased energy production, states of discomfort, and increased energy requirements (inflammatory process), possibly evidenced by reports of overwhelming lack of energy, inability to maintain usual routines, lethargy, and malaise.

acute Pain/[Discomfort] may be related to inflammation of lymphoid and organ tissues, irritation of oropharyngeal mucous membranes, and effects of circulating toxins, possibly evidenced by verbal reports, distraction behaviors, and self-focusing.

Hyperthermia may be related to inflammatory process, possibly evidenced by increased body temperature, warm/flushed skin, and tachycardia.

deficient Knowledge [Learning Need] regarding disease transmission, self-care needs, medical therapy, and potential complications may be related to lack of information/misinterpretation, possibly evidenced by statements of concern, misconceptions, and inaccurate follow-through of instructions.

Mood disorders   PSY

(Refer to Depression, major; Bipolar disorder, Premenstrual dysphoric disorder)

Mountain sickness, acute (AMS)   CH/MS

acute Pain may be related to reduced oxygen tension possibly evidenced by reports of headache.

Fatigue may be related to stress, increased physical exertion, sleep deprivation possibly evidenced by overwhelming lack of energy, inability to restore energy even after sleep, compromised concentration, decreased performance.

risk for deficient Fluid Volume: risk factors may include increased water loss (e.g., overbreathing dry air), exertion, altered fluid intake (nausea).

Multiple organ dysfunction syndrome   MS

(Also refer to specific organs involved; Sepsis; Ventilator assist/dependence)

ineffective peripheral/renal/gastrointestinal Tissue Perfusion may be related to hypovolemia, selective vasoconstriction, microvascular embolization possibly evidenced by cool skin, diminished pulses, oliguria/anuria, nausea, abdominal tenderness, hypoactive bowel sounds.

impaired Gas Exchange may be related to ventilation perfusion imbalance, alveolar hypoventilation possibly evidenced by dyspnea, irritability, confusion, abnormal ABGs.

Activity Intolerance may be related to generalized weakness, bedrest, imbalance between oxygen supply/demand, pain possibly evidenced by abnormal heart rate/BP response to activity, pallor, exertional discomfort, ECG changes (dysrhythmias, ischemia).

severe Anxiety/Fear may be related to situational crisis, change in health status, threat of death possibly evidenced by expressed concerns, apprehension, increased tension, fearful, restlessness, decreased perceptual field.

imbalanced Nutrition: less than body requirements may be related to restricted intake, inability to digest food, increased metabolic demands possibly evidenced by weight loss, poor muscle tone, decreased subcutaneous fat/muscle mass, abnormal laboratory studies.

risk for Infection: risk factors may include stasis of body fluids, immunosuppression, malnutrition, invasive devices/procedures, environmental exposure.

Multiple personality   PSY

(Refer to Dissociative Disorders)

Multiple sclerosis   CH

Fatigue may be related to decreased energy production/increased energy requirements to perform activities, psychological/emotional demands, pain/discomfort, medication side effects, possibly evidenced by verbalization of overwhelming lack of energy, inability to maintain usual routine, decreased performance, impaired ability to concentrate, increase in physical complaints.

disturbed visual/kinesthetic/tactile Sensory Perception may be related to delayed/interrupted neuronal transmission, possibly evidenced by impaired vision, diplopia, disturbance of vibratory or position sense, paresthesias, numbness, and blunting of sensation.

impaired physical Mobility may be related to neuromuscular impairment, discomfort/pain, sensoriperceptual impairments, decreased muscle strength, control and/or mass, deconditioning, as evidenced by limited ability to perform motor skills, limited range of motion, gait changes/postural instability.

Powerlessness/Hopelessness may be related to illness-related regimen and lifestyle of helplessness, possibly evidenced by verbal expressions of having no control or influence over the situation, depression over physical deterioration that occurs despite client compliance with regimen, nonparticipation in care or decision making when opportunities are provided, passivity, decreased verbalization/affect.

impaired Home Maintenance may be related to effects of debilitating disease, impaired cognitive and/or emotional functioning, insufficient finances, and inadequate support systems, possibly evidenced by reported difficulty, observed disorderly surroundings, and poor hygienic conditions.

compromised/disabled family Coping may be related to situational crises/temporary family disorganization and role changes, client providing little support in turn for SO(s), prolonged disease/disability progression that exhausts the supportive capacity of SO(s), feelings of guilt, anxiety, hostility, despair, and highly ambivalent family relationships, possibly evidenced by client expressing/confirming concern or report about SOs'(s) response to client's illness, SO(s) preoccupied with own personal reactions, intolerance, abandonment, neglectful care of the client, and distortion of reality regarding client's illness.

Mumps   PED/CH

acute Pain may be related to presence of inflammation, circulating toxins, and enlargement of salivary glands, possibly evidenced by verbal reports, guarding/distraction behaviors, self-focusing, and autonomic responses (changes in vital signs).

Hyperthermia may be related to inflammatory process (increased metabolic rate) and dehydration, possibly evidenced by increased body temperature, warm/flushed skin, and tachycardia.

risk for deficient Fluid Volume: risk factors may include hypermetabolic state and painful swallowing, with decreased intake.

Muscular dystrophy (Duchenne's)   PED/CH

impaired physical Mobility may be related to musculoskeletal impairment/weakness, possibly evidenced by decreased muscle strength, control, and mass; limited range of motion; and impaired coordination.

delayed Growth and Development may be related to effects of physical disability, possibly evidenced by altered physical growth and altered ability to perform self-care/self-control activities appropriate to age.

risk for imbalanced Nutrition: more than body requirements: risk factors may include sedentary lifestyle and dysfunctional eating patterns.

compromised family Coping may be related to situational crisis/emotional conflicts around issues about hereditary nature of condition and prolonged disease/disability that exhausts supportive capacity of family members, possibly evidenced by preoccupation with personal reactions regarding disability and displaying protective behavior disproportionate (too little/too much) to client's abilities/need for autonomy.

Myasthenia gravis   MS

ineffective Breathing Pattern/Airway Clearance may be related to neuromuscular weakness and decreased energy/fatigue, possibly evidenced by dyspnea, changes in rate/depth of respiration, ineffective cough, and adventitious breath sounds.

impaired verbal Communication may be related to neuromuscular weakness, fatigue, and physical barrier (intubation), possibly evidenced by facial weakness, impaired articulation, hoarseness, and inability to speak.

impaired Swallowing may be related to neuromuscular impairment of laryngeal/pharyngeal muscles and muscular fatigue, possibly evidenced by reported/observed difficulty swallowing, coughing/choking, and evidence of aspiration.

Anxiety [specify level]/Fear may be related to situational crisis, threat to self-concept, change in health/socioeconomic status or role function, separation from support systems, lack of knowledge, and inability to communicate, possibly evidenced by expressed concerns, increased tension, restlessness, apprehension, sympathetic stimulation, crying, focus on self, uncooperative behavior, withdrawal, anger, and noncommunication.

                                                               CH

deficient Knowledge [Learning Need] regarding drug therapy, potential for crisis (myasthenic or cholinergic) and self-care management may be related to inadequate information/misinterpretation, possibly evidenced by statements of concern, questions, and misconceptions; development of preventable complications.

impaired physical Mobility may be related to neuromuscular impairment, possibly evidenced by reports of progressive fatigue with repetitive/prolonged muscle use, impaired coordination, and decreased muscle strength/control.

disturbed visual Sensory Perception may be related to neuromuscular impairment, possibly evidenced by visual distortions (diplopia) and motor incoordination.

Myeloma, multiple   MS/CH
(Also refer to Cancer)

acute/chronic Pain may be related to destruction of tissues/bone, side effects of therapy possibly evidenced by verbal or coded reports, guarding/protective behaviors, changes in appetite/weight, sleep; reduced interaction with others.

impaired physical Mobility may be related to loss of integrity of bone structure, pain, deconditioning, depressed mood possibly evidenced by verbalizations, limited range of motion, slowed movement, gait changes.

risk for ineffective Protection: risk factors may include presence of cancer, drug therapies, radiation treatments, inadequate nutrition.

Myocardial infarction   MS
(Also refer to Myocarditis)

acute Pain may be related to ischemia of myocardial tissue, possibly evidenced by verbal reports, guarding/distraction behaviors (restlessness), facial mask of pain, self-focusing, and autonomic responses (diaphoresis, changes in vital signs).

Anxiety [specify level]/Fear may be related to threat of death, threat of change of health status/role functioning and lifestyle, interpersonal transmission/contagion, possibly evidenced by increased tension, fearful attitude, apprehension, expressed concerns/uncertainty, restlessness, sympathetic stimulation, and somatic complaints.

risk for decreased Cardiac Output: risk factors may include changes in rate and electrical conduction, reduced preload/increased SVR, and altered muscle contractility/depressant effects of some medications, infarcted/dyskinetic muscle, structural defects.

Myocarditis   MS
(Also refer to Myocardial Infarction)

Activity Intolerance may be related to imbalance in O_2 supply and demand (myocardial inflammation/damage) cardiac depressant effects of certain drugs, and enforced bedrest, possibly evidenced by reports of fatigue, exertional dyspnea, tachycardia/palpitations in response to activity, ECG changes/dysrhythmias, and generalized weakness.

risk for decreased Cardiac Output: risk factors may include degeneration of cardiac muscle.

deficient Knowledge [Learning Need] regarding pathophysiology of condition/outcomes, treatment, and self-care needs/lifestyle changes may be related to lack of information/misinterpretation, possibly evidenced by statements of concern, misconceptions, inaccurate follow-through of instructions, and development of preventable complications.

Myofascial pain syndrome   CH
(Also refer to Fibromyalgia)

acute/chronic Pain may be related to nocturnal bruxism (clenching/grinding teeth) possibly evidenced by reports of pain (temporomandibular region), headache, muscular tenderness to palpation, limitation in opening mouth.

risk for impaired Dentition: risk factors may include bruxism, ineffective oral hygiene (limitations in opening mouth).

Myringotomy   PED/MS
(Refer to Mastoidectomy)

Myxedema   CH
(Also refer to Hypothyroidism)

disturbed Body Image may be related to change in structure/function (loss of hair/thickening of skin, masklike facial expression, enlarged tongue, menstrual and reproductive disturbances), possibly evidenced by negative feelings about body, feelings of helplessness, and change in social involvement.

imbalanced Nutrition: more than body requirements may be related to decreased metabolic rate and activity level, possibly evidenced by weight gain greater than ideal for height and frame.

risk for decreased Cardiac Output: risk factors may include altered electrical conduction and myocardial contractility.

Narcolepsy   CH
disturbed Sleep Pattern may be related to medical condition possibly evidenced by hypersomnia, reports of unsatisfying nighttime sleep, vivid visual/auditory illusions/hallucinations at onset of sleep, sleep interrupted by vivid/frightening dreams.

risk for Trauma: risk factors may include sudden loss of muscle tone/momentary paralysis (cataplexy), sudden inappropriate sleep episodes.

risk for chronic low Self-Esteem: risk factors may include negative evaluation of self, personal vulnerability, chronic physical condition, impaired work/school performance, problems with social relationships, reduced quality of life.

Near drowning   MS
impaired Gas Exchange may be related to ventilation perfusion imbalance (patchy atelectasis), alveolar-capillary membrane changes, aspiration or acute reflex laryngospasm

possibly evidenced by severe hypoxia, pale/dusky skin, change in mentation (confusion to coma).

risk for excess Fluid Volume: risk factors may include aspiration of fresh water .

risk for Hypothermia: risk factors may include submersion in very cold water.

NEC   PED
(Refer to Necrotizing enterocolitis)

Necrotizing cellulitis/fasciitis   MS
(Also refer to Cellulitis; Sepsis)

Hyperthermia may be related to inflammatory process, response to circulating toxins possibly evidenced by body temperature above normal range, flushed/warm skin, tachycardia, altered mental status.

impaired Tissue Integrity may be related to inflammation/edema (infection), ischemia possibly evidenced by damaged or destroyed tissue/dermal gangrene.

Necrotizing enterocolitis   PED
(Also refer to Sepsis)

imbalanced Nutrition: less than body requirements may be related to inabililty to digest/absorb nutrients (ischemia of bowel) possibly evidenced by abdominal pain/distension, gastric residuals after feedings, failure to gain weight.

risk for deficient Fluid Volume: risk factors may include vomiting, third-space fluid losses (bowel inflammmation, peritonitis), lack of oral intake.

Neglect/Abuse   CH/PSY
(Refer to Abuse, Battered child syndrome)

Nephrectomy   MS
acute Pain may be related to surgical tissue trauma with mechanical closure (suture), possibly evidenced by verbal reports, guarding/distraction behaviors, self-focusing, and autonomic responses (changes in vital signs).

risk for deficient Fluid Volume: risk factors may include excessive vascular losses and restricted intake.

ineffective Breathing Pattern may be related to incisional pain with decreased lung expansion, possibly evidenced by tachypnea, fremitus, changes in respiratory depth/chest expansion, and changes in ABGs.

Constipation may be related to reduced dietary intake, decreased mobility, GI obstruction (paralytic ileus), and incisional pain with defecation, possibly evidenced by decreased bowel sounds, reduced frequency/amount of stool, and hard/formed stool.

Nephrolithiasis   MS/CH
(Refer to Calculi, urinary)

Nephrotic syndrome   MS/CH
(Also refer to Renal failure, acute/chronic)

excess Fluid Volume may be related to compromised regulatory mechanism with changes in hydrostatic/oncotic vascular pressure and increased activation of the renin-angiotensin-aldosterone system, possibly evidenced by edema/anasarca, effusions/ascites, weight gain, intake greater than output, and BP changes.

imbalanced Nutrition: less than body requirements may be related to excessive protein losses and inability to ingest adequate nutrients (anorexia), possibly evidenced by weight loss/muscle wasting (may be difficult to assess due to edema), lack of interest in food, and observed inadequate intake.

risk for Infection: risk factors may include chronic disease and steroidal suppression of inflammatory responses.

risk for impaired Skin Integrity: risk factors may include presence of edema and activity restrictions.

Neuralgia, trigeminal   CH

acute Pain may be related to neuromuscular impairment with sudden violent muscle spasm, possibly evidenced by verbal reports, guarding/distraction behaviors, self-focusing, and autonomic responses (changes in vital signs).

deficient Knowledge [Learning Need] regarding control of recurrent episodes, medical therapies, and self-care needs may be related to lack of information/recall and misinterpretation, possibly evidenced by statements of concern, questions, and exacerbation of condition.

Neural tube defect   PED
(Refer to Spina bifida)

Neuritis   CH

acute/chronic Pain may be related to nerve damage usually associated with a degenerative process, possibly evidenced by verbal reports, guarding/distraction behaviors, self-focusing, and autonomic responses (changes in vital signs).

deficient Knowledge [Learning Need] regarding underlying causative factors, treatment, and prevention may be related to lack of information/misinterpretation, possibly evidenced by statements of concern, questions, and misconceptions.

Newborn, growth deviations   PED
(Also refer to Newborn, premature)

disproportionate Growth may be related to maternal nutrition, substance use/abuse, multiple gestation, prematurity, maternal conditions (e.g., PIH, diabetes) possibly evidenced by birth weight at or below tenth percentile/at or above 90th percentile (considering gestational age, ethnicity, etc.)

imbalanced Nutrition: less than body requirements may be related to decreased nutritional stores, increased insulin production/hyperplasia of pancreatic beta cells possibly evidenced by weight deviation from expected, decreased muscle mass/fat stores, electrolyte imbalance.

risk for ineffective Tissue Perfusion: risk factors may include interruption of arterial/venous blood flow (hyperviscosity associated with polycythemia).

risk for Injury: risk factors may include altered growth, delayed CNS/neurologic development, abnormal blood profile.

risk for disorganized Infant Behavior: risk factors may include functional limitations related to growth deviations (restricting neonate's opportunity to seek out, recognize, and interpret stimuli), electrolyte imbalance, psychological stress, low energy reserves, poor organizational ability, limited ability to control environment.

Newborn, normal   PED

risk for impaired Gas Exchange: risk factors may include prenatal or intrapartal stressors, excess production of mucus, or cold stress.

risk for imbalanced Body Temperature: risk factors may include large body surface in relation to mass, limited amounts of insulating subcutaneous fat, nonrenewable sources of brown fat and few white fat stores, thin epidermis with close proximity of blood vessels to the skin, inability to shiver, and movement from a warm uterine environment to a much cooler environment.

risk for impaired parent/infant Attachment: risk factors may include developmental transition (gain of a family member), anxiety associated with the parent role, lack of privacy (intrusive family/visitors).

risk for imbalanced Nutrition: less than body requirements: risk factors may include rapid metabolic rate, high-caloric requirement, increased insensible water losses through pulmonary and cutaneous routes, fatigue, and a potential for inadequate or depleted glucose stores.

risk for Infection: risk factors may include inadequate secondary defenses (inadequate acquired immunity, e.g., deficiency of neutrophils and specific immunoglobulins), and inadequate primary defenses (e.g., environmental exposure, broken skin, traumatized tissues, decreased ciliary action).

Newborn at 1 week   PED
(Also refer to Newborn, normal)

risk for Injury: risk factors may include physical (hyperbilirubinemia), environmental (inadequate safety precautions), chemical (drugs in breastmilk), psychological (inappropriate parental stimulation/interaction).

risk for Constipation/Diarrhea: risk factors may include type/amount of oral intake, medications or dietary intake of lactating mother, presence of allergies, infection.

risk for impaired Skin Integrity: risk factors may include excretions (ammonia formation from urea), chemical irritation from laundry detergent/diapering material, mechanical factors (e.g., long fingernails).

Newborn, postmature   PED
risk for impaired Gas Exchange: risk factors may include ventilation perfusion imbalances (meconium aspiration/pneumonitis).

Hypothermia may be related to decreased subcutaneous fat stores, poor metabolic reserves, exposure to cool environment, decreased ability to shiver possibly evidenced by reduction in body temperature, cool skin, pallor.

risk for imbalanced Nutrition: less than body requirements: risk factors may include placental insufficiency, decreased subcutaneous fat stores, decreased glycogen stores at birth (neonatal hypoglycemia).

risk for impaired Skin Integrity: risk factors may include dry/peeling skin, long fingernails, absence of vernix caseous.

Newborn, premature   PED
impaired Gas Exchange may be related to alveolar-capillary membrane changes (inadequate surfactant levels), altered blood flow (immaturity of pulmonary arteriole musculature), altered O_2 supply (immaturity of central nervous system and neuromuscular system, tracheobronchial obstruction), altered O_2-carrying capacity of blood (anemia), and cold stress, possibly evidenced by respiratory difficulties, inadequate oxygenation of tissues, and acidemia.

ineffective Breathing Pattern may be related to immaturity of the respiratory center, poor positioning, drug-related depression and metabolic imbalances, decreased energy/fatigue, possibly evidenced by dyspnea, tachypnea, periods of apnea, nasal flaring/use of accessory muscles, cyanosis, abnormal ABGs, and tachycardia.

risk for ineffective Thermoregulation: risk factors may include immature CNS development (temperature regulation center), decreased ratio of body mass to surface area, decreased subcutaneous fat, limited brown fat stores, inability to shiver or sweat, poor metabolic reserves, muted response to hypothermia, and frequent medical/nursing manipulations and interventions.

risk for deficient Fluid Volume: risk factors may include extremes of age and weight, excessive fluid losses (thin skin, lack of insulating fat, increased environmental temperature, immature kidney/failure to concentrate urine).

risk for disorganized Infant Behavior: risk factors may include prematurity (immaturity of CNS system, hypoxia), lack of containment/boundaries, pain, overstimulation, separation from parents.

risk for Injury [CNS damage]: risk factors may include tissue hypoxia, altered clotting factors, metabolic imbalances (hypoglycemia, electrolyte shifts, elevated bilirubin).

Newborn, small for gestational age   **PED**
(Refer to Newborn, growth deviations)

Newborn, special needs   **PED**
(Also refer to specific condition)

parental/family Grieving may be related to perceived loss of the perfect child, alterations of future expectations possibly evidenced by expression of distress at loss, sorrow, guilt, anger, choked feelings; interference with life activities, crying.

deficient parental Knowledge [Learning Need] regarding condition and infant care may be related to lack of/unfamiliarity with information resources, misinterpretation possibly evidenced by questions, concerns, misconceptions, hesitancy or inadequate performance of activities.

risk for impaired parent/infant Attachment: risk factors may include delay/interruption in bonding process (separation, physical barriers), perceived threat to infant's survival, stressors (financial, family needs), lack of appropriate response of newborn, lack of support between/from SOs.

risk for ineffective family Coping: risk factors may include situational crises, temporary preoccupation of SO trying to manage emotional conflicts and personal suffering being unable to perceive or act effectively in regards to infant's needs, temporary family disorganization.

risk for parental Social Isolation: risk factors may include perceived situational crisis, assuming sole/full-time responsibility for infant's care, lack of or inappropriate use of resources.

Nicotine abuse   **CH**

impaired Adjustment may be related to lack of motivation to change behavior, low state of optimism, absence of social/SO support for change, failure to intend to change behavior possibly evidenced by denial of health problem, failure to take action, failure to achieve optimal sense of control.

risk for Injury: risk factors may include smoking habits (e.g., in bed, while driving, near combustible chemicals/O_2), children playing with cigarettes/matches.

risk for impaired Gas Exchange: risk factors may include progressive airflow obstruction, decreased oxygen supply (carbon monoxide).

risk for ineffective peripheral Tissue Perfusion: risk factors may include reduction of arterial/venous blood flow.

Nicotine withdrawal   **CH**

Health-Seeking Behaviors (smoking cessation) may be related to concern about health status, acceptance of deleterious effects of smoking possibly evidenced by expressed concerns/desire to seek higher level of wellness.

risk for imbalanced Nutrition: more than body requirements: risk factors may include return of appetite, normalization of basal metabolic rate, eating in response to internal cues (substitution of food for activity of smoking).

risk for ineffective Therapeutic Regimen Management: risk factors may include economic difficulties, lack of support from SO/friends, continued enviromental exposure to second-hand smoke/smoking activity.

Nonketotic hyperglycemic-hyperosmolar coma   MS

deficient Fluid Volume may be related to excessive renal losses, inadequate oral intake, extremes of age, presence of infection possibly evidenced by sudden weight loss, dry skin/mucous membranes, poor skin tugor, hypotension, increased pulse, fever, change in mental status (confusion to coma).

decreased Cardiac Output may be related to decreased preload (hypovolemia), altered heart rhythm (hyper/hypokalemia) possibly evidenced by decreased hemodynamic pressures (e.g., CVP), ECG changes/dysrhythmias.

imbalanced Nutrition: less than body requirements may be related to inadequate utilization of nutrients (insulin deficiency), decreased oral intake, hypermetabolic state, possibly evidenced by recent weight loss, imbalance between glucose/insulin levels.

risk for Trauma: risk factors may include weakness, cognitive limitations/altered consciousness, loss of large- or small-muscle coordination (risk for seizure activity).

Obesity   CH

imbalanced Nutrition: more than body requirements may be related to excessive intake in relation to metabolic needs, possibly evidenced by weight 20% greater than ideal for height and frame, sedentary activity level, reported/observed dysfunctional eating patterns, and excess body fat by triceps skin fold/other measurements.

Activity Intolerance may be related to imbalance between oxygen supply and demand, and sedentary lifestyle, possibly evidenced by fatigue or weakness, exertional discomfort, and abnormal heart rate/BP response.

risk for Sleep Deprivation: risk factors may include sleep apnea.

risk for ineffective Breathing Pattern: risk factors may include obesity.

PSY

disturbed Body Image/chronic low Self-Esteem may be related to view of self in contrast to societal values, family/subcultural encouragement of overeating; control, sex, and love issues; possibly evidenced by negative feelings about body, fear of rejection/reaction of others, feeling of hopelessness/powerlessness, and lack of follow-through with treatment plan.

impaired Social Interaction may be related to verbalized/observed discomfort in social situations, self-concept disturbance, possibly evidenced by reluctance to participate in social gatherings, verbalization of a sense of discomfort with others, feelings of rejection, absence of/ineffective supportive SO(s).

Obesity-hypoventilation syndrome   CH
(Refer to Pickwickian syndrome)

Obsessive-Compulsive disorder   PSY

[severe] Anxiety may be related to earlier life conflicts possibly evidenced by repetitive actions, recurring thoughts, decreased social and role functioning.

risk for impaired Skin/Tissue Integrity: risk factors may include repetitive behaviors related to cleansing (e.g., hand-washing, brushing teeth, showering.

risk for ineffective Role Performance: risk factors may include psychological stress, health-illness problems.

Opioid abuse   CH/PSY
(Refer to Depressant abuse; Heroin abuse/withdrawal)

Oppositional defiant disorder   PED/PSY
ineffective Coping may be related to situational/maturational crisis, mild neurologic deficits,
    retarded ego development, dysfunctional family system, negative role models possibly
    evidenced by inability to meet age-appropriate role expectations, hostility toward others,
    defiant response to requests/rules, inability to delay gratification.
impaired Social Interaction may be related to retarded ego development, dysfunctional family,
    negative role models, neurologic impairment possibly evidenced by discomfort in social
    situations, difficulty playing/interacting with others, aggressive behavior, bullies/bosses/
    others, refusal to comply with requests of others.
chronic low Self-Esteem may be related to retarded ego development, lack of positive/repeated
    negative feedback, mild neurologic deficits, negative role models possibly evidenced by
    lack of eye contact, lack of self-confidence, physical risk taking, distraction of others to
    cover up own failures, projection of blame.
compromised/disabled family Coping may be related to anger, excessive guilt, blaming among
    family members regarding child's behavior, parental inconsistencies/disagreements
    regarding discipline and limit-setting, exhaustion of parental resources possibly evidenced
    by unrealistic parental expectations, rejection/overprotection of child, exaggerated expres-
    sions of anger/disappointment/despair.

Organic brain syndrome   CH
(Refer to Alzheimer's disease)

Osgood-Schlatter disease   PED
acute Pain may be related to inflammation and swelling in region of patellar tendon possibly
    evidenced by verbal reports, protective behavior, change in muscle tone.
impaired Walking may be related to inflammatory process (knee) possibly evidenced by
    impaired ability to walk desired distances, climb/descend stairs.
risk for ineffective Therapeutic Regimen Management: risk factors may include age (adoles-
    cent), perceived seriousness/benefit, competitive nature/peer pressure.

Osteitis deformans   CH
(Refer to Paget's disease)

Osteoarthritis (degenerative joint disease)   CH
(Refer to Arthritis, rheumatoid)
(Although this is a degenerative process versus the inflammatory process of rheumatoid
    arthritis, nursing concerns are the same.)

Osteomalacia   CH
(Refer to Rickets)

Osteomyelitis   MS/CH
acute Pain may be related to inflammation and tissue necrosis, possibly evidenced by verbal
    reports, guarding/distraction behaviors, self-focus, and autonomic responses (changes in
    vital signs).
Hyperthermia may be related to increased metabolic rate and infectious process, possibly
    evidenced by increased body temperature and warm/flushed skin.
ineffective bone Tissue Perfusion may be related to inflammatory reaction with thrombosis of
    vessels, destruction of tissue, edema, and abscess formation, possibly evidenced by bone
    necrosis, continuation of infectious process, and delayed healing.

risk for impaired Walking: risk factors may include inflammation and tissue necrosis, pain, joint instability.

deficient Knowledge [Learning Need] regarding pathophysiology of condition, long-term therapy needs, activity restriction, and prevention of complications may be related to lack of information/misinterpretation, possibly evidenced by statements of concern, questions, and misconceptions, and inaccurate follow-through of instructions.

Osteoporosis   CH

risk for Trauma: risk factors may include loss of bone density/integrity increasing risk of fracture with minimal or no stress.

acute/chronic Pain may be related to vertebral compression on spinal nerve/muscles/ligaments, spontaneous fractures, possibly evidenced by verbal reports, guarding/distraction behaviors, self-focus, and changes in sleep pattern.

impaired physical Mobility may be related to pain and musculoskeletal impairment, possibly evidenced by limited range of motion, reluctance to attempt movement/expressed fear of reinjury, and imposed restrictions/limitations.

Otitis media   PED

acute Pain may be related to inflammation, edema/pressure possibly evidenced by verbal/coded report, guarded behavior, restlessness, crying.

disturbed auditory Sensory Perception may be related to decreased sensory reception possibly evidenced by reported change in sensory acuity, auditory distortions, change in usual response to stimuli.

risk for delayed Development: risk factors may include auditory impairment, frequent otitis media.

Ovarian cancer   MS

(Also refer to Cancer)

disturbed Body Image may be related to surgical change in reproductive organs/surgical menopause, loss of hair and weight, possibly evidenced by negative feelings about body/sense of mutilation, preoccupation with change, feelings of helplessness/hopelessness, and change in social involvement.

ineffective Sexuality Patterns/Sexual Dysfunction may be related to change in sexual organs, postoperative menopause, vulnerability possibly evidenced by verbalizations of problem, inability in achieving desired satisfaction, alterations in relationship with SO.

Paget's disease, bone   CH

acute Pain may be related to compression/entrapment of nerves, joint degeneration possibly evidenced by reports of headache, back/joint pain.

Fatigue may be related to disease state/hypermetabolic condition possibly evidenced by overwhelming lack of energy, inability to maintain usual routines, tired.

disturbed Body Image may be related to physical deformities (enlarged skull, bowing of long bones) possibly evidenced by verbalization of feelings reflecting altered view of body, negative feelings about body, fear of rejection/reaction of others, change in social involvement.

disturbed auditory Sensory Perception may be related to altered sensory reception/transmission (nerve compression) possibly evidenced by decreased auditory acuity.

risk for impaired Walking: risk factors may include bowing of long bones, hobbling gait, joint stiffness/pain, paresis/paralysis.

risk for Injury/Falls: risk factors may include bone deformity/fragility, joint stiffness/pain, altered gait.

risk for decreased Cardiac Output: risk factors may include excessive circulatory demands (metabolically active and highly vascular nature of lesions).

Palliative care   CH
(Refer to Hospice Care)

Palsy, cerebral (spastic hemiplegia)   PED/CH
impaired physical Mobility may be related to muscular weakness/hypertonicity, increased deep tendon reflexes, tendency to contractures, and underdevelopment of affected limbs, possibly evidenced by decreased muscle strength, control, mass; limited range of motion, and impaired coordination.
compromised family Coping may be related to permanent nature of condition, situational crisis, emotional conflicts/temporary family disorganization, and incomplete information/understanding of client's needs, possibly evidenced by verbalized anxiety/guilt regarding client's disability, inadequate understanding and knowledge base, and displaying protective behaviors disproportionate (too little/too much) to client's abilities or need for autonomy.
delayed Growth and Development may be related to effects of physical disability, possibly evidenced by altered physical growth, delay or difficulty in performing skills (motor, social, expressive), and altered ability to perform self-care/self-control activities appropriate to age.

Pancreas transplantation   MS/CH
(Refer to Transplantation, recipient)

Pancreatic cancer   MS
(Also refer to Cancer)
acute Pain/[Discomfort] may be related to pressure on surrounding organs/nerves possibly evidenced by verbal reports, guarding/distraction behaviors, focus on self, and autonomic responses (changes in vital signs).
imbalanced Nutrition: less than body requirements may be related to inability to ingest/digest food, absorb nutrients, increased metabolic needs possibly evidenced by inadequate food intake, anorexia, abdominal pain after eating, weight loss, cachexia.
risk for Infection: risk factors may include stasis of body fluids (biliary obstruction), malnutrition.
risk for impaired Tissue Integrity: risk factors may include poor skin turgor, skeletal prominence, presence of edema/ascites, bile salt accumulation in the tissues.

Pancreatitis   MS
acute Pain may be related to obstruction of pancreatic/biliary ducts, chemical contamination of peritoneal surfaces by pancreatic exudate/autodigestion, extension of inflammation to the retroperitoneal nerve plexus, possibly evidenced by verbal reports, guarding/distraction behaviors, self-focusing, grimacing, autonomic responses (changes in vital signs), and alteration in muscle tone.
risk for deficient Fluid Volume: risk factors may include excessive gastric losses (vomiting, nasogastric suctioning), increase in size of vascular bed (vasodilation, effects of kinins), third-space fluid transudation, ascites formation, alteration of clotting process, hemorrhage.
imbalanced Nutrition: less than body requirements may be related to vomiting, decreased oral intake as well as altered ability to digest nutrients (loss of digestive enzymes/insulin), possibly evidenced by reported inadequate food intake, aversion to eating, reported altered taste sensation, weight loss, and reduced muscle mass.

risk for Infection: risk factors may include inadequate primary defenses (stasis of body fluids, altered peristalsis, change in pH secretions), immunosuppression, nutritional deficiencies, tissue destruction, and chronic disease.

Panic disorder   PSY

Fear may be related to unfounded morbid dread of a seemingly harmless object/situation possibly evidenced by physiologic symptoms, mental/cognitive behaviors indicative of panic, withdrawal from or total avoidance of situations that place client in contact with feared object.

[severe to panic] Anxiety may be related to unidentified stressors, contact with feared object/situation, limitations placed on ritualistic behavior possibly evidenced by attacks of immobilizing apprehension, physical/mental/cognitive behaviors indicative of panic, expressed feelings of terror/inability to cope.

Paranoid personality disorder   PSY

risk for other/self-directed Violence: risk factors may include perceived threats of danger, paranoid delusions, and increased feelings of anxiety.

[severe] Anxiety may be related to inability to trust (has not mastered tasks of trust versus mistrust), possibly evidenced by rigid delusional system (serves to provide relief from stress that justifies the delusion), frightened of other people and own hostility.

Powerlessness may be related to feelings of inadequacy, lifestyle of helplessness, maladaptive interpersonal interactions (e.g., misuse of power, force; abusive relationships), sense of severely impaired self-concept, and belief that individual has no control over situation(s), possibly evidenced by paranoid delusions, use of aggressive behavior to compensate, and expressions of recognition of damage paranoia has caused self and others.

disturbed Thought Processes may be related to psychological conflicts, increased anxiety, and fear, possibly evidenced by difficulties in the process and character of thought, interference with the ability to think clearly and logically, delusions, fragmentation, and autistic thinking.

compromised family Coping may be related to temporary or sustained family disorganization/role changes, prolonged progression of condition that exhausts the supportive capacity of SO(s), possibly evidenced by family system not meeting physical/emotional/spiritual needs of its members, inability to express or to accept wide range of feelings, inappropriate boundary maintenance; SO(s) describe(s) preoccupation with personal reactions.

Paranoid schizophrenia   PSY
(Refer to Schizophrenia)

Paraphilias   PSY

ineffective Sexuality Patterns may be related to conflict with sexual orientation or variant preferences possibly evidenced by alterations in achieving sexual satisfaction, difficulty achieving desired satisfaction in socially acceptable ways.

chronic low Self-Esteem may be related to psychosocial factors (e.g., achievement of sexual satisfaction in deviant ways), substance use possibly evidenced by expressions of shame/guilt, self-destructive behaviors, feelings of powerlessness, helplessness.

interrupted Family Processes may be related to situational crisis (e.g., revelation of sexual deviance/dysfunction) possibly evidenced by expressions of confusion about/difficulty dealing with situation, inappropriate boundary maintenance, family system does not meet emotional/security needs, failure to deal with traumatic experience constructively.

Paraplegia   MS/CH

(Also refer to Quadriplegia)

impaired Transfer Ability may be related to loss of muscle function/control, injury to upper extremity joints (overuse).

disturbed kinesthetic/tactile Sensory Perception: may be related to neurologic deficit with loss of sensory reception and transmission, psychological stress, possibly evidenced by reported/measured change in sensory acuity and loss of usual response to stimuli.

reflex urinary Incontinence/impaired Urinary Elimination may be related to loss of nerve conduction above the level of the reflex arc, possibly evidenced by lack of awareness of bladder filling/fullness, absence of urge to void, uninhibited bladder contraction, urinary tract infections—UTIs, kidney stone formation.

disturbed Body Image/ineffective Role Performance may be related to loss of body functions, change in physical ability to resume role, perceived loss of self/identity, possibly evidenced by negative feelings about body/self, feelings of helplessness/powerlessness, delay in taking responsibility for self-care/participation in therapy, and change in social involvement.

Sexual Dysfunction may be related to loss of sensation, altered function, and vulnerability, possibly evidenced by seeking of confirmation of desirability, verbalization of concern, alteration in relationship with SO, and change in interest in self/others.

Parathyroidectomy   MS

acute Pain may be related to presence of surgical incision and effects of calcium imbalance (bone pain, tetany), possibly evidenced by verbal reports, guarding/distraction behaviors, self-focus, and autonomic responses (changes in vital signs).

risk for excess Fluid Volume: risk factors may include preoperative renal involvement, stress-induced release of ADH, and changing calcium/electrolyte levels.

risk for ineffective Airway Clearance: risk factors may include edema formation and laryngeal nerve damage.

deficient Knowledge [Learning Need] regarding postoperative care/complications and long-term needs may be related to lack of information/recall, misinterpretation, possibly evidenced by statements of concern, questions, and misconceptions.

Parent-child relational problem   PED/PSY

impaired Parenting may be related to lack of/ineffective role model, lack of support between/from SO, interruption in bonding process, unrealistic expectations for self/child/partner, presence of stressors, lack of appropriate response of child to parent possibly evidenced by frequent verbalization of disappointment in child, inability to care for/discipline child, lack of parental attachment behaviors, child abuse/abandonment.

chronic low Self-Esteem/ineffective Role Performance may be related to view self as "poor" or ineffective parent, belief that seeking help is an admission of defeat/failure, psychiatric/physical illness of the child possibly evidenced by change in usual patterns/responsibility, expressions of lack of information, lack of follow-through of therapy, nonparticipation in therapy.

interrupted Family Process may be related to situational crisis of child/adolescent, maturational crisis (e.g., adolescence, midlife) possibly evidenced by expressions of confusion and difficulty coping with situation, family system not meeting physical/emotional/security needs of members, difficulty accepting help, parents not respecting each other's parenting practices.

compromised/disabled family Coping may be related to individual preoccupation with own emotional conflicts and personal suffering/anxiety about the crisis, temporary family disorganization, exhausted supportive capacity of members, highly ambivalent family relationships possibly evidenced by detrimental decisions/actions, neglected relationships, intolerance, agitation, depression, hostility, aggression.

readiness for enhanced family Coping may be related to surfacing of self-actualization goals possibly evidenced by expressing interest in making contact with another person experiencing a similar situation, moving in direction of health-promoting/enriching lifestyle, auditing/negotiating therapy program.

Parenteral feeding   MS/CH

risk for Infection: risk factors may include invasive procedure/surgical placement of feeding tube, malnutrition, chronic disease.

risk for Injury [multifactor]: risk factors may include catheter-related complications (air emboli, septic thrombophlebitis).

risk for imbalanced Fluid Volume: risk factors may include active loss/failure of regulatory mechanisms (specific to underlying disease process/trauma), complications of therapy—high glucose solutions/hyperglycemia (hyperosmolar nonketotic coma and severe dehydration), inability to obtain/ingest fluids.

Fatigue may be related to decreased metabolic energy production, increased energy requirements (hypermetabolic state, healing process), altered body chemistry (medications, chemotherapy) possibly evidenced by overwhelming lack of energy, inability to maintain usual routines/accomplish routine tasks, lethargy, impaired ability to concentrate.

Parkinson's disease   CH

impaired Walking may be related to neuromuscular impairment (muscle weakness, tremors, bradykinesia) and musculoskeletal impairment (joint rigidity), possibly evidenced by inability to move about the environment as desired, increased occurrence of falls.

impaired Swallowing may be related to neuromuscular impairment/muscle weakness, possibly evidenced by reported/observed difficulty in swallowing, drooling, evidence of aspiration (choking, coughing).

impaired verbal Communication may be related to muscle weakness and incoordination, possibly evidenced by impaired articulation, difficulty with phonation, and changes in rhythm and intonation.

Caregiver Role Strain may be related to illness, severity of care receiver, psychological/cognitive problems in care receiver, caregiver is spouse, duration of caregiving required, lack of respite/recreation for caregiver, possibly evidenced by feeling stressed, depressed, worried; lack of resources/support, family conflict.

Passive-Aggressive personality disorder   PSY

[moderate to severe] Anxiety may be related to unconscious conflict, unmet needs, threat to self-concept, difficulty in asserting self directly, feelings of resentment toward authority figures possibly evidenced by difficulty resolving feelings/trusting others, passive resistence to demands made by others, extraneous movements, irritability, argumentativeness.

ineffective Coping may be related to inadequate level of confidence in ability to cope/perception of control, uncertainty, high degree of threat, inadequate social support created by characteristics of relationships, disturbance in pattern of tension release possibly evidenced by verbalizations or inability to cope/ask for help, lack of goal-directed behavior/resolution of problem, lack or assertive behavior, use of forms of coping that impede adaptive behavior, decreased use of social supports, risk taking.

chronic low Self-Esteem may be related to retarded ego development, unmet dependency needs, early rejection by SO, lack of positive feedback possibly evidenced by lack of self-confidence, feelings of inadequacy, fear of asserting self, dependency on others, directing frustrations toward others by using covert aggressive tactics, not accepting responsibility for what happens as a result of maladaptive behaviors, failing to work through negative feelings.

Powerlessness may be related to interpersonal interaction, lifestyle of helplessness, dependency feelings, difficulty connecting own passive-resistent behaviors with hostility or resentment possibly evidenced by experiencing conscious hostility toward authority figures, releasing anger/hostility through others, getting back at others through aggravation.

PCP (phencyclidine) intoxication   MS/PSY
(Also refer to Hallucinogen abuse)

risk for self/other-directed Violence: risk factors may include drug abuse, psychotic symptomology, impulsivity.

risk for Trauma/Suffocation/Poisoning: risk factors may include clouded sensorium, increased muscle strength, myoclonic jerks/convulsions, ataxia, decreased pain perception, coma.

risk for ineffective cerebral Tissue Perfusion: risk factors may include alterations in blood flow (hypertensive crisis).

Pelvic inflammatory disease   OB/GYN/CH

risk for Infection [spread]: risk factors may include presence of infectious process in highly vascular pelvic structures, delay in seeking treatment.

acute Pain may be related to inflammation, edema, and congestion of reproductive/pelvic tissues, possibly evidenced by verbal reports, guarding/distraction behaviors, self-focus, and autonomic responses (changes in vital signs).

Hyperthermia may be related to inflammatory process/hypermetabolic state, possibly evidenced by increased body temperature, warm/flushed skin, and tachycardia.

risk for situational low Self-Esteem: risk factors may include perceived stigma of physical condition (infection of reproductive system).

deficient Knowledge [Learning Need] regarding cause/complications of condition, therapy needs, and transmission of disease to others may be related to lack of information/misinterpretation, possibly evidenced by statements of concern, questions, misconceptions, and development of preventable complications.

Periarteritis nodosa   MS/CH
(Refer to Polyarteritis [nodosa])

Pericarditis   MS

acute Pain may be related to tissue inflammation and presence of effusion, possibly evidenced by verbal reports of pain affected by movement/position, guarding/distraction behaviors, self-focus, and autonomic responses (changes in vital signs).

Activity Intolerance may be related to imbalance between O_2 supply and demand (restriction of cardiac filling/ventricular contraction, reduced cardiac output), possibly evidenced by reports of weakness/fatigue, exertional dyspnea, abnormal heart rate or BP response, and signs of heart failure.

risk for decreased Cardiac Output: risk factors may include accumulation of fluid (effusion) restricted cardiac filling/contractility.

Anxiety [specify level] may be related to change in health status and perceived threat of death, possibly evidenced by increased tension, apprehension, restlessness, and expressed concerns.

Perinatal loss/death of child   OB/CH
(Refer to Fetal demise)

Peripheral arterial occlusive disease   CH
(Refer to Arterial occlusive disease)

Peripheral vascular disease (atherosclerosis)   CH
ineffective peripheral Tissue Perfusion may be related to reduction or interruption of
    arterial/venous blood flow, possibly evidenced by changes in skin temperature/color, lack
    of hair growth, BP/pulse changes in extremity, presence of bruits, and reports of claudica-
    tion.
Activity Intolerance may be related to imbalance between O_2 supply and demand, possibly
    evidenced by reports of muscle fatigue/weakness and exertional discomfort (claudication).
risk for impaired Skin/Tissue Integrity: risk factors may include altered circulation with
    decreased sensation and impaired healing.

Peritonitis   MS
risk for Infection [spread/septicemia]: risk factors may include inadequate primary defenses
    (broken skin, traumatized tissue, altered peristalsis), inadequate secondary defenses
    (immunosuppression), and invasive procedures.
deficient Fluid Volume [mixed] may be related to fluid shifts from extracellular, intravascular,
    and interstitial compartments into intestines and/or peritoneal space, excessive gastric
    losses (vomiting, diarrhea, NG suction), hypermetabolic state, and restricted intake, possi-
    bly evidenced by dry mucous membranes, poor skin turgor, delayed capillary refill, weak
    peripheral pulses, diminished urinary output, dark/concentrated urine, hypotension, and
    tachycardia.
acute Pain may be related to chemical irritation of parietal peritoneum, trauma to tissues,
    accumulation of fluid in abdominal/peritoneal cavity, possibly evidenced by verbal
    reports, muscle guarding/rebound tenderness, distraction behaviors, facial mask of pain,
    self-focus, autonomic responses (changes in vital signs).
risk for imbalanced Nutrition: less than body requirements: risk factors may include
    nausea/vomiting, intestinal dysfunction, metabolic abnormalities, increased metabolic
    needs.

Persian Gulf syndrome   CH/MS
(Refer to Gulf War syndrome)

Personality disorders   PSY
(Refer to Antisocial; Borderline; Obsessive-Compulsive; Passive-Aggressive; or Paranoid
    personality disorders)

Pertussis   PED
ineffective Airway Clearance may be related to retained secretions, excessive thick tenacious
    mucus, infection possibly evidenced by dyspnea, adventitious breath sounds,
    hacking/paroxysmal cough.
deficient Fluid Volume may be related to decreased intake/anorexia, vomiting, increased insen-
    sible losses (fever/diaphoresis) possibly evidenced by decreased urine output/increased
    specific gravity, decreased BP, increased pulse rate, decreased skin/tongue turgor, dry
    skin/mucous membranes.
risk for Infection [transmission/secondary]: risk factors may include contagious nature of
    disease, stasis of body fluids, malnutrition, insufficient knowledge to avoid exposure to
    pathogens.

risk for imbalanced Nutrition: less than body requirements: risk factors may include inability to ingest food or absorb nutrients (anorexia, vomiting), increased metabolic demands.

risk for impaired Gas Exchange: risk factors may include compromised airways (tenacious mucus, inflammation), paroxysms of coughing, ventilation perfusion imbalance (atelectasis).

Pervasive developmental disorders   PED/PSY
(Refer to Autistic disorder; Rett's syndrome; Asperger's disorder)

Pheochromocytoma   MS
Anxiety [specify level] may be related to excessive physiologic (hormonal) stimulation of the sympathetic nervous system, situational crises, threat to/change in health status, possibly evidenced by apprehension, shakiness, restlessness, focus on self, fearfulness, diaphoresis, and sense of impending doom.

deficient Fluid Volume [mixed] may be related to excessive gastric losses (vomiting/diarrhea), hypermetabolic state, diaphoresis, and hyperosmolar diuresis, possibly evidenced by hemoconcentration, dry mucous membranes, poor skin turgor, thirst, and weight loss.

decreased Cardiac Output/ineffective Tissue Perfusion (specify) may be related to altered preload/decreased blood volume, altered SVR, and increased sympathetic activity (excessive secretion of catecholamines), possibly evidenced by cool/clammy skin, change in BP (hypertension/postural hypotension), visual disturbances, severe headache, and angina.

deficient Knowledge [Learning Need] regarding pathophysiology of condition, outcome, preoperative and postoperative care needs may be related to lack of information/recall, possibly evidenced by statements of concern, questions, and misconceptions.

Phlebitis   CH
(Refer to Thrombophlebitis)

Phobia   PSY
(Also refer to Anxiety Disorder, generalized)
Fear may be related to learned irrational response to natural or innate origins (phobic stimulus), unfounded morbid dread of a seemingly harmless object/situation, possibly evidenced by sympathetic stimulation and reactions ranging from apprehension to panic, withdrawal from/total avoidance of situations that place individual in contact with feared object.

impaired Social Interaction may be related to intense fear of encountering feared object/activity or situation and anticipated loss of control, possibly evidenced by reported change of style/pattern of interaction, discomfort in social situations, and avoidance of phobic stimulus.

Physical abuse   CH/PSY
(Refer to Abuse, physical; Battered child syndrome)

Pickwickian syndrome   CH
ineffective Breathing Pattern may be related to obesity, hypoventilation possibly evidenced by decreased pulmonary function, hypercapnia, hypoxia, reduced effect of CO_2 in stimulating respirations.

PID   GYN/OB/CH
(Refer to Pelvic inflammatory disease)

Pinkeye CH
(Refer to Conjunctivitis, bacterial)

Placenta previa OB
risk for deficient Fluid Volume: risk factors may include excessive vascular losses (vessel damage and inadequate vasoconstriction).
impaired fetal Gas Exchange: may be related to altered blood flow, altered oxygen carrying capacity of blood (maternal anemia), and decreased surface area of gas exchange at site of placental attachment, possibly evidenced by changes in fetal heart rate/activity and release of meconium.
Fear may be related to threat of death (perceived or actual) to self or fetus, possibly evidenced by verbalization of specific concerns, increased tension, sympathetic stimulation.
risk for deficient Diversional Activity: risk factors may include imposed activity restrictions/bedrest.

Plague, bubonic MS
Hyperthermia may be related to illness, dehydration possibly evidenced by increased body temperature, tachycardia, chills, confusion.
acute Pain may be related to inflammatory process, enlarged lymph nodes possibly evidenced by verbal/coded reports, expressive behavior, autonomic responses.
risk for deficient Fluid Volume: risk factors may include fever, decreased oral intake.
risk for impaired Skin Integrity: risk factors may include infectious process.

Plague, pneumonic MS
risk for Infection [spread]: risk factors may include contagious nature of disease, close contact with others.
Hyperthermia may be related to illness, dehydration possibly evidenced by increased body temperature, tachycardia, chills, severe headache, confusion.
impaired Gas Exchange may be related to alveolar-capillary membrane changes possibly evidenced by tachypnea, dyspnea, stridor, hemoptysis, cyanosis.
deficient Fluid Volume may be evidenced by fever/hypermetabolic state, decreased intake, bleeding diathesis (DIC) possibly evidenced by weakness, decreased venous filling, decreased BP, decreased skin turgor, dry mucous membranes, change in mental state.

Pleural effusion CH/MS
(Also refer to Hemothorax)
acute Pain may be related to inflammation/irritation of the parietal pleura, possibly evidenced by verbal reports, guarding/distraction behaviors, self-focus, and autonomic responses (changes in vital signs).
ineffective Breathing Pattern may be related to pain on inspiration, possibly evidenced by decreased respiratory depth, tachypnea, and dyspnea.
risk for impaired Gas Exchange: risk factors may include ventilation perfusion imbalance.

Pleurisy CH
acute Pain may be related to inflammation/irritation of the parietal pleura, possibly evidenced by verbal reports, guarding/distraction behaviors, self-focus, and autonomic responses (changes in vital signs).
ineffective Breathing Pattern may be related to pain on inspiration, possibly evidenced by decreased respiratory depth, tachypnea, and dyspnea.

risk for Infection, [pneumonia]: risk factors may include stasis of pulmonary secretions, decreased lung expansion, and ineffective cough.

Pneumonia   CH/MS
(Refer to Bronchitis; Bronchopneumonia)

Pneumoconiosis (black lung)   CH
(Refer to Pulmonary fibrosis)

Pneumothorax   MS
(Also refer to Hemothorax)
ineffective Breathing Pattern may be related to decreased lung expansion (fluid/air accumulation), musculoskeletal impairment, pain, inflammatory process, possibly evidenced by dyspnea, tachypnea, altered chest excursion, respiratory depth changes, use of accessory muscles/nasal flaring, cough, cyanosis, and abnormal ABGs.
risk for decreased Cardiac Output: risk factors may include compression/displacement of cardiac structures.
acute Pain may be related to irritation of nerve endings within pleural space by foreign object (chest tube), possibly evidenced by verbal reports, guarding/distraction behaviors, self-focus, and autonomic responses (changes in vital signs).

Polyarteritis nodosa   MS/CH
ineffective Tissue Perfusion (specify) may be related to reduction/interruption of blood flow, possibly evidenced by organ tissue infarctions, changes in organ function, and development of organic psychosis.
Hyperthermia may be related to widespread inflammatory process, possibly evidenced by increased body temperature and warm/flushed skin.
acute Pain may be related to inflammation, tissue ischemia, and necrosis of affected area, possibly evidenced by verbal reports, guarding/distraction behaviors, self-focus, and autonomic responses (changes in vital signs).
anticipatory Grieving may be related to perceived loss of self, possibly evidenced by expressions of sorrow and anger, altered sleep and/or eating patterns, changes in activity level, and libido.

Polycythemia vera   CH
Activity Intolerance may be related to imbalance between O_2 supply and demand, possibly evidenced by reports of fatigue/weakness.
ineffective Tissue Perfusion (specify) may be related to reduction/interruption of arterial/venous blood flow (insufficiency, thrombosis, or hemorrhage), possibly evidenced by pain in affected area, impaired mental ability, visual disturbances, and color changes of skin/mucous membranes.

Polyradiculitis   MS
(Refer to Guillain-Barré syndrome)

Postconcussion syndrome   CH
acute/chronic Pain may be related to neuronal damage possibly evidenced by reports of headache.
disturbed Thought Processes may be related to head injury possibly evidenced by memory deficit/problems, cognitive dissonance, distractibility.
Anxiety [specify level] may be related to situational crisis, change in health status/ongoing nature of disability, stress, unmet needs possibly evidenced by expressed concerns, apprehension, uncertainty, feelings of inadequacy, focus on self, difficulty concentrating.

Postmaturity syndrome   **PED**
(Refer to Newborn, postmature)

Postmyocardial syndrome   **CH**
(Refer to Dressler's syndrome)

Postoperative recovery period   **MS**
ineffective Breathing Pattern may be related to neuromuscular and perceptual/cognitive
    impairment, decreased lung expansion/energy, and tracheobronchial obstruction, possibly
    evidenced by changes in respiratory rate and depth, reduced vital capacity, apnea, cyanosis,
    and noisy respirations.
risk for imbalanced Body Temperature: risk factors may include exposure to cool environ-
    ment, effect of medications/anesthetic agents, extremes of age/weight, and dehydra-
    tion.
disturbed Sensory Perception (specify)/disturbed Thought Processes may be related to chemical
    alteration (use of pharmaceutical agents, hypoxia), therapeutically restricted environment,
    excessive sensory stimuli and physiologic stress, possibly evidenced by changes in usual
    response to stimuli, motor incoordination; impaired ability to concentrate, reason, and
    make decisions; and disorientation to person, place, and time.
risk for deficit Fluid Volume: risk factors may include restriction of oral intake, loss of fluid
    through abnormal routes (indwelling tubes, drains) and normal routes (vomiting, loss of
    vascular integrity, changes in clotting ability), extremes of age and weight.
acute Pain may be related to disruption of skin, tissue, and muscle integrity, musculoskele-
    tal/bone trauma, and presence of tubes and drains, possibly evidenced by verbal reports,
    alteration in muscle tone, facial mask of pain, distraction/guarding behaviors, narrowed
    focus, and autonomic responses.
impaired Skin/Tissue Integrity may be related to mechanical interruption of skin/tissues,
    altered circulation, effects of medication, accumulation of drainage, and altered metabolic
    state, possibly evidenced by disruption of skin surface/layers and tissues.
risk for Infection: risk factors may include broken skin, traumatized tissues, stasis of body
    fluids, presence of pathogens/contaminants, environmental exposure, and invasive proce-
    dures.

Postpartum period, 4–48 hours   **OB/CH**
risk for impaired parent/infant Attachment/Parenting: risk factors may include lack of
    support between/from SO(s), ineffective or no role model, anxiety associated with the
    parental role, unrealistic expectations, presence of stressors (e.g., financial, housing,
    employment).
risk for deficient Fluid Volume: risk factors may include excessive blood loss during delivery,
    reduced intake/inadequate replacement, nausea/vomiting, increased urine output, and
    insensible losses.
acute Pain/[Discomfort] may be related to tissue trauma/edema, muscle contractions, bladder
    fullness, and physical/psychological exhaustion, possibly evidenced by reports of cramp-
    ing (afterpains), self-focusing, alteration in muscle tone, distraction behaviors, and auto-
    nomic responses (changes in vital signs).
impaired Urinary Elimination may be related to hormonal effects (fluid shifts/continued
    elevation in renal plasma flow), mechanical trauma/tissue edema, and effects of medica-
    tion/anesthesia, possibly evidenced by frequency, dysuria, urgency, incontinence, or reten-
    tion.
Constipation may be related to decreased muscle tone associated with diastasis recti, prenatal
    effects of progesterone, dehydration, excess analgesia or anesthesia, pain (hemorrhoids,

episiotomy, or perineal tenderness), prelabor diarrhea and lack of intake, possibly evidenced by frequency less than usual pattern, hard-formed stool, straining at stool, decreased bowel sounds, and abdominal distention.

disturbed Sleep Pattern may be related to pain/discomfort, intense exhilaration/ excitement, anxiety, exhausting process of labor/delivery, and needs/demands of family members, possibly evidenced by verbal reports of difficulty in falling asleep/ not feeling well-rested, interrupted sleep, frequent yawning, irritability, dark circles under eyes.

Postpartum period, 4–6 weeks   OB/CH

disturbed Body Image may be related to unrealistic expectations of postpartum recovery, permanency of some changes possibly evidenced by verbalization of negative feelings about body, feelings of helplessness, preoccupation with change, focus on past appearance, fear of rejection/reaction of others.

risk for Sexual Dysfunction: risk factors may include health-related transition, changes in body function (including lactation), lack of privacy, fear of pregnancy.

readiness for enhanced family Coping may be related to sufficiently meeting individual needs and adaptive tasks possibly evidenced by family members moving in direction of health-promoting and enriching lifestyle.

readiness for enhanced Parenting may be related to sufficiently mastering skills/adapting to new responsibilities possibly evidenced by expressed willingness to enhance parenting, physical and emotional needs of infant/children are met, bonding evident.

Postpartum blues   OB/PSY
(Refer to Depression, postpartum)

Postpartum period, postdischarge to 4 weeks   OB/CH

risk for Fatigue: risk factors may include physical/emotional demands of infant and other family members, psychological stressors, continued discomfort.

Breastfeeding (specify) may be related to level of knowledge/support, previous experiences, infant gestational age, physical structure/characteristics of maternal breast possibly evidenced by maternal verbalizations regarding level of satisfaction, observations of feeding process, infant response/weight gain.

risk for imbalanced Nutrition: less than body requirements: risk factors may include intake insufficient to meet metabolic demands/correct existing deficiencies (e.g., lactation, anemia/excessive blood loss, infection/excessive tissue trauma, desire to regain prenatal weight).

risk for Infection: risk factors may include tissue trauma/broken skin, decreased Hb, invasive procedures, increased environmental exposure, malnutrition.

risk for ineffective Coping: risk factors may include situational/developmental changes, temporary family disorganization/role changes, little support provided by partner/family members.

ineffective Role Performance may be related to situational crisis (addition and demands of new family member, changes in responsibilities of family members) possibly evidenced by change in usual patterns or responsibility, conflict in roles.

Postpolio syndrome   CH

Anxiety [specify]/Fear may be related to change in health status, progressive/debilitating disease, change in role function/economic status possibly evidenced by expressed concerns, uncertainty, awareness of physiologic symptoms, worried, sleep disturbance, forgetfulness.

Fatigue may be related to disease state, stress, anxiety, sleep deprivation, depression possibly evidenced by overwhelming lack of energy, inability to maintain usual routines/level of physical activity, difficulty concentrating.

chronic Pain may be related to chronic physical disability, joint degeneration possibly evidenced by reports of deep aching pain, altered ability to continue previous activities, change in sleep patterns, reduced interaction with others.

impaired Walking/physical Mobility may be related to neuromuscular impairment, decreased muscle strength/atrophy, decreased endurance, pain, inability to stand erect (flat back syndrome) possibly evidenced by gait disturbances, joint/postural instability, decreased ability to perform gross motor skills.

Sleep Deprivation may be related to sleep apnea (central and obstructive), chronic pain possibly evidenced by daytime drowsiness, decreased ability to function, inability to concentrate.

impaired Swallowing may be related to neuromuscular impairment, pharyngeal muscle weakness possibly evidenced by coughing, choking, recurrent pulmonary infections.

ineffective Airway Clearance may be related to neuromuscular dysfunction (muscle weakness/atrophy), retained secretions possibly evidenced by diminished/adventitious breath sounds (chronic microatelectasis), poor cough (decreased pulmonary compliance, increased chest wall tightness).

Post-traumatic stress disorder   PSY

Post-Trauma Syndrome related to having experienced a traumatic life event, possibly evidenced by reexperiencing the event, somatic reactions, psychological/emotional numbness, altered lifestyle, impaired sleep, self-destructive behaviors, difficulty with interpersonal relationships, development of phobia, poor impulse control/irritability, and explosiveness.

risk for other-directed Violence: risk factors may include startled reaction, an intrusive memory causing a sudden acting out of a feeling as if the event were occurring; use of alcohol/other drugs to ward off painful effects and produce psychic numbing, breaking through the rage that has been walled off, response to intense anxiety or panic state, and loss of control.

ineffective Coping may be related to personal vulnerability, inadequate support systems, unrealistic perceptions, unmet expectations, overwhelming threat to self, and multiple stressors repeated over a period of time, possibly evidenced by verbalization of inability to cope or difficulty asking for help, muscular tension/headaches, chronic worry, and emotional tension.

dysfunctional Grieving may be related to actual/perceived object loss (loss of self as seen before the traumatic incident occurred as well as other losses incurred in/after the incident), loss of physiopsychosocial well-being, thwarted grieving response to a loss, and lack of resolution of previous grieving responses, possibly evidenced by verbal expression of distress at loss, anger, sadness, labile affect; alterations in eating habits, sleep/dream patterns, libido; reliving of past experiences, expression of guilt, and alterations in concentration.

interrupted Family Processes may be related to situational crisis, failure to master developmental transitions, possibly evidenced by expressions of confusion about what to do and that family is having difficulty coping, family system not meeting physical/emotional/spiritual needs of its members, not adapting to change or dealing with traumatic experience constructively, and ineffective family decision-making process.

Preeclampsia   OB
(Refer to Pregnancy-induced hypertension; Abruptio placentae)

Pregnancy, 1st trimester   OB/CH

risk for imbalanced Nutrition: less than body requirements: risk factors may include changes in appetite, insufficient intake (nausea/vomiting, inadequate financial resources and nutritional knowledge); meeting increased metabolic demands (increased thyroid activity associated with the growth of fetal and maternal tissues).

[Discomfort]/acute Pain may be related to hormonal influences, physical changes, possibly evidenced by verbal reports (nausea, breast changes, leg cramps, hemorrhoids, nasal stuffiness), alteration in muscle tone, restlessness, and autonomic responses (changes in vital signs).

risk for fetal Injury: risk factors may include environmental/hereditary factors and problems of maternal well-being that directly affect the developing fetus (e.g., malnutrition, substance use).

[maximally compensated] Cardiac Output may be related to increased fluid volume/maximal cardiac effort and hormonal effects of progesterone and relaxin (places the client at risk for hypertension and/or circulatory failure), and changes in peripheral resistance (afterload), possibly evidenced by variations in BP and pulse, syncopal episodes, presence of pathological edema.

readiness for enhanced family Coping may be related to situational/maturational crisis with anticipated changes in family structure/roles, needs sufficiently met and adaptive tasks effectively addressed to enable goals of self-actualization to surface, as evidenced by movement toward health-promoting and enriching lifestyle, choosing experiences that optimize pregnancy experience/wellness.

risk for Constipation: risk factors may include changes in dietary/fluid intake, smooth muscle relaxation, decreased peristalsis, and effects of medications (e.g., iron).

Fatigue/disturbed Sleep Pattern may be related to increased carbohydrate metabolism, altered body chemistry, increased energy requirements to perform ADLs, discomfort, anxiety, inactivity, possibly evidenced by reports of overwhelming lack of energy/inability to maintain usual routines, difficulty falling asleep/not feeling well-rested, interrupted sleep, irritability, lethargy, and frequent yawning.

risk for ineffective Role Performance: risk factors may include maturational crisis, developmental level, history of maladaptive coping, absence of support systems.

deficient Knowledge [Learning Need] regarding normal physiologic/psychological changes and self-care needs may be related to lack of information/recall and misinterpretation of normal physiologic/psychological changes and their impact on the client/family, possibly evidenced by questions, statements of concern, misconceptions and inaccurate follow-through of instructions/development of preventable complications.

Pregnancy, 2nd trimester   OB/CH

(Also refer to Pregnancy, 1st trimester)

risk for disturbed Body Image: risk factors may include perception of biophysical changes, response of others.

ineffective Breathing Pattern may be related to impingement of the diaphragm by enlarging uterus possibly evidenced by reports of shortness of breath, dyspnea, and changes in respiratory depth.

risk for [decompensated] Cardiac Output: risk factors may include increased circulatory demand, changes in preload (decreased venous return) and afterload (increased peripheral vascular resistance), and ventricular hypertrophy.

risk for excess Fluid Volume: risk factors may include changes in regulatory mechanisms, sodium/water retention.

ineffective Sexuality Patterns may be related to conflict regarding changes in sexual desire and expectations, fear of physical injury to woman/fetus possibly evidenced by reported difficulties, limitations or changes in sexual behaviors/activities.

Pregnancy, 3ʳᵈ trimester   OB/CH

(Also refer to Pregnancy, first and second trimesters)

deficient Knowledge [Learning Need] regarding preparation for labor/delivery, infant care may be related to lack of exposure/experience, misinterpretations of information possibly evidenced by request for information, statement of concerns/misconceptions.

impaired Urinary Elimination may be related to uterine enlargement, increased abdominal pressure, fluctuation of renal blood flow, and glomerular filtration rate (GFR) possibly evidenced by urinary frequency, urgency, dependent edema.

risk for ineffective [individual/] family Coping: risk factors may include situational/maturational crisis, personal vulnerability, unrealistic perceptions, absent/insufficient support systems.

risk for maternal Injury: risk factors may include presence of hypertension, infection, substance use/abuse, altered immune system, abnormal blood profile, tissue hypoxia, premature rupture of membranes.

Pregnancy, adolescent   OB/CH

(Also refer to Pregnancy—prenatal period)

interrupted Family Processes may be related to situational/developmental transition (economic, change in roles/gain of a family member), possibly evidenced by family expressing confusion about what to do, unable to meet physical/emotional/spiritual needs of the members, family inability to adapt to change or to deal with traumatic experience constructively; does not demonstrate respect for individuality and autonomy of its members, ineffective family decision-making process, and inappropriate boundary maintenance.

Social Isolation may be related to alterations in physical appearance, perceived unacceptable social behavior, restricted social sphere, stage of adolescence, and interference with accomplishing developmental tasks, possibly evidenced by expressions of feelings of aloneness/rejection/difference from others, uncommunicative, withdrawn, no eye contact, seeking to be alone, unacceptable behavior, and absence of supportive SO(s).

disturbed Body Image/situational/chronic low Self-Esteem may be related to situational/maturational crisis, biophysical changes, and fear of failure at life events, absence of support systems, possibly evidenced by self-negating verbalizations, expressions of shame/guilt, fear of rejection/reaction of other, hypersensitivity to criticism, and lack of follow-through/nonparticipation in prenatal care.

deficient Knowledge [Learning Need] regarding pregnancy, developmental/individual needs, future expectations may be related to lack of exposure, information misinterpretation, unfamiliarity with information resources, lack of interest in learning, possibly evidenced by questions, statement of concern/misconception, sense of vulnerability/denial of reality, inaccurate follow-through of instruction, and development of preventable complications.

risk for impaired Parenting: may be related to chronological age/developmental stage, unmet social/emotional/maturational needs of parenting figures, unrealistic expectation of self/infant/partner, ineffective role model/social support, lack of role identity, and presence of stressors (e.g., financial, social).

Pregnancy, high-risk   OB/CH

(Also refer to Pregnancy, 1ˢᵗ, 2ⁿᵈ, and 3ʳᵈ trimesters)

Anxiety [specify level] may be related to situational crisis, threat of maternal/fetal death (perceived or actual), interpersonal transmission/contagion possibly evidenced by increased tension, apprehension, feelings of inadequacy, somatic complaints, difficulty sleeping.

deficient Knowledge [Learning Need] regarding high-risk situation/preterm labor may be related to lack of exposure to/misinterpretation of information, unfamiliarity with individual risks and own role in risk prevention/management possibly evidenced by request for information, statement of concerns/misconceptions, inaccurate follow-through of instructions.

risk of maternal Injury: risk factors may include preexisting medical conditions, complications of pregnancy.

risk for Activity Intolerance: risk factors may include presence of circulatory/respiratory problems, uterine irritability.

risk for ineffective Therapeutic Regimen Management: risk factors may include client value system, health beliefs/cultural influences, issues of control, presence of anxiety, complexity of therapeutic regimen, economic difficulties, perceived susceptibility.

Pregnancy-induced hypertension   OB/CH
(Also refer to Eclampsia)

deficient Fluid Volume [isotonic] may be related to a plasma protein loss, decreasing plasma colloid osmotic pressure allowing fluid shifts out of vascular compartment, possibly evidenced by edema formation, sudden weight gain, hemoconcentration, nausea/vomiting, epigastric pain, headaches, visual changes, decreased urine output.

decreased Cardiac Output may be related to hypovolemia/decreased venous return, increased SVR, possibly evidenced by variations in BP/hemodynamic readings, edema, shortness of breath, change in mental status.

ineffective [uteroplacental] Tissue Perfusion: may be related to vasospasm of spiral arteries and relative hypovolemia, possibly evidenced by changes in fetal heart rate/activity, reduced weight gain, and premature delivery/fetal demise.

deficient Knowledge [Learning Need] regarding pathophysiology of condition, therapy, self-care/nutritional needs, and potential complications may be related to lack of information/recall, misinterpretation, possibly evidenced by statements of concern, questions, misconceptions, inaccurate follow-through of instructions/development of preventable complications.

Pregnancy, postmaturity   OB

Anxiety [specify level] may be related to situational crisis, threat to maternal/fetal health status (perceived or actual), interpersonal transmission/contagion possibly evidenced by increased tension, apprehension, irritability, feelings of inadequacy, somatic complaints.

ineffective [uteroplacental] Tissue Perfusion: may be related to placental involution/mutiple infarcts and villous degeneration possibly evidenced by decrease in fetal motion, meconium staining of amniotic fluid, intrauterine growth restriction, late decelerations on fetal monitor.

risk for maternal Injury: risk factors may include dysfunctional/prolonged labor.

risk for impaired fetal Gas Exchange: risk factors may include altered placental perfusion, cord compression (oligohydramnios).

risk for fetal Injury: risk factors may include prolonged labor (tissue hypoxia/acidosis), meconium aspiration.

Premature ejaculation   CH

Sexual Dysfunction may be related to altered body function, partner-related issues possibly evidenced by reports of disruption of sexual response pattern, inability to achieve desired satisfaction.

situational low Self-Esteem may be related to functional impairment, perceived failure to perform satisfactorily, rejection of other(s) possibly evidenced by self-negating verbalizations, expressions of helplessness/powerlessness.

Premature infant   **OB/PED**
(Refer to Neonate, premature newborn)

Premenstrual dysphoric disorder   **GYN/CH/PSY**
chronic Pain may be related to cyclic changes in female hormones affecting other systems (e.g., vascular congestion/spasms), vitamin deficiency, fluid retention, possibly evidenced by increased tension, apprehension, jitteriness, verbal reports, distraction behaviors, somatic complaints, self-focusing, physical and social withdrawal.
[moderate to panic] Anxiety may be related to cyclic changes in female hormones affecting other systems, possibly evidenced by feelings of inability to cope/loss of control, depersonalization, increased tension, apprehension, jitteriness, somatic complaints, and impaired functioning.
ineffective Coping may be related to personal vulnerability, threat to self-concept, multiple stressors (premenstrual symptoms) repeated over period of time, poor nutrition possibly evidenced by verbalization of difficulty coping/problem solving, inability to meet role expectation/seek help, emotional/muscular tension, chronic fatigue, insomnia, lack of appetite/overeating, high illness rate, decreased societal participation.
excess Fluid Volume may be related to abnormal alterations of hormonal levels, possibly evidenced by edema formation, weight gain, and periodic changes in emotional status/irritability.
deficient Knowledge [Learning Need] regarding pathophysiology of condition and self-care/treatment needs may be related to lack of information/misinterpretation, possibly evidenced by statements of concern, questions, misconceptions, and continuation of condition, exacerbating symptoms.

Premenstrual tension syndrome(PMS)   **GYN/CH/PSY**
(Refer to Premenstrual dysphoric disorder)

Prenatal substance abuse   **OB**
(Refer to Substance dependence/abuse, prenatal)

Pressure ulcer or sore   **CH**
(Also refer to Ulcer, decubitus)
ineffective peripheral Tissue Perfusion may be related to reduced/interrupted blood flow, possibly evidenced by presence of inflamed, necrotic lesion.
deficient Knowledge [Learning Need] regarding cause/prevention of condition and potential complications may be related to lack of information or misinterpretation, possibly evidenced by statements of concern, questions, misconceptions, and inaccurate follow-through of instructions.

Preterm labor   **OB/CH**
(Refer to Labor, preterm)

Prostate cancer   **MS**
(Also refer to Cancer; Prostatectomy)
[acute/chronic] Urinary Retention may be related to blockage of urethra possibly evidenced by sensation of bladder fullness, dysuria, small/frequent voiding, residual urine, bladder distention.

acute Pain may be related to destruction of tissues, pressure on surrounding structures, bladder distension possibly evidenced by verbal reports, restlessness, irritability, autonomic responses.

Prostatectomy   MS

impaired Urinary Elimination may be related to mechanical obstruction (blood clots, edema, trauma, surgical procedure, pressure/irritation of catheter/balloon) and loss of bladder tone, possibly evidenced by dysuria, frequency, dribbling, incontinence, retention, bladder fullness, suprapubic discomfort.

risk for deficient Fluid Volume: risk factors may include trauma to highly vascular area with excessive vascular losses, restricted intake, postobstructive diuresis.

acute Pain may be related to irritation of bladder mucosa and tissue trauma/edema, possibly evidenced by verbal reports (bladder spasms), distraction behaviors, self-focus, and autonomic responses (changes in vital signs).

disturbed Body Image may be related to perceived threat of altered body/sexual function, possibly evidenced by preoccupation with change/loss, negative feelings about body, and statements of concern regarding functioning.

                                                                    CH

risk for Sexual Dysfunction: risk factors may include situational crisis (incontinence, leakage of urine after catheter removal, involvement of genital area) and threat to self-concept/change in health status.

Prostatitis, acute   CH
(Also refer to Cystitis)

acute Pain/[Discomfort] may be related to inflammatory response possibly evidenced by reports of low back/pelvic pain, arthralgia, myalgia.

impaired Urinary Elimination may be related to localized swelling, UTI possibly evidenced by dysuria/burning on urination, frequency, urgency, nocturia, obstructed voiding.

Hyperthermia may be related to illness possibly evidenced by high fever, flushed/warm skin, chills.

risk for ineffective Therapeutic Regimen Management: risk factors may include length of therapy, perceived seriousness/benefits.

Prostatitis, chronic   CH
(Also refer to Cystitis)

acute Pain/[Discomfort] may be related to inflammatory response possibly evidenced by reports of back/pelvic/scrotal discomfort, low-grade fever.

impaired Urinary Elimination may be related to localized swelling, UTI possibly evidenced by dysuria, frequency, urgency.

Pruritus   CH

acute Pain may be related to cutaneous hyperesthesia and inflammation, possibly evidenced by verbal reports, distraction behaviors, and self-focus.

risk for impaired Skin Integrity: risk factors may include mechanical trauma (scratching) and development of vesicles/bullae that may rupture.

Psoriasis   CH

impaired Skin Integrity may be related to increased epidermal cell proliferation and absence of normal protective skin layers, possibly evidenced by scaling papules and plaques.

disturbed Body Image may be related to cosmetically unsightly skin lesions, possibly evidenced by hiding affected body part, negative feelings about body, feelings of helplessness, and change in social involvement.

Psychological abuse **CH/PSY**
(Refer to Abuse, psychological)

PTSD **PSY**
(Refer to Post-traumatic stress disorder)

Pulmonary edema, high altitude **MS**
(Refer to High altitude pulmonary edema)

Pulmonary edema **MS**
impaired Gas Exchange may be related to alveolar-capillary membrane changes (fluid collection/shifts into interstitial space/alveoli) possibly evidenced by dyspnea, restlessness, irritability, abnormal rate/depth of respirations, lethargy, confusion.
[moderate to severe] Anxiety may be related to change in health status, threat of death, interpersonal transmission possibly evidenced by expressed concerns, distressed, apprehension, extraneous movement.
risk for impaired spontaneous Ventilation: risk factors may include respiratory muscle fatigue, problems with secretion management.

Pulmonary embolus **MS**
ineffective Breathing Pattern may be related to tracheobronchial obstruction (inflammation, copious secretions or active bleeding), decreased lung expansion, inflammatory process, possibly evidenced by changes in depth and/or rate of respiration, dyspnea/use of accessory muscles, altered chest excursion, abnormal breath sounds (crackles, wheezes), and cough (with or without sputum production).
impaired Gas Exchange may be related to altered blood flow to alveoli or to major portions of the lung, alveolar-capillary membrane changes (atelectasis, airway/alveolar collapse, pulmonary edema/effusion, excessive secretions/active bleeding), possibly evidenced by profound dyspnea, restlessness, apprehension, somnolence, cyanosis, and changes in ABGs/pulse oximetry (hypoxemia and hypercapnia).
ineffective cardiopulmonary Tissue Perfusion may be related to interruption of blood flow (arterial/venous), exchange problems at alveolar level or at tissue level (acidotic shifting of the oxyhemoglobin curve), possibly evidenced by radiology/laboratory evidence of ventilation/perfusion mismatch, dyspnea, and central cyanosis.
Fear/Anxiety [specify level] may be related to severe dyspnea/inability to breathe normally, perceived threat of death, threat to/change in health status, physiologic response to hypoxemia/acidosis, and concern regarding unknown outcome of situation, possibly evidenced by restlessness, irritability, withdrawal or attack behavior, sympathetic stimulation (cardiovascular excitation, pupil dilation, sweating, vomiting, diarrhea), crying, voice quivering, and impending sense of doom.

Pulmonary fibrosis **CH**
impaired Gas Exchange may be related to alveolar-capillary membrane changes (inflammation, development of scar tissue), ventilation perfusion imbalance (retained secretions) possibly evidenced by dyspnea, adventitious breath sounds, nonproductive cough, cyanosis.
Anxiety [specify]/Fear may be related to situational crisis, change in health status, threat of death, interpersonal transmission possibly evidenced by expressed concerns, apprehension, uncertainty, ruminations, increased tension.

Activity Intolerance may be related to imbalance between oxygen supply/demand, generalized weakness possibly evidenced by exertional dyspnea, abnormal heart rate/BP response to activity, cyanosis.

risk for Infection: risk factors may include stasis of secretions, chronic disease, drug therapies (corticosteroids, cytotoxins).

Pulmonary hypertension   CH/MS

impaired Gas Exchange may be related to changes in alveolar membrane, increased pulmonary vascular resistance possibly evidenced by dyspnea, irritability, decreased mental acuity, somnolence, abnormal ABGs.

decreased Cardiac Output may be related to increased pulmonary vascular resistance, decreased blood return to left-side of heart possibly evidenced by increased heart rate, dyspnea, fatigue.

Activity Intolerance may be related to imbalance between oxygen supply and demand possibly evidenced by reports of weakness/fatigue, abnormal vital signs with activity.

[mild to moderate] Anxiety may be related to change in health status, stress, threat to self-concept possibly evidenced by expressed concerns, uncertainty, anxious, awareness of physiologic symptoms, diminished productivity/ability to problem-solve.

Pulmonic insufficiency   MS/CH
(Refer to Valvular heart disease)

Pulmonic stenosis   MS/CH
(Refer to Valvular heart disease)

Purpura, idiopathic thrombocytopenic   CH

ineffective Protection may be related to abnormal blood profile, drug therapy (corticosteroids or immunosuppressive agents), possibly evidenced by altered clotting, fatigue, deficient immunity.

Activity Intolerance may be related to decreased oxygen-carrying capacity/imbalance between O_2 supply and demand, possibly evidenced by reports of fatigue/weakness.

deficient Knowledge [Learning Need] regarding therapy choices, outcomes, and self-care needs may be related to lack of information/misinterpretation, possibly evidenced by statements of concern, questions, and misconceptions.

Pyelonephritis   MS

acute Pain may be related to acute inflammation of renal tissues, possibly evidenced by verbal reports, guarding/distraction behaviors, self-focus, and autonomic responses (changes in vital signs).

Hyperthermia may be related to inflammatory process/increased metabolic rate, possibly evidenced by increase in body temperature, warm/flushed skin, tachycardia, and chills.

impaired Urinary Elimination may be related to inflammation/irritation of bladder mucosa, possibly evidenced by dysuria, urgency, and frequency.

deficient Knowledge [Learning Need] regarding therapy needs and prevention may be related to lack of information/misinterpretation, possibly evidenced by statements of concern, questions, misconceptions, and recurrence of condition.

Pyloric stenosis   PED

deficient Fluid Volume may be related to excessive projectile vomiting possibly evidenced by decreased/concentrated urine, poor skin turgor, dry skin/mucous membranes, lethargy.

---

imbalanced Nutrition: less than body requirements may be related to inability to digest/absorb nutrients possibly evidenced by weight loss, poor muscle tone, pale conjunctiva/mucous membranes.

Quadriplegia   MS/CH
(Also refer to Paraplegia)

ineffective Breathing Pattern may be related to neuromuscular impairment (diaphragm and intercostal muscle function), reflex abdominal spasms, gastric distention, possibly evidenced by decreased respiratory depth, dyspnea, cyanosis, and abnormal ABGs.

risk for Trauma [additional spinal injury]: risk factors may include temporary weakness/instability of spinal column.

anticipatory Grieving may be related to perceived loss of self, anticipated alterations in lifestyle and expectations, and limitation of future options/choices, possibly evidenced by expressions of distress, anger, sorrow; choked feelings; and changes in eating habits, sleep, communication patterns.

total Self-Care Deficit related to neuromuscular impairment, evidenced by inability to perform self-care tasks.

Bowel Incontinence/Constipation may be be related to disruption of nerve innervation, perceptual impairment, changes in dietary/fluid intake, change in activity level possibly evidenced by inability to evacuate bowel voluntarily, increased abdominal pressure/distention, dry/hard formed stool, change in bowel sounds.

impaired bed/wheelchair Mobility may be related to loss of muscle function/control.

risk for Autonomic Dysreflexia: risk factors may include altered nerve function (spinal cord injury at T6 or above), bladder/bowel/skin stimulation (tactile, pain, thermal).

impaired Home Maintenance may be related to permanent effects of injury, inadequate/absent support systems and finances, and lack of familiarity with resources, possibly evidenced by expressions of difficulties, requests for information and assistance, outstanding debts/financial crisis, and lack of necessary aids and equipment.

Rabies   CH/MS
Hyperthermia may be related to infection possibly evidenced by fever, malaise.

risk for ineffective Airway Clearance: risk factors may include excessive salivation, muscle spasms (laryngeal/pharyngeal).

deficient Fluid Volume related to inability to drink (severe painful pharyngeal muscle spasms), excessive salivation possibly evidenced by extreme thirst, decreased skin turgor, decreased output/concentrated urine.

risk for trauma: risk factors may include progressive restlessness, uncontrollable excitement, inability to utilize physical restraints for safety.

Radiation therapy   CH
(Refer to Radiotherapy)

Radiation syndrome/poisoning   MS
(Dependent on dose and duration of exposure)

[severe] Anxiety/Fear may be related to situational crisis, threat of death, interpersonal transmission/contagion, unmet needs possibly evidenced by expressed concerns, scared, fearful, hoplessness, restlessness, agitation, anguish, increased tension, awareness of physiologic symptoms.

deficient Fluid Volume may be related to intractable nausea, vomiting, diarrhea (GI tissue necrosis and atrophy), interference with adequate intake (stomatitis/anorexia), hemorrhagic losses (thrombocytopenia) possibly evidenced by dry skin/mucous membranes, poor skin turgor, decreased venous filling, reduced pulse volume/pressure, hypotension, weakness, change in mentation.

acute Confusion may be related to CNS inflammation, decreased circulation/hypotension, effects of circulating toxins possibly evidenced by fluctuations in cognition/level of consciousness, agitation.

ineffective Protection may be related to effects of radiation, abnormal blood profile (leukopenia, thrombocytopenia, anemia), inadequate nutrition possibly evidenced by neurosensory alterations, anorexia, deficient immunity, impaired healing, altered clotting, disorientation.

risk for Infection: risk factors may include inadequate primary defenses (traumatized/necrotic tissues, stasis of body fluids, altered peristalsis), inadequate secondary defenses (anemia, leukopenia).

Sexual Dysfunction may be related to altered body function possibly evidenced by amenorrhea, decreased libido, infertility.

risk for disturbed visual Sensory Perception: risk factors may include altered sensory reception (development of cataracts).

Radical neck surgery   MS
(Refer to Laryngectomy)

Radiation therapy   CH
(Also refer to Brachytherapy; Cancer)

Nausea may be related to therapeutic procedure, irritation to GI system possibly evidenced by verbal reports, vomiting, gastric stasis.

imbalanced Nutrition: less than body requirements may be related to inability to ingest adequate nutrients (nausea, stomatitis, and fatigue), hypermetabolic state, possibly evidenced by weight loss, aversion to eating, reported altered taste sensation, sore, inflamed buccal cavity; diarrhea.

impaired Oral Mucous Membrane may be related to side effects of radiation, dehydration, and malnutrition, possibly evidenced by ulcerations, leukoplakia, decreased salivation, and reports of pain.

ineffective Protection may be related to inadequate nutrition, radiation, abnormal blood profile, disease state (cancer), possibly evidenced by impaired healing, deficient immunity, anorexia, fatigue.

Rape   CH

deficient Knowledge [Learning Need] regarding required medical/legal procedures, prophylactic treatment for individual concerns (STDs, pregnancy), community resources/supports may be related to lack of information, possibly evidenced by statements of concern, questions, misconceptions, and exacerbation of symptoms.

Rape-Trauma Syndrome (acute phase) related to actual or attempted sexual penetration without consent, possibly evidenced by wide range of emotional reactions, including anxiety, fear, anger, embarrassment, and multisystem physical complaints.

risk for impaired Tissue Integrity: risk factors may include forceful sexual penetration and trauma to fragile tissues.

PSY

ineffective Coping may be related to personal vulnerability, unmet expectations, unrealistic perceptions, inadequate support systems/coping methods, multiple stressors repeated over time, overwhelming threat to self, possibly evidenced by verbalizations of inability to cope or difficulty asking for help, muscular tension/headaches, emotional tension, chronic worry.

Sexual Dysfunction may be related to biopsychosocial alteration of sexuality (stress of post-trauma response), vulnerability, loss of sexual desire, impaired relationship with SO, possibly evidenced by alteration in achieving sexual satisfaction, change in interest in self/others, preoccupation with self.

Raynaud's disease   CH

acute/chronic Pain may be related to vasospasm/altered perfusion of affected tissues and ischemia/destruction of tissues, possibly evidenced by verbal reports, guarding of affected parts, self-focusing, and restlessness.

ineffective peripheral Tissue Perfusion may be related to periodic reduction of arterial blood flow to affected areas, possibly evidenced by pallor, cyanosis, coolness, numbness, paresthesia, slow healing of lesions.

deficient Knowledge [Learning Need] regarding pathophysiology of condition, potential for complications, therapy/self-care needs may be related to lack of information/misinterpretation, possibly evidenced by statements of concern, questions, and misconceptions; development of preventable complications.

Raynaud's phenomenon   CH
(Refer to Raynaud's disease)

Reactive attachment disorder   PED/PSY
(Refer to Anxiety disorders—PED)

Reflex sympathetic dystrophy   CH

acute/chronic Pain may be related to continued nerve stimulation, possibly evidenced by verbal reports, distraction/guarding behaviors, narrowed focus, changes in sleep patterns, and altered ability to continue previous activities.

ineffective peripheral Tissue Perfusion may be related to reduction of arterial blood flow (arteriole vasoconstriction), possibly evidenced by reports of pain, decreased skin temperature and pallor, diminished arterial pulsations, and tissue swelling.

disturbed tactile Sensory Perception may be related to altered sensory reception (neurologic deficit, pain), possibly evidenced by change in usual response to stimuli/abnormal sensitivity of touch, physiologic anxiety, and irritability.

risk for ineffective Role Performance: risk factors may include situational crisis, chronic disability, debilitating pain.

risk for compromised family Coping: risk factors may include temporary family disorganization and role changes and prolonged disability that exhausts the supportive capacity of SO(s).

Regional Enteritis   CH
(Refer to Crohn's disease)

Renal disease, end-stage   CH/MS
(Also refer to Renal failure, chronic)

death Anxiety may be related to progressive debilitating disease, unmet needs, inadequate support system, personal vulnerability, past negative experiences possibly evidenced by fear of the process of dying/loss of abilities, concerns of unfinished business, powerlessness/loss of control, denial of impending death.

Renal failure, acute   MS

excess Fluid Volume may be related to compromised regulatory mechanisms (decreased kidney function), possibly evidenced by weight gain, edema/anasarca, intake greater than output, venous congestion, changes in BP/CVP, and altered electrolyte levels.

imbalanced Nutrition: less than body requirements may be related to inability to ingest/digest adequate nutrients (anorexia, nausea/vomiting, ulcerations of oral mucosa, and increased metabolic needs) in addition to therapeutic dietary restrictions, possibly evidenced by lack of interest in food/aversion to eating, observed inadequate intake, weight loss, loss of muscle mass.

risk for Infection: risk factors may include depression of immunologic defenses, invasive procedures/devices, and changes in dietary intake/malnutrition.

disturbed Thought Processes may be related to accumulation of toxic waste products and altered cerebral perfusion, possibly evidenced by disorientation, changes in recent memory, apathy, and episodic obtundation.

Renal failure, chronic   CH/MS
(Also refer to Dialysis, general)

risk for decreased Cardiac Output: risk factors may include fluid imbalances affecting circulating volume/myocardial workload/systemic vascular resistance, alterations in rate/rhythm/cardiac conduction (electrolyte imbalances, hypoxia), accumulation of toxins (urea), soft-calcification.

risk for ineffective Protection: risk factors may include abnormal blood profile (suppressed erythropoietin production/secretion, decreased RBC production/survival, altered clotting factors), increased capillary fragility, inadequate nutrition.

disturbed Thought Processes may be related to physiologic changes—accumulation of toxins (e.g., urea, ammonia), metabolic acidosis, hypoxia, electrolyte imbalances, calcifications in brain possibly evidenced by disorientation, memory deficit, altered attention span, decreased ability to grasp idea, impaired ability to make decisions/problem-solve, changes in sensorium, irritability, psychosis.

risk for impaired Skin Integrity: risk factors may include altered metabolic state/circulation (anemia with tissue ischemia)/sensation (peripheral neuropathy), decreased skin turgor, reduced activity/immobility, accumulation of toxins in the skin.

risk for impaired Oral Mucous Membrane: risk factors may include decreased/lack of salivation, fluid restrictions, chemical irritation (conversion of urea in saliva to ammonia).

Renal transplantation   MS
(Also refer to Transplantation, recipient)

risk for excess Fluid Volume: risk factors may include compromised regulatory mechanism (implantation of new kidney requiring adjustment period for optimal functioning).

disturbed Body Image may be related to failure and subsequent replacement of body part and medication-induced changes in appearance, possibly evidenced by preoccupation with loss/change, negative feelings about body, and focus on past strength/function.

Fear may be related to potential for transplant rejection/failure and threat of death, possibly evidenced by increased tension, apprehension, concentration on source, and verbalizations of concern.

risk for Infection: risk factors may include broken skin/traumatized tissue, stasis of body fluids, immunosuppression, invasive procedures, nutritional deficits, and chronic disease.

CH

risk for ineffective Coping/compromised family Coping: risk factors may include situational crises, family disorganization and role changes, prolonged disease exhausting supportive capacity of SO/family, therapeutic restrictions/long-term therapy needs.

Repetitive motion injury   **CH**
(Refer to Carpal tunnel syndrome)

Respiratory distress syndrome, acute (ARDS)   MS
ineffective Airway Clearance may be related to loss of ciliary action, increased amount and
    viscosity of secretions, and increased airway resistance, possibly evidenced by presence of
    dyspnea, changes in depth/rate of respiration, use of accessory muscles for breathing,
    wheezes/crackles, cough with or without sputum production.
impaired Gas Exchange may be related to changes in pulmonary capillary permeability with
    edema formation, alveolar hypoventilation and collapse, with intrapulmonary shunting;
    possibly evidenced by tachypnea, use of accessory muscles, cyanosis, hypoxia per arterial
    blood gases (ABGs)/oximetry; anxiety and changes in mentation.
risk for deficient Fluid Volume: risk factors may include active loss from diuretic use and
    restricted intake.
risk for decreased Cardiac Output: risk factors may include alteration in preload (hypovolemia,
    vascular pooling, diuretic therapy, and increased intrathoracic pressure/use of
    ventilator/positive end-expiratory pressure–PEEP).
Anxiety [specify level]/Fear may be related to physiologic factors (effects of hypoxemia); situa-
    tional crisis, change in health status/threat of death; possibly evidenced by increased
    tension, apprehension, restlessness, focus on self, and sympathetic stimulation.
risk for barotrauma Injury: risk factors may include increased airway pressure associated with
    mechanical ventilation (PEEP).

Respiratory distress syndrome (premature infant) PED
(Also refer to Neonatal, premature newborn)
impaired Gas Exchange may be related to alveolar/capillary membrane changes (inadequate
    surfactant levels), altered oxygen supply (tracheobronchial obstruction, atelectasis), altered
    blood flow (immaturity of pulmonary arteriole musculature), altered oxygen-carrying
    capacity of blood (anemia), and cold stress, possibly evidenced by tachypnea, use of acces-
    sory muscles/retractions, expiratory grunting, pallor or cyanosis, abnormal ABGs, and
    tachycardia.
impaired Spontaneous Ventilation may be related to respiratory muscle fatigue and metabolic
    factors, possibly evidenced by dyspnea, increased metabolic rate, restlessness, use of acces-
    sory muscles, and abnormal ABGs.
risk for Infection: risk factors may include inadequate primary defenses (decreased ciliary
    action, stasis of body fluids, traumatized tissues), inadequate secondary defenses (defi-
    ciency of neutrophils and specific immunoglobulins), invasive procedures, and malnutri-
    tion (absence of nutrient stores, increased metabolic demands).
risk for ineffective gastrointestinal Tissue Perfusion: risk factors may include persistent fetal
    circulation and exchange problems.
risk for impaired parent/infant Attachment: risk factors may include premature/ill infant who
    is unable to effectively initiate parental contact (altered behavioral organization), separa-
    tion, physical barriers, anxiety associated with the parental role/demands of infant.

Respiratory syncytial virus   PED
impaired Gas Exchange may be related to inflammation of airways, ventilation perfusion
    imbalance (areas of consolidation), apnea possibly evidenced by dyspnea, abnormal
    ABGs/hypoxia.
ineffective Airway Clearance may be related to infection, retained secretions, exudate in alve-
    oli, inflammation of airways possibly evidenced by dyspnea, adventitious breath sounds,
    cough.

risk for deficient Fluid Volume: risk factors may include increased insensible losses (fever/diaphoresis), decreased oral intake.

Retinal detachment   CH

disturbed visual Sensory Perception related to decreased sensory reception, possibly evidenced by visual distortions, decreased visual field, and changes in visual acuity.

[mild to moderate] Anxiety may be related to situational crisis, change in health status/role function possibly evidenced by expressed concerns, apprehension, uncertainty, focus on self.

deficient Knowledge [Learning Need] regarding therapy, prognosis, and self-care needs may be related to lack of information/misconceptions, possibly evidenced by statements of concern and questions.

risk for impaired Home Maintenance: risk factors may include visual limitations/activity/restrictions.

Rett's syndrome   PED/PSY

(Also refer to Autistic disorder)

delayed Growth and Development may be related to effects of physical/mental disability, possibly evidenced by altered physical growth; delay/inability in performing skills and self-care/self-control activities appropriate for age.

impaired Walking/physical Mobility may be related to neuromuscular impairment, joint stiffness/contractures, disuse possibly evidenced by limited range of motion, inability to perform gross motor skills/walk/reposition self.

risk for Trauma: risk factors may include cognitive deficits, lack of muscle tone/coordination, seizure activity.

imbalanced Nutrition: less than body requirements may be related to poor muscle tone, dependence on others/inability to meet own needs possibly evidenced by weak and ineffective sucking/swallowing and observed lack of adequate intake with weight loss/failure to gain.

risk for dysfunctional Grieving: risk factors may include loss of "the perfect child," chronic condition requiring long-term care, and unresolved feelings.

Reye's syndrome   PED

deficient Fluid Volume [isotonic] may be related to failure of regulatory mechanism (diabetes insipidus), excessive gastric losses (pernicious vomiting), and altered intake, possibly evidenced by increased/dilute urine output, sudden weight loss, decreased venous filling, dry mucous membranes, decreased skin turgor, hypotension, and tachycardia.

ineffective cerebral Tissue Perfusion may be related to diminished arterial/venous blood flow and hypovolemia, possibly evidenced by memory loss, altered consciousness, and restlessness/agitation.

risk for Trauma: risk factors may include generalized weakness, reduced coordination, and cognitive deficits.

ineffective Breathing Pattern may be related to decreased energy and fatigue, cognitive impairment, tracheobronchial obstruction, and inflammatory process (aspiration pneumonia), possibly evidenced by tachypnea, abnormal ABGs, cough, and use of accessory muscles.

Rheumatic fever   PED

acute Pain may be related to migratory inflammation of joints, possibly evidenced by verbal reports, guarding/distraction behaviors, self-focus, and autonomic responses (changes in vital signs).

Hyperthermia may be related to inflammatory process/hypermetabolic state, possibly evidenced by increased body temperature, warm/flushed skin, and tachycardia.

Activity Intolerance may be related to generalized weakness, joint pain, and medical restrictions/bedrest, possibly evidenced by reports of fatigue, exertional discomfort, and abnormal heart rate in response to activity.

risk for decreased Cardiac Output: risk factors may include cardiac inflammation/enlargement and altered contractility.

Rheumatic heart disease   PED/MS
(Also refer to Valvular heart disease)

Activity Intolerance may be related to imbalance between O_2 supply/demand, generalized weakness, and prolonged bedrest/sedentary lifestyle, possibly evidenced by reported/observed weakness, fatigue; changes in vital signs, presence of dysrhythmias; dyspnea, pallor.

impaired Adjustment may be related to health status requiring change in lifestyle/restriction of desired activities, unrealistic expectations, negative attitudes possibly evidenced by denial of situation, demonstration of nonacceptance of health status, failure to achieve optimal sense of control.

risk for ineffective Therapeutic Regimen Management: risk factors may include complexity/duration of therapeutic regimen, imposed restrictions or limitations, economic difficulties, family patterns of healthcare, perceived seriousness/benefits.

risk for impaired Gas Exchange: risk factors may include alveolar-capillary membrane changes (fluid collection/shifts into interstitial space/alveoli).

Rhinitis, allergic   CH
(Refer to Hay fever)

Rickets   PED
delayed Growth and Development may be related to dietary deficiencies/indiscretions, malabsorption syndrome, and lack of exposure to sunlight, possibly evidenced by altered physical growth and delay or difficulty in performing motor skills typical for age.

deficient Knowledge [Learning Need] regarding cause, pathophysiology, therapy needs and prevention may be related to lack of information, possibly evidenced by statements of concern, questions, misconceptions, and inaccurate follow-through of instructions.

Ringworm, tinea   CH
(Also refer to Athlete's Foot)

impaired Skin Integrity may be related to fungal infection of the dermis, possibly evidenced by disruption of skin surfaces/presence of lesions.

deficient Knowledge [Learning Need] regarding infectious nature, therapy, and self-care needs may be related to lack of information/misinformation, possibly evidenced by statements of concern, questions, and recurrence/spread.

Rocky Mountain spotted fever   CH/MS
(Refer to Typhus)

RSD   CH
(Refer to Reflex sympathetic dystrophy)

RSV   PED
(Refer to Respiratory syncytial virus)

Rubella   **PED/CH**

acute Pain/[Discomfort] may be related to inflammatory effects of viral infection and presence of desquamating rash, possibly evidenced by verbal reports, distraction behaviors/restlessness.

deficient Knowledge [Learning Need] regarding contagious nature, possible complications, and self-care needs may be related to lack of information/misinterpretations, possibly evidenced by statements of concern, questions, and inaccurate follow-through of instructions.

Rubeola   **PED/CH**
(Refer to Measles)

Ruptered intervertebral disk   **CH/MS**
(Refer to Herniated nucleus pulposus)

SARS (Sudden acute respiratory syndrome)   **MS**

Hyperthermia may be related to inflammatory process possibly evidenced by high fever, chills, rigors, headache.

acute Pain/[Discomfort] may be related to inflammation/circulating toxins possibly evidenced by reports of myalgia, headache, malaise.

impaired Gas Exchange may be related to ventilation perfusion imbalance (interstitial infiltrates, areas of consolidation) possibly evidenced by dyspnea, changes in mentation/level of consciousness, restlessness, hypoxemia.

risk for impaired spontaneous Ventilation: risk factors may include hypermetabolic state/infection, depletion of energy stores, respiratory muscle fatigue.

risk for ineffective Protection: risk factors may include inadequate nutrition, abnormal blood profile (leukopnea, thrombocytopnia).

Scabies   **CH**

impaired Skin Integrity may be related to presence of invasive parasite and development of pruritus, possibly evidenced by disruption of skin surface and inflammation.

deficient Knowledge [Learning Need] regarding communicable nature, possible complications, therapy, and self-care needs may be related to lack of information/misinterpretation, possibly evidenced by questions and statements of concern about spread to others.

Scarlet fever   **PED**

Hyperthermia may be related to effects of circulating toxins, possibly evidenced by increased body temperature, warm/flushed skin, and tachycardia.

Pain/[Discomfort] may be related to inflammation of mucous membranes and effects of circulating toxins (malaise, fever), possibly evidenced by verbal reports, distraction behaviors, guarding (decreased swallowing), and self-focus.

risk for deficient Fluid Volume: risk factors may include hypermetabolic state (hyperthermia) and reduced intake.

Schizoaffective disorder   **PSY**

risk for other/self-directed Violence: risk factors may include depressed mood, feelings of worthlessness, hoplessness, unsatisfactory parent/child relationship, feelings of abandonment by SOs, anger turned inward/directed at the environment, punitive superego, irrational feeelings of guilt, numerous failures, misinterpretation of reality.

Social Isolation may be related to developmental regression, depressed mood, feelings of worthlessness, egocentric behaviors (offending others and discouraging relationships), delusional thinking, fear of failure, unresolved grief possibly evidenced by sad/dull affect, absence of support systems, uncommunicative/withdrawn/catatonic behavior, absence of eye contact, preoccupation with own thoughts, repetitive/meaningless actions.

imbalanced Nutrition: less than body requirements may be related to energy ezpenditure in excess of intake, refusal/inability to take time to eat, lack of attention to/recognition of hunger cues possibly evidenced by lack of interest in food, weight loss, pale conjunctiva and mucous membranes, poor muscle tone/skin turgor, amenorrhea, abnormal laboratory studies.

Schizophrenia (schizophrenic disorders)   PSY

disturbed Thought Processes may be related to disintegration of thinking processes, impaired judgment, presence of psychological conflicts, disintegrated ego boundaries, sleep disturbance, ambivalence and concomitant dependence, possibly evidenced by impaired ability to reason/problem-solve, inappropriate affect, presence of delusional system, command hallucinations, obsessions, ideas of reference, cognitive dissonance.

Social Isolation may be related to alterations in mental status, mistrust of others/delusional thinking, unacceptable social behaviors, inadequate personal resources, and inability to engage in satisfying personal relationships, possibly evidenced by difficulty in establishing relationships with others; dull affect, uncommunicative/withdrawn behavior, seeking to be alone, inadequate/absent significant purpose in life, and expression of feelings of rejection.

risk for self/other-directed Violence: risk factors may include disturbances of thinking/feeling (depression, paranoia, suicidal ideation), lack of development of trust and appropriate interpersonal relationships, catatonic/manic excitement, toxic reactions to drugs (alcohol).

ineffective Coping may be related to personal vulnerability, inadequate support system(s), unrealistic perceptions, inadequate coping methods, and disintegration of thought processes, possibly evidenced by impaired judgment/cognition and perception, diminished problem-solving/decision-making capacities, poor self-concept, chronic anxiety, depression, inability to perform role expectations, and alteration in social participation.

CH

interrupted Family Processes/disabled family Coping may be related to ambivalent family system/relationships, change of roles, and difficulty of family member in coping effectively with client's maladaptive behaviors, possibly evidenced by deterioration in family functioning, ineffective family decision-making process, difficulty relating to each other, client's expressions of despair at family's lack of reaction/involvement, neglectful relationships with client, extreme distortion regarding client's health problem including denial about its existence/severity or prolonged overconcern.

ineffective Health Maintenance/impaired Home Maintenance may be related to impaired cognitive/emotional functioning, altered ability to make deliberate and thoughtful judgments, altered communication, and lack of/inappropriate use of material resources, possibly evidenced by inability to take responsibility for meeting basic health practices in any or all functional areas and demonstrated lack of adaptive behaviors to internal or external environmental changes, disorderly surroundings, accumulation of dirt/unwashed clothes, repeated hygienic disorders.

Self-Care Deficit [specify] may be related to perceptual and cognitive impairment, immobility (withdrawal/isolation and decreased psychomotor activity), and side effects of psychotropic medications, possibly evidenced by inability or difficulty in areas of feeding self, keeping body clean, dressing appropriately, toileting self, and/or changes in bowel/bladder elimination.

Sciatica   CH

acute/chronic Pain may be related to peripheral nerve root compression, possibly evidenced by verbal reports, guarding/distraction behaviors, and self-focus.

impaired physical Mobility may be related to neurologic pain and muscular involvement, possibly evidenced by reluctance to attempt movement and decreased muscle strength/mass.

Scleroderma   CH

(Also refer to Lupus Erythematosus, Systemic—SLE)

impaired physical Mobility may be related to musculoskeletal impairment and associated pain, possibly evidenced by decreased strength, decreased range of motion, and reluctance to attempt movement.

ineffective Tissue Perfusion, (specify) may be related to reduced arterial blood flow (arteriolar vasoconstriction), possibly evidenced by changes in skin temperature/color, ulcer formation, and changes in organ function (cardiopulmonary, GI, renal).

imbalanced Nutrition: less than body requirements may be related to inability to ingest/digest/absorb adequate nutrients (sclerosis of the tissues rendering mouth immobile, decreased peristalsis of esophagus/small intestines, atrophy of smooth muscle of colon), possibly evidenced by weight loss, decreased intake/food, and reported/observed difficulty swallowing.

impaired Adjustment may be related to disability requiring change in lifestyle, inadequate support systems, assault to self-concept, and altered locus of control, possibly evidenced by verbalization of nonacceptance of health status change and lack of movement toward independence/future-oriented thinking.

disturbed Body Image may be related to skin changes with induration, atrophy, and fibrosis, loss of hair, and skin and muscle contractures, possibly evidenced by verbalization of negative feelings about body, focus on past strength/function or appearance, fear of rejection/reaction by others, hiding body part, and change in social involvement.

Scoliosis   PED

disturbed Body Image may be related to altered body structure, use of therapeutic device(s), and activity restrictions, possibly evidenced by negative feelings about body, change in social involvement, and preoccupation with situation or refusal to acknowledge problem.

deficient Knowledge [Learning Need] regarding pathophysiology of condition, therapy needs, and possible outcomes may be related to lack of information/misinterpretation, possibly evidenced by statements of concern, questions, misconceptions, and inaccurate follow-through of instructions.

impaired Adjustment may be related to lack of comprehension of long-term consequences of behavior, possibly evidenced by failure to adhere to treatment regimen/keep appointments and evidence of failure to improve.

Seasonal affective disorder   PSY

(Refer to Affective disorder, seasonal)

Sedative intoxication/abuse   CH/PSY

(Refer to Depressant abuse)

Seizure disorder   CH

deficient Knowledge [Learning Need] regarding condition and medication control may be related to lack of information/misinterpretations, scarce financial resources, possibly evidenced by questions, statements of concern/misconceptions, incorrect use of anticonvulsant medication, recurrent episodes/uncontrolled seizures.

chronic low Self-Esteem/disturbed Personal Identity may be related to perceived neurologic functional change/weakness, perception of being out of control, stigma associated with condition, possibly evidenced by negative feelings about "brain"/self, change in social involvement, feelings of helplessness, and preoccupation with perceived change or loss.

impaired Social Interaction may be related to unpredictable nature of condition and self-concept disturbance, possibly evidenced by decreased self-assurance, verbalization of concern, discomfort in social situations, inability to receive/communicate a satisfying sense of belonging/caring, and withdrawal from social contacts/activities.

risk for Trauma/Suffocation: risk factors may include weakness, balancing difficulties, cognitive limitations/altered consciousness, loss of large- or small-muscle coordination (during seizure).

Separation anxiety disorder   PED/PSY
(Refer to Anxiety disorders—PED)

Sepsis   MS
(Also refer to Sepsis, Puerperal)

ineffective Tissue Perfusion (specify) may be related to changes in arterial/venous blood flow (selective vasoconstriction, presence of microemboli) and hypovolemia, possibly evidenced by changes in skin temperature/color, changes in blood/pulse pressure; changes in sensorium, and decreased urinary output.

risk for deficient Fluid Volume: risk factors may include marked increase in vascular compartment/massive vasodilation, vascular shifts to interstitial space, and reduced intake.

risk for decreased Cardiac Output: risk factors may include decreased preload (venous return and circulating volume), altered afterload (increased SVR), negative inotropic effects of hypoxia, complement activation, and lysosomal hydrolase.

Sepsis, puerperal   OB
(Also refer to Septicemia)

risk for Infection [spread/septic shock]: risk factors may include presence of infection, broken skin, and/or traumatized tissues, rupture of amniotic membranes, high vascularity of involved area, stasis of body fluids, invasive procedures, and/or increased environmental exposure, chronic disease (e.g., diabetes mellitus, anemia, malnutrition), altered immune response, and untoward effect of medications (e.g., opportunistic/secondary infection).

Hyperthermia may be related to inflammatory process/hypermetabolic state, possibly evidenced by increase in body temperature, warm/flushed skin, and tachycardia.

risk for impaired parent/infant Attachment: risk factors may include interruption in bonding process, physical illness, perceived threat to own survival.

risk for ineffective peripheral Tissue Perfusion: risk factors may include interruption/reduction of blood flow (presence of infectious thrombi).

Septicemia   MS
(Refer to Sepsis)

Serum sickness   CH

acute Pain may be related to inflammation of the joints and skin eruptions, possibly evidenced by verbal reports, guarding/distraction behaviors, and self-focus.

deficient Knowledge [Learning Need] regarding nature of condition, treatment needs, potential complications, and prevention of recurrence may be related to lack of information/misinterpretation, possibly evidenced by statements of concern, questions, misconceptions, and inaccurate follow-through of instructions.

Sexual desire disorder   **PSY**

Sexual Dysfunction may be related to boredom/conflict in relationship, depression, hormonal imbalance, harmful relationships/traumatic events in childhood possibly evidenced by loss of sexual desire, disruption of sexual response pattern, alteration in relationship with SO.

Anxiety (specify) may be related to situational crisis, stress, unconscious conflict about essential values, unmet needs possibly evidenced by expressed concerns, distressed, feelings of inadequacy, fear of unspecific consequences.

situational low Self-Esteem may be related to perceived functional impairment, emotional insecurity, rejection by SO possibly evidenced by expressions of helplessness, self-negating verbalizations, change in involvement with partner.

Severe acute respiratory syndrome   **MS**
(Refer to SARS)

Sexual dysfunctions   **PSY**
(Refer to Dyspareunia; Erectile dysfunction; Sexual desire disorder; Vaginismus)

Sexually transmitted disease   **GYN/CH**

risk for Infection [transmission]: risk factors may include contagious nature of infecting agent and insufficient knowledge to avoid exposure to/transmission of pathogens.

impaired Skin/Tissue Integrity may be related to invasion of/irritation by pathogenic organism(s), possibly evidenced by disruptions of skin/tissue and inflammation of mucous membranes.

deficient Knowledge [Learning Need] regarding condition, prognosis/complications, therapy needs, and transmission may be related to lack of information/misinterpretation, lack of interest in learning, possibly evidenced by statements of concern, questions, misconceptions; inaccurate follow-through of instructions, and development of preventable complications.

Shingles   **CH**
(Refer to Herpes zoster)

Shock   **MS**
(Also refer to Shock, cardiogenic; Shock, hypovolemic/hemorrhagic; Sepsis)

ineffective Tissue Perfusion (specify) may be related to changes in circulating volume and/or vascular tone, possibly evidenced by changes in skin color/temperature and pulse pressure, reduced blood pressure, changes in mentation, and decreased urinary output.

Anxiety [specify level] may be related to change in health status and threat of death, possibly evidenced by increased tension, apprehension, sympathetic stimulation, restlessness, and expressions of concern.

Shock, cardiogenic   **MS**
(Also refer to Shock)

decreased Cardiac Output may be related to structural damage, decreased myocardial contractility, and presence of dysrhythmias, possibly evidenced by ECG changes, variations in hemodynamic readings, jugular vein distention, cold/clammy skin, diminished peripheral pulses, and decreased urinary output.

risk for impaired Gas Exchange: risk factors may include ventilation perfusion imbalance, alveolar-capillary membrane changes.

Shock, hypovolemic/hemorrhagic   **MS**
(Also refer to Shock)

deficient Fluid Volume [isotonic] may be related to excessive vascular loss, inadequate intake/replacement, possibly evidenced by hypotension, tachycardia, decreased pulse volume and pressure, change in mentation, and decreased/concentrated urine.

Shock, septic   **MS**
(Refer to Sepsis)

Sick sinus syndrome   **MS**
(Also refer to Dysrhythmia, cardiac)
decreased Cardiac Output may be related to alterations in rate, rhythm, and electrical conduction, possibly evidenced by ECG evidence of dysrhythmias, reports of palpitations/weakness, changes in mentation/consciousness, and syncope.
risk for Trauma: risk factors may include changes in cerebral perfusion with altered consciousness/loss of balance.

SIDS   **PED**
(Refer to Sudden infant death syndrome)

Sinusitis, chronic   **CH**
acute/chronic Pain may be related to inflammatory process possibly evidenced by reports of headache/facial pain, irritability, change in sleep, fatigue.
risk for Infection [spread]: risk factors may include chronic irritation/inflamed tissues, stasis of body fluids, improper handling of infectious material.

Skin cancer   **CH**
impaired Skin Integrity may be related to invasive growth, surgical excision may be evidenced by disruption of skin surface, destruction of dermis.
risk for acute Pain: risk factors may include ulceration of skin, surgical incision.
risk for disturbed Body Image: risk factors may include skin lesion, surgical intervention.
deficient Knowledge [Learning Need] regarding condition, prognosis, treatment, prevention may be related to lack of information/misinterpretation, possibly evidenced by statements of concern, questions, misconceptions; inaccurate follow-through of instructions, and development of preventable complications/recurrence.

SLE   **CH**
(Refer to Lupus erythematosus, systemic)

Sleep apnea   **CH**
Sleep Deprivation may be related to sleep apnea (recurrent apneic episodes followed by gasping arousal) possibly evidenced by daytime drowsiness, tiredness, decreased ability to perform/slowed mentation.
impaired Gas Exchange may be related to altered oxygen supply (recurrent apneic episodes lasting 10 seconds to 2 minutes) possibly evidenced by morning headache, decreased mental acuity, abnormal ABGs (hypoxemia, hypercapnia), dysrhythmias (e.g., extreme bradycardia, ventricular tachycardia).
risk for ineffective Therapeutic Regimen Management: risk factors may include duration of therapy, associated discomfort, perceived seriousness/benefit.

Smallpox   **MS**
risk of Infection [spread]: risk factors may include contagious nature of organism, inadequate acquired immunity, presence of chronic disease, immunosuppression.

---

deficient Fluid Volume may be related to hypermetabolic state, decreased intake (pharyngeal lesions, nausea), increased losses (vomiting), fluid shifts from vascular bed possibly evidenced by reports of thirst, decreased BP, venous filling and urinary output; dry mucous membranes, decreased skin turgor, change in mental state, elevated Hct.

impaired Tissue Integrity may be related to immunological deficit possibly evidenced by disruption of skin surface, cornea, mucous membranes.

Anxiety[specify level]/Fear may be related to threat of death, interpersonal transmission/contagion, separation from support system possibly evidenced by expressed concerns, apprehension, restlessness, focus on self.

CH

interrupted Family Processes may be related to temporary family disorganization, situational crisis, change in health status of family member possibly evidenced by changes in satisfaction with family, stress-reduction behaviors, mutual support; expression of isolation from community resources.

ineffective community Coping may be related to human-made disaster (bioterrorism), inadequate resources for problem-solving possibly evidenced by deficits of community participation, high illness rate, excessive community conflicts, expressed vulnerability/powerlessness.

Snake bite, venomous   MS

[severe] Anxiety/Fear may be related to situational crisis, threat of death, interpersonal transmission possibly evidenced by expressed concerns, apprehension, irritability, jittery, increased tension, tremors.

acute Pain/[Discomfort] may be related to effects of toxins (edema formation, erythema, enlargement of lymph nodes, nausea, fever, diaphoresis, muscle fasciculations) possibly evidenced by reports of pain/paresthesias, guarded behavior, restlessness, autonomic responses.

impaired Skin Integrity may be related to trauma, inflammation, altered circulation possibly evidenced by disruption of skin surface/distruction of skin layers (skin tense, discolored, necrosis around bite).

risk for deficient Fluid Volume: risk factors may include excessive losses (vomiting, edema formation, hemorrhage from mucous membranes).

Snow blindness   CH

disturbed visual Sensory Perception may be related to altered status of sense organ (irritation of the conjunctiva, hyperemia), possibly evidenced by intolerance to light (photophobia) and decreased/loss of visual acuity.

acute Pain may be related to irritation/vascular congestion of the conjunctiva, possibly evidenced by verbal reports, guarding/distraction behaviors, and self-focus.

Anxiety [specify level] may be related to situational crisis and threat to/change in health status, possibly evidenced by increased tension, apprehension, uncertainty, worry, restlessness, and focus on self.

Somatoform disorders   PSY

ineffective Coping may be related to severe level of anxiety that is repressed, personal vulnerability, unmet dependency needs, fixation in earlier level of development, retarded ego development, and inadequate coping skills, possibly evidenced by verbalized inability to cope/problem-solve, high illness rate, multiple somatic complaints of several years' duration, decreased functioning in social/occupational settings, narcissistic tendencies with total focus on self/physical symptoms, demanding behaviors, history of "doctor shopping," and refusal to attend therapeutic activities.

chronic Pain may be related to severe level of repressed anxiety, low self-concept, unmet dependency needs, history of self or loved one having experienced a serious illness, possibly evidenced by verbal reports of severe/prolonged pain, guarded movement/protective behaviors, facial mask of pain, fear of reinjury, altered ability to continue previous activities, social withdrawal, demands for therapy/medication.

disturbed Sensory Perception (specify) may be related to psychological stress (narrowed perceptual fields, expression of stress as physical problems/deficits), poor quality of sleep, presence of chronic pain, possibly evidenced by reported change in voluntary motor or sensory function (paralysis, anosmia, aphonia, deafness, blindness, loss of touch or pain sensation), la belle indifférence (lack of concern over functional loss).

impaired Social Interaction may be related to inability to engage in satisfying personal relationships, preoccupation with self and physical symptoms, altered state of wellness, chronic pain, and rejection by others, possibly evidenced by preoccupation with own thoughts, sad/dull affect, absence of supportive SO(s), uncommunicative/withdrawn behavior, lack of eye contact, and seeking to be alone.

Spina bifida   PED
(Also refer to Paraplegia; Newborn, special needs)

Bowel Incontinence/Constipation may be be related to disruption of nerve innervation, perceptual impairment, reduced activity level possibly evidenced by inability to evacuate bowel voluntarily, increased abdominal pressure/distention, dry/hard formed stool, change in bowel sounds.

risk for impaired physical Mobility: risk factors may include neuromuscular impairment, developmental delay, musculoskeletal impairments (clubfoot, hip dislocation, joint deformities, kyphosis).

risk for decreased Intracranial Adaptive Capacity: risk factors may include structural changes (aqueductal stricture, malformation of brain stem).

risk for Infection: risk factors may include increased environmental exposure, invasive procedures, traumatized tissues (CSF leak).

Spinal cord injury (SCI)   MS/CH
(Refer to Paraplegia; Quadriplegia)

Splenectomy   MS/CH
(Refer to Surgery, general)

risk for Infection: risk factors may include inadequate secondary defenses (decreased antibody synthesis/reduced immunoglobin M), insufficient knowledge/motivation to avoid exposure to pathogens.

risk for ineffective Therapeutic Regimen Management: risk factors may include length of therapy, economic difficulties, perceived benefits.

Spongiform encephalopathy   CH
(Refer to Creutzfeldt-Jakob disease)

Sprain of ankle or foot   CH

acute Pain may be related to trauma to/swelling in joint, possibly evidenced by verbal reports, guarding/distraction behaviors, self-focusing, and autonomic responses (changes in vital signs).

impaired Walking may be related to musculoskeletal injury, pain, and therapeutic restrictions, possibly evidenced by reluctance to attempt movement, inability to move about environment easily.

Stapedectomy   MS
risk for Trauma: risk factors may include increased middle-ear pressure with displacement of prosthesis and balancing difficulties/dizziness.
risk for Infection: risk factors may include surgically traumatized tissue, invasive procedures, and environmental exposure to upper respiratory infections.
acute Pain may be related to surgical trauma, edema formation, and presence of packing, possibly evidenced by verbal reports, guarding/distraction behaviors, and self-focus.

Stasis dermatitis   CH
(Also refer to Venous insufficiency)
impaired Skin Integrity may be related to altered circulation, presence of edema, extremely fragile epidermis, pigmentation possibly evidenced by erythema, scaling, brown discoloration, disruption of skin surface.
risk for Infection: risk factors may include cirulatory stasis/edema formation (small-vessel vasoconstrictive reflexes) in lower extremities, persistent inflammation, tissue destruction.

STD   CH
(refer to Sexually transmitted disease)

Stress disorder, acute   PSY
(Refer to Post-traumatic stress disorder)

Stillbirth   OB
(Refer to Fetal demise)

Stimulant abuse   CH
(Also refer to Cocaine hydrochloride poisoning, acute; Substance dependence/abuse rehabilitation)
imbalanced Nutrition: less than body requirements may be related to anorexia, insufficient/inappropriate use of financial resources, possibly evidenced by reported inadequate intake, weight loss/less than normal weight gain; lack of interest in food, poor muscle tone, signs/laboratory evidence of vitamin deficiencies.
risk for Infection: risk factors may include injection techniques, impurities of drugs; localized trauma/nasal septum damage, malnutrition, altered immune state.
disturbed Sleep Pattern may be related to CNS sensory alterations/psychological stress possibly evidenced by constant alertness, racing thoughts preventing rest, denial of need to sleep/reported inability to stay awake, initial insomnia then hypersomnia.

                                                                                                      PSY
Fear/Anxiety [specify] may be related to paranoid delusions associated with stimulant use possibly evidenced by feelings/beliefs that others are conspiring against or are about to attack/kill client.
ineffective Coping may be related to personal vulnerability, negative role modeling, inadequate support systems; ineffective/inadequate coping skills with substitution of drug, possibly evidenced by use of harmful substance despite evidence of undesirable consequences.

---

disturbed Sensory Perception (specify) may be related to exogenous chemical, altered sensory reception/transmission/integration (hallucination), altered status of sense organs, possibly evidenced by responding to internal stimuli from hallucinatory experiences, bizarre thinking, anxiety/panic changes in sensory acuity (sense of smell/taste).

Stomatitis   CH

impaired Oral Mucous Membrane may be related to infection, vitamin deficiency, excessive alcohol/tobacco use, ill-fitting dentures, jagged teeth, orthodontic appliances, mouth breathing, nursing bottles with hard/too long nipples possibly evidenced by oral pain, lesions/ulcers, white patches/plaques, sensitive tongue.

risk for deficient Fluid Volume: risk factors may include oral pain, difficulty swallowing.

Stress disorder, acute   PSY

(Refer to Post-traumatic stress disorder)

Substance dependence/abuse, prenatal   OB

imbalanced Nutrition: less than body requirements may be related to insufficient dietary intake to meet metabolic needs, inadequate/improper use of financial resources possibly low-weight gain, decreased subcutaneous fat/muscle mass, reported altered taste sensation, lack of interest in food, protein/vitamin deficiencies.

ineffective Denial/Coping may be related to personal vulnerability, difficulty handling new situations, use of drugs for coping, inadequate support systems possibly evidenced by denial, lack of acceptance of consequences of drug use, manipulation to avoid responsibility for self, impaired adaptive behaviors.

Powerlessness may be related to substance addiction, episodic compulsive indulgence, failed attempts at recovery, lifestyle of helplessness possibly evidenced by statements of inability to stop behavior, continuous thinking about drug, alterations in personal/occupational/social life.

chronic low Self-Esteem may be related to social stigma attached to substance abuse, social expectation that one controls own behavior, continual negative evaluation of self, personal vulnerabilities possibly evidenced by not taking responsibility for self, lack of follow-through, self-destructive behavior, denial that substance use is a problem.

compromised/disabled Family Coping may be related to codependency issues, situational crisis of pregnancy and drug abuse, family disorganization, exhausted supportive capacity of family members possibly evidenced by denial or belief that all problems are due to substance use, financial difficulties, severely dysfunctional family, codependent behaviors.

Substance dependence/abuse rehabilitation   PSY/CH

(Following acute detoxification)

ineffective Denial/Coping may be related to personal vulnerability, difficulty handling new situations, learned response patterns, cultural factors, personal/family value systems, possibly evidenced by lack of acceptance that drug use is causing the present situation, use of manipulation to avoid responsibility for self, altered social patterns/participation, impaired adaptive behavior and problem-solving skills, employment difficulties, financial affairs in disarray, and decreased ability to handle stress of recent events.

Powerlessness may be related to substance addiction with/without periods of abstinence, episodic compulsive indulgence, attempts at recovery, and lifestyle of helplessness, possibly evidenced by ineffective recovery attempts, statements of inability to stop behavior/requests for help, continuous/constant thinking about drug and/or obtaining drug, alteration in personal/occupational and social life.

imbalanced Nutrition: less than body requirements may be related to insufficient dietary intake to meet metabolic needs for psychological/physiologic/economical reasons, possibly evidenced by weight less than normal for height/body build, decreased subcutaneous fat/muscle mass, reported altered taste sensation, lack of interest in food, poor muscle tone, sore/inflamed buccal cavity, laboratory evidence of protein/vitamin deficiencies.

Sexual Dysfunction may be related to altered body function (neurologic damage and debilitating effects of drug use), changes in appearance, possibly evidenced by progressive interference with sexual functioning, a significant degree of testicular atrophy, gynecomastia, impotence/decreased sperm counts in men; and loss of body hair, thin/soft skin, spider angiomas, and amenorrhea/increase in miscarriages in women.

dysfunctional Family Processes: alcoholism [substance abuse] may be related to abuse/history of alcoholism/drug use, inadequate coping skills/lack of problem-solving skills, genetic predisposition/biochemical influences, possibly evidenced by feelings of anger/frustration/responsibility for alcoholic's behavior, suppressed rage, shame/embarrassment, repressed emotions, guilt, vulnerability; disturbed family dynamics/deterioration in family relationships, family denial/rationalization, closed communication systems, triangulating family relationships, manipulation, blaming, enabling to maintain substance use, inability to accept/receive help.

OB

risk for fetal Injury: risk factors may include drug/alcohol use, exposure to teratogens.

deficient Knowledge [Learning Need] regarding condition/pregnancy, prognosis, treatment needs may be related to lack /misinterpretation of information, lack of recall, cognitive limitations/interference with learning possibly evidenced by statements of concern, questions/misconceptions, inaccurate follow-through of instructions, development of preventable complications, continued use in spite of complications.

Sudden infant death syndrome   PED

dysfunctional Grieving may be related to unexpected loss of child, lack of anticipatory grieving possibly evidenced by expressions of distress, guilt, anger; idealization of child, reliving past with little reduction of intensity of grief, labile affect, crying, prolonged interference with life functioning, withdrawal.

risk for impaired Parenting: risk factors may include recent crisis, change in family unit, maladaptive coping strategies, sleep disruption, depression.

risk for interrupted Family Processes: risk factors may include situational crisis, loss of a family member.

risk for chronic Sorrow: risk factors may include death of a loved one, anniversary dates (birth, death, etc.), trigger events (e.g., infants on TV, at play).

Suicide attempt   MS

(Also refer to specific means; e.g., Drug overdose, acute; Wound, gunshot)

PSY

Hopelessness may be related to long-term stress, abandonment (actual or perceived), deteriorating physical/mental condition, challenged value/belief system possibly evidenced by verbal cues, passivity, lack of involvement/withdrawal, angry outbursts.

risk for Suicide: risk factors may include prior/current attempt, marked changes in behavior/attitude/performance, impulsiveness, sudden euphoric recovery from major depression, living alone, loss of independence, economic instability, substance abuse, has a plan/available means.

chronic/situational low Self-Esteem may be related to losses, functional impairment, developmental changes, failures/rejection possibly evidenced by evaluateing self as unable to deal with events, expressions of helplessness/uselessness/shame/guilt, self-negating verbalizations.

compromised family Coping may be related to temporary family disorganization, role changes, prolonged disease/disability, situational/developmental crises possibly evidenced by client expressing concern about SO's response to problems, SO confirms ineffective supportive behaviors, SO withdraws from client at the time of need.

Sunstroke   MS
(Refer to Heatstroke)

Surgery, general   MS
(Also refer to Postoperative recovery period)

deficient Knowledge [Learning Need] regarding surgical procedure/expectation, postoperative routines/therapy, and self-care needs may be related to lack of information/misinterpretation, possibly evidenced by statements of concern, questions, and misconceptions.

Anxiety [specify level]/Fear may be related to situational crisis, unfamiliarity with environment, change in health status/threat of death and separation from usual support systems, possibly evidenced by increased tension, apprehension, decreased self-assurance, fear of unspecific consequences, focus on self, sympathetic stimulation, and restlessness.

risk for perioperative-positioning Injury: risk factors may include disorientation, immobilization, muscle weakness, obesity/edema.

risk for ineffective Breathing Pattern: risk factors may include chemically induced muscular relaxation, perception/cognitive impairment, decreased energy.

risk for deficient Fluid Volume: risk factors may include preoperative fluid deprivation, blood loss, and excessive GI losses (vomiting/gastric suction).

Synovitis (knee)   CH
acute Pain may be related to inflammation of synovial membrane of the joint with effusion, possibly evidenced by verbal reports, guarding/distraction behaviors, self-focus, and autonomic responses (changes in vital signs).

impaired Walking may be related to pain and decreased strength of joint, possibly evidenced by reluctance to attempt movement, inability to move about environment as desired.

Syphilis, congenital   PED
(Also refer to Sexually Transmitted Disease—STD)

acute Pain may be related to inflammatory process, edema formation, and development of skin lesions, possibly evidenced by irritability/crying that may be increased with movement of extremities and autonomic responses (changes in vital signs).

impaired Skin/Tissue Integrity may be related to exposure to pathogens during vaginal delivery, possibly evidenced by disruption of skin surfaces and rhinitis.

delayed Growth and Development may be related to effect of infectious process, possibly evidenced by altered physical growth and delay or difficulty performing skills typical of age group.

deficient Knowledge [Learning Need] regarding pathophysiology of condition, transmissibility, therapy needs, expected outcomes, and potential complications may be related to caretaker/parental lack of information, misinterpretation, possibly evidenced by statements of concern, questions, and misconceptions.

Syringomyelia   **MS**

disturbed Sensory Perception (specify) may be related to altered sensory perception (neurologic lesion), possibly evidenced by change in usual response to stimuli and motor incoordination.

Anxiety [specify level]/Fear may be related to change in health status, threat of change in role functioning and socioeconomic status, and threat to self-concept, possibly evidenced by increased tension, apprehension, uncertainty, focus on self, and expressed concerns.

impaired physical Mobility may be related to neuromuscular and sensory impairment, possibly evidenced by decreased muscle strength, control, and mass; and impaired coordination.

Self-Care Deficit [specify] may be related to neuromuscular and sensory impairments, possibly evidenced by statement of inability to perform care tasks.

Tarsal tunnel syndrome   **CH**

acute/chronic Pain may be related to pressure on posterior tibal nerve at ankle, possibly evidenced by verbal reports, reluctance to use affected extremity, guarding behaviors, expressed fear of reinjury, altered ability to continue previous activities.

impaired Walking may be related to neuromuscular impairment and increased pain with walking, possibly evidenced by inability to walk desired distances, climb stairs, navigate curbs/uneven surfaces.

Tay-Sachs disease   **PED**

delayed Growth and Development may be related to effects of physical condition, possibly evidenced by altered physical growth, loss of/failure to acquire skills typical of age, flat affect, and decreased responses.

disturbed visual Sensory Perception may be related to neurologic deterioration of optic nerve, possibly evidenced by loss of visual acuity.

                                                                     CH

anticipatory family Grieving may be related to expected eventual loss of infant/child, possibly evidenced by expressions of distress, denial, guilt, anger, and sorrow; choked feelings; changes in sleep/eating habits; and altered libido.

family Powerlessness may be related to absence of therapeutic interventions for progressive/fatal disease, possibly evidenced by verbal expressions of having no control over situation/outcome and depression over physical/mental deterioration.

risk for Spiritual Distress: risk factors may include challenged belief and value system by presence of fatal condition with racial/religious connotations and intense suffering.

compromised family Coping may be related to situational crisis, temporary preoccupation with managing emotional conflicts and personal suffering, family disorganization, and prolonged/progressive disease, possibly evidenced by preoccupations with personal reactions, expressed concern about reactions of other family members, inadequate support of one another, and altered communication patterns.

TBI   **MS/CH**

(Refer to Traumatic brain injury)

Temporal arteritis   **CH**

acute Pain may be related to arterial inflammation possibly evidenced by reports of severe headache, scalp tenderness, pain with chewing, myalgia.

risk for disturbed visual Sensory Perception: risk factors may include altered reception (arterial inflammation, ischemic optic neuropathy).

risk for ineffective Therapeutic Regimen Management: risk factors may include medication side effects, economic difficulties, perceived seriousness/benefits.

Temporomandibular joint syndrome   **CH**
chronic Pain may be related to pressure on nerves possibly evidenced by reports of pain in TMJ area worsened with chewing, muscle tension headache.
risk for imbalanced Nutrition: less than body requirements: risk factors may include inability to ingest food (pain worsened by chewing, limited movement of joint).
risk for disturbed auditory Sensory Perception: risk factors may include altered sensory reception (tinnitis, occassionally deafness).

Tendonitis   **CH**
acute/chronic Pain may be related to inflammation, swelling of tendon possibly evidenced by verbal reports, guarding/protective behavior, fear of reinjury, altered ability to continue previous activities.
impaired physical Mobility may be related to pain, joint stiffness, musculoskeletal impairment, prescribed movement restrictions possibly evidenced by limited range of motion, limited ability to perform fine/gross motor skills.
risk for ineffective Role Performance: risk factors may include health alterations, fatigue, pain.

Testicular cancer   **MS**
(Also refer to Cancer)
disturbed Body Image may be related to surgical change in reproductive organs, loss of hair and weight, possibly evidenced by negative feelings about body/sense of mutilation, preoccupation with change, feelings of helplessness/hopelessness, and change in social environment.
Sexual Dysfunction may be related to change in sexual organs, postoperative impotence, vulnerability possibly evidenced by verbalizations of problem, inability in achieving desired satisfaction, alterations in relationships.

Tetraplegia   **MS/CH**
(Refer to Quadriplegia)

Thoracotomy   **MS**
(Refer to Surgery, general; Hemothorax)

Thrombophlebitis   **CH/MS/OB**
ineffective peripheral Tissue Perfusion may be related to interruption of venous blood flow, venous stasis, possibly evidenced by changes in skin color/temperature over affected area, development of edema, pain, diminished peripheral pulses, slow capillary refill.
acute Pain/[Discomfort] may be related to vascular inflammation/irritation and edema formation (accumulation of lactic acid), possibly evidenced by verbal reports, guarding/distraction behaviors, restlessness, and self-focus.
Anxiety [specify level] may be related to change in health status, perceived/actual threat to self, situational crisis, interpersonal transmission possibly evidenced by increased tension, apprehension, restlessness, sympathetic stimulation.
risk for impaired physical Mobility: risk factors may include pain and discomfort and restrictive therapies/safety precautions.
deficient Knowledge [Learning Need] regarding pathophysiology of condition, therapy/self-care needs, and risk of embolization may be related to lack of information/misinterpretation,

possibly evidenced by statements of concern, questions, inaccurate follow-through of instructions, and development of preventable complications.

Thrombosis, venous   MS
(Refer to Thrombophlebitis)

Thrush   CH
impaired Oral Mucous Membrane may be related to presence of infection as evidenced by white patches/plaques, oral discomfort, mucosal irritation, bleeding.
risk for imbalanced Nutrition: less than body requirements: risk factors may include inability to ingest adequate amount of nutrients (oral pain).

Thyroidectomy   MS
(Also refer to Hyperthyroidism; Hypoparathyroidism, Hypothyroidism)
risk for ineffective Airway Clearance: risk factors may include hematoma/edema formation with tracheal obstruction, laryngeal spasms.
impaired verbal Communication may be related to tissue edema, pain/discomfort, and vocal cord injury/laryngeal nerve damage, possibly evidenced by impaired articulation, does not/cannot speak, and use of nonverbal cues/gestures.
risk for Injury [tetany]: risk factors may include chemical imbalance/excessive CNS stimulation.
risk for head/neck Trauma: risk factors may include loss of muscle control/support and position of suture line.
acute Pain may be related to presence of surgical incision/manipulation of tissues/muscles, postoperative edema, possibly evidenced by verbal reports, guarding/distraction behaviors, narrowed focus, and autonomic responses (changes in vital signs).

Thyrotoxicosis   MS
(Also refer to Hyperthyroidism)
risk for decreased Cardiac Output: risk factors may include uncontrolled hypermetabolic state increasing cardiac workload, changes in venous return and SVR; and alterations in rate, rhythm, and electrical conduction.
Anxiety [specific level] may be related to physiologic factors/CNS stimulation (hypermetabolic state and pseudocatecholamine effect of thyroid hormones), possibly evidenced by increased feelings of apprehension, shakiness, loss of control, panic, changes in cognition, distortion of environmental stimuli, extraneous movements, restlessness, and tremors.
risk for disturbed Thought Processes: risk factors may include physiologic changes (increased CNS stimulation/accelerated mental activity) and altered sleep patterns.
deficient Knowledge [Learning Needs] regarding condition, treatment needs, and potential for complications/crisis situation may be related to lack of information/recall, misinterpretation, possibly evidenced by statements of concern, questions, misconceptions; and inaccurate follow-through of instructions.

TIA   CH
(Refer to Transient ischemic attack)

Tic douloureux   CH
(Refer to Neuralgia, trigeminal)

TMJ syndrome   CH
(Refer to Temporomandibular joint syndrome)

Tonsillectomy   **PED/MS**
(Refer to Adenoidectomy)

Tonsillitis   **PED**
acute Pain may be related to inflammation of tonsils and effects of circulating toxins, possibly
    evidenced by verbal reports, guarding/distraction behaviors, reluctance/refusal to swallow,
    self-focus, and autonomic responses (changes in vital signs).
Hyperthermia may be related to presence of inflammatory process/hypermetabolic state and
    dehydration, possibly evidenced by increased body temperature, warm/flushed skin, and
    tachycardia.
*deficient Knowledge [Learning Need] regarding cause/transmission, treatment needs, and poten-
    tial complications* may be related to lack of information/misinterpretation, possibly
    evidenced by statements of concern, questions, inaccurate follow-through of instructions,
    and recurrence of condition.

Total joint replacement   **MS**
risk for Infection: risk factors may include inadequate primary defenses (broken skin, exposure
    of joint), inadequate secondary defenses/immunosuppression (long-term corticosteroid
    use), invasive procedures/surgical manipulation, implantation of foreign body, and
    decreased mobility.
impaired physical Mobility may be related to pain and discomfort, musculoskeletal impair-
    ment, and surgery/restrictive therapies, possibly evidenced by reluctance to attempt
    movement, difficulty purposefully moving within the physical environment, reports of
    pain/discomfort on movement, limited range of motion, and decreased muscle
    strength/control.
risk for ineffective peripheral Tissue Perfusion: risk factors may include reduced arterial/venous
    blood flow, direct trauma to blood vessels, tissue edema, improper location/dislocation of
    prosthesis, and hypovolemia.
acute Pain may be related to physical agents (traumatized tissues/surgical intervention,
    degeneration of joints, muscle spasms) and psychological factors (anxiety, advanced age),
    possibly evidenced by verbal reports, guarding/distraction behaviors, self-focus, and auto-
    nomic responses (changes in vital signs).

Tourette's syndrome   **CH**
chronic low Self-Esteem may be related to inherited disorder, continual negative evaluation of
    self/capabilities, personal vulnerability possibly evidenced by self-negating verbalizations,
    expressed shame, exaggerates negative feedback about self, hesitancy to try new situations.
Social Isolation may be related to unaccepted social behaviors, inability to engage in satisfying
    personal relationships, rejection/ridicule by others.
risk for Injury: risk factors may include adverse side effects of medications, negative response
    of uneducated individuals.

Toxemia of pregnancy   **OB**
(Refer to Pregnancy-Induced Hypertension)

Toxic enterocolitis   **PED/MS**
(Also refer to Colostomy)
deficient Fluid Volume may be related to fulminating losses into the bowel, diarrhea, lack of
    intake evidenced by decreased/concentrated urine, dry mucous membranes, poor skin
    turgor, decreased venous filling, change in mentation.
risk for decreased Cardiac Output: risk factors may include decreased venous return, altered
    heart rate/rhythm.

Toxic megacolon   **MS**

(Refer to Toxic enterocolitis)

Toxic shock syndrome   **MS**

(Also refer to Sepsis)

Hyperthermia may be related to inflammatory process/hypermetabolic state and dehydration, possibly evidenced by increased body temperature, warm/flushed skin, and tachycardia.

deficient Fluid Volume [isotonic] may be related to increased gastric losses (diarrhea, vomiting), fever/hypermetabolic state, and decreased intake, possibly evidenced by dry mucous membranes, increased pulse, hypotension, delayed venous filling, decreased/concentrated urine, and hemoconcentration.

acute Pain may be related to inflammatory process, effects of circulating toxins, and skin disruptions, possibly evidenced by verbal reports, guarding/distraction behaviors, self-focus, and autonomic responses (changes in vital signs).

impaired Skin/Tissue Integrity may be related to effects of circulating toxins and dehydration, possibly evidenced by development of desquamating rash, hyperemia, and inflammation of mucous membranes.

Traction   **MS**

(Also refer to Casts; Fractures)

acute Pain may be related to direct trauma to tissue/bone, muscle spasms, movement of bone fragments, edema, injury to soft tissue, traction/immobility device, anxiety, possibly evidenced by verbal reports, guarding/distraction behaviors, self-focus, alteration in muscle tone, and autonomic responses (changes in vital signs).

impaired physical Mobility may be related to neuromuscular/skeletal impairment, pain, psychological immobility, and therapeutic restrictions of movement, possibly evidenced by limited range of motion, inability to move purposefully in environment, reluctance to attempt movement, and decreased muscle strength/control.

risk for Infection: risk factors may include invasive procedures (including insertion of foreign body through skin/bone), presence of traumatized tissue, and reduced activity with stasis of body fluids.

deficient Diversional Activity may be related to length of hospitalization/therapeutic intervention and environmental lack of usual activity, possibly evidenced by statements of boredom, restlessness, and irritability.

Transfusion reaction, blood   **MS**

(Also refer to Anaphylaxis)

risk for imbalanced Body Temperature: risk factors may include infusion of cold blood products, systemic response to toxins.

Anxiety [specify level] may be related to change in health status and threat of death, exposure to toxins possibly evidenced by increased tension, apprehension, sympathetic stimulation, restlessness, and expressions of concern.

risk for impaired Skin Integrity: risk factors may include immunologic response.

Transient ischemic attack   **CH**

ineffective cerebral Tissue Perfusion may be related to interruption of blood flow (e.g., vasospasm) possibly evidenced by altered mental status, behavioral changes, language deficit, change in motor/sensory response.

Anxiety [specify level]/Fear may be related to change in health status, threat to self-concept, situational crisis, interpersonal contagion possibly evidenced by expressed concerns, apprehension, restlessness, irritability.

---

risk for ineffective Denial: risk factors may include change in health status requiring change in lifestyle, fear of consequences, lack of motivation.

Transplant, living donor   MS
(Also refer to Surgery, general; Nephrectomy)

decisional Conflict may be related to multiple/divergent sources of information, family system (demands/expectations/responsibilities to others), risk to self possibly evidenced by verbalized uncertainty about choices, questioning personal values/beliefs, delayed decision making, increased tension.

[moderate to severe] Anxiety/Fear may be related to situational crisis, unconscious conflict about essential beliefs/values, familial association, threat to health status/death possibly evidenced by expressed concerns, apprehension, uncertainty, increased tension, fear of failing family member (e.g., organ rejection), sympathetic stimulation.

Transplantation, recipient   MS
(Also refer to Surgery, general; Cardiac surgery)

Anxiety [specify level]/Fear may be related to unconscious conflict about essential values/beliefs, situational crisis, interpersonal contagion, threat to self concept, threat of organ rejection/death, side effects of medication possibly evidenced by increased tension, apprehension, uncertainty, expressed concerns, somatic complaints, sympathetic stimulation, insomnia.

risk for Infection: risk factors may include medically induced immunosuppression, suppressed inflammatory response, antibiotic therapy, invasive procedures, broken skin/traumatized tissue, effects of chronic/debilitating disease.

[Refer to specific conditions relative compromise/failure of individual transplanted organ; e.g., Renal failure, acute, Heart failure, chronic; Pancreatitis)

                                                                  CH

ineffective Coping/compromised family Coping may be related to situational crisis, high degree of threat, uncertainty, family disorganization/role changes, prolonged disease exhausting supportive capacity of family/SO possibly evidenced by verbalizations, sleep disturbance/fatigue, poor concentration, protective behaviors disproportionate to client's needs, SO describes preoccupation with personal reaction.

risk for ineffective Protection: risk factors may include drug therapies/compromised immune system, effects of debilitating disease.

readiness for enhanced Therapeutic Regimen Management may be related to desire to live life more fully, engage in healthy lifestyle possibly evidenced by expressed desire to manage treatment and prevention of sequelae, reduction of risk factors, no unexpected sequelae.

risk for ineffective Therapeutic Regimen Management: risk factors may include complexity of therapeutic regimen and healthcare system, economic difficulties, family patterns of healthcare.

Transurethral resection of prostate   MS
(Refer to Prostatectomy)

Traumatic brain injury (TBI)   MS

risk for decreased Intracranial Adaptive Capacity: risk factors may include brain injuries, systemic hypotension with intracranial hypertension.

risk for ineffective Breathing Pattern: risk factors may include neuromuscular dysfunction (injury to respiratory center of brain), perception/cognitive impairment.

disturbed Sensory Perception (specify) may be related to altered sensory reception, transmission and/or integration (neurologic trauma or deficit) possibly evidenced by disorientation to time, place, person; motor incoordination, altered communication patterns, restlessness/irritability, change in behavior pattern.

risk for Infection: risk factors may include traumatized tissues, broken skin, invasive procedures, decreased ciliary action, stasis of body fluids, nutritional deficits, altered integrity of closed system (CSF leak).

risk for imbalanced Nutrition: less than body requirements: risk factors may include altered ability to ingest nutrients (decreased level of consciousness), weakness of muscles for chewing/swallowing, hypermetabolic state.

CH

impaired physical Mobility may be related to perceptual/cognitive impairment, decreased strength/endurance, restrictive therapies/safety precautions possibly evidenced by inability to purposefully move within physical environment—including bed mobility, transfer, ambulation; impaired coordination, limited range of motion, decreased muscle strength/control.

disturbed Thought Processes may be related to physiologic changes, psychological conflicts possibly evidenced by memory deficits, distractibility, altered attention span/concentration, disorientation to time, place, person, circumstances, or events; impaired ability to make decisions, problem-solve, reason or conceptualize; personality changes.

interrupted Family Processes may be related to situational transition and crisis, uncertainty about ultimate outcome/expectations possibly evidenced by difficulty adapting to change, family not meeting needs of all members, difficulty accepting/receiving help, inability to express or to accept feelings of members.

Self-Care Deficit (specify) may be related to neuromuscular/musculoskeletal impairment, weakness, pain, perceptual/cognitive impairment possibly evidenced by inability to perform desired/appropriate ADLs.

Trench foot   MS
(Refer to Immersion foot)

Trichinosis   CH

acute Pain may be related to parasitic invasion of muscle tissues, edema of upper eyelids, small localized hemorrhages, and development of urticaria, possibly evidenced by verbal reports, guarding/distraction behaviors (restlessness), and autonomic responses (changes in vital signs).

deficient Fluid Volume [isotonic] may be related to hypermetabolic state (fever, diaphoresis); excessive gastric losses (vomiting, diarrhea); and decreased intake/difficulty swallowing, possibly evidenced by dry mucous membranes, decreased skin turgor, hypotension, decreased venous filling, decreased/concentrated urine, and hemoconcentration.

ineffective Breathing Pattern may be related to myositis of the diaphragm and intercostal muscles, possibly evidenced by resulting changes in respiratory depth, tachypnea, dyspnea, and abnormal ABGs.

deficient Knowledge [Learning Need] regarding cause/prevention of condition, therapy needs, and possible complications may be related to lack of information, misinterpretation, possibly evidenced by statements of concern, questions, and misconceptions.

Tricuspid insufficiency   CH
(Refer to Valvular heart disease)

Tricuspid stenosis   CH
(Refer to Valvular heart disease)

Tubal pregnancy   **OB**
(Refer to Ectopic pregnancy)

Tuberculosis (pulmonary)   **CH**
risk for Infection [spread/reactivation]: risk factors may include inadequate primary defenses (decreased ciliary action/stasis of secretions, tissue destruction/extension of infection), lowered resistance/suppressed inflammatory response, malnutrition, environmental exposure, insufficient knowledge to avoid exposure to pathogens, or inadequate therapeutic intervention.
ineffective Airway Clearance may be related to thick, viscous or bloody secretions; fatigue/poor cough effort, and tracheal/pharyngeal edema, possibly evidenced by abnormal respiratory rate, rhythm, and depth; adventitious breath sounds (rhonchi, wheezes), stridor and dyspnea.
risk for impaired Gas Exchange: risk factors may include decrease in effective lung surface, atelectasis, destruction of alveolar-capillary membrane, bronchial edema; thick, viscous secretions.
Activity Intolerance may be related to imbalance between O_2 supply and demand, possibly evidenced by reports of fatigue, weakness, and exertional dyspnea.
imbalanced Nutrition: less than body requirements may be related to inability to ingest adequate nutrients (anorexia, effects of drug therapy, fatigue, insufficient financial resources), possibly evidenced by weight loss, reported lack of interest in food/altered taste sensation, and poor muscle tone.
risk for ineffective Therapeutic Regimen Management: risk factors may include complexity of therapeutic regimen, economic difficulties, family patterns of healthcare, perceived seriousness/benefits (especially during remission), side effects of therapy.

TURP   **MS**
(Refer to Prostatectomy)

Tympanoplasty   **MS**
(Refer to Stapedectomy)

Typhoid fever   **MS**
(Also refer to Sepsis)
risk for Infection [spread]: risk factors may include presence of bacteria in excretions, inadequate knowledge to avoid exposure to pathogen (food/water, fecally contaminated objects).
risk for deficient Fluid Volume [isotonic]: risk factors may include gastric irritation/ulcers.
imbalanced Nutrition: less than body requirements: risk factors may include inability to ingest/digest/absorb nutrients, hypermetabolic state possibly evidenced by anorexia, abdominal pain, weight loss.

Typhus   **CH/MS**
Hyperthermia may be related to generalized inflammatory process (vasculitis), possibly evidenced by increased body temperature, warm/flushed skin, and tachycardia.
acute Pain may be related to generalized vasculitis and edema formation, possibly evidenced by verbal reports, guarding/distraction behaviors, self-focus, and autonomic responses (changes in vital signs).
ineffective Tissue Perfusion (specify) may be related to reduction/interruption of blood flow (generalized vasculitis/thrombi formation), possibly evidenced by reports of

headache/abdominal pain, changes in mentation, and areas of peripheral ulceration/
necrosis.

Ulcer, decubitus   CH/MS

impaired Skin/Tissue Integrity may be related to altered circulation, nutritional deficit, fluid
imbalance, impaired physical mobility, irritation of body excretions/secretions, and
sensory impairments, evidenced by tissue damage/destruction.

acute Pain may be related to destruction of protective skin layers and exposure of nerves,
possibly evidenced by verbal reports, distraction behaviors, and self-focus.

risk for Infection: risk factors may include broken/traumatized tissue, increased environmental exposure, and nutritional deficits.

Ulcer, peptic (acute)   MS/CH

deficient Fluid Volume [isotonic] may be related to vascular losses (hemorrhage), possibly
evidenced by hypotension, tachycardia, delayed capillary refill, changes in mentation, restlessness, concentrated/decreased urine, pallor, diaphoresis, and hemoconcentration.

risk for ineffective Tissue Perfusion (specify): risk factors may include hypovolemia.

Fear/Anxiety [specify level] may be related to change in health status and threat of death,
possibly evidenced by increased tension, restlessness, irritability, fearfulness, trembling,
tachycardia, diaphoresis, lack of eye contact, focus on self, verbalization of concerns, withdrawal, and panic or attack behavior.

acute Pain may be related to caustic irritation/destruction of gastric tissues, possibly
evidenced by verbal reports, distraction behaviors, self-focus, and autonomic responses
(changes in vital signs).

*deficient Knowledge [Learning Need] regarding condition, therapy/self-care needs, and poten-
tial complications* may be related to lack of information/recall, misinterpretation, possibly
evidenced by statements of concern, questions, misconceptions; inaccurate follow-
through of instructions, and development of preventable complications/recurrence of
condition.

Ulcer, pressure   CH/MS
(Refer to Ulcer, decubitus)

Ulcer, venous stasis   CH
(Also refer to Venous insufficiency)

impaired Skin/Tissue Integrity may be related to altered venous circulation, edema formation,
inflammation, decreased sensation possibly evidenced by destruction of skin layers, invasion of body structures.

decreased peripheral Tissue Perfusion may be related to interruption of venous flow (small-
vessel vasoconstrictive reflex) possibly evidenced by skin discoloration, edema formation,
altered sensation, delayed healing.

Ulnar neuropathy   CH
(Refer to Cubital tunnel syndrome)

Unconsciousness   MS
(Refer to Coma)

Upper GI bleeding   MS
(Refer to Gastritis, acute or chronic; Ulcer, peptic)

Urinary diversion   MS/CH

risk for impaired Skin Integrity: risk factors may include absence of sphincter at stoma, character/flow of urine from stoma, reaction to product/chemicals, and improperly fitting appliance or removal of adhesive.

disturbed Body Image related factors may include biophysical factors (presence of stoma, loss of control of urine flow), and psychosocial factors (altered body structure, disease process/associated treatment regimen, such as cancer), possibly evidenced by verbalization of change in body image, fear of rejection/reaction of others, negative feelings about body, not touching/looking at stoma, refusal to participate in care.

acute Pain may be related to physical factors (disruption of skin/tissues, presence of incisions/drains), biologic factors (activity of disease process, such as cancer, trauma), and psychological factors (fear, anxiety), possibly evidenced by verbal reports, self-focusing, guarding/distraction behaviors, restlessness, and autonomic responses (changes in vital signs).

impaired Urinary Elimination, may be related to surgical diversion, tissue trauma, and postoperative edema, possibly evidenced by loss of continence, changes in amount and character of urine, and urinary retention.

Urinary tract infection   CH
(Refer to Cystitis)

Urolithiasis   MS/CH
(Refer to Calculi, urinary)

Uterine bleeding, dysfunctional   GYN/MS

Anxiety [specify level] may be related to perceived change in health status and unknown etiology, possibly evidenced by apprehension, uncertainty, fear of unspecified consequences, expressed concerns, and focus on self.

Activity Intolerance may be related to imbalance between oxygen supply and demand/decreased oxygen-carrying capacity of blood (anemia), possibly evidenced by reports of fatigue/weakness.

Uterine myomas   GYN
(Also refer to Anemia)

acute Pain/[Discomfort] may be related to growth/size/degeneration or twisting of tumors possibly evidenced by reports of pressure, cramping, guarding behavior, irritability.

impaired Urinary Elimination may be related to uterine pressure on bladder possibly evidenced by frequency, urgency.

risk for deficient Fluid Volume: risk factors may include excessive/chronic blood loss.

Uterus, rupture of, in pregnancy   OB

deficient Fluid Volume [isotonic] may be related to excessive vascular losses, possibly evidenced by hypotension, increased pulse rate, decreased venous filling, and decreased urine output.

decreased Cardiac Output may be related to decreased preload (hypovolemia), possibly evidenced by cold/clammy skin, decreased peripheral pulses, variations in hemodynamic readings, tachycardia, and cyanosis.

acute Pain may be related to tissue trauma and irritation of accumulating blood, possibly evidenced by verbal reports, guarding/distraction behaviors, self-focus, and autonomic responses (changes in vital signs).

Anxiety [specify level] may be related to threat of death of self/fetus, interpersonal contagion, physiologic response (release of catecholamines), possibly evidenced by fearful/scared affect, sympathetic stimulation, stated fear of unspecified consequences, and expressed concerns.

UTI   **CH**
(Refer to Cystitis)

Vaginal hysterectomy   **MS**
(Refer to Hysterectomy)

Vaginismus   **GYN/PSY**
acute Pain may be related to muscle spasm and hyperesthesia of the nerve supply to vaginal mucous membrane, possibly evidenced by verbal reports, distraction behaviors, and self-focus.
Sexual Dysfunction may be related to physical and/or psychological alteration in function (severe spasms of vaginal muscles), possibly evidenced by verbalization of problem, inability to achieve desired satisfaction, and alteration in relationship with SO.

Vaginitis   **GYN/CH**
impaired Tissue Integrity may be related to irritation/inflammation and mechanical trauma (scratching) of sensitive tissues, possibly evidenced by damaged/destroyed tissue, presence of lesions.
acute Pain may be related to localized inflammation and tissue trauma, possibly evidenced by verbal reports, distraction behaviors, and self-focus.
deficient Knowledge [Learning Need] regarding hygienic/therapy needs and sexual behaviors/transmission of organisms may be related to lack of information/misinterpretation, possibly evidenced by statements of concern, questions, and misconceptions.

Vaginosis, bacterial   **GYN**
risk for impaired Tissue Integrity: risk factors may include vulvar/vaginal irritation, itching.
risk for [secondary] Infection: risk factors may include prescribed antibiotic therapy, insufficient knowledge to avoid exposure to pathogens.

Valvular heart disease   **MS**
decreased Cardiac Output may be related to alteration in preload/increased arterial pressure and venous congestion, increased afterload, changes in electrical conduction possibly evidenced by variations in hemodynamic parameters, dysrhythmias/ECG changes, dyspnea, adventitious breath sounds, cyanosis/pallor, jugular vein distension, fatigue.
Activity Intolerance may be related to imbalance between oxygen supply and demand (decreased/fixed cardiac output) possibly evidenced by reports of fatigue/weakness, abnormal heart rate/BP in response to activity, exertional discomfort/dyspnea.
Anxiety may be related to threat to/change in health status (chronicity of disease), physiologic effects, situational crisis (changes in lifestyle, hospitalization) possibly evidenced by expressed concerns, increased tension, apprehension, uncertainty, sympathetic stimulation, insomnia.
risk for excess Fluid Volume: risk factors may include increased sodium/water retention, changes in glomerular filtration.

risk for ineffective Tissue Perfusion (specify): risk factors may include interruption of arterial-venous flow (systemic emboli), venous thrombosis (venous stasis, decreased activity).

Varices, esophageal   **MS**
(Also refer to Ulcer, peptic [acute])
deficient Fluid Volume [isotonic] may be related to excessive vascular loss, reduced intake, and gastric losses (vomiting), possibly evidenced by hypotension, tachycardia, decreased venous filling, and decreased/concentrated urine.
Anxiety [specify level]/Fear may be related to change in health status and threat of death, possibly evidenced by increased tension/apprehension, sympathetic stimulation, restlessness, focus on self, and expressed concerns.

Varicose veins   **CH**
chronic Pain may be related to venous insufficiency and stasis, possibly evidenced by verbal reports.
disturbed Body Image may be related to change in structure (presence of enlarged, discolored tortuous superficial leg veins) possibly evidenced by hiding affected parts and negative feelings about body.
risk for impaired Skin/Tissue Integrity: risk factors may include altered circulation/venous stasis and edema formation.

Varicose Veins ligation/stripping   **MS**
risk for ineffective peripheral Tissue Perfusion: risk factors may include localized edema, vascular irritation, inadequate venous return, dressings.
impaired Skin Integrity may be related to surgical procedure, pressure dressings, tissue edema, vascular engorgement possibly evidenced by incisions, development of complications (e.g., ulcerations).

Varicose veins sclerotherapy   **MS**
risk for impaired Skin Integrity: risk factors may include pressure wraps, extravasation of sclerosing agent.
risk for ineffective Therapeutic Regimen Management: risk factors may include perceived seriousness/benefit, required lifestyle/activity changes, post procedure dressings.

Variola   **MS**
(Refer to Smallpox)

Vasculitis   **CH**
(Refer to Polyarteritis nodosa; Temporal arteritis)

Vasectomy   **CH/MS**
acute Pain/[Discomfort] may be related to manipulation of delicate tissues, edema/hematoma formation possibly evidenced by verbal reports, guarding behavior, irritability.
deficient Knowledge regarding self-care, future expectations (issues of reproduction, safety/STDs) may be related to information misinterpretation, lack of recall possibly evidenced by verbalizations, misconceptions, inaccurate follow-through of instructions.

Venereal disease   **CH**
(Refer to Sexually Transmitted Disease—STD)

Venous insufficiency   **CH**

(Also refer to Stasis dermatitis; Ulcer, venous stasis)

chronic Pain/[Discomfort] may be related to altered venous circulation, edema formation possibly evidenced by reports of aching, fullness, tiredness of lower extremities with activity.

risk for impaired Adjustment: risk factors may include health status requiring change in lifestyle, lack of motivation to change behaviors.

risk for ineffective Therapeutic Regimen Management: risk factors may include economic difficulties, perceived seriousness/benefit, social support deficit.

Ventilator assist/dependence   **MS/CH**

ineffective Breathing Pattern/impaired spontaneous Ventilation may be related to neuromuscular dysfunction, respiratory muscle fatigue, spinal cord injury, hypoventilation syndrome—possibly evidenced by dyspnea, increased work of breathing/use of accessory muscles, reduced vital capacity/total lung volume, changes in respiratory rate, decreased PO_2/SaO_2, increased PCO_2.

ineffective Airway Clearance may be related to foreign body/artificial airway in trachea, inability to cough/ineffective cough possibly evidenced by changes in rate/depth of respirations, abnormal breath sounds, anxiety/restlessness, cyanosis.

impaired verbal Communication may be related to physical barrier (artificial airway), neuromuscular weakness/paralysis possibly evidenced by inability to speak.

Fear/Anxiety [specify] may be related to situational crisis, threat to self-concept, threat of death/dependency on machine, change in health status/socioeconomic status/role functioning, interpersonal transmission possibly evidenced by increased muscle/facial tension, hypervigilance, restlessness, fearfulness, apprehension, expressed concerns, insomnia, negative self-talk.

risk for impaired Oral Mucous Membrane: risk factors may include inability to swallow oral fluids, decreased salivation, ineffective oral hygiene, presence of ET tube in mouth.

risk for imbalanced Nutrition: less than body requirements: risk factors may include inability to ingest nutrients, increased metabolic demands.

risk for dysfunctional Ventilatory Weaning Response: risk factors may include limited/insufficient energy stores, sleep disturbance, pain/discomfort, perceived inability to wean/decreased motivation, inadequate support/adverse environment, history of ventilator dependence greater than 1 week/unsuccessful weaning attempts.

Ventricular fibrillation   **MS**

(Also refer to Dysrhythmias)

decreased Cardiac Output may be related to altered electrical conduction and reduced myocardial contractility possibly evidenced by absence of measurable cardiac output, loss of consciousness, no palpable pulses.

Ventricular tachycardia   **MS**

(Also refer to Dysrhythmias)

risk for decreased Cardiac Output: risk factors may include altered electrical conduction and reduced myocardial contractility.

Vertigo   **CH**

disturbed kinesthetic Sensory Perception may be related to altered status of sensory organ (middle/inner ear), altered sensory integration possibly evidenced by visual distortions, altered sense of balance, falls.

risk for Falls: risk factors may include presence of postural hypotension, acute illness, medications, substance abuse.

West Nile Fever   CH/MS

Hyperthermia may be related to infectious process possibly evidenced by elevated body temperature, skin flushed/warm to touch, tachycardia, increased respiratory rate.

acute Pain may be related to infectious process/circulating toxins possibly evidenced by reports of headache, myalgia, eye pain, abdominal discomfort.

risk for deficient Fluid Volume: risk factors may include hypermetabolic state, decreased intake anorexia, nausea, losses from normal routes (vomiting, diarrhea).

risk for impaired Skin Integrity: risk factors may include hyperthermia, decreased fluid intake, alterations in skin turgor, bedrest, circulating toxins.

Wilms' tumor   PED

(Also refer to Cancer; Chemotherapy)

Anxiety [specify level]/Fear may be related to change in environment and interaction patterns with family members and threat of death with family transmission and contagion concerns, possibly evidenced by fearful/scared affect, distress, crying, insomnia, and sympathetic stimulation.

risk for Injury: risk factors may include nature of tumor (vascular, mushy with very thin covering) with increased danger of metastasis when manipulated.

interrupted Family Processes, may be related to situational crisis of life-threatening illness, possibly evidenced by a family system that has difficulty meeting physical, emotional, and spiritual needs of its members, and inability to deal with traumatic experience effectively.

deficient Diversional Activity may be related to environmental lack of age-appropriate activity (including activity restrictions) and length of hospitalization/treatment, possibly evidenced by restlessness, crying, lethargy, and acting-out behavior.

Withdrawal, drugs/alcohol   CH/MS

(Refer to Alcohol intoxication, acute; Drug overdose, acute; Drug withdrawal)

Whooping cough   PED

(Refer to Pertussis)

Wound, gunshot   MS

(Depends on site and speed/character of bullet)

risk for deficient Fluid Volume: risk factors may include excessive vascular losses, altered intake/restrictions.

acute Pain may be related to destruction of tissue (including organ and musculoskeletal), surgical repair, and therapeutic interventions, possibly evidenced by verbal reports, guarding/distraction behaviors, self-focus, and autonomic responses (changes in vital signs).

impaired Tissue Integrity may be related to mechanical factors (yaw of projectile and muzzle blast), possibly evidenced by damaged or destroyed tissue.

risk for Infection: risk factors may include tissue destruction and increased environmental exposure, invasive procedures, and decreased hemoglobin.

                                                                         CH

risk for Post-Trauma Syndrome: risk factors may include nature of incident (catastrophic accident, assault, suicide attempt) and possibly injury/death of other(s) involved.

Zollinger-Ellison syndrome   MS/CH

(Also refer to Ulcer, peptic)

Diarrhea may be related to intestinal irritation (hypersecretion of gastric acid) possibly evidenced by at least 3 loose liquid stools/day, abdominal pain, change in bowel sounds.

risk for impaired Skin/Tissue Integrity: risk factors include frequent bowel movements, hyperacidity of liquid stools, esophageal regurgitation.

acute/chronic Pain may be related to acidic irritation of esophageal mucosa (GERD), muscle spasm possibly evidenced by reports of heartburn, distraction behaviors.

risk for ineffective Therapeutic Regimen Management: risk factors may include length of therapy, economic difficulties, perceived susceptability.

Appendix

Definitions of Taxonomy II Axes

Axis 1 The Diagnostic Concept: Defines as the principal element or the fundamental and essential part, the root, of the diagnostic statement.

Axis 2 Time: Defined as the duration of a period or interval.

Acute: Less than 6 months
Chronic: More than 6 months
Intermittent: Stopping or starting again at intervals, periodic, cyclic
Continuous: Uninterrupted, going on without stop

Axis 3 The Unit of Care: The population to which a diagnostic concept is applied in this nursing diagnosis. Values are:

Individual: A single human being distinct from others, a person.
Family: Two or more people having continuous or sustained relationships, perceiving reciprocal obligations, sensing common meaning, and sharing certain obligations toward others; related by blood or choice.
Group: Individuals gathered, classified, or acting together
Community: "'A group of people living in the same locale under the same government.' Such as neighborhoods, cities, census tracts, and populations at risk." (Craft Rosenberg, 1999, p. 127)

When the unit of care is not explicity stated, it becomes the individual by default.

Axis 4 Age: The length of time or interval during which an individual has existed. Values are:

Fetus	*Adolescent*
Neonate	*Young adult*
Infant	*Middle-age adult*
Toddler	*Young old adult*
Pre-school child	*Middle old adult*
School-age child	*Old old adult*

Axis 5 Health status: The position or rank on the health continuum of wellness to illness (or death). Values are:

Wellness: The quality or state of being healthy, especially as a result of deliberate effort.
Risk: Vulnerability, especially as a result of exposure to factors that increase the chance of injury or loss.
Actual: Existing in fact or reality, existing at the present time.

Axis 6 Descriptor: A judgment that limits or specifies the meaning of a nursing diagnosis. Values are:

Ability: Capacity to do or act
Anticipatory: To realize beforehand, foresee
Balance: State of equilibrium
Compromised: To make vulnerable to threat
Decreased: Lessened; lesser in size, amount or degree
Deficient: Inadequate in amount, quality, or degree; not sufficient; incomplete
Defensive: To feel constantly under attack and the need to quickly justify one's actions

Delayed: To postpone, impede, and retard

Depleted: Emptied wholly or in part, exhausted of

Disproportionate: Not consistent with a standard

Disabling: To make unable or unfit, to incapacitate

Disorganized: To destroy the systematic arrangement

Disturbed: Agitated or interrupted, interfered with

Dysfunctional: Abnormal, incomplete functioning

Effective: Producing the intended or expected effect

Excessive: Characterized by the amount or quantity that is greater than necessary, desirable, or useful

Functional: Normal complete functioning

Imbalanced: State of disequilibrium

Impaired: Made worse, weakened, damaged, reduced, deteriorated

Inability: Incapacity to do or act

Increased: Greater in size, amount or degree

Ineffective: Not producing the desired effect

Interrupted: To break the continuity or uniformity

Low: Containing less than normal amount of some usual element

Organized: To form as into a systematic arrangement

Perceived: To become aware of by means of the senses; assignment of meaning

Readiness for enhanced (for use with wellness diagnoses): To make greater, to increase in quality, to attain the more desired

Axis 7: Topology: Consists of parts/regions of the body—all tissues, organs, anatomical sites or structures. Values are:

Auditory	*Oral*
Bowel	*Olfactory*
Cardiopulmonary	*Peripheral neurovascular*
Cerebral	*Peripheral vascular*
Gastrointestinal	*Renal*
Gustatory	*Skin*
Intracranial	*Tactile*
Urinary	*Visual*
Mucous membranes	

Permission from NANDA International (2002). NANDA Nursing Diagnoses: Definitions & Classification 2003–2004. Philadelphia: NANDA.

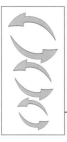

Doenges & Moorhouse's
Diagnostic Division Index

HYGIENE-Ability to perform activities of daily living
Self-care deficit: bathing/hygiene, dressing/grooming, feeding, toileting, 483–89

NEUROSENSORY-Ability to perceive, integrate, and respond to internal and external cues
Confusion, acute, 150–54
Confusion, chronic, 154–58
Infant behavior, disorganized, 330–36
Infant behavior, readiness for enhanced organized, 337–39
Infant behavior, risk for disorganized, 336–37
Memory, impaired, 368–71
Neglect, unilateral, 387–90
Peripheral neurovascular dysfunction, risk for, 437–41
Sensory perception, disturbed [specify type], 510–17
Thought processes, disturbed, 607–11

PAIN/DISCOMFORT-Ability to control internal/external environment to maintain comfort
Pain, acute, 417–22
Pain, chronic, 422–28

RESPIRATION-Ability to provide and use oxygen to meet physiologic needs
Airway clearance, ineffective, 53–58
Aspiration, risk for, 74–77
Breathing pattern, ineffective, 111–16
Gas exchange, impaired, 282–87
Ventilation, impaired spontaneous, 665–70
Ventilatory weaning response, dysfunctional, 671–75

SAFETY-Ability to provide safe, growth-promoting environment
Allergy response: latex, 58–62
Allergy response: latex, risk for, 62–64

Body temperature, risk for imbalanced, 93–96
Death syndrome, risk for sudden infant , 195–98
Environmental interpretation syndrome, impaired, 227–31
Falls, risk for, 235–39
Health maintenance, ineffective, 305–8
Home maintenance, impaired, 312–14
Hyperthermia, 319–23
Hypothermia, 323–27
Infection, risk for, 342–46
Injury, risk for, 346–50
Injury, risk for perioperative positioning, 351–54
Mobility, impaired physical, 375–80
Poisoning, risk for, 441–46
Protection, ineffective, 465–66
Self-mutilation, 503–6
Self-mutilation, risk for, 506–10
Skin integrity, impaired, 525–31
Skin integrity, risk for impaired, 531–35
Suffocation, risk for, 571–75
Suicide, risk for, 575–80
Surgical recovery, delayed, 580–83
Tissue integrity, impaired, 612–17
Trauma, risk for, 628–33
Violence, risk for other-directed, 675–83
Violence, risk for self-directed, 677
Wandering [specify sporadic or continual], 686–90

SEXUALITY-[Component of Ego Integrity and Social Interaction] Ability to meet requirements/characteristics of male/female role
Sexual dysfunction, 517–21
Sexuality patterns, ineffective, 522–25

SOCIAL INTERACTION-Ability to establish and maintain relationships
Attachment, risk for impaired parent/child/infant, 78–82
Caregiver role strain, 123–28
Caregiver role strain, risk for, 129–32
Communication, impaired verbal, 132–38

Communication, readiness for enhanced, 138–42
Coping, community: ineffective, 184–86, 184–87
Coping, community: readiness for enhanced, 190–92
Coping, family: compromised, 169–75
Coping, family: disabled, 175–79
Coping, family: readiness for enhanced, 192–95
Family processes, dysfunctional, 244–48
Family processes, dysfunctional: alcoholism, 240–44
Family processes, readiness for enhanced, 248–51
Loneliness, risk for, 365–68
Parental role conflict, 146–49
Parenting, impaired, 428–33
Parenting, readiness for enhanced, 434–37
Parenting, risk for impaired, 433–34
Role performance, ineffective, 479–82
Social interaction, impaired, 548–53
Social isolation, 553–57

TEACHING/LEARNING-Ability to incorporate and use information to achieve healthy lifestyle/optimal wellness
Development, risk for delayed, 205–8
Growth, risk for disproportionate, 295–99
Growth and development, delayed, 299–304
Health-seeking behaviors, 308–11
Knowledge, deficient [learning need] (specify), 358–63
Knowledge (specify), readiness for enhanced, 363–65
Noncompliance (specify), 391–95
Therapeutic regimen management, community: ineffective, 592–95
Therapeutic regimen management, effective, 589–92
Therapeutic regimen management: family, ineffective, 595–98
Therapeutic regimen management, ineffective, 598–601
Therapeutic regimen management, readiness for enhanced, 601–4

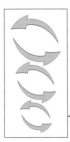

Nursing Diagnoses Index

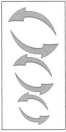

Index

Page numbers followed by "i" and "t" indicate illustrations and tables, respectively.